Probiotics in the Prevention and Management of Human Diseases
A Scientific Perspective

Edited by

Mitesh Kumar Dwivedi
C.G. Bhakta Institute of Biotechnology, Faculty of Science,
Uka Tarsadia University, Maliba Campus, Bardoli, India

N. Amaresan
C.G. Bhakta Institute of Biotechnology, Faculty of Science,
Uka Tarsadia University, Maliba Campus, Bardoli, India

A. Sankaranarayanan
Department of Life Sciences, Sri Sathya Sai University for Human Excellence,
Gulbarga, India

E. Helen Kemp
Department of Oncology and Metabolism, University of Sheffield, Sheffield,
United Kingdom

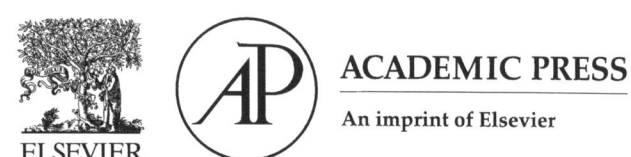

Academic Press is an imprint of Elsevier
125 London Wall, London EC2Y 5AS, United Kingdom
525 B Street, Suite 1650, San Diego, CA 92101, United States
50 Hampshire Street, 5th Floor, Cambridge, MA 02139, United States
The Boulevard, Langford Lane, Kidlington, Oxford OX5 1GB, United Kingdom

Copyright © 2022 Elsevier Inc. All rights reserved.

No part of this publication may be reproduced or transmitted in any form or by any means, electronic or mechanical, including photocopying, recording, or any information storage and retrieval system, without permission in writing from the publisher. Details on how to seek permission, further information about the Publisher's permissions policies and our arrangements with organizations such as the Copyright Clearance Center and the Copyright Licensing Agency, can be found at our website: www.elsevier.com/permissions.

This book and the individual contributions contained in it are protected under copyright by the Publisher (other than as may be noted herein).

Notices

Knowledge and best practice in this field are constantly changing. As new research and experience broaden our understanding, changes in research methods, professional practices, or medical treatment may become necessary.

Practitioners and researchers must always rely on their own experience and knowledge in evaluating and using any information, methods, compounds, or experiments described herein. In using such information or methods they should be mindful of their own safety and the safety of others, including parties for whom they have a professional responsibility.

To the fullest extent of the law, neither the Publisher nor the authors, contributors, or editors, assume any liability for any injury and/or damage to persons or property as a matter of products liability, negligence or otherwise, or from any use or operation of any methods, products, instructions, or ideas contained in the material herein.

British Library Cataloguing-in-Publication Data
A catalogue record for this book is available from the British Library

Library of Congress Cataloging-in-Publication Data
A catalog record for this book is available from the Library of Congress

ISBN: 978-0-12-823733-5

For Information on all Academic Press publications
visit our website at https://www.elsevier.com/books-and-journals

Publisher: Charlotte Cockle
Acquisitions Editor: Megan Ball
Editorial Project Manager: Moises Carlo Catain
Production Project Manager: Sruthi Satheesh
Cover Designer: Victoria Pearson Esser

Typeset by MPS Limited, Chennai, India

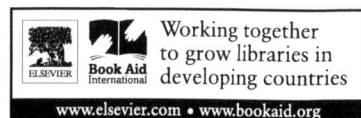

Contents

List of contributors xi
About the editors xv
Foreword xvii
Preface xix

1 The concept of probiotics, prebiotics, postbiotics, synbiotics, nutribiotics, and pharmabiotics 1
Archana Chaudhari and Mitesh Kumar Dwivedi

1.1 Introduction 1
1.2 Probiotics 1
1.3 Prebiotics 3
1.4 Synbiotics 5
1.5 Postbiotics 6
1.6 Nutribiotics 7
1.7 Pharmabiotics 7
Acknowledgments 9
References 9

2 Food or pharma: the name does make a difference 13
Magali Cordaillat-Simmons, Alice Rouanet and Bruno Pot

2.1 Introduction 13
2.2 Probiotics: a substance or a product? 13
2.3 The various regulatory statuses applicable to products containing "probiotics" 16
2.4 Comparative summary 31
2.5 Conclusion: the name does make a difference 37
Conflict of interest 38
Notice 38
References 38

3 The role of probiotics in maintaining immune homeostasis 41
Velaphi C. Thipe, Shireen Mentor, Caroline S.A. Lima, Lucas F. Freitas, Ana C.M. Fonseca, Kamila M. Nogueira, Adriana S. Rodrigues, Jorge G.S. Batista, Aryel H. Ferreira and Ademar B. Lugão

3.1 Introduction 41
3.2 Conlusion 53
Acknowledgment 53
References 53

4 Effect of intestinal microbiome, antibiotics, and probiotics in the prevention and management of ulcerative colitis 59
Ivan Kushkevych and Josef Jampílek

4.1 Introduction 59
4.2 The role of intestinal microbiota in the development of bowel diseases 61
4.3 General characteristics of drugs used in bowel diseases 70
4.4 Modification of intestinal microbiome 74
4.5 Conclusion 81
Acknowledgments 81
References 81

5 Probiotics in the prevention and management of necrotizing enterocolitis 93
Eleonora Seghesio, Charlotte De Geyter and Yvan Vandenplas

5.1 Introduction 93
5.2 The microbiome, dysbiosis, and NEC 93
5.3 Most relevant mechanisms of probiotic action in the preterm 94
5.4 Probiotics and prevention of NEC 94
5.5 Safety aspects of probiotics 96
5.6 Conclusions and challenges for future research 96
References 97

6 Probiotics in the prevention and management of irritable bowel syndrome 101
Elvira Ingrid Levy, Charlotte De Geyter, Bruno Hauser and Yvan Vandenplas

6.1 Introduction 101

6.2	Probiotics in prevention and management of IBS	102
6.3	Conclusion	103
References		104

7 Probiotics in the prevention and treatment of diarrheal disease — 107

Aruna Jyothi Kora

7.1	Introduction	107
7.2	Diarrheal diseases	109
7.3	Probiotics in prevention and treatment of diarrheal diseases	109
7.4	Mode of action of probiotics	113
7.5	Conclusions	113
Acknowledgment		114
References		114

8 Probiotics in the prevention and treatment of atopic skin diseases — 117

Archana Chaudhari, Ankit Bharti and Mitesh Kumar Dwivedi

8.1	Introduction	117
8.2	Etiology and pathophysiology of atopic dermatitis	117
8.3	Relationship between gut microbiota and atopic dermatitis	118
8.4	Intervention of probiotics in atopic dermatitis	119
8.5	Future perspectives of probiotics in prevention and treatment of AD	123
8.6	Conclusion	124
Acknowledgment		124
References		124

9 Probiotics for the treatment of other skin conditions (acne, psoriasis, seborrheic dermatitis, wounds, and skin cancer) — 129

Sophia Sangar, Michelle W. Cheng and Yang Yu

9.1	Acne vulgaris	129
9.2	Psoriasis	130
9.3	Seborrheic dermatitis	131
9.4	Wound healing	132
9.5	Skin cancer	133
References		134

10 Probiotics in the prevention and management of allergic diseases (asthma and allergic rhinitis) — 139

Lien Meirlaen, Elvira Ingrid Levy and Yvan Vandenplas

10.1	Introduction	139
10.2	Prevention of asthma	140
10.3	Probiotics for the treatment of asthma	141
10.4	Probiotics for the prevention of allergic rhinitis	141
10.5	Probiotics for the treatment of allergic rhinitis	142
10.6	Conclusions	143
Acknowledgment		143
Funding		143
Conflicts of interest		143
References		143

11 Prenatal and neonatal probiotic intake in pediatric allergy — 147

Youcef Shahali, Naheed Mojgani and Maryam Dadar

11.1	Introduction	147
11.2	Safety of probiotics and prebiotics	148
11.3	Probiotics, prebiotics, and immunity	149
11.4	Microbiota and allergic disorders	150
11.5	Mother's microbiome and child health	151
11.6	Clinical studies	152
11.7	Conclusions	156
References		156

12 Probiotics and prebiotics in the suppression of autoimmune diseases — 161

Prashant S. Giri, Firdosh Shah and Mitesh Kumar Dwivedi

12.1	Introduction	161
12.2	Autoimmune diseases	162
12.3	Relationship between gut microbiota and immune system	163
12.4	Gut microbiota associated with autoimmune diseases	165
12.5	Beneficial role of probiotics in the suppression of autoimmune diseases	167
12.6	Future perspectives	178
12.7	Conclusions	178
Acknowledgments		179
Conflict of interest		179
References		179

13 Probiotics and prebiotics in the prevention and management of human cancers (colon cancer, stomach cancer, breast cancer, and cervix cancer) — 187

Josef Jampílek, Katarína Králová and Vladimír Bella

13.1	Introduction	187
13.2	Probiotics and prebiotics in stomach cancer	191
13.3	Probiotics and prebiotics in colon cancer	193

13.4 Probiotics and prebiotics in breast cancer 198
13.5 Probiotics and prebiotics in cervical cancer 200
13.6 Conclusion 202
Acknowledgment 203
References 203

14 Probiotics in mitigation of food allergies and lactose intolerance 213

Bhuvan Shankar Vadala, Prasant Kumar and Mitesh Kumar Dwivedi

14.1 Introduction of probiotics and the gut microbiome 213
14.2 Food allergies and lactose intolerance 213
14.3 Lactose intolerance 214
14.4 Role of probiotics in mitigation of food allergies and lactose intolerance 214
14.5 Dietary management strategies 216
14.6 Therapeutic applications 216
14.7 Intake of probiotics 216
14.8 Future prospective of probiotic in food allergies 217
14.9 Conclusions 218
References 218

15 Probiotics in the prevention and treatment of nosocomial infections 223

Julie Kalabalik-Hoganson, Malgorzata Slugocki and Elif Özdener-Poyraz

15.1 Introduction 223
15.2 Hospital-acquired pneumonia and ventilator-associated pneumonia 224
15.3 *Clostridium difficile* infection 228
15.4 Conclusion 232
References 232

16 Role of probiotics in urological health 237

Santosh S. Waigankar

16.1 Introduction 237
16.2 Vaginal microbiota 237
16.3 Commensal microbial flora and preventing UTI 237
16.4 Scope of the problem 238
16.5 Urinary tract infection 238
16.6 Bacterial vaginosis 238
16.7 Yeast vaginitis 238
16.8 Modes of administration of probiotics 239
16.9 What does the evidence say? 240
16.10 Conclusion 240
References 240

17 Role of probiotics in prevention and treatment of Candida vaginitis and Bacterial vaginosis 243

Adekemi Titilayo Adesulu-Dahunsi

17.1 Introduction 243
17.2 Healthy vaginal microflora and probiotic lactobacilli 244
17.3 Vaginitis (vaginal infection) 244
17.4 Probiotic roles in the prevention and treatment of vaginal infection 245
17.5 Conclusion 246
References 247

18 Role of probiotics in the prevention and treatment of oral diseases 251

Devang Bharatkumar Khambholja, Prasant Kumar, Rushikesh G. Joshi and Hiteshkumar V. Patel

18.1 Introduction 251
18.2 Role of probiotics in prevention and treatment of dental caries 252
18.3 Role of probiotics in the prevention and treatment of periodontal diseases 253
18.4 Role of probiotics in the prevention and treatment of halitosis 255
18.5 Conclusions 259
References 259

19 Role of probiotics in infections with multidrug-resistant organisms 265

Basavaprabhu Haranahalli Nataraj and Rashmi Hogarehalli Mallappa

19.1 Introduction 265
19.2 Probiotics 266
19.3 General mechanisms of actions of probiotics against MDR bacteria 267
19.4 Probiotics in organ-specific resistant infections 272
19.5 Conclusion 274
References 275

20 Probiotics in the prevention and treatment of infections with *Helicobacter pylori*, Enterohemorrhagic *Escherichia coli*, and *Rotavirus* 281

Nilanjana Das, Mangala Lakshmi Ragavan and Sanjeeb Kumar Mandal

20.1 Introduction 281
20.2 Probiotics and their health implications 282
20.3 Infections caused by *Helicobacter pylori*, enterohemorrhagic *Escherichia coli*, and rotavirus 283

20.4	*Helicobacter pylori*	285
20.5	Enterohemorrhagic *Escherichia coli*	288
20.6	Rotavirus	291
20.7	Conclusion and future perspectives	295
References		296

21 Role of probiotics in the management of fungal infections — 305

Archana Chaudhari, Ankit Bharti and Mitesh Kumar Dwivedi

21.1	Introduction	305
21.2	Probiotics	305
21.3	Probiotics in fungal diseases	306
21.4	Future perspectives	314
21.5	Conclusions	314
Acknowledgment		315
References		315

22 Role of probiotics in the prevention and management of diabetes and obesity — 321

Rashmi Hogarehalli Mallappa, Chandrasekhar Balasubramaniam, Monica Rose Amarlapudi, Shweta Kelkar, Gbenga Adedeji Adewumi, Saurabh Kadyan, Diwas Pradhan and Sunita Grover

22.1	Introduction	321
22.2	Pathophysiology and risk factors of diabetes mellitus and obesity	322
22.3	Probiotics for the management of diabetes and obesity	327
22.4	Conclusions	332
References		332

23 Probiotics in the prevention and management of cardiovascular diseases with focus on dyslipidemia — 337

Cíntia Lacerda Ramos, Elizabethe Adriana Esteves, Rodrigo Pereira Prates, Lauane Gomes Moreno and Carina Sousa Santos

23.1	Introduction	337
23.2	Probiotic bacteria	338
23.3	Probiotic yeasts	344
23.4	Conclusion	345
References		345

24 Gut–brain axis: role of probiotics in neurodevelopmental disorders including autism spectrum disorder — 353

Ranjith Kumar Manokaran and Sheffali Gulati

24.1	Introduction	353
24.2	Colonization of the intestinal ecosystem in early life and its evolution	353
24.3	Gut microbiota	354
24.4	What are probiotics?	354
24.5	Psychobiotics, prebiotics, and synbiotics	354
24.6	Autism and probiotics	354
24.7	ASD and GI disorders	354
24.8	The gut–brain axis	355
24.9	Neurodevelopmental disorders	356
24.10	Is the gut microbiota of children with autism spectrum disorder different?	357
24.11	Literature evidence in ASD	358
24.12	Newer techniques involving microbiota	358
24.13	ADHD	360
24.14	Other neurodevelopmental disorders	360
24.15	Future perspectives	360
24.16	Conclusion	361
References		361

25 Probiotics in the prevention and control of foodborne diseases in humans — 363

Atef A. Hassan, Rasha M.H. Sayed-ElAhl, Ahmed M. El Hamaky, Noha H. Oraby and Mahmoud H. Barakat

25.1	Introduction	363
25.2	Foodborne diseases	364
25.3	Probiotics	364
25.4	Antimicrobial potential of probiotics against foodborne pathogens	367
25.5	Probiotics mechanisms of action in the control and prevention of foodborne pathogens	368
25.6	Supplementation of probiotics in food materials	372
25.7	Delivery system of probiotics	372
25.8	The safety of probiotic therapy in host	372
25.9	Health significance of probiotics in the prevention of foodborne diseases	373
25.10	Conclusion and future perspectives	374
Acknowledgment		374
References		374

26 Role of probiotics in the management of respiratory infections 383

Cristina Méndez-Malagón, Alejandro Egea-Zorrilla, Pedro Perez-Ferrer and Julio Plaza-Diaz

- 26.1 Introduction 383
- 26.2 Respiratory tract infections 384
- 26.3 In search of new therapeutic strategies: microbiota and gut-lung axis 385
- 26.4 Pulmonary microbiota in diseases 386
- 26.5 History of probiotics 386
- 26.6 Probiotic usage and safety 387
- 26.7 Probiotic administration in respiratory infections 388
- 26.8 Conclusion 393
- References 393

27 The role of probiotics in nutritional health: probiotics as nutribiotics 397

María Chávarri, Lucía Diez-Gutiérrez, Izaskun Marañón, María del Carmen Villarán and Luis Javier R. Barrón

- 27.1 Nutribiotics: ways to improve the nutritional status 397
- 27.2 Nutritional health benefits of probiotics and postbiotics 400
- 27.3 Encapsulation technology for the development of functional ingredients 405
- 27.4 Current market of probiotics and future perspectives 408
- 27.5 Conclusions 409
- References 409

28 Role of immunobiotic lactic acid bacteria as vaccine adjuvants 417

Maryam Dadar, Youcef Shahali and Naheed Mojgani

- 28.1 Introduction 417
- 28.2 Vaccine adjuvants 417
- 28.3 Probiotic lactic acid bacteria 418
- 28.4 Conclusions 425
- References 425

29 Probiotics: past, present, and future challenges 431

Marieta Georgieva, Kaloyan Georgiev and Nadezhda Hvarchanova

- 29.1 Probiotics—the concept 431
- 29.2 Probiotics—modern trends 432
- 29.3 Viability of probiotic bacteria in the gastrointestinal tract and their secondary reproduction: probiotic concentration 435
- 29.4 Dose of probiotics 437
- 29.5 Safety of probiotic bacteria 437
- 29.6 Health effects of probiotics 437
- 29.7 Probiotics and metabolic syndrome 441
- 29.8 Probiotics and urogenital infections 442
- 29.9 Probiotics and immunity 442
- 29.10 Probiotics and mental illness called Plus Ultra 443
- 29.11 The next 45 years 443
- 29.12 Summary 443
- 29.13 Probiotics and Covid-19: data supporting the use of probiotics to prevent Covid-19 444
- 29.14 Conclusion 445
- References 445

30 Probiotics: health safety considerations 449

Hemant Borase, Mitesh Kumar Dwivedi, Ramar Krishnamurthy and Satish Patil

- 30.1 Introduction 449
- 30.2 Conclusions 459
- Acknowledgments 459
- Declaration of competing interest 459
- References 459

31 Probiotics: current regulatory aspects of probiotics for use in different disease conditions 465

Maja Šikić Pogačar, Dušanka Mičetić-Turk and Sabina Fijan

- 31.1 Introduction 465
- 31.2 Current regulation bodies that include probiotics 467
- 31.3 Regulations for use of probiotics in gastrointestinal diseases 468
- 31.4 Regulations for use of probiotics in diseases other than gastrointestinal diseases 480
- 31.5 Conclusions 488
- References 489

Index 501

List of contributors

Adekemi Titilayo Adesulu-Dahunsi Food Science and Technology Programme, College of Agriculture, Engineering and Science, Bowen University, Iwo, Nigeria

Gbenga Adedeji Adewumi Department of Microbiology, Faculty of Science, University of Lagos, Lagos, Nigeria

Monica Rose Amarlapudi Molecular Biology Unit, Dairy Microbiology Division, ICAR-National Dairy Research Institute, Karnal, India

Chandrasekhar Balasubramaniam Molecular Biology Unit, Dairy Microbiology Division, ICAR-National Dairy Research Institute, Karnal, India

Mahmoud H. Barakat Faculty of Medicine, Cairo University (Al Kasr Al Ainy), Cairo, Egypt

Luis Javier R. Barrón Lactiker Research Group, Department of Pharmacy and Food Sciences, University of the Basque Country (UPV/EHU), Vitoria-Gasteiz, Spain

Jorge G.S. Batista Energy and Nuclear Research Institute (IPEN), University of São Paulo, São Paulo, Brazil

Vladimír Bella Departmentof Mammology, St. Elizabeth Cancer Institute, Bratislava, Slovakia

Ankit Bharti Aura Skin and Dental Clinic, Tapi, India

Hemant Borase C. G. Bhakta Institute of Biotechnology, Uka Tarsadia University, Maliba Campus, Bardoli, India

Archana Chaudhari Vyara Clinical Laboratory Pvt Ltd., Tapi, India; Department of Biochemistry, The Maharaja Sayajirao University of Baroda, Vadodara, India

María Chávarri Health and Food Area, Health Division, TECNALIA, Basque Research and Technology Alliance (BRTA), Parque Tecnológico de Álava, Miñano, Spain

Michelle W. Cheng Division of Dermatology and Department of Medicine, David Geffen School of Medicine at UCLA, Los Angeles, CA, United States

Magali Cordaillat-Simmons Pharmabiotic Research Institute (PRI), Narbonne, France

Maryam Dadar Razi Vaccine and Serum Research Institute, Agricultural Research, Education and Extension Organization (AREEO), Karaj, Iran

Nilanjana Das Department of Biomedical Sciences, School of Bio Sciences and Technology, Vellore, India

Charlotte De Geyter Vrije Universiteit Brussel (VUB), UZ Brussel, KidZ Health Castle, Brussels, Belgium

María del Carmen Villarán Health and Food Area, Health Division, TECNALIA, Basque Research and Technology Alliance (BRTA), Parque Tecnológico de Álava, Miñano, Spain

Lucía Diez-Gutiérrez Health and Food Area, Health Division, TECNALIA, Basque Research and Technology Alliance (BRTA), Parque Tecnológico de Álava, Miñano, Spain

Mitesh Kumar Dwivedi C.G. Bhakta Institute of Biotechnology, Faculty of Science, Uka Tarsadia University, Maliba Campus, Bardoli, India

Alejandro Egea-Zorrilla Laboratory of Cardiovascular Development and Disease, Andalusian Centre for Nanomedicine and Biotechnology (Bionand), Technological Park of Andalusia C/ Severo Ochoa, Málaga, Spain

Ahmed M. El Hamaky Mycology department, Animal Health Research Institute (AHRI), Agriculture Research Center (ARC), Giza, Egypt

Elizabethe Adriana Esteves Graduate Program in Nutrition Sciences, Faculty of Biological and Health Sciences/Federal University of Jequitinhonha and Mucuri Valeys, Diamantina, Brazil; Graduate Program in Health Sciences, Faculty of Biological and Health Sciences/Federal University of Jequitinhonha and Mucuri Valeys, Diamantina, Brazil

Aryel H. Ferreira Energy and Nuclear Research Institute (IPEN), University of São Paulo, São Paulo, Brazil

Sabina Fijan University of Maribor, Faculty of Health Sciences, Institute for Health and Nutrition, Maribor, Slovenia

Ana C.M. Fonseca Virtual University of the State of Sao Paulo (UNIVESP), São Paulo, Brazil

Lucas F. Freitas Energy and Nuclear Research Institute (IPEN), University of São Paulo, São Paulo, Brazil

Kaloyan Georgiev Department of Pharmacology, Toxicology and Pharmacotherapy, Faculty of Pharmacy, Medical University of Varna, Varna, Bulgaria

Marieta Georgieva Department of Pharmacology, Toxicology and Pharmacotherapy, Faculty of Pharmacy, Medical University of Varna, Varna, Bulgaria

Prashant S. Giri C.G. Bhakta Institute of Biotechnology, Faculty of Science, Uka Tarsadia University, Maliba Campus, Bardoli, India

Sunita Grover Molecular Biology Unit, Dairy Microbiology Division, ICAR-National Dairy Research Institute, Karnal, India

Sheffali Gulati Center of Excellence and Advanced Research for Childhood Neurodevelopmental Disorders, Child Neurology Division, Department of Pediatrics, AIIMS, New Delhi, India

Atef A. Hassan Mycology department, Animal Health Research Institute (AHRI), Agriculture Research Center (ARC), Giza, Egypt

Bruno Hauser Vrije Universiteit Brussel (VUB), UZ Brussel, KidZ Health Castle, Brussels, Belgium

Nadezhda Hvarchanova Department of Pharmacology, Toxicology and Pharmacotherapy, Faculty of Pharmacy, Medical University of Varna, Varna, Bulgaria

Josef Jampílek Department of Analytical Chemistry, Faculty of Natural Sciences, Comenius University, Bratislava, Slovakia; Institute of Neuroimmunology, Slovak Academy of Sciences, Bratislava, Slovakia

Rushikesh G. Joshi Department of Biochemistry and Forensic Science, University School of Sciences, Gujarat University, Ahmedabad, India

Saurabh Kadyan Molecular Biology Unit, Dairy Microbiology Division, ICAR-National Dairy Research Institute, Karnal, India

Julie Kalabalik-Hoganson School of Pharmacy and Health Sciences, Fairleigh Dickinson University, Florham Park, NJ, United States

Shweta Kelkar Molecular Biology Unit, Dairy Microbiology Division, ICAR-National Dairy Research Institute, Karnal, India

Devang Bharatkumar Khambholja P.G. Department of Medical Technology, B.N. Patel Institute of Paramedical and Science (Paramedical Division), Anand, India

Aruna Jyothi Kora National Centre for Compositional Characterisation of Materials (NCCCM), Bhabha Atomic Research Centre (BARC), ECIL PO, Hyderabad, India; Homi Bhabha National Institute (HBNI), Mumbai, India

Katarína Kráľová Institute of Chemistry, Faculty of Natural Sciences, Comenius University, Bratislava, Slovakia

Ramar Krishnamurthy C. G. Bhakta Institute of Biotechnology, Uka Tarsadia University, Maliba Campus, Bardoli, India

Prasant Kumar Ingress Bio-Solutions Pvt Ltd, Ahmedabad, India

Ivan Kushkevych Department of Experimental Biology, Faculty of Science, Masaryk University, Brno, Czech Republic

Elvira Ingrid Levy Vrije Universiteit Brussel (VUB), UZ Brussel, KidZ Health Castle, Brussels, Belgium

Caroline S.A. Lima Energy and Nuclear Research Institute (IPEN), University of São Paulo, São Paulo, Brazil

Ademar B. Lugão Energy and Nuclear Research Institute (IPEN), University of São Paulo, São Paulo, Brazil

Rashmi Hogarehalli Mallappa Molecular Biology Unit, Dairy Microbiology Division, ICAR-National Dairy Research Institute, Karnal, India

Sanjeeb Kumar Mandal Sri Shakthi Institute of Engineering and Technology, Coimbatore, India

Ranjith Kumar Manokaran Center of Excellence and Advanced Research for Childhood Neurodevelopmental Disorders, Child Neurology Division, Department of Pediatrics, AIIMS, New Delhi, India

Izaskun Marañón Health and Food Area, Health Division, TECNALIA, Basque Research and Technology Alliance (BRTA), Parque Tecnológico de Álava, Miñano, Spain

Lien Meirlaen Vrije Universiteit Brussel (VUB), UZ Brussel, KidZ Health Castle, Brussels, Belgium

Cristina Méndez-Malagón Center of Biomedical Research, University of Granada, Granada, Spain

Shireen Mentor Department of Medical Biosciences, University of the Western Cape, Cape Town, South Africa

Dušanka Mičetić-Turk University of Maribor, Faculty of Medicine, Maribor, Slovenia; University of Maribor, Faculty of Health Sciences, Institute for Health and Nutrition, Maribor, Slovenia

Naheed Mojgani Razi Vaccine and Serum Research Institute, Agricultural Research, Education and Extension Organization (AREEO), Karaj, Iran

Lauane Gomes Moreno Multicentre Graduate Program in Physiological Sciences, Faculty of Biological and Health Sciences/Federal University of Jequitinhonha and Mucuri Valeys, Diamantina, Brazil

Basavaprabhu Haranahalli Nataraj Molecular Biology Unit, Dairy Microbiology Division, ICAR-National Dairy Research Institute, Karnal, India

Kamila M. Nogueira Energy and Nuclear Research Institute (IPEN), University of São Paulo, São Paulo, Brazil

Noha H. Oraby Mycology department, Animal Health Research Institute (AHRI), Agriculture Research Center (ARC), Giza, Egypt

Elif Özdener-Poyraz School of Pharmacy and Health Sciences, Fairleigh Dickinson University, Florham Park, NJ, United States

Hiteshkumar V. Patel Department of Biochemistry, Shri A.N. Patel PG Institute of Science and Research, Anand, India

Satish Patil School of Life Sciences, Kavayitri Bahinabai Chaudhari North Maharashtra University, Jalgaon, India

Pedro Perez-Ferrer Department of Molecular and Cell Biology, School of Natural Sciences, University of California, Merced, Merced, CA, United States

Julio Plaza-Diaz Children's Hospital of Eastern Ontario Research Institute, Ottawa, ON, Canada

Maja Šikić Pogačar University of Maribor, Faculty of Medicine, Maribor, Slovenia

Bruno Pot Pharmabiotic Research Institute (PRI), Narbonne, France; Research Group of Industrial Microbiology and Food Biotechnology (IMDO), Vrije Universiteit Brussel (Free University Brussels), Elsene, Belgium

Diwas Pradhan Molecular Biology Unit, Dairy Microbiology Division, ICAR-National Dairy Research Institute, Karnal, India

Rodrigo Pereira Prates Multicentre Graduate Program in Physiological Sciences, Faculty of Biological and Health Sciences/Federal University of Jequitinhonha and Mucuri Valeys, Diamantina, Brazil

Mangala Lakshmi Ragavan Department of Biomedical Sciences, School of Bio Sciences and Technology, Vellore, India

Cíntia Lacerda Ramos Graduate Program in Nutrition Sciences, Faculty of Biological and Health Sciences/Federal University of Jequitinhonha and Mucuri Valeys, Diamantina, Brazil; Graduate Program in Health Sciences, Faculty of Biological and Health Sciences/Federal University of Jequitinhonha and Mucuri Valeys, Diamantina, Brazil

Adriana S. Rodrigues Energy and Nuclear Research Institute (IPEN), University of São Paulo, São Paulo, Brazil

Alice Rouanet Pharmabiotic Research Institute (PRI), Narbonne, France

Sophia Sangar Division of Dermatology and Department of Medicine, David Geffen School of Medicine at UCLA, Los Angeles, CA, United States

Carina Sousa Santos Graduate Program in Nutrition Sciences, Faculty of Biological and Health Sciences/Federal University of Jequitinhonha and Mucuri Valeys, Diamantina, Brazil

Rasha M.H. Sayed-ElAhl Mycology department, Animal Health Research Institute (AHRI), Agriculture Research Center (ARC), Giza, Egypt

Eleonora Seghesio Vrije Universiteit Brussel (VUB), UZ Brussel, KidZ Health Castle, Brussels, Belgium

Firdosh Shah C.G. Bhakta Institute of Biotechnology, Faculty of Science, Uka Tarsadia University, Maliba Campus, Bardoli, India

Youcef Shahali Razi Vaccine and Serum Research Institute, Agricultural Research, Education and Extension Organization (AREEO), Karaj, Iran; The University Hospital of Besançon, Besançon, France

Malgorzata Slugocki School of Pharmacy and Health Sciences, Fairleigh Dickinson University, Florham Park, NJ, United States

Velaphi C. Thipe Energy and Nuclear Research Institute (IPEN), University of São Paulo, São Paulo, Brazil

Bhuvan Shankar Vadala Sri Venkateswara University, Tirupati, India

Yvan Vandenplas Vrije Universiteit Brussel (VUB), UZ Brussel, KidZ Health Castle, Brussels, Belgium

Santosh S. Waigankar Kokilaben Dhirubhai Ambani Hospital, Mumbai, India

Yang Yu Division of Dermatology and Department of Medicine, David Geffen School of Medicine at UCLA, Los Angeles, CA, United States

About the editors

Dr. Mitesh Kumar Dwivedi is an assistant professor of microbiology at C.G. Bhakta Institute of Biotechnology, Uka Tarsadia University. He has published 54 research papers in reputed journals, written 16 book chapters, and is the editor of 6 books. He has an *h*-index of 21 with 1603 citations for his research papers. He has more than 14 years of experience in research and teaching in various allied fields of microbiology and immunology. His research areas include autoimmunity, probiotics in human health and disease, host−microbe interaction, and immunogenetics of human diseases. He has been serving as an editorial board member and reviewer of many international journals. He has been honored with many international and national awards for his excellent research performance [Best Researcher Award (2020), INSA Visiting Scientist Award (2019), DST-SERB Early Career Research Award (2018), Young Scientist Awards (2011, 2013, and 2018)] and secured all India rank "32" in CSIR-NET National examination (2011; Life Sciences). He has successfully completed research projects from national funding agencies such as SERB-DST, GUJCOST, UTU, and Neosciences & Research Solutions Pvt. Ltd. and guided students for their doctoral and master degrees.

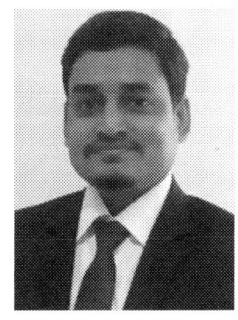

Dr. N. Amaresan is an assistant professor at C.G. Bhakta Institute of Biotechnology, Uka Tarsadia University, Gujarat. He has over 15 years of experience in teaching and research in various allied fields of microbiology. He has been awarded the Young Scientist Awards by the Association of Microbiologists of India and the National Academy of Biological Sciences. He was also awarded visiting scientist fellowship from the National Academy of India. He has published more than 100 research articles, book chapters, and books of national and international repute. He also deposited over 550 16S rDNA, 28S rDNA, and ITS rDNA sequences in the Genbank (NCBI, EMBL, and DDBJ) and also preserved over 150 microbial germplasm in various culture collection centers of India. He has successfully completed research projects from national funding agencies such as SERB-DST, GUJCOST, UTU, and GEMI and guided students for their doctoral and master's degrees.

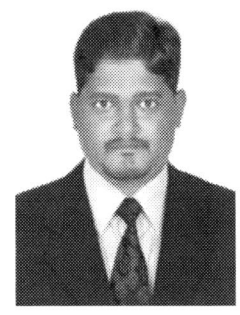

Dr. A. Sankaranarayanan is an associate professor in the Department of Life Sciences, Sri Sathya Sai University for Human Excellence, Kalaburagi, Karnataka, India from June 2021 onward. His current research focus is on fermented food products. He has published 8 books, 30 chapters, 60 research articles in international and national journals of repute; guided 5 Ph.D., and 16 M.Phil., scholars; and operated 5 minor funded projects in Microbiology. From 2002−15, he worked as an assistant professor and head in the Department of Microbiology, K.S.R. College of Arts & Science, Tiruchengode, Tamil Nadu, and from August 2015 to May 2021, he was associated with Uka Tarsadia University, Surat, Gujarat, India. He has been awarded Indian Academy of Sciences (IASc), National Academy of Sciences (NAS), and The National Academy of Sciences (TNAS) sponsored summer research fellowship for young teachers consecutively for 3 years and his name is included as a mentor in DST-Mentors/Resource persons for summer/winter camps and other INSPIRE initiatives, Department of Science & Technology, Govt. of India, New Delhi. He is a grant reviewer in the British Society of Antimicrobial Chemotherapy (BSAC), United Kingdom.

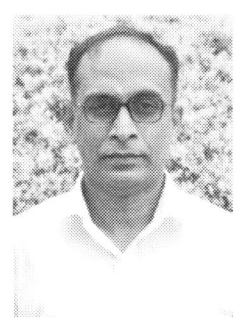

Dr. E. Helen Kemp completed her Ph.D. in microbiology at the University of Warwick and the Centre for Applied Microbiology and Research, Salisbury, in 1988. Since 1989, she has worked at the University of Sheffield as a Postdoctoral Research Fellow in the Department of Molecular Biology and Biotechnology and then in the Department of Oncology and Metabolism. She has long-standing interests in the autoimmune and genetic aspects of the depigmenting disease vitiligo, characterizing autoimmune responses against the calcium-sensing receptor in patients with parathyroid autoimmunity, and the etiology of autoimmune thyroid disease. She has published more than 70 research papers on all these areas of research and has contributed to books and review articles.

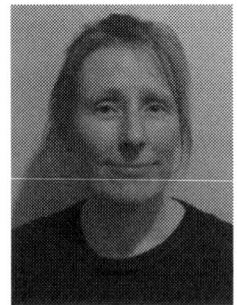

Foreword

Dear Reader,

When I became aware of a book being prepared entitled "Probiotics in the Prevention and Management of Human Diseases: A Scientific Perspective," I became really interested! Probiotics have a long history in foods that, by their WHO/FAO definition, exert health benefits. In the past, these health benefits rarely covered real *treatment* approaches for human diseases, at least not in a way known for traditional drugs. I saw this book as an opportunity to pull the focus toward a different *intended use* for probiotics: prevent or cure disease!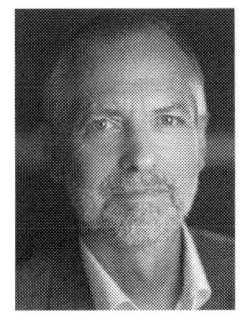

The huge progress in sequencing and metabolomic technology overwhelmingly showed the impact of the (gut) microbiota in the development of human disease, beyond microbiota quality or functionality, such as mood, anxiety, and autism spectrum disorder. The logical, but maybe unfortunate, consequence of this was the fact that expectations for foods were raised to a prophylactic and even therapeutic level! While there is of course nothing wrong with foods contributing to health, expectations for probiotics were no longer at the "food" level, and the initial absence of "drug" *results* tended to impact negatively on the use of probiotics for both types of applications.

So when the opportunity to contribute to this book came along, I was really excited. It indeed turned out to be a wonderful occasion to clarify and realistically discuss the broad application pallet of probiotics in different fields of medicine. Interestingly, these applications were often those where traditional drugs, because of side effects, can offer only short-term successes or are in the field of noncommunicable diseases, which are putting a huge burden on our current and future health care system and for which often no adequate drug solutions are available. This book shall explain that drugs are not the same as foods in terms of strain selection, clinical research strategy, intended use, or manufacturing. For that particular reason, I am very grateful to the editors to have considered chapters on regulatory differences between foods and pharma, and their efforts to clarify the concepts of prebiotics, postbiotics, synbiotics, nutribiotics, and pharmabiotics, besides probiotics. Without any doubt, this may contribute to a more correct use of the terms, help reduce confusion for both doctors and their patients, and define clear health benefits of the "biotic" family.

So here it is, a book on probiotics in medicine. Whether you are interested in how probiotics interact with the immune system, how to use probiotics in early life such as preterm infants and through the life stages, or wonder if there are specific strains for specific applications, you may find some of the answers here. The book is organized around at least 25 possible disease topics but will also try to answer current safety questions as well as highlight challenges for the probiotics of the future.

Having a keen interest in probiotics for almost 35 years as a food microbiologist, I have always welcomed the wider, medical interest in these wonderful microorganisms, but at the same time got slightly concerned about expectations that went far beyond the wildest of our scientific dreams. It is my sincere hope that this book will contribute to a better, realistic understanding of where probiotics could support, sometimes replace, and in some cases excel traditional drugs. The timing for the book is definitely right, the setting too, now it is only up to you to enjoy!

Bruno Pot is the Science Director Europe for Yakult; the Pharmabiotics Research Institute's president; a member of the Taxonomic Subcommittee for Lactobacilli, Bifidobacteria, and related taxa; and a teacher of courses in food microbiology and food hygiene at the Vrije Universiteit Brussels.

Bruno Pot[1,2]
[1]*Yakult Europe Science Department, Almere, The Netherlands*
[2]*Vrije Universiteit Brussel, Research Group of Industrial Microbiology and Food Biotechnology (IMDO), Elsene, Belgium*

Preface

Probiotics, a rapidly emerging field during the past three decades, continues to gain ground with applications in various fields, especially in human health. According to FAO and WHO reports, live microorganisms, which are administered in sufficient amounts to provide beneficial health to their host, are considered as "Probiotics." They can have beneficial and potentially therapeutic effects through their antimicrobial and immune-modulatory activities.

The major focus of this book is to highlight the current and future use of probiotics in different human diseases as addressed by relevant research studies, clinical case studies, and animal models. Probiotics are diverse, so there is a need to explain in depth their mechanism of action and to give an update on research especially in the area of human disease. Hence, the book presents invited chapters from experts in the field of probiotic research on the prevention and management of various human diseases such as life-threatening cancers, immune-mediated conditions, and infectious diseases, including the emerging multidrug-resistant infections. Collectively 31 chapters cover the basic concepts of probiotics as well as current research into their effects on human disease including cardiovascular, neurological, respiratory, allergic, autoimmune, metabolic, and diarrheal diseases as well as human cancers especially of the colon, stomach, breast, and cervix. In addition, the book addresses the novel concept of probiotics as a vaccine adjuvant and as a solution for nutritional health problems. Along with this, the chapters also deal with the current challenges and health-safety concerns in using probiotics, biosafety measures, and various regulatory aspects of probiotic usage in different disease conditions.

We, the editorial team, strongly believe that this book will be used for education and as a scientific tool among academics, clinicians, scientists, young researchers, and health professionals, as well as graduate and postgraduate students.

As the editors of this book, we would like to express our sincere gratitude to all authors for their excellent contributions to this book. We are also indebted to the publishers for all their efforts to bring out the book in a timely manner. Healthy criticism and comments are always welcome.

Mitesh Kumar Dwivedi
N. Amaresan
A. Sankaranarayanan
E. Helen Kemp

Chapter 1

The concept of probiotics, prebiotics, postbiotics, synbiotics, nutribiotics, and pharmabiotics

Archana Chaudhari[1] and Mitesh Kumar Dwivedi[2]
[1]Department of Biochemistry, The Maharaja Sayajirao University of Baroda, Vadodara, India, [2]C.G. Bhakta Institute of Biotechnology, Faculty of Science, Uka Tarsadia University, Maliba Campus, Bardoli, India

1.1 Introduction

Human health is slowly deteriorating due to the inclination toward sedentary lifestyle of people, decrease in the consumption of home-cooked foods along with rise in the consumption of poor-quality food (Christmann, 2020). This has also affected the qualitative and quantitative composition of the intestinal microbiota, which correlates with various pathological disorders. Bioactive components, such as probiotics, prebiotics, and synbiotics, have provided a new hope to human health by restoring microbial imbalance and have come out as a nonharmful cure to painful diseases, thereby improving well-being and preventing complications (Fujiya et al., 2014; Maslennikov et al., 2018; Shen et al., 2017). As a result, there is rise in interest on the consumption of food products containing bioactive components that enhance the nutritive value (Pandey et al., 2015). This chapter is focused to provide the conceptual basis of different emerging terminologies used in the probiotic field (Fig. 1.1).

1.2 Probiotics

The modern history of probiotics starts with the pioneering studies of Russian scientist Elie Metchnikoff in 1907, who first created the foundation of the concept of beneficial microorganisms that today we know as "probiotics." He studied the effect of consumption of fermented products, such as yogurt, on human health, thereby associating it with the long-life expectancy of Bulgarian people (Mackowiak, 2013). He also specified that "the dependence of the intestinal microbes on the food makes it possible to adopt measures to modify the flora in our bodies and to replace the harmful microbes by useful microbes." This clearly states the "probiotic concept." He considered the *Lactobacilli* as probiotic that could have a positive influence on health and prevent aging. Since then the precise definition of probiotic has evolved according to the development of probiotic concept. Werner Kollath in 1953 first developed the term probiotics for active substances that are essential for healthy development of life (Gasbarrini et al., 2016). In 1965 Lilly and Stillwell determined that a microorganism secrets some growth stimulators for another microorganism (Lilly & Stillwell, 1965). This positive effect may cause the application of the term probiotic for these kinds of microorganisms. The term probiotic was first used by Parker for the definition of substances and organisms, which cause the microbial balance in the gastrointestinal tract (Parker, 1974). And there were also other researchers in between who had their own different definition for probiotic. Finally, in 2014 the International Scientific Association for Probiotics and Prebiotics (ISAPP) defined probiotics as "live microorganisms, that when administered in adequate amounts, confer a health benefit on the host" (Hill et al., 2014). From that time on, this definition has been widely used by scientific community (Fig. 1.2).

Probiotics have been isolated from various sites, such as gut and traditional fermented foods. They mostly belong to genera *Lactobacillus* and *Bifidobacterium*, although there are also some members of *Bacillus* and *Escherichia coli* for bacteria and the yeast *Saccharomyces* among others. Table 1.1 shows currently used microorganisms as probiotics.

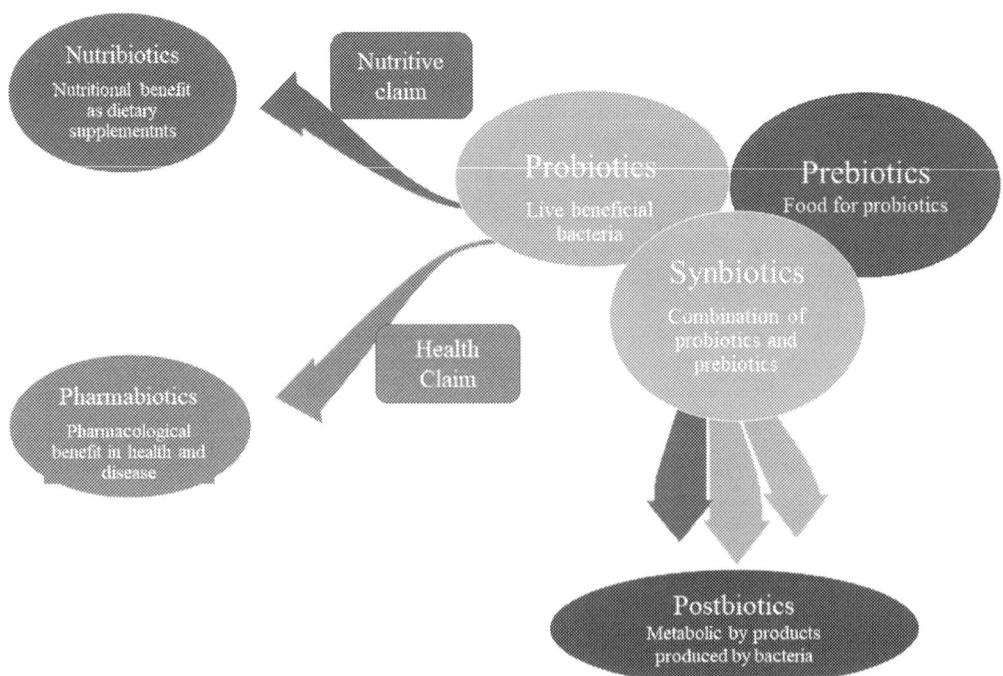

FIGURE 1.1 Different terminologies related to probiotics.

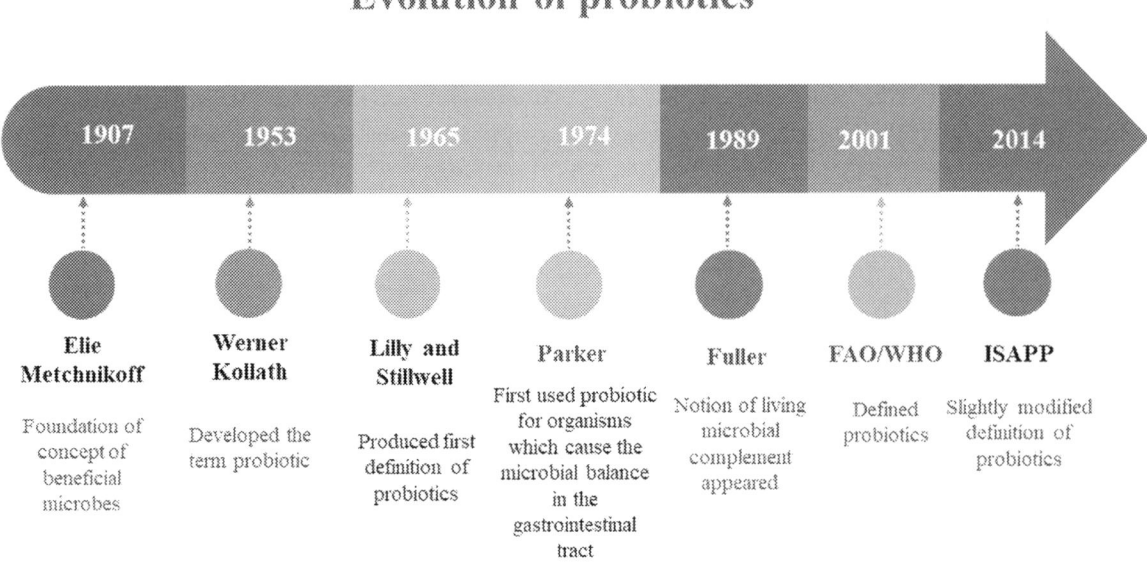

FIGURE 1.2 Evolution of the term "probiotics."

Many researchers have shown the use of probiotics in a wide variety of fields. Various studies in probiotics support the fact that probiotics are useful for the eradication of antibiotic resistance by fecal transplantation to decolonize naturally resistant bacterial strains (Crum-Cianflone et al., 2015; Millan et al., 2016). Probiotics have also been shown to play an important role in psychopathology, as studies indicate that administration of probiotics is associated with a decrease in anxiety (Bravo et al., 2011). Application of probiotics has been shown to improve the acne by reducing skin colonization, improving atopic dermatitis, aging skin, and healing burns and scars (Bowe & Logan, 2011; Krutmann, 2012). Apart from this, oral supplementation of probiotics could improve skin health by a gut—brain—skin axis reducing systemic and brain inflammation and improving nutrient absorption, which favors barrier synthesis. Probiotics also

TABLE 1.1 Current microorganisms used as probiotics.

Probiotic genus	Species
Akkermansia	Akkermansia muciniphila
Bacillus	Bacillus coagulans, Bacillus subtilis, Bacillus laterosporus
Bacteroides	Bacteroides uniformis
Bifidobacterium	Bifidobacterium breve, Bifidobacterium adolescentis, Bifidobacterium animalis, Bifidobacterium bifidum, Bifiobacterium infantis, Bifidobacterium lactis, Bifidobacterium longum, Bifidobacterium catenulatum, Bifidobacterium thermophilum
Enterococcus	Enterococcus faecium, Enterococcus faecalis
Lactobacillus	Lactobacillus plantarum, Lactobacillus paracasei, Lactobacillus acidophilus, Lactobacillus casei, Lactobacillus rhamnosus, Lactobacillus crispatus, Lactobacillus gasseri, Lactobacillus reuteri, Lactobacillus delbrueckii ssp. (Lactobacillus bulgaricus), Lactobacillus fermentum, Lactobacillus johnsonii, Lactobacillus brevis, Lactobacillus curvatus, Lactobacillus lactis, Lactobacillus cellobiosus
Leuconostoc	Leuconostoc lactis subsp. cremoris, Leuconostoc mesenteroides
Pediococcus	Pediococcus acidilactici
Peptostreptococcus	Peptostreptococcus productus
Propionibacterium	Propionibacterium jensenii, Propionibacterium freudenreichii
Saccharomyces	Saccharomyces cerevisiae, Saccharomyces boulardii
Streptococcus	Streptococcus oralis, Streptococcus uberis, Streptococcus rattus, Streptococcus salivarius, Streptococcus sanguis, Streptococcus mitis, Streptococcus thermophilus, Streptococcus diacetylactis, Streptococcus cremoris, Streptococcus intermedius

play an important role in pharmacological therapies, such as immunotherapy in patients with advanced melanoma, and reducing the side effects of therapeutics (Gopalakrishnan et al., 2018; Guthrie et al., 2017).

1.3 Prebiotics

Glenn Gibson and Marcel Roberfroid first acknowledged prebiotics in 1995 and defined the old but still valid definition of prebiotics as "a nonviable food component that confers a health benefit on the host associated with modulation of the microbiota" (Gibson & Roberfroid, 1995; Pineiro et al., 2008). According to this definition, only a few compounds of the carbohydrate group, such as short- and long-chain β-fructans [fructo-oligosaccharides (FOSs) and inulin], lactulose, and galacto-oligosaccharide (GOS), can be classified as prebiotics. The 6th Meeting of the ISAPP in 2008 defined "dietary prebiotics" as "a selectively fermented ingredient that results in specific changes in the composition and/or activity of the gastrointestinal microbiota, thus conferring benefit(s) upon host health" (Gibson & Roberfroid, 1995). However, in 2017 experts of the ISAPP described the prebiotic as "a substrate that is selectively utilized by host microorganisms conferring a health benefit" (Fig. 1.3; Gibson et al., 2017). The current definition of prebiotics comprises of substances, such as polyphenols and polyunsaturated fatty acids, converted to their respective conjugated fatty acids together with some peptides catabolized by bacteria into active ingredients apart from carbohydrate-based prebiotics. The definition requires documented beneficial health effects of potential prebiotics. Apart from this, the updated definition includes a variety of organic and inorganic substances (i.e., micronutrients necessary for the development of bacteria) used externally and internally stimulating microorganisms not only in the GI tract but also in all niches of the body, including skin, urinary tract, and vagina (Gibson et al., 2017; Tomasik & Tomasik, 2020).

There are many types of prebiotics mainly identified as inulin and subset of carbohydrate groups, mostly oligosaccharides. Oligosaccharides are further grouped into FOSs and GOSs. The most popular and widely used prebiotics include fructans, inulin, FOS, and GOS, which are generally regarded as safe (Ambalam et al., 2016; Kumar et al., 2015). Table 1.2 shows currently used different prebiotics and their sources.

Prebiotics have been gaining a great deal of attention in recent years as they provide nutritional benefit along with health and physiological benefits. Benefits of prebiotics upon health are constantly evolving; however, until now

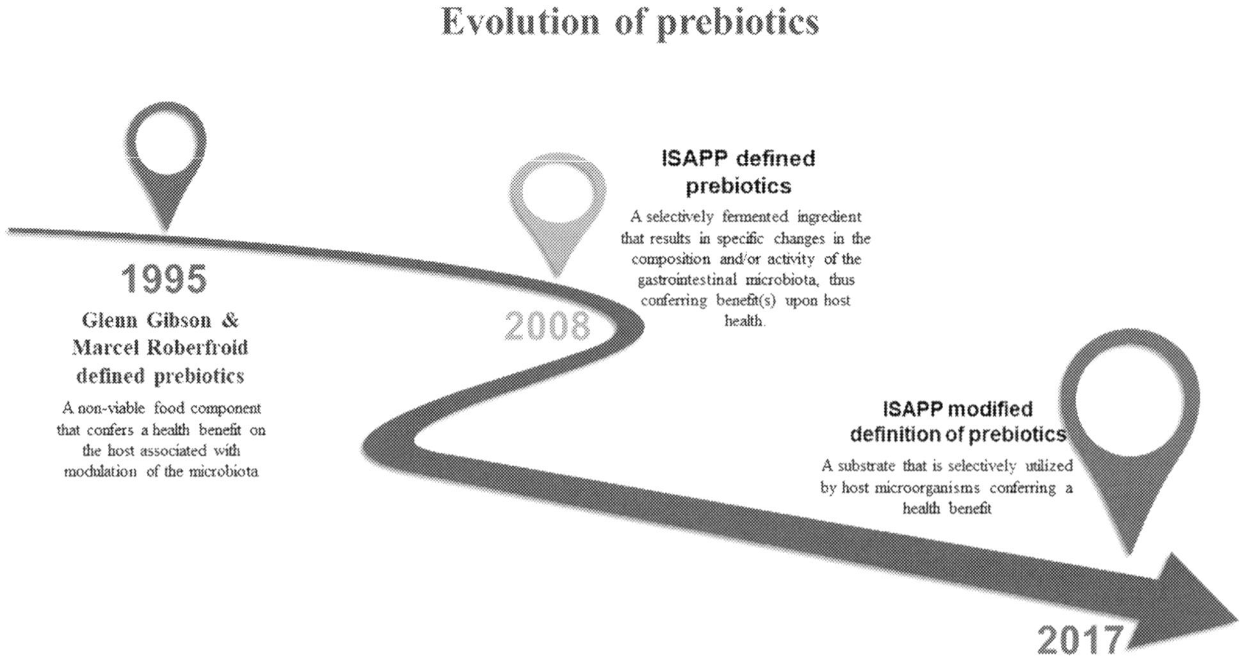

Evolution of prebiotics

1995 — Glenn Gibson & Marcel Roberfroid defined prebiotics
A non-viable food component that confers a health benefit on the host associated with modulation of the microbiota

2008 — ISAPP defined prebiotics
A selectively fermented ingredient that results in specific changes in the composition and/or activity of the gastrointestinal microbiota, thus conferring benefit(s) upon host health.

2017 — ISAPP modified definition of prebiotics
A substrate that is selectively utilized by host microorganisms conferring a health benefit

FIGURE 1.3 Evolution of term "prebiotic."

TABLE 1.2 Prebiotics and their sources.

Prebiotics	Sources
Fructo-oligosaccharides	Occur naturally in fruits and vegetables (onion, leek, asparagus, chicory, Jerusalem artichoke, garlic, oat). Other sources: cereals, wheat, barley, rye, and honey
Fructans	Naturally occurring oligosaccharides found in onions, bananas, wheat, artichokes, garlic, and other whole foods
Inulin	Present in a range of natural foods, including agave, banana/plantain, burdock camas, chicory, coneflower, costus, dandelion, elecampane, garlic, globe artichoke, Jerusalem artichoke, jicama, leopard's bane, mugwort root, onion, wild yam, and yacon
Galacto-oligosaccharides	Legumes, nuts, soy beans and soy products, peas, rapeseed meal, lentils, human milk, Chickpeas/hummus, green peas, lima beans, and kidney beans
Resistant starch 1,2,3,4	Raw potatoes, beans/legumes, starchy fruits and vegetables, whole grains, and bananas
Pectins	Apple, sugar beet pulp
β-Glucans	Oats and barley
Psyllium	Psyllium husk (plant)
Iso-maltooligosaccharides	Miso, soy, sauce, sake, and honey
Lactulose	Skim milk
Milk oligosaccharides	Human and cow's milk
Soybean oligosaccharides	Soybean
Xylo-oligosaccharides	Bamboo shoot, fruits, vegetables, milk, and honey
Arabinoxylan	Bran of grasses
Arabinoxylan oligosaccharides	Cereals

prebiotics have been shown to be beneficial for gastrointestinal tract (pathogens' inhibition or immune response stimulation), cardio metabolism (reduction of lipid levels in blood, effects on insulin resistance), mental health (metabolites with influence on brain function, energy, and cognition), bones (minerals bioavailability), skin (hydration of surface layers of the skin and normalizes its keratinization and exfoliation), and urogenital tract (reduces the level of toxins in chronic kidney diseases). They also play an important role in the reduction of metabolic diseases, such as obesity, type 1 and type 2 diabetes, and nonalcoholic fatty liver disease.

1.4 Synbiotics

Different probiotic strains require different food sources to live according to the need whereby only a single strain will be able to utilize a particular food source and remaining strains will decrease. The researchers in early 1960s had noticed the potential of synbiotics in the field of nutrition to interfere with the human intestinal microbiota (Turek, 1960). Prebiotics are utilized for the most part as a particular vehicle for the development of a probiotic strain and maturation in intestinal section. Because of the utilization of prebiotics, probiotic microorganisms secure higher resistance to ecological conditions, such as oxygenation, pH, and temperature, in the digestive tract of a specific organism. Together, synbiotics support to reestablish a healthy ecology of microflora within the gastrointestinal tract by strategically combining probiotics with prebiotics, which encourages a more profound effect on gastrointestinal ecology than probiotics or prebiotics alone. Hence, the synbiotic can be defined as, "A supplement that contains both a prebiotic and a probiotic that work together to promote 'healthy microflora' in the human intestine." Synbiotics are "next generation of probiotics." Since synbiotic refers to synergism, it should be reserved for products in which the prebiotic component selectively favors the probiotic compound (Mishra et al., 2018). Table 1.3 presents few examples of synbiotics wherein the probiotics and the respective prebiotics are shown.

Furthermore, the combination of probiotics with prebiotics brings about development of beneficial microbiota, the equilibrium of the metabolic movement in the gastrointestinal tract maintaining the intestinal structure and preventing the development of potential pathogens present in the intestinal tract (Goyal & Rastogi, 2020). In synbiotics, the probiotics use the prebiotics as a food source, which enables them to survive for an extended period within the intestine. The improvement in the viability of probiotics facilitates in delivering projected health benefits. These consequences increase the count of *Lactobacillus* and *Bifidobacterium* genera and maintain the balance of intestinal microflora. The synbiotics help to reduce undesired concentration of metabolites, including nitrosamines, to inactivate carcinogens and prevent constipation and diarrhea from various etiologies (Wasilewski et al., 2015). Their utilization prompts a huge increment in levels of short-chain unsaturated fats, ketones, carbon disulfides, and methyl acetic acid derivations, which possibly brings about a beneficial outcome on the host's well-being (Markowiak & Śliżewska, 2017).

TABLE 1.3 List of synbiotics.

Prebiotics	Probiotics
Arabinoxylan and arabinoxylan oligosaccharides	*Bifidobacterium* sp.
Fructo-oligosaccharides	*Bifidobacteria, Bacteroides fragilis, Peptostreptococcaceae, Klebsiellae*
Fructo-oligosaccharides	*Bifidobacterium bifidum, Bifidobacterium lactis*
Galacto-oligosaccharides	*Bifidobacterium longum, Bifidobacterium catenulatum*
Inulin	*Bifidobacterium animalis, Lactobacillus acidophilus, Lactobacillus paracasei*
Isomalto-oligosaccharides	*Bifidobacteria, Bacteroides fragilis* group
Lactosucrose	*Zymomonas mobilis*
Lactulose	*Bifidobacteria lactis, Lactobacillus bulgaricus, Lactobacillus acidophilus, Lactobacillus rhamnosus*
Resistant starch-1,2,3,4	*Bacteroides, Eubacterium rectal*
Xylo-oligosaccharides	*Bifidobacterium adolescentis, Lactobacillus plantarum*

1.5 Postbiotics

The research in recent years has revealed that dead or inactivated cells, cell extracts, and the cell metabolites could render significant health benefits on human (Di Lena et al., 2015). On the other hand, it is worth to mention that using living cells in some special cases might have an adverse effect on the health. For example, the administration of living probiotic cells to host with weak immune system increased the inflammatory responses (Kothari et al., 2019). Current knowledge allows stating that bacterial viability is not necessary to attain all probiotic effects, as not all mechanisms nor clinical benefits are directly related to viable bacteria (Cuevas-González et al., 2020). This was demonstrated recently, since few researchers have compared viable or inactivated microorganisms and different microbial fractions obtained from them. Research also indicates that bacterial viability is not a critical requirement for imparting health benefits and hence new terms, such as "postbiotics," were created to denote the health benefits beyond the inherent viability of probiotics, providing a broader context to the probiotic concept. The concept of postbiotics is built up on the observation that the positive effects of the microflora are facilitated by the secretion of several metabolites. Postbiotics, also known as "metabiotics" are "soluble factors secreted by live bacteria or released after bacterial lysis which confer physiological benefits to the host" (Schönfeld & Wojtczak, 2016). Most common types of postbiotics are SCFA, peptides, enzymes, teichoic acids, and vitamins (Moreno-Navarrete et al., 2018). While postbiotics do not comprise live microbes, they show a valuable health outcome through the similar mechanisms that are representative of probiotics while minimizing the risks related to their intake. So, similar to prebiotics, postbiotics appear to lack serious side effects while keeping similar efficacy to probiotics. Overall, the probiotics present in a viable state can produce postbiotics. The postbiotic is also defined as "cell-free supernatants, biogenics, metabolites, and metabolic waste of activity of probiotic." In 2013 Tsilingiri defined postbiotic as any effects obtained from metabolites of probiotics or any extracted or secreted molecule that offers health benefits to the host directly or indirectly (Tsilingiri & Rescigno, 2013). These soluble compounds include enzymes, exo and endo polysaccharides, surface proteins, vitamins, organic acids, fatty acids, and peptides (Aguilar-Toalá et al., 2018; Malashree et al., 2019; Tsilingiri & Rescigno, 2013). Table 1.4 lists out the different groups of postbiotics with certain examples.

The production methods of postbiotics involve cell rupture by heat, enzymatic, ultrasound, or solvent treatments. After extraction, cleaning steps are needed, which can be performed by centrifugation, dialysis, lyophilization, and column purification. The postbiotics may be classified into distinct categories according to the observed physiological benefits (antiinflammatory, antioxidant, antihypertensive, antiproliferative, antimicrobial, hypocholesterolemic, and immunomodulatory activities) or by their composition, which can be derived from both bacterial cell compounds and microbial action (synthesis of metabolites and products from microbial enzymatic activity over the food matrix) (Aguilar-Toalá et al., 2018; Collado et al., 2019). Postbiotics can include bacterial lysates with cell surface proteins, bacterial enzymes and peptides, metabolites produced by bacteria, such as teichoic acids, peptidoglycan-derived neuropeptides, polysaccharides, and lower organic acids, for instance, lactic acid. Table 1.5 shows different postbiotics and respective microbial sources.

Thus many health-beneficial effects acquired through the consumption of fermented foods are associated to postbiotics since they are related not only to the ingested live microorganisms but also to the microbial structures and metabolites produced during fermentation. Moreover, postbiotics can stimulate the immunological system, likely involving bowel and intestine developing antiinflammatory, immunomodulatory, antiobesogenic, antihypertensive, antiproliferative, antioxidative, and

TABLE 1.4 The main groups of postbiotics.

Postbiotic group	Examples
Carbohydrates	Galactose-rich polysaccharides, techoic acid
Proteins	Lactocepin, P40 molecule, cell surface proteins
Enzymes	GPx, SOD, NADH peroxidase
Complex molecules	Peptidoglycan-derived muropeptides, lipoteichoic acids
Vitamins	B group vitamins
Lipids	Butyrate, propionate, dimethyl acetyl-derived plasmalogen
Organic acids	Propionic, 3-phenyl lactic acid

TABLE 1.5 Postbiotics and their sources.

Postbiotics	Sources
Bacteriocins	*Lactobacillus plantarum* I-UL4
Butyrate	*Faecalibacterium prausnitzii*
Exopolysaccharides	*Lactobacillus pentosus*
Heat-killed LGG	*Lactobacillus rhamnosus*
Polyphosphate	*Lactobacillus brevis*
Short-chain fatty acids	*Lactobacillus gasseri*
Soluble mediator	*Lactobacillus paracasei*

hypocholesterolemic activity (Tomasik & Tomasik, 2020). In addition, a rise in the B vitamin content in cereal grains is another remarkable case of postbiotic fermentation.

Probiotics are considered health-promoting microbes for a range of diseases throughout the human body from the gut to nonintestinal body sites, such as brain and skin (Bowe & Logan, 2011). Accordingly, the probiotics used currently are administered not only through oral delivery but are also applied on skin for burn injury and cosmetic purposes (Huseini et al., 2012; Simmering & Breves, 2010). The classical definition of probiotics covers a broad range of probiotics in foods and medicine. However, this current categorization is vague and the differences between functional foods, medicinal foods, or pharmaceutical medicine are unclear, making proper regulation difficult (Arora & Baldi, 2015). Arora and Baldi from India suggested a new categorization of probiotics as nutribiotics and pharmabiotics.

1.6 Nutribiotics

Nutribiotics can be in the forms of a food, a food product, or a dietary supplement, which are subjected to regulatory requirements related to food safety and dietary guidelines. Specific microbial groups exhibit probiotic effects on nutritional functions by producing essential nutrients, such as vitamins and minerals, converting precursors to bioactive metabolites, or relieving health problems related to nutritional status or metabolism (Vandenplas et al., 2015).

There are various probiotics that are classified as "nutribiotics" and used for their nutraceutic functionalities. Some microbial groups produce vitamins and contribute to the availability of vitamins in the human host. These vitamins are synthesized by the gut microbiota (LeBlanc et al., 2013), and thus the nutritional requirement for individuals with low intake of these vitamins that are not synthesized in the human body and not consumed through the diet depends on gut microbial production. Ingestion of nutribiotics may improve the vitamin status, increasing their availability in the gut (Pompei et al., 2007). Various studies have claimed to improve vitamin status of riboflavin, folate, etc. (Lin & Young, 2000; Thakur & Tomar, 2015). Nutribiotics have also been claimed to be useful for lactose intolerance, a nutritional health problem with a prevalence of approximately 70% in some regions of the Mediterranean area (Corgneau et al., 2017; Roškar et al., 2017). Research has also claimed the use of nutribiotics in the production of health-beneficial metabolites, such as conjugated linoleic acid (Kim et al., 2015). Table 1.6 presents few examples of nutribiotics.

1.7 Pharmabiotics

Colin Hill from University of College Cork, Ireland, for the first time used the term "pharmabiotics" in 2002, during his work with Irish government-funded collaborative groups studying probiotics, led by Fergus Shanahan (Hill, 2010). The term probiotics fit into bigger category pharmabiotics, defined as "bacterial cells of human origin, or their products, with a proven pharmacological role in health or disease." The pharmabiotics were suggested to include pharmaceutic probiotics with specific health claims, which may show beneficial physiological effects on body functions or play a pharmacological role in disease (Hill, 2010; Sreeja & Prajapati, 2013). Table 1.7 presents few examples of pharmabiotics. The term pharmabiotics encompasses the wide potential use of microbes that are alive or dead, the components of organisms, or metabolites of microbes (Shanahan, 2010) that are not covered by the classical definition of probiotics by the FAO/WHO. Thus the term pharmabiotics is not just limited to live microorganisms but contain probiotics, bacteriocins, bacteriophages, and bioactive molecules. Therapeutic pharmabiotics have been studied for various categories of

TABLE 1.6 List of probiotics categorized as nutribiotics.

Nutribiotics	Mode of action
Bifidobacterium adolescentis MB 227, *B. adolescentis* MB 239, and *Bifidobacterium pseudocatenulatum* MB 116-added diet	Increase in folate status
Bifidobacterium bifidum LMG 10645, *Bifidobacterium breve* LMG 11040, *B. breve* LMG 11084, *B. breve* LMG 11613, *B. breve* LMG 13194, and *Bifidobacterium pseudolongum* LMG 11595	Conjugated linoleic and linolenic acid production in culture media
Lactobacillus acidophilus N1, *L. acidophilus* 4356, *Bifidobacterium longum* B6, *Lactobacillus bulgaricus* 448, *L. bulgaricus* 449, *Streptococcus thermophilus* MC, and *S. thermophilus* 573	Folate production in foods
Lactobacillus acidophilus, Lactobacillus fermentum KTLF1, *L. fermentum* MTCC8711, *L. fermentum* PBCC11.5, *Lactobacillus plantarum* CRL 725	Riboflavin production
L. plantarum S48 and P1201	Conjugated linoleic acid production in culture media
Lactobacillus reuteri Lb2 BM	Selenium production in foods
Streptococcus thermophilus LMG18311	Lactose intolerance

TABLE 1.7 Pharmabiotics and specific health claim.

Pharmabiotics	Health claim
Akkermansia muciniphila	Prevention of obesity and metabolic disorders
Bifidobacterium bifidum+*Streptococcus thermophilus*	Prevention of acute diarrhea
Bifidobacterium longum	Prevention of antibiotic associated diarrhea
Butyricicoccus pullicaecorum	Therapeutic treatment of ulcerative colitis
Enterococcus faecium SF68	Prevention of antibiotic associated diarrhea
Lactobacillus acidophilus+*Lactobacillus bulgaricus*	Prevention of antibiotic associated diarrhea
Lactobacillus casei Shirota	Therapeutic treatment of rotavirus-associated diarrhea
Lactobacillus helveticus R0052, *Bifidobacterium longum* R0175 (PF)	Treatment of depression
Lactobacillus plantarum DSM9843, *L. plantarum* 299V	Curative treatment of irritable bowel syndrome
Lactobacillus reuteri	Therapeutic treatment of acute diarrhea
Lactobacillus rhamnosus GG	Prevention of antibiotic associated diarrhea
Saccharomyces boulardii	Prevention of antibiotic associated diarrhea

diseases, typically gastrointestinal diseases, such as infectious diarrhea, inflammatory bowel diseases, and metabolic diseases, including obesity and diabetes (Lee et al., 2018). The representative fields of pharmabiotics include postbiotics, paraprobiotics, and probioceuticals (probiotaceuticals) (Sreeja & Prajapati, 2013).

The term "paraprobiotics" was proposed by Taverniti and Guglielmetti (2011). They are also known as ghosts or inactivated probiotics that are defined as "nonviable microbial cells" (ruptured or intact) or raw cellular extracts (with complex chemical composition), which when administered (topically or orally) in adequate amounts, confer a benefit on the human or animal consumer. In particular, paraprobiotics constitutes inactivated/dead/nonviable microbial cells or cell components of probiotic cells that can be intact or ruptured upon lysis. Few examples included in the list are teichoic acids, peptidoglycan-derived muropeptides, surface protruding molecules (pili, fimbriae, flagella), polysaccharides, such as exopolysaccharides, cell surface-associated proteins, and cell wall-bound biosurfactants (Shenderov, 2013; Singh et al., 2018). Moreover, paraprobiotics are microorganisms that had its viability compromised after being submitted to processes that have induced structural and metabolic changes to the bacterial cells (de Almada et al., 2016). Paraprobiotics and postbiotics provide immunomodulatory activity to the host and are a safer alternative when the use of live probiotic bacteria is not indicated, for example, in the case of immunodeficient individuals, such as seniors and transplanted or premature newborns. The use of paraprobiotics and postbiotics in aforementioned cases reduces the risks of: (1) development of opportunistic infections; (2) increased inflammatory responses to vaccine or allergens; (3) deleterious metabolic effects due to the degradation of mucine and production of deconjugated bile salts and D-lactate, which can cause gastrointestinal disorders; (4) horizontal transfer of antibiotic resistance genes to other commensals or pathogenic bacteria in the gut; and (5) microbial translocation. In addition, paraprobiotics and postbiotics do not lose bioactivity when administered together with antibacterial and antifungal agents (Aguilar-Toalá et al., 2018; Deshpande et al., 2018; Zawistowska-Rojek & Tyski, 2018).

The term "probioceuticals" (probiotaceuticals) refers to "probiotic-derived factors" which inhibit the growth of microorganisms or other infectious organisms (yeast, molds, protozoa, viruses) (Howarth, 2010). Probiotic-derived factors include products (proteinaceous molecules, carbohydrates, and cell wall components) and metabolites (short-chain fatty acids) that exert health-promoting effects on host contributing to the reinforcement of intestinal barrier function and stimulating antiinflammatory immune responses, leading to the amelioration of intestinal inflammatory disorders (Yan & Polk, 2020). Probiotic-derived factors, for example, reuterin from *Lactobacillus reuteri*, have been described to inhibit the viability and adhesion of known enteric pathogens, signifying that probiotic supernatants could be a rich source of new antipathogenic compounds. Table 1.7 presents few examples of pharmabiotics with specific health claims.

In this chapter, our goal was to discuss the emerging terms in the expanding field of probiotics during the recent years. Our aim was to shed light on the differences among all the definitions to allow a clear understanding among scientific community and general public.

Acknowledgments

We are grateful to Uka Tarsadia University, Maliba Campus, Tarsadi, Gujarat, India, for providing the facilities needed for the preparation of this book chapter.

References

Aguilar-Toalá, J. E., Garcia-Varela, R., Garcia, H. S., Mata-Haro, V., González-Córdova, A. F., Vallejo-Cordoba, B., & Hernández-Mendoza, A. (2018). Postbiotics: An evolving term within the functional foods field. *Trends in Food Science and Technology*, 75, 105–114. Available from https://doi.org/10.1016/j.tifs.2018.03.009.

Ambalam, P., Raman, M., Purama, R. K., & Doble, M. (2016). Probiotics, prebiotics and colorectal cancer prevention. *Best Practice and Research: Clinical Gastroenterology*, 30(1), 119–131. Available from https://doi.org/10.1016/j.bpg.2016.02.009.

Arora, M., & Baldi, A. (2015). Regulatory categories of probiotics across the globe: A review representing existing and recommended categorization. *Indian Journal of Medical Microbiology*, 33, S2–S10. Available from https://doi.org/10.4103/0255-0857.150868.

Bowe, W. P., & Logan, A. C. (2011). Acne vulgaris, probiotics and the gut-brain-skin axis—Back to the future? *Gut Pathogens*, 3(1). Available from https://doi.org/10.1186/1757-4749-3-1.

Bravo, J. A., Forsythe, P., Chew, M. V., Escaravage, E., Savignac, H. M., Dinan, T. G., Bienenstock, J., & Cryan, J. F. (2011). Ingestion of Lactobacillus strain regulates emotional behavior and central GABA receptor expression in a mouse via the vagus nerve. *Proceedings of the National Academy of Sciences of the United States of America*, 108(38), 16050–16055.

Christmann, M. (2020). Physical Activity in the Modern Working World. In W. Seiferlein, & C. Kohlert (Eds.), *The Networked Health-Relevant Factors for Office Buildings* (pp. 157–165). Cham: Springer.

Collado, M. C., Vinderola, G., & Salminen, S. (2019). Postbiotics: Facts and open questions. A position paper on the need for a consensus definition. *Beneficial Microbes*, 10(7), 711–719. Available from https://doi.org/10.3920/BM2019.0015.

Corgneau, M., Scher, J., Ritie-Pertusa, L., Le, D. T. L., Petit, J., Nikolova, Y., Banon, S., & Gaiani, C. (2017). Recent advances on lactose intolerance: Tolerance thresholds and currently available answers. *Critical Reviews in Food Science and Nutrition*, 57(15), 3344–3356. Available from https://doi.org/10.1080/10408398.2015.1123671.

Crum-Cianflone, N. F., Sullivan, E., & Ballon-Landa, G. (2015). Fecal microbiota transplantation and successful resolution of multidrug-resistant-organism colonization. *Journal of Clinical Microbiology*, 53(6), 1986–1989. Available from https://doi.org/10.1128/JCM.00820-15.

Cuevas-González, P. F., Liceaga, A. M., & Aguilar-Toalá, J. E. (2020). Postbiotics and paraprobiotics: From concepts to applications. *Food Research International*, 109502.

de Almada, C. N., Almada, C. N., Martinez, R. C. R., & Sant'Ana, A. S. (2016). Paraprobiotics: Evidences on their ability to modify biological responses, inactivation methods and perspectives on their application in foods. *Trends in Food Science and Technology*, 58, 96–114. Available from https://doi.org/10.1016/j.tifs.2016.09.011.

Deshpande, G., Athalye-Jape, G., & Patole, S. (2018). Para-probiotics for preterm neonates—The next frontier. *Nutrients*, 10(7), 871.

Di Lena, M., Quero, G. M., Santovito, E., Verran, J., De Angelis, M., & Fusco, V. (2015). A selective medium for isolation and accurate enumeration of Lactobacillus casei-group members in probiotic milks and dairy products. *International Dairy Journal*, *47*, 27−36. Available from https://doi.org/10.1016/j.idairyj.2015.01.018.

Fujiya, M., Ueno, N., & Kohgo, Y. (2014). Probiotic treatments for induction and maintenance of remission in inflammatory bowel diseases: A meta-analysis of randomized controlled trials. *Clinical Journal of Gastroenterology*, *7*(1), 1−13. Available from https://doi.org/10.1007/s12328-013-0440-8.

Gasbarrini, G., Bonvicini, F., & Gramenzi, A. (2016). Probiotics history. *Journal of Clinical Gastroenterology*, *50*, S116−S119. Available from https://doi.org/10.1097/MCG.0000000000000697.

Gibson, G. R., & Roberfroid, M. B. (1995). Dietary modulation of the human colonic microbiota: Introducing the concept of prebiotics. *Journal of Nutrition*, *125*(6), 1401−1412. Available from https://doi.org/10.1093/jn/125.6.1401.

Gibson, G. R., Hutkins, R., Sanders, M. E., Prescott, S. L., Reimer, R. A., Salminen, S. J., Scott, K., Stanton, C., Swanson, K. S., Cani, P. D., Verbeke, K., & Reid, G. (2017). Expert consensus document: The International Scientific Association for Probiotics and Prebiotics (ISAPP) consensus statement on the definition and scope of prebiotics. *Nature Reviews Gastroenterology and Hepatology*, *14*(8), 491−502. Available from https://doi.org/10.1038/nrgastro.2017.75.

Gopalakrishnan, V., Spencer, C. N., Nezi, L., Reuben, A., Andrews, M. C., Karpinets, T. V., Prieto, P. A., Vicente, D., Hoffman, K., Wei, S. C., Cogdill, A. P., Zhao, L., Hudgens, C. W., Hutchinson, D. S., Manzo, T., Petaccia De Macedo, M., Cotechini, T., Kumar, T., Chen, W. S., ... Wargo, J. A. (2018). Gut microbiome modulates response to anti-PD-1 immunotherapy in melanoma patients. *Science*, *359*(6371), 97−103. Available from https://doi.org/10.1126/science.aan4236.

Goyal, N., & Rastogi, M. (2020). Probiotics, prebiotics & synbiotics: A new era. *Food and Agriculture Spectrum Journal.*, *2*.

Guthrie, L., Gupta, S., Daily, J., & Kelly, L. (2017). Human microbiome signatures of differential colorectal cancer drug metabolism. *NPJ Biofilms and Microbiomes*, *3*(1). Available from https://doi.org/10.1038/s41522-017-0034-1.

Hill, C. (2010). Probiotics and pharmabiotics: Alternative medicine or an evidence-based alternative? *Bioengineered Bugs*, *1*(2), 79−84. Available from https://doi.org/10.4161/bbug.1.2.10796.

Hill, C., Guarner, F., Reid, G., Gibson, G. R., Merenstein, D. J., Pot, B., Morelli, L., Canani, R. B., Flint, H. J., Salminen, S., Calder, P. C., & Sanders, M. E. (2014). Expert consensus document: The international scientific association for probiotics and prebiotics consensus statement on the scope and appropriate use of the term probiotic. *Nature Reviews Gastroenterology and Hepatology*, *11*(8), 506−514. Available from https://doi.org/10.1038/nrgastro.2014.66.

Howarth, G. S. (2010). Probiotic-derived factors: Probiotaceuticals? *Journal of Nutrition*, *140*(2), 229−230. Available from https://doi.org/10.3945/jn.109.118844.

Huseini, H. F., Rahimzadeh, G., Fazeli, M. R., Mehrazma, M., & Salehi, M. (2012). Evaluation of wound healing activities of kefir products. *Burns*, *38*(5), 719−723. Available from https://doi.org/10.1016/j.burns.2011.12.005.

Kim, B., Lee, B. W., Hwang, C. E., Lee, Y. Y., Lee, C., Kim, B. J., Park, J. Y., Sim, E. Y., Haque, M. A., Lee, D. H., Lee, J. H., Ahn, M. J., Lee, H. Y., Ko, J. M., Kim, H. T., & Cho, K. M. (2015). Screening of conjugated linoleic acid (CLA) producing Lactobacillus plantarum and production of CLA on soy-powder milk by these stains. *Korean Journal of Microbiology*, *51*(3), 231−240. Available from https://doi.org/10.7845/kjm.2015.5045.

Kothari, D., Patel, S., & Kim, S. K. (2019). Probiotic supplements might not be universally-effective and safe: A review. *Biomedicine and Pharmacotherapy*, *111*, 537−547. Available from https://doi.org/10.1016/j.biopha.2018.12.104.

Krutmann, J. (2012). Pre- and probiotics for human skin. *Clinics in Plastic Surgery*, *39*(1), 59−64. Available from https://doi.org/10.1016/j.cps.2011.09.009.

Kumar, H., Salminen, S., Verhagen, H., Rowland, I., Heimbach, J., Bañares, S., Young, T., Nomoto, K., & Lalonde, M. (2015). Novel probiotics and prebiotics: Road to the market. *Current Opinion in Biotechnology*, *32*, 99−103. Available from https://doi.org/10.1016/j.copbio.2014.11.021.

LeBlanc, J. G., Milani, C., de Giori, G. S., Sesma, F., van Sinderen, D., & Ventura, M. (2013). Bacteria as vitamin suppliers to their host: A gut microbiota perspective. *Current Opinion in Biotechnology*, *24*(2), 160−168. Available from https://doi.org/10.1016/j.copbio.2012.08.005.

Lee, E. S., Song, E. J., Nam, Y. D., & Lee, S. Y. (2018). Probiotics in human health and disease: from nutribiotics to pharmabiotics. *Journal of Microbiology*, *56*(11), 773−782.

Lilly, D. M., & Stillwell, R. H. (1965). Probiotics: Growth-promoting factors produced by microorganisms. *Science*, *147*(3659), 747−748. Available from https://doi.org/10.1126/science.147.3659.747.

Lin, M. Y., & Young, C. M. (2000). Folate levels in cultures of lactic acid bacteria. *International Dairy Journal*, *10*(5−6), 409−413. Available from https://doi.org/10.1016/S0958-6946(00)00056-X.

Mackowiak, P. A. (2013). Recycling Metchnikoff: probiotics, the intestinal microbiome and the quest for long life. *Frontiers in Public Health*, *1*, 52.

Malashree, L., Angadi, V., Yadav, K. S., & Prabha, R. (2019). Postbiotics. One step ahead of probiotics. *Int J Curr Microbiol Appl Sci.*, *8*, 2049−2053.

Markowiak, P., & Śliżewska, K. (2017). Effects of probiotics, prebiotics, and synbiotics on human health. *Nutrients*, *9*(9), 1021.

Maslennikov, R., Pavlov, C., & Ivashkin, V. (2018). Small intestinal bacterial overgrowth in cirrhosis: Systematic review and meta-analysis. *Hepatology International*, *12*(6), 567−576. Available from https://doi.org/10.1007/s12072-018-9898-2.

Millan, B., Park, H., Hotte, N., Mathieu, O., Burguiere, P., Tompkins, T. A., Kao, D., & Madsen, K. L. (2016). Fecal microbial transplants reduce antibiotic-resistant genes in patients with recurrent clostridium difficile infection. *Clinical Infectious Diseases*, *62*(12), 1479−1486. Available from https://doi.org/10.1093/cid/ciw185.

Mishra, S. S., Behera, P. K., Kar, B., & Ray, R. C. (2018). *Advances in probiotics, prebiotics and nutraceuticals. In Innovations in technologies for fermented food and beverage industries* (pp. 121−141). Cham: Springer.

Moreno-Navarrete, J. M., Serino, M., Blasco-Baque, V., Azalbert, V., Barton, R. H., Cardellini, M., Latorre, J., Ortega, F., Sabater-Masdeu, M., Burcelin, R., Dumas, M. E., Ricart, W., Federici, M., & Fernández-Real, J. M. (2018). Gut microbiota interacts with markers of adipose tissue browning, insulin action and plasma acetate in morbid obesity. *Molecular Nutrition and Food Research*, 62(3). Available from https://doi.org/10.1002/mnfr.201700721.

Pandey, K. R., Naik, S. R., & Vakil, B. V. (2015). Probiotics, prebiotics and synbiotics—A review. *Journal of Food Science and Technology*, 52(12), 7577−7587. Available from https://doi.org/10.1007/s13197-015-1921-1.

Parker, R. B. (1974). Probiotics, the other half of the antibiotic story. *Animal Nutrition and Health*, 29, 4−8.

Pineiro, M., Asp, N. G., Reid, G., Macfarlane, S., Morelli, L., Brunser, O., & Tuohy, K. (2008). FAO Technical meeting on prebiotics. *Journal of Clinical Gastroenterology*, 42, S156−S159.

Pompei, A., Cordisco, L., Amaretti, A., Zanoni, S., Raimondi, S., Matteuzzi, D., & Rossi, M. (2007). Administration of folate-producing bifidobacteria enhances folate status in wistar rats. *Journal of Nutrition*, 137(12), 2742−2746. Available from https://doi.org/10.1093/jn/137.12.2742.

Roškar, I., Švigelj, K., Štempelj, M., Volfand, J., Štabuc, B., Malovrh, Š., & Rogelj, I. (2017). Effects of a probiotic product containing Bifidobacterium animalis subsp. animalis IM386 and Lactobacillus plantarum MP2026 in lactose intolerant individuals: Randomized, placebo-controlled clinical trial. *Journal of Functional Foods*, 35, 1−8. Available from https://doi.org/10.1016/j.jff.2017.05.020.

Schönfeld, P., & Wojtczak, L. (2016). Short- and medium-chain fatty acids in energy metabolism: The cellular perspective. *Journal of Lipid Research*, 57(6), 943−954. Available from https://doi.org/10.1194/jlr.R067629.

Shanahan, F. (2010). Gut microbes: From bugs to drugs. *American Journal of Gastroenterology*, 105(2), 275−279. Available from https://doi.org/10.1038/ajg.2009.729.

Shen, N. T., Maw, A., Tmanova, L. L., Pino, A., Ancy, K., Crawford, C. V., Simon, M. S., & Evans, A. T. (2017). Timely use of probiotics in hospitalized adults prevents Clostridium difficile infection: A systematic review with meta-regression analysis. *Gastroenterology*, 152(8), 1889−1900.

Shenderov, B. A. (2013). Metabiotics: novel idea or natural development of probiotic conception. *Microbial Ecology in Health and Disease*, 24(1), 20399.

Simmering, R., & Breves, R. (2010). Prebiotic Cosmetics. In J. Krutmann, & P. Humbert (Eds.), *Nutrition for Healthy Skin*. Berlin, Heidelberg: Springer.

Singh, A., Vishwakarma, V., & Singhal, B. (2018). Metabiotics: the functional metabolic signatures of probiotics: current state-of-art and future research priorities—metabiotics: probiotics effector molecules. *Advances in Bioscience and Biotechnology*, 9(04), 147.

Sreeja, V., & Prajapati, J. B. (2013). Probiotic formulations: Application and status as pharmaceuticals—A review. *Probiotics and Antimicrobial Proteins*, 5(2), 81−91. Available from https://doi.org/10.1007/s12602-013-9126-2.

Taverniti, V., & Guglielmetti, S. (2011). The immunomodulatory properties of probiotic microorganisms beyond their viability (ghost probiotics: Proposal of paraprobiotic concept). *Genes and Nutrition*, 6(3), 261−274. Available from https://doi.org/10.1007/s12263-011-0218-x.

Thakur, K., & Tomar, S. K. (2015). Exploring indigenous Lactobacillus species from diverse niches for riboflavin production. *Journal of Young Pharmacists*, 7(2), 126−131. Available from https://doi.org/10.5530/jyp.2015.2.11.

Tomasik, P., & Tomasik, P. (2020). Probiotics, non-dairy prebiotics and postbiotics in nutrition. *Applied Sciences*, 10(4), 1470.

Tsilingiri, K., & Rescigno, M. (2013). Postbiotics: What else? *Beneficial Microbes*, 4(1), 101−107. Available from https://doi.org/10.3920/BM2012.0046.

Turek, S. (1960). The use of fractionated deproteinization of the blood serum for the determination of the soluble protein fractions. *Clinica Chimica Acta; International Journal of Clinical Chemistry*, 5, 689−694.

Vandenplas, Y., Huys, G., & Daube, G. (2015). Probiotics: An update. *Jornal de Pediatria*, 91(1), 6−21. Available from https://doi.org/10.1016/j.jped.2014.08.005.

Wasilewski, A., Zielińska, M., Storr, M., & Fichna, J. (2015). Beneficial effects of probiotics, prebiotics, synbiotics, and psychobiotics in inflammatory bowel disease. *Inflammatory Bowel Diseases*, 21(7), 1674−1682. Available from https://doi.org/10.1097/MIB.0000000000000364.

Yan, F., & Polk, D. B. (2020). Probiotics and probiotic-derived functional factors-mechanistic insights into applications for intestinal homeostasis. *Frontiers in Immunology*, 11, 1428.

Zawistowska-Rojek, A., & Tyski, S. (2018). Are probiotic really safe for humans? *Polish Journal of Microbiology*, 67(3), 251−258. Available from https://doi.org/10.21307/pjm-2018-044.

Chapter 2

Food or pharma: the name does make a difference

Magali Cordaillat-Simmons[1], Alice Rouanet[1] and Bruno Pot[1,2]
[1]Pharmabiotic Research Institute (PRI), Narbonne, France, [2]Research Group of Industrial Microbiology and Food Biotechnology (IMDO), Vrije Universiteit Brussel (Free University Brussels), Elsene, Belgium

2.1 Introduction

As the body of knowledge on the interaction between the microbiome and its host expands, the industry is taking this opportunity to develop new approaches to improve overall and specific health management. An increasing number of stakeholders are now involved in the development of products containing living microorganisms, aimed at positively influencing health by improving the balance between the microbiome and its host. Many strategies allow targeting the microbiome, varying from fecal and vaginal microbiota transplants, the use of synthetic ecosystem, phages, all the way to highly characterized strains (single or in combination) often addressed as "probiotics," a concept the consumer is familiar with due to the large media coverage.

In this chapter, we like to dive a bit deeper than the (social) media normally do, clarifying the legal width of the term "probiotic," particularly when it is used to "prevent, cure or manage a human disease."

When a product is intended to "prevent, cure or manage a human disease," it is to be considered a drug in legal terms. The drug status is highly regulated, with multiple requirements for the product to be placed on the market. The first section of this chapter will deal with the drug status, focusing on the importance of the "disease" aspect. The second section will deal with "probiotics" in particular focusing on their different regulatory statuses. In Section 2.3, the regulations in Europe, the United States, Canada, and Japan will be compared for probiotic substances used to promote human health, again with a focus on the intended use. Finally, in this chapter, we will try to objectively describe the borders between the "scientific" and the "regulatory" statuses of probiotics, which, still today, are often not very clear.

2.2 Probiotics: a substance or a product?

2.2.1 The probiotic confusion

A definition of probiotics has been proposed about 20 years ago by an expert committee composed by the WHO/FAO (Food and Agriculture Organization of the United Nations and World Health Organization, 2001) and was revisited more recently (Hill et al., 2014). While the definition is still quite universally used, the probiotics themselves have been the subject of many discussions, mainly on their efficacy, safety, dosing, or mode of action. Despite the vast amount of scientific literature, probiotics still cause confusion in the minds of consumers, patients, medical doctors, scientists, product developers, and interestingly, also regulators. A lot of confusion and discussion derives from differences in the intended use of the probiotic, which can be present in the market as a fresh food, as a food supplement, or even as a registered drug, all of which are intended to act on human health.

While a certain level of scientific confusion between substances' intrinsic characteristics and its biological abilities is not unusual, a similar confusion on its regulatory status should not be commonly observed. In the microbiome field, however, the term "probiotic" is often used disconnected from its intended use and target population and therefore outside its regulatory framework.

Below, the different regulatory categories will be clarified, together with their implications on safety and needed levels of efficacy documentation, determining the product's development cycle and its path to market.

2.2.2 Regulations at the "product" level: how to define the product's regulatory status?

To understand the regulatory confusion mentioned above, it is necessary to go back to the actual definition provided by the WHO/FAO, being "live microorganisms which when administered in adequate amounts, confer a health benefit to the host" (Food and Agriculture Organization of the United Nations and World Health Organization, 2001). Because this definition addresses notions of quality ("live," "in adequate amounts") and efficacy ("a health benefit"), the difference between the concepts "substance" and "product" may not be clearly retained. While a "substance" in most cases refers to the probiotic strain, scientifically documented for its biological effect on human physiological functions, the "product" is, regulatory speaking, what is placed on the market and includes, besides the product matrix, the packaging, the conditions of use, etc., also the scientific and technical considerations required by the regulatory status under which the product has been placed on the market. While the WHO/FAO definition of a "probiotic" is an important milestone in the recognition of a microbiome-based strategy to maintain or improve health, the definition only applies to the probiotic *substance*, and does not define its regulatory status as a *product*. As a consequence, it is clear that various types of products, under several regulatory statuses, may contain "probiotics," but that "probiotics" themselves are not a product.

For regulators worldwide, the most important characteristic of a product is its *intended use*. Indeed, it is very important to understand that the *composition* of a product has no influence at all on its path to market, as the latter is only defined by *what the product is supposed to do, and to whom*. Regulatory speaking, different types of probiotic products, containing the same active substance, can be commercialized under various regulatory regimes, determined by the intended use and the target population (Fig. 2.1).

Each and every one of these regulatory statuses is defined by appropriate legislation, and in the lack of international harmonization (often characterized by national and regional differences leading to specific standards and rules for documentation), product development, including the demonstration of safety and efficacy, must be carried out within the limits of the intended use. As mentioned before, the latter is very important as concepts of safety and efficacy do not exist per se, but are always in relation to the disease severity and vulnerability of the target population. Consequently, comparison and extrapolation of safety and efficacy between products of different regulatory statuses (e.g., between food and drug) is not possible (Cordaillat-Simmons et al., 2020).

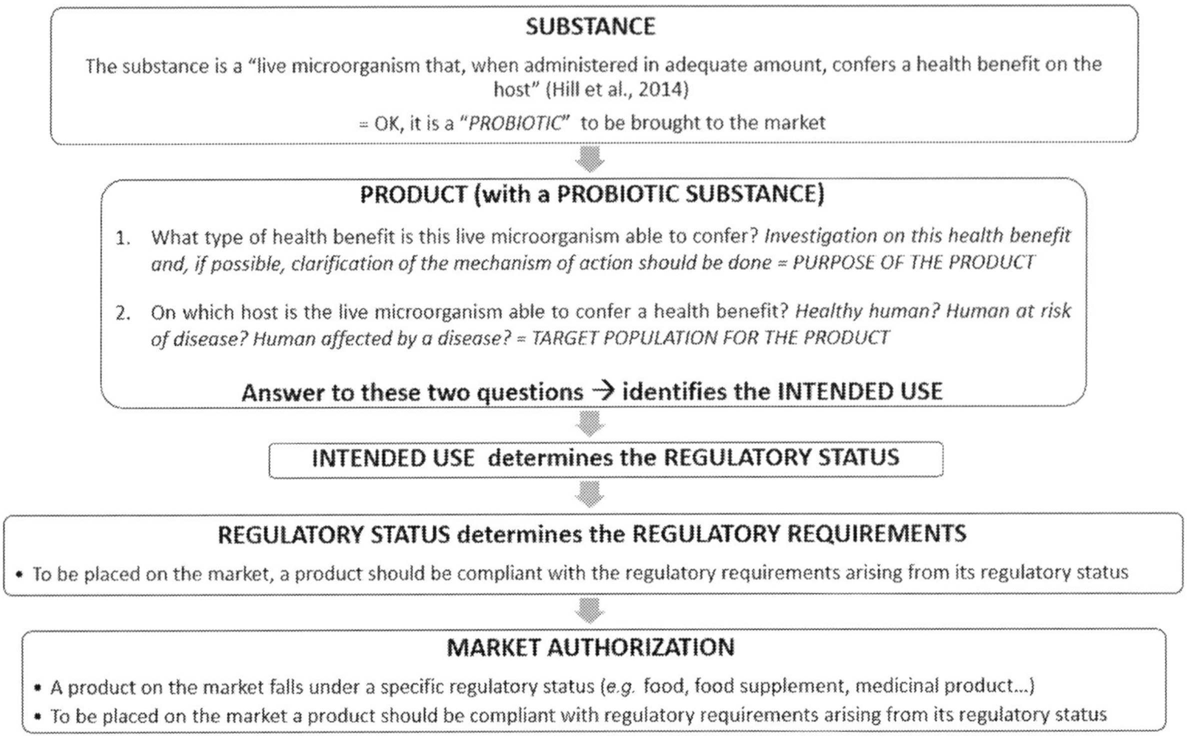

SUBSTANCE

The substance is a "live microorganism that, when administered in adequate amount, confers a health benefit on the host" (Hill et al., 2014)

= OK, it is a "*PROBIOTIC*" to be brought to the market

PRODUCT (with a PROBIOTIC SUBSTANCE)

1. What type of health benefit is this live microorganism able to confer? *Investigation on this health benefit and, if possible, clarification of the mechanism of action should be done = PURPOSE OF THE PRODUCT*

2. On which host is the live microorganism able to confer a health benefit? *Healthy human? Human at risk of disease? Human affected by a disease? = TARGET POPULATION FOR THE PRODUCT*

Answer to these two questions → identifies the INTENDED USE

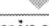

INTENDED USE determines the REGULATORY STATUS

REGULATORY STATUS determines the REGULATORY REQUIREMENTS

- To be placed on the market, a product should be compliant with the regulatory requirements arising from its regulatory status

MARKET AUTHORIZATION

- A product on the market falls under a specific regulatory status (*e.g.* food, food supplement, medicinal product...)
- To be placed on the market a product should be compliant with regulatory requirements arising from its regulatory status

FIGURE 2.1 Illustration of the difference between a substance and a product. The regulatory status is determining the path of the product to the market.

2.2.3 The drug status

Around the world, one concept is common and approved by almost all drug and health competent authorities: when a product is intended to prevent or cure a human disease, it is a drug (Government of Canada, 1985; Japan Pharmaceutical Manufacturers Association, 2018; Office of the Law Revision Counsel in the United States House of Representatives, 2016; The European Parliament and Council of the European Union, 2001). A drug can contain one or several active substance(s), intended to act on the human body to resolve or anticipate a disorder or disease. A drug is therefore intended to be administered to a sick human being, or to a person at risk of an anticipated pathology.

Consequently, drugs are rigorously regulated and drug development routines may be long, expensive, and complex. Once on the market, drug consumption will also be highly supervised by pharmacists and medical doctors. Before being placed on the market, however, drug competent authorities worldwide will evaluate and determine if a drug is efficient and safe for the targeted disease and in the targeted patient population. They will assess the risk–benefit balance of the drug before its market authorization (EMA, 2008; FDA, 2018a), based on the evidence of efficacy, safety, and quality of the drug, provided by the developer. Such evidence should be gathered according to a specific process detailed in regulatory and pharmaceutical guidelines (The International Council for Harmonisation of Technical Requirements for Pharmaceuticals for Human Use (ICH), 2002, 2016).

In short, a new active substance must first be tested in nonclinical models (e.g., in vitro and nonhuman in vivo models) before being tested in healthy humans. Results obtained from these so-called preclinical studies will be submitted to drug competent authorities before a Clinical Trial Authorisation can be obtained to enable the first-in-human use of the new active substance. This first-in-human use is normally performed in healthy humans only, at a preset dose range. In general, when found safe, the product can be tested in humans affected by the targeted pathology. However, for drugs containing live microorganisms as the active substance(s), it is not out of the ordinary to directly assess tolerability in the target population as the ecosystem of a healthy individual might not allow an optimal assessment of safety aspects, e.g. related to a patients' dysbiosis (Rouanet et al., 2020). Further testing on larger numbers of humans will require further authorization procedures, building on earlier test results. The data obtained during the different study phases will be compiled and will form the rationale for requesting marketing authorization. The format of a marketing authorization dossier is harmonized at the international level, well-known as the Common Technical Document (CTD), details of which are published by the International Council for Harmonisation of Technical Requirements for Pharmaceuticals for Human Use (ICH). In these dossiers, national and European guidelines are to be considered, as they can provide valuable information, allowing to anticipate on the competent authorities' expectations at each step of the development. While initially developed for "traditional" drugs, this procedure is valid and required for drugs that contain live microorganisms.

While the regulatory status by definition provides information on the way the product will be placed on the market, it also regulates the type of advertisement or information that can and needs to be provided to the consumer. Advertisement in relationship to drug products is highly regulated in most parts of the world, to the extent that some products, certainly for vulnerable populations, can only be obtained as prescription drugs.

2.2.4 The food status

Food and food supplements are also strictly regulated in most countries, although different from the above in terms of safety requirements and the type of claims that can be made (nutrition or health claims vs. medical claims). While in general the claim regulations for foods are much more heterogeneous in different parts of the world, a common pursuit by almost all legislators is to avoid untruthful claims or claims carrying misleading messages to the consumer, as well as to ban messages that suggest a medical or a therapeutic notion. In most cases, national competent authorities are in charge of reinforcing food claims and they may publish local, nonbinding recommendations explaining the regulatory requirements in their markets, which may help and support developers in their product development processes.

The second important difference with the drug category is that the target population for foods is a healthy or an at-risk population. As such, foods mostly address a less vulnerable population and requirements for safety and efficacy testing may be different, for example, allowing also aspects like "long history of safe use" as a safety consideration (Organisation for Economic Co-operation and Development (OECD), 1993). As discussed further in this chapter, notions of dose and efficacy, however, will still need to be addressed adequately to gain a health or nutrition claim.

It is thus of critical importance that developers consider early enough in the development cycle these two main questions "What is/are the health benefit(s) that my substance(s) is/are able to confer?" and "On which population my substance(s) is/are able to confer this/these health benefit(s)?" When in doubt it is advisable to consult the respective competent authorities.

2.3 The various regulatory statuses applicable to products containing "probiotics"
2.3.1 The general EU regulatory framework
2.3.1.1 The legal requirements

In the European Union (EU), community regulation is based on treaties (i.e., "primary law"), democratically approved by its members. EU laws (i.e., "secondary law") also exist and help to achieve the objectives of the EU treaties and to put EU policies into practice. EU laws are governing several areas, including public health. Public health regulation aims at attaining a high level of protection of consumers and patients and therefore covers different types of products, including foods and pharmaceuticals (European Commission, 2020).

EU law-making processes involve several European institutions including: the European Commission (EC), the European Parliament (EP), and the Council of the European Union (CEU). The EC is responsible for *planning, preparing*, and *proposing* new European legislation, while the EP and the CEU are in charge of *voting and implementing* EC proposals (The European Parliament and the Council of the European Union, 2002a).

The two most common types of legislation regulating foods and pharmaceuticals in the EU, among others, are the *Regulations* and *Directives*. *Regulations* are legal acts that apply automatically and uniformly as soon as they enter into force and are binding in their entirety for all EU countries. *Directives* require EU countries to achieve a certain result but leave member states free to choose how to achieve these. In general, EU countries will adopt measures by incorporating them into national law (transposition).

In Europe, there are two main regulatory statuses for human health-related products: foods and pharmaceuticals. Besides the specific regulation, laid down in the general principles and requirements of *food* law (The European Parliament and the Council of the European Union, 2002a) and applicable for all types of food products, the regulatory status of foods includes subcategories, covering different food aspects and products, leading to multiple derived legislations and laws. There is, for example:

- a regulation on the provision of *food information to consumers* (The European Parliament and the Council of the European Union, 2011), applicable to all food products, as well as,
- a directive relating to *food supplements* (The European Parliament and the Council of the European Union, 2002b), applicable only to food supplements, and
- a regulation on *nutrition and health claims* made on foods (The European Parliament and the Council of the European Union, 2006), applicable for developers wanting to claim specific health or nutritional benefits for their food product.

The drug regulatory status is regulated under the "Directive on the Community code relating to medicinal products for human use" (The European Parliament and Council of the European Union, 2001), describing all main regulatory requirements applicable to drugs intended for the European market. Additional *directives* or *regulations* were added more recently with the intention to clarify specific aspects of the registration process for *innovative products*. These legislations should be seen as complementary texts applicable during the development and registration cycle, but not aiming at replacing Directive 2001/83/EC (The European Parliament and Council of the European Union, 2001).

2.3.1.2 Complementary recommendations

Within the EU, there are separate legal entities, identified as European agencies, which are in charge of setting up and performing specific tasks under EU law and which are distinct from the EU institutions. In the context of human public health, two principal European agencies should be mentioned: the European Medicines Agency (EMA) (European Medicines Agency, 2018), closely working together with the European Directorate for Quality of Medicines (EDQM), and the European Food Safety Authority (EFSA) (European Food Safety Authority, 2020).

The EMA has to "foster scientific excellence in the evaluation and supervision of medicines, for the benefit of public and animal health in the European Union (EU)" (European Medicines Agency, 2018). For that purpose, the EMA publishes scientific guidelines in consultation with national drug regulatory authorities of the EU Member States. These guidelines are not binding (although strongly recommended by the Agency) but aim at helping applicants to prepare marketing authorization applications for medicines. These guidelines reflect the European harmonized approach on how to interpret and apply requirements stated in the Directive 2001/83/EC (The European Parliament and Council of the European Union, 2001), for the demonstration of quality, safety, and efficacy of medicinal products. The EMA is working closely together with another European entity (although with memberships extending outside the EU), namely the

EDQM (EDQM, 2020a). EDQM is a division of the Council of Europe, involved in European public health protection, enabling the development, support implementation, and monitoring of quality standards for safe medicines and their safe use (EDQM, 2020a). The EDQM is updating the European Pharmacopoeia (EDQM, 2020b), which includes monographs for medicines. These monographs establish quality standards for some category of medicines or proprietary medicines already on the European market.

The EFSA was founded in 2002. Following a series of food crises in the late 1990s, the agency was created by the European Commission to become "a source of scientific advice and communication on risks associated with the food chain" (European Food Safety Authority, 2020). This agency was legally established under the Regulation (EC) No 178/2002, also named the "General Food Law" (The European Parliament and the Council of the European Union, 2002a), which created a European food safety system. Within this system, the EFSA is mainly responsible for food risk assessment and also has a duty to communicate its scientific findings on food-related risks to the public. Later EFSA was made responsible for the scientific evaluation of health claims, according to Regulation (EC) No 1924/2006 of the European parliament and of the Council, published on December 20, 2006, and covering nutrition and health claims made on foods. While EFSA is responsible for the scientific evaluation of the dossiers submitted by the EU member states, their advice is turned into decision by the European Commission, as explained below.

2.3.1.3 Specificities of the food and the pharmaceutical regulatory framework in the EU
2.3.1.3.1 The pharma status of probiotics

The above-mentioned EC Directive (The European Parliament and Council of the European Union, 2001) clearly defines what is to be considered a medicinal product at the EU level:

(a) *Any substance or combination of substances presented as having properties for treating or preventing disease in human beings; or*
(b) *Any substance or combination of substances which may be used in or administered to human beings either with a view to restoring, correcting or modifying physiological functions by exerting a pharmacological, immunological or metabolic action, or to making a medical diagnosis.*

As mentioned above, the definition does not take into account the particular nature of the product but is based on its *intended use* (Fig. 2.1). In the EU, a medicinal product must be registered at national or at EU level, through the obtention of an appropriate marketing authorization.

Since Directive 2001/83/EC (The European Parliament and Council of the European Union, 2001, p. 83) defines "*Substance*" as:

any matter irrespective of origin which may be:

(a) *human, e.g. human blood and human blood products;*
(b) *animal, e.g.* **micro-organisms**, *whole animals, parts of organs, animal secretions, toxins, extracts, blood products;*
(c) *vegetable, e.g.* **micro-organisms**, *plants, parts of plants, vegetable secretions, extracts;*
(d) *chemical, e.g. elements, naturally occurring chemical materials and chemical products obtained by chemical change or synthesis.*

it is clear that microorganisms can be the active substance(s) of a medicinal product. Consequently, products containing probiotic substance(s) intended to prevent or treat disease through a pharmacological, immunological, or metabolic action, fall under the *medicinal product* status and should be registered as such in the EU.

In the marketing authorization application, developers must demonstrate a positive benefit/risk ratio in the intended population. Documentation on the quality, efficacy and safety of the medicinal product must be provided and pharmaceutical standards must be applied all along the development process.

The CTD and its guidelines are organized around two big categories of medicinal products: the new chemical entities and the biological/biotechnological products. For the biological products category, as explained before (Cordaillat-Simmons et al., 2020), the legislator has defined subcategories, such as vaccines, blood- and plasma-derived products, or advanced therapies medicinal products (including gene therapy, somatic cell therapy, and tissue engineered products).

In the absence of any specific regulation, probiotic substance(s) intended to prevent or treat human disease are therefore to be considered *biological medicinal products* by nature and must comply with the requirements laid out in the legislation and pharmaceutical regulatory framework for those products. In contrast to the United States, the EMA has yet to produce specific guidelines for this type of medicinal product. However, existing guidelines, relating to other types of biological products can and should be considered, applying the corresponding concepts to the development of probiotic substance(s) intended to prevent or treat human disease (Cordaillat-Simmons et al., 2020).

Importantly, in 2019, the European Pharmacopoeia (European Pharmacopoeia Commission, 2019) released the first guideline dedicated to "medicinal products containing live microorganism(s) as active substance," which are not acting as vaccines, and decided to name them "Live Biotherapeutic Products" (LBPs). This name avoids future regulatory confusion with the "probiotic" terminology and, interestingly, for producers and developers, harmonizes the terminology with the United States. The 2019 Monograph (European Pharmacopoeia Commission, 2019) now defines the category at the EU level and provides the standards applicable for the production and quality control of these products.

Overall, as for all medicinal products, but particularly for biological medicinal products, LBPs must be developed on the basis of a risk analysis that takes into account the particular characteristics of the strain(s) as well as the particular vulnerabilities of the patients. As explained before (Rouanet et al., 2020), risk analysis is the thread, which will guide and verify the entire development process from substance selection, over preclinical and human clinical studies, all the way to postmarket surveillance.

Finally, we like to highlight the necessity for an adapted, proprietary and unique approach during this entire process. All stakeholders involved, from academia to clinicians and industrial producers, need to understand that data obtained with products registered under any *other* regulatory status may at best provide "proof of concept" or may be considered "supportive evidence" but cannot be considered specific for the substantiation of the safety and efficacy of a particular LBP, even when containing a similar or even an identical "probiotic substance." Pharmaceutical standards are such that the very specific composition of the LBP, its particular production process (determined by the pharmaceutical requirements in terms of quality), its biological efficacy, and safety documentation are all fully framed by the intended use, in the intended population, and by the risk analysis, which has been made in this explicit context only.

Therefore it is important for stakeholders to use appropriate wordings and respect regulatory concepts at any time, to avoid regulatory confusion, and to consider the use of the LBP terminology for any publication or communication on products used for the prevention or treatment of human disease and containing "probiotic strain(s)" as active substance.

2.3.1.3.2 The status of "probiotic" claims for foods in Europe

2.3.1.3.2.1 Health claims made on foods In Europe, a health claim is defined as "any statement about a relationship between food and health." As mentioned above, the two main categories, the health claims and the nutrition claims, are regulated by Regulation (EC) No 1924/2006, Regulation on nutrition and health claims made on foods (The European Parliament and the Council of the European Union, 2006), legally enforced since July 1, 2007. In the frame of this chapter, we will only consider health claims (and not nutrition claims), as health claims, to a certain extent, may be confused with medical claims.

After the introduction of the new health claim regulation (The European Parliament and the Council of the European Union, 2006), nationally approved health claims were no longer valid and needed to be replaced by EU-approved health claims. In Europe, individual producers or academic institutions cannot submit health claims to the EFSA, a process that is reserved to the national authorities, besides the EU parliament and the EU Commission. EU countries initially provided the Commission with national lists containing around 44,000 claims. These were consolidated into 4637 claims that in the meantime have in part been evaluated by the EFSA. The outcomes were published as "opinions" in series; an overview of the authorized and not authorized claims can be found in Nutrition and Health Claims register (EU Register of nutrition and health claims made on foods (v.3.5), 2020).

The European Commission authorized different subtypes of health claims. "Function Health Claims," also called Article 13 claims (The European Parliament and the Council of the European Union, 2006), either relate to the role of a nutrient or substance in the growth, development, and function of the body, in psychological and behavioral functions, or in slimming and weight-control (by reducing energy intake or increasing satiety). The "Risk Reduction Claims," or Article 14(1)(a) claims (The European Parliament and the Council of the European Union, 2006), are intended to claim the reduction of a risk factor in the development of a disease. The most well-known cases are, for example, related to *plant stanol esters*, shown to reduce blood cholesterol, which is considered as a proven risk factor for the development of cardiovascular disease, or the claim related to the replacement of fast sugars by *dietary fibers*, resulting in reduced blood glucose levels and therefore potentially in reducing or delaying the development of diabetes. The third and last category covers health claims referring to "Children's development" (Article 14(1)(b) claims) (The European Parliament and the Council of the European Union, 2006), with, for example, vitamin D, accepted to be important for bone development in children.

Health claims of any of these categories can only be approved, provided "they are based on scientific evidence and can be understood by the consumers." It is the above-mentioned EFSA who is responsible for the evaluation of the scientific evidence provided by the food producer. The EFSA, however, does not have the power to adopt health claims, a task that is reserved for the European Commission. Once adopted by the Commission, approved health claims can be used in all 27 EU member states.

The procedure to adopt "Article 13" and "Article 14" health claims may slightly differ (European Commission, 2016).

For "Article 13" health claims, the Commission prepares a draft decision establishing the list of approved claims, which is submitted to the Standing Committee on the Food Chain and Animal Health, composed of representatives of the competent authorities of the EU member states. After the Standing Committee approved the list by qualified majority vote, the European Parliament and the European Council will have the final word and without further objection the Commission will adopt the draft decision. Currently, the "Article 13 list" is processed in two steps, the health claim list for botanical substances and the health claims other than those for botanical substances.

The list of permitted "Article 13" health claims (nonbotanicals) was published as a part of the Commission Regulation (EU) No 432/2012 (European Commission, 2012), applicable since December 14, 2012. In 2012, the European Commission also published a list of 2000 claims for which the scientific assessment by the EFSA was put "on hold," most of them referring to "botanicals." Early 2021, these claims are still "on hold" and can only be used nationally if they comply with national legislation or Europe-wise when they comply with other provisions of the 1924/2006 Nutrition and Health Claim regulation. The list of permitted health claims No 432/2012 (European Commission, 2012) is regularly updated with newly authorized health claims.

For "Article 14" health claims [Articles 14(1)(a) and 14(1)(b)], a slightly different authorization procedure is to be used. Individual applications should first be submitted to the competent authority of an EU member state, who will transmit the dossier to the EFSA, when found admissible. EFSA will evaluate the dossier and publish its opinion. The Commission will then prepare a draft decision, which again is submitted to the Standing Committee on Plants, Animals, Food and Feed. Upon a favorable opinion of the Standing Committee, the European Parliament and the European Council will have the last word and in the lack of any objection, the Commission will adopt the draft decision.

Important in the whole concept is the fact that stakeholders cannot apply directly for health claims but have to submit their application through a member state of the EU. To be successful, applicants should use the Commission's implementing rules, established by Commission Regulation (EC) No 353/2008 (European Commission, 2008) and using several guidance documents available on the EFSA website (EFSA, 2021).

Third parties can also only address their concerns through their country's competent authority or through the Commission but cannot communicate directly with the EFSA. Comments or questions relating to scientific issues received by the Commission will be transmitted to the EFSA and their response will be published.

Following the publication of the first health claim list, the Commission received numerous letters about the effects of the Regulation on the sector of food supplements, including those which contain probiotic substances. As mentioned above, EFSA consequently produced additional guidance documents, which helped to clarify the initial regulations, as for some conditions developers had doubts on the exact requirements for a dossier or had trouble in defining the borders with pharmaceutical products (EU Standing Committee on the Food Chain and Animal Health, 2007; European Food Safety Authority, 2011a,b). Examples of these situations are the reduction of a risk factor in the development of a human disease, or the use of probiotics for "treating" widely spread discomforts, such as irritable bowel syndrome, which, in some cases might also require a treatment as a disease.

Relevant for this chapter is that the term "probiotic" has been said to imply a health claim in itself (EU Standing Committee on the Food Chain and Animal Health, 2007). As such, food products, including food supplements, aiming to affix the word "probiotic" on their label should only do so after a health claim has been submitted and approved by the European Commission. More details on the classification of claims and the labeling in the EU can be found in the General Guidance on the implementation of Regulation No 1924/2006 on nutrition and health claims made on foods (EU Standing Committee on the Food Chain and Animal Health, 2007).

2.3.1.3.2.2 *Food for special medical purposes* Europe has also defined a "Food for special medical purposes" category, regulated by the Commission Directive 1999/21/EC (European Commission, 1999), adopted under the old legislative framework of Directive 2009/39/EC (The European Parliament and the Council of the European Union, 2009). A more recent Commission delegated Regulation (EU) 2016/128 (The European Commission, 2015) started to apply on February 22, 2019, mainly extending the scope to infants and young children.

Foods for special medical purposes are intended for the dietary management of individuals who suffer from certain diseases, disorders, or medical conditions, and whose nutritional requirements cannot be met by normal foods. These foods should be used only under medical supervision.

The above directives describe the rules for the composition and the labeling of these foods and give guidance for the minimum and maximum levels of vitamins and minerals. Nutritional substances that may be used in the manufacture of foods for special medical purposes are laid down in Commission Regulation (EC) No 953/2009 (European Commission, 2009); pro- or prebiotics are not on the list. Given, however, the increasing understanding of the potential role of the microbiota in the maintenance of health or the development of disease, it is not unlikely that they might be considered for inclusion on this foods for special medical purposes list in the future.

2.3.2 The general US regulatory framework

In the United States, regulation is based on federal laws which are compiled in the "United States Code." Federal lawmaking processes involve the Congress, which includes two legislative bodies: the US Senate and the US House of Representatives. The Congress is the legislative branch of government and passes laws, in the form of acts of Congress (United States Government, 2021). Products for human health are regulated in the US Federal Food, Drug, and Cosmetic Act (Office of the Law Revision Counsel in the United States House of Representatives, 2016) where the regulatory statuses of food, medicines, and cosmetics are defined. In comparison to Europe, all regulatory requirements are stated in the same text and all the information related to human health products can be found in this Federal Food, Drug, and Cosmetic Act (Office of the Law Revision Counsel in the United States House of Representatives, 2016). The Federal Food, Drug, and Cosmetic Act is codified into Title 21 Chapter 9 of the US Code (Office of the Law Revision Counsel in the United States House of Representatives, 2016).

Besides the Congress, as is the case in the EU, executive agencies are charged to carry out federal laws; this represents the executive branch of the American government. Executive agencies publish, in the form of specific regulations, their interpretation of the law, and what stakeholders must do to follow the law to meet the agency's requirements. The American executive agencies responsible for protecting public health in general are the National Institute of Health (NIH), the Center for Diseases Control (CDC), and the Food and Drug Administration (FDA). Among those, the FDA is the competent authority for food and drugs.

The FDA is mandated to ensure "*the safety, efficacy, and security of human and veterinary drugs, biological products, and medical devices*" and to ensure "*the safety of food supply, cosmetics, and products that emit radiation*" (FDA, 2018b). Therefore the FDA is the primary agency to promulgate the Federal Food, Drug, and Cosmetic Act. For that purpose, this agency publishes and updates regulations in the Code of Federal Regulations (CFR) Title 21 and, in addition, publishes guidance documents clarifying such regulations.

Like guidelines in the EU, guidance documents represent FDA's current thinking on a particular subject but do not create or confer any rights for, or on, any person and do not operate to bind FDA or the public. In the United States, the FDA performs the functions of both the European EMA and the EFSA, managing and controlling both drug and food regulations.

2.3.2.1 Specificities of the food and the pharmaceutical regulatory framework in the United States

Chapter 9 of the US Federal Food, Drug, and Cosmetic Act (Office of the Law Revision Counsel in the United States House of Representatives, 2016) defines and clarifies the intended use of food and pharmaceutical products.

"*Food*" means

(1) articles used for food or drink for man or other animals,
(2) chewing gum, and
(3) articles used for components of any such article.

"*Dietary supplement*" means

(1) a product (other than tobacco) intended to supplement the diet that bears or contains one or more of the following dietary ingredients:

  (A) a vitamin;
  (B) a mineral;

(C) a herb or other botanical;
(D) an amino acid;
(E) a dietary substance for use by man to supplement the diet by increasing the total dietary intake; or
(F) a concentrate, metabolite, constituent, extract, or combination of any ingredient described in clause (A), (B), (C), (D) or (E);
a product that [...] is not represented for use as a conventional food or as a sole item of a meal or the diet [...].

Dietary supplements shall be deemed to be a food within the meaning of this chapter.

"Drug" means

[...] articles intended for use in the diagnosis, cure, mitigation, treatment, or prevention of disease in man or other animals [...].

As explained above, when the intended use of a product is therapeutic or prophylactic, in the United States as well as in the EU, the product will fall under the pharmaceutical legislation and have a drug status.

2.3.2.2 The food status of probiotics in the United States

In the United States, probiotic strain(s) may be regulated as drugs, foods, dietary supplements, or medical foods, according to their intended use. Dietary supplements can be seen as a special food class and are regulated by the Dietary Supplement Health and Education Act (DSHEA) of 1994 (Office of the Law Revision Counsel in the United States House of Representatives, 1994), which amended the Food, Drug, and Cosmetic Act (Office of the Law Revision Counsel in the United States House of Representatives, 2016). The DSHEA provides information on the definition (and therefore its intended use), the composition, the form of ingestion, and the approach for the safety assessment of the dietary supplements. In addition, the FDA (who is part of the US Department of Health and Humans Services) also specifies the rules of good manufacturing practices (GMP), packaging, labeling, and holding operations for such products (FDA, 2019a).

To not add to the potential confusion, it is important to remind that the terms "functional foods" or "nutraceuticals," often used by marketers and most often well known to the consumer, do not officially "exist" in the legislative framework and stakeholders therefore should only refer to the above definitions, guidelines, and standards when developing and documenting their products with probiotic strains for market authorization.

2.3.2.2.1 Health claims in the United States

When considering health claims for foods and dietary supplements, US legislation is, furthermore, also very strict, aiming to avoid misleading the consumer.

"Health claims" are defined (FDA, 2020a) as *"any claim made on the label or in labelling of a food, including a dietary supplement, that expressly or by implication, including "third party" references, written statements (e.g., a brand name including a term such as "heart"), symbols (e.g., a heart symbol), or vignettes, characterizes the relationship of any substance to a disease or health-related condition."*

"Implied health claims" include *"those statements, symbols, vignettes, or other forms of communication that suggests, within the context in which they are presented, that a relationship exists between the presence or level of a substance in the food and a disease or health-related condition."*

In addition, and to avoid confusion, the American legislator also clarified the terms **"disease"** and **"health-related condition"** (FDA, 2020a) as *"damage to an organ, part, structure, or system of the body such that it does not function properly (e.g., cardiovascular disease), or a state of health leading to such dysfunctioning (e.g. hypertension); except that diseases resulting from essential nutrient deficiencies (e.g. scurvy, pellagra) are not included in this definition."*

In the United States, few types of health claims can be made for food products and dietary supplements.

The **"NLEA Authorized Health Claims"** characterize the relationship between a food, a food component, or a dietary ingredient and risk of diseases (FDA, 2020b). In this category, all claims must be approved by the FDA, based on an extensive review of the scientific literature and in agreement with scientific standards and will only allow the product to be placed on the market if the substance/disease relationship is well established.

The "**Health Claims based on Authoritative Statements**" can be authorized by submitting a notification from certain scientific bodies of the US government, such as the CDC or NIH, or the national academy of sciences, to the FDA. However, this type of claim is not allowed for dietary supplements (FDA, 2020b).

The "**Qualified Health Claim**" (FDA, 2020b) is based on a petition procedure that provides a mechanism to request that the FDA reviews scientific evidence and exercises enforcement discretion to permit the use of the Qualified Claim. The Qualified Health Claim is assessed based on the body of knowledge and the level of scientific evidence for a relationship between a food substance (a food, food component, or dietary ingredient), and reduced risk of a disease or health-related condition. If the FDA finds the evidence credible, it issues a letter outlining the circumstances under which the claim can be used as well as the qualifying language to indicate that the evidence supporting the claim is limited.

In addition to health claims, another type of claims can be made on food such as:

The *"structure/function claim"* also named *"statement of nutritional support"* can be made, according to DSHEA (Office of the Law Revision Counsel in the United States House of Representatives, 1994), if *"the statement claims a benefit related to a classical nutrient deficiency disease and discloses the prevalence of such disease in the United States, describes the role of a nutrient or dietary ingredient intended to affect the structure or function in humans, characterizes the documented mechanism by which a nutrient or dietary ingredient acts to maintain such structure or function, or describes general well-being from consumption of a nutrient or dietary ingredient."*

This type of claim does not require preapproval by the FDA but must be truthful and not misleading. The manufacturer, however, must submit a notification with the text of the claim to FDA no later than 30 days after marketing the product. Unlike health claims, dietary guidance statements and structure/function claims are not subject to premarket review and authorization by FDA.

When using structure function claims, DSHEA makes mandatory the insertion of the following statement: "This statement has not been evaluated by the Food and Drug Administration. This product is not intended to diagnose, treat, cure, or prevent any disease." Indeed, as reminded by the DSHEA, "a statement under this subparagraph may not claim to diagnose, mitigate, treat, cure, or prevent a specific disease or class of diseases."

Therefore in the United States as well, it is forbidden to make "disease claims" or "therapeutic claims" on foods and dietary supplements, outside of those approved through regulatory mechanisms by the FDA because they are not developed according to the appropriate standards needed for an intended use as drug.

2.3.2.2.2 Probiotics as medical foods

According to the Orphan Drug Act (FDA, 2013a), a "***Medical food***" means "a *food which is formulated to be consumed or administered enterally under the supervision of a physician and which is intended for the specific dietary management of a disease or condition for which distinctive nutritional requirements, based on recognized scientific principles, are established by medical evaluation.*"

In 2016, the FDA released a guideline with the frequently asked questions about medical foods (FDA Center for Food Safety and Applied Nutrition, 2016) in which it is stated, very similarly as in the EU, that "*medical foods are distinguished from the broader category of foods for special dietary use, by the requirement that medical food be intended to meet distinctive nutritional requirements of a disease or condition, used under medical supervision, and intended for the specific dietary management of a disease or condition.*"

The competent authority also specifies that "*they are not those (foods) simply recommended by physicians as part as an overall diet to manage the symptoms or reduce a risk of a disease or condition. [...] instead, medical foods are foods that are specially formulated and processed (as opposed to naturally occurring food stuff used in natural state) for a patient who requires use of the product as a major component of a disease or condition's specific management*" (FDA Center for Food Safety and Applied Nutrition, 2016).

In addition to this definition, the FDA has established criteria that clarify this definition by way of regulation (21 CFR 101.9(j)(8)) (FDA, 2020c):

A medical food is exempt from the nutrition labelling requirements of 21 CFR 101.9 only if:

(a) *It is a specially formulated and processed product (as opposed to a naturally occurring foodstuff used in its natural state) for the partial or exclusive feeding of a patient by means of oral intake or enteral feeding by tube, meaning a tube or catheter that delivers nutrients beyond the oral cavity directly into the stomach or small intestine;*

(b) It is intended for the dietary management of a patient who, because of therapeutic or chronic medical needs, has limited or impaired capacity to ingest, digest, absorb, or metabolize ordinary foodstuffs or certain nutrients, or who has other special medically determined nutrient requirements, the dietary management of which cannot be achieved by the modification of the normal diet alone.
(c) It provides nutritional support specifically modified for the management of the unique nutrient needs that result from the specific disease or condition, as determined by medical evaluation;
(d) It is intended to be used under medical supervision; and
(e) It is intended only for a patient receiving active and ongoing medical supervision wherein the patient requires medical care on a recurring basis for, among other things, instructions on the use of the medical food.

While enforcement of the "medical food" regulation is challenging for the FDA, a few opportunities allowed the FDA to publish their vision regarding the use of the "medical food" status for selected foods.

In 2013, the FDA sends a warning letter to a company that commercialized medical foods containing probiotics, indicated for various diseases (FDA, 2013b). They stated that *"FDA considers the statutory definition of "medical food" to narrowly constrain the types of products that fit within this category. In addition to other criteria, medical foods must be for the dietary management of a specific disorder, disease, or condition for which there are distinctive nutritional requirements and must be intended to be used under medical supervision. Patients with such a disorder, disease, or condition must have a limited capacity to ingest, digest, absorb, or metabolize ordinary foodstuffs or certain nutrients, or have other special medically determined nutrient requirements, which cannot be managed by the modification of the normal diet alone. Medical foods are not those simply recommended by a physician as part of an overall diet to reduce the risk of a disease or condition."* In this warning letter, the FDA furthermore reminded that, based on its interpretation of the limits of the medical food regulatory status, the authority is not aware of distinctive nutritional requirements for chronic fatigue syndrome, fibromyalgia, leaky gut syndrome, metabolic syndrome, inflammatory bowel diseases, type 2 diabetes, allergy-responsive asthma, eczema, rhinitis, or peripheral artery disease, which were labeled on the various medical food products (FDA, 2013b).

In the United States, medical food products are therefore equivalent to the European Food for Special Medical Purposes (FSMP) and, as discussed above, are also differently regulated from the "traditional" dietary supplements. In both cases, the intended use is very similar and, even if reinforcement is challenging for the authorities (particularly in the United States where multiple products have already been placed on the market with a medical food status), developers must understand that FSMP and medical food statuses are not appropriate for the vast majority of probiotic strains. Indeed, it would require the demonstration that such strains have a nutritional effect in patients for whom the same nutritional impact cannot be obtained by a modification of the normal diet alone.

Finally, in terms of standards, medical foods must comply with all applicable FDA requirements for foods, such as the current GMP requirements for production (FDA, 2019a). Any ingredient added to a medical food should be in compliance with the applicable provision of the Food and Drug Act and the FDA regulations. More specifically, in terms of safety, the substance should be generally recognized by qualified experts, to be safe under the condition of its intended use (Generally Recognized As Safe; status granted) (FDA, 2019b).

2.3.2.3 The pharmaceutical regulatory status for probiotics in the United States

As mentioned above and, to avoid regulatory confusion for probiotics (among others), the FDA decided to specifically clarify the regulatory status and framework to be applied to "probiotic strain(s)" used as active substances in products intended to cure, mitigate, treat, or prevent human diseases.

In a dedicated guideline from 2012 (FDA, 2016), the FDA introduced the term "**Live Biotherapeutic Product**" (LBP) as

"a biological product that

(1) contains live organisms, such as bacteria;
(2) is applicable to the prevention, treatment, or cure of a disease or condition of human beings; and,
(3) is not a vaccine."

and furthermore, *"LBPs are not filterable viruses, oncolytic bacteria, or products intended as gene therapy agents and, as a general matter, are not administered by injection."*

This guideline specifies the minimum requirements for quality as well as the expectations of the competent authority toward the assessment of safety and efficacy at the preclinical and clinical levels.

As for all drugs, LBPs are intended to prevent disease or treat human beings and the standards for their evaluation and placement on the market must take into account the fact that these products are potentially targeting populations presenting particular weaknesses, and in this context, the risks associated with their intake must be documented with appropriate studies (Cordaillat-Simmons et al., 2020).

To obtain a Biologics Licence, equivalent to a drug-marketing authorization for LBPs in the United States, developers must demonstrate a favorable benefit/risk ratio in the intended population, respecting the requirements laid out in the CTD (The International Council for Harmonisation of Technical Requirements for Pharmaceuticals for Human Use (ICH), 2002), harmonized at the ICH level as mentioned previously. As many of these "live" products have a mode of action that differs considerably from the majority of traditional drug products, including other biologics, recent guidelines have further clarified the approach to be taken for their development (Cordaillat-Simmons et al., 2020; Dreher-Lesnick et al., 2017).

As mentioned in Section 2.3, the regulatory framework for drugs is quite harmonized, and competent authorities in different parts of the world have adopted the "LBP" terminology, minimizing the confusion for drug products containing probiotic substances.

2.3.3 Canadian regulatory framework

In Canada, health products are regulated by the Ministry of Health through the Food and Drug Act (Government of Canada, 1985) and the Food and Drug Regulations (Government of Canada, 2020a). Besides, Health Canada is the competent authority in charge of the evaluation and approval of foods, drugs, and other health products for the Canadian market (Health Canada, 2016a), including the publication of guidance documents and monographs.

2.3.3.1 Details of the food regulatory framework

Under Section 2 of the Canadian Food and Drug Act (Government of Canada, 1985), a **food product** is defined as *"any article manufactured, sold, represented for use as food or drinking in human beings, chewing gum, and any ingredient that may be mixed with food for any purpose whatever."* According to this document, the intended use of a food product in Canada is therefore *"to feed or hydrate human beings."*

Under Section 5(1) of the same legislation we are reminded that *"No person shall label, package, treat, process, sell or advertise any food in a manner that is false, misleading or deceptive or is likely to create an erroneous impression regarding its character, value, quantity, composition, merit or safety."* Clearly, these provisions cover claims for food products and have been designed to avoid false claims toward consumers.

To clarify the acceptable use of health claims for probiotics, Health Canada released a dedicated guideline in 2009 (Health Canada, Food Directorate Health Products and Food Branch, 2009) as well as a list of eligible species for nonstrain-specific claims (Government of Canada, C.F.I.A., 2014). The Canadian Food Inspection Agency uses this guideline to administer and assess compliance with the Food and Drug Act (Government of Canada, 1985). This guideline specifies:

"Health Claims" are *"any representation in labelling or advertising that states, suggests or implies that a relationship exists between consumption of a food or food constituent (including an ingredient in the food) and a person's health."*

"Function Claims" are *"health claims that describe the physiological effect of foods or food constituents on normal functions or biological activities of the body associated with health or performance."*

"Therapeutic Claims" are *"claims that would bring a food into the definition of a drug or a natural health product (drug claim)."* These claims are therefore excluding the product from the food framework.

The competent authority in Canada reminds us that health claims for food products should be scientifically validated and with validation of claims is understood *"a) a systematic review of the relevant scientific evidence to support the claimed or implied effect of each of the probiotic strain(s) at their claimed intake levels; and b) when evidence from markers is used to support the claimed or implied health benefit, the markers should be recognized as being valid and biologically relevant to the claim being made."*

Under the same Food and Drug Act (Government of Canada, 1985), manufacturers and importers of food products are made legally responsible for the safety of the product(s) they place on the market, including products containing living microorganisms. With regard to safety, the guideline on the Use of Probiotic Microorganisms in Food (Health Canada, Food Directorate Health Products and Food Branch, 2009) reminds us that *"if live bacterial cultures (or*

"*Probiotics*") *added to food or food ingredients do not have a safe history of use in foods, or if the strain is genetically modified, or otherwise falls into the definition of a novel food under division 28 of Part B of the Food and Drug Regulations, it would be subjected to the requirements set out in that division,*" thereby requiring that all strain(s) placed on the market are safe for the consumer.

Like comparable legislations in Europe and the United States, the Canadian legislation and competent authorities try to ensure that within the framework of the intended use, any food product placed on the market is safe and does not carry misleading or false claims for the intended population.

2.3.3.2 The pharmaceutical regulatory framework in Canada

As mentioned above, all products with claimed therapeutic use will be qualified as drugs in Canada. Under Article 2 of the Food and Drugs Act (Government of Canada, 1985), **drugs** are defined as:

> *Any substance or mixture of substances manufactured, sold or represented for use in:*
>
> *The diagnosis, treatment, mitigation or prevention of a disease, disorder, or abnormal physical state, or its symptoms, in human beings or animals,*
> *Restoring, correcting, or modifying organic functions in human beings or animals, or*
> *Disinfection in premises in which food is manufactured prepared or kept.*

Drug products that contain living microorganisms as active substance may fall under two categories according to their specific characteristics and history of use and can therefore be placed on the market as either "**Natural Health Products**" (NHPs) or "**Biologic Drugs**."

2.3.3.2.1 Natural Health Products

The Natural Health Products Regulation (Government of Canada, 2003) defines a NHP as "*a substance set out in Schedule 1,* (in which the included NHP substances are specified, with Number 8 in the list being "A probiotic" (Government of Canada, 2020b)) *or a combination of substances in which all the medicinal ingredients are substances set out in Schedule 1, a homeopathic medicine or a traditional medicine, that is manufactured, sold or represented for use in:*

> *(a) the diagnosis, treatment, mitigation, or prevention of a disease, disorder, or abnormal physical state or its symptoms in humans,*
> *(b) restoring or correcting organic functions in humans; or*
> *(c) modifying organic functions in humans, such as modifying those functions in a manner that maintains or promotes health.*"

This definition clearly indicates that the intended use of a NHP is for prevention, treatment, or cure of a disease, therefore safety, and efficacy of NHP containing probiotics should be addressed in the context of a population presenting certain weaknesses, in contrast to food products containing probiotics. The body of knowledge to be presented to the competent authority should therefore focus on that medical aspect, and data generated will not only provide information on the safety of the strain(s) but also on the safety of the product within the targeted population.

2.3.3.2.2 Biologic Drugs

Products for which the active substance is a strain recently isolated from humans and pursuant to a prescription, could in the near future fall under Section 2(2) as well as under Schedule D of the Food and Drug Regulations, specifying "*Drugs, other than antibiotics, prepared from microorganisms*" (Government of Canada, 2020a). As such, these products would be classified as "*Biologic Drugs*" in Canada as well.

While the "*Biologic Drug*" terminology has not been officially defined yet in the Canadian legal framework, Health Canada already defines it as "*coming from living microorganisms or from their cells*" (Health Canada, 2016b) and when strains are developed as active substance of a biological drug product, safety, efficacy, and quality of the products are assessed by the Biologic and Radiopharmaceutical Drugs Directorate within the Health Product and Food Branch of Health Canada (Health Canada, 2007). This Directorate is in charge of evaluating whether developers are producing strong enough evidence to support the quality, safety, and efficacy of the product, in line with the intended fragile population.

Finally, to further clarify the differences between NHPs and Biologic Drugs according to Article C.04.002 under Schedule D, *"this division (Biologic Drugs) does not apply to a drug in oral dosage form that contains microorganisms, if the drug is recommended solely for restoring, normalizing, or stabilizing the intestinal flora"* (Government of Canada, 2020a). Such provision represents the traditional intended use for an NHP containing probiotic strains.

In conclusion, in analogy with the LBP nomenclature in the EU and the United States for products with live microorganisms as active substance, stakeholders should be encouraged to use the appropriate terminology in Canada as well and use the NHP or Biologic Drug Product qualification for drugs that contain a probiotic substance intended to prevent or treat a disease in a specific population.

2.3.3.3 Standards and constraints associated with the pharmaceutical regulatory frameworks

2.3.3.3.1 Natural Health Products

Part 2, Article 4(1) of the Natural Health Products Regulations (Government of Canada, 2003) specifies that *"no person shall sell a Natural Health Product unless a product license is issued in respect of the Natural Health Product."* In addition, Article 4(2) and (3) forbid the selling of NHPs when the license for the product has been stopped or suspended. The Natural Health Products Regulations (Government of Canada, 2003) also provide the type of information that should be provided to the competent authority, allowing the assessment of such required product license.

As for all drug products worldwide, NHPs are also to be produced under GMP conditions and clinical trials involving such product should be compliant with the Good Clinical Practices according to Part 4, Article 74 (Government of Canada, 2003).

In addition to the legal and regulatory provisions, Health Canada has released a monograph intended to serve as a guide to the industry for the preparation of a Product Licence Application for products containing probiotics (Health Canada, 2019). This document specifies the standards to be applied for the products to claim the license and, among others, specifies that microorganisms must be identified at the strain level, just as in the United States or Europe. The monograph is also listing the therapeutic claims already accepted for a dedicated list of strains, mentioning the directions of use, the cautions, warnings, and contraindications, and, the appropriate dosage in Colony-Forming Units for different populations (children 1–11 years, adolescents 12–17 years, and adults 18 years and older). While the monograph does not specify product-specific statements for, for example, the recommended duration of use, that information, along with possible adverse reactions, must be provided to the authorities to qualify for a license.

In terms of quality, all nonmedicinal ingredients must be chosen from the NHP Ingredient Database and meet the limitations outlined in the database. Cryoprotectants, as an example, must be disclosed as nonmedicinal ingredients.

The monograph lays out the mandatory documentation to be provided for the product, such as:

(1) the validation of the strain identity(ies);
(2) the phenotype and genotype allowing identification at the strain level;
(3) the survivability of the strain(s) in the human gut;
(4) the documentation or potential virulence or antimicrobial resistance AND the absence of transfer; and
(5) the lack of toxigenic activity

and reminds the need for packaging notifications for potential risks associated to the presence of allergens or antimicrobial resistances.

A final requirement specifies that the quality of the finished product must be established in accordance with the requirements described in the Natural and Non-prescription Health Product Directorate Quality of Natural Health Products Guide (Health Canada, 2015). Stability/viability measures must be put in place, ensuring that a minimum of 80% of the quantity declared on the product label is present at the end of shelf life. Moreover, details must be provided on the validated methodology used to test and identify potential microbial contaminants in the finished product.

2.3.3.3.2 Biologic Drugs

Similar to the European situation, but in contrast to the United States, Health Canada has yet to produce specific guidelines for this type of medicinal product. However, since Canada is an official member of the ICH (Health Canada, 2018), existing ICH guidelines relating to comparable types of biological products can be considered and the corresponding concepts applied, also in Canada (Cordaillat-Simmons et al., 2020).

Overall, as for drug products, the Canadian Food and Drug Act, the Food and Drug regulation, the Natural Health Products Regulations, and the Monograph on Natural Health Products containing probiotics are the four most important documents clarifying the food and pharma statuses for those products, to be placed on the Canadian market. They specify the standards for quality, safety, and efficacy that must be addressed, especially for the products intended to prevent or treat human diseases through the correction of organic function. In placing drug products on the Canadian market as well, in the absence of specific guidelines for LBPs, developers are encouraged to analyze the current guidelines referring to other biologics and to apply the spirit of the guidelines to their own products as it was recently proposed for the European framework (Cordaillat-Simmons et al., 2020; Rouanet et al., 2020).

2.3.4 The Japanese regulatory framework

In Japan, the Japanese Ministry of Health, Labour, and Welfare (MHLW) (2020) implements legally binding regulations by the way of ordinances. Japanese laws distinguish between foods and medicines/therapeutic goods.

2.3.4.1 Details of the food regulatory framework

As in many other countries, several organizations are responsible for the regulatory framework for foods in Japan.

There is, on the one hand, the Consumer Affairs Agency (CAA), which is governing, among others, the Food Labeling Act (Government of Japan, 2013), the Consumer Safety Act (Government of Japan, 2009), the Food Safety Basic Act (Government of Japan, 2003), the Food Sanitation Act (Government of Japan, 1947), and the Basic Consumer Act (CBA) (Government of Japan, 1968). Article 2 of the CBA sets out the state's role to protect consumer's right and supports his/her independency for food choices. The mission of the CAA is:

- *to protect and promote consumer's interests and benefits;*
- *to ensure a free and rational choice of goods and services*; and
- *to ensure correct labeling of the goods that are available to the consumer.*

The law that governs food labeling regulation (Consumer Affairs Agency, 2020) is the Food Labeling Act (Government of Japan, 2013), and the law governing health aspects is the Health Promotion Act (Government of Japan, 2020), promoting health through the improvement of the nutritional status of foods and therefore dealing with nutrition labeling and health claims.

The main law, however, governing food quality and integrity in Japan is the Food Sanitation Act (FSA) (Government of Japan, 1947). The FSA regulates food quality and integrity by establishing standards and specifications for food, food containers, and packaging. Under the FSA, additives and foods containing additives must not be sold unless the MHLW has declared them as having no risk for human health, after seeking the views of the Pharmaceutical Affairs and Food Sanitation (Safety) Council (PAFSC; see below). In addition, it is not allowed to add processing aids, vitamins, minerals, novel foods, or nutritive substances to foods unless they have been expressly declared by the MHLW as having no risk to human health. Accordingly, although substances are allowed to be added to food, they may only be used within the limits expressly set by the specifications and standards established by the MHLW. Besides additives, the FSA regulation also is setting forward rules about labeling of allergens, expiry dates, storage conditions, presence of GMOs, manufacturer's details, and ingredients.

Central in the regulation is the **Health Foods** category. Before April 2015, there were **Foods with Health Claims** (FHC) and non-FHC foods. In the FHC category, there was a subdivision in **Foods with Specified Health Use** (FOSHU) (Japanese Ministry of Health, Labour and Welfare, 2015a) (see below) and **Foods with Nutrient Function Claims** (FNFC). Standards and specifications for FNFCs have been established for 12 vitamins and 5 minerals and when these are met, manufacturing and distribution of FNFCs is exempted from notification to, or approval from the government. In the non-FHC category, there were also two food types, the so-called Health Foods (HF) and the General Foods (GF).

In June 2014, the Japanese government decided to allow more products on the market with specific nutritional or health functions, while maintaining a stricter control on the labeling. They created the new category **Foods with Function Claims** (FFC) for the earlier HF subcategory. The difference between this food category and the FOSHU category (see below) is the lack of an obligatory review of the individual products by the Secretary General of the CAA.

The requirements for the FFC foods, obligatory as of April 2015, relate to the quantitative and qualitative information of the functional substance, which should not be on a drug list, and for which the mode of action is known. Certification of analysis by a third-party test organization is required, as is the proof of equivalence of the functional ingredient with the substance description in the literature. The target population is people without disease, but not people below the age of 20 years, elderly and pregnant or lactating women. Safety is provided through a history of safe use by humans as well as documentation of possible interactions with drugs or, when multiple functional substances are added to a food, documentation of the interaction (or absence thereof) between these functional substances. GMP production is strongly recommended. Functionality is supported by clinical study(ies) with the finished product or by systematic review on the product or the functional substance. In the first case, the trial has to be approved by the University Hospital Medical Information Network—Clinical Trials Registry (UMIN-CTR) or by the International Clinical Trials Registry Platform (ICTRP) of the WHO, the design in agreement with the FOSHU requirements (see below) and published in a peer-reviewed journal. In the case of a systematic review, the complete procedure must be explained, but the totality of the evidence can be used, including Japanese as well as overseas sources, but with the clear analysis and explanation of publication bias, potential conflicts of interest, etc. The label should have clear contact information to be able to report adverse events.

2.3.4.1.1 Food for special dietary uses

The food category in Japan that does describe foods for patients is the **Food for Special Dietary Uses** (FOSDU) (Japanese Ministry of Health, Labour and Welfare, 2015b), intended for infants, patients, or pregnant and lactating women. Typical examples of FOSDU foods are low protein foods, lactose-free foods, infant formula, food for elderly with difficulties in masticating and/or swallowing and (see below). The respective labeling should be approved by CAA, who will routinely check the food composition by comparing with established standards, or, in lack of available standards, based on an individual case by case approval system. FOSDU must be labeled with information as prescribed in the Ministerial Ordinance under the Health Promotion Law (Government of Japan, 2020).

2.3.4.1.2 Food for Specific Health Uses

The largest and best-known category of health foods in Japan, however, is the **FOSHU** (or **TOKUHO**) category, with an estimated value of $13.2 billion in 2018 [compared to 2.3 billion for FFC products (United States Department of Agriculture—Foreign Agricultural Service, 2020)]. FOSHU refers to any food containing one or more functional components that can provide positive effects on health or bodily functions and that are approved by the CAA to mention that specific health claim on the label. To obtain an FOSHU label, an applicant will need to contact the Food Labeling Division of the CAA, who will request the Consumer Commission to make an assessment of the safety and the efficacy of the dossier. Their report will be sent to the MHLW who will express their findings about the labeling permission or the possible violation, with the Act on Securing Quality, Efficacy and Safety of Products Including Pharmaceuticals and Medical Devices (Government of Japan, 1960). Based on these two reports, the CAA will approve or not the FOSHU application. Conditions for approval are specified below and are derived from the Notification Shokuanhatsu 0201002, February 1, 2007, published by the MHLW (Japanese Ministry of Health, Labour and Welfare, 2015a):

Consumption of the product will lead to an improvement of dietary habits and contribute to health maintenance or enhancement, if:

- *Scientific evidence for the claimed health benefit is available.*
- *Clinical and nutritional intake levels of the product and/or its functional component are established.*
- *The product and/or its functional component are safe for human consumption.*

Following items are defined for the functional component:

1. *Physical, chemical, and biological characterization and the methodology used;* and
2. *Methods for its qualitative and quantitative analytical determination*
   a. *The nutrient composition of a similar type of the food is not significantly changed,*
   b. *The food is intended to be consumed on a daily basis and not on a rare occasion,* and
   c. *The product or its functional component is not listed on the medical drug list.*

The Japanese regulation discriminates between different FOSHU types (Shen, 2021):

1. *FOSHU.* Foods for specified health use, conditions defined above.
   – Requires a detailed review process with scientific evidence for each application.

2. **Standardized FOSHU.** Standards and specifications have been sufficiently established already for foods with FOSHU approval and with accumulated scientific evidence. Standardized FOSHU is approved when the product meets these standards and specifications.
   - No requirement for a detailed review process for food products meeting the established standards and specifications.
   - Must be accompanied by sufficient documentation and scientific evidence.
   - A short process can be used for products whose safety is already approved.
3. **Reduction of disease risk FOSHU.** Reduction of disease risk claim is permitted when reduction of disease risk is clinically and nutritionally established through an ingredient.
   - Requires a detailed review process with scientific evidence for each application.
   - Permitted for products whose ingredients are clinically and nutritionally established to be able to reduce a risk of certain disease (i.e., calcium for osteoporosis or folic acid for neural tube defects).
4. **Qualified FOSHU.** Food with a health function which is not substantiated on scientific evidence that meets the level of FOSHU, or the food with certain effectiveness but without established mechanism of the effective element for that function.
   - Requires a detailed review process with scientific evidence for each application.
   - Permitted for products with ingredients showing certain health effects but not reaching the established standards for FOSHU approval.
   - Labeled as "Qualified Food for Specified Health Uses."

Qualified and standardized FOSHU have been introduced to facilitate applicants to apply for FOSHU status (MHLW) (Japanese Ministry of Health, Labour and Welfare, 2015a).

In all of these regulations, there is no specific regulation or mentioning of conditions to be applied on live microorganisms. The FOSHU regulation actually covers a large set of health claims related to the improvement of gastrointestinal health using probiotics (Iwatani and Yamamoto, 2019).

2.3.4.2 Details of the pharmaceutical regulatory framework in Japan

2.3.4.2.1 Responsible authorities and structures

Similarly, as for the food regulation, it is also the MHLW (Japanese Ministry of Health, Labour, and Welfare (MHLW), 2020) that is responsible for the Japanese law that governs development of pharmaceuticals. The MHLW is the result of a merger in 2001 of the Ministry of Health and Welfare and the Ministry of Labour and has a complex structure. The Pharmaceutical Safety and Environmental Health Bureau (PSEHB) is one of the MHLW bureaus and should assure the efficacy and safety of drugs, quasi-drugs, cosmetics, medical devices, and cellular- and tissue-based products. The bureau itself has a complex structure, with five divisions, details of which are not the topic of this chapter. The PSEHB deals with clinical studies, approval reviews, and postmarketing safety measures. In 2004 the Pharmaceutical and Medical Devices Agency (PMDA) (Japanese Pharmaceuticals and Medical Devices Agency, 2020) was created to provide consultations concerning the clinical trials of new drugs and medical devices and to conduct approval reviews and surveys of the reliability of application data. Together, PSEHB and PMDA will thus be a partner for drug developers to assist them in the process of the design of clinical studies and the development of the dossier and will be responsible for the approval reviews, postmarketing stage, and pharmaceutical safety evaluations. In addition, the PAFSC, already mentioned above, serves as an advisory body for the MHLW. The experts of the Pharmaceutical Affairs Committee will meet four times a year and examine and review pharmaceutical matters, including new drug applications.

Finally, it is worth mentioning the National Institute of Health Sciences (NIHS) (Japanese National Institute of Health Sciences, 2020) who conducts testing, research, and studies to ensure the quality, safety, and efficacy of drugs, quasi-drugs, cosmetics, medical devices, foods, poisonous and deleterious substances, and the numerous chemicals in the environment, closely related to people's lives. In July 1997 the former National Institute of *Hygienic* Sciences became the National Institute of *Health* Sciences. In addition to its long-standing work in testing and research, the institute supervised the Pharmaceuticals and Medical Devices Evaluation Centre (PMDE), in charge of reviews required for approval to manufacture or import drugs, quasi-drugs, cosmetics, and medical devices, as well as the reexamination and the reevaluation of drugs and medical devices. The PMDE was incorporated into the PMDA in April 2004.

2.3.4.2.2 Pharmaceutical law in Japan

In Japan, pharmaceutical lawgiving is based on a variety of laws and regulations, including the very important Drugs and Medical Devices Law (the PMD Act or PMDA, also known as the Act on Securing Quality, Efficacy and Safety of Pharmaceuticals, Medical Devices, Regenerative and Cellular Therapy Products, Gene Therapy Products, and Cosmetics) and the Law Concerning the Establishment for Pharmaceuticals and Medical Device Organization. Other laws, less relevant for this chapter, cover, for example, the security and stability of blood products, the control of poisonous and deleterious substances, or laws on narcotics and psychotropics, cannabis, opium, or stimulants.

The PMDA affects all aspects of Japanese medical product registration, certification processes, licensing, and quality assurance, including representation in Japan. The PMDA was officially established on November 25, 2014, and replaces the old Pharmaceutical Affairs Law. It reviews new drugs, generic drugs, Over-The-Counter (OTC) drugs, Behind-The-Counter drugs, and quasi-drugs and can reevaluate previously approved drugs. In doing so, PMDA reviewers consider five main points during their evaluation:

- Are the studies conducted and documents submitted reliable?
- Has the efficacy of the drug been shown to be more effective than placebo in the studied target population and is this through properly designed clinical studies?
- Are the results clinically significant?
- Are there any unacceptable risks compared to the benefits?
- Is a continuous supply, with stable efficacy, safety, and quality assured?

English translations of the most relevant documents produced by the PMDA can be found on this website: https://www.pmda.go.jp/english/review-services/regulatory-info/0003.html.

Inevitably multiple regulations will apply to the development, manufacture, import, distribution, marketing and use of drugs (prescribed, as well as OTC), or medical devices. As mentioned, the Drugs and Medical Devices Law is offering the most important basis, supplemented with ministerial ordinances and notifications, such as the Enforcement Ordinance and the Enforcement Regulations, for their enforcement and management. Notifications and ordinances are issued by the Director General or Division Directors of the MHLW bureaus and divisions.

2.3.4.2.3 Drug definition in Japan

Drugs subjected to the regulations in the Drugs and Medical Devices Law are defined as follows (Japanese Pharmaceutical and Medical Devices Agency, 2019; Regulatory Information Task Force Japan Pharmaceutical Manufacturers Association, 2020):

1) *Substances listed in the Japanese Pharmacopoeia.*
2) *Substances (other than quasi-drugs and regenerative medicine products), which are intended for use in the diagnosis, treatment, or prevention of disease in humans or animals, and which are not equipment or instruments, including dental materials, medical supplies, sanitary materials, and programs.*
3) *Substances (other than quasi-drugs, cosmetics or regenerative medicine products) which are intended to affect the structure or functions of the body of humans or animals, and which are not equipment or instruments.*

2.3.4.2.4 Drugs classification in Japan

Drugs are classified into different ways, following the regulatory provisions in the Drugs and Medical Devices Law (Asia-Pacific Economic Cooperation (APEC)—Harmonization Center, 2015): classification may be made according to *use and supply*, *handling regulations related to safety*, *regenerative medicine products* and, relevant for this chapter, *biological products and specified biological products* (Japan Pharmaceutical Manufacturers Association, 2018).

MHLW defines "**Biological Products**" as "*drugs, quasi-drugs, cosmetics, or medical devices using materials manufactured from humans or other organisms (excluding plants) as raw materials or packaging materials, which are designated as requiring special precautions in terms of public health and hygiene*" and "**Specified Biological Products**" as "*products designated as requiring measures to prevent the onset or spread of risk to public health and hygiene due to the biological product concerned after selling, leasing or giving*" and presents measures to assure safety when a risk of infection has been designated (Japanese Pharmaceutical and Medical Devices Agency, 2019; Kishioka, 2015). Product classification is based on scientific assessment of the potential risk of infection transmission according to the Pharmaceutical Affairs and Food Sanitation Council recommendation. If the risk is estimated to be equivalent to blood and plasma-derived products in terms of dose, quantities, and duration, then the product could be classified as "Specified Biological Product" (Kishioka, 2015). However, for products containing nonpathogenic bacteria, the risk assessment could place them in the "Biological Products" (Kishioka, 2015).

2.3.4.2.5 Standards for Biological Materials

The Standards for Biological Materials were specified in Notice No. 210, issued by the MHLW in 2003. They assure the quality and safety of raw materials and packaging materials manufactured from biological materials and used in the manufacturing process for drugs, quasi-drugs, cosmetics, and medical devices based on the provisions of Article 42, Paragraph 1 (Standards of Drugs, etc.) of the Japanese Law (Japan Pharmaceutical Manufacturers Association, 2018).

However, there is again no specific mention of LBP's or probiotic strains, nor of live microbes. Therefore because nonpathogenic bacteria could fall within the "Biological Products Category" (Kishioka, 2015) and because Japan is part of the ICH, developers should rely on all relevant ICH harmonized guidelines, various appropriated Pharmacopoeia monographs from the different regions, as well as all relevant local guidelines established for other types of biologics and apply their spirit to the development of their LBPs, as also mentioned above and before for Canada and EU (Cordaillat-Simmons et al., 2020; Rouanet et al., 2020).

2.3.4.2.6 The manufacturing of bio(techno)logical products (including GMOs)

Good Manufacturing Practice (GMP) requires obtaining a manufacturing business license or an overseas manufacturer accreditation. GMP involves standards for structures and equipment, for manufacturing and quality control of all manufactured products. In particular, the GMP conditions for investigational drugs were amended on July 9, 2008, to assure the quality of the investigational drug at every stage of the clinical trial and is now harmonized in a dedicated ICH guideline [The International Council for Harmonisation of Technical Requirements for Pharmaceuticals for Human Use (ICH), 2000, p. 7].

The Pharmaceutical Inspection Cooperation Scheme (PIC/S) should guarantee a high level of the implementation of the internationally recognized GMP rules and should further promote international standardization and conformity in GMP inspection. On July 1, 2014, the MHLW, PMDA, and prefectures became members of the office of the PIC/S. The enforcement notification of the GMP was amended in August 2013 to meet the criteria of the PIC/S.

GMP compliance inspections happen at the point of application for new marketing approval or at the occasion of the application for partial changes of approved information and are conducted every 5 years following the obtainment of marketing approval (Asia-Pacific Economic Cooperation—Harmonization Center, 2015).

In Japan, as elsewhere, formal manufacturing/marketing approvals are required for individual formulations of drugs and should be obtained prior to market launch. *Product licenses* have been abolished (April 2005 amendment of the law) and replaced by *manufacturing (import) or marketing approvals*, but compliance with the criteria in GMP has been specified as an approval condition. It is the Minister of the MHLW or the prefectural governor for nonprescription drugs that allows, or not, the *marketing approval*. Data and documents should be submitted reviewing the product quality, efficacy, and safety, allowing the ministry to evaluate if the product in the application is suitable as a drug to be marketed by the marketing authorization holder and to confirm that the product has been manufactured in a GMP compliant production plant.

2.4 Comparative summary

In the lack of a uniform global regulatory situation, it is important to compare the various regional "intended use" regulations to apply the correct and appropriate local regulatory framework when considering to bring a product with live microorganisms to the market. The understanding of the regional similarities and differences might also help to design and optimize the development paths, minimizing the need for duplication and repetitions.

The following tables compare the different regulatory settings in the various regions discussed above, with a focus on the intended use.

2.4.1 Food regulatory statuses

2.4.1.1 Food regulatory statuses (Table 2.1)

TABLE 2.1 Identification of the different legal international definitions in a food setting.

Geographic area	Legal definition of the status in the relevant regulation	Intended use = purpose + target population
Europe	Relevant regulation: Regulation No 178/2002 (The European Parliament and the Council of the European Union, 2002a) "Food" (or "foodstuff") means any substance or product, whether processed, partially processed or unprocessed, intended to be, or reasonably expected to be ingested by humans. "Food" includes drink, chewing gum and any substance, including water, intentionally incorporated into the food during its manufacture, preparation or treatment. "Food" shall not include: (a) feed; (b) live animals unless they are prepared for placing on the market for human consumption; (c) plants prior to harvesting; (d) medicinal products (…); (e) cosmetics (…); (f) tobacco and tobacco products (…); (g) narcotic or psychotropic substances (…); (h) residues and contaminants. For exhaustiveness, within the same Regulation: "Feed" (or "feeding stuff") means any substance or product, including additives, whether processed, partially processed or unprocessed, intended to be used for oral feeding to animals.	Target population: humans = consumers = general healthy population.
United States	Relevant regulation: Title 21 of the US Federal Food, Drug, and Cosmetic Act [13] "Food" means (1) articles used for food or drink for man or other animals, (2) chewing gum, and (3) articles used for components of any such article.	Target population: man or other animals.
Canada	Relevant regulation: Food and Drug act (Government of Canada, 1985) "Food" includes any article manufactured, sold or represented for use as food or drink for human beings, chewing gum, and any ingredient that may be mixed with food for any purpose whatever.	Target population: human beings.

2.4.1.2 Food or dietary supplements regulatory statuses (Table 2.2)

TABLE 2.2 Identification of the different legal international definitions of food or dietary supplements.

Geographic area	Legal definition of the status in the relevant regulation	Intended use = purpose + target population
Europe	Relevant regulation: Directive 2002/46/EC (The European Parliament and the Council of the European Union, 2002b) *"Food supplements" means foodstuffs the purpose of which is to supplement the normal diet and which are concentrated sources of nutrients or other substances with a nutritional or physiological effect, alone or in combination, marketed in dose form, namely forms such as capsules, pastilles, tablets, pills and other similar forms, sachets of powder, ampoules of liquids, drop dispensing bottles, and other similar forms of liquids and powders designed to be taken in measured small unit quantities.*	Purpose (FS): supplement the normal diet. Intended health benefit (FS): nutritional or physiological effect. Target population (FS): general population = healthy population.
United States	Relevant regulation: Title 21 of the US Federal Food, Drug, and Cosmetic Act [13] *"Dietary supplement" means A product (other than tobacco) intended to supplement the diet that bears or contains one or more of the following dietary ingredients: (A) a vitamin; (B) a mineral; (C) an herb or other botanical; (D) an amino acid; (E) a dietary substance for use by man to supplement the diet by increasing the total dietary intake; or (F) a concentrate, metabolite, constituent, extract, or combination of any ingredient described in clause (A), (B), (C), (D), or (E); Is not represented for use as a conventional food or as a sole item of a meal or the diet (…) dietary supplements shall be deemed to be a food within the meaning of this chapter.*	Purpose (DS): supplement the diet. Target population (DS): general population = healthy population. Intended health benefit (DS): not a conventional food and not a sole item of a meal or the diet so the health benefit should be superior to food, meal, and diet.
Canada	To our knowledge, the Canadian Food and Drug act do not define a specific status for food or dietary supplement.	

2.4.1.3 Food for specific dietary use (Table 2.3)

TABLE 2.3 Identification of the different legal international definitions of the food for special dietary use category.

Geographic area	Legal definition of the status in the relevant regulation	Intended use = purpose + target population
Europe	Relevant regulation: Regulation (EU) No 609/2013 and Commission delegated Regulation (EU) 2016/128 *"Food for special medical purposes" means food specially processed or formulated and intended for the dietary management of patients, including infants, to be used under medical supervision; it is intended for the exclusive or partial feeding of patients with a limited, impaired or disturbed capacity to take, digest, absorb, metabolise or excrete ordinary food or certain nutrients contained therein, or metabolites, or with other medically-determined nutrient requirements, whose dietary management cannot be achieved by modification of the normal diet alone.*	Purpose (FSMP): exclusive or partial feeding of patients with a limited, impaired, or disturbed capacity to take, digest, absorb, metabolize, or excrete ordinary food or certain nutrients or metabolites or with other medically determined nutrient requirements whose dietary management cannot be achieved by modification of the normal diet alone. Target population (FSMP): patients, including infants, with a limited, impaired, or disturbed capacity to take, digest, absorb, metabolize, or excrete ordinary food or certain nutrients or metabolites or with other medically determined nutrient requirements whose dietary management cannot be achieved by modification of the normal diet alone. Intended health benefit (FSMP): Allow patients "affected by or malnourished because if a specific diagnosed disease, disorder or medical condition" to "satisfy their nutritional needs."
	This subcategory of food is often causing confusion for product developers as it balances at the borderline with the drug regulation. Indeed, compared to food or food supplements, FSMP are not intended to be administered to the general healthy population but to a population of patients. Patients are also the target population of medicinal products, which is causing the confusion. To be clear, the difference between drugs and FSMP is the health benefit they are intended to confer. Drugs will prevent or treat the disease when FSMP will "only" satisfy specific nutritional needs, linked or derived from the disease. Admittedly, FSMP will positively influence the disease evolution, through the considered nutritional support, but, regulatory speaking, it will not be targeting the cause of the disease.	
United States	Relevant regulation: Code of Federal Regulations (TITLE 21, Chapter I, Subchapter B, Part 105, Subpart a) (FDA, 2020d) "The term special dietary uses, as applied to food for man, means particular (as distinguished from general) uses of food, as follows: (i) Uses for supplying particular dietary needs which exist by reason of a physical, physiological, pathological or other condition, including but not limited to the conditions of diseases, convalescence, pregnancy, lactation, allergic hypersensitivity to food, underweight, and overweight; (ii) Uses for supplying particular dietary needs which exist by reason of age, including but not limited to the ages of infancy and childhood; (iii) Uses for supplementing or fortifying the ordinary or usual diet with any vitamin, mineral, or other dietary property. Any such particular use of a food is a special dietary use, regardless of whether such food also purports to be or is represented for general use." In the US Orphan Drug Act, there is also a subcategory of food called "medical food," defined as "food which is formulated to be consumed or administered enterally under the supervision of a physician and which is intended for the specific dietary management of a disease or condition for which distinctive nutritional requirements, based on recognized scientific principles, are established by medical evaluation." (FDA, 2020e) "Medical foods are foods that are specially formulated and processed (as opposed to naturally occurring food stuff used in natural state) for a patient who requires use of the product as a major component of a disease or condition's specific management." (FDA Center for Food Safety and Applied Nutrition, 2016)	The US regulation precises that food for special dietary uses (FOSDU) is not covered by a specific regulatory status but describes a particular use of products marketed under the food regulatory status. Purpose (FOSDU): covering particular dietary needs or supplementing or fortifying the ordinary or usual diet. Target population (FOSDU): Human beings having particular dietary needs, due to: physical, physiological, pathological, or other conditions, including the conditions of diseases, convalescence, pregnancy, lactation, allergic hypersensitivity to food, underweight, and overweight; age, including ages of infancy and childhood. Purpose (medical food): specific dietary management of a disease or condition for which distinctive nutritional requirements are established by medical evaluation. Medical foods represent a major component of the specific management of a disease or condition. Target population (medical food): patients affected by a disease or a condition for which distinctive nutritional requirements are established by medical evaluation.

(Continued)

TABLE 2.3 (Continued)

Geographic area	Legal definition of the status in the relevant regulation	Intended use = purpose + target population
	The difference between drugs and medical foods seems blurred and tiny. Once again, the difference rests on the intended health benefit. Drugs will prevent or treat the disease; medical foods will be a major component of the disease's management but (alone) will not be sufficient to manage the disease. Certainly, and in comparison, to FSDU, the medical food is essential to a positive evolution of the disease, but, regulatory speaking, will not be considered the exclusive cause of the disease's resolution.	
Canada	Relevant regulation: Food and Drug act (Government of Canada, 1985) *"Food for a special dietary purpose" means a food that has been specially processed or formulated: (a) to meet the particular requirements of an individual in whom a physical or physiological condition exists as a result of a disease, disorder or abnormal physical state, or (b) to be the sole or primary source of nutrition for an individual.*	Purpose (FOSDP): meet the particular dietary requirements of an individual in whom a physical or physiological condition exists as a result of a disease, disorder, or abnormal physical state. Be the sole or primary source of nutrition for an individual. Target population (FOSDP): individual requiring particular dietary needs due to a physical or physiological condition existing as a result of a disease, disorder, or abnormal physical state
Japan	*"Food for Special Dietary Uses" (FOSDU) refers to food that are approved/permitted to display that the food is appropriate for special dietary uses. There are five categories of FOSDU: (1) Formulas for pregnant or lactating women, (2) Infant Formulas, (3) Foods for the elderly with difficulty in masticating or swallowing, (4) Medical foods for the ill, (5) Foods for Specified Health Uses (FOSHU)* (Japanese Ministry of Health, Labour and Welfare, 2015b). *"FOSHU" refers to foods containing ingredient with functions for health and officially approved to claim its physiological effects on the human body. FOSHU is intended to be consumed for the maintenance/promotion of health or special health uses by people who wish to control health conditions, including blood pressure or blood cholesterol. In order to sell a food as FOSHU, the assessment for the safety of the food and effectiveness of the functions for health is required, and the claim must be approved by the MHLW* (Japanese Ministry of Health, Labour and Welfare, 2015a).	Target population (FOSDU): very broad target population: pregnant or lactating women, infants, elderly with difficulty in masticating or swallowing, "ill" person, but also people wanting to control or maintain health conditions. Purpose (FOSDU): meet the particular dietary requirements of an individual with specific nutritional requirements or desires. Target population (FOSHU): those people wanting to control or maintain health conditions, including blood pressure or blood cholesterol. Purpose (FOSHU): functions for health. Physiological effects on the human body. Maintenance/promotion of health.
	Even exposed differently, here again, in the Japanese regulation, FOSDU is targeting an healthy population and, when targeting an "ill" population, the purpose of the foodstuff is not to cure the disease but to satisfy the nutritional needs, incidental to the disease.	

2.4.2 Drug regulatory statuses (Table 2.4)

TABLE 2.4 Identification of the different legal international definition of the drug regulatory status.

Geographic area	Legal definition of the status in the relevant regulation	Intended use = purpose + target population
Europe	Relevant regulation: Directive 2001/83/CE (The European Parliament and Council of the European Union, 2001) *"Medicinal product": (a) Any substance or combination of substances presented as having properties for treating or preventing disease in human beings; or (b) Any substance or combination of substances which may be used in or administered to human beings either with a view to restoring, correcting or modifying physiological functions by exerting a pharmacological, immunological or metabolic action, or to making a medical diagnosis.*	Purpose: treat or prevent disease. Target population: diseased human beings. Intended use: be used or administered to restore, correct, or modify physiological functions or to make a medical diagnosis
United States	Relevant regulation: Title 21 of the US Federal Food, Drug, and Cosmetic Act *"Drug" means articles intended for use in the diagnosis, cure, mitigation, treatment, or prevention of disease in man or other animals.*	Purpose: diagnosis, cure, mitigation, treatment, or prevention of disease. Target population: diseased man or animals.
Canada	Relevant regulation: Food and Drug act (Government of Canada, 1985) *"Drug" includes any substance or mixture of substances manufactured, sold or represented for use in: (a) the diagnosis, treatment, mitigation or prevention of a disease, disorder or abnormal physical state, or its symptoms, in human beings or animals, (b) restoring, correcting or modifying organic functions in human beings or animals.* In the Canadian legislation, there is also a subcategory of drugs called "Natural Health Products" (NHP) and defined as *substance set out in Schedule 1* or a combination of substances in which all the medicinal ingredients are substances set out in Schedule 1*, a homeopathic medicine or a traditional medicine, that is manufactured, sold or represented for use in: (a) the diagnosis, treatment, mitigation or prevention of a disease, disorder or abnormal physical state or its symptoms in humans; (b) restoring or correcting organic functions in humans; or (c) modifying organic functions in humans, such as modifying those functions in a manner that maintains or promotes health* (Government of Canada, 2003). Schedule 1: plant or a plant material, an alga, a bacterium, a fungus or a nonhuman animal material or an extract or isolate of these substances, the primary molecular structure of which is identical to that which it had prior to its extraction or isolation; Any of the following vitamins: biotin, folate, niacin, pantothenic acid, riboflavin, thiamine, vitamin A, vitamin B6, vitamin B12, vitamin C, vitamin D, vitamin E, vitamin K1, and vitamin K2; an amino acid; an essential fatty acid; a synthetic duplicate of all the substances described above; a mineral; and a probiotic.	Purpose: diagnose, treatment, mitigation, or prevention of a disease, disorder, or abnormal physical state, or its symptoms. Restore, correct, or modify organic functions. Target population: human beings or animals presenting a disease, a disorder, or an abnormal physical state or abnormal organic functions.
Japan	Relevant regulation: Pharmaceutical and Medical Device Act, Article 2, Paragraph 1 (Japan Pharmaceutical Manufacturers Association, 2018). *The term "drugs" refers to the following substances: (1) Substances listed in the Japanese Pharmacopoeia. (2) Substances (other than quasi-drugs and regenerative medicine products), which are intended for use in the diagnosis, treatment, or prevention of disease in humans or animals, and which are not equipment or instruments, including dental materials, medical supplies, sanitary materials, and programs. (3) Substances (other than quasi-drugs, cosmetics or regenerative medicine products) which are intended to affect the structure or functions of the body of humans or animals, and which are not equipment or instruments.*	Purpose: use in diagnosis, treatment, or prevention of disease. Intended to affect the structure or functions of the body. Target population: diseased humans or animals.

2.5 Conclusion: the name does make a difference

Despite regulatory differences on international, national, and even regional levels, it is clear that legislators and regulators worldwide have two common concepts in mind: (1) avoid misleading the consumer and (2) ensure the safety of the product within the framework of its intended use.

The possible regulatory confusion therefore is not on the message to the consumers nor on the safety aspect, but mainly on the intended use. Regulatory confusion should be avoided, whenever possible, as it is not only negative for the consumer but for all stakeholders: healthcare professionals, authorities, academia, and industry, and leads to biased regulatory interpretations, loss of confidence in various types of products, mainly because of inappropriate expectations for the intended use of the products concerned.

Probiotics, unfortunately, are a very good example of this. With strains and applications that can be classified as foods and drugs, it is very tempting, for producers, to present foods as potentially beneficial in curing disease, or, for consumers to expect that foods will cure their disease.

Therefore it is of paramount importance that stakeholders handle the "probiotics" terminology very carefully and differently when addressing either patients or consumers, as wrong usage can raise false expectations. Avoiding to spread false expectations is exactly what regulators want, as this will almost surely lead to a "unsatisfactory" results, which neither the patient nor the medical doctor or dietician wants.

Regulators also share responsibility in this. The attempts that have been made to define "Live Biotherapeutic Products" or "Natural Health Products" have been an important step forward, but the terms are not used enough (yet) to see a positive result in practice. Also, the lack of clarity, due to the lack of effort by the various competent authorities to agree on a common interpretation of the differences/limitations associated with either a health claim or a medical claim, is perceived as one of the main obstacles, mainly caused by confusion concerning the intended use of the product and therefore the correct, corresponding framework for its evaluation. The existing confusion has made it more difficult for, for example, the medical community to keep both concepts apart (Su et al., 2020). This has led to discussions among scientists and the industry as to the value of these products and their ability to fulfill the "expectations" (Daniells, 2020). Clearly, the lack of knowledge on the specific intended use and corresponding regulatory requirements for the different categories makes it difficult to choose the right product for the right application in the right patient.

We therefore encourage academic, medical, nutritional, or industrial stakeholders to apply the correct regulatory wordings, based on appropriate regulatory concepts.

Probiotic *strains* are the biological entities and active substances of probiotic foods or drugs. They have certain biological abilities, based on physiological, immunological, microbiological, neurological, or endocrinological interactions with the host, and these interactions can be of nutritional or medical value.

These probiotic *applications* determine

- the regulatory framework (food or drug), impacting the production conditions, the supporting research level, the conditions of use, the shelf life, etc.;
- the communication by the producer, whether on pack, through websites, on TV, mainstream, or social media;
- the expectations for the consumers/patients, which in the end is the reason for researchers, doctors, and producers to perform research and invest in a reliable and safe product.

As a result of that research there are three possible levels of scientific support.

Microbial strains are present in many foods without specific proof of their biological effects, as listed above. In this case, the strains cannot be called "pro"-"biotic," as their "beneficial"-"biological" activities have not been shown or documented. Products with these strains (thousands of fermented foods all over the world) should not claim any health benefit on pack, other than their inherent nutritional value or the presence of the live microorganisms, and should not be directed to a particular part of the population.

Probiotic foods, which have been investigated for a potential beneficial health effect and for which a plausible mechanism of action (microbiological, metabolical, physiological, neurological, or endocrinological) is anticipated, and, importantly, which should be safe for the *total population* without side effects. These products should be able to mention their potential health benefits on pack and in direct communications from the producer to the consumer, although these communications might be subject to local regulatory approval.

Probiotic drugs are products that have been investigated for their potential to cure or prevent disease and that have been selected and studied in that diseased population, for that particular effect, based on an anticipated mechanism of action (microbiological, physiological, metabolical, neurological, or endocrinological), knowing that their positive medical effect will outweigh the possible side effects for the *patient* treated. Communication on these products should be directed only to the doctors and health professionals and cannot be to the general population. It would be good if in the future these products would be referred to as "Live Biotherapeutic Products."

The simple fact to associate the term "probiotic" with its product status would most likely prevent a lot of misconceptions and frustration. Consumers and healthcare professionals in the first place, but also producers will gain from a clear and open communication. It may even lead to a situation that the regulators, now very strict in their ruling about the marketing of probiotic foods (especially in Europe), might accept a certain differentiation between probiotic foods and probiotic drugs, in terms of expected scientific support and production methods. It may lead to situations that all stakeholders might understand that changing the matrix or carrier of a probiotic food (e.g., adding fruits to the probiotic yoghurt) might have less impact than changing the formula or administration mode of a probiotic drug.

We hope that the above considerations make clear that the *name does make a difference*, a perception difference, a regulatory difference, a communication difference, a real difference!

Conflict of interest

MC-S and AR are employed by the Pharmabiotic Research Institute. BP is employed by Yakult Europe BV, but the authors declare no conflict of interest for this chapter.

Notice

1. Due to the purpose of this document, most of the information was quoted directly from the respective websites or related guidelines of each country's drug regulatory agencies.
2. This document is limited only to biological products, no applicable to the broader pharmaceutical framework or herbal products.
3. As regulation and law giving is dynamic, it is advised to check the up-to-date information, including related laws and regulations, and revision of guidelines, when referring to the contents of this document.

References

Asia-Pacific Economic Cooperation—Harmonization Center. (2015). *Drug approval system in Japan*.
Consumer Affairs Agency. (2020). *Japanese Food Labelling Regulations*. https://www.caa.go.jp/en/policy/food_labeling/. (Accessed 12.08.20).
Cordaillat-Simmons, M., Rouanet, A., & Pot, B. (2020). Live biotherapeutic products: The importance of a defined regulatory framework. *Experimental & Molecular Medicine*.
Daniells, S. (2020). *AGA issues guidelines for probiotics for sick, at-risk populations*. https://www.nutraingredients-usa.com/Article/2020/06/12/AGA-issues-guidelines-for-probiotics-for-sick-at-risk-populations. (Accessed 01.20.21).
Dreher-Lesnick, S. M., Stibitz, S., & Carlson, Jr., P. E. (2017). U.S. regulatory considerations for development of live biotherapeutic products as drugs. *Microbiology Spectrum*, 5.
EDQM. (2020a). *Vision, mission and values of the EDQM*. https://www.edqm.eu/en/EDQM-mission-values-604.html. (Accessed 08.07.20).
EDQM. (2020b). *Background and Legal Framework of the European Pharmacopoeia—EDQM*. https://www.edqm.eu/en/European-Pharmacopoeia-Background-Mission. (Accessed 10.20.20).
EFSA. (2021). *Guidance and other assessment methodology documents*. European Food Safety Authority. https://www.efsa.europa.eu/en/methodology/guidance. (Accessed 01.15.21).
EMA. (2008). *Reflection paper on benefit-risk assessment methods in the context of the evaluation of marketing authorisation applications of medicinal products for human use*.
EU Register of nutrition and health claims made on foods (v.3.5). (2020). https://ec.europa.eu/food/safety/labelling_nutrition/claims/register/public/?event = search. (Accessed 01.15.21).
EU Standing Committee on the Food Chain and Animal Health. (2007). *Guidance on the implementation of Regulation No 1924/2006 on nutrition and health claims made on foods conclusions of the Standing Committee on the Food Chain and Animal Health*.
European Commission. (1999). Commission Directive 1999/21/EC on dietary foods for special medical purposes. *Official Journal of the European Communities*.
European Commission. (2008). Commission Regulation (EC) 353/2008 establishing implementing rules for applications for authorisation of health claims as provided for in Article 15 of Regulation (EC) No 1924/2006. *Official Journal of the European Union*.
European Commission. (2009). Commission Regulation (EC) No 953/2009 on substances that may be added for specific nutritional purposes in foods for particular nutritional uses. *Official Journal of the European Union*.
European Commission. (2012). Commission Regulation (EU) No 432/2012 of 16 May 2012 establishing a list of permitted health claims made on foods, other than those referring to the reduction of disease risk and to children's development and health. *Official Journal of the European Union*.

European Commission. (2015). Commission Delegated Regulation (EU) 2016/128 supplementing Regulation (EU) No 609/2013 as regards the specific compositional an information requirements for food for special medical purposes. *Official Journal of the European Union*.

European Commission. (2016). *Health claims*. European Commission. Available from https://ec.europa.eu/food/safety/labelling_nutrition/claims/health_claims_en. (Accessed 01.15.21).

European Commission. (2020). *European law-making process*. European Commission. Available from https://ec.europa.eu/info/law/law-making-process_en. (Accessed 08.06.20).

European Food Safety Authority. (2011a). *General guidance for stakeholders on the evaluation of Article 13.1, 13.5 and 14 health claims*.

European Food Safety Authority. (2011b). Guidance on the scientific requirements for health claims related to gut and immune function. *EFSA Journal*.

European Food Safety Authority. (2020). *About EFSA*. European Food Safety Authority. Available from https://www.efsa.europa.eu/en/aboutefsa. (Accessed 08.07.20).

European Medicines Agency. (2018). *EMA: What we do?* European Medicines Agency. Available from https://www.ema.europa.eu/en/about-us/what-we-do. (Accessed 08.06.20).

European Pharmacopoeia Commission. (2019). 3053E General monograph on live biotherapeutic products. *European Pharmacopoeia*, 9, 7.

FDA Center for Food Safety and Applied Nutrition. (2016). *Guidance for industry FAQs about medical foods*.

FDA. (2013a). *Orphan drugs, subpart A—General provisions, sec316.3—Definitions*, Code of Federal Regulations.

FDA. (2013b). *FDA Warning Letter regarding for misbranding of products as medical foods*. https://wayback.archive-it.org/7993/20170112190403/http://www.fda.gov/ICECI/EnforcementActions/WarningLetters/2013/ucm367142.htm. (Accessed 01.19.21).

FDA. (2016). *Early clinical trials with live biotherapeutic products: Chemistry, manufacturing, and control information*.

FDA. (2018a). *Benefit-risk assessment in drug regulatory decision-making*. Prescription Drug User Fee Act (PDUFA VI) Implementation Plan (FY 2018-2022).

FDA. (2018b). *FDA: What we do?* FDA. Available from https://www.fda.gov/about-fda/what-we-do. (Accessed 08.07.20).

FDA. (2019a). Current good manufacturing practice in manufacturing, packaging, labelling, or holding operations for dietary supplements. *Code of Federal Regulations*.

FDA. (2019b). *Food additives, subpart A—General provisions, sec170.3—Definitions*. Code of Federal Regulations.

FDA. (2020a). *Food labeling, subpart A—General provisions, sec101.4—Health claims: General requirements*. Code of Federal Regulations.

FDA. (2020b). *Label claims for conventional foods and dietary supplements*. FDA. Available from https://www.fda.gov/food/food-labeling-nutrition/label-claims-conventional-foods-and-dietary-supplements. (Accessed 12.08.20).

FDA. (2020c). *Food labeling, subpart A—General provisions, sec101.9—Nutrition labeling on food*. Code of Federal Regulations.

FDA. (2020d). *Food for special dietary use—General provisions*. Code of Federal Regulations.

FDA. (2020e). *Medical foods guidance documents & regulatory information*. FDA. Available from https://www.fda.gov/food/guidance-documents-regulatory-information-topic-food-and-dietary-supplements/medical-foods-guidance-documents-regulatory-information. (Accessed 08.10.20).

Food and Agriculture Organization of the United Nations, World Health Organization. (2001). *Probiotics in food: Health and nutritional properties and guidelines for evaluation*.

Government of Canada. (1985). *Food and Drugs Act*.

Government of Canada. (2003). *Natural Health Products Regulations*.

Government of Canada. (2020a). *Food and Drug Regulations*.

Government of Canada. (2020b). *Consolidated federal laws of canada, Natural Health Products Regulations—Schedule 1 (Subsection 1(1))*. https://laws-lois.justice.gc.ca/eng/regulations/SOR-2003-196/section-sched701180.html?txthl = schedule + 1. (Accessed 12.08.20).

Government of Canada, C.F.I.A. (2014). *List of eligible species for non-strain specific probiotic claims*. https://www.inspection.gc.ca/food-label-requirements/labelling/industry/health-claims-on-food-labels/eng/1392834838383/1392834887794?chap = 10. (Accessed 01.19.21).

Government of Japan. (1947). *Japanese Food Sanitation Act*. http://www.japaneselawtranslation.go.jp/law/detail/?id = 3524&vm = 04&re = 01. (Accessed 12.08.20).

Government of Japan. (1960). *Act on Securing Quality, Efficacy and Safety of Products Including Pharmaceuticals and Medical Devices*. http://www.japaneselawtranslation.go.jp/law/detail_main?re = &vm = 2&id = 3213. (Accessed 01.19.21).

Government of Japan. (1968). *Japanese Basic Act on Consumer Policies*. http://www.japaneselawtranslation.go.jp/law/detail/?id = 3198&vm = 04&re = 01. (Accessed 12.08.20).

Government of Japan. (2003). *Japanese Food Safety Basic Act*. http://www.japaneselawtranslation.go.jp/law/detail/?id = 1839&vm = 04&re = 01. (Accessed 12.08.20).

Government of Japan. (2009). *Japanese Consumer Safety Act*. http://www.japaneselawtranslation.go.jp/law/detail/?id = 2887&vm = 04&re = 01. (Accessed 12.08.20).

Government of Japan. (2013). *Japanese Food Labelling Act*. http://www.japaneselawtranslation.go.jp/law/detail/?id = 3586&vm = 04&re = 01. (Accessed 12.08.20).

Government of Japan. (2020). *Japanese Health Promotion Act*. https://www.mhlw.go.jp/english/////wp/wp-hw3/dl/2-063.pdf. (Accessed 12.08.20).

Health Canada. (2007). *Biologic and radiopharmaceutical drugs*. https://www.canada.ca/en/health-canada/corporate/about-health-canada/branches-agencies/health-products-food-branch/biologic-radiopharmaceutical-drugs-directorate.html. (Accessed 12.19.20).

Health Canada. (2015). *Quality of natural health products guide*.

Health Canada. (2016a). *What health Canada does as a regulator*. https://www.canada.ca/en/health-canada/corporate/mandate/regulatory-role/what-health-canada-does-as-regulator.html. (Accessed 08.08.20).

Health Canada. (2016b). *Biosimilar biologic drugs in Canada: Fact sheet*. https://www.canada.ca/en/health-canada/services/drugs-health-products/biologics-radiopharmaceuticals-genetic-therapies/applications-submissions/guidance-documents/fact-sheet-biosimilars.html#a1. (Accessed 01.19.21).

Health Canada. (2018). *Regulatory roadmap for biologic (schedule D) drugs in Canada*. https://www.canada.ca/en/health-canada/services/drugs-health-products/biologics-radiopharmaceuticals-genetic-therapies/regulatory-roadmap-for-biologic-drugs.html. (Accessed 12.19.20).

Health Canada. (2019). *Monograph on natural health products containing probiotics*.

Health Canada, Food Directorate Health Products and Food Branch. (2009). *Guidance document—The use of probiotic microorganisms in food*.

Hill, C., Guarner, F., Reid, G., Gibson, G. R., Merenstein, D. J., Pot, B., Morelli, L., Canani, R. B., Flint, H. J., Salminen, S., Calder, P. C., & Sanders, M. E. (2014). The International Scientific Association for Probiotics and Prebiotics consensus statement on the scope and appropriate use of the term probiotic. *Nature Reviews Gastroenterology & Hepatology, 11*, 506–514.

Iwatani, S., & Yamamoto, N. (2019). Functional food products in Japan: A review. *Food Science and Human Wellness, 8*, 96–101.

Japan Pharmaceutical Manufacturers Association. (2018). *Pharmaceutical administration and regulations in Japan*.

Japanese Ministry of Health, Labour and Welfare. (2015a). *Food for specified health use (FOSHU)*. https://www.mhlw.go.jp/english/topics/foodsafety/fhc/02.html. (Accessed 12.08.20).

Japanese Ministry of Health, Labour and Welfare. (2015b). *Food for special dietary use (FOSDU)*. https://www.mhlw.go.jp/english/topics/foodsafety/fhc/03.html. (Accessed 12.08.20).

Japanese Ministry of Health, Labour, and Welfare (MHLW). (2020). https://www.mhlw.go.jp/english/index.html. (Accessed 12.08.20).

Japanese National Institute of Health Sciences. (2020). http://www.nihs.go.jp/english/index.html. (Accessed 12.08.20).

Japanese Pharmaceutical and Medical Devices Agency. (2019). *Japanese Pharmaceutical Laws and Regulations*. http://www.jpma.or.jp/english/parj/pdf/2019e_ch02.pdf. (Accessed 12.08.20).

Japanese Pharmaceuticals and Medical Devices Agency. (2020). https://www.pmda.go.jp/english/. (Accessed 12.08.20).

Kishioka, Y. (2015). *Regulatory framework for biotherapeutic products including similar biotherapeutic products*. https://www.pmda.go.jp/files/000204341.pdf. (Accessed 12.08.20).

Office of the Law Revision Counsel in the United States House of Representatives. (1994). *Dietary Supplement Health and Education Act of 1994—DSHEA*, United States Code.

Office of the Law Revision Counsel in the United States House of Representatives. (2016). *Federal Food, Drug, and Cosmetic Act*, United States Code. FDA.

Organisation for Economic Co-operation and Development (OECD). (1993). *Safety evaluation of foods derived by modern biotechnology: Concepts and principles*. OECD Publications.

Regulatory Information Task Force Japan Pharmaceutical Manufacturers Association. (2020). *Pharmaceutical Regulations in Japan 2020*.

Rouanet, A., Bolca, S., Bru, A., Claes, I., Cvejic, H., Girgis, H., Harper, A., Lavergne, S.N., Mathys, S., Pane, M., Pot, B., Shortt, C., Alkema, W., Bezulowsky, C., Blanquet-Diot, S., Chassard, C., Claus, S.P., Hadida, B.,..., Cordaillat-Simmons, M. (2020). Live biotherapeutic products. A road map for safety assessment. *Frontiers in Medicine*.

Shen, R. (2021). *Health food regulatory system in Japan*. http://food.chemlinked.com/foodpedia/health-food-regulatory-system-japan. (Accessed 01.19.21).

Su, G. L., Ko, C. W., Bercik, P., Falck-Ytter, Y., Sultan, S., Weizman, A. V., & Morgan, R. L. (2020). AGA clinical practice guidelines on the role of probiotics in the management of gastrointestinal disorders. *Gastroenterology*.

The European Parliament and Council of the European Union. (2001). Directive 2001/83/EC on the Community code relating to medicinal product for human use. *Official Journal of the European Union*.

The European Parliament and the Council of the European Union. (2002a). Regulation (EC) No 178/2002 laying down the general principles and requirements of food law, establishing the European Food Safety Authority and laying down procedures in matters of food safety. *Official Journal of the European Communities*.

The European Parliament and the Council of the European Union. (2002b). Directive 2002/46/EC on the approximation of the laws of the Member States relating to food supplements. *Official Journal of the European Union*.

The European Parliament and the Council of the European Union. (2006). Regulation (EC) No 1924/2006 on nutrition and health claims made on foods. *Official Journal of the European Union*.

The European Parliament and the Council of the European Union. (2009). Directive 2009/39/EC on foodstuffs intended for particular nutritional uses (recast)Text with EEA relevance. *Official Journal of the European Union*.

The European Parliament and the Council of the European Union. (2011). Regulation (EU) No 1169/2011 on the provisions of food information to consumers. *Official Journal of the European Union*.

The International Council for Harmonisation of Technical Requirements for Pharmaceuticals for Human Use (ICH). (2000). *Guideline ICHQ7 on good manufacturing practice guide for active pharmaceutical ingredients*.

The International Council for Harmonisation of Technical Requirements for Pharmaceuticals for Human Use (ICH). (2002). *The common technical document for the registration of pharmaceuticals for human use*.

The International Council for Harmonisation of Technical Requirements for Pharmaceuticals for Human Use (ICH). (2016). *Revision of M4E guideline on enhancing the format structure of benefit-risk information in ICH Efficacy M4E(R2)*.

United States Department of Agriculture—Foreign Agricultural Service. (2020). *Japan health foods market overview*.

United States Government. (2021). *How laws are made and how to research them?* https://www.usa.gov/how-laws-are-made. (Accessed 08.07.20).

Chapter 3

The role of probiotics in maintaining immune homeostasis

Velaphi C. Thipe[1], Shireen Mentor[2], Caroline S.A. Lima[1], Lucas F. Freitas[1], Ana C.M. Fonseca[3], Kamila M. Nogueira[1], Adriana S. Rodrigues[1], Jorge G.S. Batista[1], Aryel H. Ferreira[1] and Ademar B. Lugão[1]

[1]*Energy and Nuclear Research Institute (IPEN), University of São Paulo, São Paulo, Brazil,* [2]*Department of Medical Biosciences, University of the Western Cape, Cape Town, South Africa,* [3]*Virtual University of the State of Sao Paulo (UNIVESP), São Paulo, Brazil*

3.1 Introduction

The immune system is composed of the complex architecture of the collective, coordinated, and interconnected network of cells, tissues, organs, and molecules responsible for surveillance, neutralization, and elimination of pathogens, foreign agents/molecules to maintain dynamic homeostasis of the organism. Homeostasis is referred to as the body's ability to thermodynamically maintain the internal environment in an almost constant balance, regardless of the changes that occur in the external environment (Sattler, 2017). The immune system is divided into two types of immunity characterized by their respective responses: innate or natural immunity as the first line of defense and acquired or adaptive immunity immune responses are carefully regulated pathways facilitated by the release of pro-inflammatory [interleukin (IL)-1β, IL-6, IL-18, and tumor necrosis factor-α (TNF-α)] and antiinflammatory (IL-1, IL-4, IL-10, IL-11, IL-12, and IL-13) cytokines produced by many cell populations but predominantly produced by activated macrophages and helper T cells (Th), respectively (Kany et al., 2019). The innate/adaptive cytokines play pivotal roles in the overall immunity against infected cells in the body.

A significant area of the human body, either internal or external, is colonized by resident microorganisms, and their communities in different regions that exist in symbiosis are called microbiota. The gastrointestinal tract is home to gut microbiota which is one of the most diverse and extremely microbiologically active sites, making up the digestive system, varying among individuals according to factors such as age, ethnicity, diet, stress, and etc. The gut microbiota is composed of 90% bacteria which play a fundamental role in gut-associated lymphoid tissue development, the integrity of the mucosal barrier, and overall immune homeostasis. It is well known that the human gut houses a plethora of microbes that support nutrition, physiology, metabolism, and immunity (Nicholson et al., 2012; Tremaroli & Bäckhed, 2012; van de Wouw et al., 2018; Yadav et al., 2018). An estimated 10^{14} bacteria have been reported to colonize the gut, with $\sim 10^{11}$ bacteria per gram of colon tissue (Dhar & Mohanty, 2020). The gut bacteria within healthy individuals are dominated by four phyla: *Actinobacteria*, *Bacteroidetes*, *Firmicutes*, and *Proteobacteria*. The gut microbiota offers significant stimuli (i.e., gut-brain, gut-lung, and gut-liver axis) for both innate and adaptive immunity, mediating immune and metabolic homeostasis (van Baarlen et al., 2013), apart from its importance in digestion, nutrient absorption, adiposity, satiety, energy expenditure, metabolism, and defense against pathogens (Maldonado Galdeano et al., 2019; Wang et al., 2017; Xiong et al., 2017) as shown in Fig. 3.1.

The intestinal microbiota is often reconstructed overtime by a myriad of factors including the colonization of pathogenic bacteria, constant use of antibiotics, and inflammation in relation to infections and onset of diseases (Calder, 2020). There is an intricate correlation between changes in the gut microbiota composition/activity and common diseases/disorders. The host defenses against pathogens rely on four pivotal functions: (1) creating a physical barrier to prevent the invasion of pathogens; (2) identifying pathogens in case of invasion—facilitating increased immunosurveillance; (3) neutralizing the pathogens; and (4) the generation of immunological memory. The pathological alteration of the gut microbiota is called gut dysbiosis, a condition that is often triggered by a diet rich in industrialized food, sugar, fat, and alcohol, as well as by air pollution and epigenetic factors such as stress. Since the gut microbiota impacts the

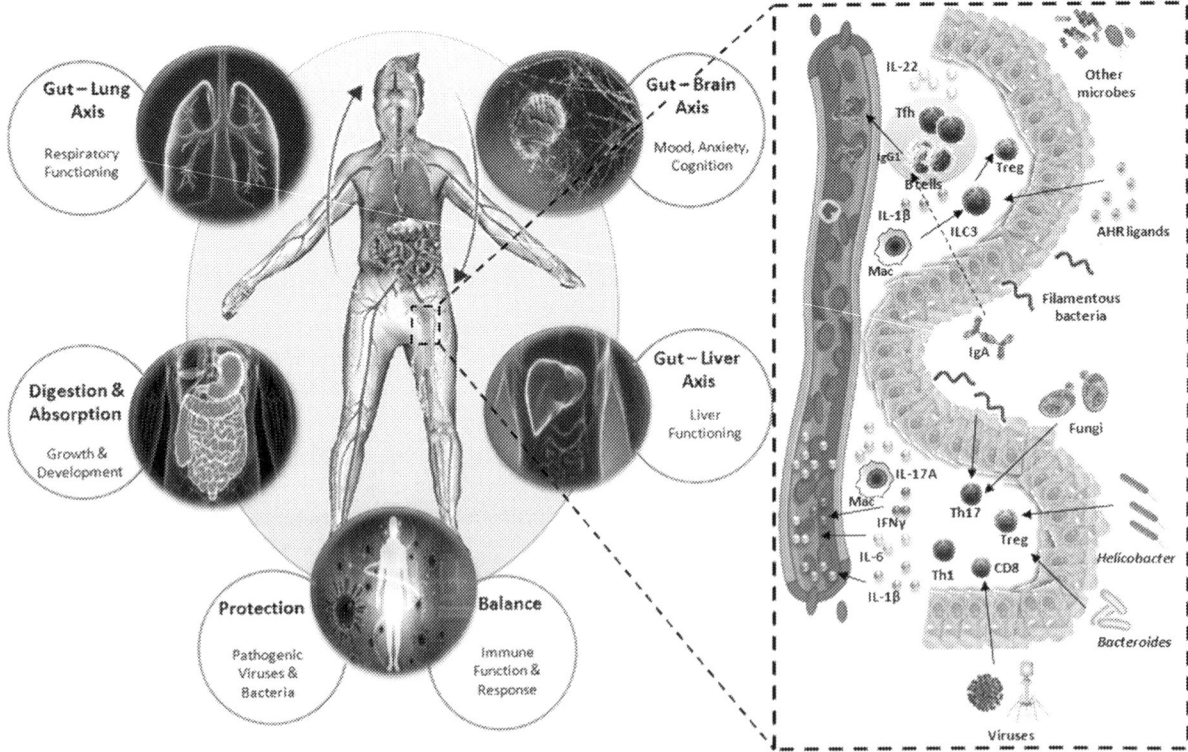

FIGURE 3.1 Gut microbiota regulates potent immunoregulators in a cascade of pathways that facilitate the differentiation of myeloid cell lineages in the bone marrow and splenic macrophages that sense microbe-associated molecular patterns (MAMPs) as well as pathogen-associated molecular patterns (PAMPs) expressed by gut microbes and activated to the release cytokines to regulate innate lymphoid cell (ILC3) and regulatory T cell (Treg) responses that maintain overall immune homeostasis. Filamentous bacteria promote immunoglobulin (IgG1) and IgA production by B cells via T follicular helper (Tfh)-dependent and independent mechanisms, respectively. Indigenous fungi dictate the balance of pro-inflammatory T helper 17 (Th17) and antiinflammatory Treg/Type 1 regulatory T (Tr1) cells in the gut, responsible for pathological implications and serve tissue-protective functions. During chronic intestinal inflammation, loss of intestinal barrier integrity to gut microbes can activate innate and adaptive immune cells to release pro-inflammatory cytokines (IL-1β, IL-6, TNF-α) into the circulatory system, leading to systemic inflammation. *AHR*, Aryl hydrocarbon receptor.

immune responses, situations of dysbiosis may lead to diarrhea, loss of appetite (Videlock & Cremonini, 2012), and to the invasion of these pathogenic bacteria into the system, leading to immunological, neurological, inflammatory, and endocrinological problems (Fioramonti et al., 2003). In addition to the influence on the severity of inflammatory diseases such as asthma, chronic peptic ulcer, tuberculosis, rheumatoid arthritis, periodontitis, ulcerative colitis, type 2 diabetes, Crohn's disease, sinusitis, active hepatitis, neurological disorders (e.g., anxiety and depression), cardiovascular diseases, and of late the coronavirus disease, Covid-19, caused by severe acute respiratory syndrome coronavirus 2 (SARS-CoV-2) (Anderson & Reiter, 2020).

Epidemiological researchers have decoded the inter-connective signaling network between the gut microbiome and diseases for understanding and maintaining immune homeostasis and integrity (Matarazzo et al., 2018). For example, individuals suffering from irritable bowel syndrome are often depressed; this also extends to individuals on the constant intake of antibiotics. In addition, individuals on the autism spectrum tend to have digestive problems. Moreover, individuals with Parkinson's disease are often prone to constipation (Pennisi, 2020), mostly all culminating from immune homeostasis imbalance. Probiotics are important for the balance of the mucosa's immune system, as they reduce its permeability and potentiate local immune responses by augmenting the expression of mediators, such as immunoglobulin G (IgG), IgA, etc. (Hardy et al., 2013; Zheng et al., 2020).

According to the World Health Organization (WHO), probiotics are classified as "live microorganisms that, when administered in adequate amounts, confer a health benefit on the host" (DuPont & DuPont, 2011; Martin Manuel et al., 2017). Probiotics temporarily colonize the gut; therefore, their supplementation must be continuous in order to be effective. Various microorganisms are beneficial for the human gut and are most commonly present in supplements and probiotic foods. These microorganisms which preferentially colonize the intestines belong to *Lactobacillus* spp., often found in the terminal ileum, and *Bifidobacterium* spp. in the colon (Mikelsaar et al., 2016; Walter, 2008). Among the lactic acid bacteria belonging to the genus *Lactobacillus* include *Lactobacillus acidophilus*, *Lactobacillus amylovorus*, *Lactobacillus casei*, *Lactobacillus gassei*, *Lactobacillus. helveticus*, *Lactobacillus johnsonii*, *Lactobacillus. pentosus*, *Lactobacillus plantarum*, *Lactobacillus reuteri*, and *Lactobacillus rhamnosus*; and the genus *Bifidobacterium* includes *Bifidobacterium adolescentis*, *Bifidobacterium animalis*, *Bifidobacterium bifidum*, *Bifidobacterium breve*, *Bifidobacterium infantis*, and *Bifidobacterium longum*. Other probiotic bacteria include *Enterococcus faecium*, *Lactococcus lactis*, *Streptococcus thermophiles*, *Bacillus clausii*, *Escherichia coli Nissle* 1917, and *Saccharomyces cerevisiae* (*boulardii*). However, not all bacteria can be classified as probiotics, as they need to belong to specific strains (Markowiak & Ślizewska, 2017).

Probiotics have been reported to play a major role in influencing the population of the gut microbiota as a means to alleviate a range of disorders such as necrotizing enterocolitis, acute infectious diarrhea, hyperuricemia, hypercholesterolemia, acute respiratory tract infections, antibiotic-associated diarrhea, intestinal disorders, allergies, obesity, epilepsy, sepsis in premature infants, infant colic, neurological conditions (autism, anxiety, AD, depression, Parkinson's disease, and schizophrenia), and influence brain activity related to emotion regulation—psychobiome (Pennisi, 2020; Sarkar et al., 2016; Wallace & Milev, 2017). The regulation of the gut microbiome through the use of probiotics may help treat and prevent several diseases linked to gut dysbiosis, especially by restoring the gut microbial balance in patients under antibiotic treatments, thereby improving their gut microbiota profile. In this context, probiotic supplementation commonly found in fermented foods (i.e., yogurt, kefir, kimchi, kombucha, pickles, miso, tempeh, sauerkraut, sourdough bread, and some cheese varieties), can assist in the rejuvenation of the gut microbiota and produce beneficial effects on the recovery of the host's immune system, thereby restoring and maintaining optimal immune homeostasis (Calder, 2020).

3.1.1 Gut microbiota and Covid-19

In light of the looming global Covid-19 pandemic, it is naturally prudent to study its broad range of effects on the overall immune homeostasis. The Covid-19 infection affects immune homeostasis which has been shown to alter gut microbiota by decreasing genera Bacteroidetes, Roseburia, Faecalibacterium, Coprococcus, and Parabacteroides composition, in addition to a higher production of pro-inflammatory cytokines (i.e., IL-18) observed in Covid-19 patients compared with both seasonal flu patients and healthy control group. This suggests that gut microbiota dysbiosis due to Covid-19 infection may contribute to disease severity (Tao et al., 2020). Covid-19 has been reported with compelling evidence that suggests this disease has the ability to affect neurological, cardiovascular, or cerebrovascular functions, primary symptoms being a loss in the sense of smell, taste, and in some cases, delirium (Yavarpour-Bali & Ghasemi-Kasman, 2020). These findings suggest that the virus has the ability to compromise the cerebrovasculature between the blood and the brain paramecium (i.e., the blood-brain barrier, BBB). The BBB functions as a regulatory interface maintaining a stable chemical brain microenvironment. A compromised BBB results in vascular leakage, and inflammation which is one of the major etiological factors associated with disease onset (Bron et al., 2017; Miller et al., 2012). Inflammatory mediators are associated with central nervous system (CNS) damage through neuroinflammation. Covid-19-related cerebrovascular-disorders are a probable link to the disruption of the homeostatic environment of the neuronal milieu, by way of brain endothelial cellular (BEC) inflammation. The BEC, thus, forms the anatomical basis of the BBB which is central to the maintenance of CNS homeostasis. CNS neurons, if compromised, will have a direct impact on the chemical composition of the neuronal milieu, implicating sensory and motor function, subsequently eliciting its negative effects on our psychological persona and hormonal homeostasis (Fisher & Mentor, 2020).

In summary, the link among preexistent conditions, dysbiosis, and the severity of Covid-19 also relies mostly on the decreased butyrate levels which lead to impaired signaling between the gut-brain, gut-lung, and gut-liver axis that results in hypercytokinemia, a hallmark of immune homeostasis imbalance (Anand & Mande, 2018). Additionally, viruses (i.e., SARS-CoV-2) must enter the host cells in order to replicate; therefore, their recognition by the immune system happens when viral antigens are presented to CD8+ cytotoxic T lymphocytes via major histocompatibility complex on the surface of the infected cells, ultimately resulting in the death of the host cell. However, when the infected cells are killed, viral particles are liberated and can infect other cells (Calder, 2020). The composition of the gut microbiota can be shifted towards an increased population of Prevotella and Oscillibacter in mice, both of which produce metabolites responsible for decreasing Th17 polarization of T cells and favoring their differentiation into Th1 regulatory T cells and type-1 T-helper cells, promoting an efficient immunity against infections (Fig. 3.2) (Maldonado Galdeano et al., 2019; Pandiyan et al., 2019).

Regarding SARS-CoV-2, diarrhea related to antibiotic administration was present in 2%–36% of Covid-19 patients in China, and probiotic supplementation was proposed in order to enhance the immunity of those patients against secondary infections (Akbari et al., 2016; Calder, 2020; Din et al., 2021; Morais et al., 2020). In fact, this resulted in a

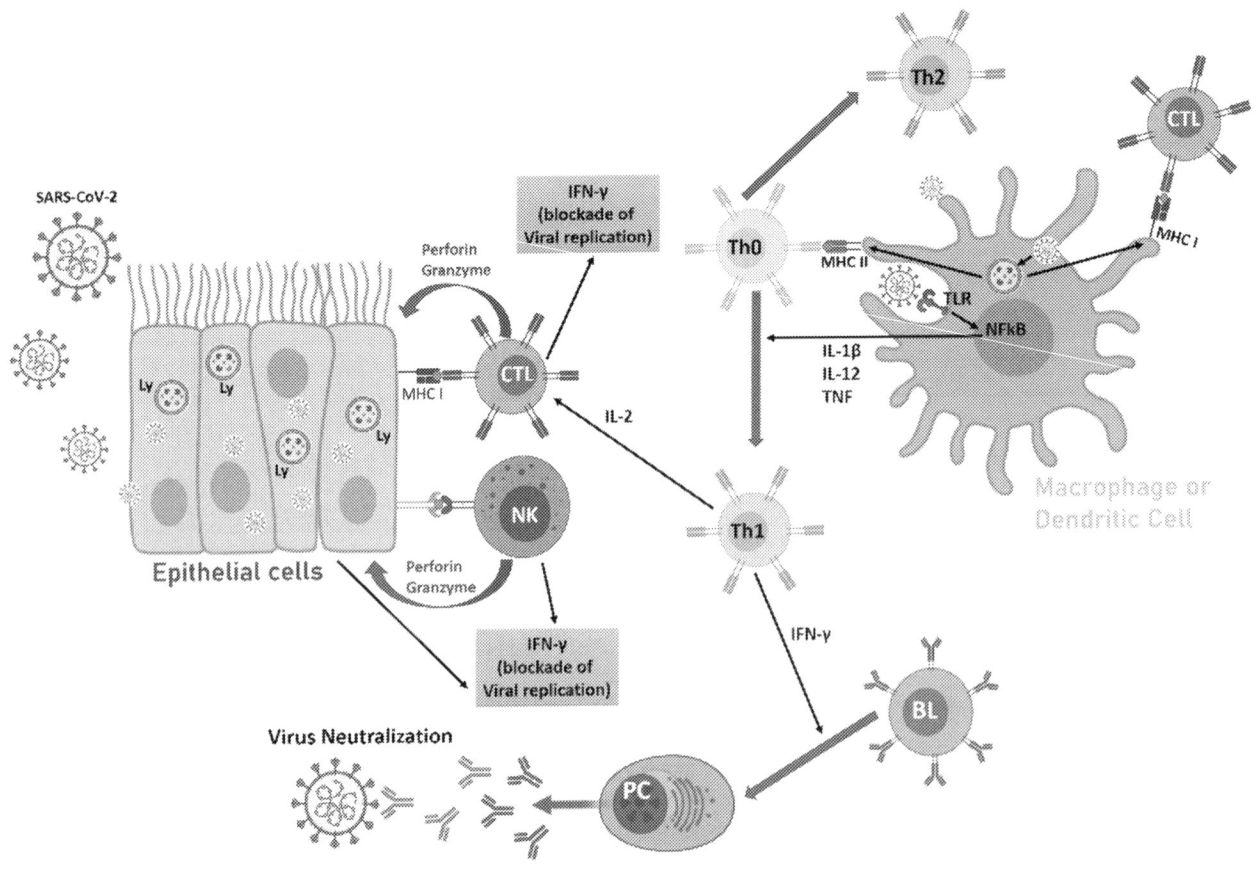

FIGURE 3.2 Innate and adaptive immunity against Covid-19 infection. The virus is digested in the lysosomes (Ly) of epithelial cells and its antigens are presented to cytotoxic T (CTL) and natural killer (NK) cells, both of which kill the host cell by secreting perforins, granzyme, and interferons (interferon-γ) that block the viral replication. This immune response is mediated by T helper type 1 (Th1) cells, which differentiate from Th0 cells after activation of toll-like receptors (TLR) from phagocytes and consequent expression of some interleukins. Th1 immunity is responsible for the differentiation of B lymphocytes (BL) into plasma cells (PC) in order to produce immunoglobulins that neutralize the virus.

reduction in the duration and the severity of Covid-19 complications in Chinese hospitalized adults and children (Akour, 2020; Morais et al., 2020). Patients with severe cases of Covid-19 often present one or more conditions that augment the risk of fatal outcomes, that is, obesity, diabetes, cardiovascular diseases, advanced age, and pulmonary conditions, and some of them are indicative of dysbiosis or can be increased during gut dysbiosis (Fig. 3.3). There is evidence suggesting that the occurrence of dysbiosis, especially when the infiltration of immune cells in the lungs in an effort to neutralize the viruses end up causing immune dysfunction, excessive inflammation, and cytokine dysregulation resulting in "cytokine storm syndrome" with fluid leakage to the alveoli, impairing the blood oxygenation, resulting in sepsis and septic shock which is associated with the higher severity of Covid-19 cases (Anderson & Reiter, 2020; Buszko et al., 2020; Datta & Bhattacharjee, 2020; Hotchkiss et al., 2016). This is attributed to angiotensin-converting enzyme 2 receptors (ACE2 receptors) abundance in the intestinal epithelium (Infusino et al., 2020), it is possible that SARS-CoV-2 can impair the absorption of nutrients (i.e., tryptophan) by the intestine epithelium and this amino acid regulates the expression of peptides with antimicrobial properties, capable of controlling the composition of the gut microbiota (elaborated further in the next section). This results in gastroenteritis symptoms that have been observed in many Covid-19 patients' cases (Infusino et al., 2020). Although the evidence pointing to the success of probiotic supplementation in enhancing the immunity of Covid-19 patients and controlling the inflammation is still mounting, more clinical studies are necessary for the development of an efficient protocol (Akour, 2020).

3.1.2 Importance of probiotic nutrition in modulating immune homeostasis

Nutrition is a cornerstone in modulating immune homeostasis and probiotic nutrition is paramount in maintaining gut microbiota subsequently regulating overall immune homeostasis. Probiotics supplementation is usually administered

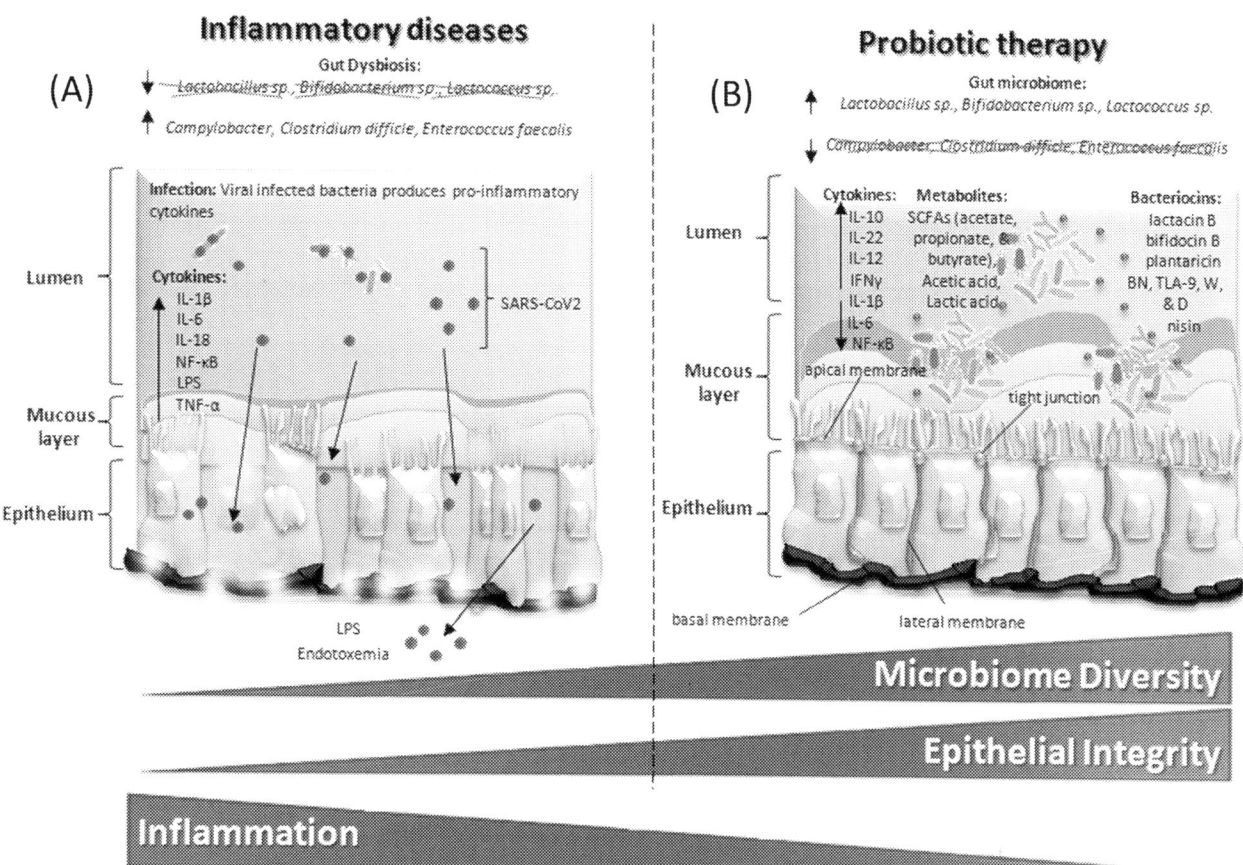

FIGURE 3.3 Influence of the gut microbiota (A) Covid-19 infection causes gut dysbiosis which results in increased proliferation of *Campylobacter, Clostridium difficle, Enterococcus faecalis* and hypercytokinemia "cytokine storm syndrome" of pro-inflammatory cytokines that ultimately impairs immune homeostasis, (B) probiotic therapy (*Lactobacillus* spp., *Bifidobacterium* spp., and *Lactococcus* spp.) that restores the gut microbiota and maintains overall immune homeostasis.

orally, whether in capsules, oil drops, water-soluble powders, or in children formulations and foods (Fenster et al., 2019; Govender et al., 2014). Orally administered probiotics may interact with approximately 200 m^2 of gut mucosa and lymphoid tissue associated with the intestines where most of the immune cells from the gut are located (Lebeer et al., 2010). This is the reason why several benefits conferred by probiotics are due to the immune system modulation affecting the host's immunity and inflammatory responses (Oelschlaeger, 2010). Furthermore, complex carbohydrates present in dietary fibers (mostly found in whole grains, fruits, vegetables, and cereals) are fermented by some bacteria species from gut microbiota, generating short-chain fatty acids (SCFAs) such as acetate, propionate, and butyrate, which are characterized to be antiinflammatory (Dhar & Mohanty, 2020). They act as signaling molecules to promote antiinflammatory cytokines production (IL-10, IL-12, IL-22, and IFN-γ), reduction of chemotaxis in the respiratory tract, immune cell adherence, increase the function of CD8 + T lymphocytes, and interferon signaling in macrophages in patients with infection and activation of Th2 effector cells in the lungs, which causes a more efficient control of external pathogens propagation (Conte & Toraldo, 2020; He et al., 2020). SCFAs also promote B-cell differentiation and antibody synthesis, thereby improving the antibody-antigen response and increases the levels of endogenous antioxidant enzyme (i.e., glutathione) which reduces oxidative stress (Park et al., 2015; Sharma & Kaur, 2020).

Besides SCFAs, bacteria from the gut microbiota produce some essential amino acids as metabolites, that is, tryptophan, which can inhibit NF-κB activation, thus reducing the expression of pro-inflammatory mediators, and can strengthen the tight junctions of the gut epithelium responsible for the impermeability of the intestinal mucosa. Finally, gut microbiota can synthesize some vitamins from complex B that can act as immune regulators (Morais et al., 2020). As mention above, butyrate is one of the main products derived from gut microbiota metabolism and is responsible for several local and systemic effects. For instance, it contributes to the barrier of the gut epithelium against external pathogens, decreases glial activity in the CNS, inhibition of histone deacetylase (action as an epigenetic regulator), and optimization of mitochondrial activity via induction of the melatonergic pathway. Furthermore, butyrate can also increase the activity of NK cells, enhancing antiviral immunity which could be useful for inflammatory diseases (Anderson & Reiter, 2020) as shown in Fig. 3.4. Moreover, with the melatonin hormone, either from the mitochondria of immune cells or from the pineal gland, melatonergic downregulation can occur in cases of stress and dysbiosis by the action of induced indoleamine 2,3-dioxygenase, which relocates tryptophan from serotonin and melatonin synthesis for the production of kynurenine products. This inhibits the activation of alpha 7 nicotinic acetylcholine receptor (α7nAChR), an important part of the cholinergic nervous system in the brain. The α7nAChR expression can be beneficial due to the regulation of autophagy in lung epithelial cells and the dampening of pulmonary immune cells; therefore, factors that inhibit α7nAChR expression, such as dysbiosis, might be detrimental to patients suffering from inflammatory diseases such as Covid-19 (Anderson & Reiter, 2020).

Gut dysbiosis itself can cause or intensify some preexistent conditions in a two-way interaction: (1) decreased melatonin levels, consequently increase circulating levels of lipopolysaccharides (LPS), a key pathogenic stimulant for inflammation in the gut; and (2) decreased butyrate levels. Butyrate suppresses platelet activation and pro-inflammatory

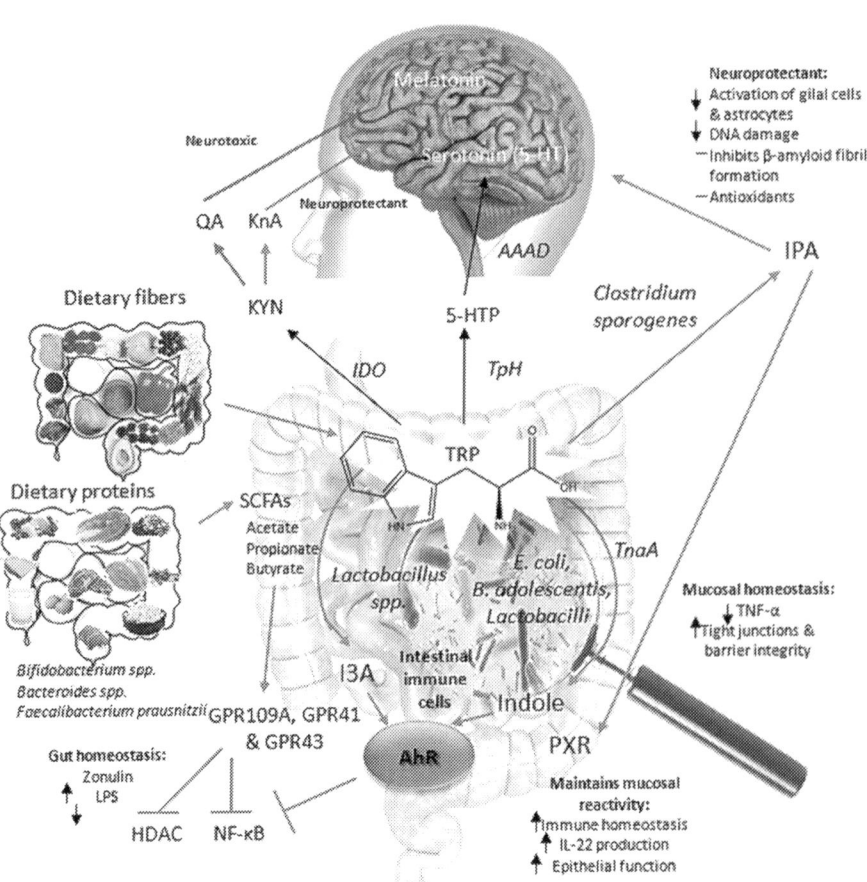

FIGURE 3.4 Probiotic nutritional interconnections from dietary fibers and proteins through a cascade of pathways to main immune homeostasis. Tryptophan (TRP) is metabolized by Clostridium sporogenes into 3-indolepropionic acid (IPA) which confers neuroprotectant activity against neurological disorders. Moreover, IPA binds to pregnane X receptor (PXR) in the intestinal cells to maintain mucosal homeostasis. Indole is produced by *E. coli*, *B. adolescentis*, and *Lactobacilli* (*L. acidophilus* and *L. reuteri*) from TRP catalyzed by tryptophanase (TnaA). TRP is further metabolized into indole-3-aldehyde (I3A) by Lactobacillus spp., and Bifidobacterium spp., in the intestinal cells to aryl hydrocarbon receptor (AhR) which maintains overall mucosal reactivity increasing the production of IL-22, immune homeostasis, and the suppression of nuclear factor-κB (NF-κB) and pro-inflammatory mediators. TRP is metabolized to 5-hydroxytryptophan (5-HTP) by tryptophan hydroxylase (TpH), then decarboxylated to 5-hydroxytryptamine (5-HT) by aromatic amino acid decarboxylase (AAAD), and to melatonin involved in sleep regulation, other cyclical bodily activities, and circadian rhythm. TRP is metabolized through the kynurenine (KYN) pathway by indoleamine-2,3-dioxygenase (IDO), KYN is further metabolized to either neuroprotective kynurenic acid (KnA) or neurotoxic quinolinic acid (QA). Dietary fibers are metabolized by some bacteria species from the gut microbiota to generate short-chain fatty acids (SCFAs) such as acetate, propionate, and butyrate, where acetate and propionate bind to G protein-coupled receptors (GPR41) and GPR43, which can modulate inflammation, and butyrate binds to GPR109A, suppressing NF-κB and inhibition of histone deacetylase (HDAC), lipopolysaccharide (LPS), and increasing the synthesis of zonulin for preventing gut permeability.

cytokines; therefore there is an increased risk of cardiovascular complications (DeGruttola et al., 2016). The BBB permeability and neuron myelination are also impaired in this case, which causes part of the neurological symptoms which is seen in some Covid-19 patients (Anderson & Reiter, 2020). The interactions of the human gut microbial flora with probiotics are far more intimate, as they facilitate an orchestrated symphony that determines the physiological, immunological, metabolic, and behavioral development that can influence future disease susceptibility (Daliri & Lee, 2015). Probiotics have also been considered in past decades as an alternative therapy for inflammatory bowel disease as they exhibited good efficacy when used as adjuvants for treating ulcerative colitis (Furrie et al., 2005; Shen et al., 2018). The use of probiotic cultures excludes potentially pathogenic microorganisms and reinforces the body's natural defense mechanisms. The modulation of the intestinal microbiota by probiotic microorganisms occurs through a mechanism called competitive exclusion. Pathogen exclusion through the production of antagonistic antimicrobial substances against pathogenic microorganisms can facilitate gut stability. This can neither be pathogenic nor trigger allergic responses even in immunocompromised hosts, thereby serving as adjuvants to stimulate and maintain immune homeostasis.

3.1.3 Probiotic mechanism of action

One of the first evidences of the interaction between the gut microbiota and the immune system was observed in germ-free mice, which tend to present reduced Peyer's patches and decreased amount of regulatory T cells and T helper 17 (Th17) cells in mesenteric lymph nodes (Shi et al., 2017). This situation was fixed rapidly after the colonization of the gut with intestinal bacteria from normal mice (Infusino et al., 2020), corroborated by further investigations which found that the modulation of T cell differentiation in Th1, Th2, Th17 helper, or T-regulatory cells by the gut microbiota, probably as a means to immunize from or to tolerate some luminal bacteria (Infusino et al., 2020; Morais et al., 2020). It is paramount for probiotics to reach the target site (the gut) for their biodistribution and optimal efficacy. This entails probiotics to endure the gastric acidity of the stomach attributed by the presence of HCl at 37°C, resistance to pancreatic enzymatic degradation, as well as navigate the bile in the upper digestive tract before reaching the small intestines (Maldonado Galdeano et al., 2019). Thereafter, allow for efficient intestinal epithelial adhesion—for immune modulation by enhanced damaged mucosa healing, followed by prolonged transient colonization—dictated by their adhesion capacity to the host gut, to other bacterial cells (coaggregation), and to some extent to the same species (auto-aggregation) in order to colonize and promote immunomodulatory effects (Piwat et al., 2015; van Tassell & Miller, 2011).

Several lines of evidence show that the antiviral adjuvant property of probiotics happens by three main mechanisms: (1) reducing the epithelium permeability by a spatial barrier, (2) reinforcement of the innate immunity in the gut mucosa, and (3) regulating the systemic immune response with an antiinflammatory effect stimulated by increased macrophages activity (Calder, 2020; Infusino et al., 2020). The regulation of inflammatory cytokines plays an important role in the modulation of the immune system due to their biological effects, that is, regulation of immunity, decrease or increase of inflammation, modulation of cell growth, and cell healing (Liu et al., 2013). Those effects are due mostly to the decreased levels of pro-inflammatory cytokines (TNF-α, IL-6, and IL-1β) and inactivation of NF-κB (Hasan et al., 2018; Jang et al., 2019; Liu et al., 2013; Xia et al., 2018).

The complexity of the interconnectivity between probiotics and gut microbiota varies in individuals. However, one major consensus revolves around the improvement of the barrier functions of the gut mucosa able to stimulate epithelial cell signaling pathways—facilitated by Paneth cells responsible for the secretion of diverse antimicrobial peptides [e.g. lysozyme, secretory phospholipase A2, defensins, defensin-like peptides (elafin and SLPI), and cathelicidins] and production of antiinflammatory cytokines (IL-10, IL-12, IL-22, and IFN-γ). Probiotics play a pivotal role in the interaction of intestinal epithelial cells and splenic macrophages in innate immune responses as a result of an increased expression of the receptors toll-like receptor 2 (TLR2) and mannose (CD206) on the surface of macrophages and dendritic cells and later stimulation of an adaptive immune response (Maldonado Galdeano et al., 2019). These results reinforce intestinal and BBBs integrity by increasing gene expression of tight junction proteins, TLR, and the proteoglycan recognition proteins, leading to activation of dendric cells and monocyte chemoattractant protein 1 which consigns signals to other immune cells, resulting in the activation of the mucosal immune system, characterized by an increase in IgA + in the lamina propria of the intestine, bronchus and mammary glands, and the activation of T cells that release IL-10 and produce SCFAs for the growth of desirable microbes (Maldonado Galdeano et al., 2019).

Another mechanism of probiotics in maintaining immune homeostasis is through the production of organic acids (acetic and lactic acids) and bacteriocins (lactacin B, bifidocin B, plantaricin, and nisin) thus inhibiting the proliferation of pathogenic bacteria and enhancing the response of the gut-associated immune repertoire (Gaspar et al., 2018). Skolnick and Greig (2019) and Yuan et al. (2019) have shown that some gut microbes convert guanine to queuine, which is described as a longevity vitamin that has been reported to improve mental well-being. The induction of a viral/LPS-induced inflammation and subsequent compromising of BBB integrity opens up an avenue of investigation into the role of probiotics as a treatment strategy to reverse the harmful effects of microbiotic-induced inflammation. Most recently, work by Cui et al. (2020) revealed that some gut microbes especially lactic acid bacteria (*Lactobacillus buchneri*, *Levilactobacillus brevis*, *Lactobacillus paracasei*, *L. plantarum*, *Lactobacillus delbrueckii* subsp. *bulgaricus*, and *L. lactis*) and *Bactereroides* (*Bacteroides fragilis*) can produce gamma-aminobutyric acid (GABA), a neurotransmitter that inhibits neural activity in the brain, also plays an important physiological function, such as antihypertensive, antidepressant activities, role in behavior, cognition, and the body's response to stress. GABA is also implicated in enhancing immunity, relieving anxiety and menopausal syndrome, regulating blood pressure, fighting obesity, and improving visual cortical function. However, the unregulation of GABA has been linked to depression and other mental health problems. Individuals with fewer *Bacteroides* bacteria exhibited a robust pattern of hyperactivity in the prefrontal cortex which is associated with severe depression (Bienenstock et al., 2015; Galland, 2014).

Complex, biochemical communication exists between the gut microbiome (weighing 2 kg) and the human brain (weighing 1.4 kg) and is denoted as the gut-brain axis, involving: the CNS, hypothalamic-pituitary-adrenal axis; autonomic nervous system, and gut microbiota linked to the brain, recently known as psychobiome which influences overall immune and brain homeostasis (Sharma & Kaur, 2020). The bacteria within the gut are tantalizing sources of untapped therapeutic potential that produce a plethora of ligands, namely glutamate (neurotransmitter), involved in cognition, learning, and memory (Baj et al., 2019). Note that glutamate levels are suppressed in individuals suffering from anxiety disorders and depression. The main action mechanism proposed for probiotics relies on the immune modulation towards the restoration of health by the influence on systemic immunological and inflammatory parameters, thus enhancing immune response and maintaining well-orchestrated immunity (Bermudez-Brito et al., 2012; Plaza-Diaz et al., 2019).

Immune gut homeostasis serves as a prerequisite for intestinal and BBB integrity which is orchestrated by the regulatory balance of pro- and antiinflammatory responses. During inflammation, enteroendocrine cells release IL-6 which acts as both a pro-inflammatory cytokine and an antiinflammatory myokine; IL-7 primarily acts on T cells (i.e., lymphocytes, produced in the thymus, central function in an immune response) that abundantly express the IL-7 receptor and are increased at the inflammatory sites, predominantly induces Th1 and Th17-associated cytokine secretion (Th2 cells secrete IL-4, IL-5, IL-6, IL-10, and IL-13 cytokines, which mediates the antiinflammatory humoral response and immune suppression via the inhibition of Th1 cytokine) (Dhar & Mohanty, 2020; Pennisi, 2020). An adjunct alternative to maintaining immune homeostasis can be through nutritional therapy which can aid in increasing immune system responsiveness. Likewise, it is also imperative to be aware of the type of food we consume over time, as in the lamina propria, probiotic functions involve the action of T helper (Th) and regulatory T (Treg) cells (Kim et al., 2018). IL-1β and IL-1α interleukins are prototypical pro-inflamed cytokines that perform pleiotropic functions on different cells and play a major role in acute, chronic, and autoimmune disorders. A probiotic formulation (*L. rhamnosus*, *B. lactis*, and *B. longum*) have demonstrated a significant increase in IL-10 and a decrease in inflammatory mediators (IL-1β and IL-6) (Sichetti et al., 2018).

Lactobacillus gasseri strains (SBT2055, TMC0356, and OLL280) have been reported to activate the human dendritic cells through an increase in the secretion of IFN-γ and IL-12 towards Type 1 T-helper polarization (Th1) responses, thereby promoting immunity against infections and other diseases attenuated by the expression of pro-inflammatory cytokines (Kumar et al., 2019; Nishihira et al., 2016) Probiotics can enhance the host defense system by increased expression of myxovirus resistance protein (Mx1) and 2′-5′ oligoadenylate synthetase 1 A, for antiviral immunity and IgA secretion, collaborating in maintaining immune homeostasis and surveillance by providing protective humoral and cellular immunity (Lemme-Dumit et al., 2018; Maldonado Galdeano et al., 2019). Additionally, probiotics have the ability to reduce purine in foods and beverages, which is essential to viral RNA synthesis during viral infections.

Moreover, in vitro investigations demonstrated that some probiotic strains (i.e., *L. paracasei*, *L. plantarum*, and *L. rhamnosus*) are able to inhibit the release of pro-inflammatory cytokines IL-6, IL-8, and prostaglandin E2 by human monocytes, and in macrophages, which modulate the production of TNF via activation of signal transducer and activator of transcription 3 and, consequently, inhibition of JunN-terminal kinases activation (Azad et al., 2018). IL-22, MAPK, and NF-κB are downregulated by various probiotics in dendritic cells, while antiinflammatory cytokines such as IL-10 are upregulated in Wistar rats with edema in the paws, with a significant improvement in the paw inflammation (de Moreno de Leblanc et al., 2011; Ding et al., 2017; Llewellyn & Foey, 2017). These findings were further supported by results reported by Dargahi et al. (2019) and Sichetti et al. (2018). They revealed that the administration of a probiotic formulation (*L. rhamnosus*, *B. lactis*, and *B. longum*) led to increased production of IL-10 and decreased production of IL-1 and IL-6 in cultured macrophages.

Various inflammatory markers (i.e., iNOS, COX-2, TNF, NF-κB, IL-6, and phosphorylated Akt) were found to decrease after the administration of probiotics in some colitis models, while there was upregulation of IL-10 and nitric oxide (Nanau & Neuman, 2012). Pro- and antiinflammatory markers were also modulated by probiotics in multiple sclerosis in vivo models, with a decreased autoreactive response from T cells contributing to the improvement in the condition (Akour, 2020). The inhibition of H1N1, HIV, rotavirus, and gastric corona by bacteria from *Lactobacillus* family has already been observed experimentally. As mentioned above, these bacteria typically secrete metabolites such as butyrate, acetic acid, lactic acid, and plantaricin, which demonstrated to enhance antiviral immunity (Anwar et al., 2020). *Lactobacillus lactis* has shown antiviral activity against influenza viruses by stimulating plasmacytoid dendritic cells via activation of TLR 9 (TLR9), which leads to an increased interferon expression and consequent antiviral immunity enhancement. Similarly, the production of interferons was augmented after the administration of *L. gasseri* in mice bearing respiratory syncytial virus, with a consequent decrease in the viral titer.

3.1.4 Probiotic interlink with immunization efficacy

The therapeutic effects of probiotics have been mostly studied in the gastrointestinal tract. Modulation of the gut-brain by probiotics has been suggested as a novel therapeutic solution for anxiety and depression. Studies have described the potential therapeutic effects of probiotics and the possible mechanisms of action to prevent and/or treat chronic airway diseases (Martens et al., 2018). Most recently compelling evidence has demonstrated that gut microbiota may influence blood pressure, and, therefore, may be important for people with hypertension. As the composition of the gut microbiota is imperative to maintain intestinal immunity and whole-body homeostasis, it is not surprising that several diseases, such as hypertension, are associated with dysbiosis. The most probable mechanism evolved in the influence of the microbiota on blood pressure is related to its influence on host-cell physiology through bacterial metabolic products or wall components. Consequently, these bacteria are able to control adiposity and inflammatory response, interacting with epithelial and dendritic cells of the gut, which are paramount for innate and adaptive immunities (Robles-Vera et al., 2017). Probiotics may be very useful for lowering cholesterol, improving atherosclerosis, or attenuate myocardial hypertrophy. Probiotics release bioactive peptides (like angiotensin-converting enzyme inhibitory peptides) when food products are being fermented that help with blood pressure regulation. A study evaluated nine controlled clinical trials about the influence of probiotics in blood pressure and concluded that it helps to lower systolic and diastolic blood pressure, especially with the ingestion of multiple species of probiotics for more than 8 weeks (Dong et al., 2019; Sabico et al., 2019).

3.1.5 Clinical translation of probiotic investigation

Albeit there are a number of probiotics in the market that are not effectively regulated by global regulatory authorities such as the FDA, WHO, etc. Probiotics research is still in its infancy with more clinical studies and investigations conducted to determine the health benefits, validity, and safety of probiotics as a function of improving "biomarker deficiency" data. Their effectiveness varies due to limited regulatory frameworks in place to monitor their efficacies. For example, probiotics *L. reuteri* NCIMB 30242 LRC, superstrain *L. acidophilus* DDS-1, *B. lactis* UABla-12, *L. gasseri* BNR17, and *L. plantarum* PPLP-217 (UAS Labs, USA; Micropharma, Canada) has been on the market as the first recognized biomarker of hypercholesterolemia and obesity by lowering cholesterol and sterol absorption, in human trials, however, there is mixed inconsistency in the outcomes.

Among the most common diseases that affect children, urinary tract infection (UTI) is detrimental because it can lead to severe conditions such as kidney ulcers or renal failure (Leung et al., 2019; Rostami et al., 2018). UTI is usually treated with antibiotics and researchers have found that probiotics may play an important role as a complementary therapy, thus increasing the effectiveness of the medication and preventing the incidence of UTIs (Rostami et al., 2018). Probiotic supplementation has also been demonstrated to play a positive impact on the treatment of depression symptoms, improving mood and cognition conditions. Major depressive disorder (MDD) is associated with high levels of pro-inflammatory cytokines (IL-6 and TNF-α) which causes several comorbidities and inflammatory conditions like rheumatoid arthritis, multiple sclerosis, and coronary heart disease, among others (Köhler et al., 2017). Furthermore, studies have shown that conventional antiinflammatories have antidepressant effects in patients, and those conventional pharmacotherapies such as selective serotonin reuptake inhibitors also have antiinflammatory properties. Inflammation may be associated with resistance to depression treatment (Bron et al., 2017; Miller et al., 2012). Accordingly, probiotics can act as an adjuvant in antidepressant treatment by reducing inflammation (Vlainić et al., 2016). Probiotics also help with metabolic complications such as obesity and diabetes which are associated with high levels of peripheral inflammatory markers and, consequently, related to mood and cognitive illnesses (Akbari et al., 2016).

TABLE 3.1 Clinical trials focusing on the role of probiotics in various diseases.

S. no	Clinical trial title	Trial no.	Probiotic formulation	Outcome	References
1	Effect of probiotic administration on gut flora composition	NCT03330678	VSL#3 capsule (a mixture of eight species— *S. thermophilus, B. breve, B. longum, B. infantis, L. acidophilus, L. plantarum, L. paracasei,* and *L. delbrueckii*)	Reduction in circulating Th17 cells, and monocyte-derived cytokines in response to LPS stimulation.	Singh et al. (2018)
2	The effect of probiotic capsule supplementation on severity depression among patients with major depressive disorder (MDD) under treatment with citalopram	IRCT2014060717993N1	Probiotic capsules containing strains of *L. acidophilus, L. casei,* and *B. bifidum*	Significantly lower Beck Depression Inventory scores in comparison to those who received the placebo. Reductions in inflammatory markers like serum insulin and serum hs-CRP were also observed in these patients	Akkasheh et al. (2016)
3	Effect of probiotic supplementation on endothelial function	NCT01952834	GoodBelly probiotic (a mixture of *L. Plantarum* 299 v (Lp299v)., *B. lactis* Bi-07, and *L. acidophilus*)	Men with stable coronary artery disease improved vascular endothelium dilation and reduced systemic inflammation attributed to reduction in cytokine (IL-8 and IL-12) expression and leptin, a biomarker of cardiovascular risk, the peptide circulates the bloodstream, and is responsible for regulating energy balance and signals to the hypothalamus in the brain.	Malik et al. (2018)
4	Effect of probiotics on gut-liver axis of alcoholic liver disease	NCT01501162	Lactowell whey permeate (*L. subtilis/ S. Faecium*)	Intestinal flora restoration and microbial LPS improvement in patients with alcoholic hepatitis, thus revealing the therapeutic effect of probiotics on the gut-liver axis of ALD disease.	Han et al. (2015)
5	Safety of BB-12 supplemented strawberry yogurt for healthy children	NCT01652287	*B. lactis* strain BB-12 (BB-12)-supplemented yogurt	No significant differences between the treatment and control group, suggesting that BB-12 is safe and well-tolerated when consumed by healthy children.	Merenstein et al. (2011)

(Continued)

TABLE 3.1 (Continued)

S. no	Clinical trial title	Trial no.	Probiotic formulation	Outcome	References
6	Impact of emergency department probiotic (LGG) treatment of pediatric gastroenteritis	NCT01773967	*L. rhamnosus* GG (ATCC 53103/LGG)	No significant outcomes between the ATCC 53103/GG group and those who received placebo.	Schnadower et al. (2018)
7	Efficacy of *Lactobacillus* GG with diosmectite in treatment children with acute gastroenteritis	NCT01657032			Schnadower et al. (2017)
8	Efficacy and safety study in the prevention of antibiotic-associated diarrhea (AAD) and *Clostridium difficile*-associated diarrhea (CDAD) in hospitalized adult patients exposed to nosocomial Infection	NCT00958308	BIO-K + CL-1285 (mixture of *L. acidophilus* CL1285 and *L. casei* LBC80R)	BIO-K + CL-1285 was well tolerated and effective for reducing risk of AAD and, in particular, CDAD in hospitalized patients on antibiotics	Gao et al. (2010)
9	Role of probiotics in recovery of children with severe acute malnutrition (SAM)	ISRCTN16454889	*B. animalis* subsp. *lactis* BB-12 and *L. rhamnosus* LGG	No effect on diarrhea in children with SAM	Grenov et al. (2017) and Lanyero et al. (2019)
10	Effect of probiotics (Bio-Three) in children's enterocolitis	NCT00463190	Bio-Three (*Bacillus mesentericus, S. faecalis* and *Clostridium butyricium*)	Bio-Three reduced the severity of diarrhea and hospital stay in children with acute diarrhea. In addition, cytokines IL-10, IFN-γ, and IL-12 were upregulated and TNF-α was downregulated in the probiotic group compared to the placebo group.	Chen et al. (2010)
11	The probiotic *Bifidobacterium breve* strain BBG-01 administrated early to preterm infants to prevent infection, necrotizing enterocolitis, and death	ISRCTN05511098	*B. breve* BBG-01	No evidence of benefit for routine use of *B. breve* BBG-001 for prevention of necrotizing enterocolitis and late-onset sepsis in very preterm infants	Costeloe et al. (2016)

Albeit microbiota composition varies from person to person, there is evidence that alteration in the enterotype of individuals with MDD, contributing to the biosignature of this condition. For example, it was found that patients with MDD present increased levels of Bacteroidetes, Proteobacteria, and Actinobacteria beyond a bigger bacterial diversity and decreased level of Firmicutes (Akkasheh et al., 2016; Jiang et al., 2015). Several studies point that the restoration of the microbiota may be related to the reduction of peripheral inflammation. This is due to the action of probiotics in the composition of the intestinal microbiota which are responsible for their antiinflammatory effects. Reducing stress-induced inflammation, obesity-and-diet-induced-inflammation and intestinal permeability are other benefits of probiotics (Lobionda et al., 2019; Miller & Raison, 2016; Vlainić et al., 2016). In the US, probiotics are rarely prescribed by physicians; however, probiotics are marketed as dietary supplements, and manufacturers suggest use while their relevance has not yet been established. The US and European government agencies remain concerned about the effectiveness and safety of probiotics. Tables 3.1 and 3.2 shows some of the probiotic clinical trials conducted for various diseases and Covid-19 listed on the WHO's International Clinical Trials Registry Platform.

TABLE 3.2 Role of probiotic in Covid-19.

S. no.	Clinical trial title	Trial no.	Probiotic formulation	Aim of the study
1	Evaluation of the complementary effect of symbiotic adjuvant on inflammatory markers and clinical manifestations in patients with Covid-19	IRCT20200923048815N1	Two lactocar brand synbiotic adjuvant capsules	Evaluation of the treatment inflammatory markers (CRP, ESR, IL-6, CBC) and clinical prognosis before and 8 weeks after treatment in patients with Covid-19
2	Effects of Lactocare synbiotic against Covid-19 infection in the staff of emergency department	IRCT20101020004976N6	Lactocare synbiotic capsule	Evaluate the effects of Lactocare synbiotic against Covid-19 infection
3	Study for the application of novel coronavirus pneumonia (Covid-19) intestinal tract toxicity in diagnosis and its prognostic effect	ChiCTR2000032686	Rifximine intervention versus probiotic intervention	Monitor the influence of treatment on changes of microbiota, virology and metabolomics
4	Stress-reduction using probiotics to promote ongoing resilience throughout Covid-19 for healthcare workers: A randomized placebo-controlled trial	ACTRN12620000480987	*L. rhamnosus* N001	To monitor mental health of nurses using the Perceived Stress Scale to evaluate their psychological stress level, cognitive function and behavior during the Covid-19 pandemic
5	Oxygen-ozone as adjuvant treatment in early control of Covid-19 progression and modulation of the gut microbial flora (PROBIOZOVID)	NCT04366089	SivoMixx composition (*S. thermophiles*) DSM322245, *B. lactis* DSM 32246, *B. lactis* DSM 32247, *L. acidophilus* DSM 32241, *L. helveticus* DSM 32242, *L. paracasei* DSM 32243, *L. plantarum* DSM 32244, *L. brevis* DSM 27961	To evaluate effectiveness of oxygen-ozone therapy accompanied by probiotics supplementation for preventing the progression of Covid-19
6	Efficacy of *L. plantarum* and *P. acidilactici* in adults with Covid-19	NCT04517422	*L. plantarum* CECT7481, *L. plantarum* CECT 7484, *L. plantarum* CECT 7485, and *P. acidilactici* CECT 7483	To evaluate safety and efficacy of the probiotics to reduce gastrointestinal Covid-19 severity and modulate the levels of IgG/IgM

A study by Nishihira et al. (2016) evaluated the efficacy of drinkable yogurt containing 1×10^9 CFU/100 g of *L. gasseri* strain SBT2055 (LG2055) in stimulating immunoglobulin production and innate immunity for influenza vaccine-specific antibody responses after trivalent influenza [A/California/7/2009(X-179A)(H1N1)pdm09, A/New York/39/2012(X-233A)(H3N2), B/Massachusetts/2/2012(BX-51B)] vaccination in healthy adult volunteers against influenza viruses A/H1N1 and B; the control group receiving the placebo (drinkable yogurt without LG2055). LG2055 (Megmilk Snow Brand Co., Ltd., Tokyo, Japan) has been reported to lower the fecal *Staphylococcus* population and p-cresol concentration (cholesterol-lowering effect in humans with mild hypercholesterolemia), and prevent abdominal adiposity in rats and humans. LG2055 was also found to confer a protective effect against influenza A virus infection through the induction of antiviral genes by type I IFN signaling and IgA production in the mouse small intestine.

This compelling evidence raises the possibility that administration of LG2055 may enhance both innate and adaptive immunity. Results from the study demonstrated that the administration of LG2055 increased hemagglutination inhibition titers and the rate of seroprotection against influenza viruses A/H1N1 and B after vaccination, in addition to elevated levels of total IgG and IgA in plasma and sIgA production in saliva as compared with the control group that received the placebo. Furthermore, LG2055 was found to enhance natural killer cell activity and myxovirus resistance A gene expression, which is one of the antiviral genes stimulated by type I or type III interferons in peripheral blood mononuclear cells. Recently, some clinical trials have shown that the administration of probiotics can prevent ventilator-associated pneumonia in patients with Covid-19, but the effectiveness in reducing deaths in these patients has yet to be proven. Table 3.2 reviewed some of the registered clinical trials focused on the role of probiotics in Covid-19. A targeted approach to the modulation of the intestinal microbiota of patients with Covid-19 in order to define the treatment with the appropriate probiotic is necessary (Kalantar-Zadeh et al., 2020; Sundararaman et al., 2020).

3.2 Conlusion

The gut microbiota functions as a motherboard for overall immune homeostasis and gut dysbiosis is linked to a variety of inflammatory diseases and disorders. Probiotics have been shown to restore gut dysbiosis to main immune homeostasis; however, biomarker deficiency data is limited to determine the health benefits, validity, and safety of probiotics as a function of improving immunity against infections. Probiotics might be useful in regulating and enhancing immune response through antiinflammatory cytokines, improve gut barrier function by antagonistic effects against pathogens bacterial strains as a result of gut dysbiosis including patients with Covid-19. The race for an effective and safe Covid-19 vaccine has been on everyone's radar worldwide. Expert virologists believe that a single dose alone would not be as effective for prolonged immunity against the virus. This is true for patients with immunosenescence; thus, the older the person becomes, the more susceptible to infections they are. In addition, immunization by vaccines is also impaired. Vaccination is an adaptive immunity through the expression of antigen-specific antibodies and cytotoxic T cells in the most effective mechanism to prevent viral infections. As demonstrated by previous influenza vaccination, immune responses are different in individuals, weakened by specific lifestyle attributes, such as obesity, stress, and smoking cigarettes which ultimately influences overall immune homeostasis. Probiotics that activate both the innate and adaptive human immune responses are imperative, especially amid the Covid-19 vaccination paradigm; it is paramount to explore any other effective intervention strategies such as probiotics as an adjuvant synergistic approach for a more effective and beneficial prolonged antibody defense against the coronavirus and future pandemics. Therefore, probiotic supplementation can serve as armament against infectious pathogens, such as viruses, and can be included in a patient's dietary nutrition, especially since it has been demonstrated that long-term probiotics consumption does not affect the intestinal homeostasis.

Acknowledgment

The authors would like to thank the Fundação de Amparo à Pesquisa do Estado de São Paulo (FAPESP) Grant No. 2019/15154-0 for support to Velaphi Clement Thipe.

References

Akbari, E., Asemi, Z., Daneshvar Kakhaki, R., Bahmani, F., Kouchaki, E., Tamtaji, O. R., Hamidi, G. A., & Salami, M. (2016). Effect of probiotic supplementation on cognitive function and metabolic status in Alzheimer's disease: A randomized, double-blind and controlled trial. *Frontiers in Aging Neuroscience*, *8*, 256. Available from https://doi.org/10.3389/fnagi.2016.00256.

Akkasheh, G., Kashani-Poor, Z., Tajabadi-Ebrahimi, M., Jafari, P., Akbari, H., Taghizadeh, M., Memarzadeh, M. R., Asemi, Z., & Esmaillzadeh, A. (2016). Clinical and metabolic response to probiotic administration in patients with major depressive disorder: A randomized, double-blind, placebo-controlled trial. *Nutrition (Burbank, Los Angeles County, Calif.)*, *32*(3), 315−320. Available from https://doi.org/10.1016/j.nut.2015.09.003.

Akour, A. (2020). Probiotics and COVID-19: Is there any link? *Letters in Applied Microbiology*, *71*(3), 229−234. Available from https://doi.org/10.1111/lam.13334.

Anand, S., & Mande, S. S. (2018). Diet, microbiota and gut-lung connection. *Frontiers in Microbiology*, *9*, 2147. Available from https://www.frontiersin.org/article/10.3389/fmicb.2018.02147.

Anderson, G., & Reiter, R. J. (2020). COVID-19 pathophysiology: Interactions of gut microbiome, melatonin, vitamin D, stress, kynurenine and the alpha 7 nicotinic receptor: Treatment implications. *Melatonin Research*, *3*(3), 322−345. Available from https://doi.org/10.32794/mr11250066.

Anwar, F., Altayb, H. N., Al-Abbasi, F. A., Al-Malki, A. L., Kamal, M. A., & Kumar, V. (2020). Antiviral effects of probiotic metabolites on COVID-19. *Journal of Biomolecular Structure and Dynamics*, 1−10. Available from https://doi.org/10.1080/07391102.2020.1775123.

Azad, M. A. K., Sarker, M., & Wan, D. (2018). Immunomodulatory effects of probiotics on cytokine profiles. *BioMed Research International*, *2018*, 8063647. Available from https://doi.org/10.1155/2018/8063647.

Baj, A., Moro, E., Bistoletti, M., Orlandi, V., Crema, F., & Giaroni, C. (2019). Glutamatergic signaling along the microbiota-gut-brain axis. *International Journal of Molecular Sciences*, *20*(6). Available from https://doi.org/10.3390/ijms20061482.

Bermudez-Brito, M., Plaza-Díaz, J., Muñoz-Quezada, S., Gómez-Llorente, C., & Gil, A. (2012). Probiotic mechanisms of action. *Annals of Nutrition and Metabolism*, *61*(2), 160−174. Available from https://doi.org/10.1159/000342079.

Bienenstock, J., Kunze, W., & Forsythe, P. (2015). Microbiota and the gut−brain axis. *Nutrition Reviews, 73*(Suppl. 1), 28−31. Available from https://doi.org/10.1093/nutrit/nuv019.

Bron, P. A., Kleerebezem, M., Brummer, R.-J., Cani, P. D., Mercenier, A., MacDonald, T. T., Garcia-Ródenas, C. L., & Wells, J. M. (2017). Can probiotics modulate human disease by impacting intestinal barrier function? *British Journal of Nutrition, 117*(1), 93−107. Available from https://doi.org/10.1017/S0007114516004037.

Buszko, M., Park, J.-H., Verthelyi, D., Sen, R., Young, H. A., & Rosenberg, A. S. (2020). The dynamic changes in cytokine responses in COVID-19: A snapshot of the current state of knowledge. *Nature Immunology, 21*(10), 1146−1151. Available from https://doi.org/10.1038/s41590-020-0779-1.

Calder, P. C. (2020). Nutrition, immunity and COVID-19. *BMJ Nutrition, Prevention and Health, 3*(1). Available from https://doi.org/10.1136/bmjnph-2020-000085, 74 LP—92.

Chen, C.-C., Kong, M.-S., Lai, M.-W., Chao, H.-C., Chang, K.-W., Chen, S.-Y., Huang, Y.-C., Chiu, C.-H., Li, W.-C., Lin, P.-Y., Chen, C.-J., & Li, T.-Y. (2010). Probiotics have clinical, microbiologic, and immunologic efficacy in acute infectious diarrhea. *The Pediatric Infectious Disease Journal, 29*(2), 135−138. Available from https://doi.org/10.1097/inf.0b013e3181b530bf.

Conte, L., & Toraldo, D. M. (2020). Targeting the gut-lung microbiota axis by means of a high-fibre diet and probiotics may have anti-inflammatory effects in COVID-19 infection. *Therapeutic Advances in Respiratory Disease, 14*. Available from https://doi.org/10.1177/1753466620937170, 1753466620937170−1753466620937170.

Costeloe, K., Hardy, P., Juszczak, E., Wilks, M., & Millar, M. R. (2016). Bifidobacterium breve BBG-001 in very preterm infants: A randomised controlled phase 3 trial. *Lancet, 387*(10019), 649−660. Available from https://doi.org/10.1016/S0140-6736(15)01027-2.

Cui, Y., Miao, K., Niyaphorn, S., & Qu, X. (2020). Production of gamma-aminobutyric acid from lactic acid bacteria: A systematic review. *International Journal of Molecular Sciences, 21*(3), 1−21. Available from https://doi.org/10.3390/ijms21030995.

Daliri, E. B.-M., & Lee, B. H. (2015). New perspectives on probiotics in health and disease. *Food Science and Human Wellness, 4*(2), 56−65. Available from https://doi.org/10.1016/j.fshw.2015.06.002.

Dargahi, N., Johnson, J., Donkor, O., Vasiljevic, T., & Apostolopoulos, V. (2019). Immunomodulatory effects of probiotics: Can they be used to treat allergies and autoimmune diseases? *Maturitas, 119*, 25−38. Available from https://doi.org/10.1016/j.maturitas.2018.11.002.

Datta, C., & Bhattacharjee, A. (2020). Cytokine storm and its implication in Coronavirus disease 2019 (COVID-19). *Journal of Immunological Sciences, 4*(3), 4−21. Available from https://doi.org/10.29245/2578-3009/2020/3.1190.

de Moreno de Leblanc, A., Del Carmen, S., Zurita-Turk, M., Santos Rocha, C., van de Guchte, M., Azevedo, V., Miyoshi, A., & Leblanc, J. G. (2011). Importance of IL-10 modulation by probiotic microorganisms in gastrointestinal inflammatory diseases. *ISRN Gastroenterology, 2011*, 892971. Available from https://doi.org/10.5402/2011/892971.

DeGruttola, A. K., Low, D., Mizoguchi, A., & Mizoguchi, E. (2016). Current understanding of dysbiosis in disease in human and animal models. *Inflammatory Bowel Diseases, 22*(5), 1137−1150. Available from https://doi.org/10.1097/MIB.0000000000000750.

Dhar, D., & Mohanty, A. (2020). Gut microbiota and Covid-19-possible link and implications. *Virus Research, 285*, 198018. Available from https://doi.org/10.1016/j.virusres.2020.198018.

Din, A. U., Mazhar, M., Wasim, M., Ahmad, W., Bibi, A., Hassan, A., Ali, N., Gang, W., Qian, G., Ullah, R., Shah, T., Ullah, M., Khan, I., Nisar, M. F., & Wu, J. (2021). SARS-CoV-2 microbiome dysbiosis linked disorders and possible probiotics role. *Biomedicine & Pharmacotherapy, 133*, 110947. Available from https://doi.org/10.1016/j.biopha.2020.110947.

Ding, Y. H., Qian, L. Y., Pang, J., Lin, J. Y., Xu, Q., Wang, L. H., Huang, D. S., & Zou, H. (2017).). The regulation of immune cells by Lactobacilli: A potential therapeutic target for anti-atherosclerosis therapy. *Oncotarget, 8*(35), 59915−59928. Available from https://doi.org/10.18632/oncotarget.18346.

Dong, Y., Xu, M., Chen, L., & Bhochhibhoya, A. (2019). Probiotic foods and supplements interventions for metabolic syndromes: A systematic review and meta-analysis of recent clinical trials. *Annals of Nutrition and Metabolism, 74*(3), 224−241. Available from https://doi.org/10.1159/000499028.

DuPont, A. W., & DuPont, H. L. (2011). The intestinal microbiota and chronic disorders of the gut. *Nature Reviews Gastroenterology & Hepatology, 8*(9), 523−531. Available from https://doi.org/10.1038/nrgastro.2011.133.

Fenster, K., Freeburg, B., Hollard, C., Wong, C., Rønhave Laursen, R., & Ouwehand, A. C. (2019). The production and delivery of probiotics: A review of a practical approach. *Microorganisms, 7*(3), 83. Available from https://doi.org/10.3390/microorganisms7030083.

Fioramonti, J., Theodorou, V., & Bueno, L. (2003). Probiotics: What are they? What are their effects on gut physiology? *Best Practice & Research. Clinical Gastroenterology, 17*(5), 711−724. Available from https://doi.org/10.1016/S1521-6918(03)00075-1.

Fisher, D., & Mentor, S. (2020). Are claudin-5 tight-junction proteins in the blood-brain barrier porous? *Neural Regeneration Research, 15*(10), 1838−1839. Available from https://doi.org/10.4103/1673-5374.280308.

Furrie, E., Macfarlane, S., Kennedy, A., Cummings, J. H., Walsh, S. V., O'neil, D. A., & Macfarlane, G. T. (2005). Synbiotic therapy (Bifidobacterium longum/Synergy 1) initiates resolution of inflammation in patients with active ulcerative colitis: A randomised controlled pilot trial. *Gut, 54*(2), 242−249. Available from https://doi.org/10.1136/gut.2004.044834.

Galland, L. (2014). The gut microbiome and the brain. *Journal of Medicinal Food, 17*(12), 1261−1272. Available from https://doi.org/10.1089/jmf.2014.7000.

Gao, X. W., Mubasher, M., Fang, C. Y., Reifer, C., & Miller, L. E. (2010). Dose-response efficacy of a proprietary probiotic formula of *Lactobacillus acidophilus* CL1285 and *Lactobacillus casei* LBC80R for antibiotic-associated diarrhea and *Clostridium difficile*-associated diarrhea prophylaxis in adult patients. *The American Journal of Gastroenterology, 105*(7), 1636−1641. Available from https://doi.org/10.1038/ajg.2010.11.

Gaspar, C., Donders, G. G., Palmeira-de-Oliveira, R., Queiroz, J. A., Tomaz, C., Martinez-de-Oliveira, J., & Palmeira-de-Oliveira, A. (2018). Bacteriocin production of the probiotic *Lactobacillus acidophilus* KS400. *AMB Express*, *8*(1), 153. Available from https://doi.org/10.1186/s13568-018-0679-z.

Govender, M., Choonara, Y. E., Kumar, P., du Toit, L. C., van Vuuren, S., & Pillay, V. (2014). A review of the advancements in probiotic delivery: Conventional vs. non-conventional formulations for intestinal flora supplementation. *AAPS PharmSciTech*, *15*(1), 29–43. Available from https://doi.org/10.1208/s12249-013-0027-1.

Grenov, B., Namusoke, H., Lanyero, B., Nabukeera-Barungi, N., Ritz, C., Molgaard, C., Fris, H., & Michaelsen, K. F. (2017). Effect of probiotics on diarrhea in children with severe acute malnutrition: A randomized controlled study in Uganda. *Journal of Pediatric Gastroenterology and Nutrition*, *64*(3), 396–403. Available from https://doi.org/10.1097/MPG.0000000000001515.

Han, S. H., Suk, K. T., Kim, D. J., Kim, M. Y., Baik, S. K., Kim, Y. D., Cheon, G. J., Choi, D. H., Ham, Y. L., Shin, D. H., & Kim, E. J. (2015). Effects of probiotics (cultured *Lactobacillus subtilis/Streptococcus faecium*) in the treatment of alcoholic hepatitis: Randomized-controlled multicenter study. *European Journal of Gastroenterology & Hepatology*, *27*(11), 1300–1306. Available from https://doi.org/10.1097/MEG.0000000000000458.

Hardy, H., Harris, J., Lyon, E., Beal, J., & Foey, A. D. (2013). Probiotics, prebiotics and immunomodulation of gut mucosal defences: Homeostasis and immunopathology. *Nutrients*, *5*(6), 1869–1912. Available from https://doi.org/10.3390/nu5061869.

Hasan, M. T., Jang, W. J., Kim, H., Lee, B.-J., Kim, K. W., Hur, S. W., Lim, S. G., Bai, S. C., & Kong, I.-S. (2018). Synergistic effects of dietary *Bacillus* sp. SJ-10 plus β-glucooligosaccharides as a synbiotic on growth performance, innate immunity and streptococcosis resistance in olive flounder (*Paralichthys olivaceus*). *Fish & Shellfish Immunology*, *82*, 544–553. Available from https://doi.org/10.1016/j.fsi.2018.09.002.

He, Y., Wang, J., Li, F., & Shi, Y. (2020). Main clinical features of COVID-19 and potential prognostic and therapeutic value of the microbiota in SARS-CoV-2 infections. *Frontiers in Microbiology*, *11*, 1302. Available from https://doi.org/10.3389/fmicb.2020.01302.

Hotchkiss, R. S., Moldawer, L. L., Opal, S. M., Reinhart, K., Turnbull, I. R., & Vincent, J.-L. (2016). Sepsis and septic shock. *Nature Reviews Disease Primers*, *2*(1), 16045. Available from https://doi.org/10.1038/nrdp.2016.45.

Infusino, F., Marazzato, M., Mancone, M., Fedele, F., Mastroianni, C. M., Severino, P., Ceccarelli, G., Santinelli, L., Cavarretta, E., Marullo, A. G. M., Miraldi, F., Carnevale, R., Nocella, C., Biondi-zoccai, G., Pagnini, C., Schiavon, S., Pugliese, F., Frati, G., & Ettorre, G. (2020). In SARS-CoV-2 infection: A scoping review. *Nutrients*, *12*(6), 1–21.

Jang, W. J., Lee, J. M., Hasan, M. T., Lee, B.-J., Lim, S. G., & Kong, I.-S. (2019). Effects of probiotic supplementation of a plant-based protein diet on intestinal microbial diversity, digestive enzyme activity, intestinal structure, and immunity in olive flounder (*Paralichthys olivaceus*). *Fish & Shellfish Immunology*, *92*, 719–727. Available from https://doi.org/10.1016/j.fsi.2019.06.056.

Jiang, H., Ling, Z., Zhang, Y., Mao, H., Ma, Z., Yin, Y., Wang, W., Tang, W., Tan, Z., Shi, J., Li, L., & Ruan, B. (2015). Altered fecal microbiota composition in patients with major depressive disorder. *Brain, Behavior, and Immunity*, *48*, 186–194. Available from https://doi.org/10.1016/j.bbi.2015.03.016.

Kalantar-Zadeh, K., Ward, S. A., Kalantar-Zadeh, K., & El-Omar, E. M. (2020). Considering the effects of microbiome and diet on SARS-CoV-2 infection: Nanotechnology roles. *ACS Nano*, *14*(5), 5179–5182. Available from https://doi.org/10.1021/acsnano.0c03402.

Kany, S., Vollrath, J. T., & Relja, B. (2019). Cytokines in inflammatory disease. *International Journal of Molecular Sciences*, *20*(23), 1–31.

Kim, H. W., Hong, R., Choi, E. Y., Yu, K., Kim, N., Hyeon, J. Y., Cho, K. K., Choi, I. S., & Yun, C.-H. (2018). A probiotic mixture regulates T Cell balance and reduces atopic dermatitis symptoms in mice. *Frontiers in Microbiology*, *9*, 2414. Available from https://www.frontiersin.org/article/10.3389/fmicb.2018.02414.

Köhler, C. A., Freitas, T. H., Maes, M., de Andrade, N. Q., Liu, C. S., Fernandes, B. S., Stubbs, B., Solmi, M., Veronese, N., Herrmann, N., Raison, C. L., Miller, B. J., Lanctôt, K. L., & Carvalho, A. F. (2017). Peripheral cytokine and chemokine alterations in depression: A meta-analysis of 82 studies. *Acta Psychiatrica Scandinavica*, *135*(5), 373–387. Available from https://doi.org/10.1111/acps.12698.

Kumar, S., Jeong, Y., Ashraf, M. U., & Bae, Y. S. (2019). Dendritic cell-mediated Th2 immunity and immune disorders. *International Journal of Molecular Sciences*, *20*(9). Available from https://doi.org/10.3390/ijms20092159.

Lanyero, B., Grenov, B., Barungi, N. N., Namusoke, H., Michaelsen, K. F., Mupere, E., Molgaard, C., Jiang, P., Frokiaer, H., Wiese, M., Muhammed, M. K., Pesu, H., Nielsen, D. S., Friis, H., Rytter, M. J., & Christensen, V. B. (2019). Correlates of gut function in children hospitalized for severe acute malnutrition, a cross-sectional study in Uganda. *Journal of Pediatric Gastroenterology and Nutrition*, *69*(30), 292–298. Available from https://doi.org/10.1097/MPG.0000000000002381.

Lebeer, S., Vanderleyden, J., & De Keersmaecker, S. C. J. (2010). Host interactions of probiotic bacterial surface molecules: Comparison with commensals and pathogens. *Nature Reviews. Microbiology*, *8*(3), 171–184. Available from https://doi.org/10.1038/nrmicro2297.

Lemme-Dumit, J. M., Polti, M. A., Perdigón, G., & Galdeano, M. M. (2018). Probiotic bacteria cell walls stimulate the activity of the intestinal epithelial cells and macrophage functionality. *Beneficial Microbes*, *9*(1), 153–164. Available from https://doi.org/10.3920/BM2016.0220.

Leung, A. K. C., Wong, A. H. C., Leung, A. A. M., & Hon, K. L. (2019). Urinary tract infection in children. *Recent Patents on Inflammation & Allergy Drug Discovery*, *13*(1), 2–18. Available from https://doi.org/10.2174/1872213X13666181228154940.

Liu, W., Ren, P., He, S., Xu, L., Yang, Y., Gu, Z., & Zhou, Z. (2013). Comparison of adhesive gut bacteria composition, immunity, and disease resistance in juvenile hybrid tilapia fed two different Lactobacillus strains. *Fish & Shellfish Immunology*, *35*(1), 54–62. Available from https://doi.org/10.1016/j.fsi.2013.04.010.

Llewellyn, A., & Foey, A. (2017). Probiotic modulation of innate cell pathogen sensing and signaling events. *Nutrients*, *9*(10). Available from https://doi.org/10.3390/nu9101156.

Lobionda, S., Sittipo, P., Kwon, H. Y., & Lee, Y. K. (2019). The role of gut microbiota in intestinal inflammation with respect to diet and extrinsic stressors. *Microorganisms*, *7*(8), 271. Available from https://doi.org/10.3390/microorganisms7080271.

Maldonado Galdeano, C., Cazorla, S. I., Lemme Dumit, J. M., Vélez, E., & Perdigón, G. (2019). Beneficial effects of probiotic consumption on the immune system. *Annals of Nutrition and Metabolism*, *74*(2), 115–124. Available from https://doi.org/10.1159/000496426.

Malik, M., Suboc, T. M., Tyagi, S., Salzman, N., Wang, J., Ying, R., Tanner, M. J., Kakarla, M., Baker, J. E., & Widlansky, M. E. (2018). Lactobacillus plantarum 299v supplementation improves vascular endothelial function and reduces inflammatory biomarkers in men with stable coronary artery disease. *Circulation Research*, *123*(9), 1091–1102. Available from https://doi.org/10.1161/CIRCRESAHA.118.313565.

Markowiak, P., & Ślizewska, K. (2017). Effects of probiotics, prebiotics, and synbiotics on human health. *Nutrients*, *9*(9). Available from https://doi.org/10.3390/nu9091021.

Martens, K., Pugin, B., De Boeck, I., Spacova, I., Steelant, B., Seys, S. F., Lebeer, S., & Hellings, P. W. (2018). Probiotics for the airways: Potential to improve epithelial and immune homeostasis. *Allergy*, *73*(10), 1954–1963. Available from https://doi.org/10.1111/all.13495.

Martin Manuel, P., Elena, B., Carolina, M. G., & Gabriela, P. (2017). Oral probiotics supplementation can stimulate the immune system in a stress process. *Journal of Nutrition & Intermediary Metabolism*, *8*, 29–40. Available from https://doi.org/10.1016/j.jnim.2017.06.001.

Matarazzo, I., Toniato, E., & Robuffo, I. (2018). Psychobiome feeding mind: Polyphenolics in depression and anxiety. *Current Topics in Medicinal Chemistry*, *18*(24), 2108–2115. Available from https://doi.org/10.2174/1568026619666181210151348.

Merenstein, D., Gonzalez, J., Young, A. G., Roberts, R. F., Sanders, M. E., & Petterson, S. (2011). Study to investigate the potential of probiotics in children attending school. *European Journal of Clinical Nutrition*, *65*, 447–453. Available from https://doi.org/10.1038/ejcn.2010.290.

Mikelsaar, M., Sepp, E., Štšepetova, J., Songisepp, E., & Mändar, R. (2016). Biodiversity of intestinal lactic acid bacteria in the healthy population. *Advances in Experimental Medicine and Biology*, *932*, 1–64. Available from https://doi.org/10.1007/5584_2016_3.

Miller, A. H., & Raison, C. L. (2016). The role of inflammation in depression: From evolutionary imperative to modern treatment target. *Nature Reviews. Immunology*, *16*(1), 22–34. Available from https://doi.org/10.1038/nri.2015.5.

Miller, F., Afonso, P. V., Gessain, A., & Ceccaldi, P.-E. (2012). Blood-brain barrier and retroviral infections. *Virulence*, *3*(2), 222–229. Available from https://doi.org/10.4161/viru.19697.

Morais, A. H. A., Passos, T. S., Maciel, B. L. L., & da Silva-Maia, J. K. (2020). Can probiotics and diet promote beneficial immune modulation and purine control in coronavirus infection? *Nutrients*, *12*(6), 1737. Available from https://doi.org/10.3390/nu12061737.

Nanau, R. M., & Neuman, M. G. (2012). Nutritional and probiotic supplementation in colitis models. *Digestive Diseases and Sciences*, *57*(11), 2786–2810. Available from https://doi.org/10.1007/s10620-012-2284-3.

Nicholson, J. K., Holmes, E., Kinross, J., Burcelin, R., Gibson, G., Jia, W., & Pettersson, S. (2012). Host-gut microbiota metabolic interactions. *Science (New York, N.Y.)*, *336*(6086). Available from https://doi.org/10.1126/science.1223813, 1262 LP—1267.

Nishihira, J., Moriya, T., Sakai, F., Kabuki, T., Kawasaki, Y., & Nishimura, M. (2016). Lactobacillus gasseri SBT2055 stimulates immunoglobulin production and innate immunity after influenza vaccination in healthy adult volunteers: A randomized, double-blind, placebo-controlled, parallel-group study. *Functional Foods in Health and Disease*, *6*(9), 544. Available from https://doi.org/10.31989/ffhd.v6i9.284.

Oelschlaeger, T. A. (2010). Mechanisms of probiotic actions—A review. *International Journal of Medical Microbiology*, *300*(1), 57–62. Available from https://doi.org/10.1016/j.ijmm.2009.08.005.

Pandiyan, P., Bhaskaran, N., Zou, M., Schneider, E., Jayaraman, S., & Huehn, J. (2019). Microbiome dependent regulation of T(regs) and Th17 cells in mucosa. *Frontiers in Immunology*, *10*, 426. Available from https://doi.org/10.3389/fimmu.2019.00426.

Park, J., Kim, M., Kang, S. G., Jannasch, A. H., Cooper, B., Patterson, J., & Kim, C. H. (2015). Short-chain fatty acids induce both effector and regulatory T cells by suppression of histone deacetylases and regulation of the mTOR–S6K pathway. *Mucosal Immunology*, *8*(1), 80–93. Available from https://doi.org/10.1038/mi.2014.44.

Pennisi, E. (2020). Meet the psychobiome. *Science (New York, N.Y.)*, *368*(6491). Available from https://doi.org/10.1126/science.368.6491.570, 570 LP—573.

Piwat, S., Sophatha, B., & Teanpaisan, R. (2015). An assessment of adhesion, aggregation and surface charges of Lactobacillus strains derived from the human oral cavity. *Letters in Applied Microbiology*, *61*(1), 98–105. Available from https://doi.org/10.1111/lam.12434.

Plaza-Diaz, J., Ruiz-Ojeda, F. J., Gil-Campos, M., & Gil, A. (2019). Mechanisms of action of probiotics. *Advances in Nutrition*, *10*(Suppl. 1), S49–S66. Available from https://doi.org/10.1093/advances/nmy063.

Robles-Vera, I., Toral, M., Romero, M., Jiménez, R., Sánchez, M., Pérez-Vizcaíno, F., & Duarte, J. (2017). Antihypertensive effects of probiotics. *Current Hypertension Reports*, *19*(4), 26. Available from https://doi.org/10.1007/s11906-017-0723-4.

Rostami, F. M., Mousavi, H., Mousavi, M. R. N., & Shahsafi, M. (2018). Efficacy of probiotics in prevention and treatment of infectious diseases. *Clinical Microbiology Newsletter*, *40*(12), 97–103. Available from https://doi.org/10.1016/j.clinmicnews.2018.06.001.

Sabico, S., Al-Mashharawi, A., Al-Daghri, N. M., Wani, K., Amer, O. E., Hussain, D. S., Ahmed Ansari, M. G., Masoud, M. S., Alokail, M. S., & McTernan, P. G. (2019). Effects of a 6-month multi-strain probiotics supplementation in endotoxemic, inflammatory and cardiometabolic status of T2DM patients: A randomized, double-blind, placebo-controlled trial. *Clinical Nutrition*, *38*(4), 1561–1569. Available from https://doi.org/10.1016/j.clnu.2018.08.009.

Sarkar, A., Lehto, S. M., Harty, S., Dinan, T. G., Cryan, J. F., & Burnet, P. W. J. (2016). Psychobiotics and the manipulation of bacteria–gut–brain signals. *Trends in Neurosciences*, *39*(11), 763–781. Available from https://doi.org/10.1016/j.tins.2016.09.002.

Sattler, S. (2017). The role of the immune system beyond the fight against infection BT. In S. Sattler, & T. Kennedy-Lydon (Eds.), *The Immunology of Cardiovascular Homeostasis and Pathology* (pp. 3–14). Springer International Publishing. Available from https://doi.org/10.1007/978-3-319-57613-8_1.

Schnadower, D., Tarr, P. I., Casper, T. C., Gorelick, M. H., Dean, J. M., O'Connell, K. J., Mahajan, P., Levine, A. C., Bhatt, S. R., Roskind, C. G., Powell, E. C., Rogers, A. J., Vance, C., Sapien, R. E., Olsen, C. S., Metheney, M., DIckey, V. P., Hall-Moore, C., & Freedman, S. B. (2018). *Lactobacillus rhamnosus* GG versus placebo for acute gastroenteritis in children. *The New England Journal of Medicine*, 379(21), 2002–2014. Available from https://doi.org/10.1056/NEJMoa1802598.

Schnadower, D., Tarr, P. I., Casper, T. C., Gorelick, M. H., Dean, M. J., O'Connell, K. J., Mahajan, P., Chun, T. H., Bhatt, S. R., Roskind, C. G., Powell, E. C., Rogers, A. J., Vance, C., Sapien, R. E., Gao, F., & Freedman, S. B. (2017). Randomised controlled trial of *Lactobacillus rhamnosus* (LGG) versus placebo in children presenting to the emergency department with acute gastroenteritis: The PECARN probiotic study protocol. *BMJ Open*, 7, e018115. Available from https://doi.org/10.1136/bmjopen-2017-018115.

Sharma, V., & Kaur, S. (2020). The effect of probiotic intervention in ameliorating the altered central nervous system functions in neurological disorders: A review. *The Open Microbiology Journal*, 14(1), 18–29. Available from https://doi.org/10.2174/1874285802014010018.

Shen, Z.-H., Zhu, C.-X., Quan, Y.-S., Yang, Z.-Y., Wu, S., Luo, W.-W., Tan, B., & Wang, X.-Y. (2018). Relationship between intestinal microbiota and ulcerative colitis: Mechanisms and clinical application of probiotics and fecal microbiota transplantation. *World Journal of Gastroenterology*, 24(1), 5–14. Available from https://doi.org/10.3748/wjg.v24.i1.5.

Shi, N., Li, N., Duan, X., & Niu, H. (2017). Interaction between the gut microbiome and mucosal immune system. *Military Medical Research*, 4(1), 14. Available from https://doi.org/10.1186/s40779-017-0122-9.

Sichetti, M., De Marco, S., Pagiotti, R., Traina, G., & Pietrella, D. (2018). Anti-inflammatory effect of multistrain probiotic formulation (*L. rhamnosus*, *B. lactis*, and *B. longum*). *Nutrition*, 53, 95–102. Available from https://doi.org/10.1016/j.nut.2018.02.005.

Singh, A., Sarangi, A. N., Goel, A., Sirvastava, R., Gaur, P., Aggarwal, A., & Aggarwal, R. (2018). Effect of administration of a probiotic preparation on gut microbiota and immune response in healthy women in India: An open-label, single-arm pilot study. *BMC Gastroenterology*, 18, 85. Available from https://doi.org/10.1186/s12876-018-0819-6.

Skolnick, S. D., & Greig, N. H. (2019). Microbes and monoamines: Potential neuropsychiatric consequences of dysbiosis. *Trends in Neurosciences*, 42(3), 151–163. Available from https://doi.org/10.1016/j.tins.2018.12.005.

Sundararaman, A., Ray, M., Ravindra, P. V., & Halami, P. M. (2020). Role of probiotics to combat viral infections with emphasis on COVID-19. *Applied Microbiology and Biotechnology*, 104(19), 8089–8104. Available from https://doi.org/10.1007/s00253-020-10832-4.

Tao, W., Zhang, G., Wang, X., Guo, M., Zeng, W., Xu, Z., Cao, D., Pan, A., Wang, Y., Zhang, K., Ma, X., Chen, Z., Jin, T., Liu, L., Weng, J., & Zhu, S. (2020). Analysis of the intestinal microbiota in COVID-19 patients and its correlation with the inflammatory factor IL-18. *Medicine in Microecology*, 5, 100023. Available from https://doi.org/10.1016/j.medmic.2020.100023.

Tremaroli, V., & Bäckhed, F. (2012). Functional interactions between the gut microbiota and host metabolism. *Nature*, 489(7415), 242–249. Available from https://doi.org/10.1038/nature11552.

van Baarlen, P., Wells, J. M., & Kleerebezem, M. (2013). Regulation of intestinal homeostasis and immunity with probiotic lactobacilli. *Trends in Immunology*, 34(5), 208–215. Available from https://doi.org/10.1016/j.it.2013.01.005.

van de Wouw, M., Boehme, M., Lyte, J. M., Wiley, N., Strain, C., O'Sullivan, O., Clarke, G., Stanton, C., Dinan, T. G., & Cryan, J. F. (2018). Short-chain fatty acids: Microbial metabolites that alleviate stress-induced brain–gut axis alterations. *The Journal of Physiology*, 596(20), 4923–4944. Available from https://doi.org/10.1113/JP276431.

van Tassell, M. L., & Miller, M. J. (2011). Lactobacillus adhesion to mucus. *Nutrients*, 3(5), 613–636. Available from https://doi.org/10.3390/nu3050613.

Videlock, E. J., & Cremonini, F. (2012). Meta-analysis: Probiotics in antibiotic-associated diarrhoea. *Alimentary Pharmacology & Therapeutics*, 35(12), 1355–1369. Available from https://doi.org/10.1111/j.1365-2036.2012.05104.x.

Vlainić, J. V., Šuran, J., Vlainić, T., & Vukorep, A. L. (2016). Probiotics as an adjuvant therapy in major depressive disorder. *Current Neuropharmacology*, 14(8), 952–958. Available from https://doi.org/10.2174/1570159x14666160526120928.

Wallace, C. J. K., & Milev, R. (2017). The effects of probiotics on depressive symptoms in humans: A systematic review. *Annals of General Psychiatry*, 16, 14. Available from https://doi.org/10.1186/s12991-017-0138-2.

Walter, J. (2008). Ecological role of lactobacilli in the gastrointestinal tract: Implications for fundamental and biomedical research. *Applied and Environmental Microbiology*, 74(16), 4985–4996. Available from https://doi.org/10.1128/AEM.00753-08.

Wang, X., Sun, Y., Wang, L., Li, X., Qu, K., & Xu, Y. (2017). Synbiotic dietary supplement affects growth, immune responses and intestinal microbiota of *Apostichopus japonicus*. *Fish & Shellfish Immunology*, 68, 232–242. Available from https://doi.org/10.1016/j.fsi.2017.07.027.

Xia, Y., Lu, M., Chen, G., Cao, J., Gao, F., Wang, M., Liu, Z., Zhang, D., Zhu, H., & Yi, M. (2018). Effects of dietary *Lactobacillus rhamnosus* JCM1136 and *Lactococcus lactis* subsp. lactis JCM5805 on the growth, intestinal microbiota, morphology, immune response and disease resistance of juvenile Nile tilapia, *Oreochromis niloticus*. *Fish & Shellfish Immunology*, 76, 368–379. Available from https://doi.org/10.1016/j.fsi.2018.03.020.

Xiong, J., Dai, W., Zhu, J., Liu, K., Dong, C., & Qiu, Q. (2017). The underlying ecological processes of gut microbiota among cohabitating retarded, overgrown and normal shrimp. *Microbial Ecology*, 73(4), 988–999. Available from https://doi.org/10.1007/s00248-016-0910-x.

Yadav, M., Verma, M. K., & Chauhan, N. S. (2018). A review of metabolic potential of human gut microbiome in human nutrition. *Archives of Microbiology*, 200(2), 203–217. Available from https://doi.org/10.1007/s00203-017-1459-x.

Yavarpour-Bali, H., & Ghasemi-Kasman, M. (2020). Update on neurological manifestations of COVID-19. *Life Sciences*, *257*, 118063. Available from https://doi.org/10.1016/j.lfs.2020.118063.

Yuan, Y., Zallot, R., Grove, T. L., Payan, D. J., Martin-Verstraete, I., Šepić, S., Balamkundu, S., Neelakandan, R., Gadi, V. K., Liu, C.-F., Swairjo, M. A., Dedon, P. C., Almo, S. C., Gerlt, J. A., & de Crécy-Lagard, V. (2019). Discovery of novel bacterial queuine salvage enzymes and pathways in human pathogens. *Proceedings of the National Academy of Sciences*, *116*(38). Available from https://doi.org/10.1073/pnas.1909604116, 19126 LP—19135.

Zheng, D., Liwinski, T., & Elinav, E. (2020). Interaction between microbiota and immunity in health and disease. *Cell Research*, *30*(6), 492–506. Available from https://doi.org/10.1038/s41422-020-0332-7.

Chapter 4

Effect of intestinal microbiome, antibiotics, and probiotics in the prevention and management of ulcerative colitis

Ivan Kushkevych[1] and Josef Jampílek[2,3]
[1]Department of Experimental Biology, Faculty of Science, Masaryk University, Brno, Czech Republic, [2]Department of Analytical Chemistry, Faculty of Natural Sciences, Comenius University, Bratislava, Slovakia, [3]Institute of Neuroimmunology, Slovak Academy of Sciences, Bratislava, Slovakia

4.1 Introduction

The lumen of the human large intestine is inhabited by approximately $10^{11}-10^{12}$ cells/g of feces of microorganisms (Barton & Hamilton, 2007; Gibson et al., 1991). They belong to the normal microbiota (Gibson, Macfarlane, & Cummings, 1993; Gibson, Macfarlane, & Macfarlane, 1993) and colonize the surface of the intestinal mucosa, forming biofilms (Kushkevych, 2016; Kushkevych, Vítězová, Fedrová, et al., 2017). On the surface of epithelial cells, the number of microorganisms is up to 10^8 cells/cm^2 (Macfarlane & Dillon, 2007; Macfarlane et al., 2000).

The normal microbiota of the human intestine includes microorganisms of the genera *Bifidobacterium*, *Bacteroides*, *Lactobacillus*, *Escherichia*, *Eubacterium*, *Enterococcus*, *Atopobium*, *Faecalibacterium*, *Clostridium*, and others. An important component of this microbiocenosis is also sulfate-reducing bacteria (SRB) of the genera *Desulfovibrio*, *Desulfobulbus*, *Desulfobacter*, *Desulfomonas*, and *Desulfotomaculum* (Barton & Hamilton, 2007; Kushkevych, 2016; Pitcher et al., 2000). An increased number of the latter are often found in people with rheumatic diseases, ankylosing spondylitis, etc. (Cummings et al., 2003). It has also been suggested that SRB may be the cause of some forms of rectal cancer due to the formation of hydrogen sulfide (Kushkevych, 2015a,b; Kushkevych, Dordević, Vítězová, et al., 2019a; Ramasamy et al., 2006), which adversely affects the metabolism of intestinal cells and causes a variety of diseases (Pitcher & Cummings, 1996; Rowan et al., 2009).

Many people, especially the so-called Western world, suffer from various chronic inflammatory diseases, which are caused by lifestyle, diet, stress, deteriorating environment. One of the most common chronic inflammatory diseases is chronic intestinal inflammation, which includes a group of inflammatory diseases of the small or large intestine [inflammatory bowel diseases (IBDs)] of various causes, which are characterized by a prolonged or recurrent course. Manifestations vary according to the type of inflammation, its severity, location, or duration. The basic manifestations include diarrhea, abdominal pain, weight loss, blood in the stool, anemia, or vomiting. They can also manifest themselves in a number of extraintestinal problems, especially skin or joint problems (Barton & Hamilton, 2007; Loftus et al., 2000; Loubinoux et al., 2000; Montgomery et al., 1998; Plachá & Jampílek, 2021). During these diseases, an increased amount of SRB is often found in the intestine (Cummings et al., 2003; Kushkevych, Cejnar, Treml, et al., 2020; Loftus et al., 2000).

Crohn's disease and ulcerative colitis (UC) are the best known. Crohn's disease manifests itself in any part of the digestive tract, but most often in the junction of the small and large intestines. The disease was named after Burrill Bernard Crohn, an American gastroenterologist who described it with colleagues Ginzberg and Oppenheimer in 1932 in patients in the area of junction of the small bowel to appendix. The inflammation penetrates the entire wall and is granulomatous in nature. The prevalence of Crohn's disease is 3–20 cases per 100,000. The disease occurs in the industrialized countries of the Northern Hemisphere, although its incidence is rising in Asia and South America. There may be a slightly higher prevalence of the disease in women and a higher incidence in kinship in families or ethnic groups (e.g., a higher incidence of the disease in Ashkenazi Jews, or people with fair skin have been found to be twice as likely as people with dark skin). In connection with age, this disease occurs most markedly in two categories, namely in teenagers and young people after the age of 20 (especially in the category of 16–35) and then again exacerbated in 50- to 70-year olds. The main symptoms are lower abdominal pain, weight loss, fatigue, fever, and diarrhea, mostly without blood. The disease can also manifest outside the digestive tract, such as skin rash, arthritis, ocular inflammation, or the occurrence of aphthae in the oral cavity. The cause of Crohn's disease is unknown. It is generally believed that the disease is associated with immunity, but it is not clear whether it is immunodeficiency or an autoimmune disease. The tendency to the disease is genetically influenced; the disease can be caused by the environment in a susceptible person (Gajendran et al., 2018).

UC is one of the most common major forms of inflammatory IBDs. UC affects the colon (mostly the rectum) and can be acute or chronic. UC damages the mucosa and causes inflammatory changes and ulcers on its surface. Quiet asymptomatic periods often alternate with disease activation phases. The emergence of UC is explained by several hypotheses, which are discussed in more detail in this chapter. In places where the mucosa is disturbed by inflammation, ulcers form that can bleed and secrete mucus and pus, so the main symptoms of UC include diarrhea and rectal bleeding. Abdominal pain, fever, loss of appetite, and extraintestinal manifestations, such as rashes, joint, liver, biliary tract, and eye disorders resulting in blindness are also common. Worldwide, the highest incidence and prevalence of UC is observed in northern Europe and North America. UC has an incidence of 9–20 cases per 100,000 people per year. Its prevalence is 156–291 cases per 100,000 people per year. UC has a bimodal pattern of occurrence. The main onset peaks at the age of 15–30 years. The second and smaller peak occurs at the age of 50–70 years. Most studies do not show any preference for gender. Interestingly, the incidence of the disease is tied to the maturity of individual states. In poor countries, its occurrence is rare. Thus the disease can be classified as the so-called diseases of civilization (Barton & Hamilton, 2007; Lynch & Hsu, 2021; Podolsky, 2002; Roediger et al., 1993a,b; Sekirov et al., 2010).

In the intestines of patients with UC, people found an increased number of SRB, compared with healthy (Florin et al., 1990; Gibson et al., 1991; Pitcher & Cummings, 1996; Pitcher et al., 2000). Gibson and coauthors found that 92% of all SRB isolated from people with UC belong to the genus *Desulfovibrio*, in particular *Desulfovibrio desulfuricans*. They are more resistant to environmental conditions compared to strains isolated from the environment (Gibson et al., 1991; Kováč et al., 2018; Kováč & Kushkevych, 2017; Kushkevych, Vítězová, Kos, et al., 2018; Kushkevych, Castro Sangrador, Dordević, et al., 2020). This caused interest in these bacteria during the study of UC. It has been established that these microorganisms are the cause of bloody diarrhea, loss of appetite, and weight in animals (Cummings et al., 2003; Fox et al., 1994). Histological examination of intestinal tissues of patients with UC revealed epithelial hyperplasia, abscesses, dysfunction of goblet cells, and inflammatory infiltrates (Barton & Hamilton, 2007). One study found that the number of viable SRB cells is higher in the feces of patients with active disease than in latent (Pitcher et al., 2000).

Physiological and biochemical characteristics of these bacteria isolated from patients with different stages of colitis were different. Approximately 30% of SRB isolated from the feces of colitis patients were characterized by increased growth rate and more active sulfate reduction, compared with SRB isolated from healthy people (Gibson, Macfarlane, & Macfarlane, 1993). Another study found that the concentration of hydrogen sulfide in the feces of patients with colitis was significantly higher than in healthy people (Florin, 1991). The most intensive sulfate reduction was found for SRB isolated from patients with acute stage of the disease (Kushkevych, 2016; Kováč et al., 2018; Kushkevych, Dordević, Kollár, 2018; Kushkevych, Dordević, Vítězová, 2019b, 2021).

There are many factors affecting UC development, some of them are as follows: environmental, microbial effect, immune response, genetic predisposition (sometimes also called genetic susceptibility), increased amounts of SRB in the intestine and their overproduction of H_2S, and decreased lactic acid bacteria (Fig. 4.1).

Inhibition of the growth of intestinal SRB causes a decrease in the concentration of hydrogen sulfide in the lumen of the human intestine (Cummings et al., 2003; Rowan et al., 2009; Dordević et al., 2021; Kushkevych, Leščanová, Dordević, et al., 2019; Kushkevych, Castro Sangrador, Dordević, et al., 2020). In addition, H_2S from the intestinal lumen is effectively neutralized by *S*-methylation with thiol *S*-methyltransferase (TMT) (Pacifici et al., 1993). The activity of this enzyme in the erythrocyte membranes of people with VC is greater than in healthy people (Pitcher et al., 2000). Probably, the increase in the concentration of endogenous hydrogen sulfide causes homeostatic protection.

Despite numerous studies of nonspecific UC, the final role of SRB in the development of this disease has been little studied (Cummings et al., 2003; Kushkevych, 2015b; Kushkevych, Dordević, Vítězová, et al., 2018; Kushkevych, Coufalová, Vítězová, et al., 2020; Pitcher & Cummings, 1996). Therefore it is necessary to study in detail the intestinal

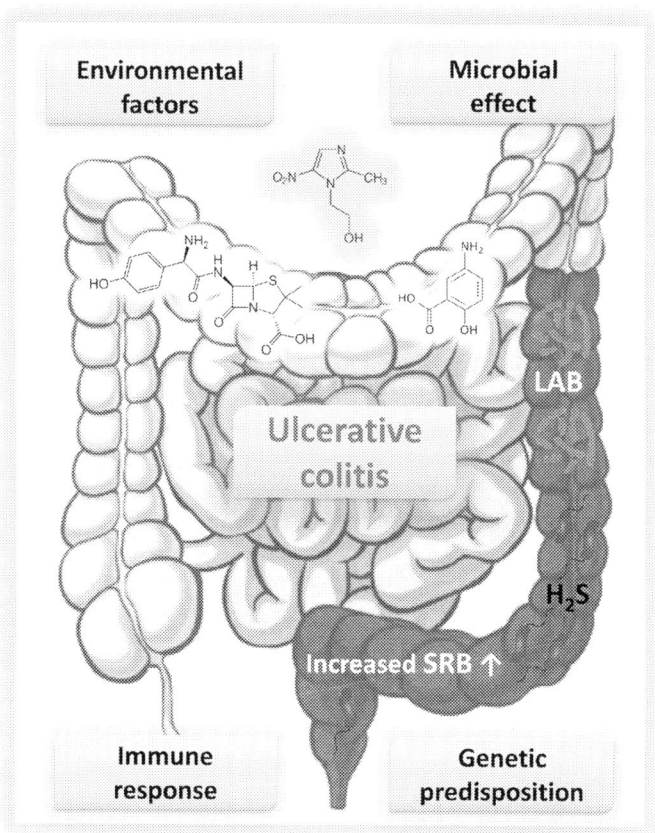

FIGURE 4.1 Main factors affecting on ulcerative colitis development: sulfate-reducing bacteria, lactic acid bacteria, and main drugs used for ulcerative colitis treatment.

SRB and their metabolism and patterns their formation of hydrogen sulfide in the intestine, to elucidate all possible mechanisms of its toxic action on epithelial cells. This will allow the development of new approaches to the treatment of UC and many other intestinal diseases.

The aim of this work was to analyze the results of modern research and summarize new scientific data on the role of SRB in the development of chronic intestinal diseases, especially UC, as well as consider possible mechanisms of hydrogen sulfide on human intestinal cells and summarize new findings of probiotic benefits.

4.2 The role of intestinal microbiota in the development of bowel diseases

The human large intestine contains approximately 200 g of digestive material (Barton & Hamilton, 2007). It often stretches during the formation of gases (CO_2, H_2, CH_4, H_2S), which are products of fermentation. Its surface area is from 1 to 2 m^2. Some parts of the mucous membrane intestinal lobes may not be in direct contact with the microbiota for several hours daily (Cummings et al., 2003; Sekirov et al., 2010). In particular, the sigmoid and rectal areas, which after defecation, remain empty and usually in these areas there is UC (Gibson et al., 1991). The probable cause of UC may be microbiota of the intestinal mucosa. As already mentioned, UC is one of the most common inflammatory diseases of the human colon. This disease is characterized by hemorrhagic-purulent inflammation of the mucous membrane, which spreads proximally from the rectum and is accompanied by the development of local and systemic complications (Cummings et al., 2003; Rowan et al., 2009). The onset of the disease is observed in people between 15 and 40 years and the second peak of the disease occurs at the age of 50–80 years (Cummings et al., 2003).

The participation of intestinal microbiota in the development of colitis is studied in animal models (Fiocchi, 1998), in the reactions of serum interaction with mucosal antibodies (Hooper et al., 2001; Macpherson et al., 1996), as well as studying the physiological and biochemical characteristics of mucosal bacteria in people with UC (Cummings et al., 2003). Some intestinal bacteria (*Escherichia coli*, members of the genera *Yersinia*, *Shigella*, *Salmonella*, *Campylobacter*, *Clostridium*, and *Aeromonas*), colonizing the intestine, can cause acute inflammatory reactions in its mucous membrane. They can be toxicogenic for the body and have invasive properties (Macfarlane & Dillon, 2007;

Macfarlane et al., 2000). The clinical symptoms of these infections are more acute than chronic. The mechanisms of pathogenesis of the disease with the participation of these microorganisms have been studied in detail (Cummings et al., 2003). However, their role in the occurrence of chronic forms of UC has not been studied enough (Marcus & Watt, 1974; Rowan et al., 2009).

It is believed that some types of bacteria that are part of the normal microbiota of the human intestine cause the development of UC (Sekirov et al., 2010). The main causative agents of IBD include bacteria *Streptococcus mobilis*, as well as some members of the genus *Fusobacterium* and *Shigella* (Sartor et al., 1996). They have the ability to penetrate the intestinal epithelium, causing various pathologies (Onderdonk et al., 1977, 1978). It is also believed that, except SRB, members of the genus *Salmonella* and *Yersinia* may be the cause of UC (Sartor et al., 1996). It has been studied that an increased number of bacteria of the genus *Bacteroides* causes inflammatory processes in the intestine (Rath et al., 2001).

It was found that the adhesive properties of *E. coli* are significantly greater in patients with UC than in strains isolated from healthy people or patients with infectious diarrhea (Burke & Axon, 1988; Kruis et al., 1997; Lobo et al., 1993; Phillips et al., 1993). Other researchers do not consider this a regularity, as it was found that the amount of *E. coli* in tissue samples from patients with UC was insignificant compared to healthy (Schultsz et al., 1997; Walmsley et al., 1998).

Bacteria devoid of cell wall (or L-form) have been found in people with UC, which is more difficult to detect when diagnosing the disease because they do not have cell wall antigens (Cummings et al., 2003). L-forms of *Enterococcus faecalis* and *E. coli* were found mainly in 42% of patients with UC ($n = 121$), in 34% of people with Crohn's disease ($n = 71$), and only in 1% of healthy people ($n = 140$). The role of these bacteria in the development of the disease has not been established. If the L-form is the cause of the disease, it is partly difficult to detect pathogenic bacteria during diagnosis or their use division from the intestinal mucosa of people with idiopathic inflammatory diseases (Burke & Axon, 1988; Cummings et al., 2003).

Studies of cell-free filtrates obtained from the feces and rectal mucosa of people with acute intestinal diseases have shown that the introduction of these filtrates into the colon of monkeys did not cause the development of the disease. UC probably cannot be of viral origin (Cummings et al., 2003). Favorable environment for the development of intestinal microbiota are the intestinal wall, which plays an important role in the disease. Commensals, which are pathogens, multiply on the surface of the intestinal epithelium and deeper penetrate into its mucosa. Adhering to the walls of the mucosa, they prevent its settlement by dangerous pathogenic species. This was found during the displacement of certain bacterial strains in people with UC by nonpathogenic *E. coli* (Rembacken et al., 1999).

It has been found that people with UC have significantly elevated levels of immunoglobulins G class (IgG) (Macpherson et al., 1996). The interaction of many bacterial proteins with IgG of the mucous membrane isolated from patients with UC has been studied and Crohn's disease (Cummings et al., 2003). Proteins were isolated from *Bacteroides fragilis*, *E. coli*, *Clostridium perfringens*, *Enterobacter faecalis*, *Staphylococcus epidermidis*, *Haemophilus influenzae*, and *Klebsiella aerogenes*, and the interactions of IgG with *B. fragilis*, *C. perfringens*, and *E. coli* were observed. However, it was absent with the bacteria of nonintestinal origin, despite the large amount of IgG in the serum (Macpherson et al., 1996).

In people with UC, there is an increase in the titer of antibodies against *Bacteroides* species (Bamba et al., 1995; Saitoh et al., 2002). *Bacteroides ovatus* has been shown to be one of the major colonial microorganisms that cause the production of immunoglobulins (IgG and IgA) in people with UC and Crohn's disease (Saitoh et al., 2002). It is believed that the disease is caused by a protein with a molecular weight of 19.5 kDa of *B. ovatus* bacteria. The ompC protein of the outer membrane of *E. coli* and a protein with a molecular weight of 100 kDa of *Bacteroides caccae* are associated with the immunity of patients with UC. These proteins interact with monoclonal antibodies (Cohavy et al., 2000; Satsangi et al., 1998).

A large number of antibodies to *Bacteroides vulgatus*, *B. fragilis*, and *Clostridium ramosum* have been detected in patients with UC (Matsuda et al., 2000). A protein with a molecular weight of 26 kDa, isolated from the membrane of *B. vulgatus*, causes the formation of IgG in 54% of patients with UC and 9% of healthy people. Probably, these proteins play an important role in the etiology of UC. A protein with a molecular weight of 50 kDa, isolated from *E. coli* bacteria, caused the formation of IgG in 29% of people with UC and in 6% of healthy people (Cummings et al., 2003). In the large intestine, bacteria are able to colonize the surfaces of epithelial cells (Giaffer et al., 1991). An experimental animal model of colitis made it possible to study the occurrence of this disease in the presence of a normal intestinal microbiota (Kushkevych, Vítězová, Fedrová, et al., 2017). Interleukin (IL)-2 mice, despite the absence of pathogenic microorganisms in the intestine, caused spontaneous inflammation of the colon. The disease was characterized by pathological and clinical features similar to UC (Sadlack et al., 1993).

Animal models of colitis where the disease can be experimentally caused in the presence of sulfate-containing compounds have increasingly been used by the scientists. The addition of carrageenan, sodium lignosulfonate, and amylopectin sulfate to drinking water in guinea pigs and rabbits caused intestinal damage resembling human UC in clinical symptoms (Marcus & Watt, 1974). Previous administration of metronidazole to animals prevented the development of colitis. However, antimicrobial drugs were not effective; they acted only on Gram-positive microorganisms and *E. coli* (Onderdonk et al., 1977). The presence of carrageenan in the intestines of mice, as well as its interaction with the normal microbiota can cause colitis (Onderdonk et al., 1978). Acute and chronic colitis in mice and hamsters have been experimentally reproduced using dextran sulfate sodium (DSS) (Okayasu et al., 1990). However, it has not yet been determined what causes the ulcer and inflammation of the colon.

Studies of animal models of intestinal inflammation, as well as studies of UC in humans, have shown that intestinal bacteria play an important role in initiating and maintaining inflammatory processes (Cummings et al., 2003). It is believed that UC arises as a result genetically indirect immune response to normal microbiota. The presence of sulfate as a product of bacterial metabolism is also important in the development of the disease (Gibson et al., 1991).

Acute colitis was found in experimental animals during the addition of sulfated polymers (partially degraded carrageenan, sulfated amylopectins, sodium lignosulfonate) to drinking water (Marcus & Watt, 1974). Clinical and pathological features of the disease resembled human UC. Inflammation was localized distal to the cecum. In humans, the disease always occurs in the distal parts of the colon. The severity of the disease correlated with the content of sulfates in the polymer. The mechanisms of these diseases have not been studied in detail, but in these animals after the introduction of sulfates in food there was an activation of the immune response, and there was damage to the intestinal mucosa (Cummings et al., 2003).

SRB are nonpathogenic symbionts of the human large intestine (Barton & Hamilton, 2007; Gibson, Macfarlane, & Cummings, 1993). However, bacteria of the genus *Desulfovibrio* have been found to cause bloody diarrhea, weight loss, and anorexia in animals and humans (Kushkevych, Fafula, et al., 2015; Kushkevych, Kollár, et al., 2015). Under these conditions, epithelial hyperplasia, abscesses, and inflammatory infiltrates can be observed (Barton & Hamilton, 2007; Fox et al., 1994). However, the isolated bacteria could not be cultured in the laboratory. The introduction of these bacteria into the hamster's intestines caused an infection clinically similar to human colitis. Bacteria of the genus *Desulfovibrio* were not detected in the samples obtained during rectal biopsy of 19 patients with UC (Pitcher & Cummings, 1996; Pitcher et al., 2000). However, in the biopsy material of a pig suffering from proliferative enteropathy, curved bacteria were found that were morphologically similar to members of the genus *Desulfovibrio*. One study analyzed the feces of 87 healthy people from the United Kingdom and found SRB in 66 people. Dominant among these bacteria were members of the genus *Desulfovibrio* (Gibson, Macfarlane, & Macfarlane, 1993). SRB were also detected in 92% of mucosal samples intestines of people with UC, and 52%—healthy (Zinkevich & Beech, 2000). The study also found an increase in the number of SRB in the feces of people with UC, compared with healthy individuals (Gibson, Macfarlane, & Macfarlane, 1993). Probably intestinal conditions during its inflammatory processes, disorder, and diarrhea are favorable for SRB. Hydrogen sulfide can be formed both by SRB and with sulfur-containing amino acids; it is toxic to mucous membranes. However, the presence of SRB and their metabolic products do not always explain the rapid development of the disease (Cummings et al., 2003).

The presence of sulfate in the colon stimulates the growth of SRB, which reduce SO_4^{2-} to H_2S (Abdulina et al., 2020; Kushkevych, Kováč, Vítězová, et al., 2018; Levitt et al., 1999; Pitcher & Cummings, 1996). Hydrogen sulfide adversely affects the intestinal mucosa, is toxic to epithelial cells, in particular inhibits the growth of colonocytes (Roediger et al., 1993b; Rowan et al., 2009), phagocytosis, causes bacterial death (Gardiner et al., 1995), and induces hyperproliferation and metabolic disorders of epithelial cells (Christl et al., 1992). It was found that the content of this metabolite and the amount of SRB increase significantly during inflammation of the ileal-anal sac (Cummings et al., 2003). The use of antibiotics (metronidazole or ciprofloxacin) and salicylamide derivatives causes a decrease in the amount of SRB and, accordingly, the formation of hydrogen sulfide (Kushkevych et al., 2016; Kushkevych, Kollár, et al., 2015; Kushkevych, Kos, Kollár, et al., 2018).

UC often occurs in genetically predisposed individuals. Their immune system cannot adequately respond to changes in the intestinal microbiota (Podolsky, 2002). As already mentioned, intestinal SRB are anaerobes that predominantly move through flagella. These microorganisms contribute to the interaction between the intestinal microbiota and the intestinal epithelium. SRB mainly colonizes the sacs of the ileum in sick people (Duffy et al., 2002; Fite et al., 2004; Zinkevich & Beech, 2000).

In patients with UC at the peak of the disease, they found SRBs, which accounted for 95% of the total intestinal microbiota content, while in patients in the recovery stage, only 55% of these bacteria were found (Pitcher et al., 2000). The number of viable SRB is three orders of magnitude higher in the active phase of the disease than in remission

(Pitcher & Cummings, 1996). Obviously, this indicates the important role of these bacteria in the development of colitis. Another study obtained opposite data on the number of SRB in healthy and patients with UC people (Loubinoux et al., 2000). After analyzing the feces of people, found more SRB cells in healthy individuals compared to patients. Among all isolated SRB, representatives of the genus *Desulfovibrio* (55%) were dominant in people with UC (Loubinoux et al., 2000). Despite the fact that the number of SRB in sick people was insignificant, the intensity of their sulfate reduction was higher than in healthy people (Gibson, Macfarlane, & Cummings, 1993; Loubinoux et al., 2000). It was also found that SRB isolated from patients with UC grew at low concentrations of sulfate. This is probably due to the composition of the intestinal environment during colitis (Gibson, Macfarlane, & Macfarlane, 1993). Therefore UC occurs mainly in the thick part, in particular straight intestines. The disease can begin and spread as a result of disruption of the intestinal structure. In severe cases, mucosal abscesses may occur. SRB and hydrogen sulfide are involved in the etiology of UC (Kushkevych, Martínková, Vítězová, et al. 2021). Hydrogen sulfide accumulation depends on the activity of SRB enzymes (Kushkevych, Abdulina, Kováč, et al., 2020). Colonization of intestine by these bacteria, their formation of hydrogen sulfide as well as the violation of homeostasis between the synthesis and utilization of H_2S are the probable path of intestinal pathogenesis.

4.2.1 Bacterial genera in the human large intestine

Bacteria living on the surface of the mucous membrane of the large intestine are in close contact with the human and animals' body. They interact more closely with the immune and neuroendocrine systems than intestinal microorganisms (Barton & Hamilton, 2007; Cummings et al., 2003; Sekirov et al., 2010). The interaction of SRB with intestinal epithelial cells has been little studied. Ninety-two percentage of SRB was found in different parts of the mucous membrane in patients with UC, while in healthy—52% of the total number of microorganisms (Zinkevich & Beech, 2000). It has also been confirmed that SRB are present in all human intestinal biopsies (Barton & Hamilton, 2007; Pathmakanthan et al., 1999; Zoetendal et al., 2002). It is believed that the species composition and number of bacteria on the surface of the intestinal mucosa differ from microorganisms in its cavity (Macfarlane & Dillon, 2007). These bacteria are in close interaction (Macfarlane et al., 2000). A large number of bacteria were found in biopsies of the intestinal mucosa of healthy people. All tissue samples were dominated by bacteria *E. coli* (Burke & Axon, 1988). Research tissues of the intestines of healthy people found different groups of bacteria on the mucous membrane. Their number was lower (10^4 cells/g biopsy) than in the intestinal cavity. Representatives of the genera *Bacteroides*, *Fusobacterium*, and *Bifidobacterium* were dominant. Microscopic analysis showed that most microorganisms were located under the upper layer of mucosa (Croucher et al., 1983). During colonoscopy, I. R. Poxton found that the number of anaerobic bacteria in the rectal area is 10–100-fold greater than the number of facultative anaerobes. The authors studied patients with UC and healthy people. In both experimental groups, the mucosal bacteria differed qualitatively and quantitatively. *Bacteroides thetaiotaomicron* (formerly *Bacillus thetaiotaomicron*) dominated in patients with UC. It was found that on the surface of the intestinal mucosa weigh approximately 69% of bacteroids (including *B. vulgatus*), compared with other microorganisms (Matsuda et al., 2000; Poxton et al., 1997). Comparison of the species composition of the microbiota isolated from intestinal biopsies of different people showed that in patients with UC the number of bacteria of the genus *Lactobacillus* and *Bifidobacterium* was significantly lower, while *B. thetaiotaomicron*—greater, comparable nanny with healthy people. The decrease in the number of bacteria of the genus *Lactobacillus* during UC led to an increase in the content of pathogenic microorganisms, as well as to their colonization on the walls of the intestinal mucosa (Pathmakanthan et al., 1999; Zoetendal et al., 2002). It was found that bacteria of the genus *Peptostreptococcus*, as well as *C. ramosum* and *Bifidobacterium breve* are found in significant quantities in patients with UC, while members of the genus *Fusobacterium*—in healthy people (Bamba et al., 1995; Matsuda et al., 2000; Schultsz et al., 1997).

The mucosa of the colon contains goblet-like secretory cells that produce mucin and colonocytes. Both cell types are formed from pluripotent cells in the colon. Goblet cells predominate and form a mucous layer, which is part of the protective barrier of the mucous membrane (Barton & Hamilton, 2007; Cummings et al., 2003; Rowan et al., 2009). The mucous layer consists of glycoproteins that are synthesized by goblet cells. Glycoproteins, containing acidic polysaccharides and are part of the secretions of all glands, called mucin. Mucin has a peptide base associated with glycosylated and nonglycosylated polysaccharides.

It is also known that approximately 20% of the peptide nucleus of mucin is nonglycosylated. The formation of glycoproteins depends on the activity of glycotransferase contained in the endoplasmic reticulum of goblet cells. This process is activated by glucocorticoids and other compounds, in particular butyrate (Rowan et al., 2009). Mucin, which is secreted by the goblet cells of the stomach, has a neutral pH (Deplancke & Gaskins, 2001). Intestinal mucin is acidic due to sialic acid residues (sialomucine) or sulfur (sulfomucine) (Rowan et al., 2009)

The ability to synthesize mucin is determined by the expression of *muc* genes in goblet cells. In humans, 21 *muc* genes have been identified. In individuals with UC, inhibition of *muc*12 gene expression has been reported (Moehle et al., 2006). The secretion of the mucous membrane creates a natural microenvironment in which bacteria can exist, forming biofilms (Macfarlane & Dillon, 2007). Such conditions ensure the retention of these microorganisms on the intestinal wall, regardless of its peristalsis. Bacteria that form biofilms are mainly resistant to antibiotics, changes in pH and mechanisms of antimicrobial protection of the body (Macfarlane & Dillon, 2007; Macfarlane et al., 2000). Bacteria of the genus *Desulfovibrio* colonize the intestine, forming biofilms and can migrate within the biofilm of the mucous layer of the colon (Macfarlane & Dillon, 2007). A large number (10^6-10^7 cells/g) of bacteria of the genus *Desulfovibrio* were found in rectal biopsies taken from colitis patients and healthy people. However, physiological and biochemical differences between these bacteria were not observed (Fite et al., 2004). Probably, the disease can be caused by certain strains of microorganisms. The study also did not find a difference between the physiological and biochemical characteristics of SRB in people with UC and the control group. In the development of the disease, the main factor in the pathogenesis is an excessive amount of hydrogen sulfide, which the human body is unable to neutralize (Fite et al., 2004). However, other researchers have found differences between SRB in people with nonspecific UC, Crohn's disease, and healthy people (Kleessen et al., 2002).

Further one study found an increase in the amount of mucin in the intestine leads to the displacement of methanogens by sulfate-reducing microorganisms (Gibson, Macfarlane, & Macfarlane, 1993). This dominance is due to the ability of the latter to use mucin sulfate as an electron acceptor during sulfate reduction. Fermentation of organic compounds by intestinal microorganisms involves many interdependent reactions in which complex polymers are first cleaved to monomers by hydrolytic enzymes synthesized by bacteria (Cummings et al., 2003; Rowan et al., 2009). The main products of fermentation are short-chain fatty acids (SCFAs), acetic, propionic and butyric acids, lactate, succinate, ethanol, butyrate, CO_2, methane, and hydrogen (Gibson, Macfarlane, & Cummings, 1993; Kristjansson et al., 1982). They play an important role in epithelial metabolism colon cells and mucosal function. Basic carbohydrates used by intestinal bacteria are polysaccharides (starch and fiber), as well as some oligosaccharides. Other substances, including proteins, can also be broken down in the large intestine (Cummings et al., 2003). Fermentation is regulated by the amount and feature of the available substrate, the chemical composition of the environment, the presence of certain types of bacteria, and the peculiarity of their metabolism. An important role in this is also played by the peculiarities of digestive mechanisms (Florin et al., 1993; Macfarlane et al., 2000). Epithelial cells of the colon receive energy during the oxidation of butyrate (Roediger, 1980; Roediger et al., 1993a,b). Epithelial cells of the small intestine mainly use glucose and glutamine as a source of energy (Cummings et al., 2003). As already mentioned butyrate is formed during the fermentation of substrates by the intestinal microbiota and provides 70% of energy for colonocytes.

For the first time, researchers showed that butyrate oxidation is significantly inhibited during all stages of UC development (Roediger, 1980). This fact was later confirmed by other scientists (Gibson, Macfarlane, & Cummings, 1993; Rowan et al., 2009). Physiological and biochemical studies of cells of the mucous membrane of the colon in people with UC have shown that at the beginning of the disease there is a violation of fatty acid metabolism (Rowan et al., 2009). This has been experimentally demonstrated in rats by induction of colitis by rectal administration of sodium 2-bromooctanoate (Roediger et al., 1993b), which is a specific inhibitor β-oxidation of fatty acids. Studies have suggested that butyrate "deficiency" in epithelial cells is likely to be important in the pathogenesis of UC (Roediger, 1980; Sekirov et al., 2010). Roediger's discovery of butyrate "deficiency" led to the hypothesis of "energy deficiency" for colonocytes, which is the cause of UC (Roediger, 1980).

It was found that mercaptoacetate and mercaptobutyrate affect the metabolism of fatty acids in colonocytes, which is characteristic of UC (Roediger et al., 1993a,b; Roediger, 1980). The effect of hydrogen sulfide on the process of inhibition of butyrate oxidation in intestinal epithelial cells was studied. It was found that the cause of inhibition of butyrate oxidation is metabolic blockade of FAD-dependent oxidation of butyryl-CoA dehydrogenase. Therefore the regulation of the concentration of hydrogen sulfide in the colon is very important for maintaining the integrity of colonocytes (Roediger et al., 1993b). SRB are able to metabolize food additives that contain oxidized sulfur compounds (Christl et al., 1993). In ruminants, dietary supplements with sulfate cause an increase in the amount of hydrogen sulfide in the rumen due to the vital activity of SRB (Kushkevych, Dordević, Vítězová, 2019a). Its toxicity is manifested clinically, in particular weight loss, fever, bloody diarrhea, intestinal inflammation (Sekirov et al., 2010). Large amounts of sulfur oxides are present in food. They are added as a preservative to extend the shelf life. Such preservatives are sulfur dioxide (E_{220}), sulfites ($E_{221-227}$), and to a lesser extent carrageenan (E_{407}), which are consumed by 98.6% of the population (Florin et al., 1991). Analysis of food and beverages for sulfate content showed that Africans consume only 2.7 mmol of sulfate per day. People who live in more developed western countries used food more than 16.6 mmol of sulfate per day (Florin et al., 1990, 1991, 1993; Florin, 1991). It has been found that the small intestine in people with ileostomy absorbs sulfate at a concentration of approximately 7 mmol sulfate per day. Its excess falls into the colon (Florin et al., 1991). Consumption of sulfate is a regulating factor of sulfate reduction in the intestine. This can play an important role in the spread of UC in developing countries (Strocchi et al., 1994).

Thus the bacteria of the mucous membrane of the large intestine are in close interaction with other microorganisms (*Bifidobacterium, Bacteroides, Lactobacillus, Escherichia, Eubacterium, Enterococcus*) of its lumen, as well as the human body. SRB are able to use food sulfates and mucin, producing hydrogen sulfide, which adversely affects colonocytes by inhibiting butyrate oxidation. Sulfate-containing dietary supplements stimulate the growth of SRB in the intestine.

4.2.2 Molecular hydrogen as a universal electron donor in intestinal SRB metabolism

An important product of bacterial fermentation in the intestine is hydrogen (Kushkevych, Vítězová, Vítěz, et al., 2017). Its formation occurs during the oxidation of carbohydrates and amino acids. In anaerobic metabolism, some bacteria form ethanol, lactate, or succinate (Kushkevych, 2016). Molecular hydrogen does not accumulate in large quantities in the intestine because some intestinal microorganisms use H_2 as an electron donor and a source of energy (Gibson, Macfarlane, & Cummings, 1993).

Hydrogen utilization occurs during dissimilation of sulfate, as well as methanogenesis and acetogenesis (Kushkevych, Cejnar, Vítězová, et al., 2020). Methanogenesis provides the formation of nontoxic to the intestine compound—methane (Vítězová et al., 2020). In the presence of sulfate, SRB is used hydrogen and accumulate toxic hydrogen sulfide (Gibson, Macfarlane, & Macfarlane, 1993). The absence of methanogens or SRB in the colon can cause excessive accumulation of H_2, which leads to bloating (Christl et al., 1992, 1993). Molecular hydrogen is also utilized during acetogenesis and dissimilation of nitrates. Acetogenic and nitrate reducing microorganisms can use H_2 as an electron donor (Kushkevych, Kobzová, Vítězová, et al., 2019). They probably metabolize H_2 more actively because during this process acetate is formed, which is an additional source of energy for the host organism (Gibson, Macfarlane, & Cummings, 1993; Gibson, Macfarlane, & Macfarlane, 1993).

Hydrogen is formed during the oxidation of pyruvate, formate, or reduction of nucleotides ($NADH^+$, $FADH^+$). In addition, clostridia are able to synthesize H_2 from pyruvate via ferredoxin, and enterobacteria—from pyruvate by fermentation using enzyme pyruvate formate lyase with the formation of formate, which is further converted to CO_2 and H_2. The presence of molecular hydrogen in the intestine does not affect its formation from pyruvate but inhibits the accumulation of H_2 from oxidized nucleotides. Using H_2 microorganisms regulates fermentation processes in the colon. In the large intestine, molecular hydrogen is present in low concentrations (Gibson, Macfarlane, & Cummings, 1993; Gibson, Macfarlane, & Macfarlane, 1993; Levitt et al., 1999). This is due to the fact that it is used by various types of microorganisms, including methanogens, acetogens, and SRB (Barton & Hamilton, 2007; Postgate, 1984).

Methanogenic microorganisms are found in the intestines of 30–50% of people (Gibson, Macfarlane, & Cummings, 1993; Gibson, Macfarlane, & Macfarlane, 1993). These bacteria grow due to the assimilation of CO_2 and H_2 (Kristjansson et al., 1982). From 4 moles of H_2 1 mol of CH_4 is formed. Methane formation is an efficient and safe way to dispose of H_2 and occurs in most animals. In people with low, the level of methanogenesis H_2 can be metabolized in another way with the participation of SRB (Černý et al., 2018; Kushkevych, Vítězová, Vítěz, et al., 2018).

As in the process of methanogenesis, 4 mol of H_2 is required for the reduction of sulfate, from which 1 mol of product (HS^-) is formed. However, in the case of methanogenesis, CH_4 is formed, which is harmless to intestinal cells, compared to hydrogen sulfide, which is cytotoxic to epithelial cells of the colon (Pitcher & Cummings, 1996). People with significant amounts of SRB in the colon have high concentrations of hydrogen sulfide in the feces compared to people with methanogenic dominance (Gibson, Macfarlane, & Cummings, 1993; Gibson, Macfarlane, & Macfarlane, 1993). The main substrates for SRB of the colon are acetate, propionate, lactate, butyrate, succinate, ethanol, pyruvate, some amino acids, and H_2/CO_2 (Macfarlane et al., 2000). It has been studied that there are types of bacteria in the human intestine that use fatty acids and polyhydric alcohols (Barton & Hamilton, 2007). They are the last link in the metabolism of organic compounds of the intestine and use sulfate as an electron acceptor in the oxidation reactions of these substances. Dominant SRB in the human intestine are members of the genera *Desulfovibrio* (66%), *Desulfobulbus* (16%), and others (18%), such as *Desulfobacter, Desulfomonas,* and *Desulfotomaculum* (Gibson, Macfarlane, & Cummings, 1993; Gibson, Macfarlane, & Macfarlane, 1993). Species that use molecular hydrogen in the gut as an electron donor belong mainly to the genera *Desulfovibrio* and *Desulfobulbus*.

It has been established that SRB are able to completely displace methanogens from the intestine, competing with them for H_2. Researchers believe that methanogens are able to displace other intestinal microorganisms that use molecular hydrogen (Strocchi et al., 1994). Competition for molecular hydrogen between SRB and methanogens largely depends on the presence and amount of sulfate in the intestine (Christl et al., 1992; Strocchi et al., 1994). The addition of sulfate and sulfated mucopolysaccharides to fecal suspensions containing metabolically active SRB products stimulates the formation of hydrogen sulfide and inhibits the intensity of methanogenesis (Gibson, Macfarlane, & Cummings, 1993; Gibson, Macfarlane, & Macfarlane, 1993). Methanogenic microorganisms are unlikely to coexist with SRB in the presence of sufficient sulphate and use a common substrate at the same time, because SRBs are able to use H_2 more intensely than methanogens (saturation constant (Ks) for *Desulfovibrio vulgaris* is 1 µmol/L, Ks for *Methanobrevibacter smithii* is 6 µmol/L) (Kristjansson et al., 1982).

Moreover, the oxidation of H_2 by SRB is thermodynamically more favorable ($\Delta G° = -152.2$ kJ/mol) than methanogens ($\Delta G° = -131$ kJ/mol) (Gibson, Macfarlane, & Cummings, 1993; Gibson, Macfarlane, & Macfarlane, 1993). It depends on the presence of sulfate and the number of SRB that compete for H_2 with methanogens (Lovley & Klug, 1983). It is likely that in the presence of sulfate in the intestine among the entire intestinal microbiota, molecular hydrogen will mainly be metabolized by SRB. Limiting the availability of sulfate may lead to an increase in methanogenic microorganisms that also use H_2. The addition of sulfate to the diet of people with elevated levels of methanogenesis causes a decrease in the number of methanogenic bacteria in 50% of people, for several days in the feces of these people detect SRB (Christl et al., 1993). It is established that the formation of H_2 during the fermentation of various carbohydrates depends on food. For example, the consumption of 15 g of lactulose by people with methanogenic communities produces 1150 mL of hydrogen, while those deprived of these bacteria, only 327 mL of H_2 is released (Christl et al., 1992; Gibson, Macfarlane, & Cummings, 1993). These data obviously indicate that there are different ways of using molecular hydrogen in the human intestine. A certain concentration of sulfates in the colon is required to displace methanogens by SRB. Their concentration in the intestine can vary greatly, depending on the food a person consumes. The amount of sulfate, which enters the colon, is from 2 to 9 mmol/day (Florin et al., 1991). The introduction of 15 mmol of sulfate per day in the diet reduces the intensity of methanogenesis; the number of methanogens is reduced by three orders of magnitude. Other sources of intestinal sulfate are also known, in particular sulfate-containing polysaccharides (chondroitin sulfate) (Gibson, Macfarlane, & Cummings, 1993).

As already mentioned, intestinal mucin is also a sulfate-containing compound (Moehle et al., 2006). Bacteria of the genus *Clostridium*, *Bifidobacterium*, and *B. fragilis* can cleave mucin, resulting in the formation of sulfate available for SRB (Macfarlane et al., 2000). The amount of mucin and its structure in humans is different. Probably, in people who have a genetic predisposition to intensive production of this polymer in the intestine, SRB are found in greater numbers. It is established that the number and variety of intestinal SRB in humans depends on geographical areas they inhabit. Different groups of the population have different amounts of SRB. No methanogens were detected in the presence of SRB (Gibson, Macfarlane, & Cummings, 1993; Lovley & Klug, 1983; Strocchi et al., 1994). Another way of utilizing H_2 is due to the activity of acetogenic microorganisms, which also grow in the colon. The process of using H_2 occurs due to the reduction of CO_2 in the presence of H_2 by acetogens (Kristjansson et al., 1982):

$$4H_2 + 2CO_2 \rightarrow CH_3COO^- + H^+ + 2H_2O$$

Significant formation of acetate with CO_2 and H_2 was found in human feces in the absence of SRB. The change in free energy H_2/CO_2 during acetogenesis is -95 kJ/mol (Kristjansson et al., 1982). This process is less energetically beneficial for SRB and methanogens compared to dissimilation of sulfate or methanogenesis. In most anaerobic ecosystems, hydrogen can be a source of energy. These processes are influenced by the pH of the medium (Gibson, Macfarlane, & Cummings, 1993; Gibson, Macfarlane, & Macfarlane, 1993). However, it is unlikely that acetogenesis is the main route of H_2 utilization in humans. The formation of acetate from CO_2 has also been found in the cecum of rats (Prins & Lankhorst, 1977) and in the intestines of termites (Breznak & Switzer, 1986). In the intestines of insects, the amount of acetate is 94% of its total content, and in humans — only 57% (Gibson, Macfarlane, & Cummings, 1993; Gibson, Macfarlane, & Macfarlane, 1993).

Therefore the use of H_2 in the large intestine can occur in several ways with the participation of SRB, methanogens and acetogenic communities. Representatives of these physiological groups of microorganisms compete with each other for molecular hydrogen. Intestinal microbiota of people living in different geographical areas is qualitatively and quantitatively different. SRB is believed to be able to displace methanogens and acetogens and that they play an important role in intestinal diseases because they produce hydrogen sulfide, which is toxic to all living organisms.

4.2.3 Hydrogen sulfide effect on intestinal cells

As already mentioned, hydrogen sulfide is the main product of SRB metabolism (Kotrsová & Kushkevych, 2019; Kushkevych, Dordević, Kollár, et al., 2019). It can also be formed endogenously during transsulfurylation and present in nontoxic concentrations in the brain, heart, blood vessels, genitourinary system, and gastrointestinal tract (Fiorucci et al., 2006; Wang, 2002). At higher concentrations, it inhibits the oxidation of butyrate, which is the main source of energy for colonocytes (Roediger et al., 1993b; Roediger, 1980), causing hyperproliferation of mucous cells and colonocyte dysfunction (Christl et al., 1993). Perfusion of the colon of rats with low concentrations of hydrogen sulfide results in the formation of intestinal ulcers (Pitcher & Cummings, 1996). The use of immunomodulators weakens the ability of polymorphonuclear leukocytes to phagocytose and inhibits bacterial growth (Gardiner et al., 1995). It is believed that SRB has a significant impact on the development of diseases. However, no less important factor is the intensity of production of SRB hydrogen sulfide in the lumen of the colon (Gibson, Macfarlane, & Cummings, 1993; Gibson, Macfarlane, & Macfarlane, 1993). It is greater in the distal intestine and much less in the proximal (Macfarlane & Dillon, 2007). This compound causes the formation ulcers of the intestinal mucosa and effects on the survival of *Lactobacillus* species (Kushkevych, Kotrsová, Dordević, et al., 2019). SRB are around the ulcer and form a dense biofilm with other microbial communities. The boundaries between ulcers and bacterial colonies are likely to be determined by the immune status of the macroorganism (host), the pH of the intestinal lumen (Kushkevych, Dordević, Vítězová, 2019b), and the foot sulfate (Rowan et al., 2009).

The toxic effect of hydrogen sulfide on intestinal cells is to disrupt their metabolism due to the inhibition of cytochrome oxidase and the destruction of disulfide bridges of intestinal organic compounds. This can lead to disruption of the structure of the protective epithelial layer (Pitcher & Cummings, 1996; Smith et al., 1977). Hydrogen sulfide has been shown to be fivefold more soluble in lipophilic solvents than in water (Barton & Hamilton, 2007). This allows it to penetrate freely through cell membranes (Fiorucci et al., 2006). For cells of the oral mucosa, hydrogen sulfide has been shown to increase epithelial permeability and disrupt cell barrier function (Kushkevych, Castro Sangrador, Dordević, et al., 2020). Incubation of a biopsy of the colon of a healthy person with 1 mm HS^- increases lability crypt, and when incubated with 1 mm HS^- and 10 mm butyrate causes the protective effect of cells to HS^- (Christl et al., 1992). It was also found that hydrogen sulfide disrupts cell proliferation. This was observed in the crypts of the epithelium during UC (Rowan et al., 2009). Perfusion of the colon of rats with physiological concentrations of NaHS leads to the development of apoptosis, destruction of goblet cells, disruption of the structure of the crypts, and superficial mucosal ulcers shell (Pitcher & Cummings, 1996). In addition, under anaerobic conditions in the colon, the intensity of cleavage of disulfide bonds in mucin increases (Sekirov et al., 2010). The action of hydrogen sulfide can also be aimed at inhibiting the phagocytic properties of polymorphonuclear leukocytes and neutralization of encapsulated bacterial strains. This is important for the spread of pathogenic bacteria in the body and for the emergence toxemia (Gardiner et al., 1995). In addition, H_2S is cytotoxic to human intestinal epithelium (Baskar et al., 2007).

Hydrogen sulfide penetrates cell membranes as well as other gaseous substances [nitrogen (II) oxide, carbon (II) oxide, and others], which do not require specific receptors on the cell. It affects adenosine-5′-triphosphate-dependent potassium channels and cytochrome c oxidase, damages DNA, inactivates intestinal cell enzymes, and as a result causes disease (Rowan et al., 2009). Enzymes of the colonic mucosa can convert methylate hydrogen sulfide to methanethiol and, subsequently, to dimethyl sulfide (Levitt et al., 1999). However, methanethiol and dimethyl sulfide were not detected in the cecum. Methanethiol is demethylated to hydrogen sulfide that oxidizes to thiosulfate. The rate of oxidation of hydrogen sulfide by enzymes of the mucous membrane of the colon is 105-fold higher than its methylation. Therefore dysfunction of the intestinal mucosa, which is able to oxidize hydrogen sulfide, can cause the accumulation of this compound in toxic concentrations (Rowan et al., 2009).

Hydrogen sulfide is also formed during the decomposition of various substrates in the intestine. In the feces of healthy people, the concentration of hydrogen sulfide is from 0.3 to 3.4 mmol/L (Attene-Ramos et al., 2007). At higher concentrations, this compound causes oxidizing stress in the cell. It forms complexes with Fe^{2+} ions, which are contained in the active centers of cytochrome c oxidase of mitochondria and, as a consequence, cell respiration is inhibited (Rowan et al., 2009; Wallace et al., 2007).

As already mentioned, hydrogen sulfide can cause DNA damage and therefore be a mutagen (Attene-Ramos et al., 2007; Baskar et al., 2007; Ramasamy et al., 2006). H_2S at a concentration of 1 μmol/L damages the DNA of isolated nuclei isolated from Chinese hamster ovary cells (Attene-Ramos et al., 2007). Hydrogen sulfide due to DNA damage can cause cell cycle arrest in the G_1 period and apoptosis (Baskar et al., 2007). Under the influence of this compound on epithelial cells, their cycle during the G_1 period slows down and the rate of phosphorylation of retinoblastoma protein decreases (Takeuchi et al., 2008).

Furthermore, researchers showed that some substances, in particular H_2S, can cause physiological and biochemical changes in the intestinal lumen and, consequently, its damage (Roediger et al., 1993b). This is most commonly seen in colon cells in human patients with UC (Rowan et al., 2009). In experiments on human colonocytes, it was found that the introduction of reduced sulfur compounds at a concentration of 2 mmol/L causes inhibition of butyrate oxidation by

75% in the distal parts of the colon and 43% in the colon. The sequence of inhibition of fatty acid oxidation is as follows: hydrogen sulfide → methanethiol → mercaptoacetate. Probably, these substances, as well as hydrogen sulfide, may also be involved in the pathogenesis of the intestine (Roediger et al., 1993a). Inhibition of fatty acid oxidation was also confirmed in a study of the effect of 0.1–0.5 mmol/L H_2S on colonocytes of healthy rats (Florin et al., 1990; Gibson, Macfarlane, & Macfarlane, 1993). Reduced sulfur compounds butyrate metabolism occurs, apparently, before NAD-dependent oxidation (Qi et al., 1993) at the level of butyryl-CoA dehydrogenase (Pitcher et al., 2000). Reduced sulfur compounds may also reduce the oxidation intensity of butyrate in the colonic epithelium because mercaptans compete with butyrate for the use of an SCFA transporter in ion exchange (Stein et al., 1995). Hypoxia is observed during IBD intracellular environment (Rowan et al., 2009).

Cysteine and methionine are sulfur-containing amino acids that are substrates for the formation of hydrogen sulfide (Kraus et al., 1998). Transsulfurylation is one of the pathways of metabolism due to the interconversion of cysteine and homocysteine through the intermediate cystathionine. Methionine is considered an essential amino acid, but when the transsulfurylation pathway is disrupted, the essential amino acid is cysteine. In some bacteria and yeasts that are able to synthesize cysteine, the process of transsulfurylation is reversed (Rowan et al., 2009). The formation of homocysteine by transsulfurylation causes the conversion of intermediate methionine through methylation with the enzyme methionine synthase (Kraus et al., 1998). Transsulfurylation occurs in stages: from homocysteine to cystathionine, cysteine and, as a result, sulfate is formed. Two pyridoxal-5′-phosphate-dependent enzymes cystathionine-β-synthase (CBS) and cystathionine-γ-lyase (CSE) reduce the rate of transsulfurylation. CBS catalyzes the first stage of this process, replacing the hydroxyl group of serine with the thiol group of L-homocysteine, forming cystathionine (Fiorucci et al., 2006). CBS is contained in the cytoplasm and consists of four identical (63 kDa) subunits (Ge et al., 2001). The human CBS gene contains 23 exons (Kraus et al., 1998).

CBS and CSE provide the formation of hydrogen sulfide. Rhodanese (thiosulfate cyanide sulfur transferase) is an enzyme mitochondria, which neutralize cyanide (CN^-), converting it to thiocyanate (SCN^-). The enzyme also utilizes H_2S, catalyzing the formation of sulfate. ATP sulfurylase, APS reductase, and sulfite reductase (DSL) are SRB enzymes that catalyze the reduction of sulfate to H_2S by anaerobic sulfate respiration (Rowan et al., 2009). Disruption of normal CBS function is due to trisomy 21 of chromosome and hyperhomocysteinuria. The latter is associated with atherosclerosis. Deficit CBS during homocysteinuria is inherited autosomal recessively (Finkelstein, 2006; Kraus et al., 1998). The formation of CBS and dysfunction of this enzyme reflects the importance of cysteine in metabolism in the body, as well as cytoprotective properties during the formation of hydrogen sulfide. The expression of the gene encoding human CBS depends on cell proliferation (Fiorucci et al., 2006).

CSE catalyzes the final stage of transsulfurylation, converting L-cystathionine to L-cysteine, α-ketobutyrate, and ammonia (Levonen et al., 2000). Two human CSE isoforms are known (Rowan et al., 2009). CSE overexpression leads to an increase in three-cell hydrogen sulfide levels, inhibition of cell proliferation and DNA synthesis (Yang et al., 2004). Inhibition of the CSE enzyme promotes healing of gastric ulcers (Wallace et al., 2007). CSE and CBS are present in neurons of the submucosal plexus of human enterocytes (Rowan et al., 2009). Sodium hydrosulfide and L-cysteine may cause the secretion of some ions in neurons of the mucous and submucosal membranes of the colon. Additions of D,L-propargylglycine and aminooxyacetyl acid inhibit CSE and CBS, respectively. The introduction of sodium hydrosulfide does not cause a secretory response by epithelial cells of the colon (Wallace et al., 2007).

In mammalian cells, hydrogen sulfide, which is not in a toxic concentration, can be oxidized to sulfate, thiocyanate, and thiosulfate. The latter is an unstable compound in an acidic environment and is converted to sulfate. The enzymes rhodanes and TMT are used to neutralize hydrogen sulfide in the intestine (Roediger et al., 1993a). Rhodanese has two isoforms: thiosulfate sulfur transferase (TST) and mercaptopyruvate sulfur transferase (MST). TST neutralizes hydrogen sulfide in colonocytes (Ramasamy et al., 2006; Rowan et al., 2009). The expression of both isoenzymes (MST and TST) is reduced in UC and colon cancer, compared with normal mucosa, which causes the possible development of the disease. However, no statistical difference was found between the activities of rhodanesis and TMT in rectal biopsies of people with nonspecific UC and healthy. It was found that in the presence of cyanide, the main product of hydrogen sulfide metabolism in the mucous membrane of the colon is thiocyanate, not thiosulfate. People who smoke cigarettes are thought to have a high concentration of cyanide in their bodies, which is likely to neutralize the effects of hydrogen sulfide. In these people, thiocyanate may be a protective mechanism against UC (Wilson et al., 2008).

The mucous membrane of the cecum and colon detoxifies hydrogen sulfide to inactive metabolites fourfold faster than other tissues (Levitt et al., 1999). The formation of butyrate in the cecum and colon increases the activity of TST (Guarner & Malagelada, 2003; Ramasamy et al., 2006). UC occurs mainly in the left side of the colon. This suggests that the formation of hydrogen sulfide SRB has a greater impact on the distal parts of the mucous membrane of the colon (Rowan et al., 2009). Hydrogen sulfide is also neutralized by reduced glutathione, which is an antioxidant. It consists of γ-glutamic acid, cysteine, and glycine residues. It can exist in oxidized (Glu-S—S-Glu) and reduced (Glu-SN) forms. The latter protects SH groups of proteins from oxidation by various oxidants. The defense mechanism is the oxidation of the SH group of glutathione with the formation of the oxidized form and the preservation of the SH groups of proteins in the active reduced form. Glutathione plays an important role in the binding of free radicals and the reduction of hydrogen peroxide and other peroxides, which prevents the development of free radical processes. It is involved in the transport of amino acids across the plasma membranes of enterocytes and other cells (γ-glutamyltransferase cycle). Glutathione acts in stages on glutamate, cysteine, and glycine with the participation of glutamate cysteine ligase and glutathione synthetase. Glutathione reductase is an enzyme that restores the disulfide bonds of oxidized glutathione (GSSG) to its sulfhydryl form of GSH. The reduction of glutathione occurs due to the energy of NADPH, which is formed in the pentose cycle (Rowan et al., 2009).

Glutathione reductase can cause oxidative stress. This enzyme is energy dependent and maintains the level of reduced glutathione. The route of utilization of hydrogen sulfide in the human body is not fully understood. It is believed that it is due to the presence of enzymes mercaptopyruvate transferase and sulfite oxidase. It was found that the activity of these enzymes is much lower in the intestinal tissues of people with UC, compared with healthy, mainly in the distal part of the intestine, where the disease progresses (Barton & Hamilton, 2007).

Thus hydrogen sulfide, which is produced by SRB in the human intestine, inhibits cytochrome oxidase and the oxidation of butyrate by colonocytes, destroys epithelial cells, and promotes the development of ulcers and, subsequently, inflammation. It is also available in nontoxic concentrations in various organs. The main antioxidant that neutralizes hydrogen sulfide is reduced glutathione.

4.3 General characteristics of drugs used in bowel diseases

The treatment of IBDs consists of nutritional, pharmacological, and surgical therapy, depending on the stage of the disease (Cummings et al., 2003; Levitt et al., 1999; Lewis et al., 2005; Lynch & Hsu, 2021). However, the patient must combine individual treatment approaches during life. Nutritional therapy, in addition to adjusting dietary habits and eliminating the consumption of inappropriate food ingredients and using the beneficial effect of probiotics and prebiotics, consists of complete enteral nutrition (elementary diet based on amino acids) for 4–6 weeks, which can induce remission and reduce inflammation. The basis of pharmacological treatment (Fig. 4.2) of UC and Crohn's disease is the administration of aminosalicylates: mesalazine (5-aminosalicylic acid, 5-ASA—a drug with a purely antiinflammatory effect) or its combination with antibacterially active sulfonamides (sulfasalazine, sulfapyridine).

The use of mesalazine leads to a decrease in the concentration of hydrogen sulfide in the feces (Pitcher & Cummings, 1996; Pitcher et al., 2000). The therapeutic dose of mesalazine, which causes a decrease in the concentration of H_2S in the intestine, is 18.75 mM (Cummings et al., 2003; Rowan et al., 2009). It should be mentioned that the occurrence of UC in animals that received both 5-ASA and N-acetylcysteine was less common compared with those receiving 5-ASA alone (Siddiqui et al., 2006). For severe and moderate attacks, corticoids are used either systemically, for example, prednisone, or locally in the form of an enema, such as budesonide. In addition, immunomodulatory treatments (azathioprine, 6-mercaptopurine, methotrexate, cyclosporin A, tacrolimus) may be administered. Antibiotics are also used (see below), their role is to reduce the harmful effects of microbiome on the course of intestinal inflammation. A modern type of therapy involves the administration of monoclonal antibodies, such as infliximab or adalimumab. This so-called biological treatment is intended for a particularly severe course of the disease. The antihistamine fexofenadine, vitamin D and iron supplements may be used as supportive therapy. Surgical therapy (resection, stricturoplasty, balloon dilatation of stenoses, drainage of abscesses, fistulotomy) is indicated for complications (perforation, bleeding, fistula, abscesses, strictures, tumors); however, even after successful surgery there is a risk of recurrence (Cummings et al., 2003; Levitt et al., 1999; Lewis et al., 2005; Lynch & Hsu, 2021).

4.3.1 Antibacterial chemotherapeutics

The main purpose of the use of antibiotics in bowel diseases is the effect of these substances on its microbiota. When antibiotics are used, it is also necessary to take into account the analysis of microbiota of feces and intestinal biopsy patients. The effect of antimicrobials is studied mainly in animal models.

For the first time, an animal model of colitis was developed by R. Marcus and J. Watt on guinea pigs, using carrageenan to cause disease. Subsequently, colitis was modeled on other animals (rats, mice, hamsters, rabbits, monkeys) using various substances [DSS, amylopectin sulfate, trinitrobenzenesulfonic acid (TNBS)], which led to the development of the disease (Fiocchi, 1998; Marcus & Watt, 1974). In 1974 Truelove and Jewell first proposed the use of

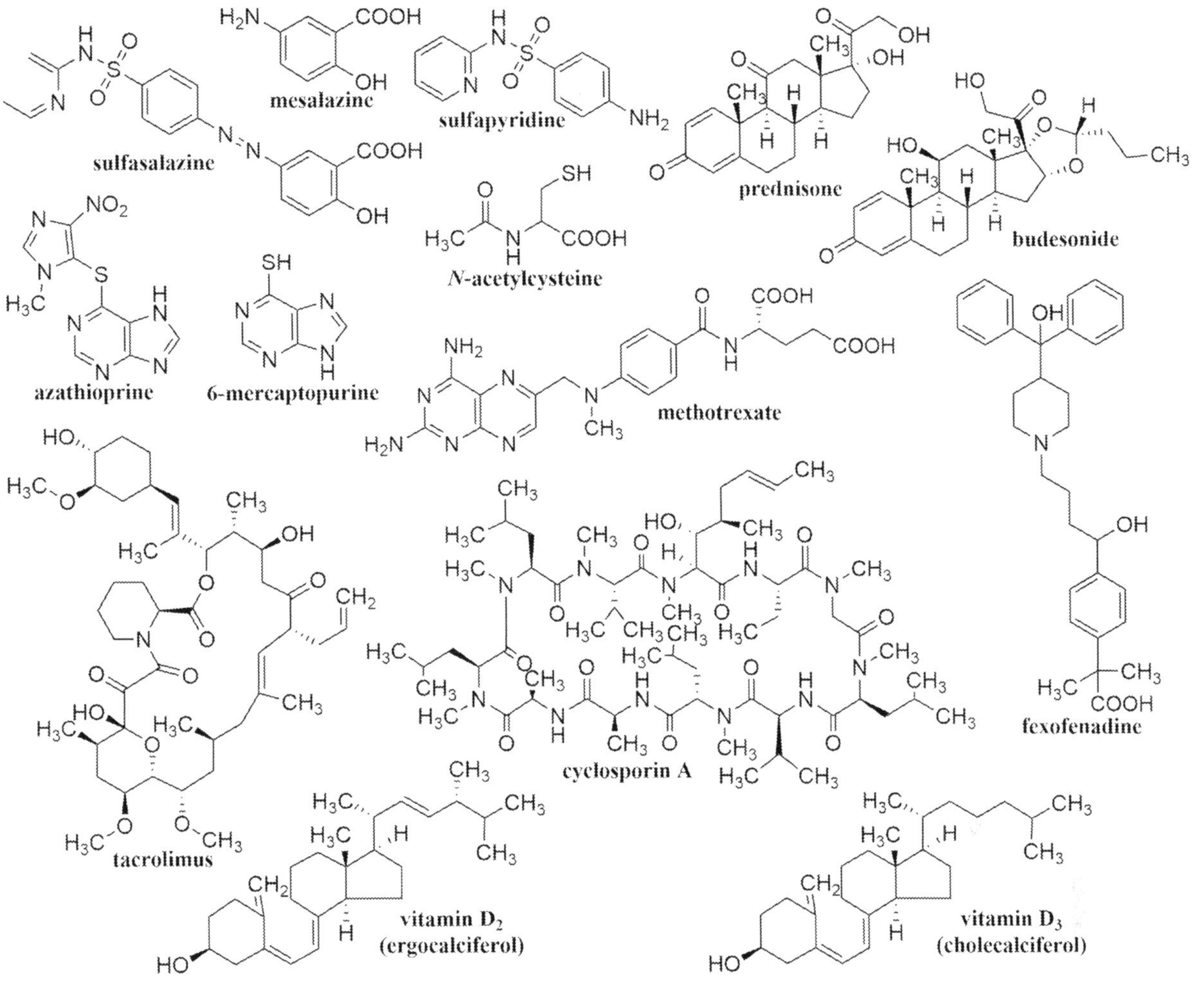

FIGURE 4.2 Drugs used in the pharmacological alleviation of inflammatory bowel disease.

antibiotics to facilitate bowel disease (Truelove & Jewell, 1974). They administered tetracycline, glucose/saline, steroids, and vitamins to patients with IR, 36 of 49 of whom observed a reduction in symptoms (Truelove & Jewell, 1974).

Antimicrobial treatment reduces the intensity of inflammation of the mucous membrane and promotes recovery. However, SRB, which play an important role in the development of UC, may be present in insignificant numbers throughout the human life. After the termination of antibiotics on SRB and the restoration of the epithelium of the colon, their colonization may again increase, leading to a likely relapse (Gibson et al., 1991; Gibson, Macfarlane, & Cummings, 1993). SRB, *D. desulfuricans*, isolated from sick people with UC, have been found to be resistant to antimicrobial agents (Fox et al., 1994). Therefore the clinical effect of these drugs during treatment may not have the expected result (Pitcher & Cummings, 1996).

In clinical practice, antibiotics are mostly not used in acute UC. Evidence of their effectiveness for animal models and humans is not convincing (Campieri & Gionchetti, 1999, 2001; Linskens et al., 2001).

Problems of antibiotic use during UC (Cummings et al., 2003):

1. The specific types of bacteria involved in colitis development are unknown, so it is difficult to find an effective antibiotic for treatment;
2. The bacteria that are likely to cause the disease may belong to the biofilm on the surface of the intestinal mucosa;
3. Therapeutic doses of antibiotics may not reach their destination;
4. The emergence of resistance of microorganisms, especially during prolonged use;
5. The effect of antibiotics on normal microbiota and disruption of the barrier resistance of the microorganism to pathogens;
6. The use of antibiotics is most effective only at the beginning of the disease;
7. Side effects of antibiotics.

The most popular drugs most commonly tested on animal models of colitis are metronidazole, ciprofloxacin, gentamicin, tobramycin, neomycin, streptomycin, vancomycin, tobramycin, imipenem, clindamycin, amoxicillin, and rifaximin (Fig. 4.3).

One of the antibiotics used for animal models and for the treatment of UC is metronidazole. However, its effectiveness is poorly understood, which has led to considerable scientific interest. Metronidazole is an antiprotozoal drug that is also active against anaerobic microorganisms. It is one of the most common antibiotics used during anaerobic infection in medical practice (Onderdonk et al., 1977, 1978). The use of enemas and suppositories, which are delivery methods for the treatment of human infections, may reduce the effect of this drug. It is also important to introduce it into the gut since the action of metronidazole, like other antibiotics, is probably most effective in the early stages of the disease (Cummings et al., 2003; Onderdonk et al., 1977). One study that gave patients orally 1.35 g/day of metronidazole or sulfasalazine during an acute UC period for 28 days observed a decrease in the symptoms of the disease in 26% and 68% of patients treated with metronidazole and sulfasalazine, respectively (Gilat et al., 1989). Over the next year, patients received 0.6 g of metronidazole or 2 g of sulfasalazine a day. Metronidazole was effective after 12 months of treatment, no side effects were observed. However, it is known that it is capable of causing peripheral neuropathy during prolonged use. Similar effect has the simultaneous use of metronidazole with tobramycin (Gilat et al., 1989;

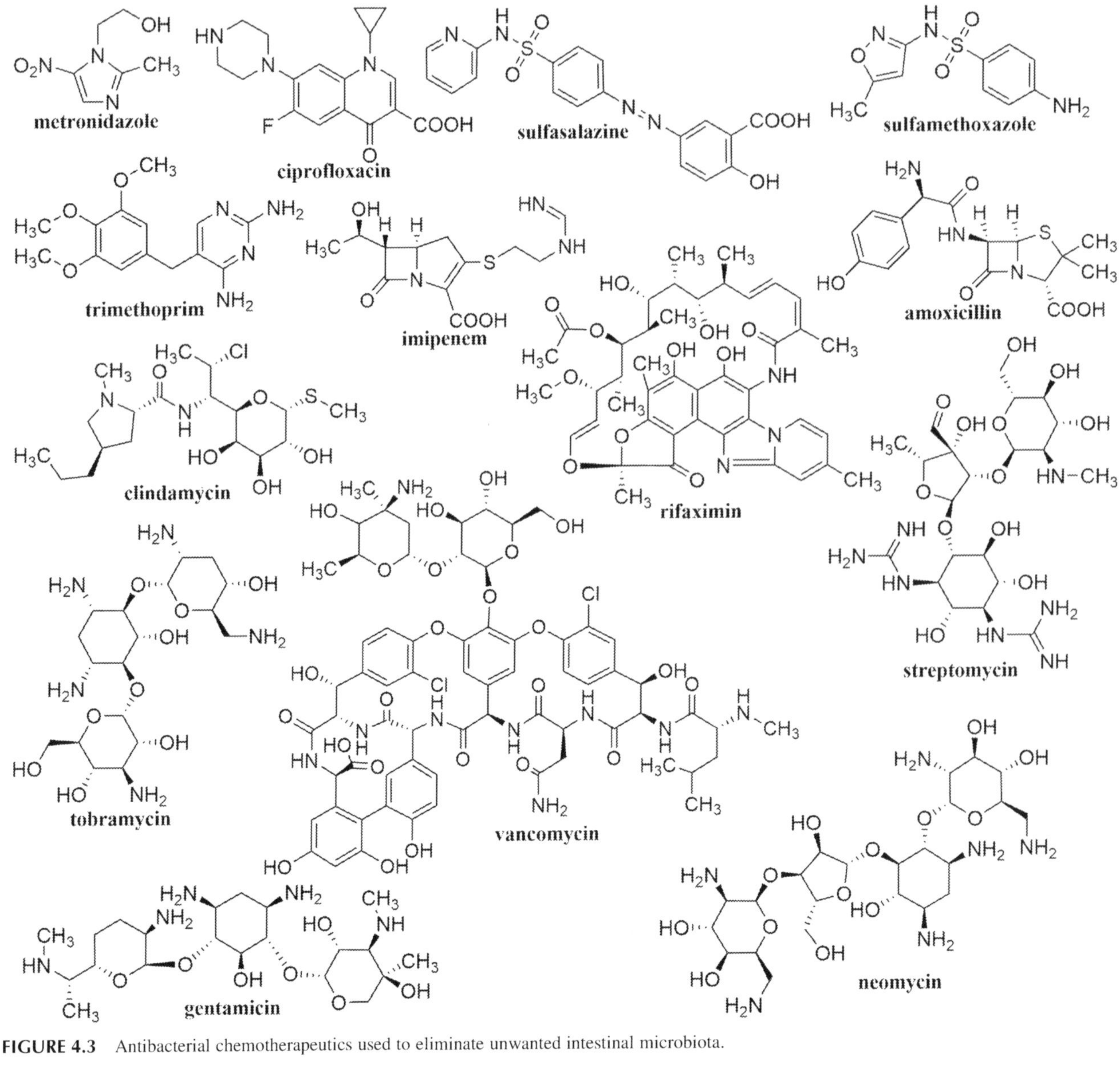

FIGURE 4.3 Antibacterial chemotherapeutics used to eliminate unwanted intestinal microbiota.

Mantzaris et al., 1997). One study showed that after the use of metronidazole in patients with UC, the content of SRB in their feces decreased (Lewis et al., 2005).

An effective antibiotic for the treatment of gastrointestinal infections is ciprofloxacin, which is used to treat Crohn's disease (Cummings et al., 2003). It is used for the prevention of animal colitis, but it is not effective for treatment (Hans et al., 2000; Madsen et al., 1999, 2000; Rath et al., 2001). Instead, the combination of this antibiotic with metronidazole has a positive effect. Ciprofloxacin is a fluoroquinolone that is well absorbed by the intestine and active against Gram-negative facultative anaerobes and microaerophiles (*Salmonella, Shigella, Campylobacter*). It is also active against Gram-positive bacteria, in particular *E. faecalis* (Cummings et al., 2003). Other studies have shown that ciprofloxacin use for six months does not cause endoscopic or histologic changes in intestinal tissues. The serum of UC patients at the beginning of treatment with ciprofloxacin contained high concentrations of IgG, IgM, and IgA to *E. coli, Proteus mirabilis*, and *Klebsiella pneumonia*. The level IgG to *E. coli* was decreased after treatment. Ciprofloxacin is probably more effective for *E. coli* than for other microorganisms (Mantzaris et al., 1997, 2001).

Among the antibiotics tested on animals, the most effective against gut microorganisms are gentamicin, tobramycin, neomycin and streptomycin (Cummings et al., 2003). They are active against Gram-negative facultative anaerobes, in particular *E. coli*, which are commensals, conditionally pathogenic bacteria of the intestine (Burke & Axon, 1988). However, these aminoglycoside antibiotics are not very effective in the treatment and prevention of human colitis. Tobramycin is used in the treatment of acute bowel disease. After a 7-day course of treatment in 74% of patients with UC who took the drug orally, on the 28th day there was a stage of remission (Burke & Axon, 1988). Other studies have shown that tobramycin for 12 and 24 months was not effective for Gram-negative species, in particular *E. coli* (Lobo et al., 1993).

Clindamycin is active against Gram-positive cocci and many anaerobic microorganisms. However, this antibiotic causes diarrhea, so its use is limited. Clindamycin adversely affects the gut microbiocenosis. It is established that it reduces the intensity of ulcer formation in the gut of the guinea pigs (Onderdonk et al., 1977, 1978).

Vancomycin is an antibacterial glycopeptide antibiotic that is not adsorbed in the gut, active against Gram-positive cocci, and some anaerobic microorganisms. Its use is not effective when combined with tobramycin, but it has a positive effect with imipenem. A study found that the simultaneous administration of vancomycin and impinem is effective in the prevention and treatment of colitis in rats and mice (Rath et al., 2001). In the treatment of acute UC with oral administration of 2 g of vancomycin per day, no positive effect has been established (Cummings et al., 2003).

Amoxicillin is a broad-spectrum antibiotic that is well adsorbed, easily diffused through tissues and active against Gram-negative and Gram-positive bacteria. There is evidence of the use of amoxicillin and clavulanic acid in rats during colitis treatment (Cummings et al., 2003) These antibiotics were administered for 5 days to treat people with acute colitis, after which they observed a decrease in the severity of the disease. Trimethoprim and sulfamethoxazole is believed to be more effective in the treatment of severe UC, probably because it exhibits antifolic (immunosuppressive) action (Mantzaris et al., 2001).

Rifaximin is a new generation antibiotic that is effective in the gut, more like rifamycin. Rifaximin is not adsorbed by the intestine (Brigidi et al., 2002; Gionchetti et al., 1999; Rizzello et al., 1998; Venturi et al., 1999), so it is found in feces at high concentrations (Jiang et al., 2000). It acts on Gram-positive and Gram-negative bacteria of the colon (Rizzello et al., 1998; Venturi et al., 1999). This antibiotic is active against *E. coli* bacteria belonging to the genera *Salmonella* and *Shigella*, so, like ciprofloxacin, it is used to treat diarrhea (Jiang et al., 2000; Steffen, 2001; Turunen et al., 1998). Rifaximin is used in combination with ciprofloxacin for the treatment of pochitis (Rizzello et al., 1998; Venturi et al., 1999). There are data on its use during UC (Guslandi, 2011; Rizzello et al., 1998). In a study of 31 people with mild to moderate, mostly left-sided UC, who were given 400 mg of the antibiotic twice daily for 10 days, observed relief from the disease (Guslandi, 2011). Researchers investigated the action of rifaximin and used it to treat UC (Rizzello et al., 1998). A 64% reduction in the incidence of the disease was reported following administration of this antibiotic. In other studies, patients were prescribed 1.8 g of rifaximin daily for 10 days (Rizzello et al., 1998). Subsequently, a significant inhibitory effect of this antibiotic on the gut microbiocenosis, including *Lactobacilli, Bifidobacteria, Bacterioides*, and *C. perfringens*, was established (Brigidi et al., 2002). However, after discontinuation of the antibiotic after 25 days, the number of these microorganisms normalized. Rifaximin is believed to be the most effective for the treatment of UC (Cummings et al., 2003).

As was mentioned, many types of microorganisms have been associated with UC in recent years, but it is not yet known exactly, which bacteria are involved in the disease (Gibson, Macfarlane, & Cummings, 1993; Gibson, Macfarlane, & Macfarlane, 1993; Rowan et al., 2009). Since the causative agent of the disease is unknown, its sensitivity to antibiotics has not been established. Another important problem with the use of antibiotics for the treatment of UC—disease-causing bacteria may be present on the surface of the epithelium, forming antibiotic-resistant biofilms (Anwar et al., 1990). In addition, it has not been established how antibiotics act on the gut mucous membrane biofilms.

Many drugs (tobramycin, rifaximin, and vancomycin) are not absorbed by the intestine, so their interaction with the mucosal surface has not been investigated. Antibiotics (such as metronidazole), which are well absorbed by the colon, have low concentrations in the intestine, and microorganisms can become resistant to them (Cummings et al., 2003).

Other important problems that cause the development of bacterial resistance to antibiotics are the long-term use of these compounds and their side effects on the human body (Campieri & Gionchetti, 1999; Farrell & LaMont, 2002). The duration of administration of a particular antibiotic and the form of the disease should be considered. Animal studies show that these substances are most effective in the early stages of UC (Farrell & Peppercorn, 2002). In addition, antibiotics adversely affect normal microbiota, disrupting its qualitative and quantitative composition. Therefore the use of probiotics is more effective for the prevention and treatment of intestinal disorders (Cummings et al., 2003). For the therapeutic purpose, they correct the gut microbiota by removing sulfate from the diet and by populating methanogenic, lactic acid bacteria, purifying it from hydrogen sulfide (Rowan et al., 2009).

Probiotics are drugs based on living microorganisms that support bowel homeostasis by normalizing the composition of microbiota. They contain beneficial bacteria or yeast, most often lactic acid bacteria (of the genus *Bifidobacterium*, *Lactobacillus*, and *Streptococcus*) (Kruis et al., 1997; Rembacken et al., 1999; Venturi et al., 1999).

The effect of probiotics on the emergence and development of UC in humans is extensively investigated. In particular, they study the effect of a drug consisting of three species of bifidobacteria, four lactobacilli and streptococci (Venturi et al., 1999). This probiotic was supplemented with food for people with UC in remission for 12 months. Patients were prescribed 6 g of probiotic per day containing 5×10^{11} cells/g of the drug. As a result of microbiological analysis of feces, the number of bacteria of the genus *Bifidobacterium*, *Lactobacillus*, and *Streptococcus* was increased by several orders of magnitude throughout the time of application. The number of other types of gut bacteria, such as *Clostridium*, *Bacteroides*, and *Enterobacteriaceae*, did not change significantly. Fifteen out of 20 people were diagnosed with disease severity and improved health status while four of them experienced relapses. This probiotic was subsequently used in other studies to treat pochitis. Seventeen out of 20 patients observed remission for 9 months with a probiotic. These individuals did not find any recurrence (Campieri & Gionchetti, 1999, 2001). In the colon biopsies of patients with pochitis, the number of lactobacilli decreased (Fabia et al., 1993).

Lactobacilli have been shown to prevent colitis in IL-10 mice (Kennedy et al., 2000; Madsen et al., 1999). They also reduce the risk of colitis induced by acetic acid or methotrexate in rats (Fabia et al., 1993; Mao et al., 1996). *Lactobacillus plantarum* 229V was used for the prophylactic and treatment of acute colitis of IL-10 mice. Studies have shown that the probiotic attenuates the inflammatory process, causing a decrease in the intestinal mucosal IgG concentration. *L. plantarum* bacteria have also been shown to exert a protective function in the gut during the development of colitis in IL-10 mice (Kennedy, 2001, 2002; Schultz et al., 2002).

In the intestines of people with UC, less lactobacilli and bifidobacteria are found than in healthy subjects. These bacteria are thought to perform a protective function and prevent the appearance of UC (Ruseler-van Embden et al., 1994). The microbiological and immunological mechanisms of action of probiotics during UC have been poorly studied. Probiotics can reduce the risk of UC (Cummings et al., 2003).

Therefore for the treatment of colitis antibiotics are used, which affect the anaerobic the intestinal microorganisms. The combination of some antibiotics (vancomycin and imipenem) is more effective. The most commonly used metronidazole, clindamycin, and ciprofloxacin. Concomitant use of vancomycin and imipenem is also effective. They are active against anaerobic microorganisms as well as Gram-positive bacteria. Antibiotic therapy does not always prevent the onset or improvement of the disease. The use of probiotics in the treatment and prevention of colitis helps to normalize the gut microbiota, facilitate the course of the disease, and reduce the risk of its occurrence.

4.4 Modification of intestinal microbiome

Although IBDs are not caused by foods, such as various allergic or enzyme-deficient diseases, a patient with IBDs finds that some foods can worsen symptoms. It is therefore important to maintain a healthy and soothing diet that helps alleviate symptoms, replace lost nutrients, and promote healing. In principle, IDBs reduce the body's ability to absorb proteins, fats, carbohydrates, water, vitamins, and minerals. Due to the diseased mucosa, it is advisable to consume soft and delicate nonspicy foods and foods rich in fiber. In the case of reduced tolerance to lactose, it is appropriate to limit the intake of dairy products (Lynch & Hsu, 2021). As indicated above, the intestinal microbiome has a great influence on the origin and development of IBDs. Antibacterial chemotherapeutics can eliminate unwanted bacterial colonization of the intestines, but then it is necessary to ensure replanting with a suitable nonpathogenic good microbiome (Alam et al., 2020; Albenberg et al., 2012; Asha & Khalil, 2020; De Musis et al., 2020; Jampílek & Králová, 2020; Jampílek et al., 2019; Khan et al., 2019; Ni et al., 2017; Nishida et al., 2018).

Probiotics, prebiotics, and synbiotics, which are becoming increasingly popular, can be used to restore or maintain a suitable microbiome. Probiotics are live nonpathogenic bacteria that are administered to colonize the large intestine and thus improve the microbial balance of the intestines. Strong probiotic cultures of microorganisms in the intestines inhibit the growth of unwanted pathogenic microorganisms, improve intestinal function, maintain proper pH and digestion of nutrient absorption, regulate body fat storage, have anticarcinogenic and immunostimulatory properties, are able to synthesize some bioactive fatty acids, some vitamins, and enzymes, have positive effect on some allergies and diseases, and improve the condition of chronic diseases (Carvalho et al., 2021; Cosme-Silva et al., 2021; Hao et al., 2021; Kechagia et al., 2013).

The most common strains of probiotic bacteria include *Lactobacillus* spp. (e.g., *L. acidophilus*, *L. brevis*, *L. casei*, *L. debrueckii*, *L. fermentum*, *L. lactis*, *L. paracasei*, *L. reuteri*, *L. rhamnosus*, *L. salivarius*, and others), *Bifidobacterium* sp. (e.g., *B. breve*, *B. bifidum*, *B. infantis*, *B. lactis*, *B. longum*, *B. thermophilus*), *Bacillus coagulans*, and *Streptococcus thermophilus* and the yeast species *Saccharomyces cerevisiae* var. *boulardii* (Banfi et al., 2021; Wilkins & Sequoia, 2017). It is necessary to distinguish between probiotic preparations and foods that contain probiotics naturally. The exact composition of the genera and strains of bacteria is known about probiotic preparations and thus their suitable optimal daily dosage is known. The preparations are adapted so that probiotic microorganisms survive in the most abundant number of stomach acids and are able to colonize the intestines. On the other hand, foods that naturally contain probiotics are fermented foods and beverages (e.g., kefir, yogurt, cheese, kimchi, and sauerkraut). The exact composition of probiotic microorganisms is not known. These are often home-made products and so may contain "wild" types of bacteria. The optimal daily dose is not known. There must be many probiotic bacteria in these foods to have a chance that at least some will survive the adverse effects of the stomach environment. On the other hand, preservatives may be present in these foods, which can completely suppress the activity of probiotic microorganisms and the food will lose its probiotic significance (Gunzburg et al., 2020; Marco et al., 2021; Terpou et al., 2019).

Prebiotics are "food" for intestinal bacteria. Thus a prebiotic is a product of a diet or dietary supplement that can induce the growth or activity of beneficial microorganisms. These are undigested fiber or other foods that contain indigestible oligosaccharides. Prebiotic fiber is found in many foods that are consumed daily, such as garlic, onions, bananas, Jerusalem artichokes, apple peels, beans, and other legumes (Asha & Khalil, 2020; Durazzo et al., 2020; Jampílek & Kráľová, 2020; Marco et al., 2021; Markowiak & Ślizewska, 2017; Rashidinejad et al., 2020).

Synbiotics are food ingredients or dietary supplements combining probiotics and prebiotics in the form of synergism. This "synbiotic concept" of a mixture of probiotics and prebiotics favorably affects the host, improves survival and facilitates the implantation of living "good" microbial organisms into the gastrointestinal tract. The Food and Agriculture Organization of the United Nations recommends that the term "synbiotic" be used only if the net health benefits are synergistic (Agnes et al., 2021; Asha & Khalil, 2020; González-Herrera et al., 2021; Jampílek & Kráľová, 2020; Johnson-Henry et al., 2016; Markowiak & Ślizewska, 2017; Newman & Arshad, 2020; Pandey et al., 2015; Pineiro et al., 2008; Salmerón, 2017).

Since these SRB can develop antimicrobial resistance toward the drugs, including antibiotics and antimicrobial agents, bacteriophages could represent an additional potential effective treatment. Since SRB can have a significant adverse influence on industry as well as on humans and animals health, phage treatment of SRB can be seen as a possible effective method of SRB inhibition. However, there are relatively few studies concerning the influence of phages on SRB strains. The current search for alternatives to chemical biocides and antibiotics has led to the renewed interest in phages as antibacterial biocontrol and therapeutic agents, including their use against SRB. Hence, phages might represent a promising treatment against SRB in the future (Kushkevych, Dordević, Vítězová, et al., 2021).

4.4.1 Probiotics

As mentioned above, probiotics have become an important part of IBD therapy (Bartlett et al., 2020; Jakubczyk et al., 2020; Picardo et al., 2020; Puvvada et al., 2020; Tarasiuk & Eibl, 2020; Yoshimatsu et al., 2021; Yue et al., 2020; Zheng & Wen, 2021) or an important dietary supplement to prevent the development of IBD (Caminero & Pinto-Sanchez, 2020; Glassner et al., 2020; Shafiee et al., 2021; Malinowski et al., 2020; Oka & Sartor, 2020; Picardo et al., 2020; Yan & Li, 2020; Yan & Polk, 2020). It should be added here that the influence of the intestinal microflora on mental and psychiatric disorders, bone and musculoskeletal disorders, respiratory problems and cancer has recently been studied (Ali et al., 2020; Bosi et al., 2020; Cardoneanu et al., 2021; Galan-Ros et al., 2020; Liu, Tran, et al., 2021; Salvo et al., 2020; Sandes et al., 2020; Singhvi et al., 2020; Thomann et al., 2020; Trivedi & Barve, 2020). A very important aspect of the whole probiotic approach is the correct selection of probiotic cultures suitable for minimizing the manifestations of IBD (De Musis et al., 2020; Ghosh et al., 2020; LeBlanc et al., 2020; Meng et al., 2020;

Tan et al., 2020) and the associated understanding of the mechanisms of the effects of probiotic cultures on the prevention or suppression of the symptoms and course of IBD. Papers describing the effects of dietary probiotics on the intestine were published recently, for example, by Ahn et al. (2020), Eveno et al. (2021), Jadhav et al. (2020), Pujo et al. (2020), and Plaza-Diaz et al. (2019).

It is important to mention briefly a slightly different approach than the administration of classical probiotic cultures. Fecal microflora transplantation (FMT) has emerged in recent years as one of the possible and very remarkable therapies for UC (de Fatima Caldeira et al., 2020; Glassner et al., 2020; Kim & Gluck, 2019; Oka & Sartor, 2020; Yan & Li, 2020; Zheng & Wen, 2021). In 11 of 12 selected patients with moderate-to-severe UC who received several FMTs and were followed for 52 weeks, a significant clinical response was observed based on colonoscopy images of the patients. However, 6 patients relapsed within 52 weeks after remission with a recurrence rate of 54.5%. Four of the six relapsed patients received FMT again, but the effectiveness of postrelapse FMT was significantly lower than that of the original FMT. But compared to the overall condition of UC before starting FMT treatment, the severity of UC was lower. It can be concluded that FMT can be used for UC therapy (Dang et al., 2020).

4.4.1.1 Effect of probiotics on UC

Statistical analysis of 21 clinical studies comparing the effects of probiotics and placebo in patients with UC showed a significant difference in clinical outcomes. Probiotics significantly reduced the levels of IL-1β, TNF-α, and IL-8. Patients taking probiotics or synbiotics also had a significant reduction in the need for systemic steroids, hospitalization, surgery, as well as histological scores and disease activity index (DAI). In addition, probiotics have improved the condition of patients with Crohn's disease (Darb Emamie et al., 2021).

The mechanism of action of *B. bifidum* ATCC 29521 in a UC-induced DSS model in male C57JBL/6 mice was studied by Din et al. (2020). Probiotics were administered orally at a concentration of 2×10^8 CFU/day. *B. bifidum* restored intestinal damage by regulating the expression of immune markers and tight junction proteins, increased the expression of reactive oxygen species (ROS)-uptake enzymes (SOD1, SOD2, CAT, and GPX2), antiinflammatory cytokines (IL-10, PPAR-γ, IL-6), and tight junction proteins (ZO-1, MUC2, Claudin-3, and E cadherin-1), and decreased TNF-α and IL-1β production. Inflammatory markers appeared to be regulated by the miRNA-associated nuclear subunit P65 NF-κB. Similar molecular-biological manifestations of the benefit of probiotically active species of *Enterococcus faecium*, *L. acidophilus*, *L. rhamnosus*, *B. bifidum*, and *B. longum* were found by Utku et al. (2020) in a large in vivo experiment with TNBS-induced colitis in female Wistar-Albino rats. Ghavami et al. (2020) exposed human dendritic cells (DCs) derived from monocytes of IBD patients to four probiotic strains of *L. salivarius*, *B. bifidum*, *B. coagulans*, and *Bacillus subtilisnatto*. It was found that CD80 and CD86 were induced by most probiotic strains in patients with UC, while only *B. bifidumin*-induced expression of CD80 and CD86 in patients with Crohn's disease. IL-10 and TGF-β production was increased regardless of dose and bacterial species, while Toll-like receptor (TLR) expression was decreased by all bacteria tested except *B. bifidumin* DC from UC patients. The expression of TLR-4 and TLR-9 was significantly downregulated, while the integrin ss8 was significantly increased in DCs from Crohn's disease patients. IL-12p40 expression was significantly downregulated only in DCs from Crohn's disease patients. These results highlight the beneficial effects of probiotics on DC immunomodulation and show the mechanism of action at the molecular-biological level.

One study evaluated the benefit of a probiotic culture of *E. coli* Nissle 1917 in a DSS-induced model of chronic colitis in mice (Souza et al., 2020). Germfree (GF) and conventional (CV) mice were used as model organisms. CV female mice were used for clinical, immunological, and permeable experiments. GF mice were used for the FMT assay. For probiotic therapy, mice were dosed with 9.0 log CFU/day. On day 10, colitis was induced. *E. coli* Nissle showed beneficial effects when prevented. The development of DAI showed a significant difference in the remission period after the first two cycles of DSS and during the third. The reduction in bacterial translocation after probiotic treatment indicated protection of the intestinal barrier. Mucosal maintenance, restoration of secretory immunoglobulin A levels and decreased levels of IL-5, IL-13, tumor necrosis factor (TNF), and interferon (IFN)-γ levels have been observed in association with *E. coli* Nissle treatment. Composition analysis showed variation of the intestinal microbiota between the control and colitis groups. Following stool transplantation with GF mice, it has been observed that treatment of *E. coli* Nissle in CV mice can lead to modulated intestinal microbiota. This was observed indirectly in the reduced daily DAI when the colitis was compared to the treated group. Finally, *E. coli* Nissle presented beneficial effects in this model, suggesting its usefulness for the treatment of UC (Souza et al., 2020).

The influence of probiotics and their mechanisms of action on the alleviation of IBD and other chronic diseases such as arthritis was also discussed in a review by Kazemi et al. (2020) and by Dore et al. (2020).

4.4.1.2 Probiotic species

Researchers have tested the anti-IBD activity of various probiotics containing *L. fermentum* CECT5716, *L. salivarius* CECT5713, *E. coli* Nissle 1917, and *S. cerevisiae* var. *boulardii* CNCMI-745 in dinitrobenzenesulfonic acid-induced UC mice (Algieri et al., 2021). Probiotics were administered for 25 days and were found to alleviate UC-associated dysbiosis and also to show intestinal antiinflammatory effects. Of the probiotic species tested, *Lactobacillus fermentum* CECT5716 was the most active and the second was *E. coli* Nissle 1917. The results of an in vitro test in a model of intestinal inflammation of Caco-2 and HT-29-MTX cells stimulated with proinflammatory IL-1β, TNF-α, IFN-γ, and lipopolysaccharide (LPS) showed that *Faecalibacterium prausnitzii*, *Roseburia intestinalis*, and *Bacteroides faecis* are able to restore damaged epithelium (Mohebali et al., 2020). However, *Firmicutes* and *Bacteroidetes* are the two most important bacterial strains in the gastrointestinal tract and *Firmicutes/Bacteroidetes* ratio affects the proper bowel function, with an increased or decreased *Firmicutes/Bacteroidetes* ratio being considered dysbiosis. An increased *Firmicutes/Bacteroidetes* ratio occurs in obesity, while a decreased *Firmicutes/Bacteroidetes* ratio in IBD. Thus orally administered probiotics may contribute to the restoration of dysbiotic microbiota and to the prevention of obesity or IBD. The most commonly tested probiotics for adjusting the F/B ratio and treating obesity and IBD are from the genus *Lactobacillus* (Stojanov et al., 2020).

4.4.1.2.1 *Lactobacillus* strains

The protective effects of the three *Lactobacillus* sp. in rats with LPS-induced CU were evaluated by Chorawala et al. (2021). *L. casei*, *L. acidophilus*, and *L. rhamnosus* (10^6 CFU/day) were administered to rats for 21 days and it was found that there was a significant improvement in the severity of UC by stopping weight loss, reducing the incidence of diarrhea and bleeding, improved food intake, and weight gain. Microscopically, the colonic mucosa healed. The treatment also reduced the levels of markers of inflammatory and oxidative stress and strengthened the antioxidant molecule. Another study evaluated *Lactobacillus* spp. in their benefit of alleviating UC symptoms in a DSS-induced Balb/c mouse model. *L. plantarum* 03 and 06, *L. brevis* 02, and *L. rhamnosus* 01a significantly prevented the shortening of the colon length and reduced DAI values (Hasannejad-Bibalan et al., 2020). Researchers also studied the benefit of *L. reuteri* R28 and *L. plantarum* AR17-1 strains in mice with DSS-induced UC. *L. plantarum* AR17-1 was found to significantly reduce colitis by reducing the levels of the proinflammatory cytokines TNF-α, IL-1β, and IL-6 (Wang et al., 2021). Evaluation of the effects of probiotics on DSS-induced UC in mice showed that *L. plantarum* AR113 and *L. casei* AR342 were two to threefold more effective than other strains in terms of alleviating indicators of epithelial damage, improving colon length and maintaining the integrity of the epithelial barrier (Xia et al., 2020). Treatment decreased the level of TNF-α, IL-1β, and IL-6 and, conversely, increased the antiinflammatory cytokine IL-10. The antiinflammatory effect of probiotics is associated with increased HO-1 expression and decreased expression of the TLR-4/MyD88/NF-κB pathway in mouse colon tissues.

Oral administration for 5 days of 10^9 CFU/mL *L. plantarum* DF68 resulted in a significant improvement in UC correlated with attenuation of macroscopic bowel damage, histopathological changes and a high significant decrease ($P < .001$) in *Enterobacteriaceae* in the intestine of Balb/c mice with DSS-induced colitis (Kefif et al., 2020). The anti-UC activity and mechanism of action of *L. plantarum* CBT LP3 was studied in vivo in DSS-induced mouse colitis. Administration of *L. plantarum* significantly improved the overall histopathological status of UC, modified the regulatory effect of T cells and helper type 2 T cells, and reduced the level of proinflammatory cytokines. These findings suggest that *L. plantarum* CBT LP3 can be used as a potent immunomodulator to alleviate IBD (Kim et al., 2020).

Further study determined a suitable strain of *L. casei* that has mitigating effects on IBD (Liu et al., 2021). Of the 29 *L. casei* strains tested, based on in vitro and in vivo tests in mice with induced colitis, it was found that only *L. casei* M2S01 alleviated UC by restoring a healthy intestinal microbiome composition. This strain restored body weight, reduced DAI and promoted the expression of antiinflammatory cytokines. *L. casei* LH23 inhibited the production of nitric oxide and inflammatory factors in the LPS-induced inflammation of the RAW264.7 cell line and DSS-induced UC in mice. This beneficial effect was manifested in the inactivation of the JNK/p38 signaling pathway, decreased number of macrophages (CD11b(+)F4/80(+)) and secretion of inflammatory cytokines, decreased myeloperoxidase activity, increased excretion of CD3(+), CD4(+), CD25(+) regulatory T cells, and restored the level of histone H3K9 acetylation in colon tissues (Liu, Ding, et al., 2020).

Administration of *L. reuteri* I5007 has been shown to be effective in suppressing DSS-induced UC in mice: compared with the control group, it prevented weight loss, colon length shortening, histopathological damage, restored mucus, and reduced levels of proinflammatory cytokines. In addition, *L. reuteri* I5007 modulates the intestinal microflora and metabolic structural and functional composition (Wang et al., 2020).

L. rhamnosus LDTM 7511 derived from Korean infant droppings showed a greater decrease in inflammatory mediator secretion and overall intestinal microbiota modification in a mouse model of UC induced by DSS compared to *L. rhamnosus* ATCC 53103, which is used for IBD studies (Yeo et al., 2020). The product of *L. rhamnosus* GG is the soluble protein HM0539, which has significant protective effects against UC in a mouse model. The protein reduced cyclooxygenase-2 (COX-2) and nitric oxide synthase (iNOS) levels, thus inhibiting the production of prostaglandin E2 (PGE2) and nitric oxide (NO) and inhibiting the production of NF-κB-associated inflammatory mediators (Li, Yang, et al., 2020). Molecular-biological mechanism of action of probiotics based on *L. rhamnosus* GG or *B. longum* spp. *infantis* S12 on intestinal epithelial cells was investigated by Huang et al. (2020). The benefit of *L. rhamnosus* 1.0320 in combination with inulin was evaluated in a BALB/c mouse model of UC induced by DSS. This combination had significantly better effects than administration of each component alone; significantly attenuated DSS-induced UC, decreased DAI, decreased myeloperoxidase activity, increased hemoglobin, and regulated the expression levels of the cytokines IL-1β, IL-6, TNF-α, and IL-10. In addition, this combination increased the diversity of the microflora and the number of beneficial bacteria (Liu, Liu, et al., 2020).

Treatment of C57BL/6 mice with azoxymethane and DDS-induced intestinal damage with *L. bulgaricus* was found to attenuate the clinical signs of UC by reducing IL-6, TNF-α, IL-17, IL-23 and IL-1β levels and also occurred to inhibit induced colon cancer (Silveira et al., 2020). In vitro and in vivo studies have shown that *L. jensenii* TL2937 suppresses the acute inflammatory response elicited by the activation of TLR-4. In a DSS-induced UC model in BALB/c mice, Sato, Garcia-Castillo, et al. (2020) found that mice-fed *L. jensenii* TL2937 had lower myeloperoxidase activity, lower production of proinflammatory substances (TNF-α, IL-1, CXCL1, MCP-1, IL-15, and IL-17), and higher levels of immunoregulatory (IL-10 and IL-27) cytokines. Thus *L. jensenii* TL2937 protects against UC. A probiotic containing *L. alimentarius* NKUSS6 and iron was tested for its ability to increase iron by its increased absorption after oral administration from the intestines of DSS-induced UC in mice. In addition to increasing the concentration of iron in the body, oral administration of *L. alimentarius* NKU556-Fe remarkably increased the expression of tight junction proteins and effectively reduced proinflammatory cytokines as well as oxidative stress, leading to a reduction in UC (Zhao et al., 2020).

4.4.1.2.2 Bifidobacterium strains

Using an in vitro porcine intestinal epithelial cell immunoassay system and DSS for UC simulation, Sato, Yuzawa, et al. (2020) demonstrated that *B. breve* M-16V and *B. longum* BB536 are able to regulate the intracellular C-jun-N-terminal kinase signaling pathway, thereby reducing DSS-induced changes in the epithelial barrier in vitro and regulating the inflammatory response by reducing the levels of proinflammatory factors, such as TNF-α and IL-1α. Zhou et al. (2019) investigated the protective effects of *B. infantis* in a DSS-induced BALB/c mouse model of colitis. *B. infantis* stopped weight loss, decreased DAI and histological damage scores, increased Foxp3 protein and cytokine IL-10 and TGF-β1 expression, and increased PD-L1 expression. *B. infantis* thus alleviated intestinal damage to UC and may therefore have potential therapeutic value for mitigating the consequences of UC.

In vitro studies testing the potential of *B. animalis*, *L. acidophilus* subsp. *lactis*, or a combination thereof were performed on HT-29 cells treated with LPS and TNF. Both species showed the ability to attenuate UC, but only a combination showed the strongest anti-UC activity by modulating TLR2-mediated NF-κB and MAPK signaling pathways in inflammatory intestinal epithelial cells (Li et al., 2019). Zhang, Guan, et al. (2021) conducted an extensive review of randomized controlled trials and confirmed that probiotic supplements (probiotics, prebiotics, and synbiotics) could help increase the number of *Bifidobacterium* in the intestinal tract of IBD patients; the UC activity index was statistically significantly ($P < .05$) reduced. A dose of $10^{10}-10^{12}$ CFU of *Lactobacillus* and *Bifidobacterium* per day may be the reference range for the use of probiotics to relieve IBD. Leccese et al. (2020) studied how *Lactobacillus* and *Bifidobacterium* strains affect UC and Crohn's disease. Both strains significantly reduced LF82 adhesion and persistence in HT-29 intestinal epithelial cells, inhibited IL-8 secretion, significantly reduced LF82 and DC survival of LF82, and reduced polarizing cytokine secretion in UC patients. It is important to note, however, that in patients with Crohn's disease, only *B. breve* Bbr8 reduced the persistence of LF82 in DCs.

4.4.1.2.3 *Bacillus* strains

Administration of *B. subtilis* caused a significant increase in body weight and decreased the DAI in the group of DSS-induced CU mice compared to the control group. Better epithelial integrity was also found and ZO-1 and occludin levels increased. The intestinal microbioma was also corrected, with a decrease in *Escherichia*, *Shigella* and *Enterococcus* strains and a significant increase in *Akkermansia*. Thus it can be concluded that long-term administration of *B. subtilis* could protect intestinal epithelial cells and adjust the presence of intestinal microorganisms (Liu, Yin, et al., 2021).

Administration of milk with *B. subtilis* JNFE0126 significantly reduced the index of IBD activity in IBD mice induced by DSS. In addition, intestinal mucosa began to heal by proliferating intestinal stem cells and inhibiting the secretion of proinflammatory cytokines (Zhang, Tong, et al., 2021). *B. subtilis* RZ001 upregulated the in vitro expression of MUC2 (the major component of intestinal mucus) and tight junction proteins in HT-29 cells. Oral administration of *B. subtilis* RZ001 to DDS-induced colitis mice significantly reduced weight loss, reduced shortening of colon length, overproduction of proinflammatory factors, and increased goblet cell counts and MUC2 and tight junction protein levels. The new probiotic strain *B. subtilis* RZ001 thus has the potential to become effective in alleviating UC (Li, Zhang, et al., 2020). Oral administration of *B. subtilis* HH2 to rabbits with IBD-induced using TNBS caused a reduction in weight loss, a reduction in histological damage and a decrease in TNF-α and IL-1β expression, and conversely an increase in IL-10 expression. *B. subtilis* HH2 also improved tight junctions of intestinal cells. In addition, *B. subtilis* HH2 caused an improvement in the microbial diversity of the colon; the proportion of the family *Bifidobacteriaceae* increased, and the amount of *Bacteroidetes* and *Proteobacteria* decreased (Luo et al., 2020).

The beneficial effects of Vivomixx^R (combination of *S. thermophilus*, *L. casei*, *B. breve*, *B. animalis* subsp. *lactis*) supplemented with *B. subtilis* were tested in a DSS-induced mouse UC model. The addition of *B. subtilis* to the commercial probiotic Vivomixx^R improved the effects of bacterial therapy, reduced UC symptoms, and decreased the expression of proinflammatory mediators (IL-6 and TNF-α) (Biagioli et al., 2020). MegaDuo containing *B. coagulans* SC208 and *B. subtilis* HU58 also had a similar effect on reduced intestinal membrane damage and reduced TNF-α and IL-6 levels in the UC model (Marzorati et al., 2020). Researchers performed an in vivo study on 42 acetic acid-induced UC rats treated with MegaSporeBiotic (MSB; 10^9 *Bacillus* sp. CFU/day) and MegaMucosa (MM; 70 mg/100 g/day) (Catinean et al., 2020). Treatment with MSB or MM alone and in combination significantly reduced inflammation and damage to the colonic mucosa. Treatment with these substances led to a reduction in proinflammatory cytokines and oxidative stress.

Spores of *B. megaterium* SF185 human isolate have antioxidant activity on Caco-2 cells exposed to hydrogen peroxide and in a mouse model of DSS-induced UC. In both model systems, the spores act as a protective state due to their cleansing: on the cells, the spores reduce the amount of intracellular ROS, while in vivo spore pretreatment protects mice from chemically induced damage. The results thus show that the treatment of *B. megaterium* SF185 spores prevents or reduces intestinal damage caused by oxidative stress, suggesting the use of spores of this strain as new probiotics (Mazzoli et al., 2019).

4.4.1.2.4 Other species

Akkermansia muciniphila ATCC BAA-835 with beneficial effects on obesity and diabetes was investigated by (Zhai et al., 2019) for the activity in alleviating IBD on DSS-induced chronic colitis in mice. Both *A. muciniphila* ATCC BAA-835 and *A. muciniphila* 139 (isolated from mice) showed in vivo effects on chronic colitis because they improved clinical parameters including colonic inflammatory index and histological findings. They also reduced the levels of proinflammatory cytokines, including TNF-α and IFN-γ. The antiinflammatory effects of the ATCC strain were stronger than strain 139. However, both strains equally normalized intestinal microbiots, but only the ATCC strain increased the production of SCFAs. It was found that while in the healthy population the colonization of *A. muciniphilais* is 48.8%, in patients with UC or Crohn's disease the colonization is significantly lower ($P < .01$). Subsequently washed microbiota transplantation of *Akkermansia*–*F. prausnitzii* in patients with IBD resulted in a clinical response in 53.7% of patients, thus reducing the incidence of IBD. It can be stated that the effectiveness of *Akkermansia* transplantation was closely correlated with the improvement of IBD (Zhang et al., 2020).

Five strains of *Parabacteroides* distasonis isolated from human adult and neonatal intestinal microflora were tested in vivo in an acute mouse model of UC for their immunomodulatory ability and ability to strengthen the intestinal barrier. In general, the beneficial activities were highly strain dependent: two strains showed strong antiinflammatory potential and restored the intestinal barrier, while the third strain restored the epithelial barrier. Some strains activated DCs to induce regulatory T cells from naive CD4(+) T cells. Unfortunately, after oral administration, it is necessary to protect the strains from adverse conditions in the stomach. Thus this study expands bacterial strains useful as probiotics (Cuffaro et al., 2020).

Pediococcus pentosaceus LI05 was administered orally once daily for 14 days to mice with DSS-induced colitis and was found to alleviate colitis, reduce the body weight loss, DAI scores, colon length shortening, modify intestinal permeability, and reduce the expression of proinflammatory cytokines. In addition, it significantly improved the composition of the intestinal microflora and caused increased production of SCFAs (Bian et al., 2020). LS 174 T goblet cells and rats with DSS-induced colitis were used to investigate the stimulation of mucin production (expression of MUC2) induced by *Propionibacterium freudenreichii* in vitro and in vivo. Following administration of *P. freudenreichii* culture supernatant, mRNA and mucin expression levels increased in LS 174 cells. Both supernatant and live *P. freudenreichii* decreased DAI in colitis rats and decreased the levels of proinflammatory cytokines and to improve histological findings (Ma et al., 2020).

A recent review has summarized the mechanisms responsible for the probiotic properties of *S. cerevisiae* var. *boulardii* CNCMI-745, such as the adhesion and elimination of enteropathogenic microorganisms and their toxins, extracellular cleavage of virulent pathogen factors, and trophic and antiinflammatory effects on the intestinal mucosa (Kaźmierczak-Siedlecka et al., 2020). The yeast is effective in treating or preventing *Helicobacter pylori* infections, diarrhea (*Clostridium difficile* infection, antibiotic-related diarrhea, and passenger diarrhea), IBDs, irritable bowel syndrome, candidiasis, dyslipidemia, and bacterial overgrowth of the small intestine in patients with multiple sclerosis. It can be stated that yeast is a widely available and safe probiotic strain.

4.4.2 Synbiotics

Bruguiera gymnorrhiza (*Rhizophoraceae*) is a tall tree growing in wet areas of the coast, where it reaches tidal seawater and forms mangroves. The species is widespread along the tropical coast of the Indian Ocean and the western part of the Pacific Ocean, where it is one of the most common tree species. Its fruits are used to treat diarrhea and also to treat UC in folk medicine. *B. gymnorrhiza* fruit is rich in pinitol and thus has strong antioxidant activity. In a model of DSS-induced colitis, fetuses effectively reduced the body weight loss and DAI, restored colon length, and improved the overall histological profile of the disease. In addition, fetal consumption decreased MDA, TNF-α, IL-6, IL-1β, and IFN-γ levels, increased IL-10 levels, and also prevented SOD and GSH depletion. Fetal consumption also increased protein levels in nuclear Nrf2 and mRNA levels in GCLC, GCLM, HO-1. and NQO1, while significantly inhibiting Keap1 and cytosolic Nrf2 protein expression. In addition, fruit consumption promoted the growth of *Bifidobacterium*, *Anaerotruncus*, and *Lactobacillus* in the gut and inhibited the growth of pathogenic bacteria of the genus *Bacteroides* and *Streptococcus*. This study provides evidence that the application of *B. gymnorrhiza* fruits may be a promising candidate in alleviating UC (Lin et al., 2020).

Lonicera japonica Thunb. (*Caprifoliaceae*) is a traditional Chinese herb used to treat IBD. In addition to the direct antiinflammatory effect, the polysaccharides extracted from this plant also had a beneficial effect on promoting the growth of *Bifidobacterium* sp. and *Lactobacilli* sp. and on the other hand antagonized pathogenic bacteria (*E. coli* and *Enterococcus*) (Zhou et al., 2021). Tea (*Camellia sinensis* L. or *Thea sinensis*, family *Theaceae*) flower polysaccharides (TFPS) have proven to be interesting prebiotics supporting the growth of probiotic cultures. In an in vitro test, the feces of IBD patients with microflora poor in good bacteria after 24 h of fermentation with TFPS under anaerobic conditions showed significant changes in microbial composition. The number of *Escherichia/Shigella*, *Enterococcus*, *Collinsella*, *Lactobacillus*, and *Bifidobacterium* species increased, while *Enterobacter*, *Streptococcus*, *Bacteroides*, *Clostridium*, *Megasphaera*, *Roseburia*, *Granulicatella*, *Akkermansia*, and *Fusobacterium* decreased. The amount of SCFAs also increased (Chen et al., 2020).

ColikindGocce® synbiotic preparation consisting of a fixed combination of *L. reuteri* DSM 25175 (2×10^9 CFU/mL), *L. acidophilus* DSM 24936 (2×10^9 CFU/mL), *Chamomilla recutita* L. oleolite (10 mg/mL), and organic extra virgin olive oil (7 mL) was evaluated on LPS-stimulated CaCo-2 cell colitis. The results showed that the preparation is able to prevent damage to the intestinal barrier function and reduce the expression of proinflammatory TNF-α and IL-8 (Borgonetti et al., 2020).

One study evaluated the synergistic effect of probiotics and omega-3 fatty acids (fish oil) on UC-induced DSS in mice (Nithya et al., 2020). The effect of treatment with UC probiotics was 27.15% after administration of organic salmon omega 47.59% and in combination 52.84%, which proves that the administration of omega-3 fatty acids together with probiotics is a suitable therapy for UC.

The synergistic effects of *B. coagulans* MTCC5856 and sugar cane fiber (PSCF) were tested for their ability to improve UC in a model of colitis MUC2 Winnie mice fed a standard diet supplemented with either one of the tested ingredients or a combination thereof for 21 days, which proved to be most effective in modulation of the overall immune profile; there was an improvement in clinical signs and histopathological findings (Shinde, Vemuri, et al., 2020). In addition, Shinde, Perera, et al. (2020) tested the probiotic efficacy of *B. coagulans* MTCC5856 in synbiotic combination with green banana-resistant starch (GBRS) to alleviate DSS-induced colitis in mice. It has been found that the combination of both components contributes significantly to the control of the disease. Synbiotic supplementation attenuated UC markers (a decrease of 67% and 94%, respectively) more than administration of *B. coagulans* (a decrease of 52% and 58%, respectively) or GBRS (a decrease of 57% and 26%, respectively) alone. In addition, the synbiotic effects represented a significant (up to 40%) decrease in IL-1β and an increase (by 29%) in IL-10 and an increase in the production of SCFAs, which was not induced by *B. coagulans* alone. Thus it can be stated that such synbiotic supplementation of *B. coagulans* and GBRS is effective in alleviating UC.

4.5 Conclusion

In recent years, the incidence of chronic IBDs especially UC has been rising. Although the pathogenesis of all these diseases is complex and probably involves a combination of various factors, patients usually experience a decrease in the diversity of the intestinal microbiome and its shift to species aggressive to the intestinal mucosa. Extensive research is focused on changing this microbiome, and therefore antibiotics, probiotics, prebiotics, synbiotics and the overall appropriate composition of the diet are studied in this context. Probiotics are gaining more and more popularity among other treatments because many studies have shown that they are effective in reducing intestinal inflammations in vitro and in vivo. Although there is no cure for chronic IBDs today, available drugs reduce intestinal inflammation and help prolong remission and reduce the rate of relapses. However, their side effects preclude their long-term use, so probiotics can be a "light at the end of the tunnel" that the choice of appropriate strains and dosages can reduce the incidence and relapse rates and improve the overall quality of life in such patients.

Acknowledgments

This study was supported by the Grant Agency of Masaryk University (MUNI/A/1425/2020) and by the Slovak Research and Development Agency (project APVV-17-0373).

References

Abdulina, D., Kováč, J., Iutynska, G., & Kushkevych, I. (2020). ATP sulfurylase activity of sulfate-reducing bacteria from various ecotopes. *3 Biotech*, *10*(2), 55. Available from https://doi.org/10.1007/s13205-019-2041-9.

Agnes, A., Puccioni, C., D'Ugo, D., Gasbarrini, A., Biondi, A., & Persiani, R. (2021). The gut microbiota and colorectal surgery outcomes: Facts or hype? A narrative review. *BMC Surgery*, *21*(1). Available from https://doi.org/10.1186/s12893-021-01087-5.

Ahn, S. I., Cho, S., & Choi, N. J. (2020). Effect of dietary probiotics on colon length in an inflammatory bowel disease-induced murine model: A *meta*-analysis. *Journal of Dairy Science*, *103*(2), 1807–1819. Available from https://doi.org/10.3168/jds.2019-17356.

Alam, M. T., Amos, G. C. A., Murphy, A. R. J., Murch, S., Wellington, E. M. H., & Arasaradnam, R. P. (2020). Microbial imbalance in inflammatory bowel disease patients at different taxonomic levels. *Gut Pathogens*, *12*(1). Available from https://doi.org/10.1186/s13099-019-0341-6.

Albenberg, L. G., Lewis, J. D., & Wu, G. D. (2012). Food and the gut microbiota in inflammatory bowel diseases: A critical connection. *Current Opinion in Gastroenterology*, *28*(4), 314–320. Available from https://doi.org/10.1097/MOG.0b013e328354586f.

Algieri, F., Garrido-Mesa, J., Vezza, T., Rodríguez-Sojo, M. J., Rodríguez-Cabezas, M. E., Olivares, M., García, F., Gálvez, J., Morón, R., & Rodríguez-Nogales, A. (2021). Intestinal anti-inflammatory effects of probiotics in DNBS-colitis via modulation of gut microbiota and microRNAs. *European Journal of Nutrition*, *60*(5), 2537–2551. Available from https://doi.org/10.1007/s00394-020-02441-8.

Ali, F., Lui, K., Wang, A., Day, A. S., & Leach, S. T. (2020). The perinatal period, the developing intestinal microbiome and inflammatory bowel diseases: What links early life events with later life disease? *Journal of the Royal Society of New Zealand*, *50*(3), 371–383. Available from https://doi.org/10.1080/03036758.2019.1706586.

Anwar, H., Dasgupta, M. K., & Costerton, J. W. (1990). Testing the susceptibility of bacteria in biofilms to antibacterial agents. *Antimicrobial Agents and Chemotherapy*, *34*(11), 2043–2046. Available from https://doi.org/10.1128/AAC.34.11.2043.

Asha, M. Z., & Khalil, S. F. H. (2020). Efficacy and safety of probiotics, prebiotics and synbiotics in the treatment of irritable bowel syndrome a systematic review and *meta*-analysis. *Sultan Qaboos University Medical Journal*, *20*(1), e13–e24. Available from https://doi.org/10.18295/squmj.2020.20.01.003.

Attene-Ramos, M. S., Wagner, E. D., Gaskins, H. R., & Plewa, M. J. (2007). Hydrogen sulfide induces direct radical-associated DNA damage. *Molecular Cancer Research*, *5*(5), 455–459. Available from https://doi.org/10.1158/1541-7786.MCR-06-0439.

Bamba, T., Matsuda, H., Endo, M., & Fujiyama, Y. (1995). The pathogenic role of Bacteroides vulgatus in patients with ulcerative colitis. *Journal of Gastroenterology*, *30*(8), 45–47.

Banfi, D., Moro, E., Bosi, A., Bistoletti, M., Cerantola, S., Crema, F., Maggi, F., Giron, M. C., Giaroni, C., & Baj, A. (2021). Impact of microbial metabolites on microbiota–gut–brain axis in inflammatory bowel disease. *International Journal of Molecular Sciences*, *22*(4), 1–42. Available from https://doi.org/10.3390/ijms22041623.

Bartlett, A., Gullickson, R. G., Singh, R., Ro, S., & Omaye, S. T. (2020). The link between oral and gut microbiota in inflammatory bowel disease and a synopsis of potential salivary biomarkers. *Applied Sciences (Switzerland)*, *10*(18), 6421. Available from https://doi.org/10.3390/APP10186421.

Barton, L. L., & Hamilton, A. W. (2007). *Sulphate-reducing bacteria: Environmental and engineered systems. Sulphate-reducing bacteria: Environmental and engineered systems* (pp. 1−538). Cambridge University Press. Available from https://doi.org/10.1017/CBO9780511541490.

Baskar, R., Li, L., & Moore, P. K. (2007). Hydrogen sulfide-induces DNA damage and changes in apoptotic gene expression in human lung fibroblast cells. *FASEB Journal*, *21*(1), 247−255. Available from https://doi.org/10.1096/fj.06-6255com.

Biagioli, M., Carino, A., Di Giorgio, C., Marchianò, S., Bordoni, M., Roselli, R., Distrutti, E., & Fiorucci, S. (2020). Discovery of a novel multi-strains probiotic formulation with improved efficacy toward intestinal inflammation. *Nutrients*, *12*(7), 1−20. Available from https://doi.org/10.3390/nu12071945.

Bian, X., Yang, L., Wu, W., Lv, L., Jiang, X., Wang, Q., Wu, J., Li, Y., Ye, J., Fang, D., Shi, D., Wang, K., Wang, Q., Lu, Y., Xie, J., Xia, J., & Li, L. (2020). Pediococcus pentosaceus LI05 alleviates DSS-induced colitis by modulating immunological profiles, the gut microbiota and short-chain fatty acid levels in a mouse model. *Microbial Biotechnology*, *13*(4), 1228−1244. Available from https://doi.org/10.1111/1751-7915.13583.

Borgonetti, V., Cocetta, V., Biagi, M., Carnevali., Governa, P., & Montopoli, M. (2020). Anti-inflammatory activity of a fixed combination of probiotics and herbal extract in an in vitro model of intestinal inflammation by stimulating Caco-2 cells with LPS-conditioned THP-1 cells medium. *Minerva Pediatrica*. Available from https://doi.org/10.23736/S0026-4946.20.05765-5.

Bosi, A., Banfi, D., Bistoletti, M., Giaroni, C., & Baj, A. (2020). Tryptophan metabolites along the microbiota-gut-brain axis: An interkingdom communication system influencing the gut in health and disease. *International Journal of Tryptophan Research*, *13*, 1178646920928984. Available from https://doi.org/10.1177/1178646920928984.

Breznak, J. A., & Switzer, J. M. (1986). Acetate synthesis from H2 plus CO_2 by termite gut microbes. *Applied and Environmental Microbiology*, *52*(4), 623−630. Available from https://doi.org/10.1128/aem.52.4.623-630.1986.

Brigidi, P., Swennen, E., Rizzello, F., Bozzolasco, M., & Matteuzzi, D. (2002). Effects of rifaximin administration on the intestinal microbiota in patients with ulcerative colitis. *Journal of Chemotherapy*, *14*(3), 290−295. Available from https://doi.org/10.1179/joc.2002.14.3.290.

Burke, D. A., & Axon, A. T. (1988). Adhesive Escherichia coli in inflammatory bowel disease and infective diarrhoea. *BMJ (Clinical Research ed.)*, *297*(6641), 102−104. Available from https://doi.org/10.1136/bmj.297.6641.102.

Caminero, A., & Pinto-Sanchez, M. I. (2020). Host immune interactions in chronic inflammatory gastrointestinal conditions. *Current Opinion in Gastroenterology*, *36*(6), 479−484. Available from https://doi.org/10.1097/MOG.0000000000000673.

Campieri, M., & Gionchetti, P. (1999). Probiotics in inflammatory bowel disease: New insight to pathogenesis or a possible therapeutic alternative? *Gastroenterology*, *116*(5), 1246−1249. Available from https://doi.org/10.1016/S0016-5085(99)70029-6.

Campieri, M., & Gionchetti, P. (2001). Bacteria as the cause of ulcerative colitis. *Gut*, *48*(1), 132−135. Available from https://doi.org/10.1136/gut.48.1.132.

Cardoneanu, A., Mihai, C., Rezus, E., Burlui, A., Popa, I., & Cijevschi Prelipcean, C. (2021). Gut microbiota changes in inflammatory bowel diseases and ankylosing spondilytis. *Journal of Gastrointestinal and Liver Diseases*, *30*(1), 46−54. Available from https://doi.org/10.15403/jgld-2823.

Carvalho, F. M., Teixeira-Santos, R., Mergulhão, F. J. M., & Gomes, L. C. (2021). The use of probiotics to fight biofilms in medical devices: A systematic review and *meta*-analysis. *Microorganisms*, *9*(1), 1−26. Available from https://doi.org/10.3390/microorganisms9010027.

Catinean, A., Neag, M. A., Krishnan, K., Muntean, D. M., Bocsan, C. I., Pop, R. M., Mitre, A. O., Melincovici, C. S., & Buzoianu, A. D. (2020). Probiotic bacillus spores together with amino acids and immunoglobulins exert protective effects on a rat model of ulcerative colitis. *Nutrients*, *12*(12), 1−18. Available from https://doi.org/10.3390/nu12123607.

Černý, M., Vítězová, M., Vítěz, T., Bartoš, M., & Kushkevych, I. (2018). Variation in the distribution of hydrogen producers from the Clostridiales order in biogas reactors depending on different input substrates. *Energies*, *11*(12), 3270. Available from https://doi.org/10.3390/en11123270.

Chen, D., Chen, G., Chen, C., Zeng, X., & Ye, H. (2020). Prebiotics effects in vitro of polysaccharides from tea flowers on gut microbiota of healthy persons and patients with inflammatory bowel disease. *International Journal of Biological Macromolecules*, *158*, 968−976. Available from https://doi.org/10.1016/j.ijbiomac.2020.04.248.

Chorawala, M. R., Chauhan, S., Patel, R., & Shah, G. (2021). Cell wall contents of probiotics (Lactobacillus species) protect against lipopolysaccharide (LPS)-induced murine colitis by limiting immuno-inflammation and oxidative stress. *Probiotics and Antimicrobial Proteins*. Available from https://doi.org/10.1007/s12602-020-09738-4.

Christl, S. U., Gibson, G. R., Murgatroyd, P. R., Scheppach, W., & Cummings, J. H. (1993). Impaired hydrogen metabolism in pneumatosis cystoides intestinalis. *Gastroenterology*, *104*(2), 392−397. Available from https://doi.org/10.1016/0016-5085(93)90406-3.

Christl, S. U., Murgatroyd, P. R., Gibson, G. R., & Cummings, J. H. (1992). Production, metabolism, and excretion of hydrogen in the large intestine. *Gastroenterology*, *102*(4), 1269−1277. Available from https://doi.org/10.1016/0016-5085(92)70022-4.

Cohavy, O., Bruckner, D., Gordon, L. K., Misra, R., Wei, B., Eggena, M. E., Targan, S. R., & Braun, J. (2000). Colonic bacteria express an ulcerative colitis pANCA-related protein epitope. *Infection and Immunity*, *68*(3), 1542−1548. Available from https://doi.org/10.1128/IAI.68.3.1542-1548.2000.

Cosme-Silva, L., Dal-Fabbro, R., Cintra, L. T. A., Ervolino, E., Do Prado, A. S., de Oliveira, D. P., de Marcelos, P. G. C. L., & Gomes-Filho, J. E. (2021). Dietary supplementation with multi-strain formula of probiotics modulates inflammatory and immunological markers in apical periodontitis. *Journal of Applied Oral Science*, *29*, e20210483. Available from https://doi.org/10.1590/1678-7757-2020-0483.

Croucher, S. C., Houston, A. P., Bayliss, C. E., & Turner, R. J. (1983). Bacterial populations associated with different regions of the human colon wall. *Applied and Environmental Microbiology*, *45*(3), 1025−1033. Available from https://doi.org/10.1128/aem.45.3.1025-1033.1983.

Cuffaro, B., Assohoun, A. L. W., Boutillier, D., Súkeníková, L., Desramaut, J., Boudebbouze, S., Salomé-Desnoulez, S., Hrdý, J., Waligora-Dupriet, A. J., Maguin, E., & Grangette, C. (2020). In vitro characterization of gut microbiota-derived commensal strains: Selection of parabacteroides distasonis strains alleviating TNBS-induced colitis in mice. *Cells*, *9*(9), 2104. Available from https://doi.org/10.3390/cells9092104.

Cummings, J. H., Macfarlane, G. T., & Macfarlane, S. (2003). Intestinal bacteria and ulcerative colitis. *Current Issues in Intestinal Microbiology, 4*(1), 9–20.

Dang, X. F., Wang, Q.-X., Yin, Z., Sun, L., & Yang, W. H. (2020). Recurrence of moderate to severe ulcerative colitis after fecal microbiota transplantation treatment and the efficacy of re-FMT: A case series. *BMC Gastroenterology, 20*(1), 401. Available from https://doi.org/10.1186/s12876-020-01548-w.

Darb Emamie, A., Rajabpour, M., Ghanavati, R., Asadolahi, P., Farzi, S., Sobouti, B., & Darbandi, A. (2021). The effects of probiotics, prebiotics and synbiotics on the reduction of IBD complications, a periodic review during 2009–2020. *Journal of Applied Microbiology, 130*(6), 1823–1838. Available from https://doi.org/10.1111/jam.14907.

de Fatima Caldeira, L., Borba, H. H., Tonin, F. S., Wiens, A., Fernandez-Llimos, F., & Pontarolo, R. (2020). Fecal microbiota transplantation in inflammatory bowel disease patients: A systematic review and *meta*-analysis. *PLoS One, 15*(9), e0238910. Available from https://doi.org/10.1371/journal.pone.0238910.

De Musis, C., Granata, L., Dallio, M., Miranda, A., Gravina, A. G., & Romano, M. (2020). Inflammatory bowel diseases: The role of gut microbiota. *Current Pharmaceutical Design, 26*(25), 2951–2961. Available from https://doi.org/10.2174/1381612826666200420144128.

Deplancke, B., & Gaskins, H. R. (2001). Microbial modulation of innate defense: Goblet cells and the intestinal mucus layer. *American Journal of Clinical Nutrition, 73*(6), 1131S–1141S. Available from https://doi.org/10.1093/ajcn/73.6.1131s.

Din, A. U., Hassan, A., Zhu, Y., Zhang, K., Wang, Y., Li, T., Wang, Y., & Wang, G. (2020). Inhibitory effect of Bifidobacterium bifidum ATCC 29521 on colitis and its mechanism. *Journal of Nutritional Biochemistry, 79*, 108353. Available from https://doi.org/10.1016/j.jnutbio.2020.108353.

Dore, M. P., Rocchi, C., Longo, N. P., Scanu, A. M., Vidili, G., Padedda, F., & Pes, G. M. (2020). Effect of probiotic use on adverse events in adult patients with inflammatory bowel disease: A retrospective cohort study. *Probiotics and Antimicrobial Proteins, 12*(1), 152–159. Available from https://doi.org/10.1007/s12602-019-9517-0.

Dordević, D., Jančíková, S., Vítězová, M., & Kushkevych, I. (2021). Hydrogen sulfide toxicity in the gut environment: *Meta*-analysis of sulfate-reducing and lactic acid bacteria in inflammatory processes. *Journal of Advanced Research, 27*, 55–69. Available from https://doi.org/10.1016/j.jare.2020.03.003.

Duffy, M., O'Mahony, L., Coffey, J. C., Collins, J. K., Shanahan, F., Redmond, H. P., & Kirwan, W. O. (2002). Sulfate-reducing bacteria colonize pouches formed for ulcerative colitis but not for familial adenomatous polyposis. *Diseases of the Colon and Rectum, 45*(3), 384–388. Available from https://doi.org/10.1007/s10350-004-6187-z.

Durazzo, A., Nazhand, A., Lucarini, M., Atanasov, A. G., Souto, E. B., Novellino, E., Capasso, R., & Santini, A. (2020). An updated overview on nanonutraceuticals: Focus on nanoprebiotics and nanoprobiotics. *International Journal of Molecular Sciences, 21*(7), 2285. Available from https://doi.org/10.3390/ijms21072285.

Eveno, M., Savard, P., Belguesmia, Y., Bazinet, L., Gancel, F., Drider, D., & Fliss, I. (2021). Compatibility, cytotoxicity, and gastrointestinal tenacity of bacteriocin-producing bacteria selected for a consortium probiotic formulation to be used in livestock feed. *Probiotics and Antimicrobial Proteins, 13*(1), 208–217. Available from https://doi.org/10.1007/s12602-020-09687-y.

Fabia, R., Ar'Rajab, A., Johansson, M. L., Andersson, R., Willén, R., Jeppsson, B., Molin, G., & Bengmark, S. (1993). Impairment of bacterial flora in human ulcerative colitis and experimental colitis in the rat. *Digestion, 54*(4), 248–255. Available from https://doi.org/10.1159/000201045.

Farrell, R. J., & LaMont, J. T. (2002). Microbial factors in inflammatory bowel disease. *Gastroenterology Clinics of North America, 31*(1), 41–62. Available from https://doi.org/10.1016/S0889-8553(01)00004-8.

Farrell, R. J., & Peppercorn, M. A. (2002). Ulcerative colitis. *The Lancet, 359*(9303), 331–340. Available from https://doi.org/10.1016/S0140-6736(02)07499-8.

Finkelstein, J. D. (2006). Inborn errors of sulfur-containing amino acid metabolism. *Journal of Nutrition, 136*(6), 1750S–1754S. Available from https://doi.org/10.1093/jn/136.6.1750s.

Fiocchi, C. (1998). Inflammatory bowel disease: Etiology and pathogenesis. *Gastroenterology, 115*(1), 182–205. Available from https://doi.org/10.1016/s0016-5085(98)70381-6.

Fiorucci, S., Distrutti, E., Cirino, G., & Wallace, J. L. (2006). The emerging roles of hydrogen sulfide in the gastrointestinal tract and liver. *Gastroenterology, 131*(1), 259–271. Available from https://doi.org/10.1053/j.gastro.2006.02.033.

Fite, A., Macfarlane, G. T., Cummings, J. H., Hopkins, M. J., Kong, S. C., Furrie, E., & Macfarlane, S. (2004). Identification and quantitation of mucosal and faecal desulfovibrios using real time polymerase chain reaction. *Gut, 53*(4), 523–529. Available from https://doi.org/10.1136/gut.2003.031245.

Florin, T. H. J. (1991). Hydrogen sulphide and total acid-volatile sulphide in faeces, determined with a direct spectrophotometric method. *Clinica Chimica Acta, 196*(2–3), 127–134. Available from https://doi.org/10.1016/0009-8981(91)90065-K.

Florin, T. H. J., Gibson, G. R., Neale, G., & Cummings, J. H. (1990). A role for sulfate reducing bacteria in ulcerative colitis. *Gastroenterology, 98*, A170.

Florin, T. H. J., Neale, G., Goretski, S., & Cummings, J. H. (1993). The sulfate content of foods and beverages. *Journal of Food Composition and Analysis, 6*(2), 140–151. Available from https://doi.org/10.1006/jfca.1993.1016.

Florin, T., Neale, G., Gibson, G. R., Christl, S. U., & Cummings, J. H. (1991). Metabolism of dietary sulphate: Absorption and excretion in humans. *Gut, 32*(7), 766–773. Available from https://doi.org/10.1136/gut.32.7.766.

Fox, J. G., Dewhirst, F. E., Fraser, G. J., Paster, B. J., Shames, B., & Murphy, J. C. (1994). Intracellular Campylobacter-like organism from ferrets and hamsters with proliferative bowel disease is a Desulfovibrio sp. *Journal of Clinical Microbiology, 32*(5), 1229–1237. Available from https://doi.org/10.1128/jcm.32.5.1229-1237.1994.

Gajendran, M., Loganathan, P., Catinella, A. P., & Hashash, J. G. (2018). A comprehensive review and update on Crohn's disease. *Disease-a-Month*, *64*(2), 20−57. Available from https://doi.org/10.1016/j.disamonth.2017.07.001.

Galan-Ros, J., Ramos-Arenas, V., & Conesa-Zamora, P. (2020). Predictive values of colon microbiota in the treatment response to colorectal cancer. *Pharmacogenomics*, *21*(14), 1045−1059. Available from https://doi.org/10.2217/pgs-2020-0044.

Gardiner, K. R., Halliday, M. I., Barclay, G. R., Milne, L., Brown, D., Stephens, S., Maxwell, R. J., & Rowlands, B. J. (1995). Significance of systemic endotoxaemia in inflammatory bowel disease. *Gut*, *36*(6), 897−901. Available from https://doi.org/10.1136/gut.36.6.897.

Ge, Y., Konrad, M. A., Matherly, L. H., & Taub, J. W. (2001). Transcriptional regulation of the human cystathionine β-synthase-1b basal promoter: Synergistic transactivation by transcription factors NF-Y and Sp1/Sp3. *Biochemical Journal*, *357*(1), 97−105. Available from https://doi.org/10.1042/0264-6021:3570097.

Ghavami, S. B., Yadegar, A., Aghdaei, H. A., Sorrentino, D., Farmani, M., Mir, A. S., Azimirad, M., Balaii, H., Shahrokh, S., & Zali, M. R. (2020). Immunomodulation and generation of tolerogenic dendritic cells by probiotic bacteria in patients with inflammatory bowel disease. *International Journal of Molecular Sciences*, *21*(17), 6266. Available from https://doi.org/10.3390/ijms21176266.

Ghosh, T. S., Arnoux, J., & O'Toole, P. W. (2020). Metagenomic analysis reveals distinct patterns of gut lactobacillus prevalence, abundance, and geographical variation in health and disease. *Gut Microbes*, *12*(1), 1822729. Available from https://doi.org/10.1080/19490976.2020.1822729.

Giaffer, M. H., Holdsworth, C. D., & Duerden, B. I. (1991). The assessment of faecal flora in patients with inflammatory bowel disease by a simplified bacteriological technique. *Journal of Medical Microbiology*, *35*(4), 238−243. Available from https://doi.org/10.1099/00222615-35-4-238.

Gibson, G. R., Cummings, J. H., & Macfarlane, G. T. (1991). Growth and activities of sulphate-reducing bacteria in gut contents of healthy subjects and patients with ulcerative colitis. *FEMS Microbiology Letters*, *86*(2), 103−112. Available from https://doi.org/10.1111/j.1574-6968.1991.tb04799.x.

Gibson, G. R., Macfarlane, G. T., & Cummings, J. H. (1993). Sulphate reducing bacteria and hydrogen metabolism in the human large intestine. *Gut*, *34*(4), 437−439. Available from https://doi.org/10.1136/gut.34.4.437.

Gibson, G. R., Macfarlane, S., & Macfarlane, G. T. (1993). Metabolic interactions involving sulphate-reducing and methanogenic bacteria in the human large intestine. *FEMS Microbiology Ecology*, *12*(2), 117−125. Available from https://doi.org/10.1111/j.1574-6941.1993.tb00023.x.

Gilat, T., Leichtman, G., Delpre, G., Eshchar, J., Meir, S. B., & Fireman, Z. (1989). A Comparison of metronidazole and sulfasalazine in the maintenance of remission in patients with ulcerative colitis. *Journal of Clinical Gastroenterology*, *11*(4), 392−395. Available from https://doi.org/10.1097/00004836-198908000-00008.

Gionchetti, P., Rizzello, F., Venturi, A., Ugolini, F., Rossi, M., Brigidi, P., Johansson, R., Ferrieri, A., Poggioli, G., & Campieri, M. (1999). Antibiotic combination therapy in patients with chronic, treatment-resistant pouchitis. *Alimentary Pharmacology and Therapeutics*, *13*(6), 713−718. Available from https://doi.org/10.1046/j.1365-2036.1999.00553.x.

Glassner, K. L., Abraham, B. P., & Quigley, E. M. M. (2020). The microbiome and inflammatory bowel disease. *Journal of Allergy and Clinical Immunology*, *145*(1), 16−27. Available from https://doi.org/10.1016/j.jaci.2019.11.003.

González-Herrera, S. M., Bermúdez-Quiñones, G., Ochoa-Martínez, L. A., Rutiaga-Quiñones, O. M., & Gallegos-Infante, J. A. (2021). Synbiotics: A technological approach in food applications. *Journal of Food Science and Technology*, *58*(3), 811−824. Available from https://doi.org/10.1007/s13197-020-04532-0.

Guarner, F., & Malagelada, J. R. (2003). Gut flora in health and disease. *Lancet*, *361*(9356), 512−519. Available from https://doi.org/10.1016/S0140-6736(03)12489-0.

Gunzburg, W. H., Aung, M. M., Toa, P., Ng, S., Read, E., Tan, W. J., Brandtner, E. M., Dangerfield, J., & Salmons, B. (2020). Efficient protection of microorganisms for delivery to the intestinal tract by cellulose sulphate encapsulation. *Microbial Cell Factories*, *19*(1), 216. Available from https://doi.org/10.1186/s12934-020-01465-3.

Guslandi, M. (2011). Rifaximin in the treatment of inflammatory bowel disease. *World Journal of Gastroenterology*, *17*(42), 4643−4646. Available from https://doi.org/10.3748/wjg.v17.i42.4643.

Hans, W., Schölmerich, J., Gross, V., & Falk, W. (2000). The role of the resident intestinal flora in acute and chronic dextran sulfate sodium-induced colitis in mice. *European Journal of Gastroenterology and Hepatology*, *12*(3), 267−273. Available from https://doi.org/10.1097/00042737-200012030-00002.

Hao, X., Shang, X., Liu, J., Chi, R., Zhang, J., & Xu, T. (2021). The gut microbiota in osteoarthritis: Where do we stand and what can we do? *Arthritis Research and Therapy*, *23*(1), 92−101. Available from https://doi.org/10.1186/s13075-021-02427-9.

Hasannejad-Bibalan, M., Mojtahedi, A., Eshaghi, M., Rohani, M., Pourshafie, M. R., & Talebi, M. (2020). The effect of selected Lactobacillus strains on dextran sulfate sodium-induced mouse colitis model. *Acta Microbiologica et Immunologica Hungarica*, *67*(2), 138−142. Available from https://doi.org/10.1556/030.2020.00834.

Hooper, L. V., Wong, M. H., Thelin, A., Hansson, L., Falk, P. G., & Gordon, J. I. (2001). Molecular analysis of commensal host-microbial relationships in the intestine. *Science (New York, N.Y.)*, *291*(5505), 881−884. Available from https://doi.org/10.1126/science.291.5505.881.

Huang, F. C., Lu, Y. T., & Liao, Y. H. (2020). Beneficial effect of probiotics on Pseudomonas aeruginosa−infected intestinal epithelial cells through inflammatory IL-8 and antimicrobial peptide human beta-defensin-2 modulation. *Innate Immunity*, *26*(7), 592−600. Available from https://doi.org/10.1177/1753425920959410.

Jadhav, P., Jiang, Y., Jarr, K., Layton, C., Ashouri, J. F., & Sinha, S. R. (2020). Efficacy of dietary supplements in inflammatory bowel disease and related autoimmune diseases. *Nutrients*, *12*(7), 2156. Available from https://doi.org/10.3390/nu12072156.

Jakubczyk, D., Leszczyńska, K., & Górska, S. (2020). The effectiveness of probiotics in the treatment of inflammatory bowel disease (Ibd)— a critical review. *Nutrients*, *12*(7), 1973. Available from https://doi.org/10.3390/nu12071973.

Jampílek, J., & Kráľová, K. (2020). Potential of nanonutraceuticals in increasing immunity. *Nanomaterials*, *10*(11), 2224. Available from https://doi.org/10.3390/nano10112224.

Jampílek, J., Kos, J., & Kráľová, K. (2019). Potential of nanomaterial applications in dietary supplements and foods for special medical purposes. *Nanomaterials*, *9*(2), 296. Available from https://doi.org/10.3390/nano9020296.

Jiang, Z. D., Ke, S., Palazzini, E., Riopel, L., & Dupont, H. (2000). In vitro activity and fecal concentration of rifaximin after oral administration. *Antimicrobial Agents and Chemotherapy*, *44*(8), 2205–2206. Available from https://doi.org/10.1128/AAC.44.8.2205-2206.2000.

Johnson-Henry, K. C., Abrahamsson, T. R., Wu, R. Y., & Sherman, P. M. (2016). Probiotics, prebiotics, and synbiotics for the prevention of necrotizing enterocolitis. *Advances in Nutrition*, *7*(5), 928–937. Available from https://doi.org/10.3945/an.116.012237.

Kazemi, A., Soltani, S., Ghorabi, S., Keshtkar, A., Daneshzad, E., Nasri, F., & Mazloomi, S. M. (2020). Effect of probiotic and synbiotic supplementation on inflammatory markers in health and disease status: A systematic review and *meta*-analysis of clinical trials. *Clinical Nutrition*, *39*(3), 789–819. Available from https://doi.org/10.1016/j.clnu.2019.04.004.

Kaźmierczak-Siedlecka, K., Ruszkowski, J., Fic, M., Folwarski, M., & Makarewicz, W. (2020). Saccharomyces boulardii CNCM I-745: A nonbacterial microorganism used as probiotic agent in supporting treatment of selected diseases. *Current Microbiology*, *77*(9), 1987–1996. Available from https://doi.org/10.1007/s00284-020-02053-9.

Kechagia, M., Basoulis, D., Konstantopoulou, S., Dimitriadi, D., Gyftopoulou, K., Skarmoutsou, N., & Fakiri, E. M. (2013). Health benefits of probiotics: A review. *ISRN Nutrition*, *2013*, 481651. Available from https://doi.org/10.5402/2013/481651.

Kefif, Y., Dib, W., Cherif., Bouferkas, Y., Kheroua, O., & Saidi, D. (2020). Potential application of Lactobacillusplantarumin the prevention of inflammatory bowel diseases in Balb/c mice. *Bioscience Research*, *17*, 1697–1705.

Kennedy, R. J. (2001). Probiotics in IBD. *Gut*, *49*, 873. Available from https://doi.org/10.1136/gut.49.6.873a.

Kennedy, R. J. (2002). Mucosal barrier function and the commensal flora. *Gut*, *50*, 441–442. Available from https://doi.org/10.1136/gut.50.3.441.

Kennedy, R. J., Hoper, M., Deodhar, K., Erwin, P. J., Kirk, S. J., & Gardiner, K. R. (2000). Interleukin 10-deficient colitis: New similarities to human inflammatory bowel disease. *British Journal of Surgery*, *87*(10), 1346–1351. Available from https://doi.org/10.1046/j.1365-2168.2000.01615.x.

Khan, I., Ullah, N., Zha, L., Bai, Y., Khan, A., Zhao, T., Che, T., & Zhang, C. (2019). Alteration of gut microbiota in inflammatory bowel disease (IBD): Cause or consequence? IBD treatment targeting the gut microbiome. *Pathogens*, *8*(3), 126. Available from https://doi.org/10.3390/pathogens8030126.

Kim, K. O., & Gluck, M. (2019). Fecal microbiota transplantation: An update on clinical practice. *Clinical Endoscopy*, *52*(2), 137–143. Available from https://doi.org/10.5946/CE.2019.009.

Kim, D. H., Kim, S., Ahn, J. B., Kim, J. H., Ma, H. W., Seo, D. H., Che, X., Park, K. C., Jeon, J. Y., Kim, S. Y., Lee, H. C., Lee, J. Y., Kim, T. I., Kim, W. H., Kim, S. W., & Cheon, J. H. (2020). Lactobacillus plantarum CBT LP3 ameliorates colitis via modulating T cells in mice. *International Journal of Medical Microbiology*, *310*(2), 151391. Available from https://doi.org/10.1016/j.ijmm.2020.151391.

Kleessen, B., Kroesen, A. J., Buhr, H. J., & Blaut, M. (2002). Mucosal and invading bacteria in patients with inflammatory bowel disease compared with controls. *Scandinavian Journal of Gastroenterology*, *37*(9), 1034–1041. Available from https://doi.org/10.1080/003655202320378220.

Kotrsová, V., & Kushkevych, I. (2019). Possible methods for evaluation of hydrogen sulfide toxicity against lactic acid bacteria. *Biointerface Research in Applied Chemistry*, *9*(4), 4066–4069. Available from https://doi.org/10.33263/BRIAC94.066069.

Kováč, J., & Kushkevych, I. (2017). New modification of cultivation medium for isolation and growth of intestinal sulfate-reducing bacteria. In *Presented at the international PhD students conference Mendel Net* (pp. 702–707).

Kováč, J., Vítězová, M., & Kushkevych, I. (2018). Metabolic activity of sulfate-reducing bacteria from rodents with colitis. *Open Medicine*, *13*(1), 344–349. Available from https://doi.org/10.1515/med-2018-0052.

Kraus, J. P., Oliveriusová, J., Sokolová, J., Kraus, E., Vlček, C., De Franchis, R., Maclean, K. N., Bao, L., Bukovská, G., Patterson, D., Pačes, V., Ansorge, W., & Kožich, V. (1998). The human cystathionine β-synthase (CBS) gene: Complete sequence, alternative splicing, and polymorphisms. *Genomics*, *52*(3), 312–324. Available from https://doi.org/10.1006/geno.1998.5437.

Kristjansson, J. K., Schönheit, P., & Thauer, R. K. (1982). Different Ks values for hydrogen of methanogenic bacteria and sulfate reducing bacteria: An explanation for the apparent inhibition of methanogenesis by sulfate. *Archives of Microbiology*, *131*(3), 278–282. Available from https://doi.org/10.1007/BF00405893.

Kruis, W., Schutz, E., Fric, P., Fixa, B., Judmaier, G., & Stolte, M. (1997). Double-blind comparison of an oral Escherichia coli preparation and mesalazine in maintaining remission of ulcerative colitis. *Alimentary Pharmacology and Therapeutics*, *11*(5), 853–858. Available from https://doi.org/10.1046/j.1365-2036.1997.00225.x.

Kushkevych, I. V. (2015a). Activity and kinetic properties of phosphotransacetylase from intestinal sulfate-reducing bacteria. *Acta Biochimica Polonica*, *62*(1), 103–108. Available from https://doi.org/10.18388/abp.2014_845.

Kushkevych, I. V. (2015b). Kinetic properties of pyruvate ferredoxin oxidoreductase of intestinal sulfate-reducing bacteria Desulfovibrio piger Vib-7 and Desulfomicrobium sp. Rod-9. *Polish Journal of Microbiology*, *64*(2), 107–114. Available from https://doi.org/10.33073/pjm-2015-016.

Kushkevych, I. V. (2016). Dissimilatory sulfate reduction in the intestinal sulfate-reducing bacteria. *Studia Biologica*, 197–228. Available from https://doi.org/10.30970/sbi.1001.560.

Kushkevych, I., Abdulina, D., Kováč, J., Dordević, D., Vítězová, M., Iutynska, G., & Rittmann, S. K. M. R. (2020). Adenosine-5′-phosphosulfate- and sulfite reductases activities of sulfate-reducing bacteria from various environments. *Biomolecules*, *10*(6), 921. Available from https://doi.org/10.3390/biom10060921.

Kushkevych, I., Cejnar, J., Treml, J., Dordević, D., Kollár, P., & Vítězová, M. (2020). Recent advances in metabolic pathways of sulfate reduction in intestinal bacteria. *Cells*, *9*(3), 698. Available from https://doi.org/10.3390/cells9030698.

Kushkevych, I., Cejnar, J., Vítězová, M., Vítěz, T., Dordević, D., & Bomble, Y. (2020). Occurrence of thermophilic microorganisms in different full scale biogas plants. *International Journal of Molecular Sciences*, *21*(1), 283. Available from https://doi.org/10.3390/ijms21010283.

Kushkevych, I., Dordević, D., Kollár, P., Vítězová, M., & Drago, L. (2019). Hydrogen sulfide as a toxic product in the small–large intestine axis and its role in IBD development. *Journal of Clinical Medicine*, *8*(7), 1054. Available from https://doi.org/10.3390/jcm8071054.

Kushkevych, I., Dordević, D., Vítězová, M., & Kollár, P. (2018). Cross-correlation analysis of the Desulfovibrio growth parameters of intestinal species isolated from people with colitis. *Biologia (Lahore, Pakistan)*, *73*(11), 1137–1143. Available from https://doi.org/10.2478/s11756-018-0118-2.

Kushkevych, I., Dordević, D., & Kollár, P. (2018). Analysis of physiological parameters of Desulfovibrio strains from individuals with colitis. *Open Life Sciences*, *13*(1), 481–488. Available from https://doi.org/10.1515/biol-2018-0057.

Kushkevych, I., Dordević, D., & Vítězová, M. (2019a). Analysis of pH dose-dependent growth of sulfate-reducing bacteria. *Open Medicine (Poland)*, *14*(1), 66–74. Available from https://doi.org/10.1515/med-2019-0010.

Kushkevych, I., Dordević, D., & Vítězová, M. (2019b). Toxicity of hydrogen sulfide toward sulfate-reducing bacteria Desulfovibrio piger Vib-7. *Archives of Microbiology*, *201*(3), 389–397. Available from https://doi.org/10.1007/s00203-019-01625-z.

Kushkevych, I., Dordević, D., & Vítězová, M. (2021). Possible synergy effect of hydrogen sulfide and acetate produced by sulfate-reducing bacteria on inflammatory bowel disease development. *Journal of Advanced Research*, *27*, 71–78. Available from https://doi.org/10.1016/j.jare.2020.03.007.

Kushkevych, I., Dordević, D., Vítězová, M., & Rittmann, S. K. M. R. (2021). Environmental impact of sulfate-reducing bacteria, their role in intestinal bowel diseases, and possible control by bacteriophages. *Applied Sciences (Switzerland)*, *11*(2), 735. Available from https://doi.org/10.3390/app11020735.

Kushkevych, I., Fafula, R., Parák, T., & Bartoš, M. (2015a). Activity of Na^+/K^+-activated Mg^{2+}-dependent ATP-hydrolase in the cell-free extracts of the sulfate-reducing bacteria Desulfovibrio piger vib-7 and Desulfomicrobium sp. Rod-9. *Acta Veterinaria Brno*, *84*(1), 3–12. Available from https://doi.org/10.2754/avb201585010003.

Kushkevych, I., Castro Sangrador, J., Dordević, D., Rozehnalová, M., Černý, M., Fafula, R., Vítězová, M., & Rittmann, S. K. M. R. (2020). Evaluation of physiological parameters of intestinal sulfate-reducing bacteria isolated from patients suffering from IBD and healthy people. *Journal of Clinical Medicine*, *9*, 1920. Available from https://doi.org/10.3390/jcm9061920.

Kushkevych, I., Kobzová, E., Vítězová, M., Vítěz, T., Dordević, D., & Bartoš, M. (2019). Acetogenic microorganisms in operating biogas plants depending on substrate combinations. *Biologia (Lahore, Pakistan)*, *74*(9), 1229–1236. Available from https://doi.org/10.2478/s11756-019-00283-2.

Kushkevych, I., Kollár, P., Ferreira, A. L., Palma, D., Duarte, A., Lopes, M. M., Bartoš, M., Pauk, K., Imramovský, A., & Jampílek, J. (2016). Antimicrobial effect of salicylamide derivatives against intestinal sulfate-reducing bacteria. *Journal of Applied Biomedicine*, *14*(2), 125–130. Available from https://doi.org/10.1016/j.jab.2016.01.005.

Kushkevych, I., Kollár, P., Suchý, P., Parák, T., Pauk, K., & Imramovsky, A. (2015b). Activity of selected salicylamides against intestinal sulfate-reducing bacteria. *Neuroendocrinology Letters*, *36*(Suppl. 1), 106–113. Available from http://www.nel.edu.

Kushkevych, I., Kos, J., Kollár, P., Kráľová, K., & Jampílek, J. (2018). Activity of ring-substituted 8-hydroxyquinoline-2-carboxanilides against intestinal sulfate-reducing bacteria Desulfovibrio piger. *Medicinal Chemistry Research*, *27*(1), 278–284. Available from https://doi.org/10.1007/s00044-017-2067-7.

Kushkevych, I., Kotrsová, V., Dordević, D., Buňková, L., Vítězová, M., & Amedei, A. (2019). Hydrogen sulfide effects on the survival of lactobacilli with emphasis on the development of inflammatory bowel diseases. *Biomolecules*, *9*(12), 752. Available from https://doi.org/10.3390/biom9120752.

Kushkevych, I., Coufalová, M., Vítězová, M., & Rittmann, S. K. M. R. (2020). Sulfate-reducing bacteria of the oral cavity and their relation with periodontitis—Recent advances. *Journal of Clinical Medicine*, *9*(8), 2347. Available from https://doi.org/10.3390/jcm9082347.

Kushkevych, I., Leščanová, O., Dordević, D., Jančíková, S., Hošek, J., Vítězová, M., Buňková, L., & Drago, L. (2019). The sulfate-reducing microbial communities and *meta*-analysis of their occurrence during diseases of small–large intestine axis. *Journal of Clinical Medicine*, *8*(10), 1656. Available from https://doi.org/10.3390/jcm8101656.

Kushkevych, I., Vítězová, M., Fedrová, P., Vochyanová, Z., Paráková, L., & Hošek, J. (2017). Kinetic properties of growth of intestinal sulphate-reducing bacteria isolated from healthy mice and mice with ulcerative colitis. *Acta Veterinaria Brno*, *86*(4), 405–411. Available from https://doi.org/10.2754/avb201786040405.

Kushkevych, I., Kováč, J., Vítězová, M., Vítěz, T., & Bartoš, M. (2018). The diversity of sulfate-reducing bacteria in the seven bioreactors. *Archives of Microbiology*, *200*(6), 945–950. Available from https://doi.org/10.1007/s00203-018-1510-6.

Kushkevych, I., Martínková, K., Vítězová, M., & Rittmann, S. K. M. R. (2021). Intestinal microbiota and perspectives of the use of *meta*-analysis for comparison of ulcerative colitis studies. *Journal of Clinical Medicine*, *10*(3), 462. Available from https://doi.org/10.3390/jcm10030462.

Kushkevych, I., Vítězová, M., Kos, J., Kollár, P., & Jampílek, J. (2018). Effect of selected 8-hydroxyquinoline-2-carboxanilides on viability and sulfate metabolism of Desulfovibrio piger. *Journal of Applied Biomedicine*, *16*(3), 241–246. Available from https://doi.org/10.1016/j.jab.2018.01.004.

Kushkevych, I., Vítězová, M., Vítěz, T., & Bartoš, M. (2017). Production of biogas: Relationship between methanogenic and sulfate-reducing microorganisms. *Open Life Sciences*, *12*(1), 82–91. Available from https://doi.org/10.1515/biol-2017-0009.

Kushkevych, I., Vítězová, M., Vítěz, T., Kováč, J., Kaucká, P., Jesionek, W., Bartoš, M., & Barton, L. (2018). A new combination of substrates: Biogas production and diversity of the methanogenic microorganisms. *Open Life Sciences*, *13*(1), 119–128. Available from https://doi.org/10.1515/biol-2018-0017.

LeBlanc, J. G., Levit, R., Savoy de Giori, G., & de Moreno de LeBlanc, A. (2020). Application of vitamin-producing lactic acid bacteria to treat intestinal inflammatory diseases. *Applied Microbiology and Biotechnology*, *104*(8), 3331–3337. Available from https://doi.org/10.1007/s00253-020-10487-1.

Leccese, G., Bibi, A., Mazza, S., Facciotti, F., Caprioli, F., Landini, P., & Paroni, M. (2020). Probiotic Lactobacillus and Bifidobacterium strains counteract adherent-invasive Escherichia coli (AIEC) virulence and hamper IL-23/Th17 axis in ulcerative colitis, but not in Crohn's disease. *Cells*, *9*(8), 1824. Available from https://doi.org/10.3390/cells9081824.

Levitt, M. D., Furne, J., Springfield, J., Suarez, F., & DeMaster, E. (1999). Detoxification of hydrogen sulfide and methanethiol in the cecal mucosa. *Journal of Clinical Investigation*, *104*(8), 1107–1114. Available from https://doi.org/10.1172/JCI7712.

Levonen, A. L., Lapatto, R., Saksela, M., & Raivio, K. O. (2000). Human cystathionine γ-lyase: Developmental and in vitro expression of two isoforms. *Biochemical Journal*, *347*(1), 291–295. Available from https://doi.org/10.1042/0264-6021:3470291.

Lewis, S., Brazier, J., Beard, D., Nazem, N., & Proctor, D. (2005). Effects of metronidazole and oligofructose on faecal concentrations of sulphate-reducing bacteria and their activity in human volunteers. *Scandinavian Journal of Gastroenterology*, *40*(11), 1296–1303. Available from https://doi.org/10.1080/00365520510023585.

Li, S. C., Hsu, W. F., Chang, J. S., & Shih, C. K. (2019). Combination of lactobacillus acidophilus and bifidobacterium animalis subsp. Lactis shows a stronger anti-inflammatory effect than individual strains in HT-29 cells. *Nutrients*, *11*(5), 969. Available from https://doi.org/10.3390/nu11050969.

Li, Y., Yang, S., Lun, J., Gao, J., Gao, X., Gong, Z., Wan, Y., He, X., & Cao, H. (2020). Inhibitory effects of the Lactobacillus rhamnosus GG effector protein HM0539 on inflammatory response through the TLR4/MyD88/NF-κB axis. *Frontiers in Immunology*, *11*, 551449. Available from https://doi.org/10.3389/fimmu.2020.551449.

Li, Y., Zhang, T., Guo, C., Geng, M., Gai, S., Qi, W., Li, Z., Song, Y., Luo, X., Zhang, T., & Wang, N. (2020). Bacillus subtilis RZ001 improves intestinal integrity and alleviates colitis by inhibiting the Notch signalling pathway and activating ATOH-1. *Pathogens and Disease*, *78*(2), ftaa016. Available from https://doi.org/10.1093/femspd/ftaa016.

Lin, Y., Zheng, X., Chen, J., Luo, D., Xie, J., Su, Z., Huang, X., Yi, X., Wei, L., Cai, J., & Sun, Z. (2020). Protective effect of Bruguiera gymnorrhiza (L.) Lam. fruit on dextran sulfate sodium-induced ulcerative colitis in mice: Role of Keap1/Nrf2 pathway and gut microbiota. *Frontiers in Pharmacology*, *10*, 1602. Available from https://doi.org/10.3389/fphar.2019.01602.

Linskens, R. K., Huijsdens, X. W., Savelkoul, P. H. M., Vandenbroucke-Grauls, C. M. J. E., & Meuwissen, S. G. M. (2001). The bacterial flora in inflammatory bowel disease: Current insights in pathogenesis and the influence of antibiotics and probiotics. *Scandinavian Journal of Gastroenterology, Supplement*, *36*(234), 29–40. Available from https://doi.org/10.1080/003655201753265082.

Liu, M., Ding, J., Zhang, H., Shen, J., Hao, Y., Zhang, X., Qi, W., Luo, X., Zhang, T., & Wang, N. (2020). Lactobacillus casei LH23 modulates the immune response and ameliorates DSS-induced colitis via suppressing JNK/p-38 signal pathways and enhancing histone H3K9 acetylation. *Food and Function*, *11*(6), 5473–5485. Available from https://doi.org/10.1039/d0fo00546k.

Liu, Y., Tran, D. Q., Lindsey, J. W., & Rhoads, J. M. (2021). The association of gut microbiota and treg dysfunction in autoimmune diseases. *Advances in Experimental Medicine and Biology*, *1278*, 191–203. Available from https://doi.org/10.1007/978-981-15-6407-9_10, Springer.

Liu, Y., Li, Y., Yu, X., Yu, L., Tian, F., Zhao, J., Zhang, H., Zhai, Q., & Chen, W. (2021). Physiological characteristics of Lactobacillus casei strains and their alleviation effects against inflammatory bowel disease. *Journal of Microbiology and Biotechnology*, *31*, 92–103. Available from https://doi.org/10.4014/jmb.2003.03041.

Liu, Y., Yin, F., Huang, L., Teng, H., Shen, T., & Qin, H. (2021). Long-term and continuous administration of Bacillus subtilis during remission effectively maintains the remission of inflammatory bowel disease by protecting intestinal integrity, regulating epithelial proliferation, and reshaping microbial structure and function. *Food and Function*, *12*(5), 2201–2210. Available from https://doi.org/10.1039/d0fo02786c.

Liu, Z., Liu, F., Wang, W., Sun, C., Gao, D., Ma, J., Hussain, M. A., Xu, C., Jiang, Z., & Hou, J. (2020). Study of the alleviation effects of a combination of: Lactobacillus rhamnosus and inulin on mice with colitis. *Food and Function*, *11*(5), 3823–3837. Available from https://doi.org/10.1039/c9fo02992c.

Lobo, A. J., Burke, D. A., Sobala, G. M., & Axon, A. T. R. (1993). Oral tobramycin in ulcerative colitis: Effect on maintenance of remission. *Alimentary Pharmacology & Therapeutics*, *7*(2), 155–158. Available from https://doi.org/10.1111/j.1365-2036.1993.tb00084.x.

Loftus, E. V., Silverstein, M. D., Sandborn, W. J., Tremaine, W. J., Harmsen, W. S., & Zinsmeister, A. R. (2000). Ulcerative colitis in Olmsted County, Minnesota, 1940–1993: Incidence, prevalence, and survival. *Gut*, *46*(3), 336–343. Available from https://doi.org/10.1136/gut.46.3.336.

Loubinoux, J., Mory, F., Pereira, I. A. C., & Le Faou, A. E. (2000). Bacteremia caused by a strain of Desulfovibrio related to the provisionally named Desulfovibrio fairfieldensis. *Journal of Clinical Microbiology*, *38*(2), 931–934. Available from https://doi.org/10.1128/jcm.38.2.931-934.2000.

Lovley, D. R., & Klug, M. J. (1983). Sulfate reducers can outcompete methanogens at freshwater sulfate concentrations. *Applied and Environmental Microbiology*, *45*(1), 187–192. Available from https://doi.org/10.1128/aem.45.1.187-192.1983.

Luo, R., Zhang, J., Zhang, X., Zhou, Z., Zhang, W., Zhu, Z., Liu, H., Wang, L., Zhong, Z., Fu, H., Jing, B., & Peng, G. (2020). Bacillus subtilis HH2 ameliorates TNBS-induced colitis by modulating gut microbiota composition and improving intestinal barrier function in rabbit model. *Journal of Functional Foods*, *74*, 104167. Available from https://doi.org/10.1016/j.jff.2020.104167.

Lynch, W. D., & Hsu, R. (2021). *Ulcerative colitis*. *StatPearls*. Treasure Island (FL): StatPearls Publishing. Available from https://www.ncbi.nlm.nih.gov/books/NBK459282/.

Ma, S., Yeom, J., & Lim, Y. H. (2020). Dairy Propionibacterium freudenreichii ameliorates acute colitis by stimulating MUC2 expression in intestinal goblet cell in a DSS-induced colitis rat model. *Scientific Reports*, *10*(1), 5523. Available from https://doi.org/10.1038/s41598-020-62497-8.

Macfarlane, S., & Dillon, J. F. (2007). Microbial biofilms in the human gastrointestinal tract. *Journal of Applied Microbiology, 102*(5), 1187−1196. Available from https://doi.org/10.1111/j.1365-2672.2007.03287.x.

Macfarlane, S., Hopkins, M. J., & Macfarlane, G. T. (2000). Bacterial growth and metabolism on surfaces in the large intestine. *Microbial Ecology in Health and Disease, 12*(2), 64−72. Available from https://doi.org/10.1080/089106000750060314.

Macpherson, A., Khoo, U. Y., Forgacs, I., Philpott-Howard, J., & Bjarnason, I. (1996). Mucosal antibodies in inflammatory bowel disease are directed against intestinal bacteria. *Gut, 38*(3), 365−375. Available from https://doi.org/10.1136/gut.38.3.365.

Madsen, K. L., Doyle, J. S., Jewell, L. D., Tavernini, M. M., & Fedorak, R. N. (1999). Lactobacillus species prevents colitis in interleukin 10 gene-deficient mice. *Gastroenterology, 116*(5), 1107−1114. Available from https://doi.org/10.1016/S0016-5085(99)70013-2.

Madsen, K. L., Doyle, J. S., Tavernini, M. M., Jewell, L. D., Rennie, R. P., & Fedorak, R. N. (2000). Antibiotic therapy attenuates colitis in interleukin 10 gene-deficient mice. *Gastroenterology, 118*(6), 1094−1105. Available from https://doi.org/10.1016/S0016-5085(00)70362-3.

Malinowski, B., Wiciński, M., Sokołowska, M. M., Hill, N. A., & Szambelan, M. (2020). The rundown of dietary supplements and their effects on inflammatory bowel disease—A review. *Nutrients, 12*(5), 1423. Available from https://doi.org/10.3390/nu12051423.

Mantzaris, G. J., Archavlis, E., Christoforidis, P., Kourtessas, D., Amberiadis, P., Florakis, N., Petraki, K., Spiliadi, C., & Triantafyllou, G. (1997). A prospective randomized controlled trial of oral ciprofloxacin in acute ulcerative colitis. *American Journal of Gastroenterology, 92*(3), 454−456.

Mantzaris, G. J., Petraki, K., Archavlis, E., Amberiadis, P., Kourtessas, D., Christidou, A., & Triantafyllou, G. (2001). A prospective randomized controlled trial of intravenous ciprofloxacin as an adjunct to corticosteroids in acute, severe ulcerative colitis. *Scandinavian Journal of Gastroenterology, 36*(9), 971−974. Available from https://doi.org/10.1080/003655201750305503.

Mao, Y., Nobaek, S., Kasravi, B., Adawi, D., Stenram, U., Molin, G., & Jeppsson, B. (1996). The effects of Lactobacillus strains and oat fiber on methotrexate-induced enterocolitis in rats. *Gastroenterology, 111*(2), 334−344. Available from https://doi.org/10.1053/gast.1996.v111.pm8690198.

Marco, M. L., Sanders, M. E., Gänzle, M., Arrieta, M. C., Cotter, P. D., De Vuyst, L., Hill, C., Holzapfel, W., Lebeer, S., Merenstein, D., Reid, G., Wolfe, B. E., & Hutkins, R. (2021). The International Scientific Association for Probiotics and Prebiotics (ISAPP) consensus statement on fermented foods. *Nature Reviews Gastroenterology and Hepatology, 18*(3), 196−208. Available from https://doi.org/10.1038/s41575-020-00390-5.

Marcus, R., & Watt, J. (1974). Ulcerative disease of the colon in laboratory animals induced by pepsin inhibitors. *Gastroenterology, 67*(3), 473−483. Available from https://doi.org/10.1016/s0016-5085(19)32849-5.

Markowiak, P., & Ślizewska, K. (2017). Effects of probiotics, prebiotics, and synbiotics on human health. *Nutrients, 9*(9), 1021. Available from https://doi.org/10.3390/nu9091021.

Marzorati, M., Van den Abbeele, P., Bubeck, S. S., Bayne, T., Krishnan, K., Young, A., Mehta, D., & Desouza, A. (2020). Bacillus subtilis HU58 and Bacillus coagulans SC208 probiotics reduced the effects of antibiotic-induced gut microbiome dysbiosis in an M-SHIME® model. *Microorganisms, 8*(7), 1028. Available from https://doi.org/10.3390/microorganisms8071028.

Matsuda, H., Fujiyama, Y., Andoh, A., Ushijima, T., Kajinami, T., & Bamba, T. (2000). Characterization of antibody responses against rectal mucosa-associated bacterial flora in patients with ulcerative colitis. *Journal of Gastroenterology and Hepatology (Australia), 15*(1), 61−68. Available from https://doi.org/10.1046/j.1440-1746.2000.02045.x.

Mazzoli, A., Donadio, G., Lanzilli, M., Saggese, A., Guarino, A. M., Rivetti, M., Crescenzo, R., Ricca, E., Ferrandino, I., Iossa, S., Pollice, A., & Isticato, R. (2019). Bacillus megaterium SF185 spores exert protective effects against oxidative stress in vivo and in vitro. *Scientific Reports, 9*(1), 12082. Available from https://doi.org/10.1038/s41598-019-48531-4.

Meng, X., Zhang, G., Cao, H., Yu, D., Fang, X., Vos, W. M., & Wu, H. (2020). Gut dysbacteriosis and intestinal disease: Mechanism and treatment. *Journal of Applied Microbiology, 129*(4), 787−805. Available from https://doi.org/10.1111/jam.14661.

Moehle, C., Ackermann, N., Langmann, T., Aslanidis, C., Kel, A., Kel-Margoulis, O., Schmitz-Madry, A., Zahn, A., Stremmel, W., & Schmitz, G. (2006). Aberrant intestinal expression and allelic variants of mucin genes associated with inflammatory bowel disease. *Journal of Molecular Medicine, 84*(12), 1055−1066. Available from https://doi.org/10.1007/s00109-006-0100-2.

Mohebali, N., Ekat, K., Kreikemeyer, B., & Breitrück, A. (2020). Barrier protection and recovery effects of gut commensal bacteria on differentiated intestinal epithelial cells in vitro. *Nutrients, 12*(8), 2251. Available from https://doi.org/10.3390/nu12082251.

Montgomery, S. M., Morris, D. L., Thompson, N. P., Subhani, J., Pounder, R. E., & Wakefield, A. J. (1998). Prevalence of inflammatory bowel disease in British 26 year olds: National longitudinal birth cohort. *British Medical Journal, 316*(7137), 1058−1059. Available from https://doi.org/10.1136/bmj.316.7137.1058.

Newman, A. M., & Arshad, M. (2020). The role of probiotics, prebiotics and synbiotics in combating multidrug-resistant organisms. *Clinical Therapeutics, 42*(9), 1637−1648. Available from https://doi.org/10.1016/j.clinthera.2020.06.011.

Ni, J., Wu, G. D., Albenberg, L., & Tomov, V. T. (2017). Gut microbiota and IBD: Causation or correlation? *Nature Reviews Gastroenterology and Hepatology, 14*(10), 573−584. Available from https://doi.org/10.1038/nrgastro.2017.88.

Nishida, A., Inoue, R., Inatomi, O., Bamba, S., Naito, Y., & Andoh, A. (2018). Gut microbiota in the pathogenesis of inflammatory bowel disease. *Clinical Journal of Gastroenterology, 11*(1), 1−10. Available from https://doi.org/10.1007/s12328-017-0813-5.

Nithya, J., Jayashree, S., Kumar, G. K., & Kumar, S. P. (2020). Comparative analysis of probiotics and fish oil against dss induced colitis model in rodents. *International Journal of Life Science and Pharma Research, 8*, 103−108.

Oka, A., & Sartor, R. B. (2020). Microbial-based and microbial-targeted therapies for inflammatory bowel diseases. *Digestive Diseases and Sciences, 65*(3), 757−788. Available from https://doi.org/10.1007/s10620-020-06090-z.

Okayasu, I., Hatakeyama, S., Yamada, M., Ohkusa, T., Inagaki, Y., & Nakaya, R. (1990). A novel method in the induction of reliable experimental acute and chronic ulcerative colitis in mice. *Gastroenterology, 98*(3), 694−702. Available from https://doi.org/10.1016/0016-5085(90)90290-H.

Onderdonk, A. B., Hermos, J. A., & Bartlett, J. G. (1977). The role of the intestinal microflora in experimental colitis. *American Journal of Clinical Nutrition, 30*(11), 1819–1825. Available from https://doi.org/10.1093/ajcn/30.11.1819.

Onderdonk, A. B., Hermos, J. A., Dzink, J. L., & Bartlett, J. G. (1978). Protective effect of metronidazole in experimentalulcerative colitis. *Gastroenterology, 74*(3), 521–526. Available from https://doi.org/10.1016/0016-5085(78)90289-5.

Pacifici, G. M., Romiti, P., Santerini, S., & Giuliani, L. (1993). S-methyltransferases in human intestine: Differential distribution of the microsomal thiol methyltransferase and cytosolic thiopurine methyltransferase along the human bowel. *Xenobiotica; the Fate of Foreign Compounds in Biological Systems, 23*(6), 671–679. Available from https://doi.org/10.3109/00498259309059404.

Pandey, K. R., Naik, S. R., & Vakil, B. V. (2015). Probiotics, prebiotics and synbiotics—A review. *Journal of Food Science and Technology, 52*(12), 7577–7587. Available from https://doi.org/10.1007/s13197-015-1921-1.

Pathmakanthan, S., Thornley, J. P., & Hawkey, C. J. (1999). Mucosally associated bacterial flora of the human colon: Quantitative and species specific differences between normal and inflamed colonic biopsies. *Microbial Ecology in Health and Disease, 11*(3), 169–174. Available from https://doi.org/10.1080/089106099435754.

Phillips, S. F., Pemberton, J. H., Shorter, R. G., & Talbot, I. C. (1993). The large intestine: Physiology, pathophysiology and disease. *Histopathology, 23*(5), 505. Available from https://doi.org/10.1111/j.1365-2559.1993.tb00509.x.

Picardo, S., Altuwaijri, M., Devlin, S. M., & Seow, C. H. (2020). Complementary and alternative medications in the management of inflammatory bowel disease. *Therapeutic Advances in Gastroenterology, 13*, 1756284820927550. Available from https://doi.org/10.1177/1756284820927550.

Pineiro, M., Asp, N. G., Reid, G., Macfarlane, S., Morelli, L., Brunser, O., & Tuohy, K. (2008). FAO technical meeting on prebiotics. *Journal of Clinical Gastroenterology, 42*, S156–S159.

Pitcher, M. C. L., Beatty, E. R., & Cummings, J. H. (2000). The contribution of sulphate reducing bacteria and 5-aminosalicylic acid to faecal sulphide in patients with ulcerative colitis. *Gut, 46*(1), 64–72. Available from https://doi.org/10.1136/gut.46.1.64.

Pitcher, M. C., & Cummings, J. H. (1996). Hydrogen sulphide: A bacterial toxin in ulcerative colitis? *Gut*, 1–4. Available from https://doi.org/10.1136/gut.39.1.1.

Plachá, D., & Jampílek, J. (2021). Chronic inflammatory diseases, anti-inflammatory agents and their delivery nanosystems. *Pharmaceutics, 13*(1), 64. Available from https://doi.org/10.3390/pharmaceutics13010064.

Plaza-Diaz, J., Ruiz-Ojeda, F. J., Gil-Campos, M., & Gil, A. (2019). Mechanisms of action of probiotics. *Advances in Nutrition, 10*, S49–S66. Available from https://doi.org/10.1093/advances/nmy063.

Podolsky, D. K. (2002). Inflammatory bowel disease. *New England Journal of Medicine, 347*(6), 417–429. Available from https://doi.org/10.1056/NEJMra020831.

Postgate, J., The suphate-reducing bacteria, 2nd ed. Cambridge University, Cambridge, UK, 1984.

Poxton, I. R., Brown, R., Sawyerr, A., & Ferguson, A. (1997). Mucosa-associated bacterial flora of the human colon. *Journal of Medical Microbiology, 46*(1), 85–91. Available from https://doi.org/10.1099/00222615-46-1-85.

Prins, R. A., & Lankhorst, A. (1977). Synthesis of acetate from CO_2 in the cecum of some rodents. *FEMS Microbiology Letters, 1*(5), 255–258. Available from https://doi.org/10.1111/j.1574-6968.1977.tb00627.x.

Pujo, J., Petitfils, C., Le Faouder, P., Eeckhaut, V., Payros, G., Maurel, S., Perez-Berezo, T., Van Hul, M., Barreau, F., Blanpied, C., Chavanas, S., Van Immerseel, F., Bertrand-Michel, J., Oswald, E., Knauf, C., Dietrich, G., Cani, P. D., & Cenac, N. (2020). Bacteria-derived long chain fatty acid exhibits anti-inflammatory properties in colitis. *Gut, 70*(6), 1088–1097. Available from https://doi.org/10.1136/gutjnl-2020-321173.

Puvvada, S. R., Luvsannyam, E., Patel, D., Hassan, Z., & Hamid, P. (2020). Probiotics in inflammatory bowel disease: Are we back to square one? *Cureus, 12*(9), e10247. Available from https://doi.org/10.7759/cureus.10247.

Qi, K., Lu, C. D., & Owens, F. N. (1993). Sulfate supplementation of Angora goats: Sulfur metabolism and interactions with zinc, copper and molybdenum. *Small Ruminant Research, 11*(3), 209–225. Available from https://doi.org/10.1016/0921-4488(93)90046-K.

Ramasamy, S., Singh, S., Taniere, P., Langman, M. J. S., & Eggo, M. C. (2006). Sulfide-detoxifying enzymes in the human colon are decreased in cancer and upregulated in differentiation. *American Journal of Physiology - Gastrointestinal and Liver Physiology, 291*(2), G288–G296. Available from https://doi.org/10.1152/ajpgi.00324.2005.

Rashidinejad, A., Bahrami, A., Rehman, A., Rezaei, A., Babazadeh, A., Singh, H., & Jafari, S. M. (2020). Co-encapsulation of probiotics with prebiotics and their application in functional/synbiotic dairy products. *Critical Reviews in Food Science and Nutrition*. Available from https://doi.org/10.1080/10408398.2020.1854169.

Rath, H. C., Schultz, M., Freitag, R., Dieleman, L. A., Li, F., Linde, H. J., Schölmerich, J., & Sartor, R. B. (2001). Different subsets of enteric bacteria induce and perpetuate experimental colitis in rats and mice. *Infection and Immunity, 69*(4), 2277–2285. Available from https://doi.org/10.1128/IAI.69.4.2277-2285.2001.

Rembacken, B. J., Snelling, A. M., Hawkey, P. M., Chalmers, D. M., & Axon, A. T. R. (1999). Non-pathogenic Escherichia coli vs mesalazine for the treatment of ulcerative colitis: A randomised trial. *The Lancet, 354*(9179), 635–639. Available from https://doi.org/10.1016/S0140-6736(98)06343-0.

Rizzello, F., Gionchetti, P., Venturi, A., Ferretti, M., Peruzzo, S., Raspanti, X., Picard, M., Canova, N., Palazzini, E., & Campieri, M. (1998). Rifaximin systemic absorption in patients with ulcerative colitis. *European Journal of Clinical Pharmacology, 54*(1), 91–93. Available from https://doi.org/10.1007/s002280050426.

Roediger, W. E. W. (1980). The colonic epithelium in ulcerative colitis: An energy-deficiency disease? *The Lancet, 316*(8197), 712–715. Available from https://doi.org/10.1016/S0140-6736(80)91934-0.

Roediger, W. E. W., Duncan, A., Kapaniris, O., & Millard, S. (1993a). Reducing sulfur compounds of the colon impair colonocyte nutrition: Implications for ulcerative colitis. *Gastroenterology, 104*(3), 802–809. Available from https://doi.org/10.1016/0016-5085(93)91016-B.

Roediger, W. E. W., Duncan, A., Kapaniris, O., & Millard, S. (1993b). Sulphide impairment of substrate oxidation in rat colonocytes: A biochemical basis for ulcerative colitis? *Clinical Science*, *85*(5), 623–627. Available from https://doi.org/10.1042/cs0850623.

Rowan, F. E., Docherty, N. G., Coffey, J. C., & O'Connell, P. R. (2009). Sulphate-reducing bacteria and hydrogen sulphide in the aetiology of ulcerative colitis. *British Journal of Surgery*, *96*(2), 151–158. Available from https://doi.org/10.1002/bjs.6454.

Ruseler-van Embden, J. G., Schouten, W. R., & van Lieshout, L. M. (1994). Pouchitis: Result of microbial imbalance? *Gut*, *35*(5), 658–664. Available from https://doi.org/10.1136/gut.35.5.658.

Sadlack, B., Merz, H., Schorle, H., Schimpl, A., Feller, A. C., & Horak, I. (1993). Ulcerative colitis-like disease in mice with a disrupted interleukin-2 gene. *Cell*, *75*(2), 253–261. Available from https://doi.org/10.1016/0092-8674(93)80067-O.

Saitoh, S., Noda, S., Aiba, Y., Takagi, A., Sakamoto, M., Benno, Y., & Koga, Y. (2002). Bacteroides ovatus as the predominant commensal intestinal microbe causing a systemic antibody response in inflammatory bowel disease. *Clinical and Diagnostic Laboratory Immunology*, *9*(1), 54–59. Available from https://doi.org/10.1128/CDLI.9.1.54-59.2002.

Salmerón, I. (2017). Fermented cereal beverages: From probiotic, prebiotic and synbiotic towards Nanoscience designed healthy drinks. *Letters in Applied Microbiology*, *65*(2), 114–124. Available from https://doi.org/10.1111/lam.12740.

Salvo, E., Stokes, P., Keogh, C. E., Brust-Mascher, I., Hennessey, C., Knotts, T. A., Sladek, J. A., Rude, K. M., Swedek, M., Rabasa, G., & Gareau, M. G. (2020). A murine model of pediatric inflammatory bowel disease causes microbiota-gut-brain axis deficits in adulthood. *American Journal of Physiology - Gastrointestinal and Liver Physiology*, *319*(3), G361–G374. Available from https://doi.org/10.1152/ajpgi.00177.2020.

Sandes, S., Figueiredo, N., Pedroso, S., Sant'Anna, F., Acurcio, L., Abatemarco, M., Junior, Barros, P., Oliveira, F., Cardoso, V., Generoso, S., Caliari, M., Nicoli, J., Neumann, E., & Nunes, Á. (2020). Weissella paramesenteroides WpK4 plays an immunobiotic role in gut-brain axis, reducing gut permeability, anxiety-like and depressive-like behaviors in murine models of colitis and chronic stress. *Food Research International*, *137*, 109741. Available from https://doi.org/10.1016/j.foodres.2020.109741.

Sartor, R. B., Rath, H. C., & Sellon, R. K. (1996). Microbial factors in chronic intestinal inflammation. *Current Opinion in Gastroenterology*, *12*(4), 327–333. Available from https://doi.org/10.1097/00001574-199607000-00003.

Sato, N., Garcia-Castillo, V., Yuzawa, M., Islam, M. A., Albarracin, L., Tomokiyo, M., Ikeda-Ohtsubo, W., Garcia-Cancino, A., Takahashi, H., Villena, J., & Kitazawa, H. (2020). Immunobiotic Lactobacillus jensenii TL2937 alleviates dextran sodium sulfate-induced colitis by differentially modulating the transcriptomic response of intestinal epithelial cells. *Frontiers in Immunology*, *11*, 2174. Available from https://doi.org/10.3389/fimmu.2020.02174.

Sato, N., Yuzawa, M., Aminul, M. I., Tomokiyo, M., Albarracin, L., Garcia-Castillo, V., Ideka-Ohtsubo, W., Iwabuchi, N., Xiao, J. Z., Garcia-Cancino, A., Villena, J., & Kitazawa, H. (2020). Evaluation of porcine intestinal epitheliocytes as an in vitro immunoassay system for the selection of probiotic bifidobacteria to alleviate inflammatory bowel disease. *Probiotics and Antimicrobial Proteins*, *13*(3), 824–836. Available from https://doi.org/10.1007/s12602-020-09694-z.

Satsangi, J., Landers, C. J., Welsh, K. I., Koss, K., Targan, S., & Jewell, D. P. (1998). The presence of anti-neutrophil antibodies reflects clinical and genetic heterogeneity within inflammatory bowel disease. *Inflammatory Bowel Diseases*, *4*(1), 18–26. Available from https://doi.org/10.1097/00054725-199802000-00004.

Schultsz, C., Moussa, M., van Ketel, R., Tytgat, G. N., & Dankert, J. (1997). Frequency of pathogenic and enteroadherent Escherichia coli in patients with inflammatory bowel disease and controls. *Journal of Clinical Pathology*, *50*(7), 573–579. Available from https://doi.org/10.1136/jcp.50.7.573.

Schultz, M., Veltkamp, C., Dieleman, L. A., Grenther, W. B., Wyrick, P. B., Tonkonogy, S. L., & Balfour Sartor, R. (2002). Lactobacillus plantarum 299V in the treatment and prevention of spontaneous colitis in interleukin-10-deficient mice. *Inflammatory Bowel Diseases*, *8*(2), 71–80. Available from https://doi.org/10.1097/00054725-200203000-00001.

Sekirov, I., Russell, S. L., Antunes, L. C. M., & Finlay, B. B. (2010). Gut microbiota in health and disease. *Physiological Reviews*, *90*(3), 859–904. Available from https://doi.org/10.1152/physrev.00045.2009.

Shafiee, N. H., Manaf, Z. A., Mokhtar, N. M., & Raja Ali, R. A. (2021). Anti-inflammatory diet and inflammatory bowel disease: What clinicians and patients should know? *Intestinal Research*, *19*(2), 171–185. Available from https://doi.org/10.5217/ir.2020.00035.

Shinde, T., Perera, A. P., Vemuri, R., Gondalia, S. V., Beale, D. J., Karpe, A. V., Shastri, S., Basheer, W., Southam, B., Eri, R., & Stanley, R. (2020). Synbiotic supplementation with prebiotic green banana resistant starch and probiotic Bacillus coagulans spores ameliorates gut inflammation in mouse model of inflammatory bowel diseases. *European Journal of Nutrition*, *59*(8), 3669–3689. Available from https://doi.org/10.1007/s00394-020-02200-9.

Shinde, T., Vemuri, R., Shastri, S., Perera, A. P., Gondalia, S. V., Beale, D. J., Karpe, A. V., Eri, R., & Stanley, R. (2020). Modulating the microbiome and immune responses using whole plant fibre in synbiotic combination with fibre-digesting probiotic attenuates chronic colonic inflammation in spontaneous colitic mice model of IBD. *Nutrients*, *12*(8), 2380. Available from https://doi.org/10.3390/nu12082380.

Siddiqui, A., Ancha, H., Tedesco, D., Lightfoot, S., Stewart, C. A., & Harty, R. F. (2006). Antioxidant therapy with N-acetylcysteine plus mesalamine accelerates mucosal healing in a rodent model of colitis. *Digestive Diseases and Sciences*, *51*(4), 698–705. Available from https://doi.org/10.1007/s10620-006-3194-z.

Silveira, D. S. C., Veronez, L. C., Lopes-Júnior, L. C., Anatriello, E., Brunaldi, M. O., & Pereira-Da-Silva, G. (2020). Lactobacillus bulgaricus inhibits colitis-associated cancer via a negative regulation of intestinal inflammation in azoxymethane/dextran sodium sulfate model. *World Journal of Gastroenterology*, *26*(43), 6782–6794. Available from https://doi.org/10.3748/wjg.v26.i43.6782.

Singhvi, N., Gupta, V., Gaur, M., Sharma, V., Puri, A., Singh, Y., Dubey, G. P., & Lal, R. (2020). Interplay of Human Gut Microbiome in Health and Wellness. *Indian Journal of Microbiology*, *60*(1), 26–36. Available from https://doi.org/10.1007/s12088-019-00825-x.

Smith, L., Kruszyna, H., & Smith, R. P. (1977). The effect of methemoglobin on the inhibition of cytochrome c oxidase by cyanide, sulfide or azide. *Biochemical Pharmacology*, *26*, 90287–90288. Available from https://doi.org/10.1016/0006-2952(77)90287-8.

Souza, E. L. S., Campos, C. L. V., Reis, D. C., Cassali, G. D., Generoso, S. V., Cardoso, V. N., Azevedo, V., Medeiros, J. D., Fernandes, G. R., Nicoli, J. R., & Martins, F. S. (2020). Beneficial effects resulting from oral administration of Escherichia coli Nissle 1917 on a chronic colitis model. *Beneficial Microbes*, *11*(8), 779–790. Available from https://doi.org/10.3920/BM2020.0045.

Steffen, R. (2001). Rifaximin: A nonabsorbed antimicrobial as a new tool for treatment of travelers' diarrhea. *Journal of Travel Medicine*, *8*(2), s34–s39. Available from https://doi.org/10.1111/j.1708-8305.2001.tb00545.x.

Stein, J., Schröder, O., Milovic, V., & Caspary, W. F. (1995). Mercaptopropionate inhibits butyrate uptake in isolated apical membrane vesicles of the rat distal colon. *Gastroenterology*, *108*(3), 673–679. Available from https://doi.org/10.1016/0016-5085(95)90438-7.

Stojanov, S., Berlec, A., & Štrukelj, B. (2020). The influence of probiotics on the firmicutes/bacteroidetes ratio in the treatment of obesity and inflammatory bowel disease. *Microorganisms*, *8*(11), 1715. Available from https://doi.org/10.3390/microorganisms8111715.

Strocchi, A., Ellis, C. J., Furne, J. K., & Levitt, M. D. (1994). Study of constancy of hydrogen-consuming flora of human colon. *Digestive Diseases and Sciences*, *39*(3), 494–497. Available from https://doi.org/10.1007/BF02088333.

Takeuchi, H., Setoguchi, T., MacHigashira, M., Kanbara, K., & Izumi, Y. (2008). Hydrogen sulfide inhibits cell proliferation and induces cell cycle arrest via an elevated p21Cip1 level in Ca9–22 cells. *Journal of Periodontal Research*, *43*(1), 90–95. Available from https://doi.org/10.1111/j.1600-0765.2007.00999.x.

Tan, Y., Shen, J., Si, T., Ho, C. L., Li, Y., & Dai, L. (2020). Engineered live biotherapeutics: Progress and challenges. *Biotechnology Journal*, *15*(10), 2000155. Available from https://doi.org/10.1002/biot.202000155.

Tarasiuk, A., & Eibl, G. (2020). Nutritional support and probiotics as a potential treatment of IBD. *Current Drug Targets*, *21*(14), 1417–1427. Available from https://doi.org/10.2174/1389450121666200504075519.

Terpou, A., Papadaki, A., Lappa, I. K., Kachrimanidou, V., Bosnea, L. A., & Kopsahelis, N. (2019). Probiotics in food systems: Significance and emerging strategies towards improved viability and delivery of enhanced beneficial value. *Nutrients*, *11*(7), 1591. Available from https://doi.org/10.3390/nu11071591.

Thomann, A. K., Mak, J. W. Y., Zhang, J. W., Wuestenberg, T., Ebert, M. P., Sung, J. J. Y., Bernstein, Ç. N., Reindl, W., & Ng, S. C. (2020). Review article: Bugs, inflammation and mood—A microbiota-based approach to psychiatric symptoms in inflammatory bowel diseases. *Alimentary Pharmacology and Therapeutics*, *52*(2), 247–266. Available from https://doi.org/10.1111/apt.15787.

Trivedi, R., & Barve, K. (2020). Gut microbiome a promising target for management of respiratory diseases. *Biochemical Journal*, *477*(14), 2679–2696. Available from https://doi.org/10.1042/BCJ20200426.

Truelove, S. C., & Jewell, D. P. (1974). Intensive intravenous regimen for severe attacks of ulcerative colitis. *The Lancet*, *303*(7866), 1067–1070. Available from https://doi.org/10.1016/S0140-6736(74)90552-2.

Turunen, U. M., Farkkila, M. A., Hakala, K., Seppala, K., Sivonen, A., Ogren, M., Vuoristo, M., Valtonen, V. V., & Miettinen, T. A. (1998). Long-term treatment of ulcerative colitis with ciprofloxacin: A prospective, double-blind, placebo-controlled study. *Gastroenterology*, *115*(5), 1072–1078. Available from https://doi.org/10.1016/S0016-5085(98)70076-9.

Utku, Ö. G., Karatay, E., Ergül, B., Yılmaz, C., Ekinci, Ö., & Arhan, M. (2020). Is the probiotic mixture effective in the treatment of TNBS-induced experimental colitis? *Journal of Academic Research in Medicine*, *10*(1), 41–47. Available from https://doi.org/10.4274/jarem.galenos.2019.2247.

Venturi, A., Gionchetti, P., Rizzello, F., Johansson, R., Zucconi, E., Brigidi, P., Matteuzzi, D., & Campieri, M. (1999). Impact on the composition of the faecal flora by a new probiotic preparation: Preliminary data on maintenance treatment of patients with ulcerative colitis. *Alimentary Pharmacology and Therapeutics*, *13*(8), 1103–1108. Available from https://doi.org/10.1046/j.1365-2036.1999.00560.x.

Vítězová, M., Kohoutová, A., Vítěz, T., Hanišáková, N., & Kushkevych, I. (2020). Methanogenic microorganisms in industrial wastewater anaerobic treatment. *Processes*, *8*(12), 1546. Available from https://doi.org/10.3390/pr8121546.

Wallace, J. L., Dicay, M., McKnight, W., & Martin, G. R. (2007). Hydrogen sulfide enhances ulcer healing in rats. *FASEB Journal*, *21*(14), 4070–4076. Available from https://doi.org/10.1096/fj.07-8669com.

Walmsley, R. S., Anthony, A., Sim, R., Pounder, R. E., & Wakefield, A. J. (1998). Absence of Escherichia coli, Listeria monocytogenes, and Klebsiella pneumoniae antigens within inflammatory bowel disease tissues. *Journal of Clinical Pathology*, *51*(9), 657–661. Available from https://doi.org/10.1136/jcp.51.9.657.

Wang, R. (2002). Two's company, three's a crowd: Can H2S be the third endogenous gaseous transmitter? *FASEB Journal*, *16*(13), 1792–1798. Available from https://doi.org/10.1096/fj.02-0211hyp.

Wang, G., Chen, Y., Fei, S., Xie, C., Xia, Y., & Ai, L. (2021). Colonisation with endogenous Lactobacillus reuteri R28 and exogenous Lactobacillus plantarum AR17-1 and the effects on intestinal inflammation in mice. *Food & Function*, *12*(6), 2481–2488. Available from https://doi.org/10.1039/d0fo02624g.

Wang, G., Huang, S., Cai, S., Yu, H., Wang, Y., Zeng, X., & Qiao, S. (2020). Lactobacillus reuteri ameliorates intestinal inflammation and modulates gut microbiota and metabolic disorders in dextran sulfate sodium-induced colitis in mice. *Nutrients*, *12*(8), 2298. Available from https://doi.org/10.3390/nu12082298.

Wilkins, T., & Sequoia, J. (2017). Probiotics for Gastrointestinal Conditions: A Summary of the Evidence. *American Family Physician*, *96*(3), 170–178.

Wilson, K., Mudra, M., Furne, J., & Levitt, M. (2008). Differentiation of the roles of sulfide oxidase and rhodanese in the detoxification of sulfide by the colonic mucosa. *Digestive Diseases and Sciences*, *53*(1), 277–283. Available from https://doi.org/10.1007/s10620-007-9854-9.

Xia, Y., Chen, Y., Wang, G., Yang, Y., Song, X., Xiong, Z., Zhang, H., Lai, P., Wang, S., & Ai, L. (2020). Lactobacillus plantarum AR113 alleviates DSS-induced colitis by regulating the TLR4/MyD88/NF-κB pathway and gut microbiota composition. *Journal of Functional Foods*, *67*, 103854. Available from https://doi.org/10.1016/j.jff.2020.103854.

Yan, F., & Polk, D. B. (2020). Probiotics and probiotic-derived functional factors—Mechanistic insights into applications for intestinal homeostasis. *Frontiers in Immunology*, *11*, 1428. Available from https://doi.org/10.3389/fimmu.2020.01428.

Yan, P. G., & Li, J. N. (2020). Advances in the understanding of the intestinal micro-environment and inflammatory bowel disease. *Chinese Medical Journal*, *133*(7), 834–841. Available from https://doi.org/10.1097/CM9.0000000000000718.

Yang, G., Cao, K., Wu, L., & Wang, R. (2004). Cystathionine γ-lyase overexpression inhibits cell proliferation via a H2S-dependent modulation of ERK1/2 phosphorylation and p21 Cip/WAK-1. *Journal of Biological Chemistry*, *279*(47), 49199–49205. Available from https://doi.org/10.1074/jbc.M408997200.

Yeo, S., Park, H., Seo, E., Kim, J., Kim, B. K., Choi, I. S., & Huh, C. S. (2020). Anti-inflammatory and gut microbiota modulatory effect of Lactobacillus rhamnosus strain ldtm 7511 in a dextran sulfate sodium-induced colitis murine model. *Microorganisms*, *8*(6), 845. Available from https://doi.org/10.3390/microorganisms8060845.

Yoshimatsu, Y., Mikami, Y., & Kanai, T. (2021). Bacteriotherapy for inflammatory bowel disease. *Inflammation and Regeneration*, *41*(1), 3. Available from https://doi.org/10.1186/s41232-020-00153-4.

Yue, B., Yu, Z. L., Lv, C., Geng, X. L., Wang, Z. T., & Dou, W. (2020). Regulation of the intestinal microbiota: An emerging therapeutic strategy for inflammatory bowel disease. *World Journal of Gastroenterology*, *26*(30), 4378–4393. Available from https://doi.org/10.3748/WJG.V26.I30.4378.

Zhai, R., Xue, X., Zhang, L., Yang, X., Zhao, L., & Zhang, C. (2019). Strain-specific anti-inflammatory properties of two Akkermansia muciniphila strains on chronic colitis in mice. *Frontiers in Cellular and Infection Microbiology*, *9*, 239. Available from https://doi.org/10.3389/fcimb.2019.00239.

Zhang, T., Li, P., Wu, X., Lu, G., Marcella, C., Ji, X., Ji, G., & Zhang, F. (2020). Alterations of Akkermansia muciniphila in the inflammatory bowel disease patients with washed microbiota transplantation. *Applied Microbiology and Biotechnology*, *104*(23), 10203–10215. Available from https://doi.org/10.1007/s00253-020-10948-7.

Zhang, X. F., Guan, X. X., Tang, Y. J., Sun, J. F., Wang, X. K., Wang, W. D., & Fan, J. M. (2021). Clinical effects and gut microbiota changes of using probiotics, prebiotics or synbiotics in inflammatory bowel disease: A systematic review and *meta*-analysis. *European Journal of Nutrition*, *60*(5), 2855–2875. Available from https://doi.org/10.1007/s00394-021-02503-5.

Zhang, X., Tong, Y., Lyu, X., Wang, J., Wang, Y., & Yang, R. (2021). Prevention and alleviation of dextran sulfate sodium salt-induced inflammatory bowel disease in mice with Bacillus subtilis-fermented milk via inhibition of the inflammatory responses and regulation of the intestinal flora. *Frontiers in Microbiology*, *11*, 622354. Available from https://doi.org/10.3389/fmicb.2020.622354.

Zhao, N., Liu, J. M., Yang, F. E., Ji, X. M., Li, C. Y., Lv, S. W., & Wang, S. (2020). A novel mediation strategy of DSS-induced colitis in mice based on an iron-enriched probiotic and in vivo bioluminescence tracing. *Journal of Agricultural and Food Chemistry*, *68*(43), 12028–12038. Available from https://doi.org/10.1021/acs.jafc.0c05260.

Zheng, L., & Wen, X. L. (2021). Gut microbiota and inflammatory bowel disease: The current status and perspectives. *World Journal of Clinical Cases*, *9*(2), 321–333. Available from https://doi.org/10.12998/wjcc.v9.i2.321.

Zhou, L., Liu, D., Xie, Y., Yao, X., & Li, Y. (2019). Bifidobacterium infantis induces protective colonic PD-L1 and Foxp3 regulatory T cells in an acute murine experimental model of inflammatory bowel disease. *Gut and Liver*, *13*(4), 430–439. Available from https://doi.org/10.5009/gnl18316.

Zhou, X., Lu, Q., Kang, X., Tian, G., Ming, D., & Yang, J. (2021). Protective role of a new polysaccharide extracted from lonicera japonica thunb in mice with ulcerative colitis induced by dextran sulphate sodium. *BioMed Research International*, *2021*, 8878633. Available from https://doi.org/10.1155/2021/8878633.

Zinkevich, V. V., & Beech, I. B. (2000). Screening of sulfate-reducing bacteria in colonoscopy samples from healthy and colitic human gut mucosa. *FEMS Microbiology Ecology*, *34*(2), 147–155. Available from https://doi.org/10.1111/j.1574-6941.2000.tb00764.x.

Zoetendal, E. G., Von Wright, A., Vilpponen-Salmela, T., Ben-Amor, K., Akkermans, A. D. L., & De Vos, W. M. (2002). Mucosa-associated bacteria in the human gastrointestinal tract are uniformly distributed along the colon and differ from the community recovered from feces. *Applied and Environmental Microbiology*, *68*(7), 3401–3407. Available from https://doi.org/10.1128/AEM.68.7.3401-3407.2002.

Chapter 5

Probiotics in the prevention and management of necrotizing enterocolitis

Eleonora Seghesio*, Charlotte De Geyter* and Yvan Vandenplas
Vrije Universiteit Brussel (VUB), UZ Brussel, KidZ Health Castle, Brussels, Belgium

5.1 Introduction

Necrotizing enterocolitis (NEC) is a severe and potentially lethal intestinal disease and occurs almost exclusively in preterm infants. It is characterized by mucosal inflammation, epithelial cell death, and transmural perforation of the intestinal wall with the leakage of intestinal fluids as a consequence. In severe cases, it leads to sepsis and multiorgan failure whereby surgical removal of the necrotized intestine is the only treatment option. The symptoms of NEC are often nonspecific, varying from temperature instability, changes in vital parameters to feeding intolerance, distention of the abdominal wall and bloody stools.

The prevalence is around 7% in preterm babies with a weight of less than 1500 g and has a mortality rate of 20%–30% (Sanchez & Kadrofske, 2019). NEC is predominantly seen in infants born at a gestational age younger than 32 weeks whereby the incidence is inversely proportional related to the gestational age (Battersby et al., 2017). NEC usually develops between the second week and the second month of life and rarely occurs in utero or prior to the first feeding (Boccia et al., 2001). Many risk factors have been identified, such as small for gestational age, premature rupture of membranes, assisted ventilation, sepsis, and hypotension (Samuels et al., 2017). Other risk factors include formula feeding, exposure to acid suppression medication, and the use of antibiotics (Carrion & Egan, 1990; Kuppala et al., 2011). The latter category of modifiable risk factors have in common that they alter the intestinal microbiome, which supports the hypothesis that dysbiosis is an important determinant factor leading to NEC. As a consequence, probiotics are more frequently used in neonatal intensive care units (NICUs). In the United States, out of 78,076 infants, 3626 (4.6%) received probiotics. Probiotic use increased over the study period, 1997–2016, and varied among NICUs (Gray et al., 2020).

The effect of evidence-based strategies to decrease NEC includes: (1) standardized feeding protocol, (2) early initiation of enteral feeding using human milk, (3) optimizing the osmolality of preterm milk feeds using standardized dilution guidelines for additives, and (4) promotion of healthy microbiome by the use of probiotics, early oral care with colostrum and by restricting high-risk medications and prolonged use of empirical antibiotics were tested during four consecutive years on one center. Baseline characteristics of the patients, including sex, gestational age, and birth weight, were similar during the study period. Incidence of NEC in very low birth weight (VLBW) infants was 7% in 2014 and dropped to 0% ($P < .001$) in 2018. Duration of parenteral nutrition, use of central line, and days to full feeds were also reduced significantly ($P < .05$) (Chandran & Mammen, 2020).

5.2 The microbiome, dysbiosis, and NEC

The number of species growing in the gut increases significantly with gestational age. The abundance of species and their diversity is, other than by gestational age, also influenced by the use of (intrapartum) antibiotics, method of feeding, and mode of delivery. The presence and abundance of *Clostridium perfringens* that produces alpha toxin and

---

*ES and CD contributed equally to this chapter.

Bacteroides dorei in meconium is associated with NEC, suggesting that factors during pregnancy, delivery, and the first moments of life may contribute to the formation of an NEC-associated microbiota (Sharif et al., 2020).

Studies found that preterm babies being formula fed had an increased abundance of *Proteobacteria*, including *Klebsiella* and *Enterobacter*, and a decreased abundance of *Firmicutes*. Moreover, *Bifidobacterium* species, beneficial commensal bacteria abundant present in breastfed term infants, seem to be less common and especially less abundant in preterm infants who go on to develop NEC (Underwood et al., 2015; Underwood, 2019).

The use of antibiotics led to an increased abundance of *Proteobacteria* and decreased relative abundances of *Firmicutes* and *Actinobacteria*. Infants not receiving antibiotics showed increased abundance of genus *Clostridium* and unclassified Clostridiaceae. According to a meta-analysis (Pammi et al., 2017), infants that would develop NEC had an increased abundance of *Proteobacteria* and a decreased abundance of *Firmicutes* and *Bacteroides* compared to healthy controls. Even though no association was found between the mode of delivery and the development of NEC, a meta-analysis found that children born by cesarean section showed an increased abundance of *Firmicutes*, while an increased abundance of *Bacteroidetes* was found in infants born through vaginal delivery (Pammi et al., 2017).

Interestingly, the absence of *Clostridia*, in particular of *Clostridium difficile*, was associated with the development of NEC (McMurtry et al., 2015). Even though this seems in contrast with the fact that infants with an abundant amount of *C. perfringens* in meconium are associated with NEC, the hypothesis is that the nontoxinogenic *C. difficile* provides effective protection against the enterotoxin-mediated diseases of the *Clostridium perfringens* (Jangi & Lamont, 2010). Similarly, newborns are frequently colonized with *C. difficile* without suffering from any illness, while they become more prone for *Clostridium*-related diseases when they are no longer *Clostridium* carriers (Wilson & Sheagren, 1983).

As said, NEC occurs almost exclusively in preterm, a group in which cesarean section and perinatal antibiotic administration are extremely frequent compared to term infants. Many preterm infants are formula fed, and if mother's milk can be given, it has to be acknowledged that mother's milk that has been banked has lost some of its benefits (Meier et al., 2017). In mice, maternal administration of *Lactobacillus acidophilus* and *Bifidobacterium infantis* (during pregnancy and lactation) promotes intestinal development, improves small intestinal barrier function, and decreases inflammatory responses of the preweaned pups (Yu et al., 2020).

5.3 Most relevant mechanisms of probiotic action in the preterm

Probiotics have different sites of action that enable them to protect the premature intestine for the development of NEC. One of the most important mechanisms is the modulation of the Toll-like receptors (TLRs) whose essential function is to recognize components of pathogenic microbes and trigger a specific inflammatory response (Underwood, 2019). The immature gut has a propensity to inflame, whereby TLR4 is thought to play a crucial role in the regulation of the injury and repair balance in the intestine epithelium (Hackam et al., 2019; Sodhi et al., 2012). Animal studies showed an increased TLR4 expression in the immature comparing to the full term gut. This is probably due to the fact that TLR4 is also essential for the activation of Notch signaling pathway leading to activation of the intestinal stem cells, which is required for the normal proliferation and differentiation (Sodhi et al., 2012). In utero, TLR4 expression is downregulated by the epithelial growth factor (EGF) present in the amniotic fluid, which is continuously swallowed by the fetus. Mother's milk also contains EGF (Dvorak et al., 2002; Good et al., 2012, 2015; Herrmann & Carroll, 2014; Newburg et al., 2005; Peng et al., 2009). The activation of TLR4 in the premature gut leads to death of the intestinal epithelium leading to NEC. Probiotics stimulate the production of TLR9, which prevents TLR4 signaling (Gribar et al., 2009). *Proteobacteria* are, for example, known to be activators of TLR4 (Lu et al., 2014).

Furthermore, the immature intestine is constantly being exposed to newly colonizing commensals and pathogens. When the intestine of the preterm infant is colonized with pathogenic bacteria, probiotics compete and may limit the overgrowth of such pathogens (Mathipa & Thantsha, 2017). Lactate-producing *Bacilli*, including *Staphylococci* and *Streptococci*, lower the pH via the production of lactate impairing the overgrowth of pathogenic Enterobacteriaceae (Kumar et al., 2009; Rivera-Chávez et al., 2017). Also, probiotics are known to support the barrier maturation and function of the intestinal wall (Martinez et al., 2013; Patel et al., 2012).

5.4 Probiotics and prevention of NEC

As described above, probiotic bacteria are present in mother's milk and maternal milk has a protective effect for NEC. However, breast milk is not always available, especially not in mothers of preterm infants, hence a poor maternal production due to premature delivery. The administration of probiotics seems therefore a logical step in the prevention of NEC.

Angela Hoyos, a neonatologist in Bogota Colombia, was the first person investigating the role of probiotics in the prevention of NEC. Twenty years ago, she decided to treat preterm in the NICU with the probiotic Infloran, containing *B. infantis* and *L. acidophilus* for the duration of their hospital stay, saw a highly significant decrease in both NEC and NEC-related death ($P < .0002$ and $P < .005$, respectively) (Hoyos, 1999). From then on, many investigators started clinical trials including more than 40,000 infants (Underwood, 2019).

A wide variety of probiotic preparations have been studied, including *Bacillus*, *Bifidobacterium* spp., *Lactobacillus* spp., and *Saccharomyces* and probiotic combinations. However, the most commonly used preparation was *Lactobacillus* spp., *Bifidobacterium* spp., or the combination of those two. Most randomized controlled trials (RCTs) compared the supplementation of a probiotic versus placebo or no supplementation at all. Also, most trials started the supplementation within the first week of birth, usually with the first enteral feed. The supplementation was usually continued until at 28 days postpartum or discharge from the hospital (Patel & Denning, 2013; Sawh et al., 2016).

Jacobs et al. (2013) reported in 2013 that the combination of *B. infantis*, *Streptococcus thermophilus*, and *Bifidobacterium lactis* was effective in the reduction of NEC. A large trial of probiotic supplementation investigating the effect of the single-strain *Bifidobacterium breve* found no effect in the reduction of NEC (Costeloe et al., 2016). According to data from Spain, between 2005 and 2017, the incidence of NEC remained stable at 8.8% among the 25,821 included infants during the whole study period and remained stable when comparing 4-year subperiods. Prophylactic probiotics were implemented during the 12-year study period in some units, reaching 18.6% of the patients in 2015–17. However, when all trials with different protocols and different strains were grouped together, the incidence of NEC remained stable despite the increase in protective factors (Zozaya et al., 2020).

The most recent Cochrane review by Sharif et al. (2020) performed a meta-analysis comparing different probiotic preparations. The reviewed population included 10.812 prematures distributed over 56 trials with an average gestational age of 28–32 weeks and an average birth weight of 1000–1200 g. The overall conclusion was that the supplementation of probiotics indeed reduced the risk of NEC {risk ratio (RR) 0.54 [95% credible interval (CI) 0.54–0.65]} with the combination of *Bifidobacterium* spp. and *Lactobacillus* spp. being the most effective [RR 0.36 (95% CI 0.23–0.59)]. Other effective combinations were *Bifidobacterium* spp. plus *Streptococcus* spp. [RR 0.35 (95% CI 0.19–0.68)] and *Bifidobacterium* spp. plus *Lactobacillus* spp. plus *Streptococcus* spp. [RR 0.42 (95% CI 0.22–0.77)]. Single genus *Bifidobacterium* spp. was also found effective [RR 0.72 (95% CI 0.54–0.96)] like *Lactobacillus* spp. [RR 0.45 (95% CI 0.28–0.71)] but less effective than the combination. Few data (from seven of the trials) were available for extremely preterm or extremely low birth weight infants. Meta-analyses did not show effects on NEC, death, or infection (low-certainty evidence). Sensitivity meta-analyses of 16 trials (4597 infants) at the low risk of bias did not show an effect on mortality or infection. Evidence was assessed as low certainty because of the limitations in trial design, and the presence of funnel plot asymmetry consistent with publication bias (Sharif et al., 2020).

Studies comparing the efficacy of different strains with each other are lacking and as a consequence, conclusions should be interpreted cautiously. Therefore different network meta-analyses on probiotics and NEC were published in 2020. A network analysis allows to compare the efficacy of different strains tested in different studies. According to van den Akker et al. (2020), provided all safety issues are met, there is currently a conditional recommendation (with low certainty of evidence) to provide either *Lactobacillus rhamnosus* GG ATCC53103 or the combination of *B. infantis* Bb-02, *B. lactis* Bb-12, and *Streptococcus thermophilus* TH-4 to reduce NEC rates. Chi et al. (2020) included 45 trials with 12,320 participants. *Bifidobacterium* plus *Lactobacillus* was associated with lower rates of mortality (RR 0.56; 95% CI 0.34–0.84) and NEC morbidity (RR 0.47; 95% CI 0.27–0.79) in comparison to placebo; *Lactobacillus* plus prebiotic was associated with lower rates of NEC morbidity (RR 0.06; 95% CI 0.01–0.41) in comparison to placebo; *Bifidobacterium* plus prebiotic had the highest probability of having the lowest rate of mortality (surface under the cumulative ranking curve 83.94%); and *Lactobacillus* plus prebiotic had the highest probability of having the lowest rate of NEC (surface under the cumulative ranking curve 95.62%) (Chi et al., 2020). An important limitation is that only in a few studies authors reported the data of infants with a lower birth weight or gestational age (Chi et al., 2020). According to a recent matched cohort study in 23- to 29-week-old infants, probiotic administration was associated with a decrease in NEC (OR 0.62, 95% CI 0.48–0.80) and death (OR 0.52, 95% CI 0.39–0.70), an increase in *Candida* infection (OR 2.23, 95% CI 1.29–3.85), but no increase in bloodstream infection (OR 0.86, 95% CI 0.70–1.05) or meningitis (OR 1.18, 95% CI 0.40–3.46) (Gray et al., 2020). To achieve optimal effect on premature infant health, combined use of prebiotic and probiotic, especially *Lactobacillus* or *Bifidobacterium*, is recommended (Chi et al., 2020). In a systematic review and network meta-analysis performed by Morgan et al. (2020) of the McMaster Probiotic, Prebiotic, and Synbiotic Work Group to determine the effects of single-strain and multistrain probiotic formulations on outcomes of preterm, low birth weight neonates, a moderate to high evidence for the superiority of combinations of one or more *Lactobacillus* spp. and one or more *Bifidobacterium* spp. versus single- and other multiple-strain probiotic treatments was reported. The combinations of *Bacillus* spp. and *Enterococcus* spp., and one or more *Bifidobacterium* spp. and *Streptococcus salivarius* spp. *thermophilus* might produce the largest reduction in NEC development (Morgan et al., 2020).

5.5 Safety aspects of probiotics

Since preterm is a fragile and immunocompromised population and probiotics are live bacteria supplement, it is extremely important to be aware of the possible risks. The most feared side effect is probiotic sepsis whereby it is important to realize that it may be hard to diagnose since the traditional pediatric culture bottle impairs the growth of anaerobic strains. Probiotic sepsis may be not only the result of intestinal translocation but also because of contamination of central lines after the preparation of the probiotic (van den Akker et al., 2020).

Probiotic sepsis has been described in several single or multiple case studies, mostly associated with *B. infantis* and *L. rhamnosus* GG. However, also other probiotic strains have been cultured, including *Lactobacillus reuteri*, *Saccharomyces boulardii*, *B. breve*, and *Echerichia coli* Nissle. Two recent papers described *L. rhamnosus* bacteremia in infants with a central line that were not receiving the probiotic but were just sharing the same room of the infant receiving this probiotic (Carlo et al., 2016; Yelin et al., 2019). However, even though the case reports should be taken seriously, it is also important to note that in all the 56 trials included in the most recent Cochrane no probiotic-related sepsis was found (Sharif et al., 2020).

Lactic acidosis is another potential adverse effect, specifically relevant for this age group since preterm has the tendency to be acidotic and is more prone to suffer from conditions that make them more acidotic, such as sepsis and renal insufficiency. Lactate may be produced by *Lactobacilli* strains in two different isoforms: D-lactate and/or L-lactate. Some strains, such as *L. rhamnosus* GG ATCC53103 produces mainly L-lactate, but for example, *L. reuteri* DSM 17938 or *L. acidophilus* NCDO 1748 produces larger proportions of D-lactate. Especially the production of D-lactate could be problematic in preterm infants since D-lactate is difficult to dispose of after enteral uptake and therefore possibly leading to acidosis (Mack, 2004). Moreover, in contrast to L-lactate, D-lactate cannot routinely be measured in blood gases with as consequence that it may be hard to be identified as the cause of metabolic acidosis. Even though, *L. reuteri* DSM 17938 has been approved for the use in term infant formula by the Food and Drug Administration (FDA, 2012) and despite that in term born infants an elevated urinary D-lactate concentrations after being fed a *L. reuteri DSM 17938*-containing formula was not associated with blood acidosis (Konstantinos et al., 2014), it may be wise not to take risks for the premature population because of the above listed reasons. Moreover, several case reports have described D-lactate acidosis in infants suffering from short bowel syndrome (Munakata et al., 2010; Reddy et al., 2013). Therefore it may be wise follow the statement of the Codex Alimentarius, saying that preterm infants should only receive probiotics that mainly produce L-lactate, until more research about this topic is available (International Food Standards Codex Commission, 2016).

Another important safety issue is related to the quality control of the probiotic supplementation whereby difference has been found between the label and the actual content. A recent report found that only 1 out of 16 tested commercial probiotic products matched exactly the label, including probiotics marketed specifically for infants (Lewis et al., 2016). Since probiotics are usually marked as food supplements instead of drugs, they fall under the regulatory framework of food with as consequence that manufactures may change the product content or production process without the obligation to properly address those issues (de Simone, 2019).

Also, limited amount of follow-up studies is available assessing the long-term efficacy or safety from probiotics used in preterm infants. A randomized trial of 400 VLBW infants with follow up of 18–24 months showed that the use of *L. reuteri* did not increase nor decrease the risk of adverse neurocognitive outcomes (Akar et al., 2017). A large trial called the "ProPrems" is currently ongoing and will hopefully provide additional data regarding long-term benefits of probiotics (Garland et al., 2011).

5.6 Conclusions and challenges for future research

NEC is a devastating disease responsible for morbidity and mortality of the premature infant. Since early dysbiosis has been associated with the development of NEC, a lot of research has been conducted in the past decades studying the role of probiotics in the prevention of this disease. Different (network) meta-analyses have been performed reviewing clinical trials including a total of more than 10,000 infants leading to the overall conclusion that probiotics could play a role in the prevention of NEC. The most recent Cochrane review (Sharif et al., 2020) dating from October 2020 including 56 trials found an overall beneficial effect of probiotics in the prevention of NEC whereby most effect was observed for *Bifidobacterium* spp. and for *Lactobacillus* spp. but even more for mixtures of *Bifidobacterium* spp. plus *Streptococcus* spp. and *Bifidobacterium* spp. plus *Streptococcus* spp. Besides that the effect of probiotics is strongly species specific, the effect of a single strain might also differ from combined strains in NEC (Guthmann et al., 2010). Despite the promising results of the Cochrane review and other (network) meta-analyses, the implementation into the clinical practice has been difficult so far due to concerns about the efficacy and safety of probiotics (Adams et al., 2019).

Since the efficacy of probiotics is highly strain specific, more studies should be performed comparing individual strain face to face with each other. So far, only network analyses have been used to compare the different strains, but it is important to realize that as indirect comparisons are not randomized, the effect size may be confounded by other factors than purely difference between the strains (Sharif et al., 2020). Moreover, there is a lack of studies investigating the optimal dose and duration of therapy. Within RCTs there is variability in the doses, age at initiation and duration of the therapy. It has been suggested that at least 1×10^9 colony-forming units are required to guarantee the passage through the gastrointestinal tract and the gut colonization for exerting a measurable beneficial effect (Bertazzoni et al., 2013). However, the majority of the trials vary in dose from 1 to 6×10^9 per day showing mixed results, leading to the conclusion that the dose-dependent effects are in fact strain dependent. Therefore studies should be performed investigating the optimal dose related to specific probiotic strains. Also, studies systemically investigating possible adverse effects, such as D-lactate acidosis and probiotic sepsis, would be of great value. Preferably, the studies should be performed with products whereby it will be guaranteed that the actual content of the probiotic product matches its label. A model demonstrated that prophylactic probiotics are a cost-effective strategy in NEC reduction. Sensitivity analysis confirmed that the model is customizable to various clinical settings and thus can aid in understanding the economic impact of this intervention (Craighead et al., 2020). Uncertainty about the therapeutic role of probiotics to prevent NEC is in part due to the wide range of bacterial strains with no previous evidence of efficacy used in clinical trials (Paul et al., 2020).

References

Adams, M., Bassler, D., Darlow, B. A., Lui, K., Reichman, B., Hakansson, S., Norman, M., Lee, S. K., Helenius, K. K., Lehtonen, L., San Feliciano, L., Vento, M., Moroni, M., Beltempo, M., Yang, J., & Shah, P. S. (2019). Preventive strategies and factors associated with surgically treated necrotising enterocolitis in extremely preterm infants: An international unit survey linked with retrospective cohort data analysis. *BMJ Open*, 9(10). Available from https://doi.org/10.1136/bmjopen-2019-031086.

Akar, M., Eras, Z., Oncel, M. Y., Arayici, S., Guzoglu, N., Canpolat, F. E., Uras, N., & Oguz, S. S. (2017). Impact of oral probiotics on neurodevelopmental outcomes in preterm infants. *Journal of Maternal-Fetal and Neonatal Medicine*, 30(4), 411–415. Available from https://doi.org/10.1080/14767058.2016.1174683.

Battersby, C., Longford, N., Mandalia, S., Costeloe, K., & Modi, N. (2017). Incidence and enteral feed antecedents of severe neonatal necrotising enterocolitis across neonatal networks in England, 2012–13: A whole-population surveillance study. *The Lancet Gastroenterology and Hepatology*, 2(1), 43–51. Available from https://doi.org/10.1016/S2468-1253(16)30117-0.

Bertazzoni, E., Donelli, G., Midtvedt, T., Nicoli, J., & Sanz, Y. (2013). Probiotics and clinical effects: Is the number what counts? *Journal of Chemotherapy*, 25(4), 194–212. Available from https://doi.org/10.1179/1973947813Y.0000000078.

Boccia, D., Stolfi, I., Lana, S., & Moro, M. L. (2001). Nosocomial necrotising enterocolitis outbreaks: Epidemiology and control measures. *European Journal of Pediatrics*, 160(6), 385–391. Available from https://doi.org/10.1007/s004310100749.

Carlo, D., Caterina, C. C., Iuri, C. I., Fabio, A., Alberto, A., & Gian, R. (2016). Lactobacillus sepsis and probiotic therapy in newborns: Two new cases and literature review. *American Journal of Perinatology Reports*, 6(1), e25–e29. Available from https://doi.org/10.1055/s-0035-1566312.

Carrion, V., & Egan, E. A. (1990). Prevention of neonatal necrotizing enterocolitis. *Journal of Pediatric Gastroenterology and Nutrition*, 11(3), 317–323. Available from https://doi.org/10.1097/00005176-199010000-00006.

Chandran, K., & Mammen, S. C. (2020). Effect of early enteral feeding on recovery profile in mild acute pancreatitis. *International Surgery Journal*, 7(6), 1969–1976. Available from https://doi.org/10.18203/2349-2902.isj20202414.

Chi, C., Li, C., Buys, N., Wang, W., Yin, C., & Sun, J. (2020). Effects of probiotics in preterm infants: A network meta-analysis. *Pediatrics*, 147(1), e20200706.

Costeloe, K., Bowler, U., Brocklehurst, P., Hardy, P., Heal, P., Juszczak, E., King, A., Panton, N., Stacey, F., Whiley, A., Wilks, M., & Millar, M. R. (2016). A randomised controlled trial of the probiotic Bifidobacterium breve BBG-001 in preterm babies to prevent sepsis, necrotising enterocolitis and death: The probiotics in preterm infantS (PiPS) trial. *Health Technology Assessment*, 20(66), vii–83. Available from https://doi.org/10.3310/hta20660.

Craighead, A. F., Caughey, A. B., Chaudhuri, A., Yieh, L., Hersh, A. R., & Dukhovny, D. (2020). Cost-effectiveness of probiotics for necrotizing enterocolitis prevention in very low birth weight infants. *Journal of Perinatology*, 40(11), 1652–1661. Available from https://doi.org/10.1038/s41372-020-00790-0.

de Simone, C. (2019). The unregulated probiotic market. *Clinical Gastroenterology and Hepatology*, 17(5), 809–817. Available from https://doi.org/10.1016/j.cgh.2018.01.018.

Dvorak, B., Halpern, M. D., Holubec, H., Williams, C. S., Mcwilliam, D. L., Dominguez, J. A., Stepankova, R., Payne, C. M., & Mccuskey, R. S. (2002). Epidermal growth factor reduces the development of necrotizing enterocolitis in a neonatal rat model. *American Journal of Physiology—Gastrointestinal and Liver Physiology*, 282(1), G156–G164. Available from https://doi.org/10.1152/ajpgi.00196.2001.

FDA (2012). *FDA GRAS notification: Lactobacillus reuteri strain DSM 17938*.

Garland, S. M., Tobin, J. M., Pirotta, M., Tabrizi, S. N., Opie, G., Donath, S., Tang, M. L., Morley, C. J., Hickey, L., Ung, L., Jacobs, S. E., & Group, P. S. (2011). The ProPrems trial: Investigating the effects of probiotics on late onset sepsis in very preterm infants. *BMC Infectious Diseases*, 11, 210. Available from https://doi.org/10.1186/1471-2334-11-210.

Good, M., Siggers, R. H., Sodhi, C. P., Afrazi, A., Alkhudari, F., Egan, C. E., Neal, M. D., Yazji, I., Jia, H., Lin, J., Branca, M. F., Ma, C., Prindle, T., Grant, Z., Shah, S., Slagle, D., Paredes, J., Ozolek, J., Gittes, G. K., & Hackam, D. J. (2012). Amniotic fluid inhibits Toll-like receptor 4 signaling in the fetal and neonatal intestinal epithelium. *Proceedings of the National Academy of Sciences of the United States of America*, 109(28), 11330–11335. Available from https://doi.org/10.1073/pnas.1200856109.

Good, M., Sodhi, C. P., Egan, C. E., Afrazi, A., Jia, H., Yamaguchi, Y., Lu, P., Branca, M. F., Ma, C., Prindle, T., Mielo, S., Pompa, A., Hodzic, Z., Ozolek, J. A., & Hackam, D. J. (2015). Breast milk protects against the development of necrotizing enterocolitis through inhibition of Toll-like receptor 4 in the intestinal epithelium via activation of the epidermal growth factor receptor. *Mucosal Immunology*, 8(5), 1166–1179. Available from https://doi.org/10.1038/mi.2015.30.

Gray, K. D., Messina, J. A., Cortina, C., Owens, T., Fowler, M., Foster, M., Gbadegesin, S., Clark, R. H., Benjamin, D. K., Zimmerman, K. O., & Greenberg, R. G. (2020). Probiotic use and safety in the neonatal intensive care unit: A matched cohort study. *Journal of Pediatrics*, 222, 59–64. e1. Available from https://doi.org/10.1016/j.jpeds.2020.03.051.

Gribar, S. C., Sodhi, C. P., Richardson, W. M., Anand, R. J., Gittes, G. K., Branca, M. F., Jakub, A., Shi, X. H., Shah, S., Ozolek, J. A., & Hackam, D. J. (2009). Reciprocal expression and signaling of TLR4 and TLR9 in the pathogenesis and treatment of necrotizing enterocolitis. *Journal of Immunology*, 182(1), 636–646. Available from https://doi.org/10.4049/jimmunol.182.1.636.

Guthmann, F., Kluthe, C., & Bührer, C. (2010). Probiotics for prevention of necrotising enterocolitis: An updated meta-analysis. *Klinische Padiatrie*, 222(5), 284–290. Available from https://doi.org/10.1055/s-0030-1254113.

Hackam, D. J., Sodhi, C. P., & Good, M. (2019). New insights into necrotizing enterocolitis: From laboratory observation to personalized prevention and treatment. *Journal of Pediatric Surgery*, 54(3), 398–404. Available from https://doi.org/10.1016/j.jpedsurg.2018.06.012.

Herrmann, K., & Carroll, K. (2014). An exclusively human milk diet reduces necrotizing enterocolitis. *Breastfeeding Medicine*, 9(4), 184–190. Available from https://doi.org/10.1089/bfm.2013.0121.

Hoyos, A. B. (1999). Reduced incidence of necrotizing enterocolitis associated with enteral administration of Lactobacillus acidophilus and Bifidobacterium infantis to neonates in an intensive care unit. *International Journal of Infectious Diseases*, 3(4), 197–202. Available from https://doi.org/10.1016/S1201-9712(99)90024-3.

International Food Standards Codex Commission (2016). *Stan 72–1981: Standard for infant formula and formulas for special medical purposes intended for infants* (Vol. 2, pp. 1–17).

Jacobs, S. E., Tobin, J. M., Opie, G. F., Donath, S., Tabrizi, S. N., Pirotta, M., Morley, C. J., & Garland, S. M. (2013). Probiotic effects on late-onset sepsis in very preterm infants: A randomized controlled trial. *Pediatrics*, 132(6), 1055–1062. Available from https://doi.org/10.1542/peds.2013-1339.

Jangi, S., & Lamont, J. T. (2010). Asymptomatic colonization by Clostridium difficile in infants: Implications for disease in later life. *Journal of Pediatric Gastroenterology and Nutrition*, 51(1), 2–7. Available from https://doi.org/10.1097/MPG.0b013e3181d29767.

Konstantinos, P., Aikaterini, F., Delphine, E., Liên-Anh, T., & Philippe, S. (2014). A randomized double blind controlled safety trial evaluating D-lactic acid production in healthy infants fed a Lactobacillus reuteri-containing formula. *Nutrition and Metabolic Insights*, 7. Available from https://doi.org/10.4137/nmi.s14113.

Kumar, A., Wu, H., Collier-Hyams, L. S., Kwon, Y. M., Hanson, J. M., & Neish, A. S. (2009). The bacterial fermentation product butyrate influences epithelial signaling via reactive oxygen species-mediated changes in cullin-1 neddylation. *Journal of Immunology*, 182(1), 538–546. Available from https://doi.org/10.4049/jimmunol.182.1.538.

Kuppala, V. S., Meinzen-Derr, J., Morrow, A. L., & Schibler, K. R. (2011). Prolonged initial empirical antibiotic treatment is associated with adverse outcomes in premature infants. *Journal of Pediatrics*, 159(5), 720–725. Available from https://doi.org/10.1016/j.jpeds.2011.05.033.

Lewis, Z. T., Shani, G., Masarweh, C. F., Popovic, M., Frese, S. A., Sela, D. A., Underwood, M. A., & Mills, D. A. (2016). Validating bifidobacterial species and subspecies identity in commercial probiotic products. *Pediatric Research*, 79(3), 445–452. Available from https://doi.org/10.1038/pr.2015.244.

Lu, P., Sodhi, C. P., & Hackam, D. J. (2014). Toll-like receptor regulation of intestinal development and inflammation in the pathogenesis of necrotizing enterocolitis. *Pathophysiology*, 21(1), 81–93. Available from https://doi.org/10.1016/j.pathophys.2013.11.007.

Mack, D. R. (2004). D(-)-Lactic acid-producing probiotics, D(-)-lactic acidosis and infants. *Canadian Journal of Gastroenterology*, 18(11), 671–675. Available from https://doi.org/10.1155/2004/342583.

Martinez, F. A. C., Balciunas, E. M., Converti, A., Cotter, P. D., & De Souza Oliveira, R. P. (2013). Bacteriocin production by Bifidobacterium spp. A review. *Biotechnology Advances*, 31(4), 482–488. Available from https://doi.org/10.1016/j.biotechadv.2013.01.010.

Mathipa, M. G., & Thantsha, M. S. (2017). Probiotic engineering: Towards development of robust probiotic strains with enhanced functional properties and for targeted control of enteric pathogens. *Gut Pathogens*, 9(1). Available from https://doi.org/10.1186/s13099-017-0178-9.

McMurtry, V. E., Gupta, R. W., Tran, L., Blanchard, E. E., Penn, D., Taylor, C. M., & Ferris, M. J. (2015). Bacterial diversity and Clostridia abundance decrease with increasing severity of necrotizing enterocolitis. *Microbiome*, 3(1). Available from https://doi.org/10.1186/s40168-015-0075-8.

Meier, P. P., Johnson, T. J., Patel, A. L., & Rossman, B. (2017). Evidence-based methods that promote human milk feeding of preterm infants: An expert review. *Clinics in Perinatology*, 44(1), 1−22. Available from https://doi.org/10.1016/j.clp.2016.11.005.

Morgan, R. L., Preidis, G. A., Kashyap, P. C., Weizman, A. V., Sadeghirad, B., & Mcmaster Probiotic, P. E.Synbiotic Work Group. (2020). Probiotics reduce mortality and morbidity in preterm, low-birth-weight infants: A systematic review and network meta-analysis of randomized trials. *Gastroenterology*, 159, 467−480.

Munakata, S., Arakawa, C., Kohira, R., Fujita, Y., Fuchigami, T., & Mugishima, H. (2010). A case of D-lactic acid encephalopathy associated with use of probiotics. *Brain and Development*, 32(8), 691−694. Available from https://doi.org/10.1016/j.braindev.2009.09.024.

Newburg, D. S., Ruiz-Palacios, G. M., & Morrow, A. L. (2005). Human milk glycans protect infants against enteric pathogens. *Annual Review of Nutrition*, 25, 37−58. Available from https://doi.org/10.1146/annurev.nutr.25.050304.092553.

Pammi, M., Cope, J., Tarr, P. I., Warner, B. B., Morrow, A. L., Mai, V., Gregory, K. E., Kroll, J. S., Mcmurtry, V., Ferris, M. J., Engstrand, L., Lilja, H. E., Hollister, E. B., Versalovic, J., & Neu, J. (2017). Intestinal dysbiosis in preterm infants preceding necrotizing enterocolitis: A systematic review and meta-analysis. *Microbiome*, 5(1), 31. Available from https://doi.org/10.1186/s40168-017-0248-8.

Patel, R. M., & Denning, P. W. (2013). Therapeutic use of prebiotics, probiotics, and postbiotics to prevent necrotizing enterocolitis. What is the current evidence? *Clinics in Perinatology*, 40(1), 11−25. Available from https://doi.org/10.1016/j.clp.2012.12.002.

Patel, R. M., Myers, L. S., Kurundkar, A. R., Maheshwari, A., Nusrat, A., & Lin, P. W. (2012). Probiotic bacteria induce maturation of intestinal claudin 3 expression and barrier function. *American Journal of Pathology*, 180(2), 626−635. Available from https://doi.org/10.1016/j.ajpath.2011.10.025.

Paul, F., Mark, W., Simon, E., Nicola, P., Richard, H., Abena, A., Pollyanna, H., Millar, M. R., & Kate, C. (2021). Bifidobacterium breve BBG-001 and intestinal barrier function in preterm babies: Exploratory studies from the PiPS trial. *Pediatric Research*, 189, 1818−1824.

Peng, L., Li, Z. R., Green, R. S., Holzman, I. R., & Lin, J. (2009). Butyrate enhances the intestinal barrier by facilitating tight junction assembly via activation of AMP-activated protein kinase in Caco-2 cell monolayers. *Journal of Nutrition*, 139(9), 1619−1625. Available from https://doi.org/10.3945/jn.109.104638.

Reddy, V. S., Patole, S. K., & Rao, S. (2013). Role of probiotics in short bowel syndrome in infants and children—A systematic review. *Nutrients*, 5(3), 679−699. Available from https://doi.org/10.3390/nu5030679.

Rivera-Chávez, F., Lopez, C. A., & Bäumler, A. J. (2017). Oxygen as a driver of gut dysbiosis. *Free Radical Biology and Medicine*, 105, 93−101. Available from https://doi.org/10.1016/j.freeradbiomed.2016.09.022.

Samuels, N., van de Graaf, R. A., de Jonge, R. C. J., Reiss, I. K. M., & Vermeulen, M. J. (2017). Risk factors for necrotizing enterocolitis in neonates: A systematic review of prognostic studies. *BMC Pediatrics*, 17(1). Available from https://doi.org/10.1186/s12887-017-0847-3.

Sanchez, J. B., & Kadrofske, M. (2019). Necrotizing enterocolitis. *Neurogastroenterology and Motility*, 31, e13569. Available from https://doi.org/10.1111/nmo.13569.

Sawh, S. C., Deshpande, S., Jansen, S., Reynaert, C. J., & Jones, P. M. (2016). Prevention of necrotizing enterocolitis with probiotics: A systematic review and meta-analysis. *PeerJ*, 2016(10). Available from https://doi.org/10.7717/peerj.2429.

Sharif, S., Meader, N., Oddie, S. J., Rojas-Reyes, M. X., & McGuire, W. (2020). Probiotics to prevent necrotising enterocolitis in very preterm or very low birth weight infants. *The Cochrane Database of Systematic Reviews*, 10, CD005496. Available from https://doi.org/10.1002/14651858.CD005496.pub5.

Sodhi, C. P., Neal, M. D., Siggers, R., Sho, S., Ma, C., Branca, M. F., Prindle, T., Russo, A. M., Afrazi, A., Good, M., Brower-Sinning, R., Firek, B., Morowitz, M. J., Ozolek, J. A., Gittes, G. K., Billiar, T. R., & Hackam, D. J. (2012). Intestinal epithelial Toll-like receptor 4 regulates goblet cell development and is required for necrotizing enterocolitis in mice. *Gastroenterology*, 143(3), 708−718. Available from https://doi.org/10.1053/j.gastro.2012.05.053.

Underwood, M. A. (2019). Probiotics and the prevention of necrotizing enterocolitis. *Journal of Pediatric Surgery*, 54(3), 405−412. Available from https://doi.org/10.1016/j.jpedsurg.2018.08.055.

Underwood, M. A., German, J. B., Lebrilla, C. B., & Mills, D. A. (2015). Bifidobacterium longum subspecies infantis: Champion colonizer of the infant gut. *Pediatric Research*, 77, 229−235. Available from https://doi.org/10.1038/pr.2014.156.

van den Akker, C. H. P., van Goudoever, J. B., Shamir, R., Domellöf, M., Embleton, N. D., Hojsak, I., Lapillonne, A., Mihatsch, W. A., Berni Canani, R., Bronsky, J., Campoy, C., Fewtrell, M. S., Fidler Mis, N., Guarino, A., Hulst, J. M., Indrio, F., Kolaček, S., Orel, R., Vandenplas, Y., ... Szajewska, H. (2020). Probiotics and preterm infants: A position paper by the European Society for Paediatric Gastroenterology Hepatology and Nutrition Committee on Nutrition and the European Society for Paediatric Gastroenterology Hepatology and Nutrition Working Group for Probiotics and Prebiotics. *Journal of Pediatric Gastroenterology and Nutrition*, 70(5), 664−680. Available from https://doi.org/10.1097/MPG.0000000000002655.

Wilson, K. H., & Sheagren, J. N. (1983). Antagonism of toxigenic Clostridium difficile by nontoxigenic C. difficile. *Journal of Infectious Diseases*, 147(4), 733−736. Available from https://doi.org/10.1093/infdis/147.4.733.

Yelin, I., Flett, K. B., Merakou, C., Mehrotra, P., Stam, J., Snesrud, E., Hinkle, M., Lesho, E., McGann, P., McAdam, A. J., Sandora, T. J., Kishony, R., & Priebe, G. P. (2019). Genomic and epidemiological evidence of bacterial transmission from probiotic capsule to blood in ICU patients. *Nature Medicine*, 25(11), 1728−1732. Available from https://doi.org/10.1038/s41591-019-0626-9.

Yu, Y., Lu, J., Oliphant, K., Gupta, N., Claud, K., & Lu, L. (2020). Maternal administration of probiotics promotes gut development in mouse offsprings. *PLoS One*, 15(8). Available from https://doi.org/10.1371/journal.pone.0237182.

Zozaya, C., García González, I., Avila-Alvarez, A., Oikonomopoulou, N., Sánchez Tamayo, T., Salguero, E., Saenz de Pipaón, M., García-Muñoz Rodrigo, F., & Couce, M. L. (2020). Incidence, treatment, and outcome trends of necrotizing enterocolitis in preterm infants: A multicenter cohort study. *Frontiers in Pediatrics*, 8. Available from https://doi.org/10.3389/fped.2020.00188.

Chapter 6

Probiotics in the prevention and management of irritable bowel syndrome

Elvira Ingrid Levy, Charlotte De Geyter, Bruno Hauser and Yvan Vandenplas

Vrije Universiteit Brussel (VUB), UZ Brussel, KidZ Health Castle, Brussels, Belgium

6.1 Introduction

Pediatric functional abdominal disorders comprise irritable bowel syndrome (IBS), functional dyspepsia, abdominal migraine, and functional abdominal pain not otherwise specified (Thapar et al., 2020). More than half of new pediatric gastrointestinal (GI) clinic patients fulfill Rome 3 criteria for at least one functional gastrointestinal disorder (FGID) (Rouster et al., 2016). Pain intensity, pain frequency, quality of life, school attendance, anxiety/depression, adequate relief, defecation pattern (disease specific, IBS), and adverse events were included in the final core outcome set for functional abdominal pain disorders in children (Zeevenhooven et al., 2020). Children with IBS suffer chronic abdominal pain related to defecation (Table 6.1) (Hyams et al., 2016; Thapar et al., 2020). Functional abdominal pain disorders are common and occur in 3%–16% of children depending on age, sex, and region (Thapar et al., 2020). Recurrent abdominal pain (RAP) was reported by 26.2% of children on at least one of different assessment timings: 1–2 years, 12 years, and 16 years, and 11.3% reported symptoms more than once (Sjölund et al., 2020).

IBS is considered to be a disorder of the gut–brain or brain–gut axis. The incidence of IBS varies in different regions of the world with a reported prevalence between 1.2% and 5.4% (Hyams et al., 2016). Children with RAP at 12 years had persistent symptoms at 16 years in 44.9% of cases and increased risks for RAP [relative risk (RR), 2.2; 95% confidence interval (CI): 1.7–2.8] and IBS (RR, 3.2; 95% CI: 2.0–5.1) at 16 years (Sjölund et al., 2020). However, RAP pain at 1–2 years was not significantly associated with any later outcome (Sjölund et al., 2020).

The subtypes of IBS reported in adults are also valid in children: IBS with constipation, IBS with diarrhea, mixed IBS with constipation and diarrhea, and unspecified IBS (Hyams et al., 2016; Thapar et al., 2020). The difference between functional constipation and IBS with constipation depends on the persistence of pain or not if the constipation has been adequately managed (Hyams et al., 2016; Thapar et al., 2020). If the abdominal pain resolves with efficacious constipation treatment, the patient suffers functional constipation (Hyams et al., 2016). If the pain does not improve despite resolution of the constipation, IBS with constipation is then the most probable diagnosis. It is has been reported that a large number of patients labeled as IBS–diarrhea or IBS-mixed may actually present functional constipation and should be managed as such (Tosto et al., 2020).

TABLE 6.1 Definition of irritable bowel syndrome.

Disease	Definition
Irritable bowel syndrome	All criteria must be present since >2 months and
	the symptoms cannot be explained by another diagnosis after appropriate clinical evaluation
	abdominal pain >4 days/month associated with defecation and/or change in frequency and composition
	resolution of constipation does not result in sufficient decrease of pain

Source: Adapted from Thapar, N., Benninga, M. A., Crowell, M. D., Di Lorenzo, C., Mack, I., Nurko, S., Saps, M., Shulman, R. J., Szajewska, H., van Tilburg, M. A. L., & Enck, P. (2020). Paediatric functional abdominal pain disorders. *Nature Reviews Disease Primers*, 6(1), 89.

6.2 Probiotics in prevention and management of IBS

The available data are quite limited. Only few double-blind, randomized therapeutic trials were reported in pediatric patients with IBS. Moreover, most randomized pediatric studies grouped all children presenting with different subtypes of functional abdominal pain disorders. However, most of the treatment modalities have a direct or indirect impact of the GI microbiota composition.

There are also data supporting the utility of probiotics. The vast majority of the studies mix IBS, functional GI disorders, and RAP. Therefore we were not selective for this review. However, it is obvious that for future research, inclusion criteria for children with RAP, IBS, functional constipation, or other functional GI disorders should be more specific.

One of the first publications dated 2005 evaluatied that the efficacy of probiotics in children with abdominal pain was negative (Bausserman & Michail, 2005). *Lactobacillus rhamnosus* GG (LGG) was not superior to the placebo in relieving abdominal pain (40.0% response rate in the placebo versus 44.0% in the LGG group; $P = .774$). There was no difference in GI symptoms, except for a lower incidence of perceived abdominal distention ($P = .02$ favoring LGG) (Bausserman & Michail, 2005). A trial published in 2007, including children with RAP showed that the LGG group had an increased treatment success (no pain) than the placebo group [25% vs 9.6%, relative benefit 2.6, 95% CI 1.05–6.6, number needed-to-treat (NNT) 7, 95% CI: 4–123] (Gawrońska et al., 2007). Specific for IBS ($n = 37$), those in the LGG group were more likely to have treatment success than those in the placebo group (33% vs 5%, relative benefit 6.3, 95% CI: 1.2–38, NNT 4, 95% CI: 2–36) and reduced frequency of pain ($P = .02$), but not pain severity ($P = .10$) (Gawrońska et al., 2007). For the functional dyspepsia group ($n = 20$) and functional abdominal pain group ($n = 47$), no differences were found (Gawrońska et al., 2007). LGG at a concentration of 1×10^{10} colony-forming units (CFU)/mL for a period of 4 weeks can lessen the severity of the patients' pain and improve the functional scale in patients with IBS (Gawrońska et al., 2007). According to another paper from 2010, in children with IBS, VSL3 was significantly superior to placebo ($P < .05$) regarding the subjective assessment of relief of symptoms; and for the relief of abdominal pain/discomfort ($P < .05$), abdominal bloating/gassiness ($P < .05$), and family assessment of life disruption ($P < .01$). No significant difference was found ($P = .06$) in the stool pattern (Guandalini et al., 2010). However, children in the placebo group improved as well (Guandalini et al., 2010). No adverse effect were recorded for any of the patients (Guandalini et al., 2010). Francavilla and coworkers reported that 8 weeks administration of LGG resulted in a significant reduction of frequency (<0.01) and severity (<0.01) of abdominal pain, with a persistent benefit at week 12 (Francavilla et al., 2010). Intestinal permeability had a baseline increase in 59% of the children, and was reduced in the LGG but not in the placebo group (Francavilla et al., 2010). A controlled, double-blind, randomized trial performed in Iran on children with IBS diagnosed by Rome III criteria confirmed that LGG significantly reduced pain already after 1 week of treatment (Kianifar et al., 2015).

According to a meta-analysis published in 2011, there was already evidence that LGG moderately increased treatment success in children with abdominal pain-related functional GI disorders, particularly in cases of IBS (Horvath et al., 2011). In 2014, a review concluded that probiotics are more effective than placebo in the treatment of patients with abdominal pain-related FGIDs, especially with respect to patients with IBS, but not in functional constipation (Guandalini, 2014). In 2015, six randomized, placebo-controlled clinical trials were included in a meta-analysis (Tiequn et al., 2015). No heterogeneity was found (66). The pooled relative risk for clinical improvement with *Lactobacillus* treatment was 7.69 (95% CI: 2.33–25.43, $P = .0008$) (Tiequn et al., 2015). For adults, the pooled relative risk for clinical improvement with *Lactobacillus* treatment reached 17.62 (95% CI: 5.12–60.65, $P < .00001$). For children, the pooled relative risk for clinical improvement with *Lactobacillus* treatment was much lower and reached only 3.71 (95% CI:1.05–13.11, $P = .04$) (Tiequn et al., 2015). Two other meta-analyses including RCTs in children showed an improvement in abdominal pain for LGG, *Lactobacillus reuteri* DSM 17938 and the probiotic mixture VSL3 (Giannetti & Staiano, 2016; Korterink et al., 2014). The patients most benefiting from probiotics were those with predominant diarrhea or with a postinfectious IBS (Giannetti & Staiano, 2016). The systematic review by Giannetti and Staiano (2016) included 24 studies and found some evidence for beneficial effects of partially hydrolyzed guar gum, cognitive behavioral therapy, hypnotherapy and probiotics (LGG and VSL3).

In IBS, but not in functional dyspepsia, a mixture of *Bifidobacterium infantis* M-63, *Bifidobacterium breve* M-16V, and *Bifidobacterium longum* BB536 determined a complete resolution of abdominal pain in a significantly higher proportion of children, when compared with placebo ($P = .006$), and significantly decreased abdominal pain frequency ($P = .02$) (Giannetti et al., 2017). The proportion of IBS children with an improved quality of life was significantly higher after probiotics than after placebo (48% vs 17%, $P = .001$), but this finding was not confirmed in functional dyspepsia (Giannetti et al., 2017). Children receiving *L. reuteri* DSM 17938 had significantly more days without pain (median 89.5 vs 51 days, $P = .029$) than a placebo group Jadrešin et al., 2017). Abdominal pain was less severe in children taking probiotics during the second (<0.05) and fourth month (<0.01) (Jadrešin et al., 2017). Placebo and *L. reuteri* groups did not differ in the duration of abdominal pain, stool type, or absence from school (Jadrešin et al., 2017). Both groups experienced significant reduction in the severity of abdominal pain from first to the fourth month, with the reduction more prominent in the intervention group ($P < .001$ vs $P = .004$) (Jadrešin et al., 2017). Administration of *L. reuteri* DSM 17938 was associated with a possible reduction of the intensity of pain and significantly more days without pain (Jadrešin et al., 2017). A *Bacillus coagulans* Unique IS2 treated group of 4- to 12-year-old IBS children showed a greater reduction in pain scores evaluated by a weekly pain intensity scale (Sudha et al., 2018). There was a significant reduction ($P < .0001$) in pain intensity in the probiotic (7.6 ± 0.98) compared to the placebo group (4.2 ± 1.41) after 8 weeks (Sudha et al., 2018). There was also a significant improvement in stool consistency as well as reduction in abdominal discomfort, bloating, staining, urgency, incomplete evacuation, and passage of gas (Sudha et al., 2018). Bowel habit satisfaction and global assessment of relief was also observed in the *B. coagulans* Unique IS2 treated group as compared to the placebo group (Sudha et al., 2018).

Eleven randomized controlled trials for functional abdominal pain disorders and six for functional constipation were included in yet another meta-analysis, showing some evidence for LGG ($n = 3$) in reducing frequency and intensity of abdominal pain in children with IBS (Pärtty et al., 2018). According to this analysis, there was no evidence to recommend *L. reuteri* DSM 17938 ($n = 5$), a mix of *B. infantis*, *B. breve*, and *B. longum* ($n = 1$), *Bifidobacterium lactis* ($n = 1$) or VSL3 ($n = 1$) for children with functional abdominal pain (Pärtty et al., 2018). No evidence supported the use of *L. casei rhamnosus* LCR35 ($n = 1$), *B. lactis* DN173 010 ($n = 1$), *B. longum* ($n = 1$), *L. reuteri* DSM 17938 ($n = 1$), a mix of *B. infantis*, *B. breve*, and *B. longum* ($n = 1$), or Protexin mix ($n = 1$) for children with functional constipation. In general, studies had an unclear or high risk of bias (Pärtty et al., 2018). Insufficient evidence exists for the use of probiotics in functional abdominal pain and functional constipation (Pärtty et al., 2018). Only LGG seems to reduce frequency and intensity of abdominal pain but only in children with IBS (Pärtty et al., 2018). A better understanding of differences in gut microbiota in health and disease might lead to better probiotic strategies to treat disease (Pärtty et al., 2018). No single strain, combination of strains, or synbiotics can be recommended for the management of IBS, functional abdominal pain, or functional constipation in children. Limited, yet encouraging, evidence exists for LGG at the dose of 3×10^9 CFU and for a multistrain preparation for the treatment of IBS (Hojsak, 2019). In the treatment of functional abdominal pain, there is some evidence for the use of *L. reuteri* DSM 17938 at the dose of at least 108 CFU/day (Hojsak, 2019). Szajewska and Hojsak reported on 13 meta-analyses, 3 systematic reviews, and 15 randomized, controlled trials that assessed B., BB-12, and LGG, either alone or in combination, when administered to infants to improve growth or to children of any age to prevent or treat acute gastroenteritis, antibiotic-, or healthcare-associated diarrhea, respiratory infections, otitis media, and functional GI disorders including IBS (Szajewska & Hojsak, 2020). They found only moderate evidence regarding the benefits of LGG for treating respiratory infections and IBS in children and minimal evidence to support the use of BB-12 (Szajewska & Hojsak, 2020). Dietary treatment with an extensively hydrolyzed casein formula containing the probiotic *L. rhamnosus* GG was reported to prevent functional GI disorders (Nocerino et al., 2019).

The efficacy of a synbiotic treatment (5×10^9 CFUs of *B. lactis* B94 and 900 mg inulin) was compared to a probiotic (5×10^9 CFU *B. lactis* B94) or a prebiotic (900 mg inulin) twice daily for 4 weeks in 71 4- to 16-year-old children diagnosed with IBS (Başturk et al., 2016). Probiotic treatment alone improved belching-abdominal fullness ($P < .001$), bloating after meals ($P = .016$), and constipation ($P = .031$), and synbiotic treatment improved belching-abdominal fullness ($P \leq .001$), bloating after meals ($P = .004$), constipation ($P = .021$), and mucus in the feces ($P = .021$) (Başturk et al., 2016). The synbiotic group had a significantly higher percentage of patients with full recovery than the prebiotic group (39.1% vs 12.5%, $P = .036$) (Başturk et al., 2016). Administration of synbiotics and probiotics resulted in significant improvements in initial complaints when compared to prebiotics. Additionally, there was a significantly higher number of patients with full recovery from IBS symptoms in the synbiotic group than in the prebiotic group (Başturk et al., 2016). The risk–benefit plane for IBS straddles the risk–benefit threshold, so patients can expect a balance between a low chance of risk and also a low chance of benefit (Bennett, 2016).

6.3 Conclusion

Despite the evidence from the pathophysiological animal and laboratory data suggesting that an alternated microbiota plays a causative role in IBS, evidence from clinical trials that the manipulation of the GI microbiota resulting in benefits is limited. Differences in study designs and outcomes is insufficient to recommend administration of probiotics or other interventions that alter the GI microbiota composition in the management of IBS in pediatrics.

References

Bausserman, M., & Michail, S. (2005). The use of Lactobacillus GG in irritable bowel syndrome in children: A double-blind randomized control trial. *Journal of Pediatrics*, *147*(2), 197−201. Available from https://doi.org/10.1016/j.jpeds.2005.05.015.

Başturk, A., Artan, R., & Yilmaz, A. (2016). Efficacy of synbiotic, probiotic, and prebiotic treatments for irritable bowel syndrome in children: A randomized controlled trial. *Turkish Journal of Gastroenterology*, *27*(5), 439−443. Available from https://doi.org/10.5152/tjg.2016.16301.

Bennett, W. E. (2016). Quantitative risk−benefit analysis of probiotic use for irritable bowel syndrome and inflammatory bowel disease. *Drug Safety*, *39*(4), 295−305. Available from https://doi.org/10.1007/s40264-015-0349-x.

Francavilla, R., Miniello, V., Magistà, A. M., De Canio, A., Bucci, N., Gagliardi, F., Lionetti, E., Castellaneta, S., Polimeno, L., Peccarisi, L., Indrio, F., & Cavallo, L. (2010). A randomized controlled trial of lactobacillus GG in children with functional abdominal pain. *Pediatrics*, *126*(6), e1445−e1452. Available from https://doi.org/10.1542/peds.2010-0467.

Gawrońska, A., Dziechciarz, P., Horvath, A., & Szajewska, H. (2007). A randomized double-blind placebo-controlled trial of lactobacillus GG for abdominal pain disorders in children. *Alimentary Pharmacology and Therapeutics*, *25*(2), 177−184. Available from https://doi.org/10.1111/j.1365-2036.2006.03175.x.

Giannetti, E., & Staiano, A. (2016). Probiotics for irritable bowel syndrome: Clinical data in children. *Journal of Pediatric Gastroenterology and Nutrition*, *63*(1), S25−6. Available from https://doi.org/10.1097/MPG.0000000000001220.

Giannetti, E., Maglione, M., Alessandrella, A., Strisciuglio, C., De Giovanni, D., Campanozzi, A., Miele, E., & Staiano, A. (2017). A mixture of 3 bifidobacteria decreases abdominal pain and improves the quality of life in children with irritable bowel syndrome. *Journal of Clinical Gastroenterology*, *51*(1), e5−e10. Available from https://doi.org/10.1097/MCG.0000000000000528.

Guandalini, S. (2014). Are probiotics or prebiotics useful in pediatric irritable bowel syndrome or inflammatory bowel disease? *Frontiers in Medicine*, *1*. Available from https://doi.org/10.3389/fmed.2014.00023.

Guandalini, S., Magazzù, G., Chiaro, A., La Balestra, V., Di Nardo, G., Gopalan, S., Sibal, A., Romano, C., Canani, R. B., Lionetti, P., & Setty, M. (2010). VSL#3 improves symptoms in children with irritable bowel Syndrome: A multicenter, randomized, placebo-controlled, double-blind, crossover study. *Journal of Pediatric Gastroenterology and Nutrition*, *51*(1), 24−30. Available from https://doi.org/10.1097/MPG.0b013e3181ca4d95.

Hojsak, I. (2019). *Probiotics in functional gastrointestinal disorders. Advances in experimental medicine and biology* (Vol. 1125, pp. 121−137). New York LLC: Springer. Available from https://doi.org/10.1007/5584_2018_321.

Horvath, A., Dziechciarz, P., & Szajewska, H. (2011). Meta-analysis: *Lactobacillus rhamnosus* GG for abdominal pain-related functional gastrointestinal disorders in childhood. *Alimentary Pharmacology and Therapeutics*, *33*(12), 1302−1310. Available from https://doi.org/10.1111/j.1365-2036.2011.04665.x.

Hyams, J. S., Di Lorenzo, C., Saps, M., Shulman, R. J., Staiano, A., & Van Tilburg, M. (2016). Childhood functional gastrointestinal disorders: Child/adolescent. *Gastroenterology*, *150*(6), 1456−1468. Available from https://doi.org/10.1053/j.gastro.2016.02.015, e2.

Jadrešin, O., Hojsak, I., Mišak, Z., Kekez, A. J., Trbojević, T., Ivković, L., & Kolaček, S. (2017). *Lactobacillus reuteri* DSM 17938 in the treatment of functional abdominal pain in children: RCT study. *Journal of Pediatric Gastroenterology and Nutrition*, *64*(6), 925−929. Available from https://doi.org/10.1097/MPG.0000000000001478.

Kianifar, H., Jafari, S., Kiani, M., Ahanchian, H., Ghasemi, S., Grover, Z., Mahmoodi, L., Bagherian, R., & Khalesi, M. (2015). Probiotic for irritable bowel syndrome in pediatric patients: A randomized controlled clinical trial. *Electron Physician*, *7*, 1255−1260. Available from https://doi.org/10.14661/1255.

Korterink, J. J., Ockeloen, L., Benninga, M. A., Tabbers, M. M., Hilbink, M., & Deckers-Kocken, J. M. (2014). Probiotics for childhood functional gastrointestinal disorders: A systematic review and meta-analysis. *Acta Paediatrica, International Journal of Paediatrics*, *103*(4), 365−372. Available from https://doi.org/10.1111/apa.12513.

Nocerino, R., Di Costanzo, M., Bedogni, G., Cosenza, L., Maddalena, Y., Di Scala, C., Della Gatta, G., Carucci, L., Voto, L., Coppola, S., Iannicelli, A. M., & Berni Canani, R. (2019). Dietary treatment with extensively hydrolyzed casein formula containing the probiotic *Lactobacillus rhamnosus* GG prevents the occurrence of functional gastrointestinal disorders in children with cow's milk allergy. *Journal of Pediatrics*, *213*, 137−142. Available from https://doi.org/10.1016/j.jpeds.2019.06.004, e2.

Pärtty, A., Rautava, S., & Kalliomäki, M. (2018). Probiotics on pediatric functional gastrointestinal disorders. *Nutrients*, *10*(12). Available from https://doi.org/10.3390/nu10121836.

Rouster, A. S., Karpinski, A. C., Silver, D., Monagas, J., & Hyman, P. E. (2016). Functional gastrointestinal disorders dominate pediatric gastroenterology outpatient practice. *Journal of Pediatric Gastroenterology and Nutrition*, *62*(6), 847−851. Available from https://doi.org/10.1097/MPG.0000000000001023.

Sjölund, J., Uusijärvi, A., Tornkvist, N., Kull, I., Bergström, A., Alm, J., Törnblom, H., Olén, O., & Simrén, M. (2020). Prevalence and progression of recurrent abdominal pain, from early childhood to adolescence. *Clinical Gastroenterology and Hepatology*, *20*, 30592−30599. Available from https://doi.org/10.1016/j.cgh.2020.04.047.

Sudha, M. R., Jayanthi, N., Aasin, M., Dhanashri, R. D., & Anirudh, T. (2018). Efficacy of *Bacillus coagulans* unique IS2 in treatment of irritable bowel syndrome in children: A double blind, randomised placebo controlled study. *Beneficial Microbes*, *9*(4), 563−572. Available from https://doi.org/10.3920/BM2017.0129.

Szajewska, H., & Hojsak, I. (2020). Health benefits of *Lactobacillus rhamnosus* GG and *Bifidobacterium animalis* subspecies lactis BB-12 in children. *Postgraduate Medicine*, *132*(5), 441−451. Available from https://doi.org/10.1080/00325481.2020.1731214.

Thapar, N., Benninga, M. A., Crowell, M. D., Di Lorenzo, C., Mack, I., Nurko, S., Saps, M., Shulman, R. J., Szajewska, H., van Tilburg, M. A. L., & Enck, P. (2020). Paediatric functional abdominal pain disorders. *Nature Reviews. Disease Primers*, 6(1), 89. Available from https://doi.org/10.1038/s41572-020-00222-5.

Tiequn, B., Guanqun, C., & Shuo, Z. (2015). Therapeutic effects of lactobacillus in treating irritable bowel syndrome: A meta-analysis. *Internal Medicine*, 54(3), 243–249. Available from https://doi.org/10.2169/internalmedicine.54.2710.

Tosto, M., D'Andrea, P., Salamone, I., Pellegrino, S., Costa, S., Lucanto, M. C., Pallio, S., Magazzu', G., & Guandalini, S. (2020). Functional constipation masked as irritable bowel syndrome. *BMC Gastroenterology*, 20(1). Available from https://doi.org/10.1186/s12876-020-01244-9.

Zeevenhooven, J., Rexwinkel, R., Van Berge Henegouwen, V. W. A., Krishnan, U., Vandenplas, Y., Strisciuglio, C., Staiano, A., Devanarayana, N. M., Rajindrajith, S., Benninga, M. A., & Tabbers, M. M. (2020). A core outcome set for clinical trials in pediatric functional abdominal pain disorders. *Journal of Pediatrics*, 221, 115–122. Available from https://doi.org/10.1016/j.jpeds.2020.02.032, e5.

Chapter 7

Probiotics in the prevention and treatment of diarrheal disease

Aruna Jyothi Kora[1,2]

[1]*National Centre for Compositional Characterisation of Materials (NCCCM), Bhabha Atomic Research Centre (BARC), ECIL PO, Hyderabad, India,*
[2]*Homi Bhabha National Institute (HBNI), Mumbai, India*

7.1 Introduction

The term probiotics is defined by World Health Organization (WHO) and Food and Agriculture Organization of the United Nations (FAO) as "any strain/product that must contain viable microorganisms in a specific number such as billion; which are tolerant to gastric acid, bile, and pancreatic juices; and reach, multiply, and colonize at the target site of small/large intestine (digestive tract) in sufficient numbers to bestow a beneficial therapeutic effect and should be authenticated via scientific, controlled clinical trials" (Franz et al., 2011; Raghuwanshi, 2015). The probiotic microorganism should also fulfill the criteria such as human origin, nonpathogenicity, stability in bile and acid; viability in delivery vehicle, shelf life, adherence to target epithelial tissue, multiplication and colonization capability in the digestive tract; production of antimicrobial substances, immune system modulation, etc. (Jack et al., 2010; Sazawal et al., 2006). The inoculated specific probiotic strains normalize the unbalanced indigenous microbiota in the digestive tract via implantation and colonization, and exhibit beneficial effects through prevention of adhesion and replication of pathogens. The strains also control enteric diseases by means of local and systemic effects via augmentation of host's immune system (Johnston et al., 2006; Marcos & DuPont, 2007; Mego et al., 2015; Surawicz, 2003).

Based on the existing guidelines laid by various countries, the probiotics are categorized as probiotic drugs, probiotic food, probiotics for animal use, and genetically modified probiotics depending on the intended application. The probiotic foods in India should meet the guidelines laid out by Indian Council of Medical Research and Department of Biotechnology, while the probiotic drugs should conform to the standards set by Schedule V of the Drugs and Cosmetics Rules, 1945 (Indian Council of Medical Research Task et al., 2011; Sehgal et al., 2016). In India, various probiotic drugs containing different strains of *Lactobacillus* (*Lactobacillus rhamnosus*, *Lactobacillus acidophilus*, *Lactobacillus plantarum*, *Lactobacillus paracasei*, *Lactobacillus bulgaricus*, *Lactobacillus delbrueckii*); *Bifidobacterium* (*Bifidobacterium bifidum*, *Bifidobacterium longum*, *Bifidobacterium breve*, *Bifidobacterium infantis*); *Bacillus* (*Bacillus coagulans*, *Bacillus clausii*, *Bacillus subtilis*, *Bacillus mesentericus*); *C. butyricum*, *Streptococcus* (*Streptococcus thermophilus*, *Streptococcus faecalis*); *Enterococcus* (*Enterococcus faecalis*, *Enterococcus faecium*); and yeast (*S. boulardii*) are marked under different brands for treating various gastrointestinal ailments including infectious diarrhea, AAD, *C. difficile* associated diarrhea, travelers' diarrhea, rotavirus diarrhea, lactose intolerance, irritable bowel syndrome, inflammatory bowel disease, *Helicobacter pylori* infection etc. (Table 7.1) (Raghuwanshi, 2015; Surawicz, 2003). These commercial drug formulations are available in the form of powders, capsules, liquids, and syrup containing either single or a multiprobiotic strain combination (Jack et al., 2010). The above mentioned probiotic bacterial strains are Gram-positive and characterized by rod (*Lactobacillus*, *Bacillus*, *Clostridium*), branched rod (*Bifidobacterium*), or spherical (*Streptococcus*, *Enterococcus*)-shaped structures. The colony morphology and bright field microscopic image indicating the rod-shaped structure of probiotic bacteria, *L. paracasei* are shown in Fig. 7.1. Similarly, the photographic images of colonies of other probiotic bacteria, *B. subtilis* and *E. faecalis* are given in Fig. 7.2. The colonies, bright field and scanning electron micrographs indicating the ellipsoidal shape of probiotic yeast, *S. boulardii*, are depicted in Fig. 7.3.

TABLE 7.1 List of Indian probiotic drugs marketed under different brand names for treating various gastrointestinal disorders, in terms of form and microbial composition.

Brand name	Form	Microbial composition	Used for treating
Becelac PB	Powder	L. acidophilus	Diarrhea, irritable bowel syndrome, inflammatory bowel disease, H. pylori infection, colitis, dyspepsia, flatulence, impaired digestion, stomatitis
Darolac IBS	Powder	L. plantarum	Irritable bowel syndrome
Darolac	Powder	B. coagulans	Diarrhea, irritable bowel syndrome
Vizylac	Powder	B. coagulans	Antibiotic-associated diarrhea, digestive disorders
Darolac aqua	Liquid	B. clausii	Diarrhea, irritable bowel syndrome
Econorm	Powder	S. boulardii	Infectious diarrhea, antibiotic-associated diarrhea, Clostridium difficile associated diarrhea
Probio		L. acidophilus, L. bulgaricus, B. bifidum	Diarrhea, antibiotic-associated diarrhea, lactose intolerance
Sporlac	Powder	B. coagulans, B. subtilis, B. clausii	Diarrhea, antibiotic-associated diarrhea, intestinal infection, gastrointestinal problems, poor digestion
Sporelac plus	Powder	L. acidophilus, L. rhamnosus, B. coagulans, B. longum, S. boulardii	Acute diarrhea, irritable bowel syndrome, travelers' diarrhea, H. pylori and urinary tract infections
Actigut	Powder	L. acidophilus, L. rhamnosus, S. thermophilus, B. bifidum, B. longum, S. boulardii	Diarrhea, antibiotic-associated diarrhea, travelers' diarrhea, rotavirus diarrhea
Sporelac plus	Powder	L. acidophilus, L. rhamnosus, B. coagulans, B. longum, S. boulardii	Acute diarrhea, irritable bowel syndrome, travelers' diarrhea, H. pylori and urinary tract infections
Vibact	Powder, syrup	B. coagulans, B. mesentericus, S. faecalis, C. butyricum	Infectious diarrhea, antibiotic-associated diarrhea, lactose intolerance, bloating
Bifilac	Powder	B. coagulans, B. mesentericus, S. faecalis, C. butyricum	Diarrhea, gastrointestinal disorders, stomach pain
Vizyl	Powder	S. faecalis, B. coagulans, C. butyricum, B. mesentericus	Diarrhea, antibiotic-associated diarrhea, irritable bowel syndrome, lactose intolerance, abnormal digestion
Vivagut	Powder	S. faecalis, B. coagulans, C. butyricum, B. mesentericus	Acute diarrhea, antibiotic-associated diarrhea, irritable bowel syndrome, inflammatory bowel disease, travelers' diarrhea, Clostridium difficile associated diarrhea, depression
Vizylac rich		B. coagulans, B. mesentericus, S. faecalis, C. butyricum, S. boulardii	Infectious diarrhea, antibiotic-associated diarrhea, inflammatory bowel disease, lactose intolerance
VSL 3	Powder	L. acidophilus, L. plantarum, L. paracasei, L. delbrueckii, S. thermophilus, B. breve, B. longum, B. infantis	Irritable bowel syndrome, ulcerative colitis

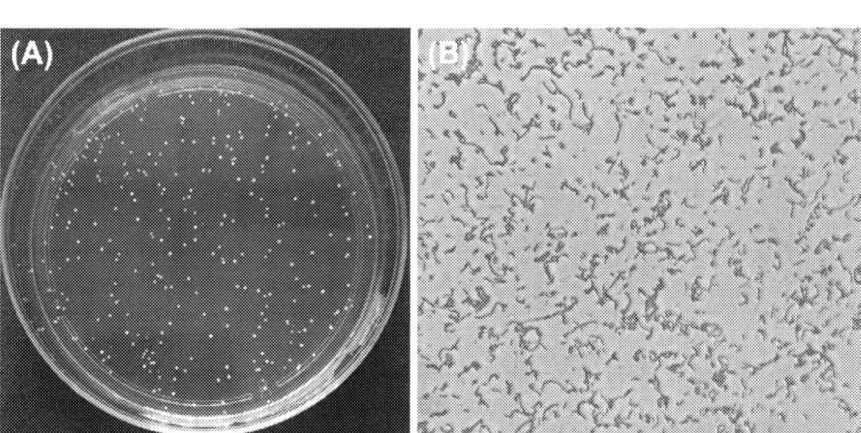

FIGURE 7.1 (A) Colony morphology, and (B) bright field microscopic image of probiotic bacteria, Lactobacillus paracasei.

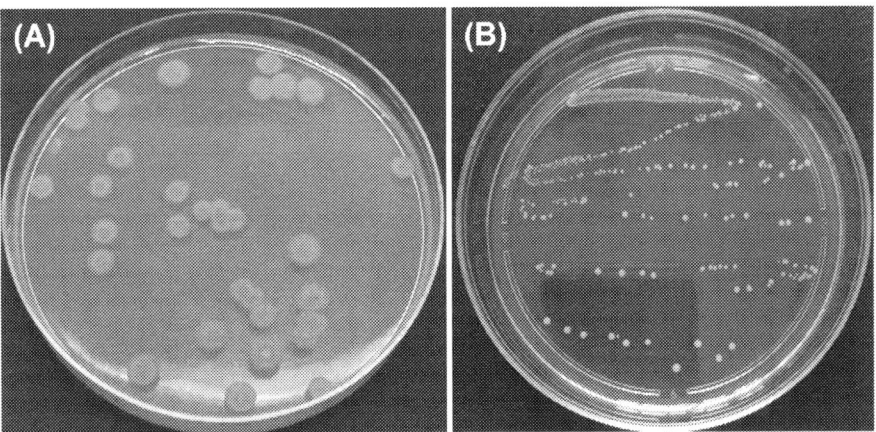

FIGURE 7.2 Photographic images of probiotic bacterial colonies of (A) *Bacillus subtilis*, and (B) *Enterococcus faecalis*.

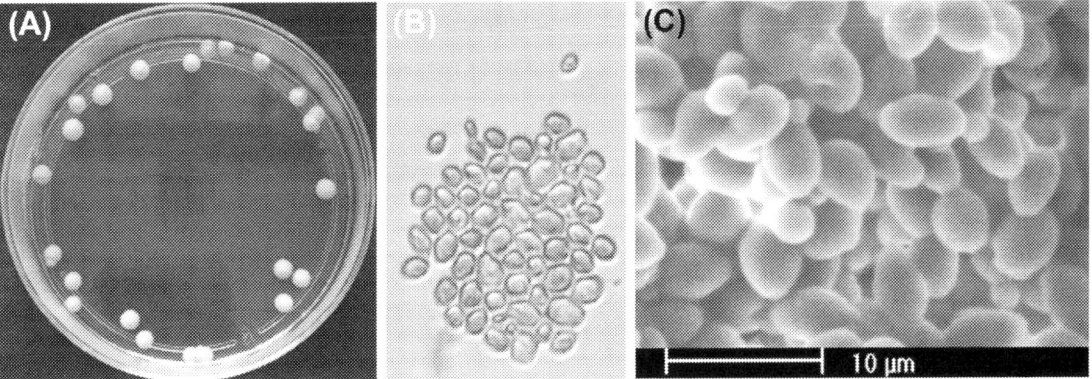

FIGURE 7.3 (A) Colony morphology, (B) bright field image, and (C) scanning electron micrograph of probiotic yeast, *Saccharomyces boulardii*.

7.2 Diarrheal diseases

Annually, around 4 billion diarrheal cases are noted worldwide, representing 4% of total deaths and 5% of day loss due to associated morbidity (Sazawal et al., 2006). According to WHO, diarrhea is a condition characterized by having a minimum of three or more liquid stools/day or more number of bowel movements which is abnormal for a person. Based on the duration, it is classified as acute, lasting for less than 14 days; persistent, lasting for more than 14 days; and chronic diarrhea lasting for more than a month (Johnston et al., 2006; Mathan, 1998). The diarrhea is graded based on number of stools/day, excess number stools/day than person's baseline and symptom severity, such as grade 1(up to 3–4 more stools/day), grade 2 (up to 4–6 more stools/day), grade 3 (up to 7–9 more stools/day) and grade 4 (up to 10 or more) (Demers et al., 2014; Johnston et al., 2006). The various gastrointestinal conditions leading to chronic diarrhea includes Crohn's disease, microscopic colitis, celiac disease, irritable bowel syndrome, bile acid malabsorption, and ulcerative colitis (Wanke & Szajewska, 2014).

7.3 Probiotics in prevention and treatment of diarrheal diseases

The current chapter briefly discusses the role of probiotics in prevention and treatment of diarrheal diseases such as infectious diarrhea, travelers' diarrhea, nosocomial diarrhea (AAD, *C. difficile* associated diarrhea), cancer therapy-induced diarrhea, lactose intolerance-induced diarrhea, enteral tube feeding diarrhea; and the mode of action of probiotics. The sub-topics such as the probiotic role in the prevention and management of inflammatory bowel diseases (Crohn's disease, ulcerative colitis, pouchitis), irritable bowel syndrome, necrotizing enterocolitis, lactose intolerance other nosocomial infections, infections caused by *H. pylori*, enterohemorrhagic *Escherichia coli* and rotavirus, food-borne diseases are covered in detail in other chapters of the book.

7.3.1 Infectious diarrhea

Infectious diarrhea, also called gastroenteritis, is a condition of the gastrointestinal tract infection caused by various pathogens which include bacteria, virus, and protozoan parasites. It is diagnosed by rapid onset of watery stools, also accompanied by vomiting, nausea, abdominal pain, and fever (Heinz, 2008). The acute diarrhea leads to malnutrition and stunted growth due to impairment of intestinal absorption of macro and micro nutrients (Demers et al., 2014). Approximately 1/3 of worldwide acute diarrhea cases in older children and adults are mediated by pathogens. In developed and developing countries, the common causative agents of diarrhea in children are bacteria (*E. coli, Salmonella, Shigella, Campylobacter jejuni*); virus (rotavirus, norovirus) and protozoan parasites (*Giardia lamblia, Entamoeba histolytic, Cryptosporidium, Cyclospora*) (Heinz, 2008; Nuraida, 2015). Bacterial pathogens account to 10% in developed countries and the important bacterial enteropathogens such as enteropathogenic *E. coli* are responsible for 50% of endemic pediatric and travellers' diarrhea in developing countries. Rotaviruses are responsible for infant diarrhea (Teran et al., 2009) and the community outbreaks of food and waterborne gastroenteritis are mediated by noroviruses in all age groups of broad genetic diversity. Also, putative agents such as enterotoxigenic *Bacteroides fragilis, Klebsiella oxytoca*, and *Laribacter hongkongensis* are associated with acute diarrhea in children (Marcos & DuPont, 2007).

The acute diarrhea is effectively treated with oral rehydration treatment and broad spectrum antiparasitic agent, nitazoxanide; the travelers' diarrhea is controlled with antibiotics, rifaximin and azithromycin (Marcos & DuPont, 2007). Various clinical trials demonstrated the efficiency of probiotics such as *L. rhamnosus, Lactobacillus reuteri, Lactobacillus casei* and *S. boulardii* in prevention and treatment of infectious diarrhea both in children and adults (Teran et al., 2009). A mixture of probiotic strains including *B. mesentericus, E. faecalis*, and *C. butyricum* efficiently reduced both severity and hospital stay duration in acute diarrhea-effected children (Franz et al., 2011). In another study, *E. faecium* was efficient in the treatment of enteritis both in adults and children, in terms of diarrhea duration and stool normalization time (Franz et al., 2011). An earlier research investigation indicated that regular intake of a probiotic or a probiotic/prebiotic combination reduces both the incidence and duration of diarrhea in childcare centers' attending children (Binns & Lee, 2010). In India, the leaves of *Plectranthus amboinicus* along with buttermilk, a rich source of probiotics, are consumed for treating pathogen-induced diarrhea to reduce the number of episodes and duration. The aqueous leaf extract of *P. amboinicus* is known to inhibit the growth of foodborne pathogens; *E. coli* and *Salmonella typhimurium* and stimulate the growth of *L. plantarum* by acting as a prebiotic (Shubha & Bhatt, 2015).

In developing countries, mass vaccination reduces the rotavirus mediated morbidity and mortality in infants, which is quite expensive (Marcos & DuPont, 2007; Teran et al., 2009; Wanke & Szajewska, 2014). Based on clinical studies, treatment with mixed probiotic preparation (*L. acidophilus, L. rhamnosus, B. longum, S. boulardii*) and nitazoxanide were proven to be effective in management of acute rotavirus gastroenteritis in children in terms of duration of diarrhea and hospitalization when compared with the control group (Isolauri et al., 2004; Marcos & DuPont, 2007; Teran et al., 2009).

7.3.2 Travelers' diarrhea

Travelers' diarrhea is a syndrome affecting healthy travelers, mostly in endemic and developing countries due to the exposure of naive gastrointestinal tract to enteric pathogens of a different environment. The incidences range from 20% to 50% based on the origin and destination of the traveler, mode of travel, etc. The temporary, infectious diarrhea is mostly foodborne and waterborne and generally caused by bacterial pathogens (*E. coli, Campylobacter*); virus (norovirus) and protozoan (*Giardia*). It is prevented by improving personal hygiene, drinking clean water and eating hot foods. Studies have shown the effectiveness of probiotic strains such as *L. rhamnosus, L. acidophilus, L. bulgaricus, B. bifidum* and *S. thermophilus* in reduction of travelers' diarrhea in comparison with a placebo (Gismondo et al., 1999; Mathan, 1998).

7.3.3 Nosocomial diarrhea

The AAD and *C. difficile*-associated diarrhea are the prominent causes of nosocomial/hospital acquired outbreaks of diarrhea and colitis. The risk factors favoring nosocomial infections are severe debilitation, prolonged stay in intensive care units, extended use of antibiotics, immunosuppression, poor environment, and inadequate waste disposal in healthcare units (Khan et al., 2017; Marcos & DuPont, 2007; Wanke & Szajewska, 2014).

7.3.3.1 Antibiotic-associated diarrhea

Based on the disclosed, pediatric prescription information from the Canadian Paediatric Society, the number of antibiotics was 14 among the 20 most regularly prescribed drugs for children. In the studied pediatric population, 76% of the children were prescribed a minimum of one antibiotic. As the antibiotic treatment does not differentiate pathogens and beneficial microbes, it results in diarrhea due to the disruption of gastrointestinal biota (Johnston et al., 2006; Raghuwanshi, 2015). The AAD is more prominent in patients treated with broad spectrum antibiotics such as cephalosporin, β lactam, macrolide, fluoroquinolone and lincosamides, and the incidence rates range from 5% to 39% based on antibiotic type, age, host's health condition, and hospital environment. The AAD is reported in outpatients, hospitalized patients, and long-term care residents and results in prolonged hospital stay, enhances medication costs, and diagnostics (McFarland, 2009; Surawicz, 2003; Xie et al., 2015).

A comparative table is given here to mention the role of probiotic strains in the management of AAD (Table 7.2). In the case of broad spectrum antibiotic-treated children, the incidence of diarrhea ranges from 11% to 62% (Polage et al., 2012). In an evaluation research on utilization of probiotics in acute diarrhea prevention, the probiotics considerably reduced the risk of AAD by 52%, travelers' diarrhea by 8%, and acute diarrhea of diverse causes by 34%. The probiotic treatment diminished the linked risk of acute diarrhea in children by 57% and adults by 26%. The protective effect with treatment of probiotic strains such as *L. rhamnosus, L. acidophilus, L. bulgaricus*, and *S. boulardii* either alone or in combination treatment is more or less similar. However, it is dependent on the host age and genus of the strain (Sazawal et al., 2006). The probiotic strains *L. rhamnosus, S. boulardii, B. lactis* and *S. thermophilus* were found to reduce the risk of AAD in children by 11.9%, in comparison with placebo-controlled randomized trials (28.5%) (Szajewska et al., 2006). The administration of probiotic strains, *L. rhamnosus, B. bifidum* and *S. thermophilus* in comparison with placebo diminished the risk of nosocomial diarrhea and rotavirus gastroenteritis (Wanke & Szajewska, 2014). The administration of probiotic strains such as *L. rhamnosus, B. lactis, S. thermophilus* and *S. boulardii* along with antibiotics reduced the risk of AAD in children (Szajewska et al., 2006). The protective effect of *L. rhamnosus* and *S. boulardii* at 5—40 billion CFU/day in prevention of AAD in children was also confirmed from randomized, parallel, controlled trials (Hayes & Vargas, 2016; Mantegazza et al., 2018).

Based on various randomized, controlled trials, the effectiveness of different probiotic strains coadministered with antibiotic for specified period (7—14 days) in prevention and controlling the pediatric AAD was determined in comparison with a placebo. It was found that a minimum 5 billion CFU daily dose of probiotic strains such as *L. rhamnosus, B. coagulans* and *S. boulardii* provide substantial protective/preventive effect on AAD (Johnston et al., 2006). Based on the human data on utilization of specific probiotics for the prevention or treatment of diarrheal diseases, three probiotic strains—*S. boulardii, L. rhamnosus*, and probiotic mixtures—notably diminished the onset of AAD (McFarland, 2006). The effectiveness of enterococci probiotic strain such as *E. faecium* was proven to be effective in controlling of AAD

TABLE 7.2 A comparative table on the role of probiotic strains in the management of antibiotic-associated diarrhea, in terms of probiotic strain, dose, duration and effect.

Antibiotic	Probiotic strain	Dose (10^{10} CFU/day)	Duration (days)	Effect	References
Pantoprazole, clarithomycin, tinidazole	L. rhamnosus	1	14	Adequate	McFarland (2006)
Varied	L. rhamnosus	1—2	10	Adequate	McFarland (2006)
Varied	L. rhamnosus	2	14	Adequate	Szajewska et al. (2006)
Amoxicillin, cefprozil, clarithromycin	L. rhamnosus	1—2	7—10	Adequate	Johnston et al. (2006)
Clindamycin	L. acidophilus B. longum	0.02—0.05	7	Adequate	Sazawal et al. (2006)
Amoxicillin	L. acidophilus, L. bulgaricus	0.3	10	Adequate	Johnston et al. (2006)
Mixture	S. boulardii	1	7—9	Adequate	Johnston et al. (2006)
β lactam	S. boulardii	2	28	Adequate	McFarland (2006)
Broad spectrum	S. boulardii	1	7—14	Adequate	McFarland (2006)
Clindamycin, cephalosporin, trimethoprim-sulfamethoxazole	S. boulardii	2	14	Adequate	McFarland (2006)

in comparison with placebo group. It is significant that only 3% of *E. faecium* administered patients developed AAD compared to 18% of placebo treated subjects (Franz et al., 2011). The beneficial effect of *S. boulardii* coadministration with antibiotics in reduction of AAD was also reported in another study. Further, a 24% reduction in AAD was noted in patients fed with 8 ounces of yogurt for 8 days, against no yogurt fed patients (12%) who were hospitalized and received oral or intravenous antibiotics (Raghuwanshi, 2015).

7.3.3.2 *Clostridium difficile* associated *diarrhea*

The *C. difficile* associated diarrhea (CDD) is one of the most regular nosocomial infections in aged patients, especially observed in intensive care units, long term care units, patients with renal diseases, orthopedic patients with proximal femoral fractures and immunocompromized adults such as cancer and transplant patients, as a result of continuous/prolonged antibiotic therapy. *C. difficile* is an exotoxin producing Gram-positive anaerobic bacteria, transmits from infected patients through healthcare staff. It is usually CDD is usually treated with vancomycin and metronidazole and results in enhanced healthcare cost, morbidity and sometimes morality (Khan et al., 2017; Mallina et al., 2018; McFarland, 2009; Polage et al., 2012; Sukhwani, 2018; Surawicz, 2003; Xie et al., 2015). The data was collected from randomized, controlled, blinded efficacy human trials on utilization of specific probiotics for the prevention or treatment of diarrheal diseases based on sample size, population characteristics, treatments and outcomes. The probiotic strain such as *S. boulardii* was efficient in controlling the clinically difficult, recurrent CDD due to the production of toxin inactivating proteases, stimulation of IgA production and competition, and steric blockage for attachment sites; it also serves as adjunctive therapy (McFarland, 2006; Sullivan & Nord, 2002; Surawicz, 2003). The probiotic strain combination of *L. acidophilus*, *L. paracasei* and *B. lactis* was found to lower the risk of AAD, *C. difficile* associated diarrhea, and other gastrointestinal symptoms in a dose dependent manner, in adult patients receiving antibiotic therapy (Ouwehand et al., 2014).

7.3.4 Cancer therapy-induced diarrhea

The frequently associated toxicity linked with chemotherapy/radiotherapy of cancers is induced diarrhea. The therapy modifies the host's normal protective gastrointestinal microbiota and affects the chemotherapy regime and tolerance towards therapy; due to morbidity associated with induced diarrhea (Redman et al., 2014). The potent anticancer drug irinotecan is known to induce diarrhea (60%−90%) in patients receiving treatment for metastatic colorectal cancer. The chemotherapy induced diarrhea is due to the production of drug metabolites, damage of intestinal mucosa, change in the intestinal mucin composition, induction of pro-inflammatory cytokines, alteration of intestinal microbiota (dysmicrobia) and predisposition to infectious diarrhea. It was found that the administration of probiotics such as *B. breve*, *B. bifidum*, *B. longum*, *B. infantis*, *L. rhamnosus*, *L. acidophilus*, *L. casei*, *L. plantarum*, *L. brevis* and *S. thermophilus* lead to a decrease in occurrence and severity of irinotecan induced diarrhea in metastatic colorectal cancer patients through the reduction of intestinal β glucuronidase activity (Mego et al., 2015). The results of the various studies showed that the probiotics may reduce both the requirement of antidiarrheal medication and the severity and rate of antibiotic-associated and chemotherapy-induced diarrhea in cancer patients. The studies included, either alone or in combination of, probiotic strains including *L. acidophilus, L. casei, L. delbrueckii, L. plantarum, S. thermophilus, B. bifidum, B. longum, B. breve* and *B. infantis* (Redman et al., 2014). Studies were carried out with immunodeficient mice models on induced diarrhea by 5-Fluorouracil, an antineoplastic drug. It was shown that oral administration of probiotics including *L. rhamnosus, L. acidophilus* and *B. bifidum* could improve diarrhea, body weight, restore jejunal crypt depth, and inhibit cytokines. In addition, probiotic use was found to be therapeutically safe with no apparent bacteremia in blood cultures (Huang et al., 2019).

Another study evaluated the effectiveness and safety of probiotics in prevention of radiotherapy induced diarrhea in cervical cancer patients. The probiotic supplementation was found to be useful in prevention of radiotherapy induced grade ≥ 2 or 3 diarrhea in cervical cancer patients and decreased the dependence of antidiarrheal medication. As often the cancer patients are immunocompromised, the probiotics are mostly safe and rarely associated with adverse effects during treatment (Qiu et al., 2019). In the case of pelvic cancer patients, the standard dose of *L. acidophilus* and *B. longum* may reduce radiation induced grade 2-3-4 diarrhea at treatment completion. For patients operated on or before radiotherapy, the probiotic dose may reduce radiation induced grade 4 diarrhea (Demers et al., 2014). Also, probiotics such as *Lactobacillus* can be used for the prevention of chemo and radiotherapy induced diarrhea in pelvic cancer patients due to their low toxicity and high tolerability (Mego et al., 2015).

7.3.5 Lactose intolerance induced diarrhea

The gastrointestinal disorder lactose intolerance is a characterized by symptoms such as diarrhea, abdominal pain, vomiting, flatulence, and rumble due to the impaired generation of the enzyme β galactosidase during childhood and after weaning (Roškar et al., 2017). Thus, the lactose intolerant person is unable to digest lactose sugar present in dairy products such as milk. A study carried out on lactose intolerant subjects revealed that consumption of lactose in yogurt form results in a more efficient assimilation than milk lactose. Thus, it resulted in reduced diarrhea due to the synthesis of β galactosidase from probiotic microbes in yogurt (Raghuwanshi, 2015). The results of randomized, placebo-controlled clinical trials indicated that the consumption of probiotics such as *L. acidophilus* notably alleviated the symptoms such as diarrhea, abdominal pain, vomiting, and flatulence in lactose intolerant subjects (Roškar et al., 2017). The subtopic is covered in detailed in Chapter 13, Probiotics and Prebiotics in the Prevention and Management of Human Cancers (Colon Cancer, Stomach Cancer, Breast Cancer, and Cervix Cancer).

7.3.6 Enteral tube feeding diarrhea

The enteral nutrition is standard care offered for hospitalized critically ill patients; 60% of the intensive care patients receive it during their stay. However, a regular gastrointestinal problem encountered is enteral tube feeding diarrhea and the incident ranges from 2% to 68%. It is attributed to multifactorial etiology including antibiotic usage, medication side effects, *C. difficile* infection, increased diet osmoloarity, elevated infusion rate, malnutrition condition, and feeding contamination. The enteral tube feeding (ETF) diarrhea results in complications such as dehydration, electrolyte imbalance, intestinal microbiota alteration, wound contamination psychological disturbance and augmented healthcare costs (de Castro Soares et al., 2017; Jack et al., 2010). The supportive evidence on probiotic administration for critically ill patients towards the management of ETF diarrhea is not conclusive (Jack et al., 2010). But, the standard protocol to treat ETF diarrhea is administration of soluble fibers. An assessment study was carried out on the efficacy of a sporulated *Bacillus cereus* in reducing ETF diarrhea in comparison with a soluble fiber by considering parameters such as antibiotic usage, nutritional status, and diet type. It was established that the probiotic *B. cereus* was more effective than the prebiotic in diminishing the diarrhea in malnourished ETF patients receiving antibiotic therapy (de Castro Soares et al., 2017).

7.4 Mode of action of probiotics

The probiotic organisms are known to act on the host by diverse mechanisms such as adhesion competition, colonization resistance, nutrient competition, mucin gene expression, improved nutrient absorption (calcium), antagonistic activity, mucosal defence stimulation, immunomodulation via cytokine production, and nutrient (B complex vitamin) production. One of them is the antipathogenic strategy is pathogen colonization resistance, a characteristic of normal gut microbiota in preventing pathogen growth which is mediated by volatile fatty acid production and lowering luminal pH. It is reported that probiotic *L. rhamnosus* adheres to mucosal cells by competing with pathogens for nutrients and receptors by steric hindrance; synthesizing antimicrobial compounds such as bacteriocins, nitric oxide, hydrogen peroxide; preventing cytokine induced intestinal epithelial apoptosis; and modifying β glucuronidase activity. Probiotics such as *L. rhamnosus* and *S. boulardii* are shown to stimulate both innate and humoral immunity by enhancing IgA levels towards rotavirus and *C. difficile*, respectively (Cremonini et al., 2002; Gill, 2003; Isolauri et al., 2004; Jack et al., 2010; Mantegazza et al., 2018; McFarland, 2009; Mekonnen et al., 2020; Penner et al., 2005; Raghuwanshi, 2015; Surawicz, 2003). The multiple modes of action of probiotics against pathogens still require detailed studies and understanding.

7.5 Conclusions

Probiotics are proven to be efficient in prevention and treatment of rotavirus gastroenteritis, pediatric infectious diarrhea, AAD, nosocomial diarrhea mediated by *C. difficile*, travelers' diarrhea, radiotherapy induced diarrhea, and they have a beneficial therapeutic or prophylactic effect (Gismondo et al., 1999; Mantegazza et al., 2018; Marcos & DuPont, 2007; Penner et al., 2005). The advantages of probiotics in terms of low cost, organism diversity, ease of administration, lack of drug interactions, multifaceted antipathogenic action, modulation of host's mucosal and systemic immunity, survival in target organ and excellent risk to benefit ratio, should be compared with reference to efficacy and safety (McFarland, 2009). In the case of immunocompromised, hospitalized adults, probiotic translocation risk and associated bacteremia, fungemia, etc., has to be evaluated. Further evaluation studies on strain-specific effects and community-based trials in developing countries are needed in preventing infectious diarrhea. Also, heterogeneous trials mandate the requirement of standardized protocols, quality control guidelines, strain specific confirmatory studies, adequate dose optimization, test strain type expansion, documentation risks/benefits, and cost/benefit analysis (Isolauri et al., 2004; McFarland, 2009; Polage et al., 2012; Sazawal et al., 2006).

Acknowledgment

The author would like to thank Dr. M. V. Balarama Krishna, Head, Environmental Science and Nanomaterials Section and Dr. Sanjiv Kumar, Head, NCCCM/BARC, for their constant support and encouragement throughout the work.

References

Binns, C., & Lee, M. K. (2010). The use of probiotics to prevent diarrhea in young children attending child care centers: A review. *Journal of Experimental & Clinical Medicine*, 2(6), 269–273.

Cremonini, F., Di Caro, S., Santarelli, L., Gabrielli, M., Candelli, M., Nista, E. C., Lupascu, A., Gasbarrini, G., & Gasbarrini, A. (2002). Probiotics in antibiotic-associated diarrhoea. *Digestive and Liver Disease*, 34(Suppl. 2), S78–S80.

de Castro Soares, G. G., Marinho, C. H., Pitol, R., Andretta, C., Oliveira, E., Martins, C., & Riella, M. C. (2017). Sporulated Bacillus as alternative treatment for diarrhea of hospitalized adult patients under enteral nutrition: A pilot randomized controlled study. *Clinical Nutrition ESPEN*, 22, 13–18.

Demers, M., Dagnault, A., & Desjardins, J. (2014). A randomized double-blind controlled trial: Impact of probiotics on diarrhea in patients treated with pelvic radiation. *Clinical Nutrition*, 33(5), 761–767.

Franz, C. M., Huch, M., Abriouel, H., Holzapfel, W., & Galvez, A. (2011). Enterococci as probiotics and their implications in food safety. *International Journal of Food Microbiology*, 151(2), 125–140.

Gill, H. S. (2003). Probiotics to enhance anti-infective defences in the gastrointestinal tract. *Best Practice & Research Clinical Gastroenterology*, 17(5), 755–773.

Gismondo, M. R., Drago, L., & Lombardi, A. (1999). Review of probiotics available to modify gastrointestinal flora. *International Journal of Antimicrobial Agents*, 12(4), 287–292.

Hayes, S. R., & Vargas, A. J. (2016). Probiotics for the prevention of pediatric antibiotic-associated diarrhea. *Explore*, 12(6), 463–466.

Heinz, P. (2008). Management of acute gastroenteritis in children. *Paediatrics and Child Health*, 18(10), 453–457.

Huang, L., Chiau, J.-S. C., Cheng, M.-L., Chan, W.-T., Jiang, C.-B., Chang, S.-W., Yeung, C.-Y., & Lee, H.-C. (2019). SCID/NOD mice model for 5-FU induced intestinal mucositis: Safety and effects of probiotics as therapy. *Pediatrics and Neonatology*, 60, 252–260.

Indian Council of Medical Research Task, F., Co-ordinating Unit, I., & Co-ordinating Unit, D. B. T. (2011). ICMR-DBT guidelines for evaluation of probiotics in food. *The Indian Journal of Medical Research*, 134(1), 22–25.

Isolauri, E., Salminen, S., & Ouwehand, A. C. (2004). Probiotics. *Best Practice & Research Clinical Gastroenterology*, 18(2), 299–313.

Jack, L., Coyer, F., Courtney, M., & Venkatesh, B. (2010). Probiotics and diarrhoea management in enterally tube fed critically ill patients-what is the evidence? *Intensive & Critical Care Nursing*, 26(6), 314–326.

Johnston, B. C., Supina, A. L., & Vohra, S. (2006). Probiotics for pediatric antibiotic-associated diarrhea: A meta-analysis of randomized placebo-controlled trials. *CMAJ: Canadian Medical Association Journal*, 175(4), 377–383.

Khan, H. A., Baig, F. K., & Mehboob, R. (2017). Nosocomial infections: Epidemiology, prevention, control and surveillance. *Asian Pacific Journal of Tropical Biomedicine*, 7(5), 478–482.

Mallina, R., Craik, J., Briffa, N., Ahluwalia, V., Clarke, J., & Cobb, A. G. (2018). Probiotic containing *Lactobacillus casei*, *Lactobacillus bulgaricus*, and *Streptococcus thermophiles* (ACTIMEL) for the prevention of *Clostridium difficile* associated diarrhoea in the elderly with proximal femur fractures. *Journal of Infection and Public Health*, 11(1), 85–88.

Mantegazza, C., Molinari, P., D'Auria, E., Sonnino, M., Morelli, L., & Zuccotti, G. V. (2018). Probiotics and antibiotic-associated diarrhea in children: A review and new evidence on *Lactobacillus rhamnosus* GG during and after antibiotic treatment. *Pharmacological Research*, 128, 63–72.

Marcos, L. A., & DuPont, H. L. (2007). Advances in defining etiology and new therapeutic approaches in acute diarrhea. *The Journal of Infection*, 55(5), 385–393.

Mathan, V. I. (1998). Diarrhoeal diseases. *British Medical Bulletin*, 54(2), 407–419.

McFarland, L. V. (2006). Meta-analysis of probiotics for the prevention of antibiotic associated diarrhea and the treatment of *Clostridium difficile* disease. *The American Journal of Gastroenterology*, 101(4), 812–822.

McFarland, L. V. (2009). Evidence-based review of probiotics for antibiotic-associated diarrhea and *Clostridium difficile* infections. *Anaerobe*, 15(6), 274–280.

Mego, M., Chovanec, J., Vochyanova-Andrezalova, I., Konkolovsky, P., Mikulova, M., Reckova, M., Miskovska, V., Bystricky, B., Beniak, J., Medvecova, L., Lagin, A., Svetlovska, D., Spanik, S., Zajac, V., Mardiak, J., & Drgona, L. (2015). Prevention of irinotecan induced diarrhea by probiotics: A randomized double blind, placebo controlled pilot study. *Complementary Therapies in Medicine*, 23(3), 356–362.

Mekonnen, S. A., Merenstein, D., Fraser, C. M., & Marco, M. L. (2020). Molecular mechanisms of probiotic prevention of antibiotic-associated diarrhea. *Current Opinion in Biotechnology*, 61, 226–234.

Nuraida, L. (2015). A review: Health promoting lactic acid bacteria in traditional Indonesian fermented foods. *Food Science and Human Wellness, 4* (2), 47–55.

Ouwehand, A. C., DongLian, C., Weijian, X., Stewart, M., Ni, J., Stewart, T., & Miller, L. E. (2014). Probiotics reduce symptoms of antibiotic use in a hospital setting: A randomized dose response study. *Vaccine, 32*(4), 458–463.

Penner, R., Fedorak, R. N., & Madsen, K. L. (2005). Probiotics and nutraceuticals: Non-medicinal treatments of gastrointestinal diseases. *Current Opinion in Pharmacology, 5*(6), 596–603.

Polage, C. R., Solnick, J. V., & Cohen, S. H. (2012). Nosocomial diarrhea: Evaluation and treatment of causes other than *Clostridium difficile*. *Clinical Infectious Diseases, 55*(7), 982–989.

Qiu, G., Yu, Y., Wang, Y., & Wang, X. (2019). The significance of probiotics in preventing radiotherapy-induced diarrhea in patients with cervical cancer: A systematic review and meta-analysis. *International Journal of Surgery, 65*, 61–69.

Raghuwanshi, S. (2015). The Indian perspective for probiotics: A review. *Indian journal of Dairy Science, 68*(3), 195–205.

Redman, M. G., Ward, E. J., & Phillips, R. S. (2014). The efficacy and safety of probiotics in people with cancer: A systematic review. *Annals of Oncology, 25*(10), 1919–1929.

Roškar, I., Švigelj, K., Štempelj, M., Volfand, J., Štabuc, B., Malovrh, Š., & Rogelj, I. (2017). Effects of a probiotic product containing *Bifidobacterium animalis* subsp. animalis IM386 and *Lactobacillus plantarum* MP2026 in lactose intolerant individuals: Randomized, placebo-controlled clinical trial. *Journal of Functional Foods, 35*, 1–8.

Sazawal, S., Hiremath, G., Dhingra, U., Malik, P., Deb, S., & Black, R. E. (2006). Efficacy of probiotics in prevention of acute diarrhoea: A meta-analysis of masked, randomised, placebo-controlled trials. *The Lancet. Infectious diseases, 6*(6), 374–382.

Sehgal, S., Dhewa, T., Bansal, N., & Thakur, M. (2016). Probiotic drugs and labeling practices in Indian market. *DU Journal of Undergraduate Research and Innovation, 2*(1), 166–170.

Shubha, J. R., & Bhatt, P. (2015). *Plectranthus amboinicus* leaves stimulate growth of probiotic *L. plantarum*: Evidence for ethnobotanical use in diarrhea. *Journal of Ethnopharmacology, 166*, 220–227.

Sukhwani, K. (2018). Clinical profile of *Clostridium difficile* associated diarrhea: A study from tertiary care centre of South India. *Tropical Gastroenterology, 39*(3), 135–141.

Sullivan, Å., & Nord, C. E. (2002). The place of probiotics in human intestinal infections. *International Journal of Antimicrobial Agents, 20*(5), 313–319.

Surawicz, C. M. (2003). Probiotics, antibiotic-associated diarrhoea and *Clostridium difficile* diarrhoea in humans. *Best Practice & Research Clinical Gastroenterology, 17*(5), 775–783.

Szajewska, H., Ruszczyński, M., & Radzikowski, A. (2006). Probiotics in the prevention of antibiotic-associated diarrhea in children: A meta-analysis of randomized controlled trials. *The Journal of Pediatrics, 149*(3), 367–372, e1.

Teran, C. G., Teran-Escalera, C. N., & Villarroel, P. (2009). Nitazoxanide vs. probiotics for the treatment of acute rotavirus diarrhea in children: A randomized, single-blind, controlled trial in Bolivian children. *International Journal of Infectious Diseases, 13*(4), 518–523.

Wanke, M., & Szajewska, H. (2014). Probiotics for preventing healthcare-associated diarrhea in children: A meta-analysis of randomized controlled trials. *Pediatria Polska, 89*(1), 8–16.

Xie, C., Li, J., Wang, K., Li, Q., & Chen, D. (2015). Probiotics for the prevention of antibiotic-associated diarrhoea in older patients: A systematic review. *Travel Medicine and Infectious Disease, 13*(2), 128–134.

Chapter 8

Probiotics in the prevention and treatment of atopic skin diseases

Archana Chaudhari[1], Ankit Bharti[2] and Mitesh Kumar Dwivedi[3]

[1]Vyara Clinical Laboratory Pvt Ltd., Tapi, India, [2]Aura Skin and Dental Clinic, Tapi, India, [3]C.G. Bhakta Institute of Biotechnology, Faculty of Science, Uka Tarsadia University, Maliba Campus, Bardoli, India

8.1 Introduction

Atopic dermatitis (AD) is a chronic or recurrent inflammatory skin disease characterized by dry skin, intense itching, recurrent eczematous lesions, and loss of sleep, which affects the patients' quality of life. It is associated with reduced quality of life, increased health care expenditures, and increased risk of developing other allergic diseases. It is common among infants and children (Emilia et al., 2019; Huang et al., 2017; Sung et al., 2017; Zhao et al., 2018). However, AD is also known as eczema, according to the World Allergy Organization, to refer to the clinical phenotype of the pathology (Ridd et al., 2019). AD is characterized by the presence of skin lesions, excoriation, lichenification, papules, exudation, and crusts, the pathology of which varies according to age. It can vary according to the darker skin type and also to follicular accentuation, hyper- or hypopigmentation. And finally, itching, which is a very frequent feature of AD, leads to the appearance of abrasions causing an increase in inflammation (Sharma & Im, 2018). This is related to other hypersensitivity reactions, such as high risks of allergy, especially food, asthma, rhinitis, and mental health problems (Huang et al., 2017; Rather et al., 2016). It is also associated with other pathologies, such as cardiovascular disease and obesity (Sharma & Im, 2018).

The incidence of AD has increased rapidly in the world in the last decades with a prevalence of 1%–3% in adults and approximately 10%–20% of infants and children experience the disease in developed countries with 60% of the cases that start during the first year of life (Dissanayake & Shimojo, 2016; Li et al., 2020; Weidinger & Novak, 2016). Distribution of disease severity was studied among those participants who met the strictest UKWP criteria (including age at onset <2 years) using the Patient-Oriented Eczema Measure (POEM). On the basis of POEM, 60.1% (95% confidence interval = 56.1–64.1) had mild disease, whereas 28.9% (25.3–32.7) and 11.0% (8.6–13.7) had moderate-to-severe disease (Chiesa Fuxench et al., 2019). In addition, other studies show that its prevalence has tripled in industrialized countries, affecting 2%–10% of adults and 15%–30% of children worldwide, with 20% being infants, in which 45% of cases the disease starts in the first 6 months of life, 60% during the first year, and 85% starts before the age of 5 (Lara et al., 2015). Furthermore, it is verified that AD is higher in urban areas than in rural areas (Choi et al., 2016).

8.2 Etiology and pathophysiology of atopic dermatitis

At the pathophysiological level, AD is a multifactorial disease with an interrelation between the skin barrier, genetic predisposition, immune development, and the microbiota composition of the skin. In addition, it involves environmental, nutritional, pharmacological, and psychological factors, which contribute to the worsening or development of AD (Emilia et al., 2019; Hulshof et al., 2017; Lise et al., 2018). The pathological chain of phenomena in AD begins with (1) weakened skin barrier function, through (2) decreased bacterial diversity of the skin, and (3) susceptibility to skin infections (including *Staphylococcus aureus* predomination and colonization), toward (4) immune dysregulation (Kong et al., 2012).

AD is classified as a biphasic disease, presenting two phases—acute and chronic phases, mainly caused by the responses of T helper 1 (Th1) and T helper 2 (Th2) cells. However, AD is more diverse in the acute phase, which consists of the responses Th2 [interleukin (IL) 4, IL5, IL13, IL31 and CCL-18] and Th22 (proteins IL-22 and S-100A). In contrast, the chronic phase comprises the accentuated acute phase pathways, together with Th1 cells [interferon (IFN)-ʎ, CXCL-9 and CXCL-10] (Sharma & Im, 2018). In AD, there are two possible causes that validate the existence, such as the extrinsic or mediated by immunoglobulin E (IgE), with high levels of IgE, and the intrinsic or non-IgE mediated, with normal serum levels of IgE. FLG encodes a protein filaggrin that is responsible for retaining moisture and protecting the skin, from environmental allergens (Rather et al., 2016). This way, FLG is an essential component for the balance of the skin barrier, as its deficiency is associated with an increase in pH, which makes the colonization of *S. aureus* favorable (Kim & Hei, 2019; Silverberg & Silverberg, 2015). Hence, it occurs that a decrease in FLG and claudin 1 leads to an imbalance in the barrier. Thus there is an increase in the permeability of the skin barrier and the consequent penetration of allergens and microorganisms (Machado, 2018).

Apart from this, there is still some controversy about AD, based on two possible hypotheses: "Inside-Out," due to the dysfunction and systemic inflammation of the epidermal barrier. And "Outside-In," with an epidermal rupture of the skin barrier, activating an immune imbalance (Guttman-Yassky et al., 2017; Silverberg & Silverberg, 2015). In the "Inside-out" hypothesis, there is a skin inflammation, as there is a weakening of the barrier. This happens because there was a decrease in the production of filaggrin. The breakage of the skin barrier is due to the transcutaneous penetration of allergens that leads to an increase in *S. aureus* (Silverberg & Silverberg, 2015). Microbial pathogens, including *S. aureus*, *Candida*, and *Trichophyton*, promote the flares of AD, creating local injury and inflammation, and contributing to systemic allergic responses (Williams et al., 2019). Almost all patients with AD are colonized by *S. aureus*. Nevertheless, topical antibiotics have been unsuccessful in showing beneficial effect and are not suggested by any consensus management guidelines. Recent evidence suggests that commensal coagulase-negative staphylococci produce peptides capable of preventing *S. aureus*-mediated epithelial damage and skin inflammation. In the "Outside-In" hypothesis, there is an immunological dysregulation because it occurs in filaggrin gene mutation. These mutations in the filaggrin gene occur due to environmental factors, such as temperature and humidity, jeopardizing its production. The rupture of the skin barrier results from an increase in cutaneous and systemic responses of Th2 cells and IL-4 and IL-a3, with thymic stromal lymphopoietin. Thus they are responsible for generating allergic diseases, such as asthma, and for the progression of AD to other forms of atopy, such as food allergy (Hulshof et al., 2017; Silverberg & Silverberg, 2015).

Another theory that justifies the prevalence of AD is the "hygiene hypothesis," which implants the colonization pattern and the diversity of the intestinal microbiota (Reddel et al., 2019; Simpson et al., 2015). Thus this theory states that in the modern hygienic living conditions, there is a reduction in exposure to microorganisms early in life, which results in inadequate immunological priming (Kim & Hei, 2019).

8.3 Relationship between gut microbiota and atopic dermatitis

Some researchers have found that gut microbiota composition differs between infants with and without AD (Hong et al., 2010; Zheng et al., 2016). Thus the exposure to bacteria and viruses in the children's environment is a crucial factor in the development of allergy (Rather et al., 2016; Yamamoto et al., 2016). The amalgamation of immune dysregulation and epidermal barrier dysfunction in AD promotes pathogenic bacterial colonization. There is an increase in *S. aureus* count in AD skin with global reduction in microbial diversity (Baviera et al., 2014; Bjerre et al., 2017; Kong et al., 2012; Williams & Gallo, 2015). A recent study established lower bacterial diversity in both nonlesional and lesional skin of patients with AD, suggesting an altogether affected skin microflora in AD (Clausen et al., 2018). Bacterial diversity is also inversely correlated with disease severity. A dramatic decrease in the skin bacterial diversity is detected in more severe disease conditions and during AD flares, whereas treatment of AD lesional skin leads to bacterial rediversification. Specifically, staphylococcal species including *Staphylococcus* epidermis increase during AD flares (Bjerre et al., 2017; Clausen et al., 2018; Kong et al., 2012; Williams & Gallo, 2015). Indeed, an investigation of AD flares showed an increase in *S. aureus* in patients with more severe disease, while *S. epidermidis* dominated in patients with less severe disease (Byrd et al., 2017). Furthermore, the intestinal environment may impact the pathogenesis of AD. Infants with IgE associated eczema have a reduced proportion of bifidobacterial species and low microflora diversity early in life (Abrahamsson et al., 2012).

Such evidence supports the idea that appropriate microbial colonization of the gut might lower the risk of developing atopic diseases. Several preclinical observations on the quorum sensing between microbial species on the skin generated a hypothesis that interventions targeting the microbiome could offer a promising, safe, and attractive approach to the topical add-on treatment in patients with AD (Ambrożej et al., 2020). The modern approach of the associations between human health and body's microbiomes has extended far beyond the novel hygiene hypothesis. Living bacteria, as well as their products, have already been successfully applied as add-on therapy in various clinical situations (Makrgeorgou et al., 2018). Therefore modulation of the microflora may be a promising new preventive and therapeutic approach in treatment of AD.

Numerous nonpharmacological interventions (e.g., bathing practices, moisturizers) and topical pharmacotherapies (e.g., topical corticosteroids, calcineurin inhibitors, antihistamines) have been used routinely as first-line therapies to manage the diseases (Eichenfield et al., 2017). However, nonpharmacological interventions mainly aim to reduce transepidermal water loss, thereby increasing skin hydration, and are used to treat mild disease. Furthermore, the safety issues related to the long-term use of topical corticosteroids (the first-line topical pharmacotherapy in treating AD) are gaining increasing attention, especially when the subjects are children. Other therapies, such as antihistamines, have been tried for the treatment of AD but unfortunately have demonstrated little utility (Eichenfield et al., 2014). Given the high prevalence of AD, its potential long-term health effects, and the safety concerns surrounding existing AD medicines, it is worth developing new therapies with promising effects and safety for use in both prevention and treatment. Here, we will see the use of probiotics as a new therapeutic approach in AD.

8.4 Intervention of probiotics in atopic dermatitis

Probiotics are live microorganisms that confer health benefits to the host when administered in adequate quantities. Probiotics play a beneficial role in the gastrointestinal tract and in the intestine−brain−skin axis and, activate several immunological mechanisms, when the response is aggravated in the atopic individual. AD diagnosis is based on clinical signs and Scoring for Atopic Dermatitis (SCORAD) index, which is a confirmed by clinical scoring system that measures the intensity, severity of disease, and quality of life parameters linked with AD symptoms. This aids physicians to evaluate severity on a regular basis (Antunes et al., 2017). The primary result selected is often a change in SCORAD index. AD usually occurs at around 3−4 months of age and resolves in about 50% of the AD subjects by 2−3 years of age.

The main aim of probiotic trials in the management of AD is reducing the severity of AD, and they are relatively of shorter duration typically 4−12 weeks. The prevention and treatment of AD is mostly based on skin care through the use of emollients and moisturizers. Immunomodulation exerted by probiotics has a better response and less adverse effects than the application of corticosteroids (Lara et al., 2015). In addition, probiotic supplementation can accelerate the favorable evolution of atopy and cause children to remain asymptomatic for a period, even after the end of treatment.

8.4.1 Animal model studies

Animal models can offer valuable information about the ability of specific probiotic strain to prevent or treat AD and to explain their cellular and molecular mechanisms of action, even though they do not completely recapitulate all clinical, histological, and immunological features of human AD. Certainly, assessing the effect of probiotic strains directly in human trials is expensive and time-consuming. Moreover, there are number of parameters, such as the dose, routes, and possible administration schedules, along with the mechanism of action of potential probiotics that should be evaluated before to a clinical trial are performed. Since blood is the only accessible biological materials in case of humans, research on use of probiotics in AD may benefit from preclinical animal models (Kalliomäki, 2010). In the context of AD, several animal models are used to evaluate the capacity of probiotic strains to prevent or manage the AD. With the increasing interest in the field of probiotics, various strains are reported to display potential benefit for AD management. Alternative models, such as the canine model of AD, are also used in studies as they display features similar to human AD. Of note, Park et al. evaluated the efficacy of probiotic *Lactobacillus helveticus* HY7801 in the prevention of AD in Beagle dogs (Park, 2020). Probiotics have been used in several studies for the treatment of AD, using animal models (Table 8.1).

8.4.2 Human studies/clinical trials

Several clinical trials have explored the efficiency of probiotic in prevention or treatment of AD. First, Simpson et al., in 2016 performed a study in which 415 pregnant women were randomly supplemented with 250 mL of probiotic milk per day or placebo from 36 weeks of gestation until 3 months after labor. Probiotic milk contained *Bifidobacterium animalis* subsp. *lactis* Bb-12 (Bb-12), 5×10^{10} colony-forming units (CFU) of *Lactobacillus rhamnosus* GG (LGG) and 5×10^9 CFU of *Lactobacillus acidophilus* La-5 (La-5) per serving. The placebo was pasteurized skim-fermented milk

TABLE 8.1 Treatment studies of probiotics using animal model.

References	Probiotics strain/s	Animal model used	Observations	Clinical/Histopathological scores
Shin et al. (2016)	*Lactobacillus acidophilus* CBT LA1, *Lactobacillus rhamnosus* CBT LR5, *Lactobacillus plantarum* CBT LP3, *Bifidobacterium bifidum* CBT BR3, *Bifidobacterium breve* CBT BR3, *Lactococcus lactis* CBT SL6, *Streptococcus thermophilus* CBT ST3	DNCB induced AD in Nc/NgA mice	Generation of CD4$^+$ Foxp3$^+$ T cells in mLN, low serum IgE, IL-4 and IL-5, high Th1 IFN-γ, IL12p40	Improved
Kim et al. (2016)	*Lactobacillus casei, L. plantarum, L. rhamnosus* and *Bifidobacterium lactis*	DNCB induced AD in Nc/NgA mice	Low serum IgE, IL-4 and IL-5, high Th1 cytokines IFN-γ, IL12p40	Improved
Lee et al. (2016)	*Lactobacillus rhamnosus* IDCC 3201	BALB mouse	An atopic therapeutic effect through immune-balance	Improved
Lim et al. (2017)	*Weissella cibaria* WIKIM28	DNCB induced AD in BALB/c mice	Reduced Th2 cytokines, generation of CD4$^+$ Foxp3$^+$ T cells and increased IL-10 levels in mLN	Improved
Choi et al. (2017)	Heat killed *Lactobacillus brevis* NS1401	House dust mice induced AD in Nc/NgA mice	Reduced serum IgE, eosinophil and mast cell infiltration, allergen specific IgG1 and Th1/Th2 cytokines	Improved
Park Mi-Sung et al. (2017)	*Lactobacilli* isolated from Jeotgal	Female BALB/c mice	*Lactobacilli* isolated from Jeotgal inhibited atopic cytokines such as IL-4 and IFN-γ in skin lesions of mice with atopic dermatitis	Improved
Kim Han-Wool et al., 2018	Duolac ATP (mixture of *L. casei* CBTLC5, *L. pantarum* CBT LP3, *L. rhamnosus* CBTLR5, *B. lactis* CBT BL3)	Balb/c mice and NC/Nga mice	Antiinflammatory cytokines IL-10 and TGF-3 increased	Improved
Kwon Min-Sung et al. (2018)	*Lactobacillus sakei* WIKIM30	Balb/c mice	Oral administration of *L. sakei* WIKIM30 reduced the atopic dermatological lesions and IgE and IL-4 levels in lymph nodes. It also lowered cytokine levels of Th2 and increased IL-10 in peripheral lymph nodes. WIKIM 30 modulated the intestinal microbiota in the mice with atopic dermatitis	Improved
Yoshihiro Tokudome et al. (2018)	Lactic acid bacteria metabolites	Mice	Oral administration of liquid *Lactobacillus* metabolites to the mice with atopic dermatitis improved the water content of the stratum corneum, the transdermal moisture loss, the AP of ceramide, and the epidermal thickness	Improved
Kim Jong-Hwa et al. (2018)	Cream cheese-derived *Lactococcus chungangensis* CAU 28	BALB/c mice	It showed the atopic dermatitis improvements, such as the immune response related to single-chain fatty acids and the intestinal environment	Improved
Holowacz et al. (2018)	*B. longum* LA 101, *L. helveticus* LA 102, *L. lactis* LA 103, *S. thermophilus* LA104, *L. rhamnosus* LA 801	Hairless SKH-1 mice	Help in preserving skin integrity and homeostasis	Improved
Park et al. (2020)	*Lactobacillus helveticus* HY7801	Beagle dogs	The epidermal hyper-proliferation and collagen deposition were inhibited compared to the placebo group, and the secretion amount of the inflammatory factors, such as TNF-α, IL-4 were reduced	Improved

AD, atopic dermatitis; *DNCB*, dinitrochlorobenzene; *IFN*, interferon; *IgE*, immunoglobulin E; *IL*, interleukin; *mLN*, mesenteric lymph node; *Th1*, type 1 helper T cell; *Th2*, type 2 helper T cell.

that did not contain probiotic bacteria. The probiotic group encouraged intestinal immune homeostasis by promoting regulatory differentiation of regulatory T (Treg) cells through IL-10, which is advantageous for the development of the neonatal immune system and prevention of AD (Simpson et al., 2016). The community probiotic and an environment rich in transforming growth factor β (TGF-β) created by probiotics promotes the expansion and differentiation of Treg cells. Few of the other studies have been summarized in Table 8.2.

A study performed by Addor et al., in 2016, evaluated the efficiency and tolerability of the *Bifidobacterium lactis* HN019, *L. acidophilus* NCFM, *L. rhamnosus* HN001, and *Lactobacillus paracasei* Lpc-37 probiotics in children with AD aged between 6 months and 12 years. *L. rhamnosus* probiotic is known to have a modulating effect on the Th1 response and induce the synthesis of IL-10 that prevents the development of AD along with the decrease of SCORAD in the AD patients. *B. lactis* also displayed an immunomodulatory effect on the lymphocyte response. *L. paracasei* induced TNF-α, IL-10, and IFN-λ production leading to the modulation of Th1 and Th2 immune responses and thereby production of secretory IgA. *L. acidophilus* also promotes the expression of cytokines that leads to the activation of the Th1 response and regulation of Th2 activity. This leads to the inhibition of the growth of *S. aureus*. As a result, the positive effects were obtained in the study that leads to the improvement of AD symptoms along with the absence of adverse effects. Thus this study promises the safe consumption of these probiotics (Addor, 2015).

Li et al., in 2018, demonstrated that supplementation with pre- and postnatal probiotics reduced the incidence of AD in babies and children. Along with this they also concluded that the treatment can be effective, despite significant heterogeneity found among the studies (Li et al., 2019). This can be described by the fact that there are differences in the various probiotic species selected and regions at the time of supplementation. This in turn influences the overall results, due to the ethnicity and immunological mechanisms of the host that may be responsible for different responses to probiotics according to the geographic area and the population. Consequently, the treatment with probiotics in early stages of pregnancy till the first 6 months of life may be more advantageous in preventing the disease conditions.

Reddel et al., in 2019, evaluated the persistence of probiotic bacteria in the age range of the study population between 0 and 6 years with diagnosis of AD. Patients with AD exhibited a decrease in some bacteria that produce short-chain fatty acid (SCFA), such as *Blautia*, *Bifidobacterium*, *Eubacteria*, *Coprococcus*, and *Propionibacterium*. The SCFAs help in preserving narrow junctions thereby maintaining epithelial integrity and the maintenance of the mucus layer. The *Bifidobacterium* spp. has several benefits like the stimulation of the immune system, the production of vitamins, improved digestion of food ingredients and inhibition of potentially pathogenic bacteria. In addition, several studies have emphasized the role of *Bifidobacterium* in inducing the production of antiinflammatory cytokines, reducing inflammation along with the suppression of the Th2 immune response and the production of IgE. Thus the absence of *Bifidobacterium* in children with AD may lead to a lack of antiinflammatory effects (Reddel et al., 2019).

Numerous studies have demonstrated that the combination of probiotics has more advantageous effects than a single probiotic (Navarro-López et al., 2018). Fooland and Armstrong, in 2014, showed the efficacy of the probiotic combination in AD. Dotterud et al. (2010) conducted a study to evaluate the possibility of a protective effect in babies, irrespective of family history of atopy. Supplementation of mothers with specific probiotic mixture of *L. acidophilus* La-5, LGG, and *B. animalis* subsp. *lactis* Bb-12 during the pre- and postnatal period leads to the prevention of AD in children at 2 years of age due to the antiinflammatory properties that resulted in less epidermal penetration

Notay et al., in 2017, conducted a randomized clinical trial in adults over the age of 18 years using the combination of probiotics *Lactobacillus salivarius* LS01 DSM 2275 and brief *Bifidobacterium* BR03 DSM 16604 that lead to an improvement in AD in the probiotic group (Notay et al., 2017).

Han et al. (2012) performed a randomized, double-blind, placebo-controlled study in which they supplemented *Lactobacillus plantarum* CJLP133 in children with AD aged between 1 and 12 years for twelve weeks. They showed SCORAD improvement and a significant decrease in IFN-γ, IL-4, and eosinophil's number. In other study, Wang et al. evaluated the effect of *Lactobacillus fermentum* alone, *L. paracasei* alone, and the combination of both strains in AD patients (Wang & Wang, 2015). The authors observed reduction of SCORAD in all groups that received probiotics as compared to the placebo group even four months after the treatment was discontinued. In another meta-analysis including 1070 children receiving oral probiotics containing *L. fermentum*, *L. salivarius*, and a mixture of different strains, significant reductions were observed in SCORAD values in patients (Huang et al., 2017). A daily oral dose of a mixture of probiotics composed of *B. lactis* CECT 8145, *Bifidobacterium longum* CECT 7347, and *Lactobacillus casei* CECT 9104 for 12 weeks in a double-blind, placebo-controlled clinical trial conducted with children and adolescents between 4 and 17 years of age with moderate AD for 12 weeks led to a reduction in SCORAD as compared with control patients (Navarro-López et al., 2018). Another double-blind, placebo-controlled study conducted with a mixture of probiotics (*L. rhamnosus*, *L. acidophilus*, *L. paracasei*, and *B. lactis*) for 6 months found a significant reduction of SCORAD after treatment with a mixture of probiotics as compared to the placebo group (Maria et al., 2020).

TABLE 8.2 Clinical trials for treatment of atopic dermatitis using probiotics.

References	Probiotics strain/s	Clinical patients	Observations	Clinical outcome (SCORAD index, clinical symptoms)
Wang et al. (2015)	*Lactobacillus paracasei, Lactobacillus fermentum*, and mixture	Pediatric	Reduced IL-4, marginally increased TGF-β, IFN-γ	Improved
Jo et al. (2015)	Mixture of *Lactobacillus plantarum* culture solution	Children	AD symptoms improved when mixed culture solution was repeatedly applied to the atopic lesion of patients	Improved
Nakatsuji et al. (2017)	*Staphylococci epidermidis* and *S. hominis*	Adults	Significant decrease in *S. aureus* abundance compared to vehicle	Improved
Blanchet-Réthoré et al. (2017)	*Lactobacillus johnsonii* NCC 533 (HT La1)	Adults	Significant decrease in mean SCORAD values. Significant decrease in *S. aureus* abundance of the treated target lesions compared with lesions not treated with *HT La1* lotion	Improved
Myles et al. (2018)	*Roseomonas mucosa*	Adults and children	In both age groups, significant decrease in mean SCORAD values in adults and children, significant decrease in subjective pruritus, significant decrease in topical steroid applications	Improved
Wickens et al. (2018)	*L. rhamnosus* HN001	Adults	Probiotic treatment did not reduce eczema	No change from placebo
Navarro-López et al. (2018)	*Bifidobacterium lactis* CECT 8145, *Bifidobacterium longum* CECT 7347, and *Lactobacillus casei* CECT 9104	Pediatric	Reduced use of topical corticosteroids	Improved
Lise et al. (2018)	Lactobacillus mixtures (*Bifidobacterium lactis* HN019, *Lactobacillus acidophilus* NCFm, *Lactobacillus rhamnosus* HN001, *Lactobacillus paracasei* LPC37)	18-Month-old female patients	SCORAD, body surface area, and Family Dermatology Life Quality Index were all improved	Improved
Ibanes et al. (2018)	Synbiotic supplementation (*Lb. casei, Bd. lactis, Lb. rhamnosus, Lb. plantarum*, fructooligosaccharides, galactooligosaccharides, biotin)	Children	Both SCORAD and VAS were reduced	Improved
Navarro-López et al. (2018)	A mixture of *Bifidobacterium lactis* CECT 8145, *B. longum* CECT 7347, and *Lactobacillus casei* CECT 9104	Children	Significantly lower levels of SCORAD	Improved
Reddel et al. (2019)	*B. breve* BR03 and *L. salivarius* LS01	Children	Consuming the probiotics alone does not improve the atopic dermatitis	No change
Schmidt et al. (2019)	Mixture of *L. rhamnosus* and *B. animalis* subsp. *lactis*	Children	No significant difference in the incidence of eczema between the mixed *Lactobacillus* intake group and the placebo control group	No change
Suzuki et al. (2020)	Yogurt containing *Lactococcus lactis* 11/19-B1 strain	Female Balb/c mice and children	*L. lactis* 11/19-B1-containing yogurt reduces SCORAD scores in AD patients. The intake of dead *L. lactis* 11/19-B1 improves AD pathology in a mouse model through the suppression of the percentage of Th1, Th2, and Th17 in T cells and the inhibition of eosinocyte infiltration into the AD lesion site	Improved
Plummer et al. (2020)	*Bifidobacterium infantis* + *Streptococcus thermophiles* + *B. lactis*	Adults and/or infants	Probiotic treatment did not reduce eczema	No change from placebo

The decrease in SCORAD continued until 3 months after treatment was discontinued, which suggested a short-term beneficial effect.

Oral probiotics have been explored for the treatment and prevention of AD through several controlled studies. In a meta-analysis, *Lactobacillus* alone and *Lactobacillus* with *Bifidobacterium bifidum* have been used which supported the role of oral probiotics in preventing the development of AD (Chang et al., 2016; Panduru et al., 2015). Application of *Escherichia coli* at an early age of 2 months might result into long-term health benefits, as it was accompanied with reduced occurrence of AD by the age of 6 years (Orivuori et al., 2015). Nevertheless, probiotics with *L. rhamnosus* and *L. paracasei* have yielded mixed results as some effects may be strain or species specific (Damm et al., 2017; Fölster-Holst et al., 2006; Rosenfeldt et al., 2003; Wu et al., 2017). Till date, only limited number of studies has exploited live bacteria in topical probiotics for treatment of AD. Topical application of commensal skin bacteria has been proved to protect against pathogens (Nakatsuji et al., 2017). A commensal Coagulase-negative staphylococci decreases *S. aureus* colonization as it selectively attacks it by the secretion of highly potent antimicrobial peptides, which is also associated with reduced local inflammation and improvement in clinical features (Nakatsuji et al., 2018). The skin commensal, the Gram-negative species *Roseomonas mucosa* have been demonstrated to significantly decrease pruritus, SCORAD, and steroid usage in adults and pediatric patients, without any adverse complications (Myles et al., 2018). Gut commensal has also been explored in several topical probiotic studies with favorable results. Topical application of *Streptococcus thermophilus* cream for 2 weeks in patients with AD led to significant improvement in pruritus, erythema, and scaling (Di Marzio et al., 2003). Moreover, a topical application of lysate of a Gram-negative bacterium *Vitreoscilla filiformis*, found in thermal spring water, have been proved to reduce clinical features in patients with AD (Gueniche et al., 2009). Topical application of *Lactobacillus johnsonii* to AD lesions twice daily for 3 weeks has been demonstrated to reduce *S. aureus* load (Blanchet-Réthoré et al., 2017). Even though only few research studies have been performed on probiotics for AD, many trials performed so far have shown positive results.

8.4.3 Mechanism of probiotics in amelioration of AD

Probiotics are now emerging as an exceptionally beneficial possibility in AD and other diseases. It has been observed to produce beneficial effects, when administered in appropriate quantities. It has been established that it has a vital role in the gastrointestinal tract and in the intestine–brain–skin axis (Huang et al., 2017; Rather et al., 2016; Yamamoto et al., 2016). The advantages in form of immunological mechanisms are immense, that are exacerbated in the atopic individual (Lara et al., 2015). Probiotics have displayed an essential role in modulation of the activation of Th cells and the production of cytokines; induction of the response of Treg cells and improvement in the barrier function (Dissanayake & Shimojo, 2016). These act in the inhibition of Th2 cells (Lara et al., 2015). The reduction in Th2 cells affects the cytokines, such as IL-4, IL-5, IL-6, and IL-13, to not release and thus causes an INF-λ reduction (cytokine released by Th1 cells). Also, probiotics kindle the secretion of IL-10 and the TGF-β (Yamamoto et al., 2016). In addition, they can decrease inflammation, by causing a decrease in cytokines, IL-4, IL-6, tumor necrosis factor-α, INF-λ, and an increasing presence of IL-10 (Emilia et al., 2019). This way, there are several mechanisms of action (Fig. 8.1), where probiotics can act in atopy specifically in: restoration of Th1 or Th2 cytokines and cause an upsurge of CD4$^+$ Foxp3 Treg cells. An additional mechanism includes the decrease in IgE. In addition, probiotics exert the function of preserving homeostasis and intestinal epithelial integrity, increasing antimicrobial antibody production and thus reducing the number of pathogens on epidermis (Sharma & Im, 2018).

8.5 Future perspectives of probiotics in prevention and treatment of AD

It has been possible to carry out comprehensive research on the human microflora due to the recent advancement in molecular and microbiological techniques. This has led to in depth understanding of the importance of the microbiome in maintaining skin health. This has revealed that alterations in the community structure of the microbiome, both within and across body habitats, and in the metabolic function of the skin microbiome are key factors in the pathophysiology of AD (Li et al., 2020). Alterations in the function of the microbiome appear to play a role in skin homeostasis and inflammation, with reductions in the microbiome derived metabolite, that has been shown to play a role in AD. Further research is required to identify other potentially important microbiome-derived metabolites involved in preserving skin health and to determine how these metabolites interact with the other cell present in skin microenvironment, such as Langerhans cells, keratinocytes, and peripheral nerves. Further understanding of the relation between the microflora and skin will offer new targets for the next generation of treatments for inflammation and barrier function in AD.

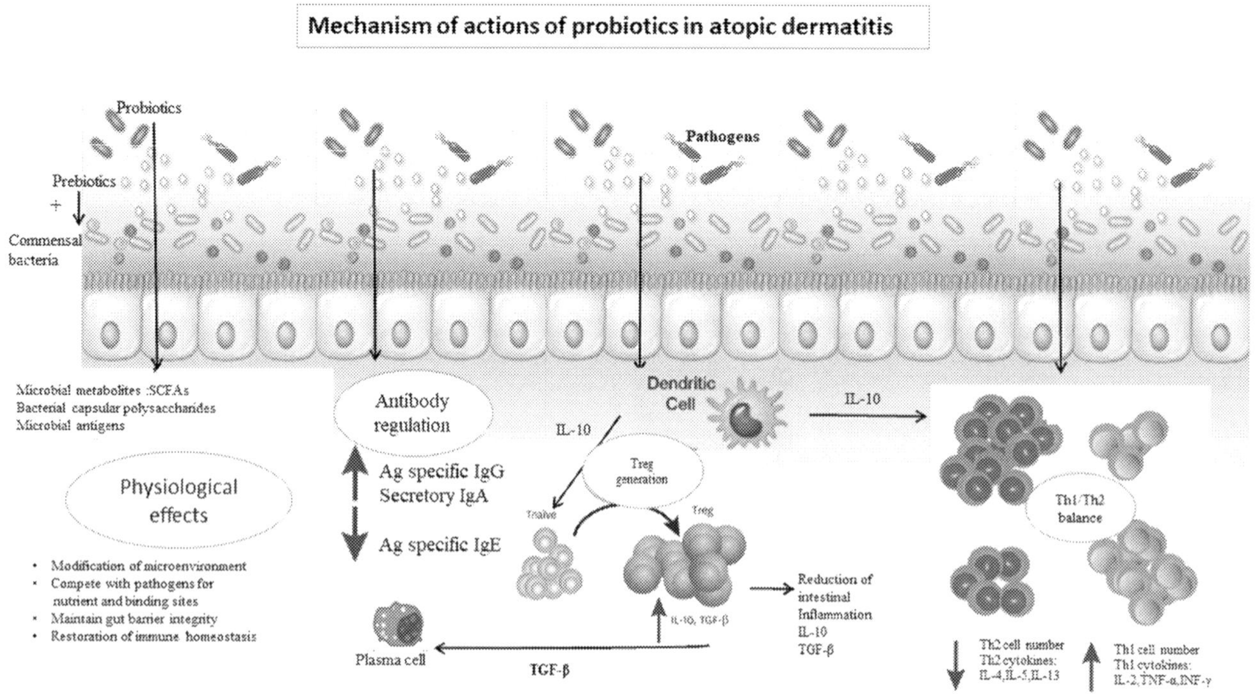

FIGURE 8.1 Overview of mechanisms of action of probiotics in atopic dermatitis. Primary mode of action of probiotics in atopic dermatitis includes restoration of Th1/Th2 cytokine balance. Other specific mechanisms include reduction in allergen specific IgE and increased SCFA levels. Probiotics also aids in constant homeostasis by maintaining intestinal epithelial integrity, increased antimicrobial production, and competitively inhibiting survival of pathogens. *Ig*, Immunoglobulin; *IL*, interleukin; *SCFA*, short-chain fatty acid; *TGF*, transforming growth factor; *Th1*, T helper 1 cell; *Th2*, T helper 2 cell; *Treg*, regulatory T cell.

8.6 Conclusion

In summary, the microbiome plays an important role in the dermatological treatment of AD and serves as a probable target for treatment. Thus probiotics may be helpful in promoting a healthy balance of microflora that may contribute to reducing inflammation, thereby preventing colonization of pathogenic bacteria. There is growing interest in the use of probiotics that have confirmed their excellent safety profile, but data regarding long-term safety are still limited. Therefore clinical trials with topical and oral probiotics with particular species combinations, doses, treatment durations, and larger samples are necessary to characterize the safety and effectiveness of probiotics.

Acknowledgment

We are grateful to Uka Tarsadia University, Maliba Campus, Tarsadi, Gujarat, India, for providing the facilities needed for the preparation of this chapter.

References

Abrahamsson, T. R., Jakobsson, H. E., Andersson, A. F., Björkstén, B., Engstrand, L., & Jenmalm, M. C. (2012). Low diversity of the gut microbiota in infants with atopic eczema. *Journal of Allergy and Clinical Immunology*, *129*(2), 434-e2. Available from https://doi.org/10.1016/j.jaci.2011.10.025.

Addor, F. A. S. (2015). Clinical improvement of atopic dermatitis in children aged 6 months to 12 years with the use of a combination of oral probiotics. *Brazilian Journal of Allergy and Immunology (BJAI)*, *3*(3), 99–105. Available from https://doi.org/10.5935/2318-5015.20150020.

Ambrożej, D., Kunkiel, K., Dumycz, K., & Feleszko, W. (2020). The use of probiotics and bacteria-derived preparations in topical treatment of atopic dermatitis—A systematic review. *The Journal of Allergy and Clinical Immunology: In Practice*, 9(1), 570–575.

Antunes, A. a, Solé, D., Carvalho, V. O., Bau, A., Kuschnir, F. C., Mallozi, M. C., Markus, J. R., Nascimento, M. G., Pires, M. C., Mello, R., & Filho. (2017). Practical guide update on atopic dermatitis—Part I: Etiopathogenesis, clinic and diagnosis. Joint positioning of the Brazilian Association of Allergy and Immunology and the Brazilian Society of Pediatrics. *Asthma, Allergy and Immunology Archives*, *1*(2), 131–156.

Baviera, G., Leoni, M. C., Capra, L., Cipriani, F., Longo, G., Maiello, N., Ricci, G., & Galli, E. (2014). Microbiota in healthy skin and in atopic eczema. *BioMed Research International*, *2014*. Available from https://doi.org/10.1155/2014/436921.

Bjerre, R. D., Bandier, J., Skov, L., Engstrand, L., & Johansen, J. D. (2017). The role of the skin microbiome in atopic dermatitis: A systematic review. *British Journal of Dermatology*, *177*(5), 1272−1278. Available from https://doi.org/10.1111/bjd.15390.

Blanchet-Réthoré, S., Bourdès, V., Mercenier, A., Haddar, C. H., Verhoeven, P. O., & Andres, P. (2017). Effect of a lotion containing the heat-treated probiotic strain Lactobacillus johnsonii NCC 533 on Staphylococcus aureus colonization in atopic dermatitis. *Clinical, Cosmetic and Investigational Dermatology*, *10*, 249−257. Available from https://doi.org/10.2147/CCID.S135529.

Byrd, A. L., Deming, C., Cassidy, S. K. B., Harrison, O. J., Ng, W. I., Conlan, S., Belkaid, Y., Segre, J. A., & Kong, H. H. (2017). Staphylococcus aureus and Staphylococcus epidermidis strain diversity underlying pediatric atopic dermatitis. *Science Translational Medicine*, *9*(397). Available from https://doi.org/10.1126/scitranslmed.aal4651.

Chang, Y. S., Trivedi, M. K., Jha, A., Lin, Y. F., Dimaano, L., & García-Romero, M. T. (2016). Synbiotics for prevention and treatment of atopic dermatitis: A meta-analysis of randomized clinical trials. *JAMA Pediatrics*, *170*(3), 236−242. Available from https://doi.org/10.1001/jamapediatrics.2015.3943.

Chiesa Fuxench, Z. C., Block, J. K., Boguniewicz, M., Boyle, J., Fonacier, L., Gelfand, J. M., Grayson, M. H., Margolis, D. J., Mitchell, L., Silverberg, J. I., Schwartz, L., Simpson, E. L., & Ong, P. Y. (2019). Atopic dermatitis in America study: A cross-sectional study examining the prevalence and disease burden of atopic dermatitis in the United States adult population. *Journal of Investigative Dermatology*, *139*(3), 583−590. Available from https://doi.org/10.1016/j.jid.2018.08.028.

Choi, C. Y., Kim, Y. H., Oh, S., Lee, H. J., Kim, J. H., Park, S. H., Kim, H. J., Lee, S. J., & Chun, T. (2017). Anti-inflammatory potential of a heat-killed *Lactobacillus* strain isolated from Kimchi on house dust mite-induced atopic dermatitis in NC/Nga mice. *Journal of Applied Microbiology*, *123*(2), 535−543.

Choi, W. J., Konkit, M., Kim, Y., Kim, M. K., & Kim, W. (2016). Oral administration of Lactococcus chungangensis inhibits 2,4-dinitrochlorobenzene-induced atopic-like dermatitis in NC/Nga mice. *Journal of Dairy Science*, *99*(9), 6889−6901. Available from https://doi.org/10.3168/jds.2016-11301.

Clausen, M. L., Agner, T., Lilje, B., Edslev, S. M., Johannesen, T. B., & Andersen, P. S. (2018). Association of disease severity with skin microbiome and filaggrin gene mutations in adult atopic dermatitis. *JAMA Dermatology*, *154*(3), 293−300. Available from https://doi.org/10.1001/jamadermatol.2017.5440.

Damm, J. A., Smith, B., Greisen, G., Krogfelt, K. A., Clausen, M. L., & Agner, T. (2017). The influence of probiotics for preterm neonates on the incidence of atopic dermatitis—Results from a historically controlled cohort study. *Archives of Dermatological Research*, *309*(4), 259−264. Available from https://doi.org/10.1007/s00403-017-1725-4.

Di Marzio, L., Centi, C., Cinque, B., Masci, S., Giuliani, M., Arcieri, A., Zicari, L., De Simone, C., & Cifone, M. G. (2003). Effect of the lactic acid bacterium Streptococcus thermophilus on stratum corneum ceramide levels and signs and symptoms of atopic dermatitis patients. *Experimental Dermatology*, *12*(5), 615−620. Available from https://doi.org/10.1034/j.1600-0625.2003.00051.x.

Dissanayake, E., & Shimojo, N. (2016). Probiotics and prebiotics in the prevention and treatment of atopic dermatitis. *Pediatric, Allergy, Immunology, and Pulmonology*, *29*(4), 174−180. Available from https://doi.org/10.1089/ped.2016.0708.

Dotterud, C. K., Storrø, O., Johnsen, R., & Øien, T. (2010). Probiotics in pregnant women to prevent allergic disease: a randomized, double-blind trial. *British Journal of Dermatology*, *163*(3), 616−623.

Eichenfield, L. F., Jusleen, A., Andrea, W., Jenna, B., Jeremy, U., & Mark, B. (2017). Current guidelines for the evaluation and management of atopic dermatitis—A comparison of the Joint Task Force Practice Parameter and American Academy of Dermatology Guidelines. *Alergologia Polska—Polish Journal of Allergology*, *4*(4), 158−168. Available from https://doi.org/10.1016/j.alergo.2017.11.001.

Eichenfield., Tom, W. L., Berger, T. G., Krol, A., Paller, A. S., Schwarzenberger, K., Bergman, J. N., Chamlin, S. L., Cohen, D. E., Cooper, K. D., Cordoro, K. M., Davis, D. M., Feldman, S. R., Hanifin, J. M., Margolis, D. J., Silverman, R. A., Simpson, E. L., Williams, H. C., Elmets, C. A., … Sidbury, R. (2014). Guidelines of care for the management of atopic dermatitis: Section 2. Management and treatment of atopic dermatitis with topical therapies. *Journal of the American Academy of Dermatology*, *71*(1), 116−132. Available from https://doi.org/10.1016/j.jaad.2014.03.023.

Emilia, R., Georgiana, E., Raluca, C., Alexandra, A., Raluca, R., Oana, O., Teodora, C., Florin, R., Mihaela, P., Mariana, J., & Gabriela, R. (2019). Prebiotics and probiotics in atopic dermatitis. *Experimental and Therapeutic Medicine*, *18*(2), 926−931. Available from https://doi.org/10.3892/etm.2019.7678.

Fölster-Holst, R., Müller, F., Schnopp, N., Abeck, D., Kreiselmaier, I., Lenz, T., Von Rüden, U., Schrezenmeir, J., Christophers, E., & Weichenthal, M. (2006). Prospective, randomized controlled trial on Lactobacillus rhamnosus in infants with moderate to severe atopic dermatitis. *British Journal of Dermatology*, *155*(6), 1256−1261. Available from https://doi.org/10.1111/j.1365-2133.2006.07558.x.

Gueniche, A. G., Knaudt, B., Schuck, E., Volz, T., Bastien, P., Martin, R., Röcken, M., Breton, L., & Biedermann, T. (2009). Effects of nonpathogenic gram-negative bacterium Vitreoscilla filiformis lysate on atopic dermatitis—Does this make a real difference? Authors' reply. *British Journal of Dermatology*, *161*(2), 478−479. Available from https://doi.org/10.1111/j.1365-2133.2009.09269.x.

Guttman-Yassky, E., Waldman, A., Ahluwalia, J., Ong, P. Y., & Eichenfield, L. F. (2017). Atopic dermatitis: Pathogenesis. *Seminars in Cutaneous Medicine and Surgery*, *36*(3), 100−103. Available from https://doi.org/10.12788/j.sder.2017.036.

Han, Y., Kim, B., Ban, J., Lee, J., Kim, B. J., Choi, B. S., Hwang, S., Ahn, K., & Kim, J. (2012). A randomized trial of *Lactobacillus plantarum* CJLP 133 for the treatment of atopic dermatitis. *Pediatric Allergy and Immunology*, *23*(7), 667−673.

Holowacz, S., Guinobert, I., Guilbot, A., Hidalgo, S., & Bisson, J. F. (2018). A mixture of five bacterial strains attenuates skin inflammation in mice. *Anti-Inflammatory & Anti-Allergy Agents in Medicinal Chemistry (Formerly Current Medicinal Chemistry-Anti-Inflammatory and Anti-Allergy Agents)*, *17*(2), 125−137.

Hong, P. Y., Lee, B. W., Aw, M., Shek, L. P. C., Yap, G. C., Chua, K. Y., & Liu, W. T. (2010). Comparative analysis of fecal microbiota in infants with and without eczema. *PLoS One*, 5(4), e9964. Available from https://doi.org/10.1371/journal.pone.0009964.

Huang, R., Ning, H., Shen, M., Li, J., Zhang, J., & Chen, X. (2017). Probiotics for the treatment of atopic dermatitis in children: A systematic review and meta-analysis of randomized controlled trials. *Frontiers in Cellular and Infection Microbiology*, 7, 392. Available from https://doi.org/10.3389/fcimb.2017.00392.

Hulshof, L., van't Land, B., Sprikkelman, A. B., & Garssen, J. (2017). Role of microbial modulation in management of atopic dermatitis in children. *Nutrients*, 9(8), 854. Available from https://doi.org/10.3390/nu9080854.

Ibanes, M. D., Rodriguez, D. R. P., GonzalezSegura, A. D., & Villegas, I. V. (2018). Effect of synbiotic supplementation on children with atopic dermatitis: an observational prospective study. *European Journal of Pediatrics*, 177(12), 1851–1858.

Jo, E. H., Kim, T. K., Hong, S. J., Jung, D. Y., Hwang, S. Y., & Ahn, S. H. (2015). The case study of *Lactobacillus* mixture culture fluid on atopic dermatitis. *The Journal of Korean Medicine*, 36(3), 135–143.

Kalliomäki, M. (2010). Guidance for substantiating the evidence for beneficial effects of probiotics: Prevention and management of allergic diseases by probiotics. *The Journal of Nutrition*, 140(3), 713S–721S.

Kim, J., & Hei, K. (2019). Microbiome of the skin and gut in atopic dermatitis (AD): Understanding the pathophysiology and finding novel management strategies. *Journal of Clinical Medicine*, 8(4), 444. Available from https://doi.org/10.3390/jcm8040444.

Kim, H. W., Hong, R., Choi, E. Y., Yu, K., Kim, N., Hyeon, J. Y., Cho, K. K., Choi, I. S., & Yun, C. H. (2018). A probiotic mixture regulates T cell balance and reduces atopic dermatitis symptoms in mice. *Frontiers in Microbiology*, 9, 2414.

Kim, J. H., Kim, K., Kanjanasuntree, R., & Kim, W. (2019). *Kazachstania turicensis* CAU Y1706 ameliorates atopic dermatitis by regulation of the gut–skin axis. *Journal of Dairy Science*, 102(4), 2854–2862.

Kim, M. S., Kim, J. E., Yoon, Y. S., Seo, J. G., Chung, M. J., & Yum, D. Y. (2016). A probiotic preparation alleviates atopic dermatitis-like skin lesions in murine models. *Toxicological Research*, 32(2), 149–158.

Kong, H. H., Oh, J., Deming, C., Conlan, S., Grice, E. A., Beatson, M. A., Nomicos, E., Polley, E. C., Komarow, H. D., Mullikin, J., Thomas, J., Blakesley, R., Young, A., Chu, G., Ramsahoye, C., Lovett, S., Han, J., Legaspi, R., Sison, C., . . . Segre, J. A. (2012). Temporal shifts in the skin microbiome associated with disease flares and treatment in children with atopic dermatitis. *Genome Research*, 22(5), 850–859. Available from https://doi.org/10.1101/gr.131029.111.

Kwon, M. S., Lim, S. K., Jang, J. Y., Lee, J., Park, H. K., Kim, N., Yun, M., Shin, M. Y., Jo, H. E., Oh, Y. J., & Roh, S. W. (2018). *Lactobacillus sakei* WIKIM30 ameliorates atopic dermatitis-like skin lesions by inducing regulatory T cells and altering gut microbiota structure in mice. *Frontiers in Immunology*, 9, 1905.

Lara, M. F., Costa, M. R. D., Júnior, R. V. S., Mendes, P. A., Moreira, P. L., Freitas, P. C. A. D., Queiroz, V. B. D. S., Andrade, V. L. A., & Araújo, L. A. D. (2015). There is a place for the use of probiotics in the prevention and treatment of pediatric atopic dermatitis? *Revista Medica de Minas Gerais*.

Lee, S. H., Kang, J. H., & Kang, D. J. (2016). Anti-allergic effect of *Lactobacillus rhamnosus* IDCC 3201 isolated from breast milk-fed Korean infant. *Korean Journal of Microbiology*, 52(1), 18–24.

Li, L., Han, Z., Niu, X., Zhang, G., Jia, Y., Zhang, S., & He, C. (2019). Probiotic supplementation for prevention of atopic dermatitis in infants and children: A systematic review and meta-analysis. *American Journal of Clinical Dermatology*, 20(3), 367–377. Available from https://doi.org/10.1007/s40257-018-0404-3.

Li, W., & Yosipovitch, G. (2020). The role of the microbiome and microbiome-derived metabolites in atopic dermatitis and non-histaminergic itch. *American Journal of Clinical Dermatology*, 1–7.

Lim, S. K., Kwon, M. S., Lee, J., Oh, Y. J., Jang, J. Y., Lee, J. H., Park, H. W., Nam, Y. D., Seo, M. J., Roh, S. W., & Choi, H. J. (2017). *Weissella cibaria* WIKIM28 ameliorates atopic dermatitis-like skin lesions by inducing tolerogenic dendritic cells and regulatory T cells in BALB/c mice. *Scientific Reports*, 7(1), 1–9.

Lise, M., Mayer, I., & Silveira, M. (2018). Use of probiotics in atopic dermatitis. *Revista da Associacao Medica Brasileira*, 64(11), 997–1001. Available from https://doi.org/10.1590/1806-9282.64.11.997.

Machado, C. (2018). *New therapeutic approaches in atopic dermatitis* (Doctoral dissertation).

Makrgeorgou, A., Leonardi-Bee, J., Bath-Hextall, F. J., Murrell, D. F., Tang, M. L. K., Roberts, A., & Boyle, R. J. (2018). Probiotics for treating eczema. *Cochrane Database of Systematic Reviews*, 2018(11). Available from https://doi.org/10.1002/14651858.CD006135.pub3.

Maria, J., Carregaro, V., Sacramento, L., Roberti, L., Aragon, D., & Roxo-Junior, P. (2020). Probiotics improve atopic dermatitis in children and adolescents: A double blind, placebo-controlled study. Authorea Preprints

Myles, I. A., Earland, N. J., Anderson, E. D., Moore, I. N., Kieh, M. D., Williams, K. W., Saleem, A., Fontecilla, N. M., Welch, P. A., Darnell, D. A., Barnhart, L. A., Sun, A. A., Uzel, G., & Datta, S. K. (2018). First-in-human topical microbiome transplantation with Roseomonas mucosa for atopic dermatitis. *JCI Insight*, 3(9). Available from https://doi.org/10.1172/jci.insight.120608.

Nakatsuji, T., Chen, T. H., Narala, S., Chun, K. A., Two, A. M., Yun, T., Shafiq, F., Kotol, P. F., Bouslimani, A., Melnik, A. V., Latif, H., Kim, J. N., Lockhart, A., Artis, K., David, G., Taylor, P., Streib, J., Dorrestein, P. C., Grier, A., & Gallo, R. L. (2017). Antimicrobials from human skin commensal bacteria protect against Staphylococcus aureus and are deficient in atopic dermatitis. *Science Translational Medicine*, 9(378). Available from https://doi.org/10.1126/scitranslmed.aah4680.

Nakatsuji, T., Yun, T., Butcher, A., Hayashi, A., Chun, K., Shafiq, F., Kim, J., Zaramela, L., Zengler, K., Hata, T., & Gallo, R. L. (2018). 426 Clinical improvement in atopic dermatitis following autologous application of microbiome therapy targeting Staphylococcus aureus. *Journal of Investigative Dermatology*, 138(5), S72. Available from https://doi.org/10.1016/j.jid.2018.03.433.

Navarro-López, V., Ana, R.-B., Daniel, R.-V., Beatriz, R.-C., Salvador, G.-M., Empar, C.-C., Miguel, C.-G., José, HdelaP., David, P.-M., & Francisco, M. C.-C. (2018). Effect of oral administration of a mixture of probiotic strains on SCORAD index and use of topical steroids in young patients with moderate atopic dermatitis. *JAMA Dermatology, 37*. Available from https://doi.org/10.1001/jamadermatol.2017.3647.

Navarro-López, V., Ramírez-Boscá, A., Ramón-Vidal, D., Ruzafa-Costas, B., Genovés-Martínez, S., Chenoll-Cuadros, E., Carrión-Gutiérrez, M., de la Parte, J. H., Prieto-Merino, D., & Codoñer-Cortés, F. M. (2018). Effect of oral administration of a mixture of probiotic strains on SCORAD index and use of topical steroids in young patients with moderate atopic dermatitis: a randomized clinical trial. *JAMA Dermatology, 154*(1), 37–43.

Notay, M., Foolad, N., Vaughn, A. R., & Sivamani, R. K. (2017). Probiotics, prebiotics, and synbiotics for the treatment and prevention of adult dermatological diseases. *American Journal of Clinical Dermatology, 18*(6), 721–732. Available from https://doi.org/10.1007/s40257-017-0300-2.

Orivuori, L., Mustonen, K., de Goffau, M. C., Hakala, S., Paasela, M., Roduit, C., Dalphin, J. C., Genuneit, J., Lauener, R., Riedler, J., Weber, J., von Mutius, E., Pekkanen, J., Harmsen, H. J. M., Vaarala, O., Hirvonen, M. R., Hyvärinen, A., Karvonen, A. M., ... Remes, S. (2015). High level of fecal calprotectin at age 2 months as a marker of intestinal inflammation predicts atopic dermatitis and asthma by age 6. *Clinical and Experimental Allergy, 45*(5), 928–939. Available from https://doi.org/10.1111/cea.12522.

Panduru, M., Panduru, N. M., Sălăvăstru, C. M., & Tiplica, G.-S. (2015). Probiotics and primary prevention of atopic dermatitis: A meta-analysis of randomized controlled studies. *Journal of the European Academy of Dermatology and Venereology, 29*(2), 232–242. Available from https://doi.org/10.1111/jdv.12496.

Park, Y. G. (2020). Oral administration on immune response and skin improvement in animal model of atopic dermatitis. *The Korean Journal of Food And Nutrition, 33*(2), 174–182.

Park, M. S., Song, N. E., Baik, S. H., Pae, H. O., & Park, S. H. (2017). Oral administration of lactobacilli isolated from Jeotgal, a salted fermented seafood, inhibits the development of 2, 4-dinitrofluorobenzene-induced atopic dermatitis in mice. *Experimental and Therapeutic Medicine, 14*(1), 635–641.

Park, Y. G., Cho, J. H., Choi, J., Kim, Y., Yu, S. J., Kim, O., & Oh, H. G. (2020). Effect of *Lactobacillus helveticus* HY7801 oral administration on immune response and skin improvement in animal model of atopic dermatitis. *The Korean Journal of Food and Nutrition, 33*(2), 174–182.

Plummer, E. L., Chebar Lozinsky, A., Tobin, J. M., Uebergang, J. B., Axelrad, C., Garland, S. M., Jacobs, S. E., & Tang, M. L.ProPrems Study Group. (2020). Postnatal probiotics and allergic disease in very preterm infants: Sub-study to the ProPrems randomized trial. *Allergy, 75*(1), 127–136.

Rather, I. A., Bajpai, V. K., Kumar, S., Lim, J., Paek, W. K., & Park, Y. H. (2016). Probiotics and atopic dermatitis: An overview. *Frontiers in Microbiology, 7*, 507. Available from https://doi.org/10.3389/fmicb.2016.00507.

Reddel, S., Del Chierico, F., Quagliariello, A., Giancristoforo, S., Vernocchi, P., Russo, A., Fiocchi, A., Rossi, P., Putignani, L., & El Hachem, M. (2019). Gut microbiota profile in children affected by atopic dermatitis and evaluation of intestinal persistence of a probiotic mixture. *Scientific Reports, 9*(1), 1–10. Available from https://doi.org/10.1038/s41598-019-41149-6.

Ridd, M. J., Wells, S., Edwards, L., Santer, M., Macneill, S., Sanderson, E., Sutton, E., Shaw, A. R. G., Banks, J., Garfield, K., Roberts, A., Barrett, T. J., Baxter, H., Taylor, J., Lane, J. A., Hay, A. D., Williams, H. C., & Thomas, K. S. (2019). Best emollients for eczema (BEE)—Comparing four types of emollients in children with eczema: Protocol for randomised trial and nested qualitative study. *BMJ Open, 9*(11), e033387. Available from https://doi.org/10.1136/bmjopen-2019-033387.

Rosenfeldt, V., Benfeldt, E., Nielsen, S. D., Michaelsen, K. F., Jeppesen, D. L., Valerius, N. H., & Paerregaard, A. (2003). Effect of probiotic Lactobacillus strains in children with atopic dermatitis. *Journal of Allergy and Clinical Immunology, 111*(2), 389–395. Available from https://doi.org/10.1067/mai.2003.389.

Schmidt, R., Pilmann, L. R., Bruun, S., Larnkiaer, A., Michaelsen, K. F., & Host, A. (2019). Probiotics in late infancy reduce the incidence of eczema: A randomized controlled trial. *Pediatr Allergy Immunol, 30*(3), 335–340.

Sharma, G., & Im, S. H. (2018). Probiotics as a potential immunomodulating pharmabiotics in allergic diseases: Current status and future prospects. *Allergy, Asthma and Immunology Research, 10*(6), 575–590. Available from https://doi.org/10.4168/aair.2018.10.6.575.

Shin, J. H., Chung, M. J., & Seo, J. G. (2016). A multistrain probiotic formulation attenuates skin symptoms of atopic dermatitis in a mouse model through the generation of CD4 + Foxp3 + T cells. *Food & Nutrition Research, 60*(1), 32550.

Silverberg, N. B., & Silverberg, J. I. (2015). Inside out or outside in: Does atopic dermatitis disrupt barrier function or does disruption of barrier function trigger atopic dermatitis? *Cutis; Cutaneous Medicine for the Practitioner, 96*(6), 359–361. Available from http://www.cutis.com//Archive/ArchivePage.aspx.

Simpson, M. R., Dotterud, C. K., Storrø, O., Johnsen, R., & Øien, T. (2015). Perinatal probiotic supplementation in the prevention of allergy related disease: 6 year follow up of a randomised controlled trial. *BMC Dermatology, 15*(1), 1–8. Available from https://doi.org/10.1186/s12895-015-0030-1.

Simpson, M. R., Rø, A. D. B., Grimstad, Ø., Johnsen, R., Storrø, O., & Øien, T. (2016). Atopic dermatitis prevention in children following maternal probiotic supplementation does not appear to be mediated by breast milk TSLP or TGF-β. *Clinical and Translational Allergy, 6*(1), 1–9. Available from https://doi.org/10.1186/s13601-016-0119-6.

Sung, M., Lee, K. S., Ha, E. G., Lee, S. J., Kim, M. A., Lee, S. W., Jee, H. M., Sheen, Y. H., Jung, Y. H., & Han, M. Y. (2017). An association of periostin levels with the severity and chronicity of atopic dermatitis in children. *Pediatric Allergy and Immunology, 28*(6), 543–550. Available from https://doi.org/10.1111/pai.12744.

Suzuki, T., Nishiyama, K., Kawata, K., Sugimoto, K., Isome, M., Suzuki, S., Nozawa, R., Ichikawa, Y., Watanabe, Y., & Suzutani, T. (2020). Effect of the *Lactococcus lactis* 11/19-B1 strain on atopic dermatitis in a clinical test and mouse model. *Nutrients, 12*(3), 763.

Tokudome, Y. (2018). Influence of oral administration of lactic acid bacteria metabolites on skin barrier function and water content in a murine model of atopic dermatitis. *Nutrients, 10*(12), 1858.

Wang, I. J., & Wang, J. Y. (2015). Children with atopic dermatitis show clinical improvement after *Lactobacillus* exposure. *Clinical & Experimental Allergy*, *45*(4), 779−787. Available from https://doi.org/10.1111/cea.12489.

Wickens, K., Barthow, C., Mitchell, E. A., Stanley, T. V., Purdie, G., Rowden, J., Kang, J., Hood, F., van den Elsen, L., Forbes-Blom, E., & Franklin, I. (2018). Maternal supplementation alone with *Lactobacillus rhamnosus* HN 001 during pregnancy and breastfeeding does not reduce infant eczema. *Pediatric Allergy and Immunology*, *29*(3), 296−302.

Weidinger, S., & Novak, N. (2016). Atopic dermatitis. *The Lancet*, *387*(10023), 1109−1122. Available from https://doi.org/10.1016/S0140-6736(15)00149-X.

Williams, M. R., & Gallo, R. L. (2015). The role of the skin microbiome in atopic dermatitis. *Current Allergy and Asthma Reports*, *15*(11), 1−10.

Williams, M. R., Costa, S. K., Zaramela, L. S., Khalil, S., Todd, D. A., Winter, H. L., Sanford, J. A., O'Neill, A. M., Liggins, M. C., Nakatsuji, T., Cech, N. B., Cheung, A. L., Zengler, K., Horswill, A. R., & Gallo, R. L. (2019). Quorum sensing between bacterial species on the skin protects against epidermal injury in atopic dermatitis. *Science Translational Medicine*, *11*(490). Available from https://doi.org/10.1126/scitranslmed.aat8329.

Wu, Y. J., Wu, W. F., Hung, C. W., Ku, M. S., Liao, P. F., Sun, H. L., Lu, K. H., Sheu, J. N., & Lue, K. H. (2017). Evaluation of efficacy and safety of Lactobacillus rhamnosus in children aged 4−48 months with atopic dermatitis: An 8-week, double-blind, randomized, placebo-controlled study. *Journal of Microbiology, Immunology and Infection*, *50*(5), 684−692. Available from https://doi.org/10.1016/j.jmii.2015.10.003.

Yamamoto, K., Yokoyama, K., Matsukawa, T., Kato, S., Kato, S., Yamada, K., & Hirota, T. (2016). Efficacy of prolonged ingestion of Lactobacillus acidophilus L-92 in adult patients with atopic dermatitis. *Journal of Dairy Science*, *99*(7), 5039−5046. Available from https://doi.org/10.3168/jds.2015-10605.

Zhao, M., Shen, C., & Ma, L. (2018). Treatment efficacy of probiotics on atopic dermatitis, zooming in on infants: A systematic review and meta-analysis. *International Journal of Dermatology*, *57*(6), 635−641. Available from https://doi.org/10.1111/ijd.13873.

Zheng, H., Liang, H., Wang, Y., Miao, M., Shi, T., Yang, F., Liu, E., Yuan, W., Ji, Z. S., & Li, D. K. (2016). Altered gut microbiota composition associated with eczema in infants. *PLoS One*, *11*(11), e0166026. Available from https://doi.org/10.1371/journal.pone.0166026.

Chapter 9

Probiotics for the treatment of other skin conditions (acne, psoriasis, seborrheic dermatitis, wounds, and skin cancer)

Sophia Sangar, Michelle W. Cheng and Yang Yu
Division of Dermatology and Department of Medicine, David Geffen School of Medicine at UCLA, Los Angeles, CA, United States

9.1 Acne vulgaris

Acne vulgaris is one of the most common skin diseases worldwide, affecting up to 85% of individuals among 12–24-year olds (Bhate & Williams, 2013). Acne is considered a disease of the pilosebaceous unit with four main factors contributing to development: increased sebum production, follicular hyperkeratinization, inflammation, and colonization of skin bacteria (Bolognia et al., 2012). Recent advances in research on the skin microbiome have shed light on our understanding of the pathophysiology of acne. *Cutibacterium acnes* (*C. acnes*), formerly known as *Propionibacterium acnes*, is predominant in sebaceous sites of the skin (Scholz & Kilian, 2016). As a commensal of the skin microbiome, it contributes to homeostasis by preventing colonization from other harmful pathogens (Christensen & Bruggemann, 2014). Contrary to previous schools of thought, proliferation and overgrowth of *C. acnes* is not a trigger in disease development, nor does it correlate with disease severity. Genomic analyses have demonstrated no significant difference in the relative abundance of *C. acnes* in the pilosebaceous units across acne patients and individuals with normal skin (Fitz-Gibbon et al., 2013). Despite this, *C. acnes* is still implicated as a pathogenic factor in acne. *C. acnes* phylotypes and the host–microbiome interactions, affecting both the innate and adaptive immune responses, may play a critical role (Yu et al., 2016).

The identification of distinct *C. acnes* phylogenic groups through DNA-based methods has allowed the detection of phenotypic characteristics and disease association patterns with significant clinical relevance. It appears that while the majority of commensal phylotypes are distributed equally between patients with acne and individuals with normal skin, there are specific *C. acnes* phylotypes more highly associated with acne, and others more exclusively associated with healthy skin (Fitz-Gibbon et al., 2013; Gehse et al., 1983; Lomholt et al., 2017). Type I *C. acnes* are more associated with acne than type II (Gehse et al., 1983). McDowell et al. (2013) showed that Phylotype type III bacteria composed approximately 20% of isolates from healthy skin but were not found in acne lesions. Fitz-Gibbon et al. (2013) found that certain ribotypes, classified based on the 16S rDNA sequence, were statistically significantly enriched in acne patients, whereas one Ribotype was strongly associated with healthy skin. It is likely that virulence-associated genomic elements, differential protein expression, and distinct capabilities to elicit inflammation may account for these disease associations (Barnard et al., 2016; Yu et al., 2016).

These discoveries have set the stage for unique therapies involving probiotics for the treatment of acne. While antibiotics to reduce *C. acnes* numbers on the skin have been a mainstay of acne treatment for 50 years, this has led to antibiotic resistance worldwide (Walsh et al., 2016). Studies have shown that resistant *C. acnes* can even spread to the skin of untreated close contacts (McDowell et al., 2012). Furthermore, antibiotic therapy is not selective and can be detrimental to other skin microbiome commensals, including coagulase-negative staphylococci (Eady et al., 1990; Harkaway et al., 1992). Instead, probiotics can be utilized as a targeted antimicrobial therapeutic strategy. One idea, specific to the pathogenesis of acne, is to utilize nonpathogenic strains of *C. acnes* that share the same ecological niche with their pathogenic counterparts. For example, healthy skin-associated *C. acnes* phylotypes may be used in a topical probiotic therapy or preventative regimen, designed to replace the acne-associated and other potentially opportunistic phylotypes

(Yu et al., 2016). Investigations have already shown that bacteriophages, or viruses that infect and kill host bacteria, can lyse acne-associated phylotypes but are often ineffective against healthy skin-associated phylotypes (Liu et al., 2015; Marinelli et al., 2012). Consequently, when formulated in a topical cream, bacteriophages may be utilized for highly specific strain replacement (Brown et al., 2016). Unfortunately, the utilization of skin commensals in a topical probiotic for acne treatment has yet to be as well explored.

In vitro studies have demonstrated that several bacterial species can directly inhibit the growth of *C. acnes* via the production of antimicrobial substances. Wang et al. (2014) showed *Staphylococcus epidermidis*, especially when cultured with glycerol, interfered with *C. acnes* proliferation from healthy individuals' skin. *Lactococcus* sp. HY 449 inhibits the growth of *C. acnes*, as well as *Staphylococcus aureus* and *Streptococcus pyogenes* through the secretion of bacteriocins (Oh et al., 2006). *Streptococcus salivarius*, a prominent component of the oropharynx, also inhibits *C. acnes* and group A *streptococci's growth* through the production of a bacteriocin-like substance (Bowe et al., 2006).

In vivo topical probiotic-based clinical studies exist but are few in number with small sample sizes. Di Marzio et al. (1999) examined the effects of sonicated *Streptococcus thermophilus* formulated in a topical probiotic cream on stratum corneum ceramide levels. They showed significant increases in ceramide levels of 17 healthy volunteers after the application of the experimental cream for 7 days, when compared to the base cream alone. These results are of particular interest because phytosphingosine, a ceramide sphingolipid, exhibits direct antiinflammatory and antimicrobial activity against *C. acnes* in vivo. A double-blind, randomized control trial found that the application of a topical *Enterococcus faecalis* SL-5 lotion for 8 weeks significantly reduced the number of pustules in individuals with mild-to-moderate acne, compared to the vehicle control group (Kang et al., 2009). Another study demonstrated that daily application of 5% *Lactobacillus plantarum* extract significantly reduced acne lesion size and erythema in 10 individuals (Muizzuddin et al., 2012). A recent, randomized, double-blinded, phase IIb/III study has demonstrated that 12-week application of *Nitrosomonas eutropha* led to a 2-point reduction in an Investigator's Global Assessment of acne severity compared to the control and a trend in the reduction of the number of inflammatory lesions (AOBiome, 2017). The results of a preprint show that twice daily application of a cream containing a mixture of *Lactobacillus rhamnosus* GG, *L. plantarum* WCFS1, and *Lactobacillus pentosus* KCA in patients with mild-to-moderate acne led to significant reduction in inflammatory lesions over an 8-week period (Lebeer et al., 2018). Unfortunately, this study lacked a control, and when treatment was stopped, exogenously applied lactobacilli could not permanently colonize the skin, and acne scores increased concomitantly. This highlights the importance of rationally selecting for skin commensals in a topical probiotic.

Oral probiotics for modulation of the gut microbiome have also been studied in acne patients. One study compared an oral probiotic mixture of *Lactobacillus acidophilus*, *Lactobacillus delbrueckii bulgaricus*, and *Bifidobacterium bifidum* to minocycline therapy over a 12-week course. The investigators found that the oral probiotic arm alone was as effective a therapy for acne as the systemic antibiotic treatment, resulting in a 67% decreased lesion count after 12 weeks. Interestingly, a combination of the oral probiotic and minocycline resulted in even greater efficacy (Jung et al., 2013). Another 12-week study utilized an oral liquid formulation of *L. rhamnosus* SP1 and demonstrated significant improvement in the appearance of back acne with concomitant normalization in the skin expression of insulin signaling genes compared to the placebo (Fabbrocini et al., 2016). Kim et al. (2010) showed that daily consumption of fermented milk containing *Lactobacillus bulgaricus* and *S. thermophilus* for 12 weeks led to a 30% reduction in inflammatory lesions in patients with mild-to-moderate acne. Sebum content and free fatty acid concentration also substantially decreased. However, this study lacked a true control.

In summary, probiotics represent a promising new therapeutic option for acne vulgaris. Topical probiotics can lead to a very targeted skin microbiome replacement strategy, replacing an "acne" microbiome with a "healthy" one, whereas restoration of a healthy gut microbiome indirectly can positively affect the skin. More robust translational and clinical trials are needed to further evaluate the efficacy of probiotics for the treatment of acne.

9.2 Psoriasis

Psoriasis is a common, chronic skin disease of polygenic susceptibility associated with several different triggers, including infection, medications, stressors, and more. Recent studies have shown alterations in the skin and gut microbiome of psoriasis patients, yet the extent of the microbiome's role has not been completely elucidated. Abnormal immune responses to microbes have been shown to be significant to its pathogenesis; thus probiotics may be a promising therapeutic addition (Notay et al., 2017).

Several studies have shown that the cutaneous microbiota of psoriatic lesions differs from that of unaffected skin. It is noteworthy that there are few studies with limited samples and different sampling methods that may account for varying results. Quan et al. (2020) showed that, when compared to unaffected adjacent skin and healthy skin controls, psoriatic lesional skin had statistically significantly higher bacterial load and a trend towards less richness in the diversity of bacteria. It was found that there was decreased *Cutibacterium* in psoriatic lesions, which is supported by similar findings in other studies (Fahlén et al., 2012; Gao et al., 2008). One known function of *Cutibacterium* is by suppressing the growth of *S. aureus* through fermentation of glycerol. In prior studies, *S. aureus* has been shown to be implicated in the pathogenesis of psoriasis (Skov & Baadsgaard, 2000). Interestingly, however, additional studies have shown decreased levels of *Staphylococci* (Fahlén et al., 2012; Gao et al., 2008). A proposed explanation for the decrease in *Cutibacterium* is the decreased size and number of sebaceous glands, which may create an inhospitable environment for *Cutibacterium* (Rittié et al., 2016; Shi et al., 2015). In addition, *Corynebacterium* has been shown to be increased in psoriatic plaques and to correlate with PASI severity (Quan et al., 2020). In mouse studies, *Corynebacterium* has been shown to induce IL-23 response, which is likely to play a central role in psoriasis pathogenesis. It has been observed that S*treptococcus* genus is commonly identified from psoriatic plaques as well (Fry et al., 2013).

In addition to dysbiosis of the skin microbiome, gut dysbiosis has been associated with psoriasis. The gut microbiota includes a large diversity of bacteria, fungi, viruses, and protozoa, which interact with the host to influence various functions, such as metabolism and immunity. There is evidence to suggest that this host–microbe interaction not only exerts local influence but may affect distant-organ systems, such as the skin as well. From a mechanistic standpoint, the gut microbiome has been shown to be important in maintaining balance between effector and regulatory T cells, which is implicated in chronic inflammatory skin conditions such as psoriasis (Alesa et al., 2019). Studies examining the makeup of the gut microbiota via surrogate stool studies of patients with psoriasis have shown decreased diversity of the fecal microbiota compared to those of patients without psoriasis (Myers et al., 2019). In addition, bacterial DNA from gut microbes has been isolated from the peripheral blood of patients with active psoriasis and is associated with longer duration of disease, earlier onset, and increased levels of inflammatory cytokines (Ramírez-Boscá et al., 2015).

There have been few studies evaluating the effect of oral probiotics in psoriasis. Navarro-López et al. (2019) sought to examine the effects of oral probiotics in psoriasis in a prospective study. In this randomized control trial of 90 patients with mild–moderate psoriasis (PASI > 70), patients with psoriasis were either administered a probiotic mix of *Bifidobacterium longum, Bifidobacterium lactis, L. rhamnosus*, or placebo over a 12-week period. At the end of the study period, there was a statistically significant increased rate of PASI 75 response rate in the treatment group. Another study showed decreased inflammatory markers such as CRP and TNFa in patients treated with oral *Bifidobacterium infantis*, though it was unclear if clinical improvement was observed (Chen et al., 2017). Similarly, decreased IL23/IL17 axis cytokines and TNFa levels were seen in a mouse study evaluating the effect of *L. pentosus* GMNL-77 on psoriasis. Improvement in clinical skin lesions was seen in mice as well (Gao et al., 2008).

9.3 Seborrheic dermatitis

Seborrheic dermatitis is a common chronic inflammatory cutaneous condition that affects 1%–3% of the general and 30%–33% of immunocompromised populations (Tamer et al., 2018). Seborrheic dermatitis characteristically presents with patches and plaques of mild-to-moderate erythema and greasy yellow scales with associated pruritus and burning. Lesions are found on sebum-rich areas of the skin, such as the scalp, eyebrows, nasolabial folds, chest, intertriginous areas, axilla, groin, and buttocks (Gupta et al., 2004). In patients with darker skin phototypes, seborrheic dermatitis can present with hypopigmented or hyperpigmented plaques and patches (Adalsteinsson et al., 2020). Seborrheic dermatitis has largely been thought to be due to an inflammatory reaction to *Malassezia* spp., predominantly *Malassezia restricta* and *Malassezia globosa*, which is a lipophilic yeast and normal member of the human cutaneous flora (Falk et al., 2005; Lee et al., 2013; Sandström et al., 2005). As a result, seborrheic dermatitis treatment has centered around the use of antifungals and antiinflammatory agents (Reygagne et al., 2017). Although the improvement of seborrheic dermatitis has been associated with a decrease in the yeast burden, the number of *Malassezia* spp. has not been shown to correlate with the severity of the disease (Gupta et al., 2004; Pierard et al., 1997). In addition, comparable numbers of *Malassezia* spp. have been reported in both patients with seborrheic dermatitis and control groups (Tamer et al., 2018).

In recent years the bacteria of the skin microbiome, such as facultative anaerobic bacteria, such as *C. acnes*, and aerobic bacteria, such as *S. aureus, Acinetobacter*, and *Corynebacterium*, have been suggested to also contribute to the pathogenesis of seborrheic dermatitis (Park et al., 2017; Tamer et al., 2018; Xu et al., 2016). *Acinetobacter, Staphylococcus*, and *Streptococcus* have been shown to be present on lesions of seborrheic dermatitis, but not in normal skin sites (Tanaka et al., 2016). Furthermore, decreased bacterial diversity relative to the fungal species predicts the severity of seborrheic dermatitis more effectively (Park et al., 2017; Tanaka et al., 2016; Xu et al., 2016). It has also been suggested that the coinhabiting bacteria on the scalp may provide nutrients to promote the proliferation of *Malassezia* spp (Tamer et al., 2018).

Consequently, several studies have investigated the role and efficacy of probiotics in the management of seborrheic dermatitis. In a randomized, double-blinded study of 60 patients with moderate seborrheic dermatitis, topical application of the gram-negative bacterium, *Vitreoscilla filiformis*, for 4 weeks resulted in a significant decrease in erythema, scaling, and pruritus (Guniche et al., 2008). *V. filiformis* lysate activates dendritic cells leading to effective induction of high levels of interleukin (IL)-10 and type 1 regular T cell low production of interferon-gamma (IFN-γ) (Volz et al., 2014). In another randomized, double-blinded study of 60 patients with moderate-to-severe dandruff, an oral supplement containing *Lactobacillus paracasei* ST11 consumed for 56 days was found to be safe and effective when compared to the placebo. Patients experienced significant improvement in pruritus and erythema and the severity of the dandruff (Reygagne et al., 2017). Comparable to *V. filiformis*, *L. paracasei* has been observed to induce substantial reduction of regulatory cytokines, such as IL-10 and transforming growth factor-beta, and suppression of the IFN-γ (Reygagne et al., 2017). As a result, these studies support the use of topical and oral probiotics in optimizing the treatment and management of seborrheic dermatitis.

9.4 Wound healing

In an era where the abuse of antibiotics has led to global antimicrobial drug resistance, the use of probiotics, with known antiinflammatory benefits and a capacity to boost innate immune mediators, continues to be investigated for wound healing (Oelschlaeger, 2010). The phases of wound healing are typically classified as: inflammation, proliferation, and maturation. Delayed wound healing is most commonly due to a prolonged inflammatory phase with a delayed progression to proliferation (Charles Brunicardi et al., 2019). The respective role of inflammatory mediators, such as neutrophils, macrophages, and fibroblasts, is well documented. However, the impact of the skin's commensal microbiota on these inflammatory mediators and wound healing is much less well understood (Canesso et al., 2014).

Importantly, whether acute or chronic, all wounds are colonized. Our understanding of how variability in microbial communities affects wound healing continues to be researched (Scales & Huffnagle, 2013). A 2017 meta-analysis of probiotic use in the treatment of cutaneous wounds demonstrated the effectiveness of various *Lactobacillus* spp. as an adjunct to pharmacological treatment in wound healing (Tsiouris et al., 2017).

9.4.1 Diabetic ulcers

Chronic diabetic foot ulcers, in particular, exist in a perpetual state of inflammation (Charles Brunicardi et al., 2019). While multifactorial, one of the factors hypothesized to prevent wound healing is the development of a biofilm within the ulcer. Overcoming this polymicrobial biofilm is the basis of many current "antibiofilm" therapies, including honey, silver, and iodine-based topical treatments (Hall-Stoodley & Stoodley, 2009; Lavery et al., 2019). Similarly, topical probiotics may also be effective. The primary known mediator of healing chronic diabetic ulcers with probiotic supplementation is IL-8 protein, coded from the CXCL8 gene in humans. The effects of IL-8 are mediated through improved neutrophil migration and phagocytosis of pathogenic microbiota (Modi et al., 1990; Peral et al., 2010). Topically applied *L. plantarum*, specifically, has been shown to have the strongest potential to aid wound healing through this mechanism. This is especially true for wounds that are chronically infected with *Pseudomonas aeruginosa*. In a prospective clinical trial of 34 patients with chronic infected venous ulcers, topical application of *L. plantarum* cultures for 8 days led to greater than 90% area coverage with granulation tissue formation in 50% of patients with type 2 diabetes mellitus (T2DM) and 55% nondiabetic patients. Furthermore, treatment for 30 days led to a greater than 90% lesion area reduction in 43% of patients with T2DM and 50% in nondiabetics (Peral et al., 2010). Oral probiotics, with multiple strains of *Lactobacillus*, have demonstrated improved healing in diabetic foot ulcers in a randomized, double-blind, placebo-controlled trial conducted among 60 patients. After 12 weeks of treatment, oral probiotic supplementation compared to the control led to statistically significant reduction in ulcer length (-1.3 ± 0.9 vs -0.8 ± 0.7 cm), width (-1.1 ± 0.7 vs -0.7 ± 0.7 cm), and depth (-0.5 ± 0.3 vs -0.3 ± 0.3 cm). This was hypothesized to be due to a combination of improved systemic illness as well as local inflammatory mediators (Mohseni et al., 2017).

9.4.2 Burn patients

Chronic wounds from burn injury provide a unique challenge in wound healing. In particular, burn patients require excellent management of patient's nutritional support, micronutrient supplementation, and infection control (Charles Brunicardi et al., 2019). Burn patients are susceptible to *P. aeruginosa* infections at both the graft donor site and the burn injury. These donor and graft sites can have catastrophic effects on wound healing as well as catalyze the likelihood of sepsis with potentially mortal consequences (Charles Brunicardi et al., 2019; Greenhalgh, 2017).

The literature supports the use of both oral and topical probiotics in the management of burn wounds (El-Ghazely et al., 2016; Peral et al., 2009). Sepsis in critically ill patients is at least in part due to the transmigration of gut flora into the systemic circulation. Oral probiotics are proposed to aid gut equilibrium and therefore prevent systemic illness in the critically ill. Improved systemic homeostasis then allows an appropriate localized inflammatory response to burn injury and wound healing (El-Ghazely et al., 2016). In a clinical trial of 40 acutely burned pediatric patients with total body surface burns between 20% and 50% and depth between 5% and 10%, oral probiotic supplementation of a mixture of *Lactobacillus fermentum* and *Lactobacillus delbruekii* led to a significant decrease in the need for grafting in the probiotic group vs. control group. In addition, when grafting was not performed, a significant decrease in the time to full burn wound healing was found in the probiotics group versus control group (6.5 ± 0.23 vs 20.7 ± 0.51 days) (El-Ghazely et al., 2016).

Locally, burn wounds fail to heal in part due to a disturbance in regional skin microflora. This has led to research into the role of topical probiotics (Cogen et al., 2010; Lopes et al., 2017; Paharik et al., 2017; Peral et al., 2009; Valdéz et al., 2005). As seen with chronic diabetic ulcers, *L. plantarum* has demonstrated the greatest role in topical probiotic treatment of burn wounds (Peral et al., 2009). In a clinical trial including 60 patients, the efficacy of topical treatment in an infected second-degree burn group treated with *L. plantarum* versus silver sulfadiazine was found to be 71% and 73%, respectively, with regard to a reduction in the bacterial load, separation of necrotic tissue, promotion of granulation tissue, and complete wound healing. Similarly, the efficacy of topical treatment in an infected third-degree burn group, treated with *L. plantarum* versus silver sulfadiazine, was found to be 83% and 71%, respectively, in reducing the risk of infection and induction of granulation tissue. The *L. plantarum* treatment group also demonstrated 75% complete wound healing compared to 64% for silver sulfadiazine. Furthermore, both treatment groups showed a 90% rate of successful skin grafting. As a result, *L. plantarum* was shown to be an efficacious alternative for the topical treatment of second- and third-degree burns when compared to silver sulfadiazine. *L. plantarum*'s positive impact in the setting of burn wounds has been demonstrated to be due to its ability to interrupt quorum-signaling molecules of *P. aeruginosa*, thereby disrupting its ability to form a biofilm and overall virulence. This provides an advantage for a patient's white blood cells to phagocytize the offending bacteria (Lopes et al., 2016; Valdéz et al., 2005).

Finally, topical probiotics have also been demonstrated to improve wound healing by making local flora resemble a more natural state. This is particularly effective in preventing chronic wound infections with *S. aureus* (Cogen et al., 2010; Paharik et al., 2017). The topical administration of peptides naturally synthesized by *S. epidermidis* and *Staphylococcus caprae*, natural residents of skin flora, has been shown to disrupt pathogenic *S. aureus* colonization. Again, this is primarily due to a disruption in *S. aureus* quorum sensing and biofilm formation (Cogen et al., 2010; Paharik et al., 2017).

9.5 Skin cancer

The role of immune surveillance has been well established in the prevention of skin cancers. It has been postulated that the microflora of the gut and skin may be involved in the development of cutaneous neoplasms given their roles in the regulation of Th17, Treg, and innate immune pathways in the promotion of carcinogenesis (Yu et al., 2015).

Dysbiosis of cutaneous microflora has been associated with cutaneous neoplasms, which can result from an increase in pathogenic, cancer-promoting microorganisms or a loss of cancer-protective microorganisms. For example, highly pathogenic *S. aureus* colonization has been associated with cutaneous T-cell lymphoma (CTCL) and other not yet defined microbial triggers have been shown to be necessary for CTCL disease progression (Fanok et al., 2018; Jackow et al., 1997; Mirvish et al., 2013; Nguyen et al., 2008; Tokura et al., 1995; Willerslev-Olsen et al., 2013). On the other hand, commensal skin bacteria reduce inflammation in wound healing as well as increase immune surveillance via activation of the innate immune system and inflammatory cytokines (Chen & Tsao, 2013). Furthermore, Nakatsuji et al. (2018) showed that strains of *S. epidermidis* isolated from healthy human skin produce 6-*N*-hydroxyaminopurine, which decreased the tumor burden of melanoma and keratinocyte neoplasms in mouse models via inhibition of DNA synthesis.

The gut microbiome has been shown to play a role in the pathogenesis of cancer in distant organs. For example, it has been shown to promote hepatocellular carcinoma via several possible mechanisms, including systemic inflammation and translocation of bacterial components (Dapito et al., 2012). The mechanism by which the gut microbiota affects cancer progression is incompletely elucidated, but it is possible that bacterial products may activate the IL23/17 axis through pattern recognition receptors (Sethi et al., 2018; Sivan et al., 2015).

Few studies have examined the effect of probiotics or probiotic products in UV radiation-associated cutaneous tumors. In a study by Weill et al. (2013), administration of lipoteichoic acid (LTA) from *L. rhamnosus GG* to UV-irradiated mice decreased time to tumor development, though the tumor burden was similar when compared to the control group. The authors additionally found increased activation in dendritic cells in the mesenteric lymph nodes, which they postulated might be indicative of a protective effect of LTA via the gut–skin axis.

In mouse models, manipulating gut microbiota has been shown to decrease the tumor burden of metastatic cancers, including melanoma (Grivennikov et al., 2012). Recently published studies have shown that gut microflora impacts outcomes of metastatic melanoma treated with anti-PDL1 immunotherapy (Gopalakrishnan et al., 2018; Matson et al., 2018; Routy et al., 2018). Three of these studies examined the stool microbiota of approximately 110 patients undergoing treatment with anti-PD-1 inhibitors in melanoma (Chaput et al., 2017; Gopalakrishnan et al., 2018; Matson et al., 2018). Increased diversity of Firmicutes, Actinobacteria, Proteobacteria, Bacteroidetes, and Verrucomicrobia were associated with improved outcomes. On the other hand, decreased diversity and colonization with *Bacteroides*, *Ruminococci*, and *Roseburia* were associated with poorer responses to immunotherapy. To take this one step further, three studies treated germ-free mice or antibiotic-treated mice with modeled metastatic melanoma with a human-fecal microbiome transfer. The human stool donors were indicated to either be responders to immunotherapy or nonresponders. Mice treated with stool transplants from responders had improved responses compared to mice treated with nonresponder fecal transplant. The authors of these papers found that strains of bacteria that may be beneficial to immunotherapy responses include *Ruminococci*, *Bifidobacteria*, *Enterococci*, and *Akkermansia* (Sears & Pardoll, 2018). Indeed, Routy et al. (2018) demonstrated that oral treatment of mice initially treated with nonresponder fecal microbiota transplant was able to restore response to treatment with PD-1 inhibitors.

References

Adalsteinsson, J. A., Kaushik, S., Muzumdar, S., Guttman-Yassky, E., & Ungar, J. (2020). An update on the microbiology, immunology and genetics of seborrheic dermatitis. *Experimental Dermatology*, 29(5), 481–489.

Alesa, D. I., Alshamrani, H. M., Alzahrani, Y. A., Alamssi, D. N., Alzahrani, N. S., & Almohammadi, M. E. (2019). The role of gut microbiome in the pathogenesis of psoriasis and the therapeutic effects of probiotics. *Journal of Family Medicine and Primary Care*, 8(11), 3496–3503.

AOBiome. AOBiome Therapeutics Reports Positive Efficacy Results from Phase 2b Clinical Trial of Ammonia Oxidizing Bacteria (AOB) for the Treatment of Acne Vulgaris. Accessed July 29, 2021. https://www.aobiome.com/pressreleases/aobiome-therapeutics-reports-positive-efficacy-results-from-phase-2b-clinical-trial-of-ammonia-oxidizing-bacteria-aob-for-the-treatment-of-acne-vulgaris/.

Barnard, E., Shi, B., Kang, D., Craft, N., & Li, H. (2016). The balance of metagenomic elements shapes the skin microbiome in acne and health. *Scientific Reports*, 6(1).

Bhate, K., & Williams, H. C. (2013). Epidemiology of acne vulgaris. *British Journal of Dermatolology*, 168, 474–485.

Bolognia, J., Jorizzo, J. L., & Schaffer, J. V. (2012). *Dermatology*. Philadelphia: Elsevier Saunders, Internet resource.

Bowe, W. P., Filip, J. C., DiRienzo, J. M., Volgina, A., & Margolis, D. J. (2006). Inhibition of Propionibacterium acnes by bacteriocin-like inhibitory substances (BLIS) produced by Streptococcus salivarius. *Journal of Drugs in Dermatology*, 5(9), 868–870.

Brown, T. L., Petrovski, S., Dyson, Z. A., Seviour, R., & Tucci, J. (2016). The Formulation of Bacteriophage in a Semi Solid Preparation for Control of Propionibacterium acnes Growth. *PLoS One*, 11(3), e0151184.

Canesso, M. C. C., Vieira, A. T., Castro, T. B. R., Schirmer, B. G. A., Cisalpino, D., Martins, F. S., Rachid, M. A., Nicoli, J. R., Teixeira, M. M., & Barcelos, L. S. (2014). Skin wound healing is accelerated and scarless in the absence of commensal microbiota. *The Journal of Immunology*, 193(10), 5171–5180.

Chaput, N., Lepage, P., Coutzac, C., Soularue, E., Le Roux, K., Monot, C., Boselli, L., Routier, E., Cassard, L., Collins, M., Vaysse, T., Marthey, L., Eggermont, A., Asvatourian, V., Lanoy, E., Mateus, C., Robert, C., & Carbonnel, F. (2017). Baseline gut microbiota predicts clinical response and colitis in metastatic melanoma patients treated with ipilimumab. *Annals of Oncology*, 28(6), 1368–1379.

Charles Brunicardi, F., Andersen, D. K., Billiar, T. R., Dunn, D. L., Hunter, J. G., Kao, L. S., Matthews, J. B., & Pollock, R. E. (2019). *Schwartz's principles of surgery* (pp. 357–424). New York: Mcgraw-Hill.

Chen, Y. E., & Tsao, H. (2013). The skin microbiome: Current perspectives and future challenges. *Journal of the American Academy of Dermatology*, 69(1), 143–155, e3.

Chen, Y.-H., Wu, C.-S., Chao, Y.-H., Lin, C.-C., Tsai, H.-Y., Li, Y.-R., Chen, Y.-Z., Tsai, W.-H., & Chen, Y.-K. (2017). Lactobacillus pentosus GMNL-77 inhibits skin lesions in imiquimod-induced psoriasis-like mice. *Journal of Food and Drug Analysis*, 25(3), 559–566.

Christensen, G. J., & Bruggemann, H. (2014). Bacterial skin commensals and their role as host guardians. *Beneficial Microbes*, 5, 201–215.

Cogen, A. L., Yamasaki, K., Sanchez, K. M., Dorschner, R. A., Lai, Y., MacLeod, D. T., Torpey, J. W., Otto, M., Nizet, V., Kim, J. E., & Gallo, R. L. (2010). Selective antimicrobial action is provided by phenol-soluble modulins derived from Staphylococcus epidermidis, a normal resident of the skin. *Journal of Investigative Dermatology*, 130(1), 192–200.

Dapito, D. H., Mencin, A., Gwak, G.-Y., Pradere, J.-P., Jang, M.-K., Mederacke, I., Caviglia, J. M., Khiabanian, H., Adeyemi, A., Bataller, R., Lefkowitch, J. H., Bower, M., Friedman, R., Sartor, R. B., Rabadan, R., & Schwabe, R. F. (2012). Promotion of hepatocellular carcinoma by the intestinal microbiota and TLR4. *Cancer Cell*, *21*(4), 504–516.

Di Marzio, L., Cinque, B., De Simone, C., & Cifone, M. G. (1999). Effect of the lactic acid bacterium Streptococcus thermophilus on ceramide levels in human keratinocytes in vitro and stratum corneum in vivo. *Journal of Investigative Dermatology*, *113*(1), 98–106.

Eady, E. A., Cove, J. H., Holland, K. T., & Cunliffe, W. J. (1990). Superior antibacterial action and reduced incidence of bacterial resistance in minocycline compared to tetracycline-treated acne patients. *British Journal of Dermatology*, *122*(2), 233–244.

El-Ghazely, M. H., Mahmoud, W., Atia, M. A., & Eldip, E. M. (2016). Effect of probiotic administration in the therapy of pediatric thermal burn. *Annals of Burns and Fire Disasters*, *29*(4), 268–272.

Fabbrocini, G., Bertona, M., Picazo, Ó., Pareja-Galeano, H., Monfrecola, G., & Emanuele, E. (2016). Supplementation with Lactobacillus rhamnosus SP1 normalises skin expression of genes implicated in insulin signalling and improves adult acne. *Beneficial Microbes*, *7*(5), 625–630.

Fahlén, A., Engstrand, L., Baker, B. S., Powles, A., & Fry, L. (2012). Comparison of bacterial microbiota in skin biopsies from normal and psoriatic skin. *Archives of Dermatological Research*, *304*(1), 15–22.

Falk, M. H. S., Linder, M. T., Johansson, C., Bartosik, J., Bäck, O., Särnhult, T., Wahlgren, C.-F., Scheynius, A., & Faergemann, J. (2005). The prevalence of Malassezia yeasts in patients with atopic dermatitis, seborrhoeic dermatitis and healthy controls. *Acta Dermato-Venereologica*, *85*(1), 17–23.

Fanok, M. H., Sun, A., Fogli, L. K., Narendran, V., Eckstein, M., Kannan, K., Dolgalev, I., Lazaris, C., Heguy, A., Laird, M. E., Sundrud, M. S., Liu, C., Kutok, J., Lacruz, R. S., Latkowski, J.-A., Aifantis, I., Ødum, N., Hymes, K. B., Goel, S., & Koralov, S. B. (2018). Role of dysregulated cytokine signaling and bacterial triggers in the pathogenesis of cutaneous T-cell lymphoma. *Journal of Investigative Dermatology*, *138*(5), 116–1125.

Fitz-Gibbon, S., Tomida, S., Chiu, B.-H., Nguyen, L., Du, C., Liu, M., Elashoff, D., Erfe, M. C., Loncaric, A., Kim, J., Modlin, R. L., Miller, J. F., Sodergren, E., Craft, N., Weinstock, G. M., & Li, H. (2013). Propionibacterium acnes strain populations in the human skin microbiome associated with acne. *The Journal of Investigative Dermatology*, *133*(9), 2152–2160.

Fry, L., Baker, B. S., Powles, A. V., Fahlen, A., & Engstrand, L. (2013). Is chronic plaque psoriasis triggered by microbiota in the skin? *The British Journal of Dermatology*, *69*(1), 47–52.

Gao, Z., Tseng, C., Strober, B. E., Pei, Z., & Blaser, M. J. (2008). Substantial alterations of the cutaneous bacterial biota in psoriatic lesions. *PLoS One*, *3*(7), e2719.

Gehse, M., Hoffer, U., Gloor, M., & Pulverer, G. (1983). Propionibacteria in patients with acne vulgaris and in healthy persons. *Archives of Dermatological Research*, *275*(2), 100–104.

Gopalakrishnan, V., Spencer, C. N., Nezi, L., Reuben, A., Andrews, M. C., Karpinets, T. V., Prieto, P. A., Vicente, D., Hoffman, K., Wei, S. C., Cogdill, A. P., Zhao, L., Hudgens, C. W., Hutchinson, D. S., Manzo, T., Petaccia de Macedo, M., Cotechini, T., Kumar, T., Chen, W. S., ... Wargo, J. A. (2018). Gut microbiome modulates response to anti–PD-1 immunotherapy in melanoma patients. *Science (New York, N.Y.)*, *359*(6371), 97–103.

Greenhalgh, D. G. (2017). Sepsis in the burn patient: A different problem than sepsis in the general population. *Burns & Trauma*, *5*(1).

Grivennikov, S. I., Wang, K., Mucida, D., Stewart, C. A., Schnabl, B., Jauch, D., Taniguchi, K., Yu, G.-Y., Österreicher, C. H., Hung, K. E., Datz, C., Feng, Y., Fearon, E. R., Oukka, M., Tessarollo, L., Coppola, V., Yarovinsky, F., Cheroutre, H., Eckmann, L., ... Karin, M. (2012). Adenoma-linked barrier defects and microbial products drive IL-23/IL-17-mediated tumour growth. *Nature*, *491*(7423), 254–258.

Guniche, A., Cathelineau, A.-C., Bastien, P., Esdaile, J., Martin, R., Queille Roussel, C., & Breton, L. (2008). Vitreoscilla filiformisbiomass improves seborrheic dermatitis. *Journal of the European Academy of Dermatology and Venereology*, *22*(8), 1014–1015.

Gupta, A. K., Batra, R., Bluhm, R., Boekhout, T., & Dawson, T. L. (2004). Skin diseases associated with Malassezia species. *Journal of the American Academy of Dermatology*, *51*(5), 785–798.

Hall-Stoodley, L., & Stoodley, P. (2009). Evolving concepts in biofilm infections. *Cellular Microbiology*, *11*(7), 1034–1043.

Harkaway, K. S., McGinley, K. J., Foglia, A. N., Lee, W. L., Fried, F., Shalita, A. R., & Leyden, J. J. (1992). Antibiotic resistance patterns in coagulase-negative staphylococci after treatment with topical erythromycin, benzoyl peroxide, and combination therapy. *British Journal of Dermatology*, *126*(6), 586–590.

Jackow, C. M., Cather, J. C., Hearne, V., Asano, A. T., Musser, J. M., & Duvic, M. (1997). Association of erythrodermic cutaneous T-cell lymphoma, superantigen-positive Staphylococcus aureus, and oligoclonal T-cell receptor V beta gene expansion. *Blood*, *89*(1), 32–40.

Jung, G. W., Tse, J. E., Guiha, I., & Rao, J. (2013). Prospective, randomized, open-label trial comparing the safety, efficacy, and tolerability of an acne treatment regimen with and without a probiotic supplement and minocycline in subjects with mild to moderate acne. *Journal of Cutaneous Medicine and Surgery*, *17*(2), 114–122.

Kang, B. S., Seo, J.-G., Lee, G.-S., Kim, J.-H., Kim, S. Y., Han, Y. W., Kang, H., Kim, H. O., Rhee, J. H., Chung, M.-J., & Park, Y. M. (2009). Antimicrobial activity of enterocins from Enterococcus faecalis SL-5 against Propionibacterium acnes, the causative agent in acne vulgaris, and its therapeutic effect. *The Journal of Microbiology*, *47*(1), 101–109.

Kim, J., Ko, Y., Park, Y. K., Kim, N. I., Ha, W. K., & Cho, Y. (2010). Dietary effect of lactoferrin-enriched fermented milk on skin surface lipid and clinical improvement of acne vulgaris. *Nutrition*, *26*(9), 902–909. Available from https://doi.org/10.1016/j.nut.2010.05.011.

Lavery, L. A., Bhavan, K., & Wukich, D. K. (2019). Biofilm and diabetic foot ulcer healing: All hat and no cattle. *Annals of Translational Medicine*, *7*(7), 159.

Lebeer, S., Oerlemans, E., Claes, I., Wuyts, S., Henkens, T., Spacova, I., van den Broek, M., et al. *Topical cream with live lactobacilli modulates the skin microbiome and reduce acne symptoms*, Preprint. Clinical Trials, November 19, 2018. Accessed July 29, 2021. http://biorxiv.org/lookup/doi/10.1101/463307.

Lee, Y. W., Lee, S. Y., Lee, Y., & Jung, W. H. (2013). Evaluation of expression of lipases and phospholipases of Malassezia restricta in patients with seborrheic dermatitis. *Annals of Dermatology*, 25(3), 310.

Liu, J., Yan, R., Zhong, Q., Ngo, S., Bangayan, N. J., Nguyen, L., Lui, T., Liu, M., Erfe, M. C., Craft, N., Tomida, S., & Li, H. (2015). Erratum: The diversity and host interactions of Propionibacterium acnes bacteriophages on human skin. *The ISME Journal*, 9(9), 2116.

Lomholt, H. B., Scholz, C. F. P., Brüggemann, H., Tettelin, H., & Kilian, M. (2017). A comparative study of Cutibacterium (Propionibacterium) acnes clones from acne patients and healthy controls. *Anaerobe*, 47, 57–63.

Lopes, E. G., Moreira, D. A., Gullón, P., Gullón, B., Cardelle-Cobas, A., & Tavaria, F. K. (2017). Topical application of probiotics in skin: Adhesion, antimicrobial and antibiofilmin vitroassays. *Journal of Applied Microbiology*, 122(2), 450–461.

Marinelli, L. J., Fitz-Gibbon, S., Hayes, C., Bowman, C., Inkeles, M., Loncaric, A., Russell, D. A., Jacobs-Sera, D., Cokus, S., Pellegrini, M., Kim, J., Miller, J. F., Hatfull, G. F., & Modlin, R. L. (2012). Propionibacterium acnes bacteriophages display limited genetic diversity and broad killing activity against bacterial skin isolates. *mBio*, 3(5).

Matson, V., Fessler, J., Bao, R., Chongsuwat, T., Zha, Y., Alegre, M.-L., Luke, J. J., & Gajewski, T. F. (2018). The commensal microbiome is associated with anti-PD-1 efficacy in metastatic melanoma patients. *Science (New York, N.Y.)*, 359(6371), 104–108.

McDowell, A., Barnard, E., Nagy, I., Gao, A., Tomida, S., Li, H., Eady, A., Cove, J., Nord, C. E., & Patrick, S. (2012). An expanded multilocus sequence typing scheme for Propionibacterium acnes: Investigation of 'pathogenic', 'commensal' and antibiotic resistant strains. *PLoS One*, 7(7).

McDowell, A., Nagy, I., Magyari, M., Barnard, E., & Patrick, S. (2013). The opportunistic pathogen Propionibacterium acnes: Insights into typing, human disease, clonal diversification and CAMP factor evolution. *PLoS One*, 8(9), 70897.

Mirvish, J. J., Pomerantz, R. G., Falo, L. D., & Geskin, L. J. (2013). Role of infectious agents in cutaneous T-cell lymphoma: Facts and controversies. *Clinics in Dermatology*, 31(4), 423–431.

Modi, W. S., Dean, M., Seuanez, H. N., Mukaida, N., Matsushima, K., & O'Brien, S. J. (1990). Monocyte-derived neutrophil chemotactic factor (MDNCF/IL-8) resides in a gene cluster along with several other members of the platelet factor 4 gene superfamily. *Human Genetics*, 84(2).

Mohseni, S., Bayani, M., Bahmani, F., Tajabadi-Ebrahimi, M., Bayani, M. A., Jafari, P., & Asemi, Z. (2017). The beneficial effects of probiotic administration on wound healing and metabolic status in patients with diabetic foot ulcer: A randomized, double-blind, placebo-controlled trial. *Diabetes/Metabolism Research and Reviews*, 34(3), e2970.

Muizzuddin, N., Maher, W., Sullivan, M., Schnittger, S., & Mammone, T. (2012). Physiological effect of a probiotic on skin. *Journal of Cosmetic Science*, 63(6), 385–395.

Myers, B., Brownstone, N., Reddy, V., Chan, S., Thibodeaux, Q., Truong, A., Bhutani, T., Chang, H.-W., & Liao, W. (2019). The gut microbiome in psoriasis and psoriatic arthritis. *Best Practice & Research. Clinical Rheumatology*, 33(6), 101494.

Nakatsuji, T., Chen, T. H., Butcher, A. M., Trzoss, L. L., Nam, S.-J., Shirakawa, K. T., Zhou, W., Oh, J., Otto, M., Fenical, W., & Gallo, R. L. (2018). A commensal strain of Staphylococcus epidermidis protects against skin neoplasia. *Science Advances*, 4(2), eaao4502.

Navarro-López, V., Martínez-Andrés, A., Ramírez-Boscá, A., Ruzafa-Costas, B., Núñez-Delegido, E., Carrión-Gutiérrez, M., Prieto-Merino, D., Codoñer-Cortés, F., Ramón-Vidal, D., Genovés-Martínez, S., Chenoll-Cuadros, E., Pérez-Orquín, J., Picó-Monllor, J., & Chumillas-Lidón, S. (2019). Efficacy and safety of oral administration of a mixture of probiotic strains in patients with psoriasis: A randomized clinical trial. *Acta Dermato Venereologica*, 99(12), 1078–1084.

Nguyen, V., Huggins, R. H., Lertsburapa, T., Bauer, K., Rademaker, A., Gerami, P., & Guitart, J. (2008). Cutaneous T-cell lymphoma and Staphylococcus aureus colonization. *Journal of the American Academy of Dermatology*, 59(6), 949–952.

Notay, M., Foolad, N., Vaughn, A. R., & Sivamani, R. K. (2017). Probiotics, Prebiotics, and Synbiotics for the Treatment and Prevention of Adult Dermatological Diseases. *Am J Clin Dermatol*, 18(6), 721–732. Available from https://doi.org/10.1007/s40257-017-0300-2, PMID: 28681230.

Oelschlaeger, T. A. (2010). Mechanisms of probiotic actions—A review. *International Journal of Medical Microbiology*, 300(1), 57–62.

Oh, S., Kim, S.-H., Ko, Y., Sim, J.-H., Kim, K. S., Lee, S.-H., Park, S., & Kim, Y. J. (2006). Effect of bacteriocin produced by Lactococcus sp. HY 449 on skin-inflammatory bacteria. *Food and Chemical Toxicology*, 44(8), 1184–1190.

Paharik, A. E., Parlet, C. P., Chung, N., Todd, D. A., Rodriguez, E. I., Van Dyke, M. J., Cech, N. B., & Horswill, A. R. (2017). Coagulase-negative staphylococcal strain prevents Staphylococcus aureus colonization and skin infection by blocking quorum sensing. *Cell Host & Microbe*, 22(6), 746–756, e5.

Park, T., Kim, H.-J., Myeong, N. R., Lee, H. G., Kwack, I., Lee, J., Kim, B. J., Sul, W. J., & An, S. (2017). Collapse of human scalp microbiome network in dandruff and seborrhoeic dermatitis. *Experimental Dermatology*, 26(9), 835–838.

Peral, M. C., Huaman Martinez, M. A., & Valdez, J. C. (2009). Bacteriotherapy with Lactobacillus plantarumin burns. *International Wound Journal*, 6(1), 73–81.

Peral, M. C., Rachid, M. M., Gobbato, N. M., Martinez, M. A. H., & Valdez, J. C. (2010). Interleukin-8 production by polymorphonuclear leukocytes from patients with chronic infected leg ulcers treated with Lactobacillus plantarum. *Clinical Microbiology and Infection*, 16(3), 281–286.

Pierard, G. E., Arrese, J. E., Pierard-Franchimont, C., & De Doncker, P. (1997). Prolonged effects of antidandruff shampoos—Time to recurrence of Malassezia ovalis colonization of skin. *International Journal of Cosmetic Science*, 19(3), 111–117.

Quan, C., Chen, X.-Y., Li, X., Xue, F., Chen, L.-H., Liu, N., Wang, B., Wang, L.-Q., Wang, X.-P., Yang, H., & Zheng, J. (2020). Psoriatic lesions are characterized by higher bacterial load and imbalance between Cutibacterium and Corynebacterium. *Journal of the American Academy of Dermatology*, 82(4), 955–961.

Ramírez-Boscá, A., Navarro-López, V., Martínez-Andrés, A., Such, J., Francés, R., Horga de la Parte, J., & Asín-Llorca, M. (2015). Identification of bacterial DNA in the peripheral blood of patients with active psoriasis. *JAMA Dermatology*, 151(6), 670.

Reygagne, P., Bastien, P., Couavoux, M. P., Philippe, D., Renouf, M., Castiel-Higounenc, I., & Gueniche, A. (2017). The positive benefit of Lactobacillus paracasei NCC2461 ST11 in healthy volunteers with moderate to severe dandruff. *Beneficial Microbes, 8*(5), 671–680.

Rittié, L., Tejasvi, T., Harms, P. W., Xing, X., Nair, R. P., Gudjonsson, J. E., Swindell, W. R., & Elder, J. T. (2016). Sebaceous gland atrophy in psoriasis: An explanation for psoriatic alopecia? *Journal of Investigative Dermatology, 136*(9), 1792–1800.

Routy, B., Le Chatelier, E., Derosa, L., Duong, C. P. M., Alou, M. T., Daillère, R., Fluckiger, A., Messaoudene, M., Rauber, C., Roberti, M. P., Fidelle, M., Flament, C., Poirier-Colame, V., Opolon, P., Klein, C., Iribarren, K., Mondragón, L., Jacquelot, N., Qu, B., . . . Zitvogel, L. (2018). Gut microbiome influences efficacy of PD-1-based immunotherapy against epithelial tumors. *Science (New York, N.Y.), 359*(6371), 91–97.

Sandström Falk, M. H., Tengvall Linder, M., Johansson, C., et al. (2005). The prevalence of Malassezia yeasts in patients with atopic dermatitis, seborrhoeic dermatitis and healthy controls. *Acta Derm Venereol, 85*(1), 17–23. Available from https://doi.org/10.1080/00015550410022276.

Scales, B. S., & Huffnagle, G. B. (2013). The microbiome in wound repair and tissue fibrosis. *The Journal of Pathology, 229*(2), 323–331.

Scholz, C. F., & Kilian, M. (2016). The natural history of cutaneous propionibacteria, and reclassification of selected species within the genus Propionibacterium to the proposed novel genera Acidipropionibacterium gen. nov., Cutibacterium gen. nov. and Pseudopropionibacterium gen. nov. *International Journal of Systematic and Evolutionary Microbiology, 66*, 4422–4432.

Sears, C. L., & Pardoll, D. M. (2018). The intestinal microbiome influences checkpoint blockade. *Nature Medicine, 24*(3), 254–255.

Sethi, V., Kurtom, S., Tarique, M., Lavania, S., Malchiodi, Z., Hellmund, L., Zhang, L., Sharma, U., Giri, B., Garg, B., Ferrantella, A., Vickers, S. M., Banerjee, S., Dawra, R., Roy, S., Ramakrishnan, S., Saluja, A., & Dudeja, V. (2018). Gut microbiota promotes tumor growth in mice by modulating immune response. *Gastroenterology, 155*(1), 33–37, e6.

Shi, V. Y., Leo, M., Hassoun, L., Chahal, D. S., Maibach, H. I., & Sivamani, R. K. (2015). Role of sebaceous glands in inflammatory dermatoses. *Journal of the American Academy of Dermatology, 73*(5), 856–863.

Sivan, A., Corrales, L., Hubert, N., Williams, J. B., Aquino-Michaels, K., Earley, Z. M., Benyamin, F. W., Man Lei, Y., Jabri, B., Alegre, M.-L., Chang, E. B., & Gajewski, T. F. (2015). Commensal Bifidobacterium promotes antitumor immunity and facilitates anti-PD-L1 efficacy. *Science (New York, N.Y.), 350*(6264), 1084–1089.

Skov., & Baadsgaard. (2000). Bacterial superantigens and inflammatory skin diseases. *Clinical and Experimental Dermatology, 25*(1), 57–61.

Tamer, F., Yuksel, M., Sarifakioglu, E., & Karabag, Y. (2018). Staphylococcus aureus is the most common bacterial agent of the skin flora of patients with seborrheic dermatitis. *Dermatology Practical & Conceptual, 8*(2), 80–84.

Tanaka, A., Cho, O., Saito, C., Saito, M., Tsuboi, R., & Sugita, T. (2016). Comprehensive pyrosequencing analysis of the bacterial microbiota of the skin of patients with seborrheic dermatitis. *Microbiology and Immunology, 60*(8), 521–526.

Tokura, Y., Yagi, H., Ohshima, A., Kurokawa, S., Wakita, H., Yokote, R., Shirahama, S., Furukawa, F., & Takigawa, M. (1995). Cutaneous colonization with staphylococci influences the disease activity of Sézary syndrome: A potential role for bacterial superantigens. *British Journal of Dermatology, 133*(1), 6–12.

Tsiouris, C. G., Kelesi, M., Vasilopoulos, G., Kalemikerakis, I., & Papageorgiou, E. G. (2017). The efficacy of probiotics as pharmacological treatment of cutaneous wounds: Meta-analysis of animal studies. *European Journal of Pharmaceutical Sciences, 104*, 230–239.

Valdéz, J. C., Peral, M. C., Rachid, M., Santana, M., & Perdigón, G. (2005). Interference of Lactobacillus plantarum with Pseudomonas aeruginosa in vitro and in infected burns: The potential use of probiotics in wound treatment. *Clinical Microbiology and Infection, 11*(6), 472–479.

Volz, T., Skabytska, Y., Guenova, E., Chen, K.-M., Frick, J.-S., Kirschning, C. J., Kaesler, S., Röcken, M., & Biedermann, T. (2014). Nonpathogenic bacteria alleviating atopic dermatitis inflammation induce IL-10-producing dendritic cells and regulatory Tr1 cells. *Journal of Investigative Dermatology, 134*(1), 96–104.

Walsh, T. R., Efthimiou, J., & Dréno, B. (2016). Systematic review of antibiotic resistance in acne: An increasing topical and oral threat. *The Lancet Infectious Diseases, 16*(3), e23–e33.

Wang, Y., Kuo, S., Shu, M., Yu, J., Huang, S., Dai, A., Two, A., Gallo, R. L., & Huang, C.-M. (2014). Staphylococcus epidermidis in the human skin microbiome mediates fermentation to inhibit the growth of Propionibacterium acnes: Implications of probiotics in acne vulgaris. *Applied Microbiology and Biotechnology, 98*(1), 411–424.

Weill, F. S., Cela, E. M., Paz, M. L., Ferrari, A., Leoni, J., & Maglio, D. H. G. (2013). Lipoteichoic acid from Lactobacillus rhamnosus GG as an oral photoprotective agent against UV-induced carcinogenesis. *British Journal of Nutrition, 109*(3), 457–466.

Willerslev-Olsen, A., Krejsgaard, T., Lindahl, L., Bonefeld, C., Wasik, M., Koralov, S., Geisler, C., Kilian, M., Iversen, L., Woetmann, A., & Odum, N. (2013). Bacterial toxins fuel disease progression in cutaneous T-cell lymphoma. *Toxins, 5*(8), 1402–1421.

Xu, Z., Wang, Z., Yuan, C., Liu, X., Yang, F., Wang, T., Wang, J., Manabe, K., Qin, O., Wang, X., Zhang, Y., & Zhang, M. (2016). Dandruff is associated with the conjoined interactions between host and microorganisms. *Scientific Reports, 6*(1).

Yu, Y., Champer, J., Agak, G. W., Kao, S., Modlin, R. L., & Kim, J. (2016). Different Propionibacterium acnes phylotypes induce distinct immune responses and express unique surface and secreted proteomes. *Journal of Investigative Dermatology, 136*(11), 2221–2228.

Yu, Y., Champer, J., Beynet, D., Kim, J., & Friedman, A. J. (2015). The role of the cutaneous microbiome in skin cancer: Lessons learned from the gut. *Journal of drugs in dermatology, 14*(5), 461–465.

Chapter 10

Probiotics in the prevention and management of allergic diseases (asthma and allergic rhinitis)

Lien Meirlaen*, Elvira Ingrid Levy* and Yvan Vandenplas

Vrije Universiteit Brussel (VUB), UZ Brussel, KidZ Health Castle, Brussels, Belgium

10.1 Introduction

Asthma is one of the most common chronic noncommunicable diseases, with around 339 million people affected worldwide (GBD 2016 Disease and Injury and Incidence and Prevalence Collaborators, 2016). The global prevalence of allergic diseases, such as allergic rhinitis, asthma, and atopic dermatitis, is significant and has been increasing over the past few decades (Asher et al., 2006). Allergic rhinitis occurs in 10%–30% of adults and up to 40% in children and its prevalence is increasing (Meltzer, 2016). The global prevalence of doctor-diagnosed asthma in adults is 4.3% [95% confidence interval (CI) 4.2%–4.4%], with a wide variation between countries: the highest prevalence is found in developed countries, such as Australia (21%), and the lowest in developing countries, such as Ethiopia (2%) (To et al., 2012). In children, asthma is more common in boys than in girls due to their smaller airways relative to their lung size, with a switch during puberty, as the prevalence in women is 20% higher than in men (Leynaert et al., 2012). Asthma prevalence is stable or even shrinking in many developed countries, but as lifestyles become more westernized in developing countries there is a fast increase in the prevalence in these parts of the world (Papi et al., 2018). The interaction between the genomic background, changing environmental conditions, such as more pollution (Kuang et al., 2021), increasing obesity, the "hygiene hypothesis", and less breastfeeding (Enilari & Sinha, 2019), are likely to play a major role. Parental reduction of smoking has proven to reduce asthma (Molero et al., 2018). Important to mention is that in less developed countries the detection rate of allergic disease is likely to be lower, what may result in an underestimation of its prevalence (Arokiasamy et al., 2017). By identifying and characterizing more of these conditions and the involved lifestyle factors, epidemiological studies try to deduce potential strategies for prevention of allergic diseases (von Mutius & Matsui, 2020). Asthma causes impaired quality of life, substantial disability, and avoidable deaths in children and young adults, combined with important health care costs (Papi et al., 2018).

10.1.1 Rationale for using probiotics in atopic diseases

Epidemiological studies have shown that Western living conditions are associated with the rise in allergic diseases. This includes a reduced consumption of fermented food, use of antibiotics and other drugs, and increased hygiene (Kalliomäki et al., 2010). In those who spend their childhood on a farm, allergic diseases are less common (Braun-Fahrländer et al., 1999). The comparison between the composition of microbiota of farm children and the microbiota of children with other lifestyles shows a significant difference (Dicksved et al., 2007). The so-called hygiene hypothesis suggests that a lack of exposure to microbial stimuli early in childhood is a major factor involved in the steep increase in allergy (Kalliomäki et al., 2010). Another important difference in composition of the microbiota was observed between healthy and allergic infants in countries with the high or low prevalence of allergies, pointing to the importance of the gut microbiota in the development of allergic diseases (Kalliomäki et al., 2010).

*These authors contributed equally to this chapter.

In the first week of life, the composition of the intestinal microbiota changes rapidly. In contrary to what long time has been believed, an amniotic microbiome has been reported, and as a consequence, the fetal intestine may not be sterile since there is presence of microbial deoxyribonucleic acid in meconium (Valdes et al., 2018). The first altering factor of the neonatal microbiome is the contact with vaginal, fecal, and skin bacteria of the mother. Therefore in cesarean section-born babies, a less diversified microbiome developed. The second altering factor is feeding. Human milk is rich in human milk oligosaccharides, which have prebiotic properties (a substrate that is selectively utilized by host microorganisms conferring a health benefit; Swanson et al., 2020) and promote the growth of selected species of bacteria. Human milk is also a natural bacterial inoculum. The third altering factor are environmental influenced alterations, which may undo the first two beneficial gut alterations: environments, such as neonatal intensive care units, and medication, such as antibiotics or proton pump inhibitors administered perinatal or during early life (Buccigrossi et al., 2013; Goulet, 2015).

Dysbiosis of the young intestinal microbiome can contribute to immune disorders later in childhood because commensal gut bacteria stimulate the development of a balanced immune system, through the gut–lung axis (Elazab et al., 2013). While the microbiota hypothesis may not conclusively explain all observations and does not provide specific guidelines for reducing the allergy epidemic, it does provide a rationale for using probiotics (live microorganisms that, when administered in adequate amounts, confer a health benefit on the host) (Swanson et al., 2020) to modify the gut microbiota to shape the host's immune response (Kalliomäki et al., 2010). Since a child's microbiota is not believed to reflect adult patterns until they are 2 years old, the infant microbiota may be more susceptible to manipulation (Sepp et al., 1993).

More knowledge is needed on the mechanisms behind dysbiosis, translocation of microbiota from the gut–lung axis through various mechanisms and for a better evaluation of the therapeutic possibilities to correct this dysbiosis, which in turn can be used to manage various respiratory diseases (Trivedi & Barve, 2020).

The aim of this article is to answer the question if probiotics supplementation can alter the micriobiome sufficient to have an efficacious prevention and/or treatment of allergic rhinitis and asthma.

10.2 Prevention of asthma

The increased social and economic burden of asthma makes asthma prevention an important public health goal (Wei et al., 2020).

10.2.1 Animal studies for prevention of asthma through probiotics

The administration of oral probiotic *Lactococcus lactis* NZ9000 resulted to be beneficial to rats. This probiotic showed to have a preventive effect or relief of inflammatory processes by a decrease of infiltration of pro-inflammatory leukocytes, mainly eosinophils and a decreased lung interleukin (IL)-4 and IL-5 expression in the bronchoalveolar lavage and a reduced level of serum allergen-specific immunoglobulin E (IgE) (Cervantes-García et al., 2020). The probiotic *Lactobacillus rhamnosus* GR-1 used in another study with mice showed significantly prevented airway hyperreactivity development and prevented microbiome disturbance in the asthmatic animals, supporting the existence of the gut–lung axis (Spacova et al., 2020). An interesting aspect is that most probiotics are given orally; however, a new approached was tested by giving probiotics (*Lactobacillus paracasei* NCC2461 (Pellaton et al., 2012) and *Lactobacillus rhamnosus* GG (LGG) (Spacova et al., 2019) in mice through the nasal and showed benefits in reducing inflammation of the lungs (Jamalkandi et al., 2020). One study administrated a probiotic *Bifidobacterium breve* M-16V to pregnant mice and was effective in lowering eosinophils in the bronchoalveolar lavage fluid of neonatal mice and reduced allergic lung inflammation in mice exposed to air pollution (Terada-Ikeda et al., 2020). In another animal study, the intranasal administration of LGG, but not *Lactobacillus rhamnosus* GR-1, suppressed airway hyperreactivity and reduced the counts of eosinophils, IL-13 and IL-5 in bronchoalveolar fluid (Spacova et al., 2019). In addition to inhibiting inflammatory cell infiltration in lung tissue, LGG was shown to decrease MMP9 expression, a class of enzymes that are involved in the degradation of the extracellular matrix and of which levels were significantly increased in asthma (Mennini et al., 2017). LGG and *Bifidobacterium lactis* were shown to increase natural regulatory T cells in the lungs of asthmatic mice in another animal study (Feleszko et al., 2007). Furthermore, four Lactobacillus species had markedly different immunomodulatory effects in animal studies (Jeongmin et al., 2013). *Lactobacillus salivarius* and *Lactobacillus fermentum* were effective, but there was no effect of *Lactobacillus plantarum* against allergy demonstrated (Huang et al., 2017). Probiotic strain-specific induction of Foxp3þ T regulatory cells was found in mouse allergy models (Lyons et al., 2010).

10.2.2 Human studies for prevention of asthma through probiotics

Preventive agents for respiratory allergies in children compared to animal studies were reported to be low (Wang et al., 2020). A meta-analysis of 2013 showed that the administration of probiotics (*Lactobacillus* spp. and/or *Bifidobacerium* spp.) early in life is effective in reducing IgE levels and the risk of atopic sensitization in young children but not the risk of asthma or wheeze (Elazab et al., 2013). There was no difference based on the timing of administration (prenatal to mothers plus postnatal vs. only postnatal) with regard to IgE, but the decrease in the risk of atopy was significant only when probiotics were started during pregnancy and continued after birth (Elazab et al., 2013).

Like in the animal studies, prenatal start of the probiotics might be crucial to colonize mothers so that they transfer them to their offspring during vaginal delivery. Administration of pro- and prebiotics during pregnancy can affect the maternal gut microbiome, potentially resulting in the transmission of tolerogenic mediators, such as regulatory cytokines, antibodies, and growth factors across the placenta, stimulating the development of the fetal immune system (West et al., 2017). This could help to prevent asthma or allergic rhinitis. The findings in pregnant mice are of interest to human since up to now knowledge was restricted to the fact that *Bifidobacterium breve* M-16V in infants can suppress T helper type 2 immune responses and modulating the systemic type 1 T helper/type 2 T helper balance (Terada-Ikeda et al., 2020). It is well known, that exposure to air pollution during pregnancy increases asthma susceptibility in the offspring. So *Bifidobacterium breve* M-16V might contribute in reducing asthma in a population living in highly polluted areas (Terada-Ikeda et al., 2020). In 2014, after a long-term follow-up of a randomized placebo-controlled trial (RCT), the Panda study could not demonstrate a beneficial effect on the development of allergic diseases at the age of 6 years from prenatal and 1-year long postnatal use of a probiotic mixture (two *Bifidobacterium* spp. and *Lactococcus lactis*) (Gorissen et al., 2014). Unfortunately, after a follow-up of 11 years, the same negative outcome of no association [relative risk (RR) 0.59, 95% CI 0.36–0.96, $P = .059$], was found (Wickens et al., 2018). This study was a two-center RCT using *Lactobacillus rhamnosus* HN001 or *Bifidobacterium lactis* HN019 taken daily from 35-week gestation to 6 months postpartum in mothers while breastfeeding and from birth to age 2 years in infants (Wickens et al., 2018). A more recent meta-analysis including 19 RCT ($n = 5157$ children) also showed that probiotic supplementation during pregnancy or early life was not significantly associated with a lower incidence of asthma or wheeze in infants (Wei et al., 2020). Subgroup analysis by asthma risk showed that probiotics significantly reduced wheeze incidence among infants with atopic disease (RR 0.61, 95% CI 0.42–0.90) (Wei et al., 2020). In view of the small sample size in this subgroup analysis, the result should be interpreted with caution. Future powerful trials are needed to confirm if infants with atopic disease could be most likely to benefit from probiotics (*Lactobacillus* spp. and/or *Bifidobacerium* spp., *Propionibacterium freudenreichii* ssp. shermanii JS) (Wei et al., 2020).

However, further research is needed to optimize the selection of probiotic species and the configuration of intervention regimens (Wei et al., 2020) because beneficial effects of specific strains might get lost by pooling probiotic strains together since the effects are strain specific. Therefore meta-analysis should be strain specific. Due to the wide heterogeneity of strains, combinations, and doses administered, the efficacy of specific probiotic strains has been difficult to evaluate.

10.3 Probiotics for the treatment of asthma

Unfortunately therapeutic effects of probiotics in asthmatic patients are not well established (Sharma & Im, 2018). A recent study in baby mice showed that *Bifidobacterium infantis* was able to reduce the infiltration of inflammatory cells by promoting Type 1 T helper and inhibiting Type 2 T helper immune responses (Wang et al., 2020). In a systematic review, the RCTs that studied the effect of probiotic administration on the treatment of asthma showed no positive effects (Vliagoftis et al., 2008). A more recent meta-analysis (including 12 studies) from Das et al. (2013) showed no improvement in quality-of-life scores in asthmatics. However, reduced asthma attacks with probiotics were found. Although some studies suggest some benefit and harm was not reported, the current evidence does not support use of probiotics in treatment of asthma (Sharma & Im, 2018).

10.4 Probiotics for the prevention of allergic rhinitis

The incidences of both perennial allergic rhinitis and seasonal allergic rhinitis have been increasing worldwide and their management is costly (Broek et al., 2010). Currently there is no strong evidence that probiotics are effective in the prevention of allergic rhinitis (Zuccotti et al., 2015), with even some studies suggesting that there may even be an increased prevalence of allergic rhinoconjunctivitis in those taking probiotics in the perinatal period and in childhood

(Peldan et al., 2017). In a systematic review published in 2014 five RCTs that addressed the preventive role of probiotics in allergic rhinitis were evaluated. The outcome revealed no difference in the incidence of allergic rhinitis between the probiotic and placebo groups [odds ratio (OR) 1.07, 95% CI 0.81−1.42, $P = .64$, fixed-effects model], and no significant difference in the prevention of allergic rhinitis (Peng et al., 2015). A 2019 meta-analysis of 17 RCTs including 5264 children, failed to identify that probiotic supplementary therapy during pre- and postnatal periods has a clear benefit in the prevention of allergic rhinitis (Du et al., 2019). However, similar as for the prevention of asthma, the absence of evidence for benefit may be related to shortcomings the study designs and the presence of multiple confounding variables. Research indicates that patients with different chronic rhinosinusitis phenotypes possess distinct nasal microbiota profiles, which influence immune response (Dimitri-Pinheiro et al., 2020). Probiotic intervention may have a promising role in the prevention and adjunctive treatment of allergic rhinitis, although results up to now are disappointing.

10.5 Probiotics for the treatment of allergic rhinitis

The treatment of allergic rhinitis continues to be based on allergen avoidance, symptomatic medication, antiinflammatory therapies, and allergy immunotherapy (Juniper et al., 2005). Intranasal corticosteroid sprays are first-line treatment for moderate-to-severe allergic rhinitis and are quite effective (May & Dolen, 2017). However, current medications may have undesirable side effects that may affect quality of life (Juniper et al., 2005). In addition, patient compliance is a main concern. Therefore it is of interest to continue to look for alternatives. It has been proposed that oral administration of probiotics improve the microbial balance in the gut and can modulate immune responses, although this paper discussed synbiotic administration and not probiotic as the title suggests (Jalali et al., 2019). A review from 2010 (seven trials, $n = 616$, children and adults mixed) suggested that probiotics (*Lactobacillus* spp. and *Bifidobacterium* spp.) can have significant beneficial effects on allergic rhinitis treatment, with the potential to improve the patient's quality of life and reduce medication use (Das et al., 2010). Similar results were reported in a 2014 meta-analysis including 11 RCTs showing that probiotic intake was associated with a significant overall improvement of the quality-of-life scores and nasal symptom scores of patients with allergic rhinitis [standard mean difference (SMD) −2.97, 95% CI −4.77 to −1.16), $P = .001$] (Peng et al., 2015). No improvements of immunologic parameters were noted. However, this meta-analysis was criticized for its methodology (Peng et al., 2015; Turner et al., 2015). The same year, a meta-analysis on the same topic identified 23 studies with 1919 patients, including 21 double-blind RCTs and two crossover RCTs, again including children and adults (Zajac et al., 2015). Seventeen studies showed a significant clinical benefit in at least one outcome measure, whereas six trials showed no benefit (Zajac et al., 2015). Probiotic administration resulted in a significant improvement in quality-of-life scores compared to placebo (SMD −2.23, $P = .02$) (Zajac et al., 2015). Probiotics had no effect on rhinitis total symptom scores (SMD −0.36, $P = .13$) or total IgE levels (SMD 0.01, $P = .94$), although there was a trend toward a reduction in antigen-specific IgE (SMD 0.20, $P = .06$) in the placebo group compared to probiotic (Zajac et al., 2015). A 2016 Meta-analysis of 22 RCTs also came up with evidence of a potential benefit of probiotics in the treatment of allergic rhinitis. Even though probiotics significantly improved the total scores of quality-of-life questionnaires, more high-quality studies are needed to prove the effectiveness of probiotics with validated quality-of-life tools and objective measurements (Güvenç et al., 2016). Among the trials eligible for meta-analysis, the use of probiotics resulted in a significant improvement in Rhinoconjunctivitis Quality of Life Questionnaire scores compared to placebo (SMD −2.23, $P = .02$). Probiotics had no effect on Rhinitis Total Symptom Scores (SMD −0.36, $P = 0.13$) or total IgE levels (SMD 0.01, $P = 0.94$), although there was a trend toward a reduction in antigen-specific IgE (SMD 0.20, $P = 0.06$) in the placebo group compared to probiotic (Güvenç et al., 2016). All meta-analyses report that evidence remains limited due to study heterogeneity and variable outcome measures and that additional high-quality studies are needed to establish appropriate recommendations (May & Dolen, 2017).

In 212 children under 5 years from Pakistan, a probiotic product administered as a single dose of a chewable tablet, containing 2×10^9 CFU of *Lactobacillus Paracasei* (LP-33) was administered daily during 6 weeks while the control group was treated with cetirizine tablet 2.5 mg (<2 years) or 5 mg (2−5 years) once daily (Ahmed et al., 2019). Significant improvement from baseline symptoms (rhinorrhea, sneezing, nasal blocking, coughing, feeding difficulties, and sleeping difficulties) was reported equally in both groups in almost all children (Ahmed et al., 2019). Although the title of the paper mentions probiotics, the study was in fact performed with postbiotics since they were lyophilized extracts of bifidobacteria, which were shown to suppress allergic rhinitis in mice via inducing IL-10-producing B cells (Xue et al., 2019). Another study showed that *Clostridium butyricum* extracts so again postbiotics can efficiently inhibit experimental allergic rhinitis by increasing IL-10 expression in the B cells (Zeng et al., 2019).

A pilot study in only 20 adult patients (18−65 years) suggests that probiotics-impregnated bed linen with five different probiotic and natural not genetically modified bacterial strains of Bacillus species (strains of *Bacillus subtilis*,

Bacillus amyloliquefaciens, and *Bacillus pumilus*) can improve symptoms and quality of life of patients with dust mite allergic rhinitis (Verheijden et al., 2016). A large-scale study is warranted to further investigate this probiotics-based method (Berings et al., 2017).

10.6 Conclusions

Meta-analyses have shown that marked heterogeneity as well in inclusion criteria, studied products, and primary outcomes between studies makes direct comparison difficult (Papi et al., 2018). Current guidelines from prominent medical societies including the American Academy of Pediatrics, the European Academy of Allergy and Clinical Immunology, the National Institute of Allergy and Infectious Disease, and the European Society for Pediatric Gastroenterology, Hepatology and Nutrition do not recommend the use of probiotics for primary prevention of allergic disease (Kalliomäki et al., 2010). Due to the heterogeneities, the optimal strains, dosages, timing, and duration of probiotic administration remain unknown. However, research in this area is under way and will hopefully give better insights into how probiotics may contribute to the prevention or treatment of atopic diseases (Wang et al., 2020). While data from studies evaluating the role of the gastrointestinal microbiota on allergic disease of the respiratory tract performed in well-controlled conditions suggest a causal relation, data from clinical human studies remain disappointing. Multiple confounding factors influencing the clinical situation are likely to interfere with these outcomes. As an overall conclusion, there is insufficient evidence to recommend administration of probiotics in prevention or treatment of respiratory tract allergies, although there are animal data suggesting benefit and harm have not been demonstrated. It is important to emphasize that future studies require thoughtful prospective considerations in study design and execution with a special focus on clinical phenotyping, sample collection, and processing procedures for microbiome-specific analyses (Huang, Marsland, et al., 2017). There is a need to develop international standards for study designs to ensure uniformity across clinical trials. Future studies are warranted to refine the effector molecules of probiotics and to identify their mode of action in healthy and diseased conditions (Sharma & Im, 2018).

Acknowledgment

None.

Funding

This study did not receive any specific funding.

Conflicts of interest

We have no conflict of interest to declare.

References

Ahmed, M., Billoo, A. G., & Iqbal, K. (2019). Efficacy of probiotic in perennial allergic rhinitis undefive year children: A randomized controlled trial. *Pakistan Journal of Medical Sciences*, *35*(6), 1538–1543. Available from https://doi.org/10.12669/pjms.35.6.744.

Arokiasamy, P., Uttamacharya., Kowal, P., Capistrant, B. D., Gildner, T. E., Thiele, E., Biritwum, R. B., Yawson, A. E., Mensah, G., Maximova, T., Wu, F., Guo, Y., Zheng, Y., Kalula, S. Z., Rodríguez, A. S., Espinoza, B. M., Liebert, M. A., Eick, G., Sterner, K. N., ... Chatterji, S. (2017). Chronic noncommunicable diseases in 6 low- and middle-income countries: Findings from wave 1 of the world health organization's Study on Global Ageing and Adult Health (SAGE). *American Journal of Epidemiology*, *185*(6), 414–428. Available from https://doi.org/10.1093/aje/kww125.

Asher, M. I., Montefort, S., Björkstén, B., Lai, C. K., Strachan, D. P., Weiland, S. K., & Williams, H. (2006). Worldwide time trends in the prevalence of symptoms of asthma, allergic rhinoconjunctivitis, and eczema in childhood: ISAAC Phases One and Three repeat multicountry cross-sectional surveys. *Lancet*, *368*(9537), 733–743. Available from https://doi.org/10.1016/S0140-6736(06)69283-0.

Berings, M., Jult, A., Vermeulen, H., De Ruyck, N., Derycke, L., Ucar, H., Ghekiere, P., Temmerman, R., Ellis, J., Bachert, C., Lambrecht, B. N., Dullaers, M., & Gevaert, P. (2017). Probiotics-impregnated bedding covers for house dust mite allergic rhinitis: A pilot randomized clinical trial. *Clinical and Experimental Allergy*, *47*(8), 1092–1096. Available from https://doi.org/10.1111/cea.12937.

Braun-Fahrländer, C., Gassner, M., Grize, L., Neu, U., Sennhauser, F. H., Varonier, H. S., Vuille, J. C., & Wüthrich, B. (1999). Prevalence of hay fever and allergic sensitization in farmer's children and their peers living in the same rural community. *Clinical and Experimental Allergy*, *29*(1), 28–34. Available from https://doi.org/10.1046/j.1365-2222.1999.00479.x.

Broek, J. L., Bousquet, J., Baena-Cagnani, C. E., Bonini, S., Canonica, G. W., Casale, T. B., VanWijk, R. G., Ohta, K., Zuberbier, T., & Schünemann, H. J. (2010). Allergic Rhinitis and its Impact on Asthma (ARIA) guidelines: 2010 revision. *Journal of Allergy and Clinical Immunology*, *126*(3), 466−476. Available from https://doi.org/10.1016/j.jaci.2010.06.047.

Buccigrossi, V., Nicastro, E., & Guarino, A. (2013). Functions of intestinal microflora in children. *Current Opinion in Gastroenterology*, *29*(1), 31−38. Available from https://doi.org/10.1097/MOG.0b013e32835a3500.

Cervantes-García, D., Jiménez, M., Rivas-Santiago, C. E., Gallegos-Alcalá, P., Hernández-Mercado, A., Santoyo-Payán, L. S., Loera-Arias, M. D. J., Saucedo-Cardenas, O., De Oca-Luna, R. M., & Salinas, E. (2020). Lactococcus lactis NZ9000 prevents asthmatic airway inflammation and remodelling in rats through the improvement of intestinal barrier function and systemic TGF-β production. *International Archives of Allergy and Immunology*. Available from https://doi.org/10.1159/000511146.

Das, R. R., Naik, S. S., & Singh, M. (2013). Probiotics as additives on therapy in allergic airway diseases: A systematic review of benefits and risks. *BioMed Research International*, *2013*. Available from https://doi.org/10.1155/2013/231979.

Das, R. R., Singh, M., & Shafiq, N. (2010). Probiotics in treatment of allergic rhinitis. *World Allergy Organization Journal*, *3*(9), 239−244. Available from https://doi.org/10.1097/WOX.0b013e3181f234d4.

Dicksved, J., Flöistrup, H., Bergström, A., Rosenquist, M., Pershagen, G., Scheynius, A., Roos, S., Alm, J. S., Engstrand, L., Braun-Fahrländer, C., Von Mutius, E., & Jansson, J. K. (2007). Molecular fingerprinting of the fecal microbiota of children raised according to different lifestyles. *Applied and Environmental Microbiology*, *73*(7), 2284−2289. Available from https://doi.org/10.1128/AEM.02223-06.

Dimitri-Pinheiro, S., Soares, R., & Barata, P. (2020). The microbiome of the nose—Friend or foe? *Allergy & Rhinology*, *11*. Available from https://doi.org/10.1177/2152656720911605, 215265672091160.

Du, X., Wang, L., Wu, S., Yuan, L., Tang, S., Xiang, Y., Qu, X., Liu, H., Qin, X., & Liu, C. (2019). Efficacy of probiotic supplementary therapy for asthma, allergic rhinitis, and wheeze: A meta-analysis of randomized controlled trials. *Allergy and Asthma Proceedings*, *40*(4), 250−260. Available from https://doi.org/10.2500/aap.2019.40.4227.

Elazab, N., Mendy, A., Gasana, J., Vieira, E. R., Quizon, A., & Forno, E. (2013). Probiotic administration in early life, atopy, and asthma: A meta-analysis of clinical trials. *Pediatrics*, *132*(3), e666−e676. Available from https://doi.org/10.1542/peds.2013-0246.

Enilari, O., & Sinha, S. (2019). The global impact of asthma in adult populatio. *Annals of Global Health*, *85*(1), 1−7. Available from https://doi.org/10.5334/aogh.2412.

Feleszko, W., Jaworska, J., Rha, R.-D., Steinhausen, S., Avagyan, A., Jaudszus, A., Ahrens, B., Groneberg, A., Wahn, U., & Hamelmann, E. (2007). Probiotic-induced suppression of allergic sensitization and airway inflammation is associated with an increase of T regulatory-dependent mechanisms in a murine model of asthma. *Clinical & Experimental Allergy*, *37*, 498−505. Available from https://doi.org/10.1111/j.1365-2222.2006.02629.x.

GBD 2016 Disease and Injury and Incidence and Prevalence Collaborators. (2016). Global, regional, and national incidence, prevalence, and years lived with disability for 328 diseases and injuries for 195 countries, 1990−2016: A systematic analysis for the Global Burden of Disease Study. *Global Health Metrics*, *390*, 32154. Available from https://doi.org/10.1016/s0140-6736, 2.

Gorissen, D. M. W., Rutten, N. B. M. M., Oostermeijer, C. M. J., Niers, L. E. M., Hoekstra, M. O., Rijkers, G. T., & van der Ent, C. K. (2014). Preventive effects of selected probiotic strains on the development of asthma and allergic rhinitis in childhood. The Panda study. *Clinical and Experimental Allergy*, *44*(11), 1431−1433. Available from https://doi.org/10.1111/cea.12413.

Goulet, O. (2015). Potential role of the intestinal microbiota in programming health and disease. *Nutrition Reviews*, *73*, 32−40. Available from https://doi.org/10.1093/nutrit/nuv039.

Güvenç, I. A., Muluk, N. B., Mutlu, F. Ş., Eşki, E., Altintoprak, N., Oktemer, T., & Cingi, C. (2016). Do probiotics have a role in the treatment of allergic rhinitis? A comprehensive systematic review and meta-analysis. *American Journal of Rhinology and Allergy*, *30*(5), e157−e175. Available from https://doi.org/10.2500/ajra.2016.30.4354.

Huang, R., Ning, H., Shen, M., Li, J., Zhang, J., Chen, X., & Huang, R., et al., (2017). Probiotics for the treatment of atopic dermatitis in children: A systematic review and meta-analysis of randomized controlled trials. *Frontiers in Cellular and Infection Microbiology*, *7*, 392.

Huang, Y. J., Marsland, B. J., Bunyavanich, S., O'Mahony, L., Leung, D. Y. M., Muraro, A., & Fleisher, T. A. (2017). The microbiome in allergic disease: Current understanding and future opportunities—2017 PRACTALL document of the American Academy of Allergy, Asthma & Immunology and the European Academy of Allergy and Clinical Immunology. *Journal of Allergy and Clinical Immunology*, *139*(4), 1099−1110. Available from https://doi.org/10.1016/j.jaci.2017.02.007.

Jalali, M. M., Soleimani, R., Alavi Foumani, A., & Ganjeh Khosravi, H. (2019). Add-on probiotics in patients with persistent allergic rhinitis: A randomized crossover clinical trial. *The Laryngoscope*, *129*(8), 1744−1750. Available from https://doi.org/10.1002/lary.27858.

Jamalkandi, S., Ahmadi, A., Ahrari, I., Salimian, J., Karimi, M., & Ghanei, M. (2020). Oral and nasal probiotic administration for the prevention and alleviation of allergic diseases, asthma and chronic obstructive pulmonary disease. *Nutrition Research Reviews*, *13*, 1−16. Available from https://doi.org/10.1017/S0954422420000116.

Jeongmin, L., Bang, J., & Woo, H. J. (2013). Immunomodulatory and anti-allergic effects of orally administered Lactobacillus species in ovalbumin-sensitized mice. *Journal of Microbiology and Biotechnology*, *23*(5), 724−730. Available from https://doi.org/10.4014/jmb.1211.11079.

Juniper, E. F., Ståhl, E., Doty, R. L., Simons, F. E. R., Allen, D. B., & Howarth, P. H. (2005). Clinical outcomes and adverse effect monitoring in allergic rhinitis. *Journal of Allergy and Clinical Immunology*, *115*(3), S390−S413. Available from https://doi.org/10.1016/j.jaci.2004.12.014.

Kalliomäki, M., Antoine, J. M., Herz, U., Rijkers, G. T., Wells, J. M., & Mercenier, A. (2010). Guidance for substantiating the evidence for beneficial effects of probiotics: Prevention and management of allergic diseases by probiotics. *Journal of Nutrition*, *140*(3). Available from https://doi.org/10.3945/jn.109.113761.

Kuang, H., Li, Z., Lv, X., Wu, P., Tan, J., Wu, Q., Li, Y., Jiang, W., Pang, Q., Wang, Y., & Fan, R. (2021). Exposure to volatile organic compounds may be associated with oxidative DNA damage-mediated childhood asthma. *Ecotoxicology and Environmental Safety*, *210*. Available from https://doi.org/10.1016/j.ecoenv.2020.111864.

Leynaert, B., Sunyer, J., Garcia-Esteban, R., Svanes, C., Jarvis, D., Cerveri, I., Dratva, J., Gislason, T., Heinrich, J., Janson, C., Kuenzli, N., De Marco, R., Omenaas, E., Raherison, C., Real, F. G., Wjst, M., Zemp, E., Zureik, M., Burney, P. G. J., & Neukirch, F. (2012). Gender differences in prevalence, diagnosis and incidence of allergic and non-allergic asthma: A population-based cohort. *Thorax*, *67*(7), 625–631. Available from https://doi.org/10.1136/thoraxjnl-2011-201249.

Lyons, A., O'Mahony, D., O'Brien, F., MacSharry, J., Sheil, B., Ceddia, M., Russell, W. M., Forsythe, P., Bienenstock, J., Kiely, B., Shanahan, F., & O'Mahony, L. (2010). Bacterial strain-specific induction of Foxp3 + T regulatory cells is protective in murine allergy models. *Clinical & Experimental Allergy*, *40*, 811–819. Available from https://doi.org/10.1111/j.1365-2222.2009.03437.x.

May, J. R., & Dolen, W. K. (2017). Management of allergic rhinitis: A review for the community pharmacist. *Clinical Therapeutics*, *39*(12), 2410–2419. Available from https://doi.org/10.1016/j.clinthera.2017.10.006.

Meltzer, E. O. (2016). Allergic rhinitis. Burden of illness, quality of life, comorbidities, and control. *Immunology and Allergy Clinics of North America*, *36*(2), 235–248. Available from https://doi.org/10.1016/j.iac.2015.12.002.

Mennini, M., Dahdah, L., Artesani, M. C., Fiocchi, A., & Martelli, A. (2017). Probiotics in asthma and allergy prevention. *Frontiers in Pediatrics*, *5*. Available from https://doi.org/10.3389/fped.2017.00165.

Molero, Y., Zetterqvist, J., Lichtenstein, P., Almqvist, C., & Ludvigsson, J. F. (2018). Parental nicotine replacement therapy and offspring bronchitis/bronchiolitis and asthma—A nationwide population-based cohort study. *Clinical Epidemiology*, *10*, 1339–1347. Available from https://doi.org/10.2147/CLEP.S171401.

Papi, A., Brightling, C., Pedersen, S. E., & Reddel, H. K. (2018). Asthma. *The Lancet*, *391*(17), 33311. Available from https://doi.org/10.1016/s0140-6736.

Peldan, P., Kukkonen, A. K., Savilahti, E., & Kuitunen, M. (2017). Perinatal probiotics decreased eczema up to 10 years of age, but at 5–10 years, allergic rhino-conjunctivitis was increased. *Clinical & Experimental Allergy*, *47*, 975–979. Available from https://doi.org/10.1111/cea.12924.

Pellaton, C., Nutten, S., Thierry, A. C., Boudousquié, C., Barbier, N., Blanchard, C., Corthésy, B., Mercenier, A., & Spertini, F. (2012). Intragastric and intranasal administration of lactobacillus paracasei NCC2461 modulates allergic airway inflammation in mice. *International Journal of Inflammation*, *2012*. Available from https://doi.org/10.1155/2012/686739.

Peng, Y., Li, A., Yu, L., & Qin, G. (2015). The role of probiotics in prevention and treatment for patients with allergic rhinitis: A systematic review. *American Journal of Rhinology and Allergy*, *29*(4), 292–298. Available from https://doi.org/10.2500/ajra.2015.29.4192.

Sepp, E., Mikelsaar, M., & Salminen, S. (1993). Effect of administration of Lactobacillus casei strain GG on the gastrointestinal microbiota of newborns. *Microbial Ecology in Health and Disease*, *6*(6), 309–314. Available from https://doi.org/10.3109/08910609309141340.

Sharma, G., & Im, S. H. (2018). Probiotics as a potential immunomodulating pharmabiotics in allergic diseases: Current status and future prospects. *Allergy, Asthma and Immunology Research*, *10*(6), 575–590. Available from https://doi.org/10.4168/aair.2018.10.6.575.

Spacova, I., Petrova, M. I., Fremau, A., Pollaris, L., Vanoirbeek, J., Ceuppens, J. L., Seys, S., & Lebeer, S. (2019). Intranasal administration of probiotic Lactobacillus rhamnosus GG prevents birch pollen-induced allergic asthma in a murine model. *Allergy: European Journal of Allergy and Clinical Immunology*, *74*(1), 100–110. Available from https://doi.org/10.1111/all.13502.

Spacova, I., Van Beeck, W., Seys, S., Devos, F., Vanoirbeek, J., Vanderleyden, J., Ceuppens, J., Petrova, M., & Lebeer, S. (2020). Lactobacillus rhamnosus probiotic prevents airway function deterioration and promotes gut microbiome resilience in a murine asthma model. *Gut Microbes*, *11*(6), 1729–1744. Available from https://doi.org/10.1080/19490976.2020.1766345.

Swanson, K. S., Gibson, G. R., Hutkins, R., Reimer, R. A., Reid, G., Verbeke, K., Scott, K. P., Holscher, H. D., Azad, M. B., Delzenne, N. M., & Sanders, M. E. (2020). The International Scientific Association for Probiotics and Prebiotics (ISAPP) consensus statement on the definition and scope of synbiotics. *Nature Reviews Gastroenterology and Hepatology*, *17*(11), 687–701. Available from https://doi.org/10.1038/s41575-020-0344-2.

Terada-Ikeda, C., Kitabatake, M., Hiraku, A., Kato, K., Yasui, S., Imakita, N., Ouji-Sageshima, N., Iwabuchi, N., Hamada, K., & Ito, T. (2020). Maternal supplementation with Bifidobacterium breve M-16V prevents their offspring from allergic airway inflammation accelerated by the prenatal exposure to an air pollutant aerosol. *PLoS One*, *15*(9). Available from https://doi.org/10.1371/journal.pone.0238923.

To, T., Stanojevic, S., Moores, G., Gershon, A. S., Bateman, E. D., Cruz, A. A., & Boulet, L. P. (2012). Global asthma prevalence in adults: Findings from the cross-sectional world health survey. *BMC Public Health*, *12*(1). Available from https://doi.org/10.1186/1471-2458-12-204.

Trivedi, R., & Barve, K. (2020). Gut microbiome a promising target for management of respiratory diseases. *Biochemical Journal*, *477*(14), 2679–2696. Available from https://doi.org/10.1042/BCJ20200426.

Turner, J. H., Adams, A. S., Zajac, A., & Qin, G. (2015). Probiotics in prevention and treatment of allergic rhinitis. *American Journal of Rhinology and Allergy*, *29*(6), e224. Available from https://doi.org/10.2500/ajra.2015.29.4257.

Valdes, A. M., Walter, J., Segal, E., & Spector, T. D. (2018). Role of the gut microbiota in nutrition and health. *BMJ (Online)*, *361*, 36–44. Available from https://doi.org/10.1136/bmj.k2179.

Verheijden, K. A. T., Willemsen, L. E. M., Braber, S., Leusink-Muis, T., Jeurink, P. V., Garssen, J., Kraneveld, A. D., & Folkerts, G. (2016). The development of allergic inflammation in a murine house dust mite asthma model is suppressed by synbiotic mixtures of non-digestible oligosaccharides and Bifidobacterium breve M-16V. *European Journal of Nutrition*, *55*(3), 1141–1151. Available from https://doi.org/10.1007/s00394-015-0928-8.

Vliagoftis, H., Kouranos, V. D., Betsi, G. I., & Falagas, M. E. (2008). Probiotics for the treatment of allergic rhinitis and asthma: Systematic review of randomized controlled trials. *Annals of Allergy, Asthma and Immunology*, *101*(6), 570−579. Available from https://doi.org/10.1016/S1081-1206(10)60219-0.

von Mutius, E., & Matsui, E. C. (2020). Prevention is the best remedy: What can we do to stop allergic disease? *Journal of Allergy and Clinical Immunology: In Practice*, *8*(3), 890−891. Available from https://doi.org/10.1016/j.jaip.2020.01.010.

Wang, W., Luo, X., Zhang, Q., He, X., Zhang, Z., & Wang, X. (2020). Bifidobacterium infantis relieves allergic asthma in mice by regulating Th1/Th2. *Medical Science Monitor*, *26*. Available from https://doi.org/10.12659/MSM.920583.

Wei, X., Jiang, P., Liu, J., Sun, R., & Zhu, L. (2020). Association between probiotic supplementation and asthma incidence in infants: A meta-analysis of randomized controlled trials. *Journal of Asthma*, *57*(2), 167−178. Available from https://doi.org/10.1080/02770903.2018.1561893.

West, C. E., Dzidic, M., Prescott, S. L., & Jenmalm, M. C. (2017). Bugging allergy; role of pre-, pro- and synbiotics in allergy prevention. *Allergology International*, *66*(4), 529−538. Available from https://doi.org/10.1016/j.alit.2017.08.001.

Wickens, K., Barthow, C., Mitchell, E. A., Kang, J., van Zyl, N., Purdie, G., Stanley, T., Fitzharris, P., Murphy, R., & Crane, J. (2018). Effects of Lactobacillus rhamnosus HN001 in early life on the cumulative prevalence of allergic disease to 11 years. *Pediatric Allergy and Immunology*, *29*(8), 808−814. Available from https://doi.org/10.1111/pai.12982.

Xue, J. M., Ma, F., An, Y. F., Suo, L. M., Geng, X. R., Song, Y. N., Mo, L. H., Luo, X. Q., Zhang, X. W., liu, D. B., Zhao, C. Q., & Yang, P. C. (2019). Probiotic extracts ameliorate nasal allergy by inducing interleukin-35-producing dendritic cells in mice. *International Forum of Allergy and Rhinology*, *9*(11), 1289−1296. Available from https://doi.org/10.1002/alr.22438.

Zajac, A. E., Adams, A. S., & Turner, J. H. (2015). A systematic review and meta-analysis of probiotics for the treatment of allergic rhinitis. *International Forum of Allergy and Rhinology*, *5*(6), 524−532. Available from https://doi.org/10.1002/alr.21492.

Zeng, X. H., Yang, G., Liu, J. Q., Geng, X. R., Cheng, B. H., Liu, Z. Q., & Yang, P. C. (2019). Nasal instillation of probiotic extracts inhibits experimental allergic rhinitis. *Immunotherapy*, *11*(15), 1315−1323. Available from https://doi.org/10.2217/imt-2019-0119.

Zuccotti, G., Meneghin, F., Aceti, A., Barone, G., Callegari, M. L., Di Mauro, A., Fantini, M. P., Gori, D., Indrio, F., Maggio, L., Morelli, L., & Corvaglia, L. (2015). Probiotics for prevention of atopic diseases in infants: Systematic review and meta-analysis. *Allergy*, *70*, 1356−1371. Available from https://doi.org/10.1111/all.12700.

Chapter 11

Prenatal and neonatal probiotic intake in pediatric allergy

Youcef Shahali[1], Naheed Mojgani[2] and Maryam Dadar[2]
[1]The University Hospital of Besançon, Besançon, France, [2]Razi Vaccine and Serum Research Institute, Agricultural Research, Education and Extension Organization (AREEO), Karaj, Iran

11.1 Introduction

In the late 19th century microbiologists identified microflora in the gastrointestinal tracts of healthy individuals that differed from those found in diseased individuals. The beneficial microflora found in the gastrointestinal tract was termed probiotics. FAO and WHO experts defined the term probiotics as "Live microorganisms which when administered in adequate amounts confer health benefit on the host" (Sánchez et al., 2017; Sanders et al., 2007). In other words, probiotics are living microorganisms used to restore gut health by changing the intestinal microbiota (Aureli et al., 2011; Didari et al., 2014). Lilly and Stillwell (1965) first coined the term probiotic in 1965 in reference to substances produced by protozoa, which stimulated the growth of other organisms. The largest group of probiotic bacteria in the intestine is lactic acid bacteria (LAB). Elie Metchnikoff, the father of modern immunology spoke highly about the possible health benefits of the LAB (Stambler, 2015). In his book, the prolongation of life, he wrote that consumption of live bacteria, such as *Streptococcus thermophilus* and *Lactobacillus bulgaricus*, in the form of yogurt are beneficial for gastro intestinal as well general health and could lead to long life (Anukam & Reid, 2007). The most common types of microbes used as probiotics are lactobacilli and bifidobacteria. Selection criteria for probiotic bacteria include that the bacterial strain: (1) must be able to survive in the gastrointestinal tract and to proliferate in the gut; (2) should exert benefits to the host through growth and/or activity in the human body; (3) should be nonpathogenic and nontoxic; (4) provide protection against pathogenic microorganisms by means of multiple mechanisms; and (5) should be lacking transferable antibiotic resistance (Aureli et al., 2011; Azad et al., 2018). Different bacterial strains of the same genus and species, verified also by genomic information, may exert completely different effects on the host. Probiotics are likely to have an impact through gut mucosa by balancing the local microbiota by inhibiting the growth of pathogenic microorganisms (Belizário & Napolitano, 2015; Marchesi & Ravel, 2015), and by enhancing local and systemic immune responses (Belizário & Napolitano, 2015). They may also influence the composition and activity of microbiota in the intestinal contents. In recent years it has been proven that the digestive system has an impact on the entire body; therefore if the digestive system is not functioning optimally, other parts of body are also affected. Probiotics provide the beneficial bacteria our bodies need to maintain healthy digestion and to counteract some of the side effects of antibiotics. Thus probiotics product is an invaluable asset to the body as it is able to provide benefits to multiple parts of the body, where other supplements simply focus on specific sites and parts (Adams, 2010; Amara & Shibl, 2015; Chi et al., 2021). Clearly, using high-dose probiotics to repopulate the intestinal flora with healthy bacteria can have some powerful health benefits, especially for those who have had medium or broad-spectrum antibiotic therapy in the past (Ghosh et al., 2004). In an in vivo trial, animals given bifidobacteria showed improved immune function of the epithelial barrier in allergic mice (Zhang et al., 2010). In another study in mice, oral supplementation with *Lactobacillus* alleviated the allergic airway response seen in asthma (Wang et al., 2017). Probiotics have also shown significant effects in treatment of eczema in children, especially IgE associated eczema. In a study, of 88 children, 45 supplemented with *Lactobacillus* daily for 12 weeks showed improvement in symptoms and a decrease in the activity of eczema (Boyle et al., 2009; Doege et al., 2012). Prebiotics as a not digestible food ingredient is composed of oligosaccharides that show several profitable impacts on host health by selective induction of the growth and/or function of particular microbes present in the gut microbiota (Gibson, 1998).

The use of probiotics and prebiotics as preventive and therapeutic approach in pediatric allergy is attracting great interest, especially in the perinatal period. This fact is partly due to recent studies revealing that microbiota colonization of the human body begins during pregnancy, thereby changing the paradigm of the fetus as a sterile entity (Milani et al., 2017). Perinatal period starts at the 5th month of gestation and ends a month after birth, thus including a part of pregnancy and the neonatal period. During the postnatal period, breastfeeding plays a key role and represents the main route by which probiotics are transferred from mother to infants. Thus maternal diet and habits will significantly influence the gut microbiota of neonates. Although the bacterial composition of healthy infant microbiota is not completely known, the standard profile used as control in most studies corresponds to the fecal microbiota of full-term infants, vaginally delivered and exclusively breastfed. While probiotic consumption in adults generally does not lead to sustainable changes in microbiota composition, the bacterial colonization of the newborn body changes rapidly in the first weeks of life and does not reflect adult patterns before 2 years of age (Adlerberth & Wold, 2009). This may partly explain the outcome of clinical studies in human showing that the use of probiotic and prebiotic supplementations for the prevention and treatment of allergy seems to be more effective during the perinatal period (Boyle & Tang, 2006).

The current chapter is devoted to providing an overview of the scientific and clinical experimentations investigating the potential effects of prenatal and neonatal probiotic intake in pediatric allergy. A number of factors, such as environmental pollution, inappropriate fat and carbohydrate rich diets, misuse of antibiotics and immunosuppressive drugs, stress, depression, and anxiety, are known as main causes of impaired immunity. In addition, a decline in cellular immunity is observed with aging. The role of probiotics in regulating the mucosal immune system by stimulating the antigen-presenting cells, such as dendritic cells, has been investigated by numerous in vivo studies. These studies showed that probiotics act on both the innate and acquired immune systems and have the potency to decrease the severity of infections in the gastrointestinal (Kanauchi et al., 2018) and upper respiratory tracts (Lehtoranta et al., 2020). A study showed that elderly volunteers with milk containing bifidus consumption experienced an increase in their white blood cells (Silva et al., 1999). As probiotics help building up the immune system, thus they also contribute in the fight against infection. A 7-month study on more than 570 children in day care centers found that drinking a probiotic milk reduced the number and severity of respiratory infections and the need for antibiotics (Hojsak et al., 2010; Wang et al., 2016). In 2003 Clancy (2003) proposed a new term for defining probiotic bacteria that specifically promote health by bolstering of the local and systemic immune responses. Hence, the term immunobiotics was coined for immune modulating probiotic bacteria. In other words, immunobiotics refers to beneficial bacteria which confer health benefits on the host via immunoregulatory functions, including upregulating immune mechanisms, downregulating the inflammatory responses, maturation of dendritic cells, and production of antiviral agents, such as lactic acid, hydrogen peroxide, and bacteriocins. The immunostimulant properties of LAB have been proved to be strain and dose dependent (Mojgani et al., 2020; Racedo et al., 2006; Villena et al., 2014). Numerous animal studies showed that oral administration of proper dosage of probiotic LAB not only increased the clearance rate of *Streptococcus pneumonia* in the lung and blood of the tested animals but also led to progressive decline in lung injuries (Racedo et al., 2006; Villena et al., 2014).

11.2 Safety of probiotics and prebiotics

The safety of probiotics and prebiotics is an important benefit leading to its extensive consumption in different forms (Castellazzi et al., 2013). In recent years the use of probiotics among pregnant women and infants considerably increased. Probiotics are also commonly consumed to ameliorate genitourinary and gastrointestinal conditions during antibiotics consumption. LAB are among the most extensively studied probiotics, and numerous investigations showed that they can be safely added to food, thereby exempting them from usual rigorous tolerance requirements for food additives. Several safety properties have been taken into accounts, such as the absence of associated disease, including endocarditis or bacteremia; the absence of antibiotic resistance gene transformation in the gastrointestinal flora as well as the absence of metabolic or toxic impacts on the gastrointestinal system (Aureli et al., 2011). Principally, the safe properties of a probiotic strain are associated with the absence of virulence factors and the absence of clinical or veterinary resistance to antibiotics (Daliri et al., 2019). Many probiotics, such as *Bifidobacteria*, *Lactococci* and *Lactobacilli*, are a natural part of the beneficial gut microbiota and have been reported as safe by the United States Food and Drug Administration (Doron & Snydman, 2015). Prebiotic carbohydrates, such as inulin and fructooligosaccharides (FOS), are natural vegetable components (Sheth & Gupta, 2014). The global market of probiotic and prebiotic products has a growing expansion and a wide range of people around the world consume probiotics daily because of their proven and purpoted beneficial effects on health (Novik & Savich, 2020). One of the most important factors for strains selection of effective probiotic bacterial is their safety. Some live microorganisms have a long history of use as probiotics without causing illness in people. Food and Drug Association has designated many probiotics to be generally recognized as safe (GRAS). Even for those without GRAS status, the industry has used probiotic bacteria in food fermentations with the assumption that their history of use implies their safety (Donohue & Salminen, 1996; Doron & Snydman, 2015). Although a number of epidemiological and safety data on probiotics exist, which shows their noninvolvement in human infections, yet it is considered necessary to assess the efficacy of all new species and strains of probiotics before incorporating them into food products. Some risk factors for probiotic sepsis have been identified including: bypassing the gastric processes (e.g., following jejunostomy or gastrostomy), gut inflammation, and the presence of a foreign body, such as an indwelling catheter. However, these risks are very low as probiotics have been safely given to premature infants and to babies with HIV without any adverse effects (Chi et al., 2021). Antibiotics resistance represents another potential risk. A number of antibiotic-resistant probiotic bacteria have been reported by Temmerman et al. (2003). According to their studies, out of 268 bacteria isolated from 55 European probiotics products, 187 of the isolates demonstrated antibiotic resistance against kanamycin (79% of the isolates), vancomycin (65%), tetracycline (26%), penicillin G (23%), erythromycin (16%), and chloramphenicol (11%) whereas 68.4% showed resistance against multiple antibiotics including intrinsic resistances. In Europe, according to the Qualified Presumption of Safety (QPS) approach, established by the European Food Safety Authority (EFSA, 2008), the nature of any antibiotic resistance determinants present in a candidate microorganism should be specified prior to its approval for QPS status. Therefore antibiotic resistance per se is not a safety issue; it only becomes such when the risk of resistance transfer is present. Thus the potential health risks that could result from the transfer of antibiotic resistance genes from LAB reservoir strains to bacteria in the resident microflora of the human gastrointestinal tract or pathogenic bacteria cannot be overlooked. As yet, the safety of probiotics has not been thoroughly studied scientifically and detailed information is yet required especially for their use in young children, elderly people, and people with compromised immune systems (Sharma et al., 2014). As a practitioner, it may be prudent to advise clients to incorporate well-known species into their diet gradually, building up to the recommended daily levels needed over a period of 2–3 weeks, to minimize any potentially deleterious effects. It is worth noting that probiotics should not be used in place of conventional medicine. Besides, the Italian Ministry of Health, as well as the Scientific Committee on Animal Nutrition of the EU (SCAN), the EFSA Panel on additives, products, and substances used in animal feed (FEEDAP), proposed to add "the absence of evidence regarding the possible transfer of genes related to antibiotic-resistant" as an essential parameter for microorganism safety confirmation (Ahanchian et al., 2016; Snydman, 2008). Furthermore, the confirmation of the safety and efficacy of probiotic strains are important for different bacterial strains of the same species, which may reveal variable effects on the host immune system (Aureli et al., 2011). In recent years the administration of probiotic products has increased in different medical conditions, because of their efficacy and safety in clinical practice. No adverse effects have been reported in preterm infants and the strain *Lactobacillus* GG was reported as safe in pediatric studies (Saxelin, 1997; Wang et al., 2014). Different studies also showed that the supplements of probiotics to critically ill neonates could decrease the occurrence of nosocomial pneumonia, increase immune activity, and decrease days in the hospital without any side effects (Wang et al., 2014). However, different strains of probiotics have different safety profiles (Gupta & Garg, 2009). Finally, pre- and probiotics are also applied as supplementation in infant formula that may be beneficial in managing the infant health (Bertelsen et al., 2016).

11.3 Probiotics, prebiotics, and immunity

The terms prebiotics and probiotics are comprehensive, and different genera, species, and strains show different effects on the immune system (Bron et al., 2012). Several effective confounding factors, including commensal diet and bacteria, could influence the gut immune system. Although specific live microorganisms (probiotics) and food components (prebiotics) may modulate the gut microbial composition, accurate knowledge of the associated molecular pathways behind their impacts on the immune system may provide insights into the therapeutic potential for many immune response-related diseases, such as allergy and eczema (Vieira et al., 2013). Several studies reported that Nod-like receptors (NLRs), Toll-like receptors (TLRs), and pattern recognition receptors (PRRs) play an important role in the improvement of immune tolerance regulated by probiotics and prebiotics (Abreu, 2010; Kamada et al., 2013). The consequence of TLRs stimulation is the overexpression of pro-inflammatory modulators that develop the host's immune system responses. Moreover, some cytoplasmic proteins and NLRs could regulate the induction of inflammatory responses and PRRs by the commensal microbiota that is directly contributed in the gut homeostasis (Yeretssian, 2012). However, disarrangement in the PRR related-microbiota interactions of different cell types and gut mucosal compartment, often lead to the development of intensified inflammation and associated diseases (Lavelle et al., 2010; Maynard et al., 2012). The beneficial effects of probiotics and prebiotics in the host have been supported through numerous in vivo investigations based on animal models or clinical experiments, indicating their effectiveness in postantibiotic-related diarrhea; necrotizing enterocolitis; prevention or treatment of acute viral gastroenteritis; inflammatory bowel disease (IBD); and certain pediatric allergic disorders (Cruchet et al., 2015). The critical role of probiotics and prebiotics in the alleviation of different dysfunctions of the gastrointestinal system has also been documented (Vieira et al., 2013). One of the main pathways by which probiotics and prebiotics may decline gut disorder symptoms is by elevating the production of short-chain fatty acids (SCFAs) in the colon that declines the intestinal permeability and the invasion of pathogenic microorganisms (Morais & Jacob, 2006; Szajewska & Kołodziej, 2015). The cell wall components of probiotics, such as peptidoglycan and lipoteichoic acid, along with specific proteins are actively involved in the immune pathways (Klaenhammer et al., 2012). Furthermore, the modulation of different receptor-regulator signaling cascades has a critical effect on the regulation of the human immune system and represents one of the most effective roles of probiotic effector molecules (Bron et al., 2012). Probiotics also modulate the activation of dendritic cells, epithelial cells, and natural killer cells (Rizzello et al., 2011; Yahfoufi et al., 2018). Also, probiotics could regulate the polarization of the immune pathways and Treg cells toward Th1 (Ceccarelli et al., 2019; Irvine et al., 2010). Prebiotics as nondigestible food ingredients showed different profitable effects on host health through the selective stimulation of the growth and/or function of specific microbes present in the gut microbiota (Gibson, 1998). Fiber carbohydrates, such as pectin, gums, lignin, beta-glucan, and cellulose, as not digested in the upper gastrointestinal tract could be fermented by residential anaerobes gut bacteria into SCFAs, particularly acetate, propionate, butyrate, and lactate, which are fermented when reaching the colon (Horrocks & De Dombal, 1978). Another profitable role of prebiotics is the induction of the immune responses by the modulation of the "beneficial microbes" population in the gut, especially LAB and bifidobacteria. Also, cytokine expression is another critical pathway which is highly influenced by the consumption of specific prebiotics and probiotics (Shokryazdan et al., 2017). The prebiotics metabolites also contribute to the regulation of chemokines, and Treg cells cytokines (Yahfoufi et al., 2018). Also, prebiotic fibers could regulate the hepatic lipogenic enzymes by promoting SCFA, such as propionate. It was fund that the supplementation of inulin could increase the levels of SCFA in the cecum of treated animals (Artiss et al., 2006; Vieira et al., 2013). Other possible roles of prebiotics are the regulation of mucin production, an increase in the number of leukocytes and/or lymphocytes in gut-associated lymphoid tissues (GALT) and peripheral blood as well as increased IgA secretion by the GALT (Schley & Field, 2002). However, the different mechanism for the effective role of prebiotics on the functions of the immune system is still largely unknown. Finally, among numerous proposed health effects of probiotics, only a few have been supported by sound research claims. The most marked health benefits of probiotics supplements studied up to date include their ability to strengthen immunity or in other words their immune-modulating role. Probiotics have significant potential to reduce mortality and morbidity in preterm neonates, by helping fight off infection and by increasing their immunity (Deshpande et al., 2017, 2018). A seven-month study on more than 570 children in daycare centers found that drinking probiotic milk reduced the number and severity of respiratory infections and the need for antibiotics.

11.4 Microbiota and allergic disorders

The term microbiota was for the first time defined by Lederberg and McCray (2001), as the assemblage of trillions of multispecies microbes (commensal, symbiotic, and pathogenic microorganisms) including bacteria, fungi, archaea, and protozoans residing in the human body within a particular niche. Later viruses were also added to this list of microbes present within the host body (Lederberg & McCray, 2001). On other hand, microbiome has been defined as the collection of genes and genomes of member of a microbiota (Marchesi & Ravel, 2015). The bacterial species found in the human gut microbiome include mostly three phyla: *Bacteroidetes* (*Porphyromonas*, *Prevotella*), *Firmicutes* (*Ruminococcus*, *Clostridium*, and *Eubacteria*), and *Actinobacteria* (*Bifidobacterium*). *Lactobacilli*, *Streptococci*, and *Escherichia coli* are facultative anaerobes found in small numbers in the gut (Belizário & Napolitano, 2015). With the progress of research on the relationship between the microbiota and diseases, commensal intestinal bacteria have been investigated for their ability to modulate the host immune system, not only in healthy individuals but also in those who are suffering from a wide range of diseases (Carding et al., 2015; Sekirov et al., 2010). It has been revealed that commensal bacteria regulate regulatory T cells, type 3 innate lymphoid cells, and T helper 17 cells through the recognition of the bacteria themselves or their metabolites/products by the immune cells and greatly affect mucosal immunity (Hepworth et al., 2013, 2015). According to reports, any imbalance in the gut microbiome compositions might result in disorders, such as cancer, malignancy, IBD, irritable bowel syndrome, fatty liver diseases, obesity, type 2 diabetes mellitus, asthma, cardiovascular, psychiatric disorders, and immune-mediated diseases (Carding et al., 2015; Sánchez et al., 2017; Sekirov et al., 2010). Such modification of the gut microbiota is referred to as dysbiosis is of paramount importance as they play potential role in initiation and progression of several diseases in humans and animals (Azad et al., 2018). Moreover, several investigations based on both animal and clinical experimentations reported that the dysbiosis (abnormalities in the microbiota composition) can lead to allergic disorders through their impacts on immune responses. The associations of developmental/genetic/environmental effects contribute to different allergic diseases. Furthermore, the key role of microbiome in the development of allergic disorders is now well documented (Bunyavanich, 2019). A modified susceptibility to allergic disorders could therefore be related to the different microbial exposure in early childhood (Cahenzli et al., 2013). Moreover, the comparison of genetically similar populations in Russia and Finland supported more insights into the close relation between the allergy, environment, and host microbiome (Haahtela et al., 2015). Experiments on animals showed that the gut microbiota of mice with food allergy have a specific signature that could be linked to increased allergic susceptibility (Rivas et al., 2013). It has thus been documented that specific composition of microbiota associated to food allergy could lead to life-threatening anaphylaxis reaction and allergic sensitization. Several studies also showed that intestinal microbiota dysregulations of infants may contributed to the pathogenesis of allergy, although the accurate composition of the human intestinal microbiota associated with allergy still need to be clarified (Matsui et al., 2019). A study based on 454 sequencing of hypervariable V1−V3 regions of the 16S rRNA gene in the feces of 34 infants with food allergy explored the microbial composition and diversity among the atopic population. The results of this study highlighted significant changes in the fecal microbiota of infants suffering from food allergy, suggesting a possible interaction with the development of food allergy (Ling et al., 2014). Food allergies are reported frequently in preschool children of developing and developed countries with a prevalence reaching 7% and 10%, respectively (Kałużna-Czaplińska et al., 2017; Prescott et al., 2013). In the food allergy population, the concentration of *Actinobacteria*, *Bacteroidetes*, and *Proteobacteria* phyla significantly decreased, while the abundance of *Firmicutes* phylum dramatically increased. Furthermore, the phyla of Clostridiaceae were regularly detected in infants suffering from food allergy. Detailed microbiota analysis revealed that the dysbiosis of fecal microbiota is related to different food allergies and may play an important role in the progress of the disease. Another investigation also reported that infants and mice with food allergy had decreased IgA and increased IgE binding to fecal bacteria (Abdel-Gadir et al., 2019). Marschan et al. (2008) showed that probiotic bacteria consumption may lead to increased level of IL-10 and total IgA in in the plasma of children with an allergic predisposition in vivo (Marschan et al., 2008). Surprisingly, bacteriotherapy induced the upregualtion of the transcription factor ROR-γt by Treg cells in a MyD88-dependent manner. These results highlight the deficient and ineffective production of transcription factor ROR-γt by the microbiota of infants and mice affected by food allergy. However, the protection by bacteriotherapy is revoked following the removal of Rorc or Myd88 in Treg cells. Thus by stimulation of a pathway of MyD88/ROR-γt in nascent Treg cells, commensal microbiota is capable to alleviate food allergy, while, inversely, dysbiosis and microbial imbalance may develop the allergy (Abdel-Gadir et al., 2019; Aitoro et al., 2017). Therefore the development of the allergy could be related to a particular microbiota composition confirmed by the comparison of the fecal microbiota in a murine model of food allergy (Diesner et al., 2016; Hussain et al., 2019). Different animal studies investigated the possible association of food allergy with intestinal microbiota. For example, a study reported that germ-free (GF) mice are more likely susceptible to oral sensitization with cow's milk protein and ovalbumin compared to wild type control mice (Cahenzli et al., 2013). Moreover, mice with antibiotic-related modifications in their microbiota were more severely affected by food allergy when compared to untreated mice (Bashir et al., 2004). However, the regulation of the microbiota of GF mice with commensals, such as prebiotics and short-chain fatty acids or *Bacteroides fragilis* and *Clostridia*, promoted the induction of Treg cells and decrease allergic sensitization (Geuking et al., 2011; Lathrop et al., 2011; Smith et al., 2013). Interestingly, significant reduction in allergic diarrhea and increased levels of Treg cells were also reported among mice exposed to the human microbiota, thereby suggesting that protection or susceptibility to food allergy could be transmitted (Atarashi et al., 2013). In human, the pathogenesis of food allergy, atopic dermatitis and asthma has been associated with altered microbiota composition (Marrs et al., 2013). However, the human gut is a complex ecosystem in which the nutrients, microbes, and host cells interact extensively. All these interactions are known to have strong impact on host homeostasis and immunostasis, and hence essential for maintaining the health condition. Undeniably, further investigations are needed to determine the implication of different microbial species and their influence on the development of allergies.

11.5 Mother's microbiome and child health

The infant microbiota takes shape in early pregnancy and varies depending on maternal nutritional habits, infections, and gestational age. Furthermore, the delivery mode, as well as breastfeeding or formula feeding strongly contribute to the diversity of infant microbiota. Microbial species, such as *Propionibacterium*, *Escherichia*, *Shigella*, and

Enterobacteriaceae, have been identified in the placenta (Collado et al., 2016; Jiménez et al., 2008), *Bifidobacterium* and *Staphylococcus* in the meconium of neonates and *Fusobacterium nucleatum* and *Streptococcus* spp. in the amniotic fluid (Bearfield et al., 2002) of healthy pregnant women. The microbiota is established in early pregnancy and varies depending on gestational age as well as maternal infections and nutrition. In addition, breastfeeding or formula feeding and the mode of delivery are strongly involved in the diversity of infant microbiota, which further influences the immune system response. The effective role of probiotics has been reported in promoting premature infants' health, although the efficacy of single probiotic supplements is limited when compared to the use of a combination of several probiotics and prebiotics. Therefore a mixture of prebiotics and probiotics is proposed for optimal healing effects on premature infants (Chi et al., 2021). The role of the intestinal microbiota in the development of food allergy is important, especially in early age, due to the immaturity of the mucosal barrier and immune system (del Giudice et al., 2010). The oligosaccharides in human breast milk cause an increase in the number of beneficial bacteria (such as bifidobacteria and lactobacilli) in the gut microflora of infants that are breast-fed (Sherman et al., 2009). Though allergic mothers had significantly lower counts of bifidobacteria in their breast milk in comparison with nonallergic mothers and therefore their infants had concomitant lower amounts of bifidobacteria in their feces (Grönlund et al., 2007). Accordingly, a reduced ratio of bifidobacteria to clostridia has been reported in the gut microflora of allergic infants (Kalliomäki et al., 2001).

11.6 Clinical studies

There are a few well-designed experiments investigating the effects of probiotics and prebiotics in the prevention of allergy. The outcome of some clinical studies is summarized in Table 11.1.

In a randomized double-blind study, probiotic bacteria were given for 1 month before delivery to mothers and for 6 months to infants with a family history of allergy. The findings of this study highlighted the action of Th2-regulating microbes capable to stimulate regulatory T cells in the prevention of allergic diseases (Marschan et al., 2008). A cohort of 237 allergy-prone infants received a combination of 4 probiotic strains or placebos prenatally during 6 months from birth. The highest fecal IgA in the probiotics group was a marker of immune maturation, which was associated with reduced risk for atopic diseases during the first 2 years of life (Kukkonen et al., 2010).

11.6.1 Atopic eczema

A number of studies investigated the effects of prenatal and neonatal probiotics intake on eczema. It was shown that children with higher severity of symptoms and type 1 allergic sensitization (Rosenfeldt et al., 2003; Sistek et al., 2006; Viljanen et al., 2005) showed a better improvement in their eczema following probiotic consumption (Sistek et al., 2006; Weston et al., 2005). Some other studies evaluated the combined prenatal and postnatal probiotic treatment in children with a high risk of allergy as suggested by their family history. Different probiotic strains were experimented and some probiotics supplementations reduced symptoms associated to IgE-mediated atopic eczema symptoms (Abrahamsson et al., 2007; Kalliomäki et al., 2001; Wickens et al., 2008). Interestingly, breastfeeding during the first 3 months reduced the risks of eczema in atopic infants treated with LGG (Rautava et al., 2002). No significant change was observed in the majority of other studies, while promising results were obtained using *L. reuteri* (Abrahamsson et al., 2007) and *L. rhamnosus* HN001 (Wickens et al., 2008). *Bifidobacterium animalis* subsp. *lactis* HN019 intake had no significant effect on the occurrence of eczema in atopic infants (Wickens et al., 2008).

11.6.2 Food allergy

Only one study reported a remarkable decrease in sensitization to cow's milk among newborns with a high risk of allergy because of using during 1 year a nonhydrolyzed formula fermented with *Streptococcus thermophilus* 06 and *Bifidobacterium breve* C50 (Campeotto et al., 2011). A significant decline was also observed in the levels of specific IgE against numerous foods, including codfish, wheat flour, hen's eggs, peanuts, and soy flour. Another research showed that the addition of the probiotic LGG to the extensively hydrolyzed casein formula is able to accelerate immune tolerance acquisition in infants with cow's milk allergy (Paparo et al., 2019). The importance of the intestinal microbiota in the development of food allergy is important especially in early age, due to the immature mucosal barrier and immune system (Del Giudice & Belsky, 2010; del Giudice et al., 2010). The oligosaccharides in human breast milk cause an increase in the number of beneficial bacteria (such as bifidobacteria and lactobacilli) in the gut microflora of infants that are breast-fed (Sherman et al., 2009). Kuitunen et al. (2009) evaluated the role of probiotics in allergic

TABLE 11.1 The outcome of some clinical studies.

Author, year	Study details	Study population number of patients completed the follow-up Mean age	Intervention strain-dose (D)—start of treatment (S)—end of treatment (E)	Placebo	Outcomes evaluation	Results
Basturk et al. (2020)	Double-blind placebo-controlled study	48 infants in probiotic group and 52 in placebo group Mean age 12 months	*Lactobacillus rhamnosus* GG; D: 1×10^9 cfu/day each probiotic; S: 4 weeks	Dietary supplement without probiotics	Physical examination	Infants in the probiotic group have showed statistically significant improvement in symptoms of bloody stool, diarrhea, restiveness, and abdominal distension
D'Auria et al. (2020)	A randomized, double-blind, placebo-controlled trial	58 infants and young children (age 6–36 months) aged 6–36 months	*Lactobacillus paracasei* CBA L74; D: 8 g of *Lactobacillus paracasei* CBA L74; S: 12 weeks	Rice-dried powder	Gut microbiota, serum cytokines	Gut microbiota at the phylum and class taxonomic levels resulted very similar, at baseline and after intervention, in both groups. No significant differences for cytokines levels, no effective role in reducing the severity of atopic dermatitis
Rautava et al. (2012)	Prospective double-blind, randomized, controlled	High-risk infants for atopy 62 placebo 73 LPR + BL99970 ST11 + BL999 Mean age 2 years	*L. rhamnosus* LPR and *Bifidobacterium longum* BL999, *Lactobacillus paracasei* ST11, and *B. longum* BL999; D: 1×10^9 cfu/day each probiotic; S: 2 months before delivery; E: 2 months of age of breastfed infants	Dietary supplement without probiotics	Physical examination and skin prick test until 24 months of age	Modulating early host–microbe interaction by maternal probiotic intervention
Ou et al. (2012)	Prospective double-blind, randomized, controlled	High-risk infants for atopy 65 LGG 63 placebo Mean age 36 months	*Lactobacillus* GG; D: 1×10^{10} cfu/day; S: from gestational week 24; E: 6 months of age of infants	Microcrystalline cellulose	ISAAC questionnaire, physical examination, blood examinations (total and specific IgE)	No significant effects of prenatal and postnatal probiotics supplementation on sensitization, development of allergic diseases
Boyle et al. (2011)	Prospective double-blind, randomized, controlled	High-risk infants for atopy 103 + placebo 109 LGG Mean age 12 months	*L. rhamnosus* GG (LGG); D: 1.8×10^{10} cfu/day; S: from 36 weeks of gestation; E: until delivery	Maltodextrin	Physical examination, skin prick test only at 12 months, questionnaire about allergy and eczema symptoms	Prenatal probiotic treatment was not associated with reduced risk of eczema probiotic, placebo; or IgE-associated eczema

(Continued)

TABLE 11.1 (Continued)

Author, year	Study details	Study population number of patients completed the follow-up Mean age	Intervention strain-dose (D)—start of treatment (S)—end of treatment (E)	Placebo	Outcomes evaluation	Results
Kim et al. (2010)	Prospective double-blind, randomized, controlled	High-risk infants for atopy 35 placebo + 33 probiotics Mean age 12 months	*Bifidobacterium bifidum* BGN4, *Bifidobacterium lactis* AD011, and *Lactobacillus acidophilus* AD031; D: 1.6×10^9 cfu/day each strain; S: from 8 weeks before the expected delivery; E: from 4–6 months to infants	Maltodextrin	Physical examination, structured interviews, blood examinations (total and sIgE) at 12 months	Significantly decreased of eczema at 1 year in the probiotic group compared with the placebo group, significantly decreased of cumulative incidence of eczema during the first 12 months in probiotic group, no difference in serum total IgE level or the sensitization against food allergens between the two groups
Wickens et al. (2013)	Prospective double-blind, randomized, controlled	High-risk infants for atopy 150 placebo + 144 HN001 152 HN019 Mean age 2 years	*L. rhamnosus* HN001; D: 6 9×10^9 cfu/day *Bifidobacterium animalis* sub sp. *lactis* HN019 D: 9×10^9 cfu/day; S: from gestational week 35; E: 2 years of life	Dextran, salt, and a yeast extract	Physical examination, structured interviews and skin prick test only at 24 months of age	*Bifidobacterium animalis* subsp. *lactis* HN019 significantly lower cumulative prevalence of eczema and skin prick tests sensitization
Niers et al. (2009)	Prospective double-blind, randomized, controlled	High-risk infants for atopy 48 placebo + 50 probiotics Mean age 2 years	*Bifidobacterium bifidum* W23, *Bifidobacterium lactis* W52, *Lactobacillus lactis* W58; D: 1×10^9 cfu/day each strain; S: from 6 weeks before the expected delivery; E: 12 months of age of infants	Rice starch and maltodextran	Physical examination, questionnaire completed by parents, total, and sIgE, skin prick test only at 24 months of age	Combination of probiotic bacteria shows a preventive effect on the incidence of eczema in high-risk children
Böttcher et al. (2008)	Double-blind, randomized, placebo controlled	High-risk infants for atopy 51 *L. reuteri* + 53 placebo Mean age 2 years	*L. reuteri* strain (American Type Culture Collection 55730); D: not stated; S: from gestational week 36 until delivery; E: 12 months of age	Not stated	Physical examination, structured interviews, skin prick test, venus blood sample	Supplementation of *L. reuteri* during pregnancy was associated with low levels of TGF-β2 and slightly increased levels of IL-10 in colostrum, infants receiving breast milk with low levels of TGF-β2 were less likely to become sensitized during their first 2 years of life. The levels of total IgA, SIgA, TGF-β1, TNF, sCD14, and Na/K ratios in breast milk were not affected by the intake of *L. reuteri*

Study	Design	Population	Probiotic; Dose (D); Start (S); End (E)	Placebo	Assessment	Results
Huurre et al. (2008)	Prospective double-blind, randomized, controlled	High-risk infants for atopy 68 placebo + 72 probiotics Mean age 12 months	*L. rhamnosus* strain GG (ATCC 53103) and *Bifidobacterium lactis* Bb12; D: 1×10^{10} cfu/day each strain; S: from the first trimester of pregnancy; E: to the end of exclusive breastfeeding	Microcrystalline cellulose and dextrose anhydrate	Physical examination, skin prick test at 6–12 months	Probiotic supplementation had a protective effect against sensitization in infants with a high hereditary risk due to maternal sensitization. The concentration of TGF-$\beta2$ tended to be higher in the colostrum of the mothers in the probiotic group
Kopp et al. (2008)	Prospective double-blind, randomized, controlled	High-risk infants for atopy 44 placebo 50 LGG Mean age 24 months	*Lactobacillus* GG (American Type Culture Collection 53103); D: 5×10^9 cfu twice daily; S: 4–6 weeks before expected delivery; E: 6 months of age	Microcrystalline cellulose	Physical examination, structured interviews; total IgE and sensitization to an inhalant allergen at 2 years of age	No difference was observed between both groups in total immunoglobulin E concentrations or numbers of specific sensitization to inhalant allergens
Wickens et al. (2008)	Prospective double-blind, randomized, controlled	High-risk infants for atopy 150 placebo + 144 HN001 152 HN019 Mean age 2 years	*L. rhamnosus* HN001; D: 6.9×10^9 cfu/day *Bifidobacterium animalis* subsp. *lactis* HN019; D: 9×10^9 cfu/day; S: from gestational week 35; E: 2 years of life	Dextran, salt, and a yeast extract	Physical examination, structured interviews, and skin prick test only at 24 months of age	*L. rhamnosus* had a significantly reduced risk of eczema compared with placebo
Abrahamsson et al. (2007)	Prospective double-blind, randomized, controlled	High-risk infants for atopy 93 placebo + 95 *L. reuteri* Mean age 2 years	*L. reuteri* (American Type Culture Collection 55730); D: 1×10^8 cfu/day; S: from gestational week 36 until delivery; E: 12 months of age	Oil without bacteria	Physical examination, structured interviews, skin prick test (only at 6–12–24 months of age)	*L reuteri* group had less IgE-associated eczema during the second year of age, a reduced risk to develop later respiratory allergic disease
Taylor et al. (2007)	Prospective double-blind, randomized, controlled	High-risk infants for atopy 89 placebo + 89 LAVRI-A1 Mean age 12 months	*Lactobacillus acidophilus* LAVRI-A1; D: 3×10^9 cfu/day; S: from birth; E: 6 months of age	Maltodextrin	Physical examination, structured interviews, skin prick test (only at 12 months of age)	Fails to reduce the risk of atopic dermatitis and increases the risk of allergen sensitization in high-risk children
Rautava et al. (2002)	Prospective double-blind, randomized, controlled	High-risk infants for atopy 30 placebo + 27 LGG Mean age 24 months	*L. rhamnosus* strain GG (ATCC 53103); D: 2×10^{10} cfu/day; S: 4 weeks before the expected delivery	Microcrystalline cellulose	Physical examination, structured interviews	Immunomodulatory protection against atopic disease in the infant, elevated cord blood IgE concentration
Kalliomäki et al. (2001)	Prospective double-blind, randomized, controlled	High-risk infants for atopy 68 placebo + 64 LGG Mean age 24 months	*Lactobacillus* GG; D: 1×10^{10} cfu/day; S: 2–4 weeks before the expected delivery; E: 6 months of age	Microcrystalline cellulose	Physical examination, structured interviews; skin prick tests at ages 6, 12, and 24 months; total and ssIgE at ages 3, 12, and 24 months	The frequency of atopic eczema in the probiotic group was half that of the placebo group

diseases and IgE sensitization in a double-blinded, placebo-controlled study randomized study including 1223 mothers and their infants at high risk for allergy. Mothers received a probiotic mixture of two lactobacilli, bifidobacteria, and propionibacteria or placebo during the last month of pregnancy and the same mixture was administrated to infants from birth until their 6 months (Kuitunen et al., 2009). Infants also received a prebiotic galactooligosaccharide or placebo. They found no significant difference in frequencies of eczema, atopic eczema, allergic rhinitis, or asthma between groups, Although less IgE-associated allergic diseases occurred in cesarean delivered children receiving probiotics. In another study, 2 probiotic Lactobacillus strains (lyophilized *Lactobacillus rhamnosus* 19070−2 and *Lactobacillus reuteri* DSM 122460) were given in combination for 6 weeks to 1- to 13-year-old children with atopic dermatitis (Rosenfeldt et al., 2003).

11.7 Conclusions

A substantive number of studies showed the promising role of the neonatal and prenatal probiotics intake in the prevention of atopic eczema in infants. These beneficial effects have not been observed in other symptoms caused by food allergy where the majority of studies have not reported significant change following probiotics consumption. Further studies are necessary on other allergic conditions, such as allergic asthma and rhinitis requiring longer follow-up studies, preferably until adolescence. The working groups of the European Academy of Allergy and Clinical Immunology and the World Allergy Organization took similar positions, concluding that there is no sufficient evidence to support the use of probiotics in the prevention and treatment of allergic diseases. Some probiotics and symbiotic preparations have shown the ability to modulate the immune response in different allergic conditions. However, these effects appeared to be highly strain specific and should be confirmed in the context of further clinical studies at different perinatal stages.

References

Abdel-Gadir, A., et al. (2019). Microbiota therapy acts via a regulatory T cell MyD88/RORγt pathway to suppress food allergy. *Nature Medicine, 25,* 1164−1174.

Abrahamsson, T. R., et al. (2007). Probiotics in prevention of IgE-associated eczema: A double-blind, randomized, placebo-controlled trial. *The Journal of Allergy and Clinical Immunology, 119,* 1174−1180.

Abreu, M. T. (2010). Toll-like receptor signalling in the intestinal epithelium: How bacterial recognition shapes intestinal function. *Nature Reviews. Immunology, 10,* 131−144.

Adams, C. A. (2010). The probiotic paradox: Live and dead cells are biological response modifiers. *Nutrition Research Reviews, 23,* 37−46.

Adlerberth, I., & Wold, A. (2009). Establishment of the gut microbiota in Western infants. *Acta Paediatrica, 98,* 229−238.

Ahanchian, H., et al. (2016). Epidemiological survey of pediatric food allergy in Mashhad in Northeast Iran. *Electronic Physician, 8,* 1727.

Aitoro, R., et al. (2017). Gut microbiota as a target for preventive and therapeutic intervention against food allergy. *Nutrients, 9,* 672.

Amara, A., & Shibl, A. (2015). Role of Probiotics in health improvement, infection control and disease treatment and management. *Saudi Pharmaceutical Journal, 23,* 107−114.

Anukam, K. C., & Reid, G. (2007). Probiotics: 100 years (1907−2007) after Elie Metchnikoff's observation. *Communicating Current Research and Educational Topics and Trends in Applied Microbiology, 1,* 466−474.

Artiss, J. D., et al. (2006). The effects of a new soluble dietary fiber on weight gain and selected blood parameters in rats. *Metabolism: Clinical and Experimental, 55,* 195−202.

Atarashi, K., et al. (2013). Treg induction by a rationally selected mixture of Clostridia strains from the human microbiota. *Nature, 500,* 232−236.

Aureli, P., et al. (2011). Probiotics and health: An evidence-based review. *Pharmacological Research, 63,* 366−376.

Azad, M., et al. (2018). Probiotic species in the modulation of gut microbiota: An overview. *BioMed Research International*.

Bashir, M. E. H., et al. (2004). Toll-like receptor 4 signaling by intestinal microbes influences susceptibility to food allergy. *The Journal of Immunology, 172,* 6978−6987.

Basturk, A., et al. (2020). Investigation of the efficacy of *Lactobacillus rhamnosus* GG in infants with cow's milk protein allergy: A randomised double-blind placebo-controlled trial. *Probiotics and Antimicrobial Proteins, 12,* 138−143.

Bearfield, C., et al. (2002). Possible association between amniotic fluid micro-organism infection and microflora in the mouth. *BJOG: An International Journal of Obstetrics and Gynaecology, 109,* 527−533.

Belizário, J. E., & Napolitano, M. (2015). Human microbiomes and their roles in dysbiosis, common diseases, and novel therapeutic approaches. *Frontiers in Microbiology, 6,* 1050.

Bertelsen, R. J., et al. (2016). Use of probiotics and prebiotics in infant feeding. *Best Practice & Research. Clinical Gastroenterology, 30,* 39−48.

Böttcher, M. F., et al. (2008). Low breast milk TGF-32 is induced by Lactobacillus reuteri supplementation and associates with reduced risk of sensitization during infancy. *Pediatric Allergy and Immunology: Official Publication of the European Society of Pediatric Allergy and Immunology, 19,* 497−504.

Boyle, R., et al. (2009). Probiotics for the treatment of eczema: A systematic review. *Clinical and Experimental Allergy: Journal of the British Society for Allergy and Clinical Immunology, 39*, 1117–1127.

Boyle, R., et al. (2011). Lactobacillus GG treatment during pregnancy for the prevention of eczema: A randomized controlled trial. *Allergy, 66*, 509–516.

Boyle, R., & Tang, M. (2006). The role of probiotics in the management of allergic disease. *Clinical and Experimental Allergy: Journal of the British Society for Allergy and Clinical Immunology, 36*, 568–576.

Bron, P. A., et al. (2012). Emerging molecular insights into the interaction between probiotics and the host intestinal mucosa. *Nature Reviews. Microbiology, 10*, 66–78.

Bunyavanich, S. (2019). Food allergy: Could the gut microbiota hold the key? *Nature Reviews Gastroenterology & Hepatology, 16*, 201–202.

Cahenzli, J., et al. (2013). Intestinal microbial diversity during early-life colonization shapes long-term IgE levels. *Cell Host & Microbe, 14*, 559–570.

Campeotto, F., et al. (2011). A fermented formula in pre-term infants: Clinical tolerance, gut microbiota, down-regulation of faecal calprotectin and up-regulation of faecal secretory IgA. *The British Journal of Nutrition, 105*, 1843–1851.

Carding, S., et al. (2015). Dysbiosis of the gut microbiota in disease. *Microbial Ecology in Health and Disease, 26*, 26191.

Castellazzi, A. M., et al. (2013). Probiotics and food allergy. *Italian Journal of Pediatrics, 39*, 1–10.

Ceccarelli, G., et al. (2019). Challenges in the management of HIV infection: Update on the role of probiotic supplementation as a possible complementary therapeutic strategy for cART treated people living with HIV/AIDS. *Expert Opinion on Biological Therapy, 19*, 949–965.

Chi, C., et al. (2021). Effects of probiotics in preterm infants: A network meta-analysis. *Pediatrics, 147*.

Clancy, R. (2003). Immunobiotics and the probiotic evolution. *FEMS Immunology and Medical Microbiology, 38*, 9–12.

Collado, M. C., et al. (2016). Human gut colonisation may be initiated in utero by distinct microbial communities in the placenta and amniotic fluid. *Scientific Reports, 6*, 1–13.

Cruchet, S., et al. (2015). The use of probiotics in pediatric gastroenterology: A review of the literature and recommendations by Latin-American experts. *Pediatric Drugs, 17*, 199–216.

D'Auria, E., et al. (2020). Rice flour fermented with Lactobacillus paracasei CBA L74 in the treatment of atopic dermatitis in infants: A randomized, double-blind, placebo-controlled trial. *Pharmacological Research: The Official Journal of the Italian Pharmacological Society*, 105284.

Daliri, E. B.-M., et al. (2019). *Safety of probiotics in health and disease. The role of functional food security in global health* (pp. 603–622). Elsevier.

Del Giudice, M., & Belsky, J. (2010). Sex differences in attachment emerge in middle childhood: An evolutionary hypothesis. *Child Development Perspectives, 4*, 97–105.

del Giudice, M. M., et al. (2010). Food allergy and probiotics in childhood. *Journal of Clinical Gastroenterology, 44*, S22–S25.

Deshpande, G., et al. (2017). Benefits of probiotics in preterm neonates in low-income and medium-income countries: A systematic review of randomised controlled trials. *BMJ Open, 7*, e017638.

Deshpande, G., et al. (2018). Para-probiotics for preterm neonates—The next frontier. *Nutrients., 10*, 871.

Didari, T., et al. (2014). A systematic review of the safety of probiotics. *Expert Opinion on Drug Safety, 13*, 227–239.

Diesner, S. C., et al. (2016). A distinct microbiota composition is associated with protection from food allergy in an oral mouse immunization model. *Clinical Immunology, 173*, 10–18.

Doege, K., et al. (2012). Impact of maternal supplementation with probiotics during pregnancy on atopic eczema in childhood—a meta-analysis. *The British Journal of Nutrition, 107*, 1–6.

Donohue, D., & Salminen, S. (1996). Safety of probiotic bacteria. *Asia Pacific the Journal of Clinical Nutrition, 5*, 25–28.

Doron, S., & Snydman, D. R. (2015). Risk and safety of probiotics. *Clinical Infectious Diseases: An Official Publication of the Infectious Diseases Society of America, 60*, S129–S134.

Geuking, M. B., et al. (2011). Intestinal bacterial colonization induces mutualistic regulatory T cell responses. *Immunity, 34*, 794–806.

Ghosh, S., et al. (2004). Probiotics in inflammatory bowel disease: Is it all gut flora modulation? *Gut, 53*, 620–622.

Gibson, G. R. (1998). Dietary modulation of the human gut microflora using prebiotics. *The British Journal of Nutrition, 80*, S209–S212.

Grönlund, M. M., et al. (2007). Maternal breast-milk and intestinal bifidobacteria guide the compositional development of the Bifidobacterium microbiota in infants at risk of allergic disease. *Clinical and Experimental Allergy: Journal of the British Society for Allergy and Clinical Immunology, 37*, 1764–1772.

Gupta, V., & Garg, R. (2009). Probiotics. *Indian Journal of Medical Microbiology, 27*, 202.

Haahtela, T., et al. (2015). Hunt for the origin of allergy—Comparing the Finnish and Russian Karelia. *Clinical & Experimental Allergy, 45*, 891–901.

Hepworth, M. R., et al. (2013). Innate lymphoid cells regulate CD4 + T-cell responses to intestinal commensal bacteria. *Nature, 498*, 113–117.

Hepworth, M. R., et al. (2015). Group 3 innate lymphoid cells mediate intestinal selection of commensal bacteria-specific CD4 + T cells. *Science (New York, N.Y.), 348*, 1031–1035.

Hojsak, I., et al. (2010). Lactobacillus GG in the prevention of gastrointestinal and respiratory tract infections in children who attend day care centers: A randomized, double-blind, placebo-controlled trial. *Clinical Nutrition (Edinburgh, Scotland), 29*, 312–316.

Horrocks, J. C., & De Dombal, F. (1978). Clinical presentation of patients with "dyspepsia." Detailed symptomatic study of 360 patients. *Gut, 19*, 19–26.

Hussain, M., et al. (2019). High dietary fat intake induces a microbiota signature that promotes food allergy. *Journal of Allergy and Clinical Immunology, 144*, 157–170.e8.

Huurre, A., et al. (2008). Impact of maternal atopy and probiotic supplementation during pregnancy on infant sensitization: A double-blind placebo-controlled study. *Clinical and Experimental Allergy: Journal of the British Society for Allergy and Clinical Immunology, 38*, 1342–1348.

Irvine, S. L., et al. (2010). Probiotic yogurt consumption is associated with an increase of CD4 count among people living with HIV/AIDS. *Journal of Clinical Gastroenterology, 44*, e201–e205.

Jiménez, E., et al. (2008). Is meconium from healthy newborns actually sterile? *Research in Microbiology, 159*, 187–193.

Kalliomäki, M., et al. (2001). Distinct patterns of neonatal gut microflora in infants in whom atopy was and was not developing. *The Journal of Allergy and Clinical Immunology, 107*, 129–134.

Kałużna-Czaplińska, J., et al. (2017). Is there a relationship between intestinal microbiota, dietary compounds, and obesity? *Trends in Food Science & Technology, 70*, 105–113.

Kamada, N., et al. (2013). Role of the gut microbiota in immunity and inflammatory disease. *Nature Reviews. Immunology, 13*, 321–335.

Kanauchi, O., et al. (2018). Probiotics and paraprobiotics in viral infection: Clinical application and effects on the innate and acquired immune systems. *Current Pharmaceutical Design, 24*, 710–717.

Kim, J. Y., et al. (2010). Effect of probiotic mix (Bifidobacterium bifidum, Bifidobacterium lactis, Lactobacillus acidophilus) in the primary prevention of eczema: A double-blind, randomized, placebo-controlled trial. *Pediatric Allergy and Immunology: Official Publication of the European Society of Pediatric Allergy and Immunology, 21*, e386–e393.

Klaenhammer, T. R., et al. (2012). The impact of probiotics and prebiotics on the immune system. *Nature Reviews. Immunology, 12*, 728–734.

Kopp, M. V., et al. (2008). Randomized, double-blind, placebo-controlled trial of probiotics for primary prevention: No clinical effects of Lactobacillus GG supplementation. *Pediatrics, 121*, e850–e856.

Kuitunen, M., et al. (2009). Probiotics prevent IgE-associated allergy until age 5 years in cesarean-delivered children but not in the total cohort. *The Journal of Allergy and Clinical Immunology, 123*, 335–341.

Kukkonen, K., et al. (2010). High intestinal IgA associates with reduced risk of IgE-associated allergic diseases. *Pediatric Allergy and Immunology: Official Publication of the European Society of Pediatric Allergy and Immunology, 21*, 67–73.

Lathrop, S. K., et al. (2011). Peripheral education of the immune system by colonic commensal microbiota. *Nature, 478*, 250–254.

Lavelle, E. C., et al. (2010). The role of TLRs, NLRs, and RLRs in mucosal innate immunity and homeostasis. *Mucosal Immunology, 3*, 17–28.

Lederberg, J., & McCray, A. T. (2001). Ome SweetOmics—A genealogical treasury of words. *The Scientist, 15*, 8.

Lehtoranta, L., et al. (2020). Role of probiotics in stimulating the immune system in viral respiratory tract infections: A narrative review. *Nutrients, 12*, 3163.

Lilly, D. M., & Stillwell, R. H. (1965). Probiotics: Growth-promoting factors produced by microorganisms. *Science (New York, N.Y.), 147*, 747–748.

Ling, Z., et al. (2014). Altered fecal microbiota composition associated with food allergy in infants. *Applied and Environmental Microbiology, 80*, 2546–2554.

Marchesi, J. R., & Ravel, J. (2015). *The vocabulary of microbiome research: A proposal*. Springer.

Marrs, T., et al. (2013). Is there an association between microbial exposure and food allergy? A systematic review. *Pediatric Allergy and Immunology, 24*, 311–320.e8.

Marschan, E., et al. (2008). Probiotics in infancy induce protective immune profiles that are characteristic for chronic low-grade inflammation. *Clinical and Experimental Allergy: Journal of the British Society for Allergy and Clinical Immunology, 38*, 611–618.

Matsui, S., et al. (2019). Dysregulation of intestinal microbiota elicited by food allergy induces IgA-mediated oral dysbiosis. *Infection and Immunity, 88*.

Maynard, C. L., et al. (2012). Reciprocal interactions of the intestinal microbiota and immune system. *Nature, 489*, 231–241.

Milani, C., et al. (2017). The first microbial colonizers of the human gut: Composition, activities, and health implications of the infant gut microbiota. *Microbiology and Molecular Biology Reviews: MMBR, 81*.

Mojgani, N., et al. (2020). Immune modulatory capacity of probiotic lactic acid bacteria and applications in vaccine development. *Beneficial Microbes, 11*, 213–226.

Morais, M. B. D., & Jacob, C. M. A. (2006). The role of probiotics and prebiotics in pediatric practice. *Jornal de Pediatria, 82*, S189–S197.

Niers, L., et al. (2009). The effects of selected probiotic strains on the development of eczema (the PandA study). *Allergy, 64*, 1349–1358.

Novik, G., & Savich, V. (2020). Beneficial microbiota. Probiotics and pharmaceutical products in functional nutrition and medicine. *Microbes and Infection, 22*, 8–18.

Ou, C. Y., et al. (2012). Prenatal and postnatal probiotics reduces maternal but not childhood allergic diseases: A randomized, double-blind, placebo-controlled trial. *Clinical and Experimental Allergy: Journal of the British Society for Allergy and Clinical Immunology, 42*, 1386–1396.

Paparo, L., et al. (2019). Randomized controlled trial on the influence of dietary intervention on epigenetic mechanisms in children with cow's milk allergy: The EPICMA study. *Scientific Reports, 9*, 1–10.

Prescott, S. L., et al. (2013). A global survey of changing patterns of food allergy burden in children. *World Allergy Organization Journal, 6*, 1–12.

Racedo, S., et al. (2006). Lactobacillus casei administration reduces lung injuries in a Streptococcus pneumoniae infection in mice. *Microbes and Infection, 8*, 2359–2366.

Rautava, S., et al. (2002). Probiotics during pregnancy and breast-feeding might confer immunomodulatory protection against atopic disease in the infant. *The Journal of Allergy and Clinical Immunology, 109*, 119–121.

Rautava, S., et al. (2012). Microbial contact during pregnancy, intestinal colonization and human disease. *Nature Reviews Gastroenterology & Hepatology, 9*, 565.

Rivas, M. N., et al. (2013). A microbiota signature associated with experimental food allergy promotes allergic sensitization and anaphylaxis. *Journal of Allergy and Clinical Immunology, 131*, 201–212.

Rizzello, V., et al. (2011). Role of natural killer and dendritic cell crosstalk in immunomodulation by commensal bacteria probiotics. *Journal of Biomedicine and Biotechnology*.

Rosenfeldt, V., et al. (2003). Effect of probiotic Lactobacillus strains in children with atopic dermatitis. *The Journal of Allergy and Clinical Immunology, 111*, 389–395.

Sánchez, B., et al. (2017). Probiotics, gut microbiota, and their influence on host health and disease. *Molecular Nutrition & Food Research, 61*, 1600240.

Sanders, M. E., et al. (2007). Probiotics: Their potential to impact human health. *Council for Agricultural Science and Technology Issue Paper, 36*, 1–20.

Saxelin, M. (1997). Lactobacillus GG—A human probiotic strain with thorough clinical documentation. *Food Reviews International, 13*, 293–313.

Schley, P., & Field, C. (2002). The immune-enhancing effects of dietary fibres and prebiotics. *The British Journal of Nutrition, 87*, S221–S230.

Sekirov, I., et al. (2010). Gut microbiota in health and disease. *Physiological Reviews*.

Sharma, P., et al. (2014). Antibiotic resistance among commercially available probiotics. *Food Research International, 57*, 176–195.

Sherman, P. M., et al. (2009). Potential roles and clinical utility of prebiotics in newborns, infants, and children: Proceedings from a global prebiotic summit meeting, New York City, June 27–28, 2008. *The Journal of Pediatrics, 155*, S61–S70.

Sheth, M. K., & Gupta, N. (2014). metabolic effect of FOS (fructooligosaccharide) in terms of gut incretin (glp-1) gut microflora and weight reduction in obese adults. *International Journal of Applied Biology and Pharmaceutical Technology, 5*, 256–264.

Shokryazdan, P., et al. (2017). Effects of prebiotics on immune system and cytokine expression. *Medical Microbiology and Immunology, 206*, 1–9.

Silva, A., et al. (1999). Protective effect of bifidus milk on the experimental infection with Salmonella enteritidis subsp. typhimurium in conventional and gnotobiotic mice. *Journal of Applied Microbiology, 86*, 331–336.

Sistek, D., et al. (2006). Is the effect of probiotics on atopic dermatitis confined to food sensitized children? *Clinical and Experimental Allergy: Journal of the British Society for Allergy and Clinical Immunology, 36*, 629–633.

Smith, P. M., et al. (2013). The microbial metabolites, short-chain fatty acids, regulate colonic Treg cell homeostasis. *Science (New York, N.Y.), 341*, 569–573.

Snydman, D. R. (2008). The safety of probiotics. *Clinical Infectious Diseases, 46*, S104–S111.

Stambler, I. (2015). Elie Metchnikoff—The founder of longevity science and a founder of modern medicine: In honor of the 170th anniversary. *Advances in Gerontology, 5*, 201–208.

Szajewska, H., & Kołodziej, M. (2015). Systematic review with meta-analysis: Saccharomyces boulardii in the prevention of antibiotic-associated diarrhoea. *Alimentary Pharmacology & Therapeutics, 42*, 793–801.

Taylor, A. L., et al. (2007). Probiotic supplementation for the first 6 months of life fails to reduce the risk of atopic dermatitis and increases the risk of allergen sensitization in high-risk children: A randomized controlled trial. *The Journal of Allergy and Clinical Immunology, 119*, 184–191.

Temmerman, R., et al. (2003). Identification and antibiotic susceptibility of bacterial isolates from probiotic products. *International Journal of Food Microbiology, 81*, 1–10.

Vieira, A. T., et al. (2013). The role of probiotics and prebiotics in inducing gut immunity. *Frontiers in Immunology, 4*, 445.

Viljanen, M., et al. (2005). Probiotics in the treatment of atopic eczema/dermatitis syndrome in infants: A double-blind placebo-controlled trial. *Allergy, 60*, 494–500.

Villena, J., et al. (2014). Immunobiotic Lactobacillus rhamnosus strains differentially modulate antiviral immune response in porcine intestinal epithelial and antigen presenting cells. *BMC Microbiology, 14*, 1–14.

Wang, X., et al. (2017). Oral administration of Lactobacillus paracasei L9 attenuates PM2.5-induced enhancement of airway hyperresponsiveness and allergic airway response in murine model of asthma. *PLoS One, 12*, e0171721.

Wang, Y., et al. (2014). Efficacy of probiotic therapy in full-term infants with critical illness. *Asia Pacific Journal of Clinical Nutrition, 23*, 575.

Wang, Y., et al. (2016). Probiotics for prevention and treatment of respiratory tract infections in children: A systematic review and *meta*-analysis of randomized controlled trials. *Medicine, 95*.

Weston, S., et al. (2005). Effects of probiotics on atopic dermatitis: A randomised controlled trial. *Archives of Disease in Childhood, 90*, 892–897.

Wickens, K., et al. (2008). A differential effect of 2 probiotics in the prevention of eczema and atopy: A double-blind, randomized, placebo-controlled trial. *The Journal of Allergy and Clinical Immunology, 122*, 788–794.

Wickens, K., et al. (2013). Early supplementation with Lactobacillus rhamnosus HN 001 reduces eczema prevalence to 6 years: Does it also reduce atopic sensitization? *Clinical and Experimental Allergy: Journal of the British Society for Allergy and Clinical Immunology, 43*, 1048–1057.

Yahfoufi, N., et al. (2018). Role of probiotics and prebiotics in immunomodulation. *Current Opinion in Food Science, 20*, 82–91.

Yeretssian, G. (2012). Effector functions of NLRs in the intestine: Innate sensing, cell death, and disease. *Immunologic Research, 54*, 25–36.

Zhang, L. L., et al. (2010). Oral Bifidobacterium modulates intestinal immune inflammation in mice with food allergy. *Journal of Gastroenterology and Hepatology, 25*, 928–934.

Chapter 12

Probiotics and prebiotics in the suppression of autoimmune diseases

Prashant S. Giri*, Firdosh Shah* and Mitesh Kumar Dwivedi
C.G. Bhakta Institute of Biotechnology, Faculty of Science, Uka Tarsadia University, Maliba Campus, Bardoli, India

12.1 Introduction

The human gastrointestinal tract (GI) consists of huge population of commensal microorganisms, which are rich in the terms of complexity of the community (Ley et al., 2008). Along with the host, even the gut microbiota are said to be evolved over years to provide health benefits, such as protection against pathogens, digestion, detoxification, and regulation of the immune system (Ley et al., 2008; Wu & Wu, 2012). Immune system holds the balance between maintenance of tolerance capacity of healthy self-tissue and the eradication of invading pathogens. However, this mechanism of self-tolerance faces defeat, when we consider the cases of individuals ailing through autoimmune diseases as it inadvertently strikes and disrupts healthy self-tissue (Westerberg et al., 2008).

It would not be surprising to mention that certain members of the gut microbiota are linked to autoimmune disorders, as there is a close interplay between gut microbiota and the immune system of host. The advancements in "next-generation" sequencing technology have provided a ground-breaking foundation to have more deeper penetration into the culture-independent microbial analysis, which provides an ease in characterizing commensal microorganisms (Turnbaugh et al., 2007). Moreover, researchers have begun to penetrate deep into understanding cellular and molecular mechanism through the help of animal models to reveal interactions between the mucosal immune system and commensal microbes in autoimmunity.

The commensal bacteria emergence begins shortly within the host after the birth where they simply colonize and gradually proliferate into a diverse ecosystem. Over the years, this symbiotic relationship between host–bacteria has come out as beneficial. Probiotic bacteria not only provide essential nutrients by metabolizing indigestible compounds but also serve as savior against opportunistic pathogens (Petschow et al., 2013). These probiotic bacteria feed on specific substrates known as "prebiotics," which are the indigestible food ingredients, which upon metabolization stimulates the growth and activity of advantageous bacteria. Dietary fibers, such as xyloglucans, oligosaccharides, and fructooligosaccharides (FOS), act as a substrate, which stimulates the proliferation of intestinal microbiota. Among these prebiotics, FOS and oligosaccharides are considered as an important nondigestible fibers that are responsible for promoting growth of probiotics strains like *Lactobacilli* and *Bifidobacterium* (Yousefi et al., 2019). These probiotics are considered essential to provide immunity and maintain homeostasis within the host via production of short-chain fatty acids (SCFAs), such as acetate, butyrate, and propionate (Yousefi et al., 2019).

Currently, the research has been more focused on the natural mechanisms for managing, treating, and curing the human diseases due to the several side effects of the chemotherapeutic agents and synthetic drugs (Dwivedi, 2018). Henceforth, the chapter discuss here rapid advancements made in the direction of host–microbiota interaction with particular focus on the role of probiotics and prebiotics in the suppression of autoimmune diseases, such as rheumatoid arthritis (RA), systemic lupus erythrematosus (SLE), type-1 diabetes, multiple sclerosis (MS), and cystic fibrosis (CF), and in maintaining immune homeostasis.

---

*These authors contributed equally to this work.

12.2 Autoimmune diseases

Autoimmune diseases are a group of medical disorders, such as RA, SLE, and MS, in which the host's immune system fails to recognize the normal constituents of cells as "self," which results in an aberrant immune response against its own tissue (Wang, Wang et al., 2015). Presently in almost all autoimmune disorders a definitive cure is lacking. There is temporary symptomatic relief and arrest in the progression of lesions upon pharmacological treatment, but it fails to provide the complete remission (Chandrashekara, 2012). Therefore emerging studies are targeting on different treatment modalities apart from pharmacological approach, among which probiotics mediated immune suppression of autoimmune disorders is the blooming field of interest within the research community. Here, in this chapter, we highlight various studies, which have put forth the clinical evidence supporting role of probiotics and prebiotics in the amelioration of autoimmune disorders.

12.2.1 Rheumatoid arthritis

RA is a chronic systemic inflammatory autoimmune disease affecting larger proportion of individuals globally (Carbone et al., 2020). If we gaze upon the standard treatment, it is mostly based on antirheumatic drugs. Since the past decades several studies have been focused on exploring the role of diet in the origination and development of the rheumatic diseases. It has been suggested that practicing a healthy dietary habits and optimal consumption of foods, which are rich in bioactive compounds, such as omega-3 fatty acids and antioxidants, are considered to be lower risk of developing these diseases and also remarkably alter the clinical severity (Oliviero et al., 2015). This clearly indicates that there is an indispensable link between the clinical features of patient, gut microbiota and the diet. Therefore manipulating the gut microbiota may result into the modulation of disease progression. In accordance to this, an emerging aspect of probiotics can be attributed in RA (Hill et al., 2014). There are various studies, which have pointed out diverse strains of probiotics, such as *Lactobacilli*, *Bifidobacterium*, and *Streptococci*, which upon administration either singly or in the mixed culture resulted in the remission of the clinical severity of RA (Mandel et al., 2010; Vaghef-Mehrabany et al., 2014).

12.2.2 Systemic lupus erythematosus

Systemic lupus erythematosus (SLE) is a chronic autoimmune disease, which triggers the formation and deposition of immune complexes that causes destruction in various organs and tissues due to the aberrant production of autoantibodies, leading to the abnormal functioning of B lymphocytes (La Paglia et al., 2017). However, the exact etiology behind the cause is yet to be explored, but the most widely considered reason for the genesis of SLE is genetic and environmental factors of an individual, which result in the disruption of self-tolerance and generation of autoreactive lymphocytes (La Paglia et al., 2017). Apart from this, Lupus is also associated with the several changes in gut microbiota, which are correlated with the manifestation of pathogenesis. Upon deep analysis, the role of microbiota in SLE reveals that there is a clear increase in *Bacteroidetes*, *Propionibacterium*, and *Actinobacteria* within the SLE patients (He et al., 2016). Emerging studies suggest that an intestinal dysbiosis is observed within the SLE patients due to alteration within the bacterial genera, such as *Bifidobacterium*, *Dialister*, *Psuedobutyvibrio*, *Roseburia*, *Lactobacillus*, *Mollicutes*, *Cryptophyta*, and *Faecalobacterium*, which were reduced in the SLE patients, whereas on the other hand bacterial genera, such as *Klebsiella*, *Rhodococcus*, *Flavonifractor*, *Eggerthella*, *Blautia*, and *Eubacterium*, were increased within SLE patients (He et al., 2016; Li et al., 2019; Luo et al., 2018). A previous study on retinoic acid administration within lupus-like animal model demonstrated restoration within *Lactobacillus* species along with improvement in lupus symptoms, suggesting the role of probiotics in the amelioration of inflammation within SLE patients (Zhang et al., 2014). The SLE animal model studies showed remission in the symptoms upon oral administration of probiotics, such as *Lactobacillus paracasei* GMNL-32 and *Lactobacillus reuteri* GMNL-89; however, so far there are no clinical trials reported for investigating the therapeutic role of probiotics in the SLE patients (Hsu et al., 2017; Tzang et al., 2017).

12.2.3 Type 1 diabetes mellitus

Type 1 diabetes mellitus (T1DM) is a chronic autoimmune disease responsible for pancreatic beta (β)-cell destruction, leading to extrinsic insulin dependence to manage blood glucose levels (Hara et al., 2013). Both genetic and environmental factors are considered responsible for causing an aggressive adaptive immune response against β cells through immune system malfunction in T1DM (Rewers & Ludvigsson, 2016). Over the years, existence of T1DM is seen to be consistently increased globally and unsuccessful treatment or therapeutic strategies could be blame for the same. According to a recent report on global diabetes prevalence, it has been stated that there are nearly 9.3% of population ailing through diabetes in 2019 and it has been estimated to rise up to 10.2% by 2030 (Saeedi et al., 2019). Dysbiosis among gut microbiota is often observed in the cases of T1DM, mostly those that are detected with belligerent and adverse immune response due to positive multiple autoantibodies (Vatanen et al., 2018). The interrelated physiological functions make more sense that gut microbes share close interaction with T cells. Several studies revealed potential interactions between immune mechanisms and gut microbiota, which are involved in the genesis of T1DM. Therefore it clearly reflects prospects of utilizing probiotics and prebiotics intervention in the amelioration of T1DM. Although various reports on animal and human models have shown to improve the clinical symptoms of T1DM, so far no precise mechanisms are proposed to explain the underlying interaction between them. These studies are discussed in the later section of this chapter.

12.2.4 Multiple sclerosis

MS is considered to be chronic, inflammatory, demyelinating, and autoimmune neurological disorder majorly affecting central nervous system (CNS) that results in the symptoms, such as depression, bowel dysfunction, vision loss, and cognitive defects due to immune reactions against myelin proteins and gangliosides (Polman et al., 2011). Around 2.5 million individuals are affected by MS globally (Polman et al., 2011). There are several factors, which are considered responsible for the initiation of MS, which includes intestinal dysbiosis, vitamin D deficiency, a hypercaloric diet, and viral infection, but major factors responsible for triggering MS are genetic and environmental factors (Milo & Kahana, 2010). Studies have suggested that the gut microbiota may also be involved in the regulation of immune system and metabolism of the host (Wu & Wu, 2012). Therefore gut microbiota could be considered as an indispensable target for the management and prevention of the inflammatory and autoimmune diseases, including MS (Vieira et al., 2014). Accumulating evidence on bidirectional relationship between gut microbiota and CNS suggested the influence on the modulation of immune diseases on both human and animal studies of MS (Cekanaviciute et al., 2017). Studies have highlighted an interesting aspect of diet and gut microbiome in the modulation of MS (Salehipour et al., 2017; Tankou et al., 2018; van den Hoogen et al., 2017). Moreover, studies have revealed that probiotics, such as *Lactobacillus* and *Bifidobacterium*, possess substantial health-promoting properties, which could efficiently modulate MS disease (Salehipour et al., 2017; Tankou et al., 2018). These probiotics produce SCFAs, which in turn reduce gut permeability and decrease inflammation (Yadav et al., 2013). Presently animal studies are being focused to assess the role of probiotics in the amelioration of MS. Administration of VSL3 probiotics has been shown to impart beneficial effects on the immune and inflammatory responses within MS patients (Tankou et al., 2018). However, despite various attempts on evaluating effects of probiotics' administration on animal and human subjects, the exact mechanism behind this remains largely unexplained.

12.2.5 Cystic fibrosis

CF is a life-threatening genetic disease, which affects approximately 70,000 children and adults worldwide due to a mutation caused in transmembrane conductance regulator, which predominantly affects the lungs, gastrointestinal tract, pancreas, and liver (CF Foundation, 2021). Individuals with CF face deprived lung function due to improper growth and nutritional status (Jadin et al., 2011). Presently only half of people with CF represent adequate nutritional status (Turck et al., 2016). Despite the case that modern era has come up with the new aspects of nutrition and pulmonary care, still many children with CF do not meet up to catch-up the level of weight gain (Jadin et al., 2011). Previous studies have suggested the potential role of intestinal dysbiosis in CF patients (Nielsen et al., 2016). Currently, there is a lack of information regarding the developmental pathway of gut microbiota in early CF (Hoen et al., 2015). Dehydrated, acid luminal environment is considered to alter gut microbiota in CF (Lee et al., 2012). Inclusion of large amount of calories and fats in a diet or else frequent antibiotic therapy has been suggested to contribute to the imbalance of gut flora further leading to an intestinal inflammation (Duytschaever et al., 2011). As far as probiotics are concerned, there are not enough reports, which could suggest the role of probiotics in the amelioration of CF. Moreover, the mechanism of action of probiotics within CF individuals remains largely unexplained.

12.3 Relationship between gut microbiota and immune system

In past decades, studies focusing on the interactions between microbiota and the host immune system have revealed the fundamental importance of the microbiome in shaping host immune responses, affecting susceptibility against immune-mediated and infectious diseases (Dwivedi et al., 2017). Intestinal immune system has a remarkable feature of maintaining immune tolerance by enormously supporting the proliferation of harmless microorganisms in one hand while actively generating immune responses upon pathogenic microbes encounter (Mowat, 2018). In a healthy condition, immune responses within host are strictly compartmentailzed to the mucosal surface (Konrad et al., 2006). During an inflammatory state, MUC2 (a hyperglycosylated mucin) resulted in the immunogenicity constrainment of the intestinal antigens through imprinting enteric dendritic cells (DCs) (Belkaid & Naik, 2013; Shan et al., 2013). Microbial signals resulted in the upregulation of tight junctions and associated cytoskeletal proteins via promoting fortification of epithelial barrier (Bansal et al., 2010). Moreover, antimicrobial peptides (AMPs) and IgA antibodies were seen to maintain mucosal barrier function (Peterson et al., 2007). Thus intestinal DCs have been suggested to play an indispensable role in promoting the compartmentalization of gut microbiota through various mechanisms of antigen presentation (Macpherson & Uhr, 2004).

12.3.1 Link between gut microbiota and innate immunity

There is a bidirectional relationship between innate immunity and gut microbiota (Fig. 12.1). Antimicrobial peptides produced by intestinal microbiota play a crucial role in the maintenance of immune homeostasis (Ehmann et al., 2019). Pattern recognition receptors, such as toll-like receptors (TLRs), are expressed to sense microbial signals in case of infection, which provide protective immune response. TLRs are described as crucial proteins, which not only provide defense against pathogens but also maintain the tissue integrity while regulating the abundance of commensal microorganisms (Price et al., 2018). *Bacteroides fragilis* is among a well-studied commensal microbe, which produces polysaccharide A (PSA) that promotes symbiosis and host immunity (Ramakrishna et al., 2019). According to a study, MyD88-deficient mice model showed an altered microbial composition (Wang, Wang et al., 2015). The MyD88 acts as an adapter for innate immune receptors that induces interleukin (IL)-1 and IL-18, which further aid in recognizing

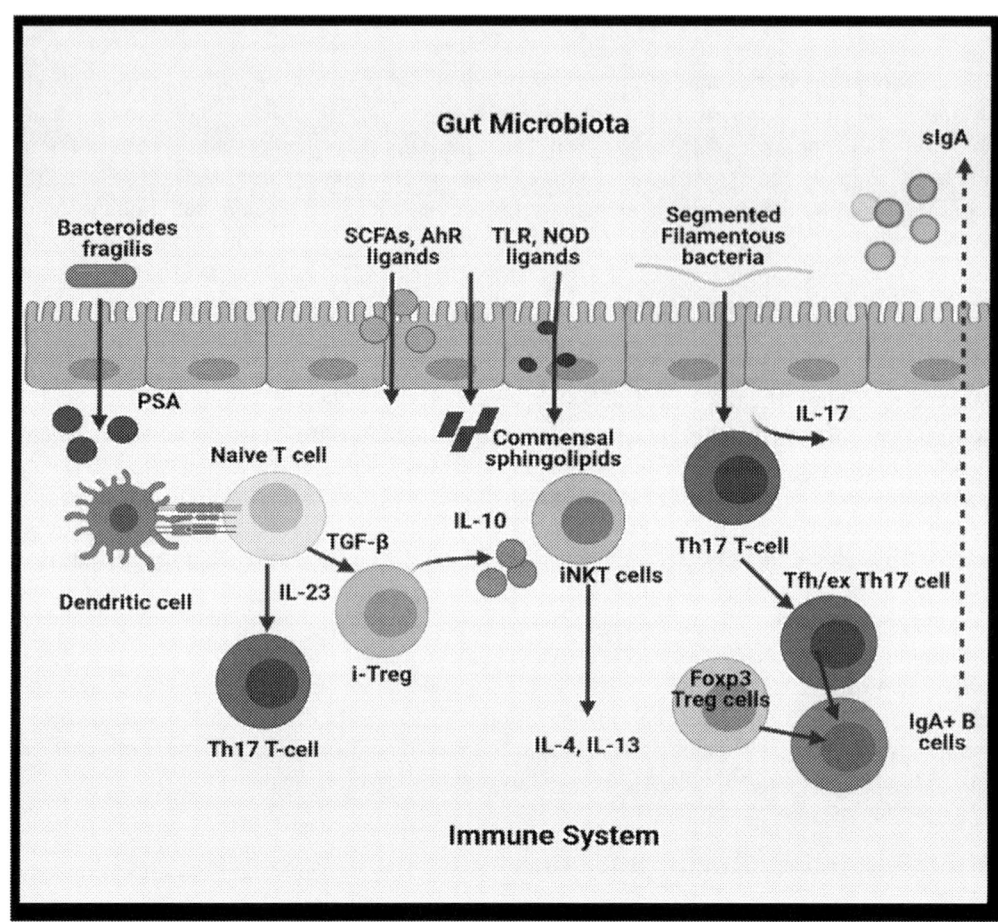

FIGURE 12.1 Relationship link between gut microbiota and immune system.

signaling pathways and microbial signals (Wang, Charbonnier, et al., 2015). Moreover, MyD88 limits the number of surface-associated gram-positive bacteria and regulates epithelial expression of different AMPs. Apart from this, MyD88 is also suggested to play an important function in T-cell differentiation and T helper 17 (Th17) cells' expansion by maintaining microbial homeostasis (Wang, Charbonnier, et al., 2015) (Fig. 12.1).

TLR and NOD ligand metabolites (e.g., SCFA, AhR ligands) produced by gut microbiota act on the intestinal immune cells. Production of B cells and secretory IgA is mediated by Foxp3$^+$ Treg cells and Tfh/ex-Th17 cells, which not only contribute in the compartmentalization of commensal microbiota but also aid in maintaining homeostasis. Differentiation of CD4$^+$ Th17 cells is promoted by the intestinal colonization of segmented filamentous bacteria. Intestinal colonization of *B. fragilis* promotes differentiation of CD4$^+$ T cell and maintains a balance between Th1 and Th2 via PSA. PSA is taken by lamina propia DCs followed by its presentation to naive CD4$^+$ T cells. This further activates TGF-β, which leads to the differentiation of iTreg cells.

Emerging studies have revealed the role of macrophages and monocytes in maintaining commensal microbiota due to their innate immune effector nature (Mosser & Edwards, 2008). Polysaccharides derived from intestinal microbiota have been reported to induce an antiinflammatory gene within murine intestinal macrophages (Danne et al., 2017). Moreover, SCFAs, such as butyrate, have been shown to enhance antimicrobial host defense through monocyte/macrophage differentiation via promoting the inhibition of histone deacetylase 3 (Schulthess et al., 2019).

12.3.2 Link between gut microbiota and adaptive immunity

Along with the innate immune functions, host–microbiota interactions are also considered to play an essential function in the adaptive immune system of the host. B cells, which are one of the crucial mediators of gut homeostasis, produce enormous amount of IgA antibodies' responses to the commensal organisms (Peterson et al., 2007). The T-cell-dependent production of IgA plays an indispensable role in shaping gut microbial communities (Fig. 12.1). This relationship between intestinal IgA and microbiota was reported to maintain both balanced and diversified microbiome, which further aids the expansion of FOXP3$^+$ regulatory T (Treg) cells regulating homeostasis (Kawamoto et al., 2014; Sterlin et al., 2020; Sutherland et al., 2016). Studies suggest that GATA4-related repression of metabolic functions depicts alteration within metabolic absorption (Shulzhenko et al., 2011). Cytokine RANKL expressing mesenchymal cells was reported to act as an intestinal M cell inducers, which resulted in the diversification of gut microbiota and promoted the IgA production (Nagashima et al., 2017).

Previously, several studies have demonstrated relationship link between CD4$^+$ Treg cells and gut microbiota. According to a study on germ-free mice, the absence of intestinal CD4$^+$ Treg cells differentiation was shown due to the lack of bacterial consortium responsible for fermenting dietary fiber into SCFAs (Arpaia et al., 2013; Atarashi et al., 2011; Smith et al., 2013). Th17 cell populations are among the most widely studied subsets of T cells as they are responsible in contributing to both inflammatory disorders and host protection (Miossec & Kolls, 2012). *Citrobacter*-induced Th17 cells are considered as a key player in flaring up inflammatory cytokines whereas Th17 cells produced by segmented filamentous bacteria are noninflammatory (Omenetti et al., 2019). Apart from Th17 cells, studies have also highlighted the role of follicular helper T cells (Tfh) in maintaining microbial homeostasis. Reports suggest that impairment within Tfh cells due to the absence of expression within ATP-gated ionotropic P2RX7 receptor or programmed cell death 1 receptor (PD-1) resulted in the alteration in gut microbial composition (Proietti et al., 2014). This impaired Tfh cells' differentiation can be restored by activating MyD88 signaling through administrating TLR2 agonists (Kubinak et al., 2015). Thus the relationship between Tfh and gut microbiota may be considered in autoimmune diseases as well (Teng et al., 2016).

Furthermore, emerging studies have revealed the underline influence of tissue resident DCs upon intestinal microbiota. A recent study on DCs has suggested the crucial role of Syk kinase-coupled signaling pathway in the microbiota-induced production of IL-17 and IL-22 by CD4$^+$ T cells (Martínez-López et al., 2019). In another study, DC-specific NF-κB-inducing kinase was reported to alter intestinal IgA secretion and microbial homeostasis (Jie et al., 2018). Moreover, gut microbiota are considered responsible for affecting phenotypic and physiological aspects of invariant natural killer T cells in mice (Gerhard et al., 2012) (Fig. 12.1).

12.4 Gut microbiota associated with autoimmune diseases

Around 100 trillion microorganisms from more than 500 bacterial genera make up the gut microbiota composition in humans (Khan & Wang, 2020). Depending on the gut microbial structure, host genetic makeup, age, and gender, the gut microbiota can direct both pro- and anti-inflammatory immune response, which can have a role in either disease promotion or disease protection (Wu & Wu, 2012). The ability of the gut microbiota to shape immune response outside the intestine is worth noting; however, the underlying mechanism by which these microbes influence the immune response is unknown (Vieira et al., 2014). Therefore the gut microbiota represents a new target in diagnosis, prognosis, and a potential therapeutic alternative in autoimmune disorders.

The gut microbiota exerts their beneficial role in protection to autoimmune diseases by several mechanisms. It has an important role in maintaining the integrity of the intestinal barrier, thus reducing the translocation of bacteria via the intestinal mucosa and reducing immune tolerance (Chelakkot et al., 2018). Dysbiosis in the gut microbiome results in altered host microbe interactions, which have been associated with inflammation in the gastrointestinal tract, irritable bowel syndrome, and inflammatory bowel disease (IBD) (Liu et al., 2020; Pittayanon et al., 2019). In addition, the leaky gut hypothesis indicates the role of altered gut barrier in the migration of mucosal lymphocytes to the liver leading to the liver autoimmune reactions (Mu, Kirby et al., 2017). Patients with autoimmune disorders, such as SLE, type 1 diabetes, and celiac disease, have also had perturbations in the gut barrier (Mu, Kirby et al., 2017; Mu, Zhang et al., 2017). These demonstrate the influence of gut microbiota and the intestinal barrier in autoimmune diseases; therefore a possible therapeutic approach in the treatment of autoimmune diseases might be able to reverse the leaky gut.

The gut microbiota also has a crucial role in maintaining the immune homeostasis in the gastrointestinal tract. The gut microbiota's role in the development and maturation of GALT has been established in germ-free mice suggesting a dynamic relationship between the gut microbiota and immune response (Round & Mazmanian, 2009). One of the hypotheses is the involvement of gut microbiota in the induction, development, and function of Treg cells, which play a crucial role in the maintenance of autoimmune diseases (Ruohtula et al., 2019). Many gut microbial species and their metabolites have the potential to induce Treg cells (Dwivedi et al., 2016). Through various mechanisms, probiotics and prebiotics have been suggested to induce Tregs to ameliorate the autoimmune conditions. These mechanisms include the activation of tolerogenic DCs and Treg-associated molecules, stimulation of TLRs, and SCFAs' induction of tregs by GPR43 and GPR109A expressions, by the inhibition of histone deacetylases and prostaglandin E2 (Dwivedi et al., 2016). Polysaccharide A produced by *Bacillus fragilis* induces Tregs through TLR2 pathways (Kayama & Takeda, 2014), whereas gut microbiota that produce SCFAs regulate Tregs by enhancing FOXP3 acetylation epigenetically (Park et al., 2015). Moreover, *Bifidobacterium* has shown to alter gut microbiota leading to the enhancement of Treg function; additionally, *Bifidobacterium* and *Lactobacillus* genera have shown to ameliorate colitis by promoting Treg cells' function (Sun et al., 2020). The Treg cells' gut microbiota have also been shown to modulate Th17 response (Chow & Mazmanian, 2009). In nonautoimmune mice, the gram-positive spore-forming segmented filamentous bacteria induces Th17 cellular immune response and has a role in the protection of T1DM (Flannigan & Denning, 2018). In contrast, in autoimmune arthritis, MS, and experimental autoimmune encephalomyelitis (EAE), the same bacterium showed a disease-promoting role (Flannigan & Denning, 2018; van den Hoogen et al., 2017). In addition, a close relationship between the gut microbiota and the IgA producing B cells has been reported where IgA deficiency has been associated with alterations in the composition of the gut microbiota (Liu and Rhoads, 2013; Pittayanon et al., 2019). Dysbiosis in gut microbiota may therefore lead to altered development of IgA leading to autoimmune diseases, such as SLE, T1DM, RA, celiac disease, and myasthenia gravis (Wang et al., 2011). Altered TLR expression on APC, Treg/Th17 balance, and antibody production by B cells has been correlated with dysbios in the gut (Omenetti & Pizarro, 2015; Wang et al., 2011); however, the precise mechanisms involving such distinct effects of gut microbiota are still unclear, unraveling that could pave a way to identify effective therapeutics for autoimmune disease.

Apart from the protective role of gut microbiota in autoimmune disease, the impairment in the gut microbiota can also promote autoimmunity by several key mechanisms. One of such mechanisms is molecular mimicry wherein autoimmune reactions can be triggered by gut microbiota by providing cross-reactive antigens to T cells (He et al., 2016; Li et al., 2019; Luo et al., 2018). One study highlighted the role of commensal bacteria in the pathogenesis of MS by mimicking several autoimmune immunogens (Westall, 2006). Moreover, the bystander activation of antigen-presenting cells leading to proinflammatory cytokine production is considered a possible mechanism in the development of autoimmunity (Li et al., 2018). Another possible mechanism is the leaky gut hypothesis; recent studies have suggested the role of bacterial translocation for the immune activation in liver, which leads to priming of gut associated T cells in the liver triggering autoimmune reactions in the liver (Mu, Kirby et al., 2017; Mu, Zhang et al., 2017). In addition, gut-associated IgA producing B cells have been associated with chronic liver diseases (Inamine & Schnabl, 2018). Overall, these studies suggest role of perturbed gut microbiota in exacerbating the autoimmune disorders.

Compelling evidence provided by the recent studies suggests the protective and disease-promoting role of gut microbiota in autoimmune diseases. However, the influence of gut microbiota on the immune system is reversible as manipulation of the microbiome restores immune function. Therefore a clear understanding of the role of the gut microbiome in autoimmune diseases is crucial in developing targeted therapeutics for the autoimmune diseases.

12.5 Beneficial role of probiotics in the suppression of autoimmune diseases

Probiotics are living microbes, beneficial to the host by exerting antimicrobial effect, enhancing mucosal barrier, and modulating the immune response (Hemarajata & Versalovic, 2013). They play a role in shaping the gut microbiome by producing metabolic and/or antimicrobial agent, which suppresses pathogenic microorganisms (Hemarajata & Versalovic, 2013). Studies have suggested that the probiotic strains of *Lactobacillus* improved gastrointestinal integrity and exerted a beneficial role in suppressing diseases, such as IBD and gastrointestinal tract inflammation (Chen et al., 2015). In addition, probiotic therapy with *Faecalibacterium prausnitzii* improved the production of butyrate, which contributed to the production of antiinflammatory cytokines, primarily by suppressing the NFkB pathway and preserving epithelial integrity by modulating the composition of gut bacteria. Therefore these studies suggest that the modulation of gut microbiota may serve as a potent therapeutic strategy for various autoimmune diseases (Table 12.1).

12.5.1 Role of probiotics in the suppression of rheumatoid arthritis

RA is a chronic systemic autoimmune condition characterized by joint synovial membrane inflammation that results in damage to the bone and cartilage, resulting in disability, discomfort, stiffness, and decreased life expectancy (Carbone et al., 2020). Studies have suggested the role of the innate and adaptive immune responses in the joint destruction (Firestein & McInnes, 2017). The exact etiology of RA is unknown, however; genetic, environmental and other factors, such as birth weight, diet, alcohol, and smoking, are extensively involved in the risk of developing RA (Deane et al., 2017). Recent evidence has suggested the role of gut microbiota in the RA pathogenesis (Horta-Baas et al., 2017). The gut microbiota maintains immune homeostasis and the dysbiosis of which leads to inflammation and several autoimmune diseases, including RA (Fig. 12.2) (Horta-Baas et al., 2017). Prolonged use of the current treatment regime causes profound side effects; therefore probiotics can be used as a potent alternative to treat RA.

The dysbiosis in gut microbiota leads to inflammation in the joint leading to pain, swelling, and bone erosion in RA patients. Probiotic treatment produces bateriocins and lactic acid, which reduce the pH of gut leading to reduced gut inflammation. The probiotics also produce SCFAs that inhibit the NFkB pathway to prevent inflammation by suppressing Th1 cytokines. In addition, probiotics suppress autoimmunity in RA by promoting Treg cells' induction, development, and function through epigenetic modifications, such as histone deacetylasation. Adenosine and retinoic acid produced by probiotics also inhibit Th1 and Th17 cells' subsets and promote Treg cells, resulting in the RA suppression.

Several human and animal model-based studies have suggested the beneficial role of probiotics in the suppression of RA (Table 12.1). Studies have highlighted the role of *Lactobacillus* and *Bifidobacterium* species in the treatment of RA (Bodkhe et al., 2019). In collagen-induced arthritis model study, the oral administration of *Lactobacillus casei* or *Lactobacillus acidophilus* controlled RA progression by downregulating proinflammatory cytokines (TNF-a, IL-6, and IL-12) while upregulating antiinflammatory cytokines (Amdekar et al., 2013). Moreover, studies have suggested that *L. casei* suppresses type II collagen reactive effector function of Th1 cells leading to the downregulation of proinflammatory cytokines (So et al., 2008). In addition, it also upregulates antiinflammatory Th2 cytokines, further suppressing the aberrant immune response in RA (So et al., 2008). Recent studies suggested that administration of the enteritis mice mode with *L. casei* increases the number and function of Treg cells, which play vital role in controlling autoimmune diseases, such as RA (Wang et al., 2017). The possible mechanism of Treg cells induction is through *trans* retinoic acid, which enhances Treg cells' function, diminishes Treg cells' apoptosis, and increases DC-mediated Treg cells' induction (Xiao et al., 2008). Overall, these studies suggest that the oral administration of *L. casei* leads to the induction of Treg cells, which then suppress the aberrant immune response, that is, proinflammatory cytokine production and humoral immune response by the production of antiinflammatory cytokines in the mouse model of collagen-induced arthritis (So, Kwon et al., 2008). Moreover, studies have suggested that *Lactobacillus heleveticus* enhances IL-10 production by CD4$^+$ T cells leading to the suppression of proinflammatory cytokines, such as TNF-α, IFN-γ, and IL-17a, and reduction of CII-reactive immunoglobulin antibodies, which leads to protection against disease activity in CIA mouse model (Kim et al., 2015). The *Lactobacillus plantarum* has also shown to have antiarthritic activity resulting in reducing pain and inflammatory molecules in the joint; however, the mechanism for the same is unknown (Gohil et al., 2018).

Randomized controlled trials have found the administration of *Bifidobacterium bifidum*, *Bacillus coagulans*, *Lactobacillus rhamnosus*, *L. reuteri*, *L. acidophilus*, and *L. casei* probiotic bacteria to be safe and effective in treating RA (de los Angeles Pineda et al., 2011; Hatakka et al., 2003; Mandel et al., 2010; Vaghef-Mehrabany et al., 2014; Zamani et al., 2016). The administration of *Lactobacillus* probiotics, *L. rhamnosus* GR-1, and *L. reuteri* RC-14 in RA

TABLE 12.1 Studies depicting role of probiotics in the suppression of various autoimmune diseases.

Probiotic strains	Key findings of the study	References
Rheumatoid arthritis		
Bacillus coagulans GBI-30, 6086	*B. coagulans* GBI-30, 6086 showed borderline statistical significance in a double-blind RCT of 45 patients with RA in decreasing pain. *B. coagulans* GBI-30, 6086 treatment resulted in greater improvement in patient global assessment and self-assessed disability; reduction in C-reactive protein (CRP); as well as the ability to walk 2 miles, reach, and participate in daily activities.	Mandel et al. (2010)
Lactobacillus rhamnosus GR-1 and *Lactobacillus reuteri* RC-14	Three month double-blind, placebo-controlled study for the probiotic treatment of *L. rhamnosus* GR-1 and *L. reuteri* RC-14 capsules administered orally in 30 patients showed significant improvement in Health Assessment Questionnaire score. Treated group showed significant reduction of proinflammatory cytokines (TNF-α, IL-1β, IL-8, IL-6, IL-12, IL-15, IL-17, and M1P-1α) in the treated group.	de los Angeles Pineda et al. (2011)
Lactobacillus casei	In the randomized double-blind clinical trial, 30 female RA patients received one capsule containing *L. casei* 01. The oral administration of *L. casei* 01 reduces serum high-sensitivity CRP (hs-CRP) levels, tender and swollen joint counts, global health score, and DAS-28-treated patients showed reduced IL-12 and TNF-α levels in RA patients.	Alipour et al. (2014)
Lactobacillus acidophilus, *Lactobacillus*, and *Bifidobacterium bifidum*	In the randomized, double-blind, placebo-controlled trial including 60 RA patients, the probiotic group received a daily capsule that contained three viable and freeze-dried strains: *L. acidophilus*, *Lactobacillus*, and *B. bifidum* for 8 weeks. The probiotic supplementation resulted in improved Disease Activity Score of 28 joints (DAS-28), a significant decrease in serum insulin levels, homeostatic model assessment B-cell function, and serum hs-CRP concentrations.	Zamani et al. (2016)
L. casei, *L. acidophilus*	Oral administration of *L. casei* and *L. acidophilus* in collagen-induced arthritis model decreased proinflammatory cytokine (IL-6, TNF-α, IL-1β, IL-17, IL-4) levels and increased antiinflammatory cytokines (IL-10) levels. *L. casei* and *L. acidophilus* reduced oxidative stress in synovial effsuate.	Amdekar et al. (2013)
L. casei	*L. casei* protects against RA by reducing the effector functions of CD4 (+) T cells. It reduces the expression of proinflammatory cytokines, such as IL-1β, IL-2, IL-6, IL-12, IL-17, IFN-γ, TNF-α, and Cox-2. Oral administration of *L. casei* reduces paw swelling, lymphocyte infiltration, and destruction of cartilage tissue. *L. casei* administration also reduced the translocation of NF-kB into nucleus and CII-reactive Th1-type IgG isotypes IgG2a and IgG2b, while upregulating immunoregulatory IL-10 levels.	So, Kwon et al. (2008)
Lactobacillus helveticus	*L. helveticus* HY7801 prevents the development of collagen-induced experimental arthritis and diminished disease progression and severity by reducing antigen-specific IgG levels and inflammatory immune response. Administration of *L. helveticus* HY7801 induces regulatory CD11c$^+$ dendritic cells, which in turn reduces proinflammatory cytokines (TNF-α, IFN-γ, and IL-17A) while enhancing antiinflammatory cytokine (IL-10) by CD4$^+$ T cells.	Kim et al. (2015)
Lactobacillus plantarum	Cell wall content of *L. plantarum* improves RA symptoms by reducing body weight, paw volume and arthritic index, joint stiffness, gait test, mobility test, erythrocyte sedimentation rate, serum CRP level, serum rheumatoid factor, and serum TNF-α levels.	Gohil et al. (2018)

(*Continued*)

TABLE 12.1 (Continued)

Probiotic strains	Key findings of the study	References
Systemic lupus erythematosus		
L. rhamnosus, Lactobacillus delbrueckii	The mix of L. rhamnosus and L. delbrueckii probiotics consumption decreased the level of lipogranuloma, antinuclear antibodies, and anti-dsDNA. In probiotics receiving groups, Tregs and the expression level of Foxp3 increased, while IL-6 decreased. The study also found a decrease in IFN-γ, IL-17, and RORγt levels in the probiotics group. The Th1–Th17 cells, the major cells subsets responsible for pathogenies of SLE, were found to be reduced in SLE group.	Khorasani et al. (2019)
Lactobacillus paracasei GMNL-32, L. reuteri GMNL-89, and L. reuteri GMNL-263	L. paracasei GMNL-32, L. reuteri GMNL-89, and L. reuteri GMNL-263 administration in NZB/W F1 mice ameliorates hepatic apoptosis and inflammatory indicators, such as matrix metalloproteinase-9 activity and CRP and inducible nitric oxide synthase expressions. Supplementation with L. paracasei GMNL-32, L. reuteri GMNL-89, and L. reuteri GMNL-263 in NZB/W F1 mice reduces the expressions of hepatic IL-1β, IL-6, and TNF-α proteins by suppressing the mitogen-activated protein kinase and NF-κB signaling pathways.	Hsu et al. (2017)
L. paracasei GMNL-32, L. reuteri GMNL-89, and L. reuteri GMNL-263	Supplementation with L. paracasei GMNL-32, L. reuteri GMNL-89, and L. reuteri GMNL-263 significantly increased antioxidant activity, reduced IL-6 and TNF-α levels and significantly decreased the toll-like receptors/myeloid differentiation primary response gene 88 signaling in NZB/W F1 mice. Notably, supplementation with GMNL-263, but not GMNL-32 and GMNL-89, in NZB/W F1 mice significantly increased the differentiation of CD4$^+$CD25$^+$FoxP3$^+$ T cells.	Tzang et al. (2017)
L. reuteri GMNL-263	L. reuteri GMNL-263 administration leads to the prevention of enlarged interstitial spaces and abnormal myocardial structures in the hearts of NZB/W F1 SLE mice model. Significant reduction in TUNEL-positive cells, Fas death receptor-related components, and apoptosis was also detected in the cardiac tissues of the NZB/W F1 SLE mice model after L. reuteri GMNL-263 treatment.	Yeh et al. (2021)
Lactobacillus oris, L. rhamnosus, L. reuteri, Lactobacillus johnsonii, and Lactobacillus gasseri	L. oris, L. rhamnosus, L. reuteri, L. johnsonii, and L. gasseri in the gut improved renal function of these mice and prolonged their survival. Leaky gut of the MRL/lpr mice was reversed by increased Lactobacillus colonization. Lactobacillus treatment contributed to an antiinflammatory environment by decreasing IL-6 and increasing IL-10 production in the gut. In the circulation, Lactobacillus treatment increased IL-10 and decreased IgG2a that is considered to be a major immune deposit in the kidney of MRL/lpr mice. Inside the kidney, Lactobacillus treatment also skewed the Treg-Th17 balance toward a Treg phenotype.	Mu, Zhang et al. (2017)
Type 1 diabetes mellitus		
L. johnsonii N6.2	In a double-blind, randomized trial in 42 healthy adults, L. johnsonii N6.2 administration significantly decreased the occurrence of abdominal pain, indigestion, and cephalic syndromes. It increased serum tryptophan levels, resulting in a decreased kynurenine:tryptophan (K:T) ratio. Monocytes and natural killer cell numbers were increased. An increase in circulating effector Th1 cells (CD45RO$^+$CD183$^+$CD196$^-$) and cytotoxic CD8$^+$ T cells' subset was observed in the L. johnsonii N6.2 group. Consumption of L. johnsonii N6.2 is well tolerated in adult control subjects, demonstrates systemic impacts on innate and adaptive immune populations, and results in a decreased K:T ratio.	Marcial et al. (2017)

(Continued)

TABLE 12.1 (Continued)

Probiotic strains	Key findings of the study	References
L. rhamnosus GG and Bifidobacterium lactis Bb12	Randomized controlled trial in 96 children probiotics treatment improved the gut mucosal barrier, preserved the β-cell function by modulating local and systemic immune responses, and reduced the risk of autoimmunity.	Groele et al. (2017)
Oligofructose prebiotics	In randomized controlled trial in young children, oligofructose prebiotics treatment treated T1D mellitus by decreasing endotoxemia and reduced insulin resistance. It improves glycemic control. It modulates gut microbiota, permeability, and inflammation.	Ho et al. (2016)
High-fiber intake	Patients in the higher-fiber intake group exhibited significantly lower systolic blood pressure (SBP) and diastolic blood pressure (DBP), higher energy intake, and lower BMI. Higher fiber intake was associated with lower SBP and DBP levels.	Beretta et al. (2018)
Bifidobacteriaceae, Lactobacillaceae, Streptococcus thermophilus	Probiotics administration inhibits IL-1β expression while enhancing the release of protolerogenic components of the inflammasome, such as indoleamine 2,3-dioxygenase and IL-33. It modulates gut immunity by promoting the differentiation of tolerogenic CD103(+) DCs and reducing the differentiation/expansion of Th1 and Th17 cells in the intestinal mucosa and pancreatic lymph nodes (PLN) in NOD mice.	Dolpady et al. (2016)
Lactobacillus brevis KLDS 1.0727 and KLDS 1.0373	Inhibits the development of T1D mellitus in diabetic mice model. By increasing γ-aminobutyric acid levels and decreasing the blood glucose level or insulin in plasma.	Abdelazez et al. (2018)
Lactobacillus species	Significant reduction in glucose-6-phosphatase and phosphoenol pyruvate carboxykinase in the liver. Significant decrease in serum inflammatory cytokines, such as IL-6, TNF-α, HbA1c, blood glucose level, and serum lipid profile. Improvement in glucose metabolism, oxidative stress, and hepatic gluconeogenesis.	Yadav et al. (2018)
Lactococcus lactis	The combination therapy of low-dose anti-CD3 with a clinical-grade self-containing L. lactis, appropriate for human application, secreting human proinsulin, and interleukin-10, cured 66% of mice with new-onset diabetes. The treatment lead to decline in insulin autoantibody positivity. The assessment of the immune changes induced by the L. lactis-based therapy revealed elevated frequencies of $CD4^+Foxp3^+$ T cells in the pancreas-draining lymph nodes, pancreas, and peripheral blood of all treated mice, independent of metabolic outcome.	Takiishi et al. (2012)
Lactobacillus kefiranofaciens and Lactobacillus kefiri	Probiotics administration increased levels in pancreas. The increased IL-10 inhibits the secretion of proinflammatory cytokines, such as TNF-α and TH1 (also IL-1β, IL-2, IL-6).	Wei et al. (2015)
Bifibobacteria, Lactobacilli, and Streptococcus salivarius	Probiotics administration leads to the prevention of autoimmune diabetes by decreasing the rate of β-cell destruction and increasing the production of IL-10 from PPs, pancreas, and spleen. Modulates GALT to antiinflammatory state. Induces immunomodulation by a reduction in insulitis severity.	Calcinaro et al. (2005)
HMOS prebiotic	Prebiotics treatment leads to beneficial alterations in fecal microbiota composition. Increases SCFA concentration in the gut. Induction of antidiabetogenic cytokine profiles. Development of tolerogenic dendritic cells (tDCs), priming of functional regulatory T cells. Changes the direct shape of the pancreatic environment, resulting in less insulitis.	Xiao et al. (2018)
Oligofructose prebiotic	Increase in levels of bifidobacteria, a dominant member of the intestinal microbiota. Oligofructose feeding significantly increased endotoxaemia. Oligofructose feeding positively correlated with improved glucose tolerance, glucose-induced insulin secretion, and normalized inflammatory tone (decreased endotoxaemia, plasma and adipose tissue proinflammatory cytokines).	Cani et al. (2007)

(Continued)

TABLE 12.1 (Continued)

Probiotic strains	Key findings of the study	References
L. johnsonii strain N6.2 (LjN6.2)	Diabetes resistance in LjN6.2-fed BBDP rodents was correlated to a Th17 cell within the mesenteric lymph nodes. LjN6.2 directly mediated enhanced Th17 differentiation of lymphocytes. Increased levels of cytokines such as IL-6 and IL-23 lead to induction and sustenance of TH17 cells.	Lau et al. (2011)
Multiple sclerosis		
Bifidobacterium animalis, *L. plantarum* A7	*B. animalis* and *L. plantarum* A7 improve experimental autoimmune encephalomyelitis condition through elevating antiinflammatory cytokines, such as IL-4, IL-10, Tregs, $CD25^+$, $CD4^+$, TGF-3, and $Foxp3^+$ in lymph nodes and spleen, with an increase in Th2, Treg, and GATA3 and a decrease in IL-6, IL-17, Th17, and Th1, resulting in the decrease in inflammation, autoreactive T cells, and demyelination.	Salehipour et al. (2017)
Oral administration of *Escherichia coli* Nissle 1917	Decrease in inflammatory cytokines, such as IFN-γ, TNF-α, and IL-17 whereas an increase in the production of autoreactive $CD4^+$ T cells, IL-10, and $CD4^+$ $Foxp3^+$ in lymph nodes. Improvement of intestinal barrier dysfunction and neuroinflammatory factors	Secher et al. (2017)
IRT5 (mixture of five probiotics containing of 10^8 CFU/g of each strain: *S. thermophilus*, *L. acidophilus*, *L. casei*, *B. bifidum*, and *L. reuteri*)	Contributed within suppression of experimental autoimmune encephalomyelitis condition.	Kwon et al. (2013)
Probiotics capsule administration containing probiotics strain of *L. casei*, *B. bifidum*, *Lactobacillus fermentum*, and *L. acidophilus*	Probiotic capsule improves depression, anxiety, and stress scale within the patients. The levels of CRP, malondialdehyde, and plasma nitric oxide were significantly changed within the placebo group	Kouchaki et al. (2017)
Probiotics capsule containing *L. fermentum*, *B. bifidum*, *L. acidophilus*, and *L. casei* with 2×10^9 CFUs/g each	Downregulation among the gene expression of TNF-α mRNA and IL-8 in the PBMCs of Ms patients. Probiotics has a modulating effect in the inflammatory cytokines of Ms patients.	Tamtaji et al. (2017)
Cystic fibrosis		
Lactobacillus GG	Reduction of pulmonary exacerbations. Probiotics may delay intestinal and pulmonary inflammation within CF.	Bruzzese et al. (2004, 2007)
L. reuteri	This report suggests that pulmonary exacerbations were significantly reduced in the *L. reuteri* group.	Di Nardo et al. (2014)

patients decreased proinflammatory cytokines, such as IL-6, IL-1α, TNF-α, and IL-12 (de los Angeles Pineda et al., 2011). Moreover, *L. casei* treatment reduced the joint swelling by lowering IL-12 and TNF-α levels in RA patients (Alipour et al., 2014). The probiotics administration also restored gut barrier, leading to reduced inflammation (Rao & Samak, 2013). The oral administration of *B. coagulans* was shown to improve RA by the production of bacteriocins and lactic acid, which reduced the pH, thereby eliminating the inflammatory response in both humans and rats (Abhari et al., 2016; Mandel et al., 2010). The proposed mechanism suggests that *B. coagulans* activates antiinflammatory response by lowering prostaglandin production (Mandel et al., 2010). Furthermore, *Lactobacillus*-associated probiotics reduced the gut dysbiosis and relieved the RA symptoms. Administration of *Bifidobacterium* probiotics in RA patients decreased the RA severity (Bodkhe et al., 2019). Probiotic treatment with *L. acidophilus*, *L. casei*, and *B. bifidum* was shown to improve the Disease Activity Score of 28 joints, and it also lowered the serum insulin and CRP levels in RA patients (Zamani et al., 2016). Moreover, the *meta*-analysis on probiotics in RA treatment suggested that the production of IL-6 (a key proinflammatory cytokine in the destruction of RA) was decreased in probiotic-treated group by the production of antiinflammatory cytokine IL-10 (Pan et al., 2017). Another *meta*-analysis suggested a reduction in C-reactive protein (CRP), TNF-α, and IL-1β levels while an increase in IL-10 production in the probiotic group (Aqaeinezhad Rudbane et al., 2018; Pan et al., 2017). Although studies assessing the effectiveness of prebiotic-based

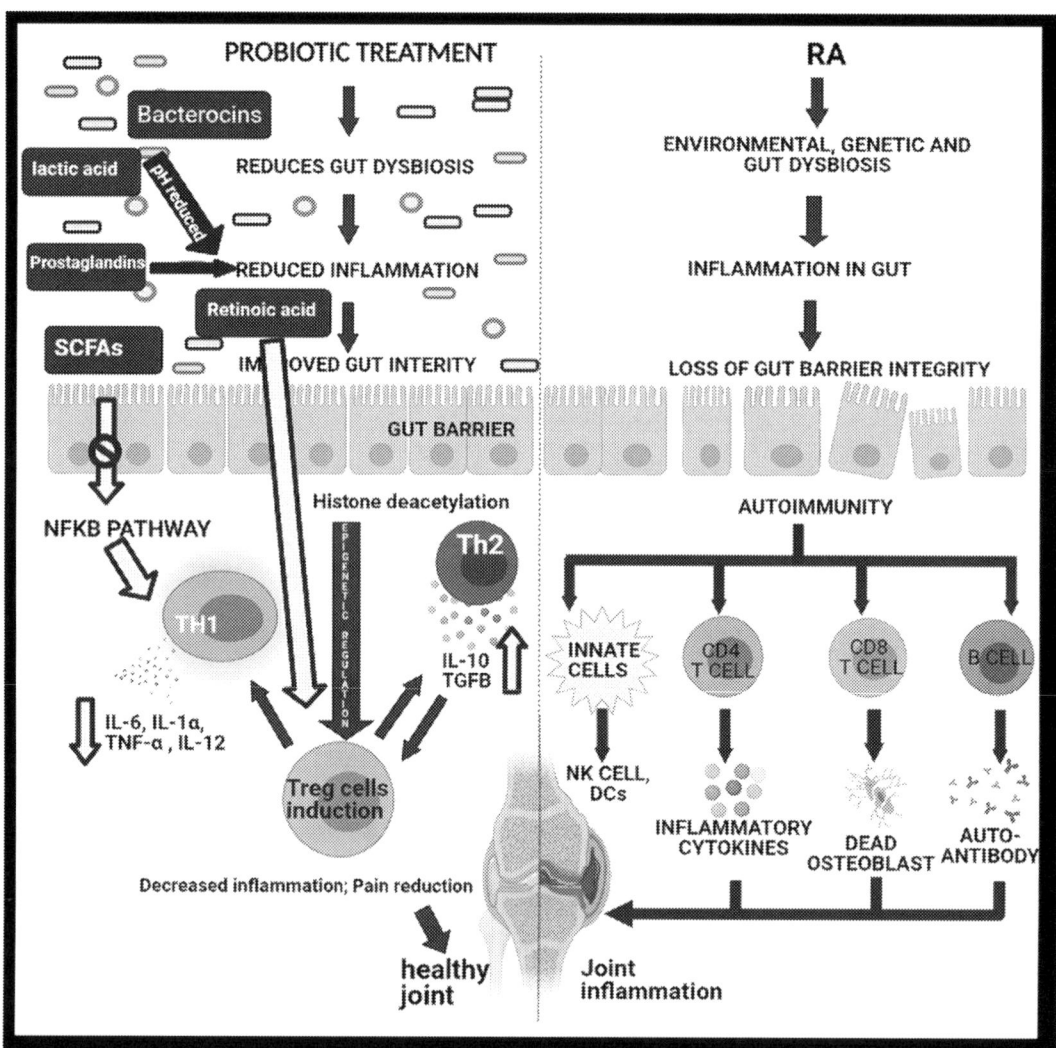

FIGURE 12.2 The role of probiotics in treatment of rheumatoid arthritis.

therapeutics in RA treatment are lacking, currently few randomized clinical trials on RA patients are exploring the effectiveness of whey protein, prebiotic supplements, and antirheumatic diet in RA treatment (ClinicalTrials.gov Identifier: NCT02881307, NCT03856190). However, detailed studies are required to delineate the role of prebiotics and probiotics in RA treatment.

The underlying mechanism of probiotic-mediated RA treatment is yet to be established; however, reports have suggested that SCFAs produced by the probiotic species inhibit the NFkB pathway to prevent inflammation (Liu et al., 2012). Moreover, studies suggested that probiotic species suppress autoimmunity in RA by promoting Treg cells' induction, development, and function through epigenetic modifications, such as histone deacetylasation (Fig. 12.2) (Park et al., 2015). In addition, probiotics also induced adenosine that suppress Th1 and Th17 cell subsets and promoted the Treg cells (Omenetti & Pizarro, 2015). Altogether, the above-mentioned studies suggest that the probiotic species suppress disease severity in RA by suppressing proinflammatory response and enhancing antiinflammatory response (Fig. 12.2).

12.5.2 Role of probiotics in suppression of systemic lupus erythematosus

SLE is an inflammatory autoimmune condition characterized by systemic damage of kidneys, skin, liver, lungs, heart, and brain (de Oliveira, 2018). It is a heterogeneous condition causing damage to multiple organs and tissue leading to clinical features involving fever, arthritis, renal disorder, hematological disorder, and cardiovascular disease

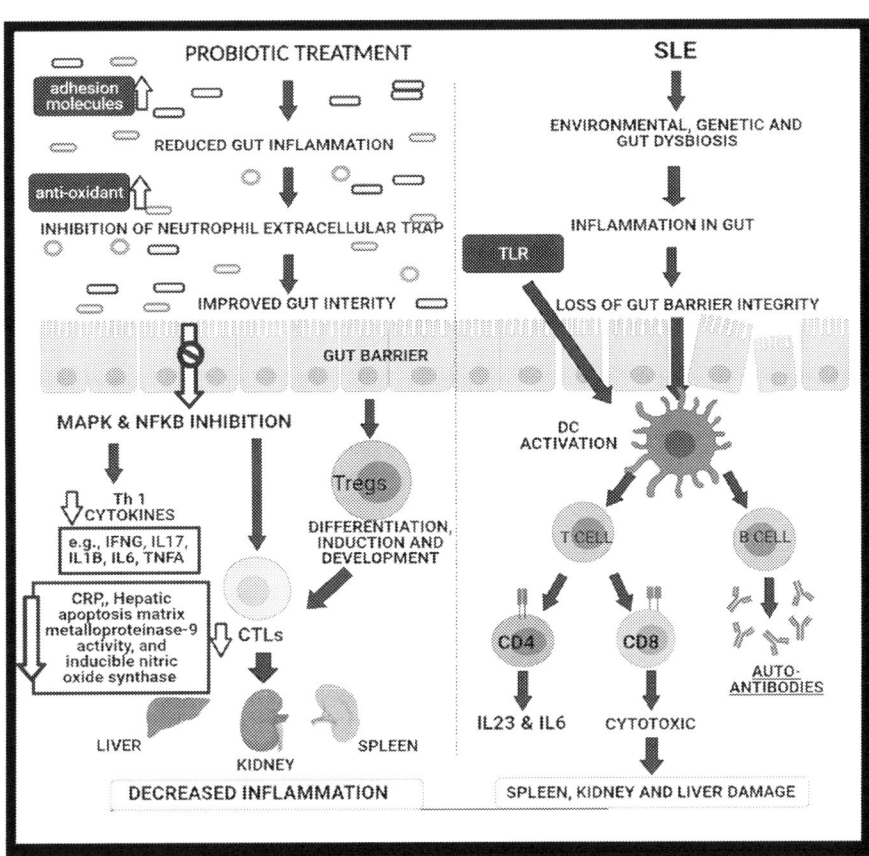

FIGURE 12.3 Beneficial role of probiotics in systemic lupus erythematosus.

(Cojocaru, 2011). Although treatment has greatly improved SLE outcome, but SLE patients still suffer from significant morbidity (Maidhof & Hilas, 2012). The etiology of SLE mainly involves genetic and environmental factors, but the exact etiology is unknown (Kamen, 2014); however, the role of immune system in pathogenesis of SLE is evident. It was suggested that TLR-mediated IFN-α production leads to the activation of innate immune cells, such as DCs (Rönnblom & Pascual, 2008). The DCs further activate autoreactive T and B cells leading to the increased production of autoantibodies. $CD4^+$ T cells play an important role in SLE pathogenesis by the production of proinflammatory cytokines, such as IL-23 and IL-6 (Fig. 12.3) (Moulton et al., 2017). Moreover, recent studies also suggest $CD4^+$ and $CD8^+$ T cells and B cells are hyporesponsive in SLE (Weißenberg et al., 2019). The role of intestinal dysbiosis in SLE development has also been implicated (Van De Wiele et al., 2016).

The beneficial role of probiotics in SLE management is enlisted in Table 12.1. Administration of probiotic species *L. rhamnosus* and *Lactobacillus delbrueckii* has shown beneficial effects in controlling SLE induction in pristane-induced SLE model (Khorasani et al., 2019). The exact mechanism is unclear but *L. rhamnosus* and *L. delbrueckii* have been found to exert antiinflammatory properties. In particular, previous reports suggest that these probiotics reduce polarization towards Th17, Th1, and cytotoxic T lymphocyte (CTL) cells, leading to the decreased proinflammatory cytokine (Khorasani et al., 2019). The study also found a decrease in IFN-γ, IL-17, and RORγt levels in the probiotics group (Khorasani et al., 2019). Moreover, recent studies have evaluated the effect of *L. reuteri* GMNL-89, *L. reuteri* GMNL-263, and *L. paracasei* GMNL-32 in SLE mouce model (Hsu et al., 2017; Tzang et al., 2017). The studies suggested reduced levels of pro-inflammatory cytokines including IL-1β, IL-6, and TNF-α along with increased antioxidant activity in serum and liver of the SLE mouse model. Furthermore, the *L. reuteri* GMNL-263 supplementation significantly increased the differentiation of Tregs in SLE (Hsu et al., 2017; Tzang et al., 2017). Moreover, the probiotic strains were found to ameliorate CRP, hepatic apoptosis matrix metalloproteinase-9 activity, and inducible nitric oxide synthase expressions (Hsu et al., 2017). In addition, the probiotic species also suppressed the MAPK and NF-κB signaling pathways leading to the reduction in proinflammatory cytokines, such as IL-1β, IL-6, and TNF-α (Hsu et al., 2017). Overall, these studies suggest that the probiotic species prevent SLE development by inducing Treg cells, which lead to the suppression of inflammatory response by suppressing proinflammatory cytokines.

Although human studies for the effect of probiotic species on SLE development are lacking but animal model studies in lupus suggest that administration of retinoic acid restores *Lactobacillus* species, resulting in the improvement of lupus symptoms by diminishing inflammation (Abdelhamid & Luo, 2018). Few studies have also suggested the use of *Lactobacillus* species in protection against cardiovascular disease in SLE (de la Visitación et al., 2019). In addition, antiapoptotic effects have been shown to inhibit SLE-induced cardiomyopathy with heat-killed *L. reuteri* GMNL-263 (Yeh et al., 2021). Another study also suggested dietary interventions, such as caloric restriction in NZB/WF1 mice promoted intestinal microbiota, which led to delayed SLE disease progression (Islam et al., 2020). Moreover, *Lactobacillus* species have been suggested to have immunomodulatory properties in gut leading to reduced gut inflammation, improved antioxidant status, inhibition of neutrophil extracellular trap formation, and increased expression of adhesion molecules in gut, finally leading to the enhancement of gastrointestinal integrity (de Oliveira et al., 2017; Hemarajata & Versalovic, 2013). In addition, oral *Lactobacillus* administration resulted in a decrease in kidney inflammation in the lupus MRL/lpr mouse model (Mu, Kirby et al., 2017). The *Lactobacillus* species also showed antiinflammatory response by suppressing the proinflammatory cytokine production and enhancing the Treg versus Th17 cells ratio (Mu, Zhang et al., 2017). Moreover, *L. rhamnosus* and *L. delbrueckii* have been reported to reduce proinflammatory cytokines (IFN-γ and IL-17) production, to inhibit autoantibodies production and Th1 and Th17 cells' production (Khorasani et al., 2019). Overall, these studies suggest the importance of probiotic in the control of SLE. Currently, no studies have been reported to assess the role of prebiotics in SLE treatment, but few studies have suggested the role of prebiotics in the treatment of two key autoimmune diseases namely IBD and type 1 diabetes (Chen et al., 2015). This suggests the importance of prebiotics in autoimmune disease and emphasizes the studies to assess the effectiveness of prebiotics in SLE treatment as well.

Although the exact mechanism of probiotics in the SLE management is obscured, but evidence suggests the unique features of probiotics in enhancing Treg cells' differentiation, development, and function as suggested by the *in vivo and in vitro* studies wherein *Lactobacillus* and *Bifidobacterium* strains induced Treg cells from naive precursors (López et al., 2011). The improvement in Treg cells' function after probiotic treatment can lead to increased antiinflammatory cytokines (TGF-β and IL-10), which then suppress the production of proinflammatory cytokines (IFN-γ, IL-6, IL-23, and IL-17, important mediators of SLE) (Azad et al., 2018) (Fig. 12.3).

Several factors, such as environmental, genetics, and gut dysbiosis, lead to inflammation in the gut and TLR-mediated DCs' activation. The activated DCs further activate autoreactive T and B cells resulting into increased proinflammatory cytokines and autoantibodies production. In the gut, the probiotic treatment increases antioxidant levels and adhesion molecules. It also inhibits neutrophil extracellular trap, which improves the gut integrity. Probiotics ameliorate SLE by enhancing Treg cells' differentiation, development, and function, which suppress proinflammatory cytokines and decrease CTL-mediated cytotoxicity. Probiotics also inhibit the MAPK and NFkB pathway to further prevent inflammation by suppressing Th1 cytokines. In addition, the probiotic strains suppress SLE by reducing CRP, hepatic apoptosis matrix metalloproteinase-9 activity, and inducible nitric oxide synthase expressions.

12.5.3 Role of probiotics in suppression of type 1 diabetes mellitus

T1DM is a chronic autoimmune condition characterized by the degradation of the insulin-producing β-cell pancreatic by immune cells (Hara et al., 2013). Early pathogenesis of T1DM is characterized by insulitis and elevated autoantibody production against β-cell antigens, followed by reduced insulin secretion and β-cell death (Pihoker et al., 2005) (Fig. 12.4). The specific environmental factors that trigger T1DM pathogenesis remain unclear, but genetic factors are also considered as responsible factors (Rewers & Ludvigsson, 2016). Interestingly, in T1DM pathology, the contribution of gut microbiota has been recently elucidated (Dedrick et al., 2020) (Fig. 12.4). However, the exact underline mechanism for this interaction is unknown.

Specific environmental and genetic factors cause gut dysbiosis, which can trigger T1DM pathogenesis characterized by insulitis and elevated autoantibody production, followed by β-cell death. The gamma amibobutyric acid and GLP-1 produced by probiotics regulates blood glucose levels and insulin production. SCFAs inhibit NFkB pathway leading to reduced Th1 cytokine levels. The probiotic treatment also modulates gut microbiota and immune signaling in GALT converting proinflammatory state to antiinflammatory state. In addition, the probiotic strains enhances Treg cells' development and function, which suppress proinflammatory cytokines and decrease CTL-mediated cytotoxicity of β-islets, resulting in the decreased blood glucose level.

Various human and animal model studies have highlighted the role of probiotics and prebiotics treatment in suppressing T1DM (Table 12.1). In a study on C57BL/6 mice, the administration of probiotic strains *Lactobacillus brevis* (*L. brevis* KLDS 1.0727 and *L. brevis* KLDS 1.0373) protected from STZ-induced T1DM symptoms by reducing blood

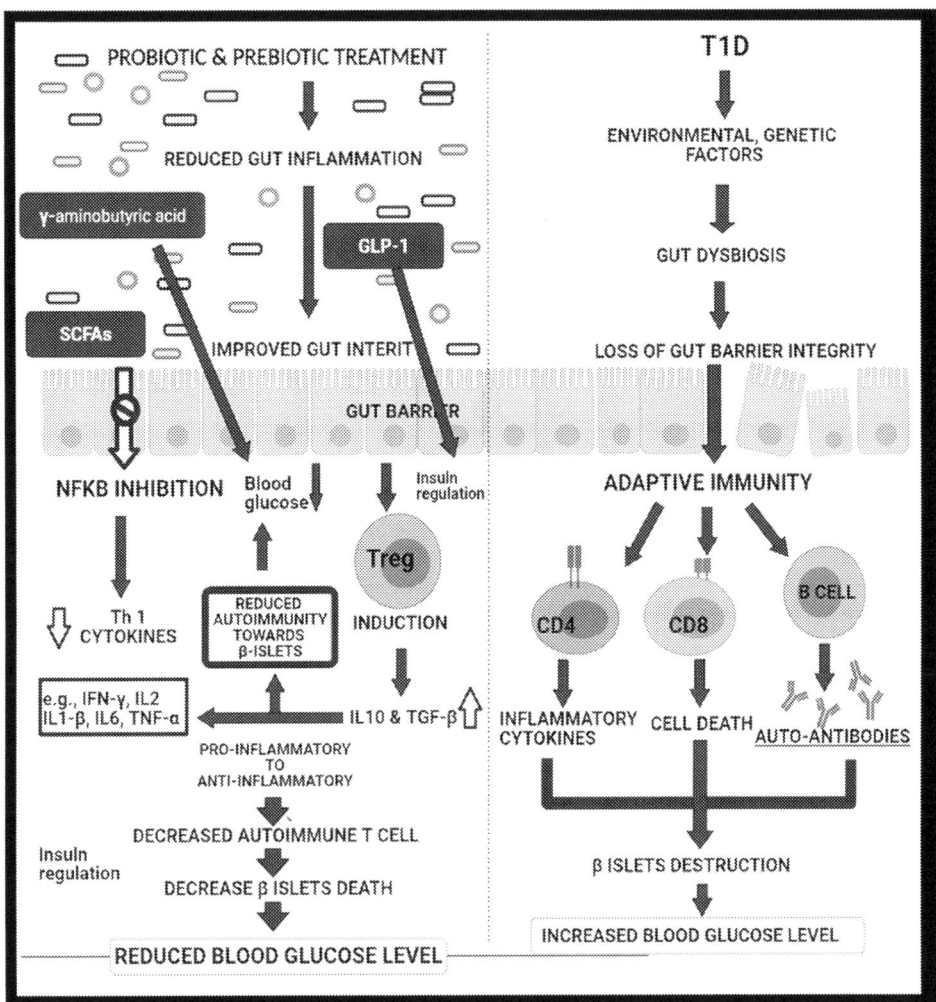

FIGURE 12.4 Role of probiotics and prebiotics in suppression of type 1 diabetes mellitus.

glucose levels by gamma-aminobutyric acid (Abdelazez et al., 2018). The *Lactococcus lactis* strain in combination with anti-CD3 showed an enhanced Tregs' development, which protected against T1DM by the production of IL-10 (Mishra et al., 2019, Takiishi et al., 2012). Moreover, *Lactobacillus kefiranofaciens* M and *Lactobacillus kefiri* K strains induced IL-10 production by pancreas (Wei et al., 2015). The production of IL-10 and development of Treg cells by these probiotic species led to the suppression of Th1-associated proinflammatory cytokines (TNF-α, IL-1β, IL-6, and IL-2) (Alejandra et al., 2011). Moreover, in the NOD mouse model, the proinflammatory state was converted to antiinflammatory state in GALT by the probiotic strains *Streptococcus salivarius*, *Streptococcus thermophilus*, *Lactobacillus* spp. and *Bifidobacterium* spp. (Calcinaro et al., 2005). Furthermore, strains belonging to *Bifidobacterium* species negatively correlated with β-cell autoimmunity in STZ-induced diabetic mice (Le et al., 2015). The probiotic species suppressed NF-κB signaling pathway thereby inhibiting the transcription of proinflammatory cytokines (Le et al., 2015). Moreover, several bacterial strains have shown to induce accountable rise in the GLP-1 production and the regulation of insulin synthesis from β-cell pancreatic islets (Wei et al., 2015).

In addition, Bifidobacteriaceae, Lactobacillaceae, and *S. thermophilus* strains modulated gut microbiota, reduced inflammation by inhibiting IL-1β, and also reduced Teff/Treg cell ratios within the gut mucosa, thereby leading to the amelioration of T1DM in NOD mice (Dolpady et al., 2016). Bacterial lipopolysaccharide (LPS) or Zymosan has also shown to increase Tregs and to suppress inflammatory immune cells by the production of IL-10 and TGF-β1 cytokines (Karumuthil-Melethil et al., 2015). Probiotic-fermented milk with *Lactobacillus* species decreased the serum inflammatory cytokines (such as IL-6 and TNF-α), HbA1c, blood glucose level, and serum lipid profile in STZ-induced albino Wistar T1DM rats (Yadav et al., 2013). Moreover, human milk oligosaccharides prebiotic increased the SCFA concentration in the gut, decreased the autoimmune T cells, and enhanced the Treg cells in NOD mice (Xiao et al., 2008).

It also increased the production of butyrate to facilitate mucin synthesis and enhanced the integrity of the intestinal barrier, which further contributed to decreased inflammation, and reduced degradation of pancreatic islets by regulating immune response (Xiao et al., 2018). Therefore a decrease in islet-specific autoimmune reaction by the probiotics confers the protection against T1DM.

A human study of the probiotic *Lactobacillus johnsonii* N6.2 in 42 healthy adult humans has found reduced risk of T1DM occurrence (Marcial et al., 2017). Another study of *L. rhamnosus* GG and *Bifidobacterium lactis* Bb12 in 96 children reported that it improved gut mucosal barrier and modulated the immune response, resulting in the suppression of autoimmunity (Groele et al., 2017). Moreover, the probiotic species also inhibited the growth of other pathogens and preserved β-cell function, thereby conferring protection to T1DM (Groele et al., 2017). Study in 1039 adult individuals suggested that probiotics led to a decrease in obesity, body mass index and regulated blood pressure, HDL cholesterol, and triglyceride components (Ahola et al., 2017). In addition, the probiotics were found to be correlated with improvement in glycemic control, suggesting their potential in controlling T1DM complications (Ahola et al., 2017).

Currently, few randomized clinical trials are studying the beneficial role of prebiotics, such as fibers, high amylose maize starch, and optimized diet supplementation in T1DM patients (ClinicalTrials.gov Identifier: NCT02442544, NCT04114357, and NCT02903615). Moreover, the administration of long-chain insulin type fructans in NOD mice regulated the gut-pancreatic immunity, resulting in delayed T1DM progression (Chen et al., 2017). In addition, SCFAs reduced the insulitis by regulating islet β-cell pathogenesis and improved the integrity of intestinal barrier, resulting in protection to T1DM (Sun et al., 2015; Knudsen et al., 2018). Study on oligofructose in diet-fed mice reported to enhance *Bifidobacterium* species, which led to glucose tolerance and insulin secretion (Cani et al., 2007). Moreover, the oligofructose-enriched inulin prebiotics may be a potential novel therapeutic against T1DM, as the study in young children resulted in changes in gut microbiota (increased number of *Bacteroidetes* and lactic acid-producing bacteria), induced hypoglycemia, and improved the glycemic control (Ho et al., 2016). In addition, *in vitro* studies have shown that fermentation of prebiotics increases abundance of *Bacteroidetes*, which decreases infection and alters the immune response to ameliorate T1DM (Falony et al., 2009). Furthermore, fermentation of fructan-like shorter-chain oligofructoses or longer-chain inulin compounds increased *Bifidobacterium* abundance, leading to increased acetate production (Falony et al., 2009). Acetate has been shown to alter immune response by increasing the antiinflammatory cytokines production, which helps in ameliorating T1DM (Fukuda et al., 2011). Altogether, the above-mentioned studies show a beneficial role of prebiotics and probiotics in controlling T1DM.

Although the exact mechanism is not yet elucidated, but studies suggest that probiotics influence the gut microbiota in developing immune signaling in GALT and mucosal immune system (Hwang et al., 2012; Nikolov, 2012). Probiotics can modulate the immune system by favoring the antiinflammatory immune response through production of IL-10 and TGF-β and in doing so, they suppress the proinflammatory immune response (Fig. 12.4) (Azad et al., 2018). Moreover, they suppress inflammation by improving the gut barrier integrity (Mishra et al., 2019). Probiotics can also enhance Treg cells to maintain the immune homeostasis of the gut (Fig. 12.4) (Mishra et al., 2019). They also modulate T1DM pathogenesis by decreasing gluconeogenesis and reducing oxidative stress and improve the blood glucose metabolism (Fig. 12.4) (Yadav et al., 2018). Overall, the above studies suggest that the probiotics modulate the immune response, which might lead to reduction in the degradation of β islet cells conferring protection against T1DM.

12.5.4 Role of probiotics in suppression of multiple sclerosis

There are several animal and human studies indicating beneficial role of probiotics and prebiotics in the suppression of MS. Presently a randomized, crossover-designed clinical trial is being designed to explore the immunological effects of prebiotics (prebiotin prebiotic fiber stick pac) supplementation along with the probiotic within the MS patients (ClinicalTrials.gov Identifier: NCT04038541). In a study, experimental animal model of MS was administered with the probiotic combination of *Bifidobacterium animalis* and *L. plantarum* A7 to investigate its effect on the amelioration of MS symptoms. The investigators reported that *B. animalis* and *L. plantarum* A7 were able to improve EAE condition by increasing antiinflammatory cytokines levels (such as IL-4, TGF-β, and IL-10), and Treg cells with increased expression of $CD25^+$, $CD4^+$, and $FOXP3^+$ in lymph nodes and spleen along with Th2 (T-helper 2) cells (Salehipour et al., 2017). Moreover, the study showed a subsequent decrease in IL-6 and IL-17 cytokines and Th17 and Th1 cells, resulting in a decrease in inflammation, autoreactive T cells, and demyelination (Salehipour et al., 2017) (Fig. 12.5).

During dysbiosis in Ms condition, LPS along with TLRs and CD14 causes disruption of enterocyte membrane leading to the lower expression of Treg cytokines (IL-10 and TGF-β), which finally results in the demyelination within the CNS. However, upon probiotic administration, SCFAs are produced, such as acetate, propionate, and butyrate. These SCFAs along with TLRs maintain the immune homeostasis. It results into the elevated levels of IL-10 and TGF-β

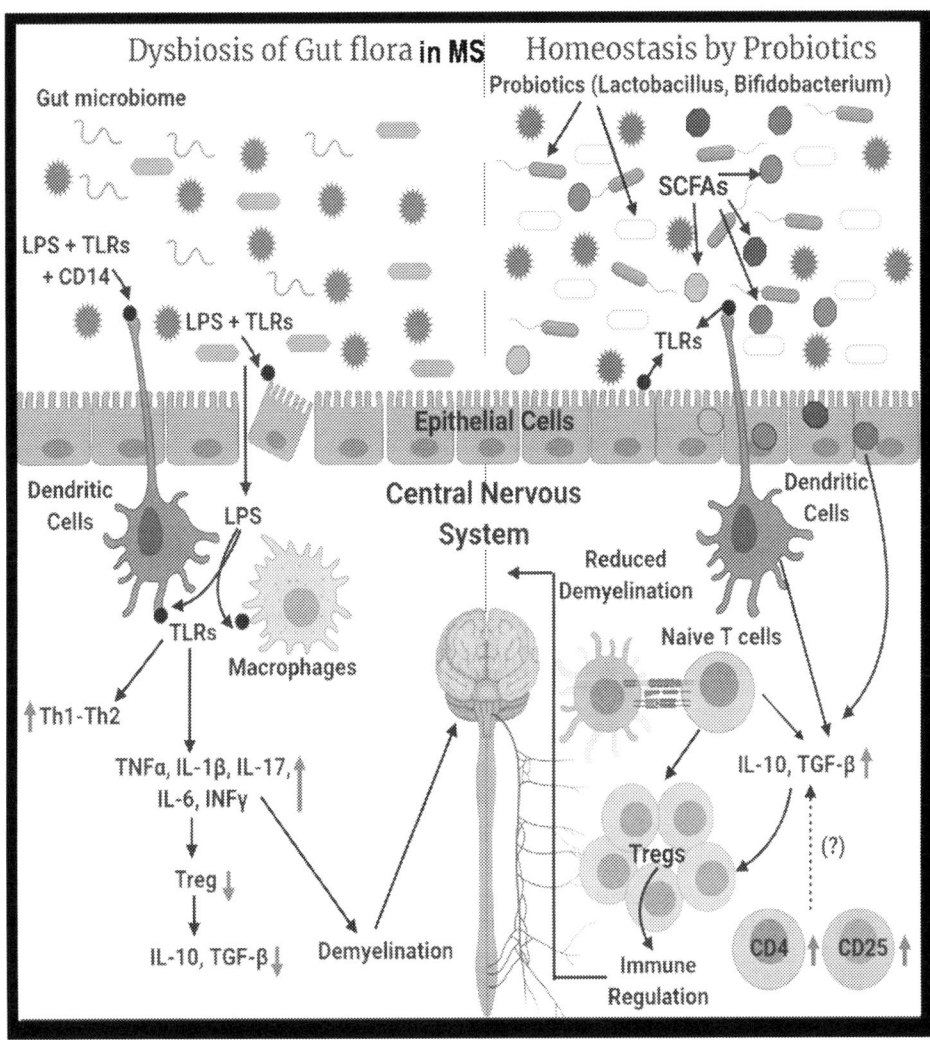

FIGURE 12.5 Role of probiotics in the suppression of multiple sclerosis.

cytokines, which further enhance Treg production and contribute to immune regulation, leading to reduced demyelination in CNS of Ms patients.

Another study on probiotic *Escherichia coli* Nissle 1917 showed a decrease in the susceptibility of neuroinflammation in EAE mice model (Secher et al., 2017). The study demonstrated a decrease in inflammatory cytokines, such as IFN-γ, TNF-α, and IL-17 whereas an increase in the production of IL-10, autoreactive CD4$^+$ T cells, IL-10, and CD4$^+$FOXP3$^+$ cells in lymph nodes. The positive aspects of oral administration of *E. coli* Nissle 1917 was consider to be associated with the lower numbers of CD4$^+$ and MOG-specific CD4$^+$ T cells (Secher et al., 2017). Oral administration of the mentioned probiotics strain contributed to the improvement of intestinal barrier dysfunction and neuroinflammatory factors (Secher et al., 2017). Moreover, treatment with IRT5 (mixture of five probiotics containing of 10^8 CFU/g of each strain: *S. thermophilus*, *L. acidophilus*, *L. casei*, *B. bifidum* and *L. reuteri*) contributed to the suppression of EAE condition (Kwon et al., 2013). The combination of *L. plantarum* DSM 15312, *L. plantarum* DSM 15312, and *L. paracasei* DSM 13434 also showed therapeutic potential in inhibiting the progression of myelin oligodendrocyte glycoprotein-induced EAE (Lavasani et al., 2010) (Fig. 12.5).

Recent human studies have also marked significant remission upon assessment of clinical and metabolic response on the effect of probiotics in MS patients. The B cells' function was observed to rapidly decline after 12 weeks of probiotics capsule administration containing probiotics strains of *L. casei*, *B. bifidum*, *Lactobacillus fermentum*, and *L. acidophilus* (Kouchaki et al., 2017). This randomized, placebo-controlled clinical trial on probiotics capsule was analyzed on 60 MS patients. The study suggested that uptake of this probiotic improved depression, anxiety and stress scale within the patients. Moreover, the levels of CRP, malondialdehyde, and plasma nitric oxide were significantly altered within the placebo group (Kouchaki et al., 2017).

Another study of randomized, double-blind, placebo-controlled clinical trial evaluated the role of probiotics on the genetic expression related to glucose, lipid, and inflammatory pathways within Ms individuals (Tamtaji et al., 2017). The study enrolled 40 Ms patients and randomly divided them into two groups, among which one group received probiotics capsule containing *L. fermentum*, *B. bifidum*, *L. acidophilus*, and *L. casei* with 2×10^9 CFU/g each and the other group was assigned as placebo for 12 weeks. The study reported downregulation of *TNFA* and *IL8* mRNA expressions in the peripheral blood mononuclear cells of Ms patients (Tamtaji et al., 2017). Overall, the human studies demonstrated positive impact on the progression and delay in the onset of the disease upon probiotic administration, suggesting that probiotics exert immunomodulatory effects in MS patients.

12.5.5 Role of probiotics in suppression of cystic fibrosis

Gastrointestinal microbiota plays an indispensable role in contributing toward immunity and metabolic function of CF (Quigley, 2013). Currently a clinical trial on prebiotics (inulin) along with high-dose vitamin D is going on in 40 participants with CF to evaluate its effect on reducing gastrointestinal dysbiosis and improving critical intestinal functions among CF individuals (ClinicalTrials.gov Identifier: NCT04118010). Emerging studies reveal that certain probiotics strains can be implemented to reduce the progression or onset of CF. A randomized, placebo-controlled study was performed to evaluate the role of probiotics *Lactobacillus* GG (LGG) in the children with CF (Bruzzese et al., 2004, 2007). In the study, a total of 19 children were administered with LGG for continuous 6 months, which resulted in the reduction of pulmonary exacerbations, suggesting that probiotics may delay intestinal and pulmonary inflammation within CF (Bruzzese et al., 2004, 2007). Similarly, another randomized, double blind, placebo controlled study assessed the role of *L. reuteri* on the gastrointestinal tract and rate of respiratory exacerbations (Di Nardo et al., 2014). The study suggested that pulmonary exacerbations were significantly reduced in the *L. reuteri* group (Di Nardo et al., 2014). Presently there is a scarcity of evidence regarding the role of probiotics and prebiotics in the amelioration of CF; therefore future studies with respect to animal model and human studies are needed for CF.

12.6 Future perspectives

Several *in vivo* and *in vitro* studies have been conducted for exploring the role of probiotics and prebiotics in improvement of autoimmune diseases. One of the major concerns associated with the probiotic field is to address its safety and efficacy. Although probiotics, such as *Lactobacillus* and *Bifidobacterium*, and prebiotics, such as inulin and GOS, do not need approval from FDA for our daily dietary uptake, few studies pointed out incidence, such as flatulence, high osmotic pressure, and bloating, that leads to gastrointestinal discomfort, indicating adverse effects of the probiotic consumption (Williams, 1999). But still probiotics are considered to be relatively safe due to low rate of adverse effects. Moreover, the effects of probiotics greatly differ from one individual to another due to the influence of diet. As of now, there is no standard guideline available for oral administration of probiotics in human. Therefore upcoming studies should be designed in such a manner that it could be able to easily analyze potential adverse reactions at specific dosages of probiotics and prebiotics in autoimmune diseases. Moreover, transmission of antibiotic resistant genes among beneficial bacteria and pathogens may cause complex microflora colony in the gastrointestinal tract leading to the development of antibiotic resistant probiotics (Mathur & Singh, 2005); hence, future studies must target these aspects of probiotics as well.

In several other autoimmue disorders, such as Myasthenia Gravis, Graves' Disease, Goodpasture's Syndrome, Autoimmune Anemias, and Hashimoto's Thyroiditis, the probiotics action has not been explored yet and/or there are scarcity of data with respect to animal model study and human clinical trials. Therefore there is need of probiotic intervention studies in such autoimmune diseases. In addition, probiotic-based mechanisms, such as induction of Tregs by probiotics and prebiotics, should be explored for the development of effective therapeutic approach toward curbing the autoimmune response and as an alternative to detrimental immunosuppressive drugs (Dwivedi et al., 2016).

12.7 Conclusions

It has become evident that the disturbances cause within gut microflora and gastrointestinal tract is responsible for contributing among exacerbation of inflammatory response in several autoimmune diseases. Rapidly emerging studies reveal new evidence for immunopathological role of autoimmune diseases. Presently probiotics are considered as one of the important approaches in restoring or maintaining immune balance for the treatment of autoimmune diseases. Several studies on the animal and human models provide evidence implicating health benefits in autoimmune diseases, such as T1D, RA, SLE, MS, and CF, upon probiotic uptake. Despite limited success in improving symptoms of the diseases, probiotics are not considered as first-line treatment in autoimmune diseases. So far, efficacy and dosages of probiotic strain remain controversial as there are incidences indicating side effects of probiotics. So far, animal and human studies' results have emphasized on the probiotic-mediated alteration in immune responses through modulating cellular immunity involving Th17, Treg, Th1, and Th2 cells. However, knowledge regarding probiotics mechanisms on the improvement of health and diseases remains a piece of mystery for the researchers, specifically in case of immunological and gastrointestinal diseases. There is lack of research on the effects of probiotics in case of MS and CF. Therefore more *in vivo* and *in vitro* studies should be incorporated to provide a solid evidence supporting the beneficial effects of probiotics in the autoimmune diseases.

Acknowledgments

We are grateful to Uka Tarsadia University, Maliba Campus, Tarsadi, Gujarat, India, for providing the facilities needed for the preparation of this chapter. This work was supported by grant to Dr. Mitesh Dwivedi {ECR/2017/000858} Science and Engineering Research Board, Department of Science; Technology (SERB-DST), New Delhi.

Conflict of interest

The authors declare no conflict of interest.

References

Abdelazez, A., Abdelmotaal, H., Evivie, S. E., Melak, S., Jia, F. F., Khoso, M. H., Zhu, Z. T., Zhang, L. J., Sami, R., & Meng, X. C. (2018). Screening potential probiotic characteristics of Lactobacillus brevis strains in vitro and intervention effect on type I diabetes in vivo. *BioMed Research International, 2018*. Available from https://doi.org/10.1155/2018/7356173.

Abdelhamid, L., & Luo, X. M. (2018). Retinoic acid, leaky gut, and autoimmune diseases. *Nutrients, 10*(8). Available from https://doi.org/10.3390/nu10081016.

Abhari, K., Shekarforoush, S. S., Hosseinzadeh, S., Nazifi, S., Sajedianfard, J., & Eskandari, M. H. (2016). The effects of orally administered Bacillus coagulans and inulin on prevention and progression of rheumatoid arthritis in rats. *Food and Nutrition Research, 60*. Available from https://doi.org/10.3402/fnr.v60.30876.

Ahola, A. J., Harjutsalo, V., Forsblom, C., Freese, R., Makimattila, S., & Groop, P. H. (2017). The self-reported use of probiotics is associated with better glycaemic control and lower odds of metabolic syndrome and its components in type 1 diabetes. *Journal of Probiotics & Health*. Available from https://doi.org/10.4172/2329-8901.1000188.

Alejandra., de, M., de, L., Silvina., del, C., Meritxell, Z.-T., Clarissa, S. R., Maarten., van de, G., Vasco, A., Anderson, M., & Guy, L. J. (2011). Importance of IL-10 modulation by probiotic microorganisms in gastrointestinal inflammatory diseases. *ISRN Gastroenterology, 1*, 1–11. Available from https://doi.org/10.5402/2011/892971.

Alipour, B., Homayouni-Rad, A., Vaghef-Mehrabany, E., Sharif, S. K., Vaghef-Mehrabany, L., Asghari-Jafarabadi, M., Nakhjavani, M. R., & Mohtadi-Nia, J. (2014). Effects of Lactobacillus casei supplementation on disease activity and inflammatory cytokines in rheumatoid arthritis patients: A randomized double-blind clinical trial. *International Journal of Rheumatic Diseases, 17*(5), 519–527. Available from https://doi.org/10.1111/1756-185X.12333.

Amdekar, S., Singh, V., Kumar, A., Sharma, P., & Singh, R. (2013). Lactobacillus casei and Lactobacillus acidophilus regulate inflammatory pathway and improve antioxidant status in collagen-induced arthritic rats. *Journal of Interferon and Cytokine Research, 33*(1), 1–8. Available from https://doi.org/10.1089/jir.2012.0034.

Aqaeinezhad Rudbane, S. M., Rahmdel, S., Abdollahzadeh, S. M., Zare, M., Bazrafshan, A., & Mazloomi, S. M. (2018). The efficacy of probiotic supplementation in rheumatoid arthritis: A meta-analysis of randomized, controlled trials. *Inflammopharmacology, 26*(1), 67–76. Available from https://doi.org/10.1007/s10787-017-0436-y.

Arpaia, N., Campbell, C., Fan, X., Dikiy, S., Van Der Veeken, J., Deroos, P., Liu, H., Cross, J. R., Pfeffer, K., Coffer, P. J., & Rudensky, A. Y. (2013). Metabolites produced by commensal bacteria promote peripheral regulatory T-cell generation. *Nature, 504*(7480), 451–455. Available from https://doi.org/10.1038/nature12726.

Atarashi, K., Tanoue, T., Shima, T., Imaoka, A., Kuwahara, T., Momose, Y., Cheng, G., Yamasaki, S., Saito, T., Ohba, Y., Taniguchi, T., Takeda, K., Hori, S., Ivanov, I. I., Umesaki, Y., Itoh, K., & Honda, K. (2011). Induction of colonic regulatory T cells by indigenous Clostridium species. *Science, 331*(6015), 337–341. Available from https://doi.org/10.1126/science.1198469.

Azad, M. A. K., Sarker, M., & Wan, D. (2018). Immunomodulatory effects of probiotics on cytokine profiles. *BioMed Research International*. Available from https://doi.org/10.1155/2018/8063647.

Bansal, T., Alaniz, R. C., Wood, T. K., & Jayaraman, A. (2010). The bacterial signal indole increases epithelial-cell tight-junction resistance and attenuates indicators of inflammation. *Proceedings of the National Academy of Sciences of the United States of America, 107*(1), 228–233. Available from https://doi.org/10.1073/pnas.0906112107.

Belkaid, Y., & Naik, S. (2013). Compartmentalized and systemic control of tissue immunity by commensals. *Nature Immunology*, *14*(7), 646–653. Available from https://doi.org/10.1038/ni.2604.

Bodkhe, R., Balakrishnan, B., & Taneja, V. (2019). The role of microbiome in rheumatoid arthritis treatment. *Therapeutic Advances in Musculoskeletal Disease*, 11. Available from https://doi.org/10.1177/1759720X19844632.

Beretta, M. V., Bernaud, F. R., Nascimento, C., Steemburgo, T., & Rodrigues, T. C. (2018). Higher fiber intake is associated with lower blood pressure levels in patients with type 1 diabetes. *Archives of endocrinology and metabolism*, *62*(1), 40–47. Available from https://doi.org/10.20945/2359-3997000000008.

Bruzzese, E., Raia, V., Gaudiello, G., Polito, G., Buccigrossi, V., Formicola, V., & Guarino, A. (2004). Intestinal inflammation is a frequent feature of cystic fibrosis and is reduced by probiotic administration. *Alimentary Pharmacology and Therapeutics*, *20*(7), 813–819. Available from https://doi.org/10.1111/j.1365-2036.2004.02174.x.

Bruzzese, E., Raia, V., Spagnuolo, M. I., Volpicelli, M., De Marco, G., Maiuri, L., & Guarino, A. (2007). Effect of Lactobacillus GG supplementation on pulmonary exacerbations in patients with cystic fibrosis: A pilot study. *Clinical Nutrition*, *26*(3), 322–328. Available from https://doi.org/10.1016/j.clnu.2007.01.004.

Calcinaro, F., Dionisi, S., Marinaro, M., Candeloro, P., Bonato, V., Marzotti, S., Corneli, R. B., Ferretti, E., Gulino, A., Grasso, F., De Simone, C., Di Mario, U., Falorni, A., Boirivant, M., & Dotta, F. (2005). Oral probiotic administration induces interleukin-10 production and prevents spontaneous autoimmune diabetes in the non-obese diabetic mouse. *Diabetologia*, *48*(8), 1565–1575. Available from https://doi.org/10.1007/s00125-005-1831-2.

Cani, P. D., Neyrinck, A. M., Fava, F., Knauf, C., Burcelin, R. G., Tuohy, K. M., Gibson, G. R., & Delzenne, N. M. (2007). Selective increases of bifidobacteria in gut microflora improve high-fat-diet-induced diabetes in mice through a mechanism associated with endotoxaemia. *Diabetologia*, *50*(11), 2374–2383. Available from https://doi.org/10.1007/s00125-007-0791-0.

Carbone, F., Bonaventura, A., Liberale, L., Paolino, S., Torre, F., Dallegri, F., Montecucco, F., & Cutolo, M. (2020). Atherosclerosis in rheumatoid arthritis: Promoters and opponents. *Clinical Reviews in Allergy and Immunology*, *58*(1). Available from https://doi.org/10.1007/s12016-018-8714-z.

Cekanaviciute, E., Yoo, B. B., Runia, T. F., Debelius, J. W., Singh, S., Nelson, C. A., Kanner, R., Bencosme, Y., Lee, Y. K., Hauser, S. L., Crabtree-Hartman, E., Sand, I. K., Gacias, M., Zhu, Y., Casaccia, P., Cree, B. A. C., Knight, R., Mazmanian, S. K., & Baranzini, S. E. (2017). Gut bacteria from multiple sclerosis patients modulate human T cells and exacerbate symptoms in mouse models. *Proceedings of the National Academy of Sciences of the United States of America*, *114*(40), 10713–10718. Available from https://doi.org/10.1073/pnas.1711235114.

CF Foundation. (2021). About cystic fibrosis. https://www.cff.org/What-is-CF/About-Cystic-Fibrosis.

Chandrashekara, S. (2012). The treatment strategies of autoimmune disease may need a different approach from conventional protocol: A review. *Indian Journal of Pharmacology*, 665. Available from https://doi.org/10.4103/0253-7613.103235.

Chelakkot, C., Ghim, J., & Ryu, S. H. (2018). Mechanisms regulating intestinal barrier integrity and its pathological implications. *Experimental and Molecular Medicine*, *50*(8). Available from https://doi.org/10.1038/s12276-018-0126-x.

Chen, K., Chen, H., Faas, M. M., de Haan, B. J., Li, J., Xiao, P., Zhang, H., Diana, J., de Vos, P., & Sun, J. (2017). Specific inulin-type fructan fibers protect against autoimmune diabetes by modulating gut immunity, barrier function, and microbiota homeostasis. *Molecular Nutrition and Food Research*, *61*(8). Available from https://doi.org/10.1002/mnfr.201601006.

Chen, L., Zou, Y., Peng, J., Lu, F., Yin, Y., Li, F., & Yang, J. (2015). Lactobacillus acidophilus suppresses colitis-associated activation of the IL-23/Th17 axis. *Journal of Immunology Research*. Available from https://doi.org/10.1155/2015/909514.

Chow, J., & Mazmanian, S. K. (2009). Getting the bugs out of the immune system: Do bacterial microbiota \Fix\ intestinal T cell responses? *Cell Host and Microbe*, *5*(1), 8–12. Available from https://doi.org/10.1016/j.chom.2008.12.006.

Cojocaru. (2011). Manifestations of systemic lupus erythematosus. *Maedica*, *6*(4), 330–336.

Danne, C., Ryzhakov, G., Martínez-López, M., Ilott, N. E., Franchini, F., Cuskin, F., Lowe, E. C., Bullers, S. J., Arthur, J. S. C., & Powrie, F. (2017). A large polysaccharide produced by Helicobacter hepaticus induces an anti-inflammatory gene signature in macrophages. *Cell Host and Microbe*, *22*(6), 733–745.e5. Available from https://doi.org/10.1016/j.chom.2017.11.002.

de la Visitación, N., Robles-Vera, I., Toral, M., & Duarte, J. (2019). Protective effects of probiotic consumption in cardiovascular disease in systemic lupus erythematosus. *Nutrients*, *11*(11). Available from https://doi.org/10.3390/nu11112676.

de los Angeles Pineda, M., Thompson, S. F., Summers, K., de Leon, F., Pope, J., & Reid, G. (2011). A randomized, double-blinded, placebo-controlled pilot study of probiotics in active rheumatoid arthritis. *Medical Science Monitor*, *17*(6), CR347–CR354. Available from https://doi.org/10.12659/MSM.881808.

de Oliveira, G. L. V. (2018). *Probiotic Applications in Autoimmune Diseases. In: Rijeka IntechOpen*. Available from https://doi.org/10.5772/intechopen.73064.

de Oliveira, G. L. V., Leite, A. Z., Higuchi, B. S., Gonzaga, M. I., & Mariano, V. S. (2017). Intestinal dysbiosis and probiotic applications in autoimmune diseases. *Immunology*, *152*(1), 1–12. Available from https://doi.org/10.1111/imm.12765.

Deane, K. D., Demoruelle, M. K., Kelmenson, L. B., Kuhn, K. A., Norris, J. M., & Holers, V. M. (2017). Genetic and environmental risk factors for rheumatoid arthritis. *Best Practice and Research: Clinical Rheumatology*, *31*(1), 3–18. Available from https://doi.org/10.1016/j.berh.2017.08.003.

Dedrick, S., Sundaresh, B., Huang, Q., Brady, C., Yoo, T., Cronin, C., Rudnicki, C., Flood, M., Momeni, B., Ludvigsson, J., & Altindis, E. (2020). The role of gut microbiota and environmental factors in type 1 diabetes pathogenesis. *Frontiers in Endocrinology*, 11. Available from https://doi.org/10.3389/fendo.2020.00078.

Di Nardo, G., Oliva, S., Menichella, A., Pistelli, R., Biase, R. V. D., Patriarchi, F., Cucchiara, S., & Stronati, L. (2014). Lactobacillus reuteri ATCC55730 in cystic fibrosis. *Journal of Pediatric Gastroenterology and Nutrition*, 58(1), 81–86. Available from https://doi.org/10.1097/MPG.0000000000000187.

Dolpady, J., Sorini, C., Di Pietro, C., Cosorich, I., Ferrarese, R., Saita, D., Clementi, M., Canducci, F., & Falcone, M. (2016). Oral probiotic VSL#3 prevents autoimmune diabetes by modulating microbiota and promoting indoleamine 2,3-dioxygenase-enriched tolerogenic intestinal environment. *Journal of Diabetes Research*. Available from https://doi.org/10.1155/2016/7569431.

Duytschaever, G., Huys, G., Bekaert, M., Boulanger, L., De Boeck, K., & Vandamme, P. (2011). Cross-sectional and longitudinal comparisons of the predominant fecal microbiota compositions of a group of pediatric patients with cystic fibrosis and their healthy siblings. *Applied and Environmental Microbiology*, 77(22), 8015–8024. Available from https://doi.org/10.1128/aem.05933-11.

Dwivedi, M. (2018). Role of probiotics in immune regulation. *Acta Scientific Microbiology*, 1(1), 29–30. Available from https://doi.org/10.31080/ASMI.2018.01.0007.

Dwivedi, M., Ansarullah., Radichev, I., & Kemp, E. (2017). Alteration of immune-mechanisms by human microbiota and development and prevention of human diseases. *Journal of Immunology Research*, 2017, 6985256. Available from https://doi.org/10.1155/2017/6985256.

Dwivedi, M., Kumar, P., Laddha, N., & Kemp, E. (2016). Induction of regulatory T cells: A role for probiotics and prebiotics to suppress autoimmunity. *Autoimmunity Reviews*, 15(4), 379–392. Available from https://doi.org/10.1016/j.autrev.2016.01.002.

Ehmann, D., Wendler, J., Koeninger, L., Larsen, I. S., Klag, T., Berger, J., Marette, A., Schaller, M., Stange, E. F., Malek, N. P., Jensen, B. A. H., & Wehkamp, J. (2019). Paneth cell α-defensins HD-5 and HD-6 display differential degradation into active antimicrobial fragments. *Proceedings of the National Academy of Sciences of the United States of America*, 116(9), 3746–3751. Available from https://doi.org/10.1073/pnas.1817376116.

Falony, G., Lazidou, K., Verschaeren, A., Weckx, S., Maes, D., & De Vuyst, L. (2009). In vitro kinetic analysis of fermentation of prebiotic inulin-type fructans by Bifidobacterium species reveals four different phenotypes. *Applied and Environmental Microbiology*, 75(2), 454–461. Available from https://doi.org/10.1128/AEM.01488-08.

Firestein, G. S., & McInnes, I. B. (2017). Immunopathogenesis of rheumatoid arthritis. *Immunity*, 46(2), 183–196. Available from https://doi.org/10.1016/j.immuni.2017.02.006.

Flannigan, K. L., & Denning, T. L. (2018). Segmented filamentous bacteria-induced immune responses: A balancing act between host protection and autoimmunity. *Immunology*, 154(4), 537–546. Available from https://doi.org/10.1111/imm.12950.

Fukuda, S., Toh, H., Hase, K., Oshima, K., Nakanishi, Y., Yoshimura, K., Tobe, T., Clarke, J. M., Topping, D. L., Suzuki, T., Taylor, T. D., Itoh, K., Kikuchi, J., Morita, H., Hattori, M., & Ohno, H. (2011). Bifidobacteria can protect from enteropathogenic infection through production of acetate. *Nature*, 469(7331), 543–549. Available from https://doi.org/10.1038/nature09646.

Gerhard, W., Marcus, H., Isaac, E., Konrad, P., Klaus, L., Hermann, H., Mitchell, K., & Sibylle, von V. (2012). Neutrophilic granulocytes modulate invariant NKT cell function in mice and humans. *The Journal of Immunology*, 3000–3008. Available from https://doi.org/10.4049/jimmunol.1101273.

Gohil, P., Patel, V., Deshpande, S., Chorawala, M., & Shah, G. (2018). Anti-arthritic activity of cell wall content of Lactobacillus plantarum in freund's adjuvant-induced arthritic rats: Involvement of cellular inflammatory mediators and other biomarkers. *Inflammopharmacology*, 26(1), 171–181. Available from https://doi.org/10.1007/s10787-017-0370-z.

Groele, L., Szajewska, H., & Szypowska, A. (2017). Effects of Lactobacillus rhamnosus GG and Bifidobacterium lactis Bb12 on beta-cell function in children with newly diagnosed type 1 diabetes: Protocol of a randomised controlled trial. *BMJ Open*, 7(10). Available from https://doi.org/10.1136/bmjopen-2017-017178.

Hara, N., Alkanani, A. K., Ir, D., Robertson, C. E., Wagner, B. D., Frank, D. N., & Zipris, D. (2013). The role of the intestinal microbiota in type 1 diabetes. *Clinical Immunology*, 146(2), 112–119. Available from https://doi.org/10.1016/j.clim.2012.12.001.

Hatakka, K., Martio, J., Korpela, M., Herranen, M., Poussa, T., Laasanen, T., Saxelin, M., Vapaatalo, H., Moilanen, E., & Korpela, R. (2003). Effects of probiotic therapy on the activity and activation of mild rheumatoid arthritis—A pilot study. *Scandinavian Journal of Rheumatology*, 32(4), 211–215. Available from https://doi.org/10.1080/03009740310003695.

He, Z., Shao, T., Li, H., Xie, Z., & Wen, C. (2016). Alterations of the gut microbiome in Chinese patients with systemic lupus erythematosus. *Gut Pathogens*, 8(1). Available from https://doi.org/10.1186/s13099-016-0146-9.

Hemarajata, P., & Versalovic, J. (2013). Effects of probiotics on gut microbiota: Mechanisms of intestinal immunomodulation and neuromodulation. *Therapeutic Advances in Gastroenterology*, 6(1), 39–51. Available from https://doi.org/10.1177/1756283X12459294.

Hill, C., Guarner, F., Reid, G., Gibson, G. R., Merenstein, D. J., Pot, B., Morelli, L., Canani, R. B., Flint, H. J., Salminen, S., Calder, P. C., & Sanders, M. E. (2014). Expert consensus document: The international scientific association for probiotics and prebiotics consensus statement on the scope and appropriate use of the term probiotic. *Nature Reviews Gastroenterology & Hepatology*, 11(8), 506–514. Available from https://doi.org/10.1038/nrgastro.2014.66.

Ho, J., Reimer, R. A., Doulla, M., & Huang, C. (2016). Effect of prebiotic intake on gut microbiota, intestinal permeability and glycemic control in children with type 1 diabetes: Study protocol for a randomized controlled trial. *Trials*, 17(1). Available from https://doi.org/10.1186/s13063-016-1486-y.

Hoen, A. G., Li, J., Moulton, L. A., O'Toole, G. A., Housman, M. L., Koestler, D. C., Guill, M. F., Moore, J. H., Hibberd, P. L., Morrison, H. G., Sogin, M. L., Karagas, M. R., & Madan, J. C. (2015). Associations between gut microbial colonization in early life and respiratory outcomes in cystic fibrosis. *Journal of Pediatrics*, 167(1), 138–147.e3. Available from https://doi.org/10.1016/j.jpeds.2015.02.049.

Horta-Baas, G., Romero-Figueroa, M. D. S., Montiel-Jarquín, A. J., Pizano-Zárate, M. L., García-Mena, J., & Ramírez-Durán, N. (2017). Intestinal dysbiosis and rheumatoid arthritis: A link between gut microbiota and the pathogenesis of rheumatoid arthritis. *Journal of Immunology Research*. Available from https://doi.org/10.1155/2017/4835189.

Hsu, T. C., Huang, C. Y., Liu, C. H., Hsu, K. C., Chen, Y. H., & Tzang, B. S. (2017). Lactobacillus paracasei GMNL-32, Lactobacillus reuteri GMNL-89 and L. reuteri GMNL-263 ameliorate hepatic injuries in lupus-prone mice. *British Journal of Nutrition, 117*(8), 1066–1074. Available from https://doi.org/10.1017/S0007114517001039.

Hwang, J.-S., Im, C.-R., & Im, S.-H. (2012). Immune disorders and its correlation with gut microbiome. *Immune Network, 12*(4), 129. Available from https://doi.org/10.4110/in.2012.12.4.129.

Inamine, T., & Schnabl, B. (2018). Immunoglobulin A and liver diseases. *Journal of Gastroenterology, 53*(6), 691–700. Available from https://doi.org/10.1007/s00535-017-1400-8.

Islam, M. A., Khandker, S. S., Kotyla, P. J., & Hassan, R. (2020). Immunomodulatory effects of diet and nutrients in systemic lupus erythematosus (SLE): A systematic review. *Frontiers in Immunology, 11*. Available from https://doi.org/10.3389/fimmu.2020.01477.

Jadin, S. A., Wu, G. S., Zhang, Z., Shoff, S. M., Tippets, B. M., Farrell, P. M., Miller, T., Rock, M. J., Levy, H., & Lai, H. J. (2011). Growth and pulmonary outcomes during the first 2y of life of breastfed and formula-fed infants diagnosed with cystic fibrosis through the Wisconsin Routine Newborn Screening Program. *American Journal of Clinical Nutrition, 93*(5), 1038–1047. Available from https://doi.org/10.3945/ajcn.110.004119.

Jie, Z., Yang, J. Y., Gu, M., Wang, H., Xie, X., Li, Y., Liu, T., Zhu, L., Shi, J., Zhang, L., Zhou, X., Joo, D., Brightbill, H. D., Cong, Y., Lin, D., Cheng, X., & Sun, S. C. (2018). NIK signaling axis regulates dendritic cell function in intestinal immunity and homeostasis. *Nature Immunology, 19*(11), 1224–1235. Available from https://doi.org/10.1038/s41590-018-0206-z.

Kamen, D. L. (2014). Environmental influences on systemic lupus erythematosus expression. *Rheumatic Disease Clinics of North America, 40*(3), 401–412. Available from https://doi.org/10.1016/j.rdc.2014.05.003.

Karumuthil-Melethil, S., Sofi, M. H., Gudi, R., Johnson, B. M., Perez, N., & Vasu, C. (2015). TLR2- and dectin 1-associated innate immune response modulates T-cell response to pancreatic β-cell antigen and prevents type 1 diabetes. *Diabetes, 64*(4), 1341–1357. Available from https://doi.org/10.2337/db14-1145.

Kawamoto, S., Maruya, M., Kato, L. M., Suda, W., Atarashi, K., Doi, Y., Tsutsui, Y., Qin, H., Honda, K., Okada, T., Hattori, M., & Fagarasan, S. (2014). Foxp3 + T cells regulate immunoglobulin A selection and facilitate diversification of bacterial species responsible for immune homeostasis. *Immunity, 41*(1), 152–165. Available from https://doi.org/10.1016/j.immuni.2014.05.016.

Kayama, H., & Takeda, K. (2014). Polysaccharide A of Bacteroides fragilis: Actions on dendritic cells and T cells. *Molecular Cell, 54*(2), 206–207. Available from https://doi.org/10.1016/j.molcel.2014.04.002.

Khan, M. F., & Wang, H. (2020). Environmental exposures and autoimmune diseases: Contribution of gut microbiome. *Frontiers in Immunology, 10*. Available from https://doi.org/10.3389/fimmu.2019.03094.

Khorasani, S., Mahmoudi, M., Kalantari, M. R., Lavi Arab, F., Esmaeili, S. A., Mardani, F., Tabasi, N., & Rastin, M. (2019). Amelioration of regulatory T cells by Lactobacillus delbrueckii and Lactobacillus rhamnosus in pristane-induced lupus mice model. *Journal of Cellular Physiology, 234*(6), 9778–9786. Available from https://doi.org/10.1002/jcp.27663.

Kim, J. E., Chae, C. S., Kim, G. C., Hwang, W., Hwang, J. s, Hwang, S. M., Kim, Y., Ahn, Y. T., Park, S. G., Jun, C. D., Rudra, D., & Im, S. H. (2015). Lactobacillus helveticus suppresses experimental rheumatoid arthritis by reducing inflammatory T cell responses. *Journal of Functional Foods, 13*, 350–362. Available from https://doi.org/10.1016/j.jff.2015.01.002.

Knudsen, K. E. B., Lærke, H. N., Hedemann, M. S., Nielsen, T. S., Ingerslev, A. K., Nielsen, D. S. G., Theil, P. K., Purup, S., Hald, S., Schioldan, A. G., Marco, M. L., Gregersen, S., & Hermansen, K. (2018). Impact of diet-modulated butyrate production on intestinal barrier function and inflammation. *Nutrients, 10*(10). Available from https://doi.org/10.3390/nu10101499.

Konrad, A., Cong, Y., Duck, W., Borlaza, R., & Elson, C. O. (2006). Tight mucosal compartmentation of the murine immune response to antigens of the enteric microbiota. *Gastroenterology, 130*(7), 2050–2059. Available from https://doi.org/10.1053/j.gastro.2006.02.055.

Kouchaki, E., Tamtaji, O. R., Salami, M., Bahmani, F., Daneshvar Kakhaki, R., Akbari, E., Tajabadi-Ebrahimi, M., Jafari, P., & Asemi, Z. (2017). Clinical and metabolic response to probiotic supplementation in patients with multiple sclerosis: A randomized, double-blind, placebo-controlled trial. *Clinical Nutrition, 36*(5), 1245–1249. Available from https://doi.org/10.1016/j.clnu.2016.08.015.

Kubinak, J. L., Petersen, C., Stephens, W. Z., Soto, R., Bake, E., O'Connell, R. M., & Round, J. L. (2015). MyD88 signaling in T cells directs IgA-mediated control of the microbiota to promote health. *Cell Host and Microbe, 17*(2), 153–163. Available from https://doi.org/10.1016/j.chom.2014.12.009.

Kwon, H. K., Kim, G. C., Kim, Y., Hwang, W., Jash, A., Sahoo, A., Kim, J. E., Nam, J. H., & Im, S. H. (2013). Amelioration of experimental autoimmune encephalomyelitis by probiotic mixture is mediated by a shift in T helper cell immune response. *Clinical Immunology, 146*(3), 217–227. Available from https://doi.org/10.1016/j.clim.2013.01.001.

La Paglia, G., Leone, M., Lepri, G., Vagelli, R., Valentini, E., Alunno, A., & Tani, C. (2017). One year in review 2017: Systemic lupus erythematosus. *Clinical and Experimental Rheumatology, 35*(4), 551–561.

Lau, K., Benitez, P., Ardissone, A., Wilson, T. D., Collins, E. L., Lorca, G., Li, N., Sankar, D., Wasserfall, C., Neu, J., Atkinson, M. A., Shatz, D., Triplett, E. W., & Larkin, J., 3rd (2011). Inhibition of Type 1 Diabetes Correlated to a Lactobacillus johnsonii N6.2-Mediated Th17 Bias. *The Journal of Immunology, 186*(6), 3538–3546. Available from https://doi:10.4049/jimmunol.1001864.

Lavasani, S., Dzhambazov, B., Nouri, M., Fåk, F., Buske, S., Molin, G., Thorlacius, H., Alenfall, J., Jeppsson, B., & Weström, B. (2010). A novel probiotic mixture exerts a therapeutic effect on experimental autoimmune encephalomyelitis mediated by IL-10 producing regulatory T cells. *PLoS One, 5*(2). Available from https://doi.org/10.1371/journal.pone.0009009.

Le, T. K. C., Hosaka, T., Nguyen, T. T., Kassu, A., Dang, T. O., Tran, H. B., Pham, T. P., Tran, Q. B., Le, T. H. H., & Da Pham, X. (2015). Bifidobacterium species lower serum glucose, increase expressions of insulin signaling proteins, and improve adipokine profile in diabetic mice. *Biomedical Research (Japan), 36*(1), 63–70. Available from https://doi.org/10.2220/biomedres.36.63.

Lee, J. M., Leach, S. T., Katz, T., Day, A. S., Jaffe, A., & Ooi, C. Y. (2012). Update of faecal markers of inflammation in children with cystic fibrosis. *Mediators of Inflammation*, 2012. Available from https://doi.org/10.1155/2012/948367.

Ley, R. E., Lozupone, C. A., Hamady, M., Knight, R., & Gordon, J. I. (2008). Worlds within worlds: Evolution of the vertebrate gut microbiota. *Nature Reviews Microbiology*, 6(10), 776–788. Available from https://doi.org/10.1038/nrmicro1978.

Li, B., Selmi, C., Tang, R., Gershwin, M. E., & Ma, X. (2018). The microbiome and autoimmunity: A paradigm from the gut–liver axis. *Cellular and Molecular Immunology*, 15(6), 595–609. Available from https://doi.org/10.1038/cmi.2018.7.

Li, Y., Wang, H. F., Li, X., Li, H. X., Zhang, Q., Zhou, H. W., He, Y., Li, P., Fu, C., Zhang, X. H., Qiu, Y. R., & Li, J. L. (2019). Disordered intestinal microbes are associated with the activity of systemic lupus erythematosus. *Clinical Science*, 133(7), 821–838. Available from https://doi.org/10.1042/CS20180841.

Liu, Y., & Rhoads, J. (2013). *Communication between B-cells and microbiota for the maintenance of intestinal homeostasis.* (4th ed., pp. 535–553). *Antibodies*, (Vol. 2, pp. 535–553). MDPI AG. Available from https://doi.org/10.3390/antib2040535.

Liu, S., Zhao, W., Lan, P., & Mou, X. (2020). The microbiome in inflammatory bowel diseases: From pathogenesis to therapy. *Protein and Cell*. Available from https://doi.org/10.1007/s13238-020-00745-3.

Liu, T., Li, J., Liu, Y., Xiao, N., Suo, H., Xie, K., Yang, C., & Wu, C. (2012). Short-chain fatty acids suppress lipopolysaccharide-induced production of nitric oxide and proinflammatory cytokines through inhibition of NF-?B pathway in RAW264.7 cells. *Inflammation*, 35(5), 1676–1684. Available from https://doi.org/10.1007/s10753-012-9484-z.

López, P., González-Rodríguez, I., Gueimonde, M., Margolles, A., & Suárez, A. (2011). Immune response to Bifidobacterium bifidum strains support Treg/Th17 plasticity. *PLoS One*, 6(9). Available from https://doi.org/10.1371/journal.pone.0024776.

Luo, X. M., Edwards, M. R., Mu, Q., Yu, Y., Vieson, M. D., Reilly, C. M., Ahmed, S. A., & Bankole, A. A. (2018). Gut microbiota in human systemic lupus erythematosus and a mouse model of lupus. *Applied and Environmental Microbiology*, 84(4). Available from https://doi.org/10.1128/AEM.02288-17.

Macpherson, A. J., & Uhr, T. (2004). Induction of protective IgA by intestinal dendritic cells carrying commensal bacteria. *Science*, 303(5664), 1662–1665. Available from https://doi.org/10.1126/science.1091334.

Maidhof, W., & Hilas, O. (2012). Lupus: An overview of the disease and management options. *P and T*, 37(4), 240–249. Available from http://www.ptcommunity.com/ptjournal/dl.cfm?file = fulltext/37/4/PTJ3704240.pdf.

Mandel, D. R., Eichas, K., & Holmes, J. (2010). Bacillus coagulans: A viable adjunct therapy for relieving symptoms of rheumatoid arthritis according to a randomized, controlled trial. *BMC Complementary and Alternative Medicine*, 10. Available from https://doi.org/10.1186/1472-6882-10-1.

Marcial, G. E., Ford, A. L., Haller, M. J., Gezan, S. A., Harrison, N. A., Cai, D., Meyer, J. L., Perry, D. J., Atkinson, M. A., Wasserfall, C. H., Garrett, T., Gonzalez, C. F., Brusko, T. M., Dahl, W. J., & Lorca, G. L. (2017). Lactobacillus johnsonii N6.2 modulates the host immune responses: A double-blind, randomized trial in healthy adults. *Frontiers in Immunology*, 8. Available from https://doi.org/10.3389/fimmu.2017.00655.

Martínez-López, M., Iborra, S., Conde-Garrosa, R., Mastrangelo, A., Danne, C., Mann, E. R., Reid, D. M., Gaboriau-Routhiau, V., Chaparro, M., Lorenzo, M. P., Minnerup, L., Saz-Leal, P., Slack, E., Kemp, B., Gisbert, J. P., Dzionek, A., Robinson, M. J., Rupérez, F. J., Cerf-Bensussan, N., & Sancho, D. (2019). Microbiota sensing by Mincle-Syk axis in dendritic cells regulates interleukin-17 and -22 production and promotes intestinal barrier integrity. *Immunity*, 50(2), 446–461.e9. Available from https://doi.org/10.1016/j.immuni.2018.12.020.

Mathur, S., & Singh, R. (2005). Antibiotic resistance in food lactic acid bacteria—A review. *International Journal of Food Microbiology*, 105(3), 281–295. Available from https://doi.org/10.1016/j.ijfoodmicro.2005.03.008.

Milo, R., & Kahana, E. (2010). Multiple sclerosis: Geoepidemiology, genetics and the environment. *Autoimmunity Reviews*, 9(5), A387–A394. Available from https://doi.org/10.1016/j.autrev.2009.11.010.

Miossec, P., & Kolls, J. K. (2012). Targeting IL-17 and TH17 cells in chronic inflammation. *Nature Reviews Drug Discovery*, 11(10), 763–776. Available from https://doi.org/10.1038/nrd3794.

Mishra, S., Wang, S., Nagpal, R., Miller, B., Singh, R., Taraphder, S., & Yadav, H. (2019). Probiotics and prebiotics for the amelioration of type 1 diabetes: Present and future perspectives. *Microorganisms*, 7(3). Available from https://doi.org/10.3390/microorganisms7030067.

Mosser, D. M., & Edwards, J. P. (2008). Exploring the full spectrum of macrophage activation. *Nature Reviews Immunology*, 8(12), 958–969. Available from https://doi.org/10.1038/nri2448.

Moulton, V. R., Suarez-Fueyo, A., Meidan, E., Li, H., Mizui, M., & Tsokos, G. C. (2017). Pathogenesis of human systemic lupus erythematosus: A cellular perspective. *Trends in Molecular Medicine*, 23(7), 615–635. Available from https://doi.org/10.1016/j.molmed.2017.05.006.

Mowat, A. M. I. (2018). To respond or not to respond—A personal perspective of intestinal tolerance. *Nature Reviews Immunology*, 18(6), 405–415. Available from https://doi.org/10.1038/s41577-018-0002-x.

Mu, Q., Kirby, J., Reilly, C. M., & Luo, X. M. (2017). Leaky gut as a danger signal for autoimmune diseases. *Frontiers in Immunology*, 8. Available from https://doi.org/10.3389/fimmu.2017.00598.

Mu, Q., Zhang, H., Liao, X., Lin, K., Liu, H., Edwards, M. R., Ahmed, S. A., Yuan, R., Li, L., Cecere, T. E., Branson, D. B., Kirby, J. L., Goswami, P., Leeth, C. M., Read, K. A., Oestreich, K. J., Vieson, M. D., Reilly, C. M., & Luo, X. M. (2017). Control of lupus nephritis by changes of gut microbiota. *Microbiome*, 5(1), 73. Available from https://doi.org/10.1186/s40168-017-0300-8.

Nagashima, K., Sawa, S., Nitta, T., Tsutsumi, M., Okamura, T., Penninger, J. M., Nakashima, T., & Takayanagi, H. (2017). Identification of subepithelial mesenchymal cells that induce IgA and diversify gut microbiota. *Nature Immunology*, 18(6), 675–682. Available from https://doi.org/10.1038/ni.3732.

Nielsen, S., Needham, B., Leach, S. T., Day, A. S., Jaffe, A., Thomas, T., & Ooi, C. Y. (2016). Disrupted progression of the intestinal microbiota with age in children with cystic fibrosis. *Scientific Reports*, 6. Available from https://doi.org/10.1038/srep24857.

Nikolov, P. (2012). *Probiotics and mucosal immune response. Probiotics*. InTech. Available from https://doi.org/10.5772/50042.

Oliviero, F., Spinella, P., Fiocco, U., Ramonda, R., Sfriso, P., & Punzi, L. (2015). How the Mediterranean diet and some of its components modulate inflammatory pathways in arthritis. *Swiss Medical Weekly*, 145. Available from https://doi.org/10.4414/smw.2015.14190.

Omenetti, S., Bussi, C., Metidji, A., Iseppon, A., Lee, S., Tolaini, M., Li, Y., Kelly, G., Chakravarty, P., Shoaie, S., Gutierrez, M. G., & Stockinger, B. (2019). The intestine harbors functionally distinct homeostatic tissue-resident and inflammatory Th17 cells. *Immunity*, 51(1), 77–89.e6. Available from https://doi.org/10.1016/j.immuni.2019.05.004.

Omenetti, S., & Pizarro, T. T. (2015). The Treg/Th17 axis: A dynamic balance regulated by the gut microbiome. *Frontiers in Immunology*, 6. Available from https://doi.org/10.3389/fimmu.2015.00639.

Pan, H., Li, R., Li, T., Wang, J., & Liu, L. (2017). Whether probiotic supplementation benefits rheumatoid arthritis patients: A systematic review and meta-analysis. *Engineering*, 3(1), 115–121. Available from https://doi.org/10.1016/J.ENG.2017.01.006.

Park, J., Kim, M., Kang, S. G., Jannasch, A. H., Cooper, B., Patterson, J., & Kim, C. H. (2015). Short-chain fatty acids induce both effector and regulatory T cells by suppression of histone deacetylases and regulation of the mTOR-S6K pathway. *Mucosal Immunology*, 8(1), 80–93. Available from https://doi.org/10.1038/mi.2014.44.

Peterson, D. A., McNulty, N. P., Guruge, J. L., & Gordon, J. I. (2007). IgA response to symbiotic bacteria as a mediator of gut homeostasis. *Cell Host and Microbe*, 2(5), 328–339. Available from https://doi.org/10.1016/j.chom.2007.09.013.

Petschow, B., Doré, J., Hibberd, P., Dinan, T., Reid, G., Blaser, M., Cani, P. D., Degnan, F. H., Foster, J., Gibson, G., Hutton, J., Klaenhammer, T. R., Ley, R., Nieuwdorp, M., Pot, B., Relman, D., Serazin, A., & Sanders, M. E. (2013). Probiotics, prebiotics, and the host microbiome: The science of translation. *Annals of the New York Academy of Sciences*, 1306(1), 1–17. Available from https://doi.org/10.1111/nyas.12303.

Pihoker, C., Gilliam, L. K., Hampe, C. S., & Lernmark, A. (2005). Autoantibodies in diabetes. *Diabetes*, 54(2), S52–S61. Available from https://doi.org/10.2337/diabetes.54.suppl_2.S52.

Pittayanon, R., Lau, J. T., Yuan, Y., Leontiadis, G. I., Tse, F., Surette, M., & Moayyedi, P. (2019). Gut microbiota in patients with irritable bowel syndrome—A systematic review. *Gastroenterology*, 157(1), 97–108. Available from https://doi.org/10.1053/j.gastro.2019.03.049.

Polman, C. H., Reingold, S. C., Banwell, B., Clanet, M., Cohen, J. A., Filippi, M., Fujihara, K., Havrdova, E., Hutchinson, M., Kappos, L., Lublin, F. D., Montalban, X., O'Connor, P., Sandberg-Wollheim, M., Thompson, A. J., Waubant, E., Weinshenker, B., & Wolinsky, J. S. (2011). Diagnostic criteria for multiple sclerosis: 2010 Revisions to the McDonald criteria. *Annals of Neurology*, 69(2), 292–302. Available from https://doi.org/10.1002/ana.22366.

Price, A. E., Shamardani, K., Lugo, K. A., Deguine, J., Roberts, A. W., Lee, B. L., & Barton, G. M. (2018). A map of toll-like receptor expression in the intestinal epithelium reveals distinct spatial, cell type-specific, and temporal patterns. *Immunity*, 49(3), 560–575. Available from https://doi.org/10.1016/j.immuni.2018.07.016, e6.

Proietti, M., Cornacchione, V., RezzonicoJost, T., Romagnani, A., Faliti, C. E., Perruzza, L., Rigoni, R., Radaelli, E., Caprioli, F., Preziuso, S., Brannetti, B., Thelen, M., McCoy, K. D., Slack, E., Traggiai, E., & Grassi, F. (2014). ATP-gated ionotropic P2X7 receptor controls follicular T helper cell numbers in peyer's patches to promote host-microbiota mutualism. *Immunity*, 41(5), 789–801. Available from https://doi.org/10.1016/j.immuni.2014.10.010.

Quigley, E. M. M. (2013). Gut bacteria in health and disease. *Gastroenterology and Hepatology*, 9(9), 560–569. Available from http://www.gastroenterologyandhepatology.net/files/2013/10/gh0913_quigley1.pdf.

Ramakrishna, C., Kujawski, M., Chu, H., Li, L., Mazmanian, S. K., & Cantin, E. M. (2019). Bacteroides fragilis polysaccharide A induces IL-10 secreting B and T cells that prevent viral encephalitis. *Nature Communications*, 10(1). Available from https://doi.org/10.1038/s41467-019-09884-6.

Rao, R. K., & Samak, G. (2013). Protection and restitution of gut barrier by probiotics: Nutritional and clinical implications. *Current Nutrition & Food Science*, 9(2), 99–107. Available from https://doi.org/10.2174/1573401311309020004.

Rewers, M., & Ludvigsson, J. (2016). Environmental risk factors for type 1 diabetes. *The Lancet*, 387(10035), 2340–2348. Available from https://doi.org/10.1016/S0140-6736(16)30507-4.

Rönnblom, L., & Pascual, V. (2008). The innate immune system in SLE: Type I interferons and dendritic cells. *Lupus*, 17(5), 394–399. Available from https://doi.org/10.1177/0961203308090020.

Round, J. L., & Mazmanian, S. K. (2009). The gut microbiota shapes intestinal immune responses during health and disease. *Nature Reviews Immunology*, 9(5), 313–323. Available from https://doi.org/10.1038/nri2515.

Ruohtula, T., de Goffau, M. C., Nieminen, J. K., Honkanen, J., Siljander, H., Hämäläinen, A. M., Peet, A., Tillmann, V., Ilonen, J., Niemelä, O., Welling, G. W., Knip, M., Harmsen, H. J., & Vaarala, O. (2019). Maturation of gut microbiota and circulating regulatory T cells and development of IgE sensitization in early life. *Frontiers in Immunology*, 10. Available from https://doi.org/10.3389/fimmu.2019.02494.

Saeedi, P., Petersohn, I., Salpea, P., Malanda, B., Karuranga, S., Unwin, N., Colagiuri, S., Guariguata, L., Motala, A. A., Ogurtsova, K., Shaw, J. E., Bright, D., & Williams, R. (2019). Global and regional diabetes prevalence estimates for 2019 and projections for 2030 and 2045: Results from the International Diabetes Federation Diabetes Atlas, 9th edition. *Diabetes Research and Clinical Practice*, 157. Available from https://doi.org/10.1016/j.diabres.2019.107843.

Salehipour, Z., Haghmorad, D., Sankian, M., Rastin, M., Nosratabadi, R., Soltan Dallal, M. M., Tabasi, N., Khazaee, M., Nasiraii, L. R., & Mahmoudi, M. (2017). Bifidobacterium animalis in combination with human origin of Lactobacillus plantarum ameliorate neuroinflammation in experimental model of multiple sclerosis by altering CD4 + T cell subset balance. *Biomedicine and Pharmacotherapy*, 95, 1535–1548. Available from https://doi.org/10.1016/j.biopha.2017.08.117.

Schulthess, J., Pandey, S., Capitani, M., Rue-Albrecht, K. C., Arnold, I., Franchini, F., Chomka, A., Ilott, N. E., Johnston, D. G. W., Pires, E., McCullagh, J., Sansom, S. N., Arancibia-Cárcamo, C. V., Uhlig, H. H., & Powrie, F. (2019). The short chain fatty acid butyrate imprints an antimicrobial program in macrophages. *Immunity*, 50(2), 432–445. Available from https://doi.org/10.1016/j.immuni.2018.12.018, e7.

Secher, T., Kassem, S., Benamar, M., Bernard, I., Boury, M., Barreau, F., Oswald, E., & Saoudi, A. (2017). Oral administration of the probiotic strain Escherichia coli Nissle 1917 reduces susceptibility to neuroinflammation and repairs experimental autoimmune encephalomyelitis-induced intestinal barrier dysfunction. *Frontiers in Immunology*, 8. Available from https://doi.org/10.3389/fimmu.2017.01096.

Shan, M., Gentile, M., Yeiser, J. R., Walland, A. C., Bornstein, V. U., Chen, K., He, B., Cassis, L., Bigas, A., Cols, M., Comerma, L., Huang, B., Blander, J. M., Xiong, H., Mayer, L., Berin, C., Augenlicht, L. H., Velcich, A., & Cerutti, A. (2013). Mucus enhances gut homeostasis and oral tolerance by delivering immunoregulatory signals. *Science*, *342*(6157), 447−453. Available from https://doi.org/10.1126/science.1237910.

Shulzhenko, N., Morgun, A., Hsiao, W., Battle, M., Yao, M., Gavrilova, O., Orandle, M., Mayer, L., Macpherson, A. J., McCoy, K. D., Fraser-Liggett, C., & Matzinger, P. (2011). Crosstalk between B lymphocytes, microbiota and the intestinal epithelium governs immunity vs metabolism in the gut. *Nature Medicine*, *17*(12), 1585−1593. Available from https://doi.org/10.1038/nm.2505.

Smith, P. M., Howitt, M. R., Panikov, N., Michaud, M., Gallini, C. A., Bohlooly-Y, M., Glickman, J. N., & Garrett, W. S. (2013). The microbial metabolites, short-chain fatty acids, regulate colonic T reg cell homeostasis. *Science*, *341*(6145), 569−573. Available from https://doi.org/10.1126/science.1241165.

So, J. S., Kwon, H. K., Lee, C. G., Yi, H. J., Park, J. A., Lim, S. Y., Hwang, K. C., Jeon, Y. H., & Im, S. H. (2008). Lactobacillus casei suppresses experimental arthritis by down-regulating T helper 1 effector functions. *Molecular Immunology*, *45*(9), 2690−2699. Available from https://doi.org/10.1016/j.molimm.2007.12.010.

So, J. S., Lee, C. G., Kwon, H. K., Yi, H. J., Chae, C. S., Park, J. A., Hwang, K. C., & Im, S. H. (2008). Lactobacillus casei potentiates induction of oral tolerance in experimental arthritis. *Molecular Immunology*, *46*(1), 172−180. Available from https://doi.org/10.1016/j.molimm.2008.07.038.

Sterlin, D., Fadlallah, J., Adams, O., Fieschi, C., Parizot, C., Dorgham, K., Rajkumar, A., Autaa, G., El-Kafsi, H., Charuel, J. L., Juste, C., Jönsson, F., Candela, T., Wardemann, H., Aubry, A., Capito, C., Brisson, H., Tresallet, C., Cummings, R. D., & Gorochov, G. (2020). Human IgA binds a diverse array of commensal bacteria. *Journal of Experimental Medicine*, *217*(3). Available from https://doi.org/10.1084/jem.20181635.

Sun, J., Furio, L., Mecheri, R., van der Does, A. M., Lundeberg, E., Saveanu, L., Chen, Y., van Endert, P., Agerberth, B., & Diana, J. (2015). Pancreatic β-cells limit autoimmune diabetes via an immunoregulatory antimicrobial peptide expressed under the influence of the gut microbiota. *Immunity*, *43*(2), 304−317. Available from https://doi.org/10.1016/j.immuni.2015.07.013.

Sun, S., Luo, L., Liang, W., Yin, Q., Guo, J., Rush, A. M., Lv, Z., Liang, Q., Fischbach, M. A., Sonnenburg, J. L., Dodd, D., Davis, M. M., & Wang, F. (2020). Bifidobacterium alters the gut microbiota and modulates the functional metabolism of T regulatory cells in the context of immune checkpoint blockade. *Proceedings of the National Academy of Sciences of the United States of America*, *117*(44), 27509−27515. Available from https://doi.org/10.1073/pnas.1921223117.

Sutherland, D. B., Suzuki, K., & Fagarasan, S. (2016). Fostering of advanced mutualism with gut microbiota by immunoglobulin A. *Immunological Reviews*, *270*(1), 20−31. Available from https://doi.org/10.1111/imr.12384.

Takiishi, T., Korf, H., Van Belle, T. L., Robert, S., Grieco, F. A., Caluwaerts, S., Galleri, L., Spagnuolo, I., Steidler, L., Van Huynegem, K., Demetter, P., Wasserfall, C., Atkinson, M. A., Dotta, F., Rottiers, P., Gysemans, C., & Mathieu, C. (2012). Reversal of autoimmune diabetes by restoration of antigen-specific tolerance using genetically modified Lactococcus lactis in mice. *Journal of Clinical Investigation*, *122*(5), 1717−1725. Available from https://doi.org/10.1172/JCI60530.

Tamtaji, O. R., Kouchaki, E., Salami, M., Aghadavod, E., Akbari, E., Tajabadi-Ebrahimi, M., & Asemi, Z. (2017). The effects of probiotic supplementation on gene expression related to inflammation, insulin, and lipids in patients with multiple sclerosis: A randomized, double-blind, placebo-controlled trial. *Journal of the American College of Nutrition*, *36*(8), 660−665. Available from https://doi.org/10.1080/07315724.2017.1347074.

Tankou, S. K., Regev, K., Healy, B. C., Tjon, E., Laghi, L., Cox, L. M., Kivisäkk, P., Pierre, I. V., Hrishikesh, L., Gandhi, R., Cook, S., Glanz, B., Stankiewicz, J., & Weiner, H. L. (2018). A probiotic modulates the microbiome and immunity in multiple sclerosis. *Annals of Neurology*, *83*(6), 1147−1161. Available from https://doi.org/10.1002/ana.25244.

Teng, F., Klinger, C. N., Felix, K. M., Bradley, C. P., Wu, E., Tran, N. L., Umesaki, Y., & Wu, H. J. J. (2016). Gut microbiota drive autoimmune arthritis by promoting differentiation and migration of Peyer's patch T follicular helper cells. *Immunity*, *44*(4), 875−888. Available from https://doi.org/10.1016/j.immuni.2016.03.013.

Turck, D., Braegger, C. P., Colombo, C., Declercq, D., Morton, A., Pancheva, R., Robberecht, E., Stern, M., Strandvik, B., Wolfe, S., Schneider, S. M., & Wilschanski, M. (2016). ESPEN-ESPGHAN-ECFS guidelines on nutrition care for infants, children, and adults with cystic fibrosis. *Clinical Nutrition*, *35*(3), 557−577. Available from https://doi.org/10.1016/j.clnu.2016.03.004.

Turnbaugh, P. J., Ley, R. E., Hamady, M., Fraser-Liggett, C. M., Knight, R., & Gordon, J. I. (2007). The human microbiome project. *Nature*, *449*(7164), 804−810. Available from https://doi.org/10.1038/nature06244.

Tzang, B. S., Liu, C. H., Hsu, K. C., Chen, Y. H., Huang, C. Y., & Hsu, T. C. (2017). Effects of oral Lactobacillus administration on antioxidant activities and CD4 + CD25 + forkhead box P3 (FoxP3) + T cells in NZB/W F1 mice. *British Journal of Nutrition*, *118*(5), 333−342. Available from https://doi.org/10.1017/S0007114517002112.

Vaghef-Mehrabany, E., Alipour, B., Homayouni-Rad, A., Sharif, S. K., Asghari-Jafarabadi, M., & Zavvari, S. (2014). Probiotic supplementation improves inflammatory status in patients with rheumatoid arthritis. *Nutrition*, *30*(4), 430−435. Available from https://doi.org/10.1016/j.nut.2013.09.007.

Van De Wiele, T., Van Praet, J. T., Marzorati, M., Drennan, M. B., & Elewaut, D. (2016). How the microbiota shapes rheumatic diseases. *Nature Reviews Rheumatology*, *12*(7), 398−411. Available from https://doi.org/10.1038/nrrheum.2016.85.

van den Hoogen, W. J., Laman, J. D., & 't Hart, B. A. (2017). Modulation of multiple sclerosis and its animal model experimental autoimmune encephalomyelitis by food and gut microbiota. *Frontiers in Immunology*, 8. Available from https://doi.org/10.3389/fimmu.2017.01081.

Vatanen, T., Franzosa, E. A., Schwager, R., Tripathi, S., Arthur, T. D., Vehik, K., Lernmark, Å., Hagopian, W. A., Rewers, M. J., She, J. X., Toppari, J., Ziegler, A. G., Akolkar, B., Krischer, J. P., Stewart, C. J., Ajami, N. J., Petrosino, J. F., Gevers, D., Lähdesmäki, H., & Xavier, R. J. (2018).

The human gut microbiome in early-onset type 1 diabetes from the TEDDY study. *Nature*, *562*(7728), 589–594. Available from https://doi.org/10.1038/s41586-018-0620-2.

Vieira, S. M., Pagovich, O. E., & Kriegel, M. A. (2014). Diet, microbiota and autoimmune diseases. *Lupus*, *23*(6), 518–526. Available from https://doi.org/10.1177/0961203313501401.

Wang, K., Dong, H., Qi, Y., Pei, Z., Yi, S., Yang, X., Zhao, Y., Meng, F., Yu, S., Zhou, T., & Hu, G. (2017). Lactobacillus casei regulates differentiation of Th17/Treg cells to reduce intestinal inflammation in mice. *Canadian Journal of Veterinary Research*, *81*(2), 122–128. Available from http://www.ingentaconnect.com/contentone/cvma/cjvr/2017/00000081/00000002/art00006.

Wang, L., Wang, F. S., & Gershwin, M. E. (2015). Human autoimmune diseases: A comprehensive update. *Journal of Internal Medicine*, *278*(4), 369–395. Available from https://doi.org/10.1111/joim.12395.

Wang, N., Shen, N., Vyse, T. J., Anand, V., Gunnarson, I., Sturfelt, G., Rantapää-Dahlqvist, S., Elvin, K., Truedsson, L., Andersson, B. A., Dahle, C., Örtqvist, E., Gregersen, P. K., Behrens, T. W., & Hammarström, L. (2011). Selective IgA deficiency in autoimmune diseases. *Molecular Medicine*, *17*(11), 1383–1396. Available from https://doi.org/10.2119/molmed.2011.00195.

Wang, S., Charbonnier, L. M., Noval Rivas, M., Georgiev, P., Li, N., Gerber, G., Bry, L., & Chatila, T. A. (2015). MyD88 adaptor-dependent microbial sensing by regulatory T cells promotes mucosal tolerance and enforces commensalism. *Immunity*, *43*(2), 289–303. Available from https://doi.org/10.1016/j.immuni.2015.06.014.

Wei, S. H., Chen, Y. P., & Chen, M. J. (2015). Selecting probiotics with the abilities of enhancing GLP-1 to mitigate the progression of type 1 diabetes in vitro and in vivo. *Journal of Functional Foods*, *18*, 473–486. Available from https://doi.org/10.1016/j.jff.2015.08.016.

Weißenberg, S. Y., Szelinski, F., Schrezenmeier, E., Stefanski, A. L., Wiedemann, A., Rincon-Arevalo, H., Welle, A., Jungmann, A., Nordström, K., Walter, J., Imgenberg-Kreuz, J., Nordmark, G., Rönnblom, L., Bachali, P., Catalina, M. D., Grammer, A. C., Lipsky, P. E., Lino, A. C., & Dörner, T. (2019). Identification and characterization of post-activated B cells in systemic autoimmune diseases. *Frontiers in Immunology*, *10*. Available from https://doi.org/10.3389/fimmu.2019.02136.

Westall, F. C. (2006). Molecular mimicry revisited: Gut bacteria and multiple sclerosis. *Journal of Clinical Microbiology*, *44*(6), 2099–2104. Available from https://doi.org/10.1128/JCM.02532-05.

Westerberg, L. S., Klein, C., & Snapper, S. B. (2008). Breakdown of T cell tolerance and autoimmunity in primary immunodeficiency-lessons learned from monogenic disorders in mice and men. *Current Opinion in Immunology*, *20*(6), 646–654. Available from https://doi.org/10.1016/j.coi.2008.10.004.

Williams, C. M. (1999). Effects of inulin on lipid parameters in humans. *Journal of Nutrition*, *129*(7). Available from https://doi.org/10.1093/jn/129.7.1471s, American Institute of Nutrition.

Wu, H. J., & Wu, E. (2012). The role of gut microbiota in immune homeostasis and autoimmunity. *Landes Bioscience*, *3*(1), 4–14. Available from https://doi.org/10.4161/gmic.19320.

Xiao, L., Van't Land, B., Engen, P. A., Naqib, A., Green, S. J., Nato, A., Leusink-Muis, T., Garssen, J., Keshavarzian, A., Stahl, B., & Folkerts, G. (2018). Human milk oligosaccharides protect against the development of autoimmune diabetes in NOD-mice. *Scientific Reports*, *8*(1). Available from https://doi.org/10.1038/s41598-018-22052-y.

Xiao, S., Jin, H., Korn, T., Liu, S. M., Oukka, M., Lim, B., & Kuchroo, V. K. (2008). Retinoic acid increases Foxp3 + regulatory T cells and inhibits development of Th17 cells by enhancing TGF-β-driven Smad3 signaling and inhibiting IL-6 and IL-23 receptor expression. *Journal of Immunology*, *181*(4), 2277–2284. Available from https://doi.org/10.4049/jimmunol.181.4.2277.

Yadav, H., Lee, J. H., Lloyd, J., Walter, P., & Rane, S. G. (2013). Beneficial metabolic effects of a probiotic via butyrate-induced GLP-1 hormone secretion. *Journal of Biological Chemistry*, *288*(35), 25088–25097. Available from https://doi.org/10.1074/jbc.M113.452516.

Yadav, R., Dey, D. K., Vij, R., Meena, S., Kapila, R., & Kapila, S. (2018). Evaluation of anti-diabetic attributes of Lactobacillus rhamnosus MTCC:5957, Lactobacillus rhamnosus MTCC:5897 and Lactobacillus fermentum MTCC:5898 in streptozotocin induced diabetic rats. *Microbial Pathogenesis*, *125*, 454–462. Available from https://doi.org/10.1016/j.micpath.2018.10.015.

Yeh, Y. L., Lu, M. C., Tsai, B. C. K., Tzang, B. S., Cheng, S. M., Zhang, X., Yang, L. Y., Mahalakshmi, B., Kuo, W. W., Xiang, P., & Huang, C. Y. (2021). Heat-killed Lactobacillus reuteri GMNL-263 inhibits systemic lupus erythematosus-induced cardiomyopathy in NZB/W F1 mice. *Probiotics and Antimicrobial Proteins*, *13*(1), 51–59. Available from https://doi.org/10.1007/s12602-020-09668-1.

Yousefi, B., Eslami, M., Ghasemian, A., Kokhaei, P., Salek Farrokhi, A., & Darabi, N. (2019). Probiotics importance and their immunomodulatory properties. *Journal of Cellular Physiology*, *234*(6), 8008–8018. Available from https://doi.org/10.1002/jcp.27559.

Zamani, B., Golkar, H. R., Farshbaf, S., Emadi-Baygi, M., Tajabadi-Ebrahimi, M., Jafari, P., Akhavan, R., Taghizadeh, M., Memarzadeh, M. R., & Asemi, Z. (2016). Clinical and metabolic response to probiotic supplementation in patients with rheumatoid arthritis: A randomized, double-blind, placebo-controlled trial. *International Journal of Rheumatic Diseases*, *19*(9), 869–879. Available from https://doi.org/10.1111/1756-185X.12888.

Zhang, H., Liao, X., Sparks, J. B., & Luo, X. M. (2014). Dynamics of gut microbiota in autoimmune lupus. *Applied and Environmental Microbiology*, *80*(24), 7551–7560. Available from https://doi.org/10.1128/AEM.02676-14.

Chapter 13

Probiotics and prebiotics in the prevention and management of human cancers (colon cancer, stomach cancer, breast cancer, and cervix cancer*)

Josef Jampílek[1,2], Katarína Kráľová[3] and Vladimír Bella[4]

[1]*Department of Analytical Chemistry, Faculty of Natural Sciences, Comenius University, Bratislava, Slovakia,* [2]*Institute of Neuroimmunology, Slovak Academy of Sciences, Bratislava, Slovakia,* [3]*Institute of Chemistry, Faculty of Natural Sciences, Comenius University, Bratislava, Slovakia,* [4]*Departmentof Mammology, St. Elizabeth Cancer Institute, Bratislava, Slovakia*

13.1 Introduction

Based on the available information from the International Agency for Research on Cancer at the WHO, the global increase in cancer in 2018 is estimated at 18.1 million new cases and 9.6 million deaths. It is reported that statistically, one in five men and one in six women developed cancer during their lifetime, with one in eight men and one in eleven women dying from the disease. Worldwide, 43.8 million people live in a so-called 5-year prevalence, which means 5 years of life since the diagnosis of the disease. The increase in the burden of cancer can be caused by several factors, including the constant growth and current aging of the population (Bray et al., 2018; IARC, 2018a–f; Irigaray et al., 2007; Khan et al., 2010; Meegan & O'Boyle, 2019).

In terms of incidence, colorectal cancer (CRC), breast cancer (BC), and lung cancer are among the three main types of cancer. Worldwide, these forms are responsible for one-third of all cancers. BC in women and lung cancer in men are the world's leading types of cancer in the number of new cases. In 2018, approximately 2.1 million new diagnoses of lung cancer as well as of BC were estimated, representing together about 23.2% of the total number of cancer cases. CRC (1.8 million cases, 10.2% of the total cancer cases) is the third most commonly diagnosed cancer, prostate cancer is the fourth (1.3 million cases, 7.1% of the total cancer cases), and gastric cancer is the fifth (1.0 million cases, 7.1% of the total cancer cases). Lung cancer is responsible for the highest number of deaths (1.8 million deaths, 18.4% of the total number of deaths) (Bray et al., 2018; IARC, 2018f).

Many treatments have been developed for the treatment of cancers, such as surgery, radiation therapy, chemotherapy, targeted therapy, and immunotherapy. One of the most common tools in the treatment of cancer is chemotherapy, that is the administration of various groups of drugs, such as alkylating or intercalating cytostatics, compounds that inhibit the mitotic apparatus of cells, kinase inhibitors, antimetabolites, or sex hormone receptor antagonists. The problem with existing drugs is their relatively low selectivity, that is, the degree of distinction between malignant and normal cells. This limited selectivity thus causes frequent and serious side effects of most clinically used antineoplastics. Research is looking for new drugs and at the same time examining existing ones for new uses. New studies have helped to improve our understanding of the development of cancer and the mechanisms of action of anticancer agents, sometimes broadening the spectrum of activity and, last but not least, finding new ways to improve patients' prognosis. The main idea of development is targeted therapy, where chemotherapeutic molecules are designed to attack only cancer cells, while normal ones damage as little as possible (Campos et al., 2019, 2020; Kauerová et al., 2016, 2020;

---

*This chapter is sincerely dedicated to all participants of Avon Walks around the world expressing support for patients with breast cancer.

Meegan & O'Boyle, 2019; Mrozek-Wilczkiewicz et al., 2010; Newton et al., 2020; Spaczyńska et al., 2019; Vettorazzi et al., 2017, 2019).

Besides targeted preparation of prodrugs and bioprecursors and antibody-directed enzyme prodrug therapy or gene-directed enzyme prodrug therapy, one of the modern ways to overcome cancer cell resistance, while ensuring higher targeted distribution and thus higher efficacy at the same or lower amount of active agents, is nanoformulation of drugs (Černíková & Jampílek, 2014; Kozik et al., 2019; Pentak et al., 2016). Such nanoformulations of anticancer drugs are usually characterized by increased bioavailability, active targeted biodistribution, and release control. The surface of nanoformulations is usually coated with specific antibodies that allow specific uptake into cells expressing cancer markers. In addition, multiple drugs or compounds that potentiate each other can be formulated together. In this way, of course, the negative side effects of the treatment on the human body can be partially suppressed (Jampílek & Králová, 2018, 2019a–c, 2020a,b; Jampílek, Kos et al., 2019; Jampílek, Králová, Campos et al., 2019; Jampílek, Králová, Novák et al., 2019; Mirhadi et al., 2020; Plachá & Jampílek, 2019).

In addition to the above strategies, drugs or special diets are used to alleviate or prevent the adverse effects of existing clinically used anticancer drugs. In addition, such dietary supplements and foods for special medical purposes may potentiate the effectiveness of drugs or even contribute to the prevention of diseases (Jampílek, Kos et al., 2019; Mirhadi et al., 2020). Probiotics are one of the most widely used over-the-counter products to prevent disease and alleviate the side effects of treatment. Ilya Ilyich Mechnikov, a Nobel Prize laureate in physiology, described the immunomodulatory function of intestinal and gastric bacterial colonies in 1908 (The Nobel Prize, 2020). Currently, interest in probiotics is on the rise due to increasing antibiotic resistance and their use in prophylactic treatment methods (Binda et al., 2020; Fiore et al., 2020; Grumet et al., 2020; Iebba et al., 2016; Jackson et al., 2019; Johnson et al., 2020; Puccetti et al., 2020; Żółkiewicz et al., 2020; Žuntar et al., 2020).

In general, the term "probiotic" refers to a living organism added to food or feed, which should have a beneficial effect on the health of the consumer by improving the balance of his intestinal microflora. Classic examples of foods containing a probiotic are yogurt, acidophilic milk or kefir. The most common probiotics are considered to be lactic bacteria of the genera *Lactobacillus*, *Bifidobacterium*, several other bacteria and yeasts (see Table 13.1). Probiotic cultures based on lactic bacteria of the genus *Lactobacillus* are referred to as passive probiotics. These probiotics (even in combination with prebiotics) can improve the environment of the stomach and intestines in the short term, but they are not resistant to physiological conditions within these organs, and therefore they are not able to multiply there. Consumption of these foods/special diets therefore brings benefits but disappears as soon as they are no longer consumed. On the other hand, active probiotics, such as *Enterococcus faecium* or *Streptococcus thermophilus* (in combination with lactobacilli and prebiotics), are able to significantly affect the body's natural metabolic processes, most often in interaction with prebiotics and in interaction with various types of probiotics. Active probiotics can be divided into: (1) probiotics supporting immunomodulatory processes (are not able to permanently colonize the digestive tract), (2) probiotics with the ability to colonize (resistant to the environment of the stomach and intestines), and (3) immunomodulatory probiotics with the ability to colonize the digestive tract. It is believed that these probiotics can promote natural metabolism/prevent the formation of toxins, promote immunity, aid healing or block unwanted enzymatic manifestations. The importance of the last "combined" group is emphasized especially in the issue of antibiotic resistance and holistic medicine, and their influence on cancer treatment is also examined. As the most important synergistic

TABLE 13.1 Microorganisms used as probiotics.

Group of microorganisms	Used as probiotics
Lactobacillus species	*L. acidophilus, L. amylovorus, L. brevis, L. bulgaricus, L. casei, L. crispatus, L. cromoris, L. delbrueckii, L. fermentum, L. gasseri, L. helveticus, L. iners, L. jensenii, L. johnsonii, L. kefiranofaciens, L. kefiri, L. lactis, L. mucosae, L. paracasei, L. pentosus, L. plantarum, L. racemosus, L. reuteri, L. rhamnosus, L. salivarius*
Bifidobacterium species	*B. adolescentis, B. animalis, B. bifidum, B. breve, B. infantis, B. lactis, B. longum, B. thermophilum*
Other bacteria	*Bacillus clausii, B. coagulans, B. cereus, B. licheniformis, Clostridium butyricum, Enterococcus faecium* SF68, *faecalis, Escherichia coli* Nissle 1917, *Lactococcus lactis, Leuconostoc cremoris, Pediococcus acidilactici, P. pentosaceus, Propionibacterium freudenreichii, Streptococcus lactis, S. thermophilus*
Yeasts	*Candida kefir, C. sphaerica, Kluyveromyces marxianus, Pichia kudriavzevii, Saccharomyces cerevisiae, S. fragilis*

immunomodulatory probiotics with the ability to replicate can be considered the genera *Lactobacillus*, *Bifidobacterium*, and the bacteria *E. faecium* and *S. thermophilus* (Cleveland Clinic, 2020; Ecosh Life OÜ, 2020; FAO, 2006; Galdeano et al., 2019; Kechagia et al., 2013; Khalighi et al., 2006; Markowiak & Śliżewska, 2017; Nazir et al., 2018; NHS, 2018b; NIH, 2019; Shi et al., 2016; Tomasik & Tomasik, 2020).

However, it is necessary to define other "biotics," such as above-mentioned prebiotics, synbiotics, and probiotics. The so-called prebiotics are indigestible components of foods, which support the growth or activity of the intestinal microflora and thus improve the health of the consumer. These oligosaccharides (most often difficult to digest or indigestible) are substrates for desirable bifidobacteria living in the large intestine. Of course, oligosaccharides that cause bloating or digestive problems must be excluded. It is therefore not possible to use oligosaccharides, such as raffinose or stachyose, from legumes. Prebiotics can be divided into natural or synthetic. The most important natural prebiotics are oligofructose and inulin; further prebiotics can be found, for example, in chicory root, Jerusalem artichoke tubers, yacon, garlic, leeks, and onions. Synthetic prebiotic oligosaccharides, for example, lactulose, maltitol, and lactitol, are prepared by the oligomerization of sucrose or lactose or by the chemical treatment of inulin or starch. Prebiotics have a beneficial effect on the microflora of the large intestine, reduce energy intake from food, increase stool volume, and suppress constipation. It is thought that they could act as a prevention and attenuation of intestinal infections and diarrhea, prevention of CRC, and prevention of osteoporosis. In addition, they could be able to reduce blood cholesterol and strengthen immunity (Ashaolu, 2020; Davani-Davari et al., 2019; de Vrese & Schrezenmeir, 2008; Guarino et al., 2020; Hutkins et al., 2016; Lockyer & Stanner, 2019; Markowiak & Śliżewska, 2017; Shah et al., 2020; Tomasik & Tomasik, 2020). It could be mentioned that natural prebiotics stimulating growth of bifidobacteria and lactobacili in the gut and reducing the incidence of allergy occur also in breast milk and infant formulas supplemented with prebiotics and can contribute to the reduction of intestinal and upper airway infections in the first year of life (Tomas, 2009). Supplementation of prebiotics, such as fructooligosaccharides, inulin, mannitol, maltodextrin, and pectin, enhanced the in vitro antihypertensive effect and production of bioactive aglycones in probiotic-fermented soymilk (Yeo & Liong, 2010). The types of prebiotics and the properties they should meet are summarized in Fig. 13.1. Fig. 13.2 presents the structures of fructooligosaccharides and galactooligosaccharides.

Synbiotics are combinations of probiotics and prebiotics with the expected synergistic effect. An example of a synbiotic food is a sour milk product containing bifidobacteria and, for example, oligofructose or inulin (Malik et al., 2016;

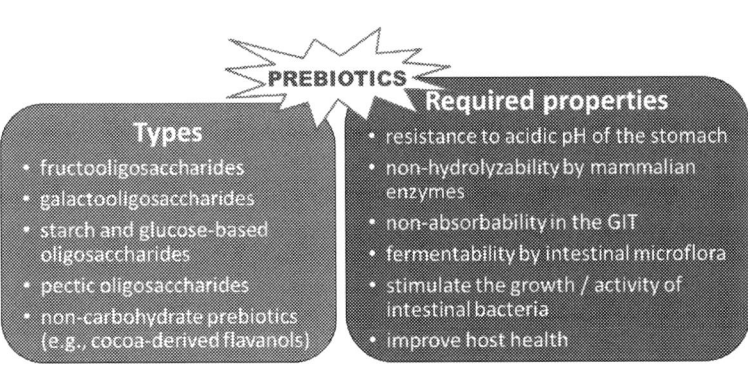

FIGURE 13.1 Types of prebiotics and properties they should meet. Source: *Adapted from Davani-Davari, D., Negahdaripour, M., Karimzadeh, I., Seifan, M., Mohkam, M., Masoumi, S. J., Berenjian, A., & Ghasemi, Y. (2019). Prebiotics: Definition, types, sources, mechanisms, and clinical applications.* Foods, 8, 92.

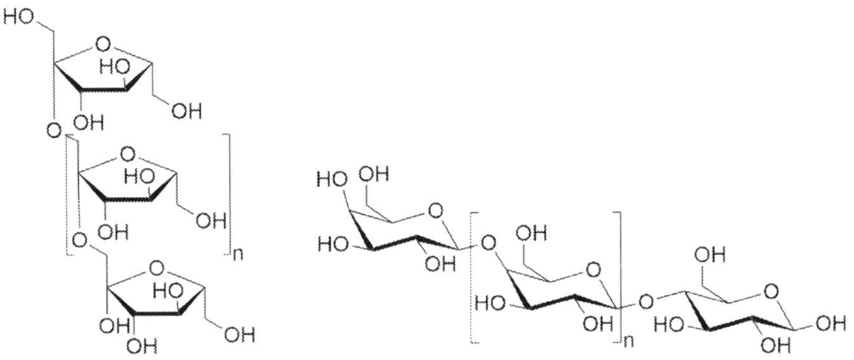

FIGURE 13.2 Structure of fructooligosaccharides and galactooligosaccharides.

Pandey et al., 2015; Pineiro et al., 2008; Swanson et al., 2020). On the other hand, postbiotics comprise metabolites and/or cell-wall components released by probiotics (Aguilar-Toalá et al., 2018).

Favorable impact of probiotics is reflected mainly in the modulation of the immune system, anti-inflammatory effect, improved intestinal functioning, and inhibition of pathogens. Although probiotics are predominantly isolated from the human microbiota pool, feces, breast milk, and fermented products, fermented fruits and vegetable belong also to the source of probiotics because they contain high amounts of functional antioxidants providing synergistically health benefits to human (James & Wang, 2019). Some gut bacterial strains at co-application with largely used anticancer drugs can exhibit synergistic effect as alkylating or immune checkpoint blockade agents resulting in improved immune response against multiple solid cancers. The most important bacteria capable to improve the immune response triggered by anticancer drugs, including their mechanism of action, which have potential to be used as novel anticancer adjuvant agents in the future therapies, were overviewed by Marinelli et al. (2017). Drago (2019) also stated in his critical review based on a study of a large amount of recent literature that some probiotics, when properly dosed and administered, can have a rebalancing effect on the intestinal microflora, which can have a positive effect on gastrointestinal (GI) immunity and inflammation of intestinal mucosa. Many findings have suggested that daily use of some selected probiotics may alleviate the adverse impact of radiation or chemotherapy.

The positive effects of probiotics are summarized in Fig. 13.3, but sometimes side effects can occur as well. The undesirable effects of probiotics are characterized mainly by microbial imbalance in the beginning of administration, when "harmful" bacteria are replaced by "good" ones, and the body gets used to the effects of the new product. The most common side effects may be diarrhea, bloating, flatulence, acne, and various rashes. However, they should not last longer than 14 days. In case of long-lasting or severe side effects, the dose can be at first reduced and subsequently gradually increased, thus stepwise getting the body used to the new product. If even this approach does not reduce the "restrictive" effects, the product should be discontinued, the body allowed to rest, and another product containing a different range of probiotics should be selected in consultation with a physician, pharmacist, or other qualified healthcare professional (Cleveland Clinic, 2020; Julson, 2017; NIH, 2019).

It is always necessary to choose probiotic products that meet the needs, the health status and age of the consumer, and especially products with guaranteed quality. As they can also be "live" products, they must be stored in accordance with the manufacturer's recommendations and purchased in premises equipped for this type of product to maintain its effectiveness (Binda et al., 2020; Grumet et al., 2020; Jackson et al., 2019; Žuntar et al., 2020).

As mentioned above, nanoforms have become a hit. In addition to the nanoformulations of drugs, nanoformulations of dietary supplements and foods for special medical purposes were developed in the laboratories of research teams and are also available on the market. It is therefore not surprising that nanoformulations of various probiotic

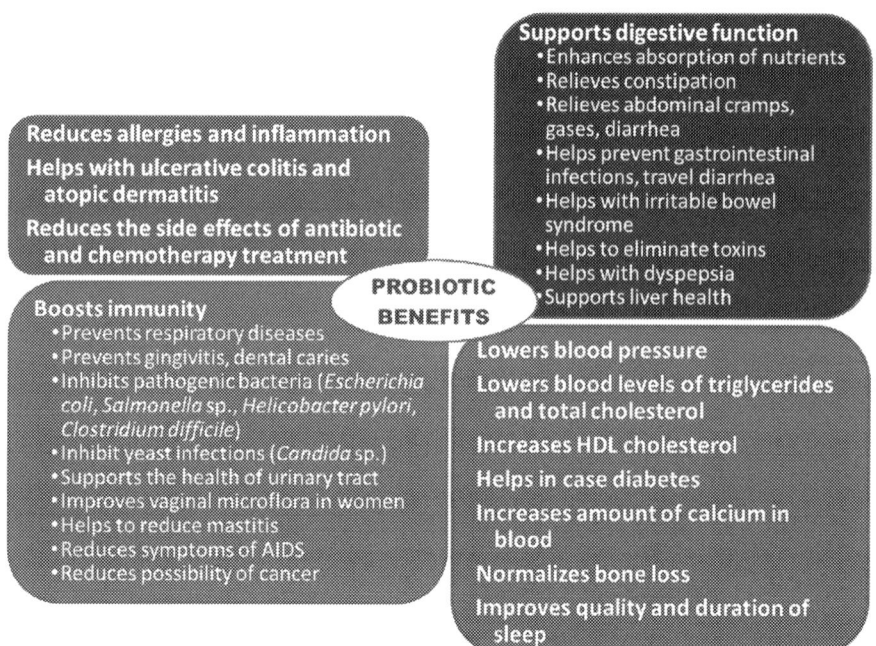

FIGURE 13.3 Beneficial effects of probiotics on human health.

microorganisms were designed as well. This contribution provides an overview of investigated formulations of microorganisms used as probiotics either alone or in combination with prebiotics or drugs that can be used to alleviate the negative effects of gastric, colon, BC and cervical cancer (CC) therapies or which are expected to have a positive effect on the prevention of these diseases. The mechanism of action of probiotics and prebiotics in cancer cells is described and the effects of nanoformulated probiotics are shortly discussed as well.

13.2 Probiotics and prebiotics in stomach cancer

Gastric cancer can be classified according to the anatomic site as cardia (the upper part of the stomach adjoining the esophagus) and noncardia (the mid and distal stomach) subtypes (Mukaisho et al., 2015). Stomach cancer (cardia and noncardia gastric cancer combined) was responsible for 1,033,701 (5.7%) new cases and 782,685 (8.2%) deaths in 2018 worldwide; it was the fifth most frequently diagnosed cancer and the third leading cause of cancer death showing two-fold higher rates in men than in women (Bray et al., 2018).

Microbiota exhibits pronounced impact on physiological homeostasis, and immune regulation. Although acidic pH and peristaltic movements of stomach represent a hostile environment for most microorganisms, various commensal microorganisms can colonize it forming a stomach niche and commensal gastric microbes or their metabolites affect the ability of *Helicobacter pylori* to colonize the stomach and regulate its pathogenicity and carcinogenic potential (Espinoza et al., 2018). The urease enzyme of *H. pylori* is crucial for the bacteria establishment in the gastric mucosa (Amar et al., 2017). Large amounts of this nickel enzyme hydrolyzing urea to ammonia produced by *H. pylori* are responsible for neutralization of the local environment and enable its survival in acidic gastric conditions (Jones et al., 2018). Hence, *H. pylori* is considered to be the main risk factor for stomach cancer and this bacterium is responsible for approx. 90% of new cases of noncardia gastric cancer. Colonization by *H. pylori*, which can be followed by inflammation of the gastric mucus layer, is also a risk factor for the development of active gastritis, peptic ulcers, and mucosa-associated lymphoid tissue lymphoma (Bray et al., 2018; Ji et al., 2018; Plummer et al., 2015; Westerik et al., 2018). As risk factors for cancers of the gastric cardia obesity (Yang et al., 2009) and gastroesophageal reflux disease (Kim, 2013) were reported. Moreover, to the risk factors of stomach cancer belong also foods preserved by salting (Strumylaite et al., 2006), low intake of fruits and vegetable (Ferro et al., 2020), alcohol consumption (Ma et al., 2017), and smoking (Li, Han et al., 2019).

While Proteobacteria, Firmicutes, Actinobacteria, Bacteroidetes, and Fusobacteria are the most abundant phyla in both *H. pylori*-positive and *H. pylori*-negative patients (Alarcon et al., 2017), gastric cancer has a great impact on the microbial diversity of the stomach reflected in enhanced number of *Streptococcus*, *Peptostreptococcus*, and *Prevotella* (pathogens) and decreasing portion of the probiotic *Bifidobacterium* (Zheng et al., 2019). The genotypes of *H. pylori*, host genetic background, lifestyle including smoking and diet may determine clinical outcomes of gastric diseases in the *H. pylori*-infected individuals, whereby natural probiotics present in traditional fermented food and beverages could ensure protection against *H. pylori*-induced gastric diseases (Nair et al., 2016). Probiotics must be able to survive during passage through GI tract and maintain their activity at different unfavorable conditions (Hakobyan et al., 2016). For the solubilization and protection of hydrophobic nutraceuticals targeting gastric tumors in clear systems digestible caseins nanoparticles (NPs) or cold-gelation based vehicles based on different crosslinking agents (e.g., rennet, transglutaminase, and genipin) can be used (Poonia, 2017). Content and functions of polyamines putrescine, spermidine, and spermine, which are required in both preneoplastic and neoplastic tissues to sustain the cell growth, can be affected by probiotics functioning as antineoplastic agents in the stomach (Russo et al., 2014).

Dietary amelioration of *Helicobacter* infection using specific foods, food components, and food products, including honey, propolis, probiotics, dairy products, vegetables, and fruits, was analyzed by Fahey et al. (2015). Mode of action of acidic hydroxylans, arabinogalactan, rhamnogalacturon, limonene, pinene, lupeol, citral, ursolic acid, and nomilin obtained from fruits, which act as prebiotics and are able to prevent the inhabitation of *H. pylori*, regulate the inflammation, inhibit growth of gastric cancer, and promote the reparative mechanisms on the affected regions was described by Khan et al. (2018). The regulation of *H. pylori*-associated gastric diseases by the intake of omega-3 polyunsaturated fatty acids (PUFAs) was reported by Park et al. (2015).

Although based on the results of some investigations it could be assumed that probiotics only retain the number of *H. pylori* at low levels inside the human stomach but cannot effectively eradicate *H. pylori*, their combined consumption with antibiotics can contribute to the eradication via altering the immune response and reducing the negative impact of antibiotics, ultimately resulting in gastroprotection (Kafshdooz et al., 2017). Mechanisms of *H. pylori* resistance to commonly used antibiotics, the mutations in the genome resulting in the resistance and the global incidence of resistant strains as well as compounds showing potential to be used in eradication therapy (e.g., probiotics, plant formulations, PUFAs and ascorbic acid) were described by Mnich et al. (2018). *H. pylori* therapy in children and the potential of the use of probiotics was discussed by Chiesa et al. (2010).

Many NPs form complexes with *H. pylori* and enteric pathogens without the need for specific functionalization. Small NPs with a negative surface charge exhibit improved binding, whereby the binding could be affected by surface modification. In the human gastric epithelial cells and 3D-organoid models of the stomach, *H. pylori*'s cellular attachment was not inhibited by NP coating. However, *H. pylori* infection was mitigated by the assembly of nonbactericidal silica NPs via reducing cytotoxin-associated gene A (CagA—a highly significant virulence factors of the *H. pylori*) phosphorylation, cytoskeletal rearrangement, and interleukin (IL)-8 secretion suggesting that NPs may modulate the pathobiology of microbes (Westmeier et al., 2018).

Thiourea and methanolic extract of *Pistacia atlantica* were found to be potent urease inhibitors, whereby the extract showed considerable bacteriostatic activity against clinical isolates of *H. pylori*, including isolates with antibiotic resistance but it was neutral against common probiotic bacteria (Amar et al., 2017).

A probiotic mixture containing *Bifidobacterium infantis*, *Lactobacillus acidophilus*, *Enterococcus faecalis*, and *Bacillus cereus* pronouncedly reduced the inflammation indices (leukocyte), while it considerably increased the immunity indices (lymphocyte) and nutrition indices (albumin and total protein) of patients who underwent gastrectomy. As mentioned above, administration of the probiotic mixture markedly increased the numbers of the probiotic bacteria *Bacteroides*, *Faecalibacterium*, and *Akkermansia* and reduced the portion of *Streptococcus* and the ratio of Firmicutes/Bacteroidetes. This ratio was greatly reduced also in patients with partial gastrectomy consuming the probiotic mixture suggesting that such treatment noticeably improved the immune response of patients and reduced the intensity of inflammation via altering of gut microbiota (Zheng et al., 2019). The *in vitro* study found that *Bifidobacterium bifidum* YIT 10347 exhibited approx. 10-fold higher adhesion rate to human gastric epithelial cells *in vitro* than the lactic acid bacteria and other bifidobacteria. One hour after ingestion of milk fermented with *B. bifidum* YIT 10347 in biopsy samples of *H. pylori*-positive subjects living *B. bifidum* YIT 10347 cells were detected (10^4 cells/g), whereby bacterial cells were situated at the interstitial mucin layer of the stomach. These results showed that the cells of probiotic adhered to the human gastric mucosa in a live state what may contribute to its favorable effects on the human stomach (Shibahara-Sone et al., 2016).

High concentrations of NO_3^- ($\geq 2.0\%$) suppressed the growth of both *Lactobacillus* and *Streptococcus* strains; however, *L. acidophilus* Ep 317/402 exhibited higher stability and adhesive properties. Even though at lower doses of NO_3^- (0.52.0%) the acid-forming activity of the strains was reduced, they coagulated milk by forming low acidity in milk compared to control (Hakobyan et al., 2016). Four probiotic *Lactobacillus* strains reduced by up to 50% the concentration of *N*-nitrosodimethylamine (NDMA), which can cause cancer of the stomach, kidney, and colon, whereby *Lactobacillus brevis* 0945 strain was found to be the most effective, reducing also the genotoxicity of NDMA up to 50% (Nowak et al., 2014). The investigation of the impact of *L. acidophilus* 1014 on the fermentation pattern of the colon microbiota using the Simulator of the Human Intestinal Microbial Ecosystem (SHIME) model showed that populations of the *Lactobacillus* spp. and *Bifidobacterium* spp. pronouncedly increased during experiment and an increase in the concentration of short-chain fatty acids (SCFAs), with considerable raising of acetic, butyric, and propionic acid levels, and reduced NH_3 concentrations were observed as well. Favorable effect of this probiotic on microbial metabolism and lactobacilli community composition can contribute to improving human health (Sivieri et al., 2013).

Lactic acid bacteria from pulque and aguamiel belonging to the genera *Lactobacillus* and *Pediococcus* were found to be were susceptible to clinical antibiotics (except to vancomycin) and 60% of them showed antimicrobial activity against *Escherichia coli* and *Staphylococcus aureus*. Moreover, they inhibited the growth and the urease activity of *H. pylori* ATCC 43504 suggesting their ability to diminish chances for survival of *H. pylori* in the stomach (Cervantes-Elizarraras et al., 2019). Administration of *L. acidophilus*, *Lactobacillus plantarum*, and *Lactobacillus rhamnosus* to mice infected with the standard strain of *H. pylori* (ATCC 43504) reduced the inflammation of stomach tissue and as most effective treatments exposure to *L. rhamnosus* or to all three *Lactobacillus* strains were estimated (Asgari et al., 2020). *L. rhamnosus* GG (ATCC 53103), which was patented in 1989, is able to survive and proliferate at gastric acid pH and in medium containing bile, and to adhere to enterocytes. It produces a biofilm that mechanically protects the mucosa as well as soluble factors favorable to gut able to reduce apoptosis of the intestinal epithelium, and preserve cytoskeletal integrity. It can stimulate type 1 immune-responsiveness via reduced expression of several activation and inflammation markers on monocytes and by increased production of IL-10, IL-12, and tumor necrosis factor-α (TNF-α) in macrophages (Capurso, 2019). The GI isolate of the probiotic bacterium *L. rhamnosus* yoba 2012 (LRY), the generic variant of *L. rhamnosus* GG, was found to inhibit *H. pylori* via competition for substrate and binding sites and by producing compounds showing antimicrobial activity (e.g., lactic acid) and was able to mitigate the host's *H. pylori*-induced apoptosis and inflammation responses and to promote angiogenesis in the gastric and duodenal epithelium.

Supplementation of yogurt with this probiotic could contribute to the reduction of gastric pathology caused by *H. pylori* and can be used in eradication therapy treatment in East Africa (Westerik et al., 2018).

Pretreatment of mice with *L. plantarum* ZDY 2013 was able to prevent gastric mucosal inflammation, avoided rising of inflammatory cytokines [e.g., IL-1 and interferon gamma (IFN-γ)] and inflammatory cell infiltration in gastric lamina propria as well as alteration of gastric microbiota induced by *H. pylori* infection. Consequently, it can be assumed that oral administration of probiotic in order to target gastric microbiota represents an alternative strategy to prevent *H. pylori* infection (Pan et al., 2016). *Lactobacillus paracasei* 06TCa19 isolated from Mongolian dairy products inhibited the growth of *H. pylori* due to rapid and excessive generation of lactic acid and after oral administration to mice infected with *H. pylori* strain no. 130 it pronouncedly decreased the number of colonizing *H. pylori* in their stomach (Takeda et al., 2015). As a superb candidate for the protection against *H. pylori* infections probiotic *Lactobacillus fermentum* UCO-979C isolated from human gut exhibiting strong inhibition of the growth and urease activity of *H. pylori* strains and *H. pylori*-induced IL-8 production in gastric adenocarcinoma human cells (AGS cells) and reducing viability of *H. pylori*, which was also susceptible to several antibiotics, can be considered; in blood agar containing red blood cells from various origins, it did not produce histamine or beta-hemolysis (Garcia et al., 2017).

13.3 Probiotics and prebiotics in colon cancer

CRC is one of the most common cancers. One of the most affected countries in the world is the Czech Republic, the Slovak Republic, and Hungary. It usually affects adults. It starts as small benign clusters of cells (so-called polyps) that are formed on the inside of the large intestine. These polyps can then turn into cancer cells. Polyps often have no symptoms. Symptoms of CRC include: weight loss, flatulence, abdominal pain, weakness, fatigue, changes in stool consistency, diarrhea or constipation, blood in the stools, and bleeding from the rectum. The exact causes of malignant transformation are unknown. Risk factors include family history, African-American race, age over 50, diabetes, obesity, chronic inflammatory bowel disease, sedentary lifestyle, eating habits (low in fiber, high in fat and calories, excessive consumption of red meat and sausages), smoking, and excessive alcohol consumption (Bray et al., 2018; IARC, 2018b,c,e,f; MFMER, 2020c).

The intestinal microbiota of patients with CRC is characterized with greater proportion of bacteria causing inflammatory diseases of GI tract and bacteria producing toxins and carcinogenic metabolites. Butyric acid-producing bacteria, probiotic bacteria, and potentially probiotic bacteria can modify the composition of the intestinal microbiota by reducing the portion of above-mentioned harmful bacteria contributing to CRC (dos Reis et al., 2019). Thus for gut microbiota modulation, to eliminate dysbiosis and ensure prevention and therapy CRC, a novel strategy utilizing probiotics, prebiotics, synbiotics or postbiotics, antibiotics, and fecal microbiota transplantation can be used. Various possible host responses to gut microbiome suggest that development of the personalized microbiome therapy may be the crucial for effective clinical medication (Fong et al., 2020). Eslami et al. (2019) in his review paper analyzed the beneficial impact of probiotics in the prevention and treatment of CRC observed in clinical trials, and in in vitro and animal model studies, emphasizing the possible immunomodulatory mechanisms. On the other hand, Farag et al. (2020) focused attention on different probiotic species, additives, and flavor-promoting compounds generated during the fermentation process contained in different fortified acidophilus milk products. For example, orally administration of probiotic Bifico cocktail improved colitis-associated cancer in mice via reducing the abundance of genera *Desulfovibrio*, *Mucispirillum*, and *Odoribacter*, and increasing the *Lactobacillus* genus as well as expression of CXCR2 ligand genes (Song et al., 2018). Also, administration of a live cocktail of several potential probiotic *Lactobacillus* species pronouncedly reduced proliferation of the HT-29 (Caucasian colon adenocarcinoma grade II cell line) and CT-26 (*N*-nitroso-*N*-methylurethane-induced, undifferentiated colon carcinoma cell line) cells and induced late apoptosis in vitro via the upregulation and downregulation of the Wnt/-catenin pathway-related genes; in vivo experiment using murine model of CRC induced by azoxymethane (AOM) and dextran sulfate sodium showed that intravenous (i.v.) administration of the probiotic considerably mitigated inflammation and tumor development in infected mice (Ghanavati et al., 2020). Probiotic *Lactobacillus* strains were reported to detoxify *N*-nitrosodimethylamine found in food products as well as synthesized in vivo by intestinal microbiota, which can cause cancer of the stomach, colon and kidney (Nowak et al., 2014). Treatment with exopolysaccharides (EPSs) from *Lactobacillus* strains pronouncedly induced G_0/G_1 cell cycle arrest and apoptosis of HT-29 cells; most effective inhibitory impact on HT-29 cells was observed using acidic EPS from the SB27 strain (Di et al., 2018). Other antitumor effects of bifidobacteria and their potential to be used in the development of cancer therapeutics were summarized by Wei et al. (2018). On the other hand, *Fusobacterium nucleatum*, oral bacterium commensal to the human oral cavity playing a role in periodontal disease, can stimulate colorectal tumor growth and inhibit T-cell-mediated immune responses against CRC, whereby the amount of *F. nucleatum* DNA in CRC tissue is associated with shorter survival, and can be used as a prognostic biomarker (Mima et al., 2016). *F. nucleatum* may preserve CRC from immune cell attack by inhibiting T cells and affecting the production of many chemokines and cytokines (Han et al., 2019).

Bile acids, which are synthesized in the liver and further metabolized by the gut microbiota, play a crucial role in maintaining the normal gut microbiota and lipid digestion and alterations of bile acid metabolism and gut microbiota can end in development of intestinal carcinogenesis. Liu et al. (2020) analyzed the role of bile acids receptors involved in CRC and emphasized that the targeting the bile acid–microbiota axis using, for example, probiotics can be used in prevention and therapy of CRC.

Supplementation of commercial probiotic to rats (1×10^9 CFU, daily/gavage) with chemically induced CRC mitigated the aggressiveness of tumor resulting in reduced count of aberrant crypt foci (ACF) and reduction of malignant neoplastic lesions (by 40% in low-grade tubular adenoma, by 40% in carcinoma in situ, and by 20% in low-grade adenocarcinoma) and at co-administration with 5-fluorouracil chemotherapy the carcinoma reduction in situ achieved even 60% (Genaro et al., 2019). Combined administration of lactic acid bacteria strains producing vitamin 9 (folate) and vitamin B_2 (riboflavin) together with immune-stimulating bacterial strains at treatments of inflammatory diseases, which was able to prevent undesirable side effects and provide nutrition value, was recommended by LeBlanc et al. (2020). However, potent anti-CRC activities do not show all probiotic strains and therefore it is desirable to perform a screen for the selection of the most suitable strains to design effective probiotic-based therapeutics to prevent the incidence and control CRC (Sivamaruthi et al., 2020). Han et al. (2019) constructed an association network of intestinal microorganisms and T lymphocytes associated with CRC and findings related to preventive role of lactobacilli supplemented per os in CRC animal models associated with reduction of oxidative stress, modulation of gut microbiota, and regulation of apoptosis and immunomodulation were summarized by Settanni et al. (2020).

Lactobacillus and *Bifidobacterium* strains can secrete compounds with anticancer activity, antioxidant enzymes, bind reactive oxygen species (ROS), release small molecular weight antioxidants and form chelates with transition metals, interact with proteins regulating the cell cycle inhibiting proliferation of cancer cells, and break the resistance of cancer cells against apoptosis via activation of procaspases and downregulation of the antiapoptotic B-cell lymphoma 2 (Bcl-2) and upregulation of proapoptotic Bax proteins; they also exhibited multipathway action in the microbiota, which contributed to their anticancer activities (Nowak et al., 2019). *Bifidobacteria* induced sevenfold higher apoptosis among human Dukes' type B, colon adenocarcinoma LS174T cells than in normal intestinal epithelial cell line (21% vs 3%) and showed pronounced anticancer properties; it also downregulated epidermal growth factor receptor (EGFR), human epidermal growth factor receptor (HER-2), and prostaglandin-endoperoxide synthase 2 (PTGS-2) or cyclooxygenase-2 (COX-2) and showed considerable anti-CRC impact on CRC mice models suggesting that this probiotic could be used as suitable nutritional supplement for the prevention and therapy of CRC (Parisa et al., 2020). Both oral and i.v. administration of probiotic *B. bifidum* to C57BL/6 mice (common inbred strain of laboratory mouse) bearing transplanted TC-1 cell of human papillomavirus (HPV)-related tumor expressing HPV-16 E6/E7 oncogenes induced antitumor immune responses, resulting in the suppression of tumor growth in mice. However, only i.v. administration of *B. bifidum* into tumor-bearing mice activated the tumor-specific IL-12 and IFN-γ, lymphocyte proliferation, and $CD8^+$ cytolytic responses controlling and destroying tumor growth suggesting immunomodulatory potential of this probiotic (Abdolalipour et al., 2020). Microencapsulation technique as a tool to ensure the protection of probiotics during the processing, which improves their transit and storage stability and prolongs their survival, was discussed by Zandu et al. (2020).

L. acidophilus CICC 6074 S-layer protein exhibited cytotoxic effect on colon cancer HT-29 cells causing arrest in the G_1 phase of the cell cycle via upregulating the expression of tumor-suppressor proteins p53, p21, and p16 and downregulating the expression of cyclin-dependent kinase 1 (CDK1) and cyclin B; it induced apoptosis via the death receptor apoptotic pathway and mitochondrial pathway and suppressed cell invasion (Zhang et al., 2020). *L. acidophilus*-fermented germinated brown rice was found to inhibit preneoplastic lesions of the colon of rats with CRC by reducing the number of ACF and decreasing serum levels of TNF-α, IL-6, and IL-1 levels and treatment with a dose of 2.5% increased expressions of proapoptotic cleaved caspase-3 and Bax, while decreased the expression of antiapoptotic Bcl-2 as well as the number of sialomucin-producing ACF. Thus such fermented rice product could be used as a dietary supplement for CRC chemoprevention (Li, Lin et al., 2019). Germinated brown rice in combination with *L. acidophilus* and/or *Bifidobacterium animalis* subsp. *lactis* able to inhibit CRC in rats via improved antioxidative capacity, inhibition of the formation of ACF-producing sialomucin (SIM-ACF), and apoptosis induction was also described by Lin et al. (2019). Administration of synbiotic combination of 10% djulis, a grain containing prebiotic dietary fiber showing anticancer property, and 5×10^6 or 5×10^7 *L. acidophilus* per gram to rats suffering on CRC induced by 1,2-dimethylhydrazine and dextran sulfate sodium, suppressed CRC by regulating proliferative, inflammatory, and apoptotic pathways

(Lee et al., 2020). Co-administration of ginger extract and *L. acidophilus* to Wistar rats reduced lipid peroxidation, increased catalase and superoxide dismutase (SOD) levels, restored colonic permeability, and reduced gut inflammation via downregulation of COX-2, inducible NO synthase (i-NOS), and regulator oncogen, c-Myc, expression (Deol et al., 2018). In male BALB/c mice receiving weekly subcutaneously 15 mg/kg AOM to induce colon cancer and subsequently treated with 1.5 g powders of *L. acidophilus* (1×10^9 CFU/g) and *B. bifidum* (1×10^9 CFU/g) in drinking water for 5 months increased expression of the tumor-suppressor miRNAs and their target genes and decreased expression of oncogenes was observed compared to the control group (Heydari et al., 2019). Weekly administration of AOM [15 mg/kg, subcutaneous (s.c.)] to male BALB/c mice caused a 74% colon lesion incidence (from mild-to-severe dysplasia and colonic adenocarcinoma) compared to control, which was suppressed by 57% and 27% at the administration of *L. acidophilus* and *B. bifidum*, respectively. Moreover, treatment with *L. acidophilus* also pronouncedly reduced the serum levels of carcinoembryonic antigen (CEA) and carbohydrate antigen 19–9 (CA19–9) tumor markers, considerably increased serum levels of IFN-γ and IL-10 as well as the number of $CD4^+$ and $CD8^+$ cells compared to AOM group suggesting that *L. acidophilus* probiotic application on mouse colon cancer was more effective than that of *B. bifidum* (Agah et al., 2019). On the other hand, oral consumption of *L. acidophilus* and *B. bifidum* probiotics significantly decreased the triglycerides, alkaline phosphatase, low-density lipoprotein cholesterol as well as the vitamin D receptor and the leptin receptor gene expression in AOM-induced mice colon cancer (Ranji et al., 2019). *L. acidophilus* and *B. animalis* subsp. *lactis* were found to exhibit powerful anti-inflammatory effect via toll-like receptor 2-mediated nuclear factor B and the mitogen-activated protein kinase (MAPK) signaling pathways in inflammatory intestinal epithelial cells and their combination has potential to be used as an adjuvant in inflammatory bowel disease therapy (Li, Hsu et al., 2019).

Cell-free extracts of *L. acidophilus* and *Lactobacillus delbrueckii* applied at doses 5 and 8 mg/mL reduced the viability of HT-29 cells to 42.2% and 19.40%, respectively, and both probiotic extracts exhibited high ROS scavenging activity. Moreover, they induced apoptosis, caused overexpression of caspase-9 and caspase-3 and an increase of Bax/Bcl-2 ratio (Baghbani-Arani et al., 2019). Administration of probiotic mixture consisting of *L. acidophilus*, *L. rhamnosus*, and *B. bifidum* to C57BL/6 mice suffering in colon cancer resulted in a decrease in average tumor size and tumor number compared to the control group, increased abundance of *Lactobacillus*, *Bifidobacterium*, *Allobaculum*, *Clostridium* XI, and *Clostridium* XVIII genera, and reduced colitis reflected in 46% reduction in the colon inflammatory index (Mendes et al., 2018).

The oral administration of the probiotic *L. rhamnosus* prevented FOLFOX (combination of the drugs consisting of folinic acid (leucovorin) "FOL," 5-fluorouracil "F," and oxaliplatin "OX") chemotherapy-induced intestinal mucositis and reduced the gravity of diarrhea in CRC-bearing mice without affecting the antitumor effect of FOLFOX (Chang et al., 2018). Long-term dietary-supplementation of *L. rhamnosus* affected gut microbiome pronouncedly enhancing the relative abundance of *Limnobacter*, *Turicibacterales*, *Enterococcus*, and *Vagococcus* and abundance of *Helicobacteraceae*, *Rikenellaceae*, *Roseburia*, *Doren*, *Anaerostipes*, *Coprococcus*, *Lachnospira*, *Oscillospira*, *Ruminococcaceae*, *Clotridiales*, *Muribaculaceae*, *Bacteroidia*, and *Bacteroidetes*. Moreover, higher level of energy production and conversion, amino acid transport and metabolism functions was observed at treatment with *L. rhamnosus* (Gamallat, Ren, Meyiah et al., 2019). *L. rhamnosus* was reported to exhibit protection against CRC in rats by inhibiting expressions of inflammatory and angiogenesis genes, and causing upregulation of apoptotic gene expression (Huang et al., 2019). Metabiotics extracted from isolated probiotic, *L. rhamnosus* MD 14, were found to be antigenotoxic and cytotoxic to Caco-2 and HT-29 human colon cancer cells (Sharma et al., 2020). Also, pretreatment of Sprague Dawley rats with *L. rhamnosus* via oral gavage considerably reduced the incidence and multiplicity of ACFs by inhibiting procarcinogenesis biomarkers and modulating the structure, composition, and functions of the gut microbiome at phylum, family, and genus levels (Gamallat, Ren, Walana et al., 2019).

Antiproliferative effects in murine (CT-26) and human (HT-29) colon carcinoma cell lines accompanied by apoptotic cell death and upregulation of TNF-related apoptosis inducing ligand (TRAIL) caused by *Lactobacillus casei* ATCC 393 were reported by Tiptiri-Kourpeti et al. (2016). Daily oral administration of live *L. casei* to BALB/c mice prior to the establishment of a syngeneic s.c. CT-26 tumor resulted in a pronounced enhancement in IFN-γ, granzyme B, and chemokine production in the tumor tissue and higher $CD8^+$ T-cell infiltration and tumor growth inhibition was observed as well. These results suggest that *L. casei* could be used as dietary immunoadjuvant suitable to improve protective anticancer immune responses (Aindelis et al., 2020). The preventive administration of *L. casei* 393 to BALB/c mouse 2 weeks before treatment with 1,2-dimethylhydrazine inducing CRC resulted in maintaining of the levels of 3 cytokines, attenuation of inflammation, modulation of splenic $CD4^+$, $CD8^+$, and natural killer T-cell subpopulations and conservation of a healthy T-cell subpopulation dynamic (Casas-Solis et al., 2020). *L. casei* Zhang isolated from naturally fermented koumiss showed high stability under amoxicillin or gentamycin exposure through 2000 generations of laboratory evolution, inhibited lipid peroxidation and increased antioxidant enzymes activities and was able to regulate cellular and humoral immunity and tumor associated immune function. Moreover, it stimulated the intestinal *Bacteroides* abundance resulting in mitigation of impaired glucose tolerance and prevention of type 2 diabetes mellitus and modulated gut microbiota composition and microbial acetic acid production leading to retardation of progression of colon cancer in mice (Zhang, 2019). Covalent conjugates of 25% galactooligosaccharides with 75% lactoferrin hydrolysate self-assembled into 0.2–1.5 m microparticles showing resistance to gastric digestion exhibited approx. double promotion of the growth rate of *L. casei* probiotic compared to the unconjugated components (0.082 vs 0.041/h) (Seifert et al., 2019). AgNPs fabricated using *L. casei* subsp. *casei* as bioreductant showed superb antibacterial activities against *S. aureus* and *Pseudomonas aeruginosa* and inhibited proliferation of human cancer cell lines HT-29 as well; it stimulated apoptosis and increased nitric oxide secretion (Leila et al., 2018).

The fermented supernatants obtained from fermentation of soluble dietary fiber from *Musa paradisiaca* inflorescence using *L. casei* and *B. bifidum* showed higher content of SCFAs and were capable to initiate apoptotic signaling in HT-29 colon cancer cells resulting in cell death. Both fermented supernatants showed cytotoxicity against HT-29 cells, induced DNA damage, and increased generation of ROS resulting in apoptosis, whereby reduction of membrane potential of mitochondria and ATP synthesis, improved delivery of cytochrome *c* (Cyto-c), and interference with the expression of pro/antiapoptotic proteins supported the apoptosis. Fermentation supernatant of *B. bifidum* was found to be more effective (Arun et al., 2019).

Cell-wall protein fractions from probiotic *L. paracasei* were found to suppress the growth of Caco-2 cells, caused a strong reduction in their viability and induced apoptosis suggesting their potential to be used as chemotherapeutic agent against human colon carcinoma cell line (Nozari et al., 2019). *L. paracasei* subsp. *paracasei* NTU 101-fermented skim milk applied as an adjuvant to uracil-tegafur treatment reduced tumor growth and metastasis compared to chemotherapy alone and improved chemotherapy side effects in an orthotopic mouse model of CRC (Chang et al., 2019). Extracellular vesicles released by *L. paracasei* consisting of a mixture of proteins, nucleic acids, and other biomolecules, which were administered to cultured HT-29 cells and to mice with induced colitis reduced the activation of inflammation-associated proteins in vitro; in an in vivo experiment they mitigated lipopolysaccharide (LPS)-induced inflammation causing reduction of proinflammatory protein activity and promoted the expression of endoplasmic reticulum stress-associated proteins (Choi et al., 2020). Heat-killed *L. brevis* and *L. paracasei* inhibited the proliferation of HT-29 cells and induced apoptosis, increased the expression of Bax, caspase-3, and caspase-9 mRNA levels, and reduced the expression of Bcl-2 in HT-29 cells, *L. brevis* being more effective (Ardestani et al., 2019). *Pediococcus pentosaceus* SP2 and *L. paracasei* SP5 isolated from kefir grains showed superb adhesion properties to HT-29 human colon cancer cells in vitro. Both viable probiotic strains caused considerable reduction of HT-29 cell growth, downregulated antiapoptotic genes, and caused overexpression of cell cycle-related genes and effectively reduced proliferation of cancer cells (Mantzourani et al., 2019).

The EPS from *L. fermentum* YL-11 containing as a main component galactose (48.0%) inhibited HT-29 cells *in vitro*, achieving $46.5 \pm 3.5\%$ and $45.6 \pm 6.1\%$ inhibition at a dose 600 and 800 g EPS/mL (Wei et al., 2019). Synergistic effect on the reduction of bacterial-glucuronidase activity in rat feces was observed at co-administration of prebiotics (EPS derived from *L. fermentum* TISTR or *Pediococcus acidilactici* TISTR 2612 as well as manno-oligosaccharides and rice syrup-oligosaccharide) with three lactobacilli strains; the highest effect showed co-administration of *L. plantarum* DSM 2648 with the EPS of *P. acidilactici* showing 57.94% and 50.72% reduction of this enzyme in male and female rats, respectively (Chaiongkarn et al., 2019). Two different isolated conjugated-linolenic acid (CLNA) isomers produced by *L. plantarum* ZS2058 suppressed the growth of 3 types of colon cancer cells and it was found that antiproliferation activity of CLNAs in Caco-2 cells was connected with oxidative stress resulting in lipid peroxidation. CLNA1 was found to activate caspase-1 and induced Caco-2 cell pyroptosis, while CLNA2 induced pyroptosis via the caspase-4/5-mediated pathway; key proteins associated with apoptosis were affected neither by CLNA1 nor by CLNA2 (Ren et al., 2020). EPS produced by probiotic *L. plantarum* C70 (accession number KX881779) isolated from camel milk with mean molecular weight of 3.8×10^5, average particle size of 525.5 nm and zeta potential of 330.71 mV applied at a dose of 10 mg/mL showed 88.1% cytotoxic activity against colon cancer lines (Ayyash et al., 2020). *L. plantarum* isolated from fermented durian (Tempoyak), a Malaysian traditional condiment, showed good tolerance against pH 2.0 and 0.3% bile salts and an adhesion index in HT-29 cells of 15910, whereby both live bacterial cells and cell-free supernatant (CFS) decreased the proliferation of HT-29 cells (Ahmad et al., 2018). Co-administration of a synbiotic consisting of *L. plantarum* MBTU-HK1 (probiotic) with acacia gum (prebiotic) to male Balb/c mice caused a decrease in cholesterol levels, increased protein and mineral content, strengthened immunoglobulin levels, and modulated phagocytosis. Such combined treatment also resulted in reduced levels of TNF-α and lowered activities of bacterial procarcinogenic fecal enzymes, suggesting the suitability of such synbiotic to prevent incidence of CRC (Chundakkattumalayil et al., 2019).

EPS produced by *Lactobacillus kefiri* MSR101 isolated from Chinese kefir grains, a heteropolymer of glucose and galactose, when applied at a dose 400 g/mL in vitro, exhibited anticancer activity on HT-29 cancer cells and upregulated the expression of Cyto-c, Bcl-2-associated X-protein (BAX), BCL-2-associated agonist of cell death (BAD), caspase-3, caspase-8, and caspase-9, suggesting that they could be used as topical medication against CRC (Rajoka et al., 2019). After the exposure of HT-29 cells to *L. kefiri* SGL 13 for 24 h, 60 differentially expressed proteins were estimated, mostly situated into the extracellular exosome, which play key roles in translation and cell adhesion; the treatment with *L. kefiri* SGL 13 increased Bax and decreased caspase-3 and mutant p53, and inhibition of IL-8 secretion from HT-29 cells stimulated with LPS was observed as well (Brandi et al., 2019).

Lactobacillus reuteri, a crucial bacterium that colonizes many mammals, was found to inhibit tumor progression, reduce inflammation, and prevent tumor progression into carcinogenesis or further metastasis (Bistas et al., 2020). Heat-killed sonicated fraction of *L. reuteri* and fractions from *L. reuteri* CFS with molecular weight >100 kDa pronouncedly increased the apoptosis percentage of human colon cancer stem-like cells (HT-29-ShE) indicating their antimetastatic and antiproliferative activities. Hence, secretory macromolecules (e.g., polysaccharides, nucleic acids, or protein) can inhibit the growth of colon cancer stem-like cells and CFS components could be used as the antimetastatic agents (Maghsood et al., 2020).

Nisin, a polycyclic antibacterial peptide produced by the bacterium *Lactococcus lactis*, inhibited the proliferation of LS180, SW48, HT-29, and Caco-2 CRC cell lines and suppressed metastatic process via downregulation of CEA, bile carcinoembryonic cell adhesion molecule 6 (CEAM6), matrix metalloproteinase-2F (MMP2F), and MMP9F genes (Norouzi et al., 2018). Recombinant *L. lactis* expressing TRAIL protein pronouncedly reduced the viability of SW480 and HCT116 cells and induced apoptosis in these colon adenocarcinoma cell lines (Bohlul et al., 2019).

Effective anticancer activity against HT-29 colon cancer cell line showed also intracellular CFS from the probiotic *Bacillus licheniformis* KT921419 (Ragul et al., 2020). Heat-inactivated bacteria of *E. coli* Nissle 1917, a probiotic showing anticancer effects against human colorectal adenocarcinoma HT-29 cells, caused their apoptosis by upregulating phosphatase and tensin homolog and Bax and downregulating AKT serine/threonine kinase 1 and Bcl-xL genes (Alizadeh et al., 2020).

Metabolites of *E. faecalis* strains, belonging to the components of the natural human GI microbiota, which were isolated from healthy donors, were reported to reduce proliferation of HCT-8 (human ileocecal adenocarcinoma) and HCT116 (human colon carcinoma) cell lines with no effects on SW620 cell line (human colorectal adenocarcinoma) or normal human diploid cell line CLR-1790. On the other hand, metabolites of *E. faecalis* strains isolated from CRC patients did not affect the cell growth of CRC cell lines (De Almeida et al., 2019). Chung et al. (2019) reported that pretreatment with a heat-killed *E. faecalis* was found to attenuate the phagocytosis required for the full activation of the NLRP3 inflammasome and the results of in vivo experiments showed that it improved gravity of intestinal inflammation resulting in protection against colitis and inflammation-associated colon carcinogenesis in wild-type mice.

Streptomycetes, soil residents producing many antiproliferative, anti-inflammatory/immunosuppressive compounds, for example, rapamycin and tacrolimus, known to act against allergy and autoimmunity as well as inflammatory bowel disease, can within gut microbiome contribute to the suppression of colon tumorigenesis. The current lifestyle, in which the exposure to nature is limited, is accompanied with a shortage of these filamentous bacteria and represents higher vulnerability to colon cancer (Bolourian & Mojtahedi, 2018a,b).

Clostridium butyricum, a butyrate-producing bacteria, pronouncedly suppressed high-fat diet-induced intestinal tumor development in Apc$^{min/+}$ mice by modulating Wnt signaling and affected the gut microbiota composition resulting in reduction of pathogenic bacteria and bile acid-biotransforming bacteria, while increasing some beneficial bacteria (e.g., SCFA-producing bacteria) (Chen et al., 2020). From various SCFAs in the colon produced by fermentation of dietary fibers especially butyrate is known to regulate the physical and functional integrity of the normal colonic mucosa via affecting mucin gene expression or the number of goblet cells. Treatment of human colon epithelial LS174T cells with butyrate resulted in changes in the adherence of gut microflora, whereby butyrate potentially promoted the MAPK signaling pathway in intestinal cells (Jung et al., 2015). The presence of extracellular lactate produced by CRC cells via "Warburg effect," where cancer cells "ferment" glucose into lactate in CRC cells, resulted in increased production of SCFAs by *Propionibacterium freudenreichii* leading to the inhibition of proliferation of CRC cells and increased cell death. *P. freudenreichii* was recommended as a probiotic suitable to be used in CRC prevention at early stages of the carcinogenesis process (Casanova et al., 2018). So it is no wonder that Richards et al. (2016) in their review paper discussed the findings related to the impact of the diet, microbiota, and gut microbial metabolites (especially SCFAs) on the modulation of the progression of inflammatory diseases and autoimmunity, and the corresponding molecular mechanisms, including metabolite-sensing G protein-coupled receptor and inhibition of histone deacetylases. Using gnotobiotic mouse models colonized with wild-type or mutant strains of a butyrate-producing bacterium

Donohoe et al. (2014) showed that dietary fibers have strong tumor-suppressive effect in a microbiota- and butyrate-dependent manner. In colorectal adenocarcinomas, higher butyrate and histone acetylation levels than in normal colonic tissues were estimated, suggesting that butyrate, which accumulated in tumors due to lower metabolization, functioned as a histone deacetylase (HDAC) inhibitor, promoted histone acetylation, and affected apoptosis and cell proliferation. The researchers emphasized that using probiotic/prebiotic strategies modulation of an endogenous HDAC inhibitor for anticancer chemoprevention can be achieved and in such way negative impact of synthetic HDAC inhibitors used in chemotherapy can be eliminated.

Heat-killed yeasts *Saccharomyces cerevisiae* induced apoptosis in SW480 colon cancer cell line via downregulation of p-Akt1, Rel A, Bcl-XL, procaspase 3, and procaspase 9 expressions and upregulation of BAX cleaved caspase-3 and caspase-9 (Shamekhi et al., 2020). Saadat et al. (2020) reported that EPSs of probiotic yeasts *Kluyveromyces marxianus* and *Pichia kudriavzevii* from dairy products prevented AKT-1, mammalian target of rapamycin, and Janus Kinase 1 pathways and induced apoptosis in different human colon cancer cell lines and recommended these probiotic yeast EPSs to be used as a molecular-targeted therapeutics against CRC.

13.4 Probiotics and prebiotics in breast cancer

BC is a malignant disease affecting women in the vast majority of cases; men make up about 1% of affected individuals. Most diseases occur after the age of 60, before the transition the disease is rather rare and before the age of 25 extremely rare. It is the second most common cancer diagnosed in women in the United States and the most common cancer diagnosed in women in Central Europe. However, the media attention and associated financial support to BC has helped to develop advanced diagnostic and treatment resulting in increasing number of cured patients and declining deaths related to the disease. Crucial to success is early diagnosis and a new personal approach to treatment and a better understanding of the disease. Symptoms of BC may include lumps or changes in the size, shape or appearance of the changes in the skin on the breasts. BC most often begins in the cells of the milk ducts (invasive ductal carcinoma) or in the glandular tissue of the lobules (invasive lobular carcinoma) or in other cells or tissues in the breast. The most common causes are hormonal factors, family predisposition (5–10%), lifestyle and environmental influences. A risk factor for BC is anything that increases the likelihood of developing BC, but on the other hand, it does not mean that the disease will actually develop. Many women who develop BC have no known risk factors other than being women. Factors associated with an increased risk of BC therefore include: being a woman, increasing age, lobular carcinoma in situ or atypical breast hyperplasia, BC in one breast, if your mother, sister or daughter was diagnosed with BC, inherited mutations of genes BRCA1 and BRCA2, radiation exposure, obesity, onset of menstruation before 12 years, onset of menopause at an older age, first birth after 30 years, absence of pregnancy, postmenopausal hormone therapy (HRT), excess alcohol (CDC, 2018; IARC, 2018a–e; MFMER, 2020a; NHS, 2019), or exposure to some environmental contaminants (Kráľová & Jampílek, 2015).

Distant organs could be affected by gut microbiota via various mechanisms, such as regulation of absorption of nutrients and/or the production of microbial metabolites, regulation and interaction with the systemic immune system, and translocation of bacteria/bacterial products through disrupted mucosal barriers (Shimizu, 2018). Dietary change and nutritional intervention can affect the human microbiome. Consumption of fiber-rich foods results in evident modifications in microbe abundances and in the production of fermentation products, for example, SCFAs and phytochemicals. Dietary change and consumption of fiber-rich foods can suppress the incidence and mortality from colon, breast, or liver cancers, westernized cardiovascular, infectious, and respiratory diseases, diabetes, and obesity (Wilson et al., 2020). Probiotics are able to modulate the GI bacteria and the systemic immune system and therefore their use in the prevention or treatment of BC is desirable. Current findings related to probiotics and their potential role in the therapy of BC was summarized by Mendoza (2019). Anticarcinogenicity of microbiota and probiotics in BC was discussed also by Malik et al. (2018). Dietary intake prior to, during, and after cancer treatment is able to affect fatigue levels of cancer survivors. Mediterranean diet and supplementation with probiotic, ginseng or ginger probiotics may improve cancer survivors' energy level and can reduce their fatigue (Inglis et al., 2019). For example, beneficial impact of the addition of probiotics (*Bifidobacterium longum* BB536, *L. rhamnosus* HN001) to a Mediterranean diet during 4 months on gut microbiota and metabolic profile in overweight BC survivors compared to Mediterranean diet alone (control) was reported by Pellegrini et al. (2020). In contrast to controls, already after 2 months of probiotic administration pronounced raise in the number of bacterial species and the bacterial diversity was observed and whereas the Bacteroidetes-to-Firmicutes ratio showed an increase in controls, its considerable increase was estimated at combined treatment with probiotics. Moreover, after 4-month treatment pronounced reductions of body weight, body mass index, fasting glucose, and homeostasis model assessment of insulin resistance was observed. The use of soy isoflavones and fermented soy beverage produced using probiotics, such as lactic acid bacteria, in the prevention of BC was discussed by Takagi et al. (2015).

As mentioned above, to risk factors associated with BC, including familial history of BC, using of hormone replacement therapy, obesity, personal habits, and environmental contaminants also patient microbiome can represent a new risk factor (CDC, 2018; Eslami-S et al., 2020; Fernández et al., 2018; Kamińska et al., 2015; Králová & Jampílek, 2015; National Breast Cancer Foundation, 2019; Parida & Sharma, 2020; Zhang & Zhang, 2020). Eslami-S et al. (2020) in a review paper discussed the role of the microbiome as a risk factor in the development of BC, analyzed the proposed mechanisms of interaction between the microbiome and human genes involved in BC, and assessed the effects of the changed composition of breast, gut, and milk microbiome in healthy and cancerous breast, examined the role of microbiome in the development and maintenance of inflammation, estrogen metabolism, and epigenetic alterations as well as application of probiotics, microbiome genome modulation, and engineered microbiome enzymes in the management of BC.

Dysbiosis can adversely affect the management of obesity and lymphedema by increasing inflammation; however, synbiotic supplementation along with a low-calorie diet showed favorable impact on the concentration of serum inflammatory markers, leptin and TNF-α, and reduced edema volume, while highly sensitive C-reactive protein and IL-1 were practically not affected in BC survivors with lymphedema (Vafa et al., 2020). On the other hand, Navaei et al. (2020) observed that following a synbiotic supplementation along with a low-calorie diet during 10 weeks to obese and overweight patients with BC-related lymphedema reduced levels of serum malonedialdehyde and elevated activity of SOD was estimated suggesting that synbiotics exhibited favorable effects via antioxidant properties, although impact on edema volume was not significant.

Kefir, fermented milk with Caucasian and Tibet origin, prepared by the incubation of kefir grains and containing a mixture of yeast and bacteria living in a symbiotic association with raw milk or water, is a powerful probiotic with anticancer properties against BC, CRC, malignant T lymphocytes, and lung carcinoma (Sharifi et al., 2017). The 48 and 72 h IC_{50} values related to kefir water cytotoxicity against 4T1 cells were estimated as 12.5 and 8.33 mg/mL, respectively. When BALB/c mice were injected with 4T1 cancer cells and treated orally with kefir water for 28 days, tumor proliferation was inhibited via cancer cell apoptosis, immunomodulation by stimulating T-helper cells and cytotoxic T cells, and anti-inflammatory, antimetastatic, and antiangiogenesis effects were observed suggesting the potential of kefir water to be used as probiotic beverage in cancer treatment (Zamberi et al., 2016).

The antiproliferative activity of water-soluble extract of Himalayan cheese (Kalari/Kradi) fermented with *L. plantarum* (NCDC 012), *L. casei* (NCDC 297), and *L. brevis* (NCDC 021) against human BC cells, colon cancer cells, and neuroblastoma was pronouncedly higher than that of cheese without added probiotics and cheese incorporating probiotics showed also enhanced antimicrobial, α-glucosidase, and α-amylase inhibitory activity and immunomodulatory activity, whereby its improved nutritional potential could be connected with the generation of bioactive peptides by the proteolytic activity of the probiotics (Mushtaq et al., 2019).

Milk fermented with *L. casei* CRL431 administered to mice in the metastatic stage of BC resulted in decreased proinflammatory cytokines and decreased $IL-10^+$ $F4/80^+$ cells in the lungs resulting in diminished metastasis in the lungs and increasing survival of the animals suggesting that modulation of immune cells in the lungs by *L. casei* could be utilized in suppression of tumor cells in the metastatic sites (Utz et al., 2019). The administration of milk fermented by *L. casei* CRL431 to mice suffering on mammary carcinogenesis reduced or inhibited tumor growth and less tumor vascularity, extravasation of tumor cells, and lung metastasis were observed what could be connected with the modulation of the immune response by reducing infiltration of macrophages in both the tumor and the lungs. Administration of fermented milk preserved an increased antitumor response associated to $CD8^+$ lymphocytes and enhanced $CD4^+$ lymphocytes that can be involved in the modulation of the immune response in BC model (Aragon et al., 2015). Inhibition of tumor growth and reduced tumor size as well as immunomodulatory, antiangiogenesis, and antimetastatic activities of probiotics in animal studies were observed and it was shown that BC incidence in humans can be reduced by the intake of *L. casei* Shirota, whereby consumption of fermented milk products and yogurt can suppress the BC incidence (Ranjbar et al., 2019). CuO NPs green synthesized using probiotic bacteria *L. casei* subsp. *casei* exhibited beside antibacterial effects also cytotoxic effects on cancer cells resulting in growth inhibition, increased oxidative stress and induction of apoptosis (Kouhkan et al., 2020).

EPSs produced by probiotic *L. plantarum* C70 (accession number KX881779) isolated from camel milk containing as the major monosaccharide constituents 13.3% arabinose, 7.1% mannose, 74.6% glucose, and 5.0% galactose exhibited cytotoxic activity against BC (73.1% at a dose of 10 mg/mL) (Ayyash et al., 2020). Co-treatment of rats, in which mammary carcinogenesis was induced by procarcinogen 7,12-dimethylbenz[a]anthracene, by probiotic *L. plantarum* LS/07 and prebiotic inulin, exhibited prodifferentiating, antiproliferative, and immunomodulatory activities; the tumor growths were not affected, but pronounced reductions in the ratio of high-/low-grade carcinomas and in tumoral Ki-67 expression were observed. These effects were further amplified by adding melatonin what was reflected in increased $CD4^+$ and $CD8^+$ T-cell tumor infiltration and increasing numbers of $CD25^+FoxP3^+$ regulatory T cells in tumors (Kassayova et al., 2016). Long-term administration of *L. plantarum* LS/07 with and without oligofructose-enriched inulin was found to be effective against BC in rats, at least partially, via immunomodulatory mechanisms (Kassayova et al., 2014)

Inhibitory effect of tamoxifen, an antiestrogenic drug inhibiting the progression of BC via competing with estrogen for binding to the estrogen receptor, on the proliferation of MCF-7, a BC cell line, synergistically increased at coadministration with *L. brevis* supernatant. Levels of Bcl-2 mRNA in the cells exposed to combined treatment with probiotic were lower than in those treated with tamoxifen suggesting that *L. brevis* could be used as an adjuvant therapy in BC treatment and prevention (Nasiri et al., 2021).

Combination of *L. rhamnosus* Heriz I (2×10^7 CFU/mL) and glucan (two 10-mg capsules) improved functional scales and symptoms in patients with BC who underwent chemotherapy (Monshikarimi et al., 2019).

Health properties of grains could be enhanced by probiotic fermentation and it was shown that solid-state fermented lupin using *Bifidobacterium* spp. exhibited threefold and fivefold greater cytotoxic activity against BC cells (MCF-7) and colon cancer cells (Caco-2) than fermented quinoa and wheat. The fermented cereals with high total phenolic contents considerably increased glucosidase inhibition and enhanced angiotensin-converting enzyme (ACE) activities (Ayyash et al., 2018).

Live and heat-killed cells of *E. faecalis* and *Staphylococcus hominis* isolated from human breast milk as well as the cytoplasmic fractions of *E. faecalis* and *S. hominis* caused up to 33.29% reduction in MCF-7 cell proliferation in a concentration- and time-dependent manner and cell shrinkage and membrane blebbing were observed. Their powerful antiproliferative activity was induced via sub-G_1 accumulation (up to 83.17%) in treated MCF-7 cells and decreased number in the G_0/G_1 phase by 74.39%, while treated nontumorigenic epithelial MCF-10A cells showed comparable viability than the control ($>90\%$). *E. faecalis* and *S. hominis* could be considered as good alternative nutraceuticals without cytotoxic effects to normal cells (Hassan et al., 2016).

13.5 Probiotics and prebiotics in cervical cancer

CC is a type of cancer that occurs in the cells of the cervix (the lower part of the uterus that attaches to the vagina). CC is the 4th common cancer in women and the 2nd most common cancer in less developed regions. In 2018, approximately 570,000 women with CC were newly diagnosed worldwide and approximately 311,000 women died from the disease; then, more than 85% of deaths account for low- and middle-income countries. The main types of CC are: squamous cell carcinoma (starting in the squamous cells lining the outer part of the cervix that protrudes into the vagina) and adenocarcinoma (starting in the columnar glandular cells that line the cervical canal), or a combination of both. Rarely, cancer occurs in other cells in the cervix. Various strains of HPV and sexually transmitted infections have been shown to be crucial for the development of CC; therefore the risk of developing CC can be reduced by vaccination that protects against HPV infection. However, other factors are likely to contribute to the likelihood of developing CC, such as the environment, lifestyle, or nutrition. CC generally does not cause any symptoms in the early stages. Symptoms of more advanced stages include: vaginal bleeding after intercourse, between periods, or after menopause, bloody, foul-smelling vaginal discharge, pelvic pain, or pain during intercourse. Risk factors for CC include: sexual promiscuity, early sexual activity, HPV, and other sexually transmitted infections (e.g., chlamydia, gonorrhea, syphilis, and HIV/AIDS), immunodeficiency, smoking, and exposure to diethylstilbestrol (CDC, 2019, 2020; MFMER, 2020b; NHS, 2018a).

The microbiota of the lower female reproductive tract (vagina and cervix) microenvironment in the majority of women of reproductive age contains *Lactobacillus* spp. as predominant species. At dysbiosis, changes in immune and metabolic signaling may result in chronic inflammation, changes in cellular proliferation and apoptosis, angiogenesis, genome instability, and metabolic dysregulation and ultimately in gynecological cancer. Moreover, genital dysbiosis and/or specific bacteria might contribute to the development and/or progression and metastasis of cervical, endometrial, and ovarian cancers, through direct and indirect mechanisms, including modulation of estrogen metabolism. Probiotics or microbiota transplants can modulate the microbiome resulting in improved responsiveness to cancer treatment (Laniewski et al., 2020). Li et al. (2020) discussed critical immune factors in lower genital tract health, highlighted the role of the vaginal microbiota in cervical carcinogenesis, and stressed the potential of the use of probiotics in treatment of CC. Changes in vaginal microbiome have great impact on the occurrence and development of CC. The role of the vaginal microbiome in gynecological cancer was comprehensively described also by Champer et al. (2018). The anticancer effect of cervicovaginal bacteria and their potential for CC treatment was overviewed by Pourmollaei et al. (2020). In addition, changes in the cervical microbiota could be used as potential biomarkers of premalignant cervical intraepithelial neoplasia and development of invasive CC in the context of HPV infection (Curty et al., 2020).

Some members of the cervical microbiota were found to be possible modifiers of the cytokine profile of the cervical microenvironment during the development of cervical lesions and CC and therefore it is important to investigate potential impact of microbiome dysbiosis on cancer evolution as well as prospective use of microbiome profiles as biomarkers for prevention and early diagnosis. Considering that microbiota may be modified by the use of pre- and probiotics it is necessary to recognize whether they prevent cancer evolution or even potentiate cancer treatment (Aviles-Jimenez et al., 2017).

The effectiveness of dietary supplements (probiotics, vitamin E, retinoids, indoles, multivitamin preparations, folic acid, and Se) used for the treatment of women with CC and some degree of cervical intraepithelial neoplasia was discussed by Ortiz et al. (2013). Common vaginal lactobacilli, *Lactobacillus gasseri* and *Lactobacillus crispatus*, exhibited cytotoxic effects on cervical HeLa cancer cells, but not on normal cells, and this cytotoxicity did not depend on pH and lactate. Apoptosis was suppressed by supernatants, which corresponded to higher human chorionic gonadotropin (hCG) beta expression because apoptosis is inhibited by hCG (Motevaseli, Shirzad, Akrami et al., 2013). *Lactobacillus* strains (*Lactobacillus mucosae* K76, *L. fermentum* K81, *L. fermentum* K85, *L. reuteri* K97 and *L. reuteri* K99) collected from the vaginal environment of the healthy Northeast Indian women showed cytotoxic activities on three cancer cell lines, which decreased in following order: A549 (lung cancer) > HeLa (cervical) > AGS (gastric cancer). *L. mucosae* K76, which was evaluated as safer based on the antibiotic resistance profile, exhibited also the best cytotoxic activity against all tested cancer cell lines and can be considered as a probiotic candidate (Das Purkayastha et al., 2020). Vaginal flora of Iranian healthy women is dominated by *Lactobacillus* species (*L. crispatus*, *L. gasseri*, *L. iners*, *L. jensenii*, *L. acidophilus* and *L. rhamnosus*), which can prevent bacterial vaginosis. On the other hand, *L. crispatus* and *L. jensenii* were significantly higher in the normal than in the bacterial vaginosis of infected women, whereby the cytotoxic effect of *L. crispatus* on CC cells exceeded that of other lactobacilli or commercial probiotics (Motevaseli, Shirzad, Raoofian et al., 2013). Women with a HPV and low-grade squamous intraepithelial lesion diagnosis, which consumed daily probiotic drink for 6 months, had twofold higher clearance of cytological abnormalities compared to control group (60% vs 31%) and HPV was cleared in 29% of probiotic users compared to 19% of control patients suggesting beneficial effects of probiotics (Verhoeven et al., 2013). Based on the preliminary study of Hodaei et al. (2019), the expression of the L1 protein-coding gene from HPV genotype 16 in the probiotic strain *Lactobacillus cromoris* could be considered as an immunogen.

Most CCs are associated with anogenital region infection with high-risk HPV. Antiviral activity of *Bifidobacterium adolescentis* SPM1005-A in the SiHa CC cell line expressing HPV type 16 was reflected in suppression E6 and E7 oncogene expression (Cha et al., 2012). Antitumor immune responses and inhibition of tumor growth in C57BL/6 mice bearing transplanted TC-1 cells of HPV-related tumor expressing HPV-16 E6/E7 oncogenes were observed after the intravenous or oral administration of *B. bifidum*, whereby only intravenous administration of probiotic resulted in the activation of tumor-specific IL-12 and IFN-γ, lymphocyte proliferation, and CD8$^+$ cytolytic responses that control and eradicate tumor growth. Consequently, the probiotic *B. bifidum* has potential to be used as an immunomodulator in the treatment of CC (Abdolalipour et al., 2020).

In the experiment of de Loera-Rodriguez et al. (2018) patients with CC ingested 20 g biogels supplemented with synbiotics or placebo three times a day for 7 weeks. Treatment with symbiotic containing 1×10^7 CFU/g biogel of *L. acidophilus* NCFM, 1×10^6 CFU/g biogel of *Bifidobacterium lactis*, and blue agave inulin considerably decreased the levels of fecal calprotectin and the frequency and intensity of vomiting.

Oral or intravaginal administration of the mixture of *L. rhamnosus* HN001 (L1), *L. acidophilus* La-14 (L2), and lactoferrin RCXTM to mice, in which bacterial vaginosis was induced via estradiol-3-benzoate-induced immunosuppression and intravaginal inoculation with *Gardnerella vaginalis*, resulted in the colonization of L1 and L2 in the vagina; the individual probiotics or their mixture pronouncedly inhibited *G. vaginalis*-induced epithelial cell disruption, myeloperoxidase activity, NF-κB activation, and IL-1β and TNF-α expression as well as IL-17 and retinoic acid receptor-related orphan receptor gamma t expression but increased IL-10 and the forkhead box P3 (Foxp3, scurfin) expression, oral administration being more effective. Both lactobacilli considerably suppressed the adherence of *G. vaginalis* to HeLa cells and growth of *G. vaginalis in vitro* as well as lipopolysaccharide-induced NF-κB activation in macrophages and the differentiation of splenocytes into Th17 cells in vitro. The probiotic formulations were able to mitigate *G. vaginalis*-induced vaginosis via regulating vaginal systemic innate and adaptive immune responses rather than direct competition or killing of *G. vaginalis* in the vagina (Jang et al., 2017).

Supernatants of *L. rhamnosus* and *L. crispatus* were found to be cytotoxic to HeLa cells, they reduced caspase-3 gene expression, and the supernatants of two studied lactobacilli could be considered as effective probiotics in the prevention of metastasis potency in HeLa cells causing decreased expression of MMP2 and MMP9 and increased expression of their inhibitors; they can be administrated to postpone late stage of cancer disease (Nouri et al., 2016).

Cell-free extracts of *L. casei* applied to Caski and HeLa cells adhering to tissue culture plates did not affect considerably their growth rate and not even synergistic effect on the suppression of the growth of cancer cells in the presence of anticancer drugs was observed (Kim et al., 2015).

EPS produced by *L. gasseri* strains (G10 and H15), isolated from a healthy human vagina applied to HeLa cells in the form of live culture (10^8 CFU/mL) or in lyophilized form (L-EPS; 100–400 g/mL), inhibited cell proliferation, whereby the L-EPS induced apoptosis in HeLa cells in a strain dependent manner. G10 was found as the most adhesive strain and induced apoptosis via an upregulation of Bax and caspase-3. However, both strains of *L. gasseri* decreased the production of TNF-α and increasing of the IL-10 production was reflected in anti-inflammatory effect on HeLa cells (Sungur et al., 2017).

Kefiran produced by the fermentation of *Lactobacillus kefiranofaciens* pronouncedly affected the viability human cervical HeLa cells with IC_{50} values of 358.8 ± 1.65 g/mL and showed negative impact on morphological characteristics of the cells, whereby exhibited safer profiles in zebrafish embryos with LC_{50} value of 279.76 g/mL suggesting its potential as anticancer agent showing no effect on normal tissue growth (Elsayed et al., 2017).

Vaginal bacterium *L. plantarum* 5BL isolated from vaginal secretions of adolescent and young adult women showed probiotic properties including low pH and high bile salt concentration tolerance, antibiotic susceptibility and antimicrobial activity against some pathogenic bacteria as well as superb anticancer activity against cervical (HeLa), breast (MCF-7), gastric (AGS), and colon (HT-29) human cancer cell lines without pronounced cytotoxic impact on normal human umbilical vein endothelial cells suggesting its potential to be used as a bioactive therapeutic agent (Nami et al., 2014). From fermented beverage Marcha of north eastern Himalayas Das and Goyal (2014a) isolated *L. plantarum* DM5 producing EPSs showed extracellular glucansucrase activity of 0.48 U/mg by synthesizing natural EPS glucan (1.87 mg/mL) from sucrose. *L. plantarum* DM5 showed bacteriocin activity against several major food-borne pathogens and its bacteriocin (plantaricin DM5) was stable in a wide pH range (2.010.0), although it was sensitive to proteolytic enzymes. Moreover, it was resistant to high temperature (121°C for 15 min), maintained its activity also at treatment with surface active agents and was not cytotoxic to mammalian cells (Das & Goyal, 2014b).

Gut microbial dysbiosis contributes to the development and progression of radiation enteritis (RE) during pelvic radiotherapy. Based on microbiota profiles of fecal samples collected from 18 CC patients during radiotherapy it was found that dysbiosis was characterized by pronouncedly reduced α-diversity and enhanced β-diversity, relative higher abundance of *Proteobacteria* and *Gammaproteobacteria* and lower abundance of *Bacteroides*. In patients with mild enteritis as more abundant *Virgi bacillus* and *Alcanivorax* was estimated. In an experiment with bacterial-epithelial cocultures, it was shown that compared with control microbiota, the microbiota derived from patients with RE induced epithelial inflammation and barrier dysfunction, and enhanced TNF-α and IL-1 expression (Wang et al., 2019).

Beneficial effect of probiotics *L. acidophilus* LA-5 plus *B. animalis* subsp. *lactis* BB-12 (1.75 billion lyophilized live bacteria per capsule taken daily during the whole period of radiotherapy) for the prevention of acute radiation-induced diarrhea (RID) among CC patients was reflected in significant reduction of the incidence and severity of diarrhea (Linn et al., 2019). Also, a systematic review and *meta*-analysis performed by Qiu et al. (2019) showed the beneficial effect of probiotics in the prevention of RID, particularly for Grade 2 or 3 diarrhea, which only rarely caused severe adverse events during treatment.

New probiotic strain-por1 isolated from intestinal food content of porcupine and identified as an *E. faecium* (por1) possessed three different bacteriocins genes (ent-A, ent-B, and ent-P), from which the expressed and purified bacteriocin enterocin-A showed superb antibacterial and antibiofilm activity against bacterial pathogens and exhibited anticancer activity not only against cervical (HeLa) cancer cells but also against human colon and gastric cancer cells (HT-29, Caco-2, and AGS), whereby showed no cytotoxicity to normal intestinal epithelial cells (Ankaiah et al., 2017).

Oncoprotective effects of SCFAs produced by fermentation from prebiotics on uterine cervical neoplasia via expression of free fatty acid receptor 2 was reported by Matsuya-Ogawa et al. (2019).

13.6 Conclusion

As mentioned above, cancer has become a part of our lives and there is probably no family in the western countries where there is no any cancer patient. This is undoubtedly closely connected with an unhealthy lifestyle, increased consumption of fast foods, insufficient physical activity even from childhood, and increased levels of everyday stress. There are only a few types of cancer that can be well and completely cured, and many types of cancer lead to the death of the patient at the first occurrence or subsequent recurrence. Unfortunately, current anticancer drugs usually cause serious side effects that could be alleviated by co-administration of many other drugs. One of the ways to try to prevent cancer is the consumption of probiotics composed of the so-called "good" microorganisms, and a balanced diet should undoubtedly contain sufficient amounts of prebiotics supporting beneficial impact of probiotics on human health. It has been found that in addition to a positive effect on many physiological processes, probiotics can sometimes potentiate the effect of treatment or reduce the side effects of anticancer drugs and radiation therapy. Recently, probiotics can also be found in the form of NPs/nanoformulations in various combinations of species/strains or with other bioactive substances, which aim to increase the biological effect and overall benefit of these "smart" food supplements. Thus probiotics in nanoformulations may have a "stronger" beneficial effect on a healthy individual, can more effectively alleviate the side effects of existing drugs used to treat cancer, and may be used as an adjunct to the therapy but it should be emphasized that the administration of probiotics alone does not cure any type of cancer.

Acknowledgment

This study was supported by the Slovak Research and Development Agency (projects APVV-17-0373 and APVV-17-0318).

References

Abdolalipour, E., Mahooti, M., Salehzadeh, A., Torabi, A., Mohebbi, S. R., Gorji, A., & Ghaemi, A. (2020). Evaluation of the antitumor immune responses of probiotic Bifidobacterium bifidum in human papillomavirus-induced tumor model. *Microbial Pathogenesis, 145*, 104207.

Agah, S., Alizadeh, A. M., Mosavi, M., Ranji, P., Khavari-Daneshvar, H., Ghasemian, F., Bahmani, S., & Tavassoli, A. (2019). More protection of Lactobacillus acidophilus than Bifidobacterium bifidum probiotics on azoxymethane-induced mouse colon cancer. *Probiotics and Antimicrobial Proteins, 11*, 857–864.

Aguilar-Toalá, J. E., Garcia-Varela, R., Garcia, H. S., Mata-Haro, V., González-Córdova, A. F., Vallejo-Cordoba, B., & Hernández-Mendoza, A. (2018). Postbiotics: An evolving term within the functional foods field. *Trends in Food Science & Technology, 75*, 105–114.

Ahmad, A., Yap, W. B., Kofli, N. T., & Ghazali, A. R. (2018). Probiotic potentials of Lactobacillus plantarum isolated from fermented durian (Tempoyak), a Malaysian traditional condiment. *Food Science & Nutrition, 6*, 1370–1377.

Aindelis, G., Tiptiri-Kourpeti, A., Lampri, E., Spyridopoulou, K., Lamprianidou, E., Kotsianidis, I., Ypsilantis, P., Pappa, A., & Chlichlia, K. (2020). Immune responses raised in an experimental colon carcinoma model following oral administration of Lactobacillus casei. *Cancers, 12*, 368.

Alarcon, T., Llorca, L., & Perez-Perez, G. (2017). Impact of the microbiota and gastric disease development by Helicobacter pylori. In N. Tegtmeyer, & S. Backert (Eds.), *Molecular Pathogenesis and signal transduction by Helicobacter pylori* (pp. 253–275). Springer International Publishing.

Alizadeh, S., Esmaeili, A., & Omidi, Y. (2020). Anti-cancer properties of Escherichia coli Nissle 1917 against HT-29 colon cancer cells through regulation of Bax/Bcl-xL and AKT/PTEN signaling pathways. *Iranian Journal of Basic Medical Sciences, 23*, 886–893.

Amar, N., Peretz, A., & Gerchman, Y. (2017). A cheap, simple high throughput method for screening native Helicobacter pylori urease inhibitors using a recombinant Escherichia coli, its validation and demonstration of Pistacia atlantica methanolic extract effectivity and specificity. *Journal of Microbiologucal Methods, 133*, 4045.

Ankaiah, D., Palanichamy, E., Perumal, V., Ayyanna, R., & Venkatesan, A. (2017). Probiotic characterization of Enterococcus faecium por1: Cloning, over expression of Enterocin-A and evaluation of antibacterial, anti-cancer properties. *Journal of Functional Foods, 38*(Part A), 280–292.

Aragon, F., Carino, S., Perdigon, G., & de LeBlanc, A. D. (2015). Inhibition of growth and metastasis of breast cancer in mice by milk fermented with Lactobacillus casei CRL 431. *Journal of Immunotherapy, 38*, 185–196.

Ardestani, S. K., Tafvizi, F., & Ebrahimi, M. T. (2019). Heat-killed probiotic bacteria induce apoptosis of HT-29 human colon adenocarcinoma cell line via the regulation of Bax/Bcl2 and caspases pathway. *Human & Experimental Toxicology, 38*, 1069–1081.

Arun, K. B., Madhavan, A., Reshmitha, T. R., Thomas, S., & Nisha, P. (2019). Short chain fatty acids enriched fermentation metabolites of soluble dietary fibre from Musa paradisiaca drives HT29 colon cancer cells to apoptosis. *PLoS One, 14*, e0216604.

Asgari, B., Kermanian, F., Yaghoobi, M. H., Vaezi, A., Soleimanifar, F., & Yaslianifard, S. (2020). The anti-Helicobacter pylori effects of Lactobacillus acidophilus, L. plantarum, and L. rhamnosus in stomach tissue of C57BL/6 mice. *Visceral Medicine, 36*, 137–143.

Ashaolu, T. J. (2020). Immune boosting functional foods and their mechanisms: A critical evaluation of probiotics and prebiotics. *Biomedicine & Pharmacotherapy, 130*, 110625.

Aviles-Jimenez, F., Yu, G. Q., Torres-Poveda, K., Madrid-Marina, V., & Torres, J. (2017). On the search to elucidate the role of microbiota in the genesis of cancer: The cases of gastrointestinal and cervical cancer. *Archives of Medical Research, 48*, 754–765.

Ayyash, M., Abu-Jdayil, B., Itsaranuwat, P., Galiwango, E., Tamiello-Rosa, C., Abdullah, H., Esposito, G., Hunashal, Y., Obaid, R. S., & Hamed, F. (2020). Characterization, bioactivities, and rheological properties of exopolysaccharide produced by novel probiotic Lactobacillus plantarum C70 isolated from camel milk. *International Journal of Biological Macromolecules, 144*, 938–946.

Ayyash, M., Johnson, S. K., Liu, S. Q., Al-Mheiri, A., & Abushelaibi, A. (2018). Cytotoxicity, antihypertensive, antidiabetic and antioxidant activities of solid-state fermented lupin, quinoa and wheat by Bifidobacterium species: In-vitro investigations. *LWT—Food Science and Technolgy, 95*, 295–302.

Baghbani-Arani, F., Asgary, V., & Hashemi, A. (2019). Cell-free extracts of Lactobacillus acidophilus and Lactobacillus delbrueckii display antiproliferative and antioxidant activities against HT-29 cell line. *Nutrition and Cancer, 72*, 1390–1399.

Binda, S., Hill, C., Johansen, C., Obis, D., Pot, B., Sanders, M. E., Tremblay, A., & Ouwehand, A. C. (2020). Criteria to qualify microorganisms as "probiotic" in foods and dietary supplements. *Frontiers in Microbiology, 11*, 1662.

Bistas, K. G., Bistas, E., & Mogaka, E. N. (2020). Lactobacillus reuteri's role in the prevention of colorectal cancer: A review of literature. *University of Toronto Medical Journal, 97*, 2936.

Bohlul, E., Hasanlou, F., Taromchi, A. H., & Nadri, S. (2019). TRAIL-expressing recombinant Lactococcus lactis induces apoptosis in human colon adenocarcinoma SW480 and HCT116 cells. *Journal of Applies Microbiology, 126*, 1558–1567.

Bolourian, A., & Mojtahedi, Z. (2018a). Immunosuppressants produced by Streptomyces: Evolution, hygiene hypothesis, tumour rapalog resistance and probiotics. *Environmental Microbiology Reports, 10*, 123–126.

Bolourian, A., & Mojtahedi, Z. (2018b). Streptomyces, shared microbiome member of soil and gut, as 'old friends' against colon cancer. *FEMS Microbiology Ecology, 94*(8). Available from https://doi.org/10.1093/femsec/fiy120.

Brandi, J., Di Carlo, C., Manfredi, M., Federici, F., Bazaj, A., Rizzi, E., Cornaglia, G., Manna, L., Marengo, E., & Cecconi, D. (2019). Investigating the proteomic profile of HT-29 colon cancer cells after Lactobacillus kefiri SGL 13 exposure using the SWATH method. *Journal of the American Society for Mass Spectrometry, 30*, 1690–1699.

Bray, F., Ferlay, J., Soerjomataram, I., Siegel, R. L., Torre, L. A., & Jemal, A. (2018). Global cancer statistics 2018: GLOBOCAN estimates of incidence and mortality worldwide for 36 cancers in 185 countries. *CA: A Cancer Journal or Clinicians, 68*, 394–424.

Campos, L. E., Garibotto, F., Angelina, E., Kos, J., Goněc, T., Marvanova, P., Vettorazzi, M., Oravec, M., Jendrzejewska, I., Jampilek, J., Alvarez, S., & Enriz, R. D. (2020). Hydroxynaphthalenecarboxamides and substituted piperazinylpropandiols, two new series of BRAF inhibitors. A theoretical and experimental study. *Bioorganic Chemistry, 103*, 104–145.

Campos, L. E., Garibotto, F. M., Angelina, E., Kos, J., Tomasic, T., Zidar, N., Kikelj, D., Goněc, T., Marvanová, P., Mokrý, P., Jampílek, J., Alvarez, S. E., & Enriz, R. D. (2019). Searching new structural scaffolds for BRAF inhibitors. integrative study using theoretical and experimental techniques. *Bioorganic Chemistry, 91*, 103–125.

Capurso, L. (2019). Thirty years of Lactobacillus rhamnosus GG: A review. *Journal of Clinical Gastroenterology, 53*, S1–S41.

Casanova, M. R., Azevedo-Silva, J., Rodrigues, L. R., & Preto, A. (2018). Colorectal cancer cells increase the production of short chain fatty acids by Propionibacterium freudenreichii impacting on cancer cells survival. *Frontiers in Nutrition, 5*, 44.

Casas-Solis, J., Huizar-Lopez, M. D., Irecta-Najera, C. A., Pita-Lopez, M. L., & Santerre, A. (2020). Immunomodulatory effect of Lactobacillus casei in a murine model of colon carcinogenesis. *Probiotics and Antimicrobial Proteins, 12*, 1012–1024.

CDC. (2019). WHO—Human papillomavirus (HPV) and cervical cancer. Retrieved from https://www.who.int/news-room/fact-sheets/detail/human-papillomavirus-(hpv)-and-cervical-cancer. Accessed September 11, 2020.

CDC. (2018). Division of Cancer Prevention and Control, Centers for Disease Control and Prevention—Breast cancer, Retrieved from https://www.cdc.gov/cancer/breast/basic_info/what-is-breast-cancer.htm. Accessed September 11, 2020.

CDC (2020). Division of Cancer Prevention and Control, Centers for Disease Control and Prevention—Cervical cancer. Retrieved from https://www.cdc.gov/cancer/cervical/basic_info/index.htm. Accessed July 29, 2020.

Černíková, A., & Jampílek, J. (2014). Structure modification of drugs influencing their bioavailability and therapeutic effect. *Chemicke Listy, 108*, 716.

Cervantes-Elizarraras, A., Cruz-Cansino, N. D., Ramirez-Moreno, E., Vega-Sanchez, V., Velazquez-Guadarrama, N., Zafra-Rojas, Q. Y., & Piloni-Martini, J. (2019). In vitro probiotic potential of lactic acid bacteria isolated from aguamiel and pulque and antibacterial activity against pathogens. *Applied Sciences, 9*, 601.

Cha, M. K., Lee, D. K., An, H. M., Lee, S. W., Shin, S. H., Kwon, J. H., Kim, K. J., & Ha, N. J. (2012). Antiviral activity of Bifidobacterium adolescentis SPM1005-A on human papillomavirus type 16. *BMC Medicine, 10*, 72.

Chaiongkarn, A., Dathong, J., Phatvej, W., Saman, P., Kuancha, C., Chatanon, L., & Moonmungmee, S. (2019). Characterization of prebiotics and their synergistic activities with Lactobacillus probiotics for β-glucuronidase reduction. *ScienceAsia, 45*, 538–546.

Champer, M., Wong, A. M., Champer, J., Brito, I. L., Messer, P. W., Hou, J. Y., & Wright, J. D. (2018). The role of the vaginal microbiome in gynaecological cancer. *BJOG—An International Journal of Obstetrics & Gynaecology, 125*, 309–315.

Chang, C. W., Liu, C. Y., Lee, H. C., Huang, Y. H., Li, L. H., Chiau, J. S. C., Wang, T. E., Chu, C. H., Shih, S. C., Tsai, T. H., & Chen, Y. J. (2018). Lactobacillus casei variety rhamnosus probiotic preventively attenuates 5-fluorouracil/oxaliplatin-induced intestinal injury in a syngeneic colorectal cancer model. *Frontiers in Microbiology, 9*, 983.

Chang, C. Y., Ho, B. Y., & Pan, T. M. (2019). Lactobacillus paracasei subsp. paracasei NTU 101-fermented skim milk as an adjuvant to uracil-tegafur reduces tumor growth and improves chemotherapy side effects in an orthotopic mouse model of colorectal cancer. *Journal of Functional Foods, 55*, 3647.

Chen, D. F., Jin, D. C., Huang, S. M., Wu, J. Y., Xu, M. Q., Liu, T. Q., Dong, W. X., Liu, X., Wang, S. A., Zhong, W. L., & Cao, H. L. (2020). Clostridium butyricum, a butyrate-producing probiotic, inhibits intestinal tumor development through modulating Wnt signaling and gut microbiota. *Cancer Letters, 469*, 456–467.

Chiesa, C., Pacifico, L., Anania, C., Poggiogalle, E., Chiarelli, F., & Osborn, J. F. (2010). Helicobacter pylori therapy in children: Overview and challenges. *International Journal of Immunopathology and Pharmacology, 23*, 405–416.

Choi, J. H., Moon, C. M., Shin, T. S., Kim, E. K., McDowell, A., Jo, M. K., Joo, Y. H., Kim, S. E., Jung, H. K., Shim, K. N., Jung, S. A., & Kim, Y. K. (2020). Lactobacillus paracasei-derived extracellular vesicles attenuate the intestinal inflammatory response by augmenting the endoplasmic reticulum stress pathway. *Experimental & Molecular Medicine, 52*, 423–437.

Chundakkattumalayil, H. C., Kumar, S., Narayanan, R., & Raghavan, K. T. (2019). Role of L. plantarum KX519413 as probiotic and acacia gum as prebiotic in gastrointestinal tract strengthening. *Microorganisms, 7*, 659.

Chung, I. C., OuYang, C. N., Yuan, S. N., Lin, H. C., Huang, K. Y., Wu, P. S., Liu, C. Y., Tsai, K. J., Loi, L. K., Chen, Y. J., Chung, A. K., Ojcius, D. M., Chang, Y. S., & Chen, L. C. (2019). Pretreatment with a heat-killed probiotic modulates the NLRP3 inflammasome and attenuates colitis-associated colorectal cancer in mice. *Nutrients, 11*, 516.

Cleveland Clinic. (2020). Probiotics. Retrived from https://my.clevelandclinic.org/health/articles/14598-probiotics. Accessed September 3, 2020.

Curty, G., de Carvalho, P. S., & Soares, M. A. (2020). The role of the cervicovaginal microbiome on the genesis and as a biomarker of premalignant cervical intraepithelial neoplasia and invasive cervical cancer. *International Journal of Molecular Sciences, 21*, 222.

Das Purkayastha, S., Bhattacharya, M. K., Prasad, H. K., Bhattacharjee, M. J., De Mandal, S., Mathipi, V., & Kumar, N. S. (2020). Probiotic and cytotoxic potential of vaginal Lactobacillus isolated from healthy northeast indian women. *Journal of Pure and Applied Microbiology, 14*, 205−214.

Das, D., & Goyal, A. (2014a). Characterization and biocompatibility of glucan: A safe food additive from probiotic Lactobacillus plantarum DM5. *Journal of the Sciences of Food and Agriculture, 94*, 683−690.

Das, D., & Goyal, A. (2014b). Characterization of a noncytotoxic bacteriocin from probiotic Lactobacillus plantarum DM5 with potential as a food preservative. *Food & Function, 5*, 2453−2462.

Davani-Davari, D., Negahdaripour, M., Karimzadeh, I., Seifan, M., Mohkam, M., Masoumi, S. J., Berenjian, A., & Ghasemi, Y. (2019). Prebiotics: Definition, types, sources, mechanisms, and clinical applications. *Foods, 8*, 92.

De Almeida, C. V., Lulli, M., di Pilato, V., Schiavone, N., Russo, E., Nannini, G., Baldi, S., Borrelli, R., Bartolucci, G., Menicatti, M., Taddei, A., Ringressi, M. N., Niccolai, E., Prisco, D., Rossolini, G. M., & Amedei, A. (2019). Differential responses of colorectal cancer cell lines to Enterococcus faecalis' strains isolated from healthy donors and colorectal cancer patients. *Journal of Clinical Medicine, 8*, 388.

de Loera-Rodriguez, L. H., Ortiz, G. G., Rivero-Moragrega, P., Velazquez-Brizuela, I. E., Santoscoy, J. F., Rincon-Sanchez, A. R., Charles-Nino, C., Cruz-Serrano, J. A., Celis-de la Rosa Ade J., Pacheco-Moises, F. P., & Gonzalez, M. D. R. M. (2018). Effect of symbiotic supplementation on fecal calprotectin levels and lactic acid bacteria, Bifidobacteria, Escherichia coli and Salmonella DNA in patients with cervical cancer. *Nutricion Hospitalaria, 35*, 1394−1400.

de Vrese, M., & Schrezenmeir, J. (2008). Probiotics, prebiotics, and synbiotics. In U. Stahl, U. E. B. Donalies, & E. Nevoigt (Eds.), *Food biotechnology* (p. 166). Springer-Verlag Berlin and Heidelberg GmbH & Co. KG.

Deol, P. K., Khare, P., Bishnoi, M., Kondepudi, K. K., & Kaur, I. P. (2018). Coadministration of ginger extract-Lactobacillus acidophilus (cobiotic) reduces gut inflammation and oxidative stress via downregulation of COX-2, i-NOS, and c-Myc. *Phytotherapy Research, 32*, 1950−1956.

Di, W., Zhang, L. W., Yi, H. X., Han, X., Zhang, Y. C., & Xin, L. (2018). Exopolysaccharides produced by Lactobacillus strains suppress HT-29 cell growth via induction of G_0/G_1 cell cycle arrest and apoptosis. *Oncology Letters, 16*, 3577−3586.

Donohoe, D. R., Holley, D., Collins, L. B., Montgomery, S. A., Whitmore, A. C., Hillhouse, A., Curry, K. P., Renner, S. W., Greenwalt, A., Ryan, E. P., Godfrey, V., Heise, M. T., Threadgill, D. S., Han, A., Swenberg, J. A., Threadgill, D. W., & Bultman, S. J. (2014). A gnotobiotic mouse model demonstrates that dietary fiber protects against colorectal tumorigenesis in a microbiota- and butyrate-dependent manner. *Cancer Discovery, 4*, 1387−1397.

dos Reis, S. A., da Conceicao, L. L., & Peluzio, M. D. G. (2019). Intestinal microbiota and colorectal cancer: Changes in the intestinal microenvironment and their relation to the disease. *Journal of Medical Microbiology, 68*, 1391−1407.

Drago, L. (2019). Probiotics and colon cancer. *Microorganisms, 7*, 66.

Ecosh Life OÜ. (2020). 17 types of good bacteria—The list of most beneficial species of probiotics lactobacillus and bifidobacteria. Retrieved from: https://ecosh.com/17-types-of-good-bacteria-the-list-of-most-beneficial-species-of-probiotics-lactobacillus-and-bifidobacteria/. Accessed September 3, 2020.

Elsayed, E. A., Farooq, M., Dailin, D., El-Enshasy, H. A., Othman, N. Z., Malek, R., Danial, E., & Wadaan, M. (2017). In vitro and in vivo biological screening of kefiran polysaccharide produced by Lactobacillus kefiranofaciens. *Biomedical Research India, 28*, 594−600.

Eslami, M., Yousefi, B., Kokhaei, P., Hemati, M., Nejad, Z. R., Arabkari, V., & Namdar, A. (2019). Importance of probiotics in the prevention and treatment of colorectal cancer. *Journal of Cell Physiology, 234*, 17127−17143.

Eslami-S, Z., Majidzadeh-A, K., Halvaei, S., Babapirali, F., & Esmaeili, R. (2020). Microbiome and breast cancer: New role for an ancient population. *Frontiers in Oncology, 10*, 120.

Espinoza, J. L., Matsumoto, A., Tanaka, H., & Matsumura, I. (2018). Gastric microbiota: An emerging player in Helicobacter pylori-induced gastric malignancies. *Cancer Letters, 414*, 147−152.

Fahey, J. W., Stephenson, K. K., & Wallace, A. J. (2015). Dietary amelioration of Helicobacter infection. *Nutrition Research, 35*, 461−473.

FAO. (2006). Probiotics in food. Health and nutritional properties and guidelines for evaluation. Retrieved from: http://www.fao.org/3/a-a0512e.pdf. Accessed September 11, 2020.

Farag, M. A., El Hawary, E. A., & Elmassry, M. M. (2020). Rediscovering acidophilus milk, its quality characteristics, manufacturing methods, flavor chemistry and nutritional value. *Critical Reviews in Food Science and Nutrition, 60*(18), 3024−3041.

Fernández, M. F., Reina-Pérez, I., Manuel Astorga, J., Rodríguez-Carrillo, A., Plaza-Díaz, J., & Fontana, L. (2018). Breast cancer and its relationship with the microbiota. *International Journal of Environmental Research and Public Health, 15*, 1747.

Ferro, A., Costa, A. R., Morais, S., Bertuccio, P., Rota, M., Hu, J. F., et al. (2020). Fruits and vegetables intake and gastric cancer risk: A pooled analysis within the stomach cancer pooling project. *International Journal of Cancer, 147*(11), 3090−3101.

Fiore, W., Arioli, S., & Guglielmetti, S. (2020). The neglected microbial components of commercial probiotic formulations. *Microorganisms, 8*, 1177.

Fong, W. N., Li, Q., & Yu, J. (2020). Gut microbiota modulation: A novel strategy for prevention and treatment of colorectal cancer. *Oncogene, 39*, 4925−4943.

Galdeano, C. M., Cazorla, S. I., Lemme Dumit, J. M., Vélez, E., & Perdigón, G. (2019). Beneficial effects of probiotic consumption on the immune system. *Annals of Nutrition and Metabolism, 74*, 115−124.

Gamallat, Y., Ren, X. M., Meyiah, A., Li, M. Q., Ren, X. X., Jamalat, Y., Song, S. Y., Xie, L. H., Ahmad, B., Shopit, A., Mousa, H., Ma, Y. F., & Ding, D. P. (2019). The immune-modulation and gut microbiome structure modification associated with long-term dietary supplementation of Lactobacillus rhamnosus using 16S rRNA sequencing analysis. *Journal of Functional Foods, 53*, 227−236.

Gamallat, Y., Ren, X. M., Walana, W., Meyiah, A., Ren, X. X., Zhu, Y. Y., Li, M. Q., Song, S. Y., Xie, L. H., Jamalat, Y., Saleem, M. Z., Ma, Y. F., Xin, Y., & Shang, D. (2019). Probiotic Lactobacillus rhamnosus modulates the gut microbiome composition attenuates preneoplastic colorectal Aberrant crypt foci. *Journal of Functional Foods, 53*, 146−156.

Garcia, A., Navarro, K., Sanhueza, E., Pineda, S., Pastene, E., Quezada, M., Henriquez, K., Karlyshev, A., Villena, J., & Gonzalez, C. (2017). Characterization of Lactobacillus fermentum UCO-979C, a probiotic strain with a potent anti-Helicobacter pylori activity. *Electronic Journal of Biotechnology, 25*, 75−83.

Genaro, S. C., Reis, L. S. L. S., Reis, S. K., Socca, E. A. R., & Favaro, W. J. (2019). Probiotic supplementation attenuates the aggressiveness of chemically induced colorectal tumor in rats. *Life Sciences, 237*, 116895.

Ghanavati, R., Akbari, A., Mohammadi, F., Asadollahi, P., Javadi, A., Talebi, M., & Rohani, M. (2020). Lactobacillus species inhibitory effect on colorectal cancer progression through modulating the Wnt/-catenin signaling pathway. *Molecular and Cellular Biochemistry, 470*, 113.

Grumet, L., Tromp, Y., & Stiegelbauer, V. (2020). The development of high-quality multispecies probiotic formulations: From bench to market. *Nutrients, 12*, 2453.

Guarino, M. P. L., Altomare, A. M., Emerenziani, S., Di Rosa, C., Ribolsi, M., Balestrieri, P., Iovino, P., Rocchi, G., & Cicala, M. (2020). Mechanisms of action of prebiotics and their effects on gastro-intestinal disorders in adults. *Nutrients, 12*, 1037.

Hakobyan, L., Harutyunyan, K., Harutyunyan, N., Melik-Andreasyan, G., & Trchounian, A. (2016). Adhesive properties and acid-forming activity of lactobacilli and streptococci under inhibitory substances, such as nitrates. *Current Microbiology, 72*, 776−782.

Han, S. W., Yang, X., Qi, Q., Pan, Y. F., Da, M., & Zhou, Q. (2019). Relationship between intestinal microorganisms and T lymphocytes in colorectal cancer. *Future Oncology, 15*, 1655−1666.

Hassan, Z., Mustafa, S., Rahim, R. A., & Isa, N. M. (2016). Anti-breast cancer effects of live, heat-killed and cytoplasmic fractions of Enterococcus faecalis and Staphylococcus hominis isolated from human breast milk. *In Vitro Cellular & Developmental Biology—Animal, 52*, 337−348.

Heydari, Z., Rahaie, M., Alizadeh, A. M., Agah, S., Khalighfard, S., & Bahmani, S. (2019). Effects of Lactobacillus acidophilus and Bifidobacterium bifidum probiotics on the expression of microRNAs 135b, 26b, 18a and 155, and their involving genes in mice colon cancer. *Probiotics and Antimicrobial Proteins, 11*, 1155−1162.

Hodaei, M. H., Anduhjerdi, R. B., Mehrabadi, J. F., & Esmaeili, D. (2019). Cloning and expression of the L1 immunogenic protein of human papillomavirus genotype 16 by using Lactobacillus expression system. Geneń Rep. 17, UNSP 100521.

Huang, J., Wang, D., Zhang, A. Y., Zhong, Q. L., & Huang, Q. (2019). Lactobacillus rhamnosus confers protection against colorectal cancer in rats. *Tropical Journal of Pharmaceutical Research, 18*, 1449−1454.

Hutkins, R. W., Krumbeck, J. A., Bindels, L. B., Cani, P. D., Fahey, G., Jr., Goh, Y. J., Hamaker, B., Martens, E. C., Mills, D. A., Rastal, R. A., Vaughan, E., & Sanders, M. E. (2016). Prebiotics: Why definitions matter. *Current Opinion in Biotechnology, 37*, 1−7.

IARC (2018a). Austria. Retrieved from: https://gco.iarc.fr/today/data/factsheets/populations/40-austria-fact-sheets.pdf. Accessed September 3, 2020.

IARC (2018b). Czechia. Retrieved from: https://gco.iarc.fr/today/data/factsheets/populations/203-czechia-fact-sheets.pdf. Accessed September 3, 2020.

IARC (2018c). Hungary. Retrieved from: https://gco.iarc.fr/today/data/factsheets/populations/348-hungary-fact-sheets.pdf. Accessed September 3, 2020.

IARC (2018d). Poland. Retrieved from: https://gco.iarc.fr/today/data/factsheets/populations/616-poland-fact-sheets.pdf. Accessed September 3, 2020.

IARC (2018e). Slovakia. Retrieved from: https://gco.iarc.fr/today/data/factsheets/populations/703-slovakia-fact-sheets.pdf. Accessed September 3, 2020.

IARC. (2018f). The International Agency for Research on Cancer. Retrieved from: https://www.who.int/cancer/PRGlobocanFinal.pdf. Accessed September 3, 2020.

Iebba, V., Totino, V., Gagliardi, A., Santangelo, F., Cacciotti, F., Trancassini, M., Mancini, C., Cicerone, C., Corazziari, E., Pantanella, F., & Schippa, S. (2016). Eubiosis and dysbiosis: The two sides of the microbiota. *New Microbiologica, 39*, 112.

Inglis, J. E., Lin, P. J., Kerns, S. L., Kleckner, I. R., Kleckner, A. S., Castillo, D. A., Mustian, K. M., & Peppone, L. J. (2019). Nutritional interventions for treating cancer-related fatigue: A qualitative review. *Nutrition and Cancer, 71*, 2140.

Irigaray, P., Newby, J.A., Clapp, R., Hardell, L., Howard, V., Montagnier, L., Epstein, S., Belpomme, D., 2007. Lifestyle-related factors and environmental agents causing cancer: An overview. Biomedicine & Pharmacotherapy. 61, 640−658.

Jackson, S. A., Schoeni, J. L., Vegge, C., Pane, M., Stahl, B., Bradley, M., Goldman, V. S., Burguière, P., Atwater, J. B., & Sanders, M. E. (2019). Improving end-user trust in the quality of commercial probiotic products. *Frontiers in Microbiology, 10*, 739.

James, A., & Wang, Y. (2019). Characterization, health benefits and applications of fruits and vegetable probiotics. *CyTA—Journal of Food, 17*, 770−780.

Jampílek, J., Kos, J., & Králová, K. (2019). Potential of nanomaterial applications in dietary supplements and foods for special medical purposes. *Nanomaterials, 9*, 296.

Jampílek, J., & Králová, K. (2018). Application of nanobioformulations for controlled release and targeted biodistribution of drugs. In A. K. Sharma, R. K. Keservani, & R. K. Kesharwani (Eds.), *Nanobiomaterials: Applications in drug delivery* (pp. 131−208). Warentown, NJ, USA: CRC Press.

Jampílek, J., & Králová, K. (2019a). Nanoformulations—Valuable tool in therapy of viral diseases attacking humans and animals. In M. Rai, & B. Jamil (Eds.), *Nanotheranostic—Applications and limitations* (pp. 137–178). Cham, Switzerland: Springer Nature.

Jampílek, J., & Králová, K. (2019b). Nanotechnology based formulations for drug targeting to central nervous system. In R. K. Keservani, & A. K. Sharma (Eds.), *Nanoparticulate drug delivery systems* (pp. 151–220). Warentown, NJ, USA: Apple Academic Press & CRC Press.

Jampílek, J., & Králová, K. (2019c). Recent advances in lipid nanocarriers applicable in the fight against cancer. In A. M. Grumezescu (Ed.), *Nanoarchitectonics in biomedicine* (pp. 219–294). Amsterdam, Netherlands: Elsevier.

Jampílek, J., & Králová, K. (2020a). Nanoweapons against tuberculosis. In S. Talegaonkar, & M. Rai (Eds.), *Nanoformulations in human health—Challenges and approaches* (pp. 469–502). Cham, Switzerland: Springer Nature Switzerland.

Jampílek, J., & Králová, K. (2020b). Natural biopolymeric nanoformulations for brain drug delivery. In R. K. Keservani, A. K. Sharma, & R. K. Kesharwani (Eds.), *Nanocarriers for brain targeting: Principles and applications* (pp. 131–203). Warentown, NJ, USA: Apple Academic Press & CRC Press.

Jampílek, J., Králová, K., Campos, E. V. R., & Fraceto, L. F. (2019). Bio-based nanoemulsion formulations applicable in agriculture, medicine and food industry. In R. Prasad, V. Kumar, M. Kumar, & D. K. Choudhary (Eds.), *Nanobiotechnology in bioformulations* (pp. 33–84). Cham, Switzerland: Springer.

Jampílek, J., Králová, K., Novák, P., & Novák, M. (2019). Nanobiotechnology in neurodegenerative diseases. In M. Rai, & A. Yadav (Eds.), *Nanobiotechnology in neurodegenerative diseases* (pp. 65–138). Cham, Switzerland: Springer Nature Switzerland AG.

Jang, S. E., Jeong, J. J., Choi, S. Y., Kim, H., Han, M. J., & Kim, D. H. (2017). Lactobacillus rhamnosus HN001 and Lactobacillus acidophilus La-14 attenuate Gardnerella vaginalis-infected bacterial vaginosis in mice. *Nutrients, 9*, 531.

Ji, W., Chen, W. Q., & Tian, X. (2018). Efficacy of compound Lactobacillus acidophilus tablets combined with quadruple therapy for Helicobacter pylori eradication and its correlation with pH value in the stomach: A study protocol of a randomised, assessor-blinded, single-centre study. *BMJ Open, 8*, e023131.

Johnson, D., Letchumanan, V., Thurairajasingam, S., & Lee, L. H. (2020). A revolutionizing approach to autism spectrum disorder using the microbiome. *Nutrients, 12*, 1983.

Jones, M. D., Li, Y. J., & Zamble, D. B. (2018). Acid-responsive activity of the Helicobacter pylori metalloregulator NikR. *Proceedings of the National Academy of the Sciences of the United States of America, 115*, 8966–8971.

Julson, E. (2017). *Possible side effects of probiotics*. Healthline Media a Red Ventures Company. Retrieved from: https://www.healthline.com/nutrition/probiotics-side-effects. Accessed September 11, 2020.

Jung, T. H., Park, J. H., Jeon, W. M., & Han, K. S. (2015). Butyrate modulates bacterial adherence on LS174T human colorectal cells by stimulating mucin secretion and MAPK signaling pathway. *Nutrition Research and Practice, 9*, 343–349.

Kafshdooz, T., Akbarzadeh, A., Seghinsara, A. M., Pourhassan, M., Nasrabadi, H. T., & Milani, M. (2017). Role of probiotics in managing of Helicobacter pylori infection: A review. *Drug Research, 67*, 8893.

Kamińska, M., Ciszewski, T., Łopacka-Szatan, K., Miotła, P., & Starosławska, E. (2015). Breast cancer risk factors. *Przeglad Menopauzalny, 14*, 196–202.

Kassayova, M., Bobrov, N., Strojny, L., Kiskova, T., Mikes, J., Demeckova, V., Orendas, P., Bojkova, B., Pec, M., Kubatka, P., & Bomba, A. (2014). Preventive effects of probiotic bacteria Lactobacillus plantarum and dietary fiber in chemically-induced mammary carcinogenesis. *Anticancer Research, 34*, 4969–4975.

Kassayova, M., Bobrov, N., Strojny, L., Orendas, P., Demeckova, V., Jendzelovsky, R., Kubatka, P., Kiskova, T., Kruzliak, P., Adamkov, M., Bomba, A., & Fedorocko, P. (2016). Anticancer and immunomodulatory effects of Lactobacillus plantarum LS/07, inulin and melatonin in NMU-induced rat model of breast cancer. *Anticancer Research, 36*, 2719–2728.

Kauerová, T., Goněc, T., Jampílek, J., Hafner, S., Gaiser, A. K., Syrovets, T., Fedr, R., Souček, K., & Kollár, P. (2020). Ring-substituted 1-hydroxynaphthalene-2-carboxanilides inhibit proliferation and trigger mitochondria-mediated apoptosis. *International Journal of Molecular Sciences, 21*, 3416.

Kauerová, T., Kos, J., Goněc, T., Jampílek, J., & Kollár, P. (2016). Antiproliferative and pro-apoptotic effect of novel nitro-substituted hydroxynaphthanilides on human cancer cell lines. *International Journal of Molecular Sciences, 17*, 1219.

Kechagia, M., Basoulis, D., Konstantopoulou, S., Dimitriadi, D., Gyftopoulou, K., Skarmoutsou, N., & Fakiri, E. M. (2013). Health benefits of probiotics: A review. *ISRN Nutrition, 2013*, 481651.

Khalighi, A., Behdani, R., & Kouhestani, S. (2006). Probiotics: A comprehensive review of their classification, mode of action and role in human nutrition. In V. Rao, & K. Rao (Eds.), *Probiotics and prebiotics in human nutrition and health* (pp. 19–39). Rijeka, Croatia: InTech.

Khan, M. S. A., Khundmiri, S. U. K., Khundmiri, S. R., Al-Sanea, M. M., & Mok, P. L. (2018). Fruit-derived polysaccharides and terpenoids: Recent update on the gastroprotective effects and mechanisms. *Frontiers in Pharmacology, 9*, 569.

Khan, N., Afaq, F., & Mukhtar, H. (2010). Lifestyle as risk factor for cancer: Evidence from human studies. *Cancer Letters, 293*, 133–143.

Kim, J. J. (2013). Upper gastrointestinal cancer and reflux disease. *Journal of Gastric Cancer, 13*, 79–85.

Kim, S. N., Lee, W. M., Park, K. S., Kim, J. B., Han, D. J., & Bae, J. (2015). The effect of Lactobacillus casei extract on cervical cancer cell lines. *Wspolczesna Onkologia, 19*, 306–312.

Kouhkan, M., Ahangar, P., Babaganjeh, L. A., & Allahyari-Devin, M. (2020). Biosynthesis of copper oxide nanoparticles using Lactobacillus casei subsp. casei and its anticancer and antibacterial activities. *Current Nanoscience, 16*, 101–111.

Kozik, V., Bąk, A., Pentak, D., Hachuła, B., Pytlakowska, K., Rojkiewicz, M., Jampílek, J., Sieroń, K., Jazowiecka-Rakus, J., & Sochanik, A. (2019). Derivatives of graphene oxide as potential drug carriers. *Journal of Nanoscience and Nanotechnology, 19*, 2489–2492.

Kràlovà, K., & Jampílek, J. (2015). Impact of environmental contaminants on breast cancer. *Ecological Chemistry and Engineering S, 22*, 94.

Laniewski, P., Ilhan, Z. E., & Herbst-Kralovetz, M. M. (2020). The microbiome and gynaecological cancer development, prevention and therapy. *Nature Revews, 17*, 232−250.

LeBlanc, J. G., Levit, R., de Giori, G. S., & de LeBlanc, A. D. (2020). Application of vitamin-producing lactic acid bacteria to treat intestinal inflammatory diseases. *Applied Microbiology and Biotechnology, 104*, 3331−3337.

Lee, C. W., Chen, H. J., Chien, Y. H., Hsia, S. M., Chen, J. H., & Shih, C. K. (2020). Synbiotic combination of djulis (Chenopodium formosanum) and Lactobacillus acidophilus inhibits colon carcinogenesis in rats. *Nutrients, 12*, 103.

Leila, A. B., Parinaz, A., Zarei, L., & Mehri, K. (2018). Biofabrication of silver nanoparticles using Lactobacillus casei subsp. casei and its efficacy against human pathogens bacteria and cancer cell lines. *Medical Science, 22*, 99110.

Li, S. C., Hsu, W. F., Chang, J. S., & Shih, C. K. (2019). Combination of Lactobacillus acidophilus and Bifidobacterium animalis subsp. lactis shows a stronger anti-inflammatory effect than individual strains in HT-29 cells. *Nutrients, 11*, 969.

Li, S. C., Lin, H. P., Chang, J. S., & Shih, C. K. (2019). Lactobacillus acidophilus-fermented germinated brown rice suppresses preneoplastic lesions of the colon in rats. *Nutrients, 11*, 2718.

Li, W. Y., Han, Y., Xu, H. M., Wang, Z. N., Xu, Y. Y., Song, Y. X., et al. (2019). Smoking status and subsequent gastric cancer risk in men compared with women: A *meta*-analysis of prospective observational studies. *BMC Cancer, 19*, 377.

Li, Y. Y., Yu, T., Yan, H., Li, D. D., Yu, T., Yuan, T., Rahaman, A., Ali, S., Abbas, F., Dian, Z. Q., Wu, X. M., & Baloch, Z. (2020). Vaginal microbiota and HPV infection: Novel mechanistic insights and therapeutic strategies. *Infection and Drug Resistance., 13*, 1213−1220.

Lin, P. Y., Li, S. C., Lin, H. P., & Shih, C. K. (2019). Germinated brown rice combined with Lactobacillus acidophilus and Bifidobacterium animalis subsp. lactis inhibits colorectal carcinogenesis in rats. *Food Science & Nutrition, 7*, 216−224.

Linn, Y. H., Thu, K. K., & Win, N. H. H. (2019). Effect of probiotics for the prevention of acute radiation-induced diarrhoea among cervical cancer patients: A randomized double-blind placebo-controlled study. *Probiotics and Antimicrobial Proteins, 11*, 638−647.

Liu, T. Y., Song, X. L., Khan, S., Li, Y., Guo, Z. X., Li, C. Q., Wang, S. A., Dong, W. X., Liu, W. T., Wang, B. M., & Cao, H. L. (2020). The gut microbiota at the intersection of bile acids and intestinal carcinogenesis: An old story, yet mesmerizing. *International Journal of Cancer, 146*, 1780−1790.

Lockyer, S., & Stanner, S. (2019). Prebiotics—An added benefit of some fibre types. *Nutrition Bulletin, 44*, 74−91.

Ma, K., Baloch, Z., He, T. T., & Xia, X. S. (2017). Alcohol consumption and gastric cancer risk: A *meta*-analysis. *Medical Science Monitor, 23*, 238−246.

Maghsood, F., Johari, B., Rohani, M., Madanchi, H., Saltanatpour, Z., & Kadivar, M. (2020). Anti-proliferative and anti-metastatic potential of high molecular weight secretory molecules from probiotic Lactobacillus reuteri cell-free supernatant against human colon cancer stem-like cells (HT29-ShE). *International Journal of Peptides Research and Therapeutics, 26*, 2619−2631.

Malik, J. K., Ahmad, A. H., Kalpana, S., Prakash, A., & Gupta, R. C. (2016). Synbiotics: Safety and toxicity considerations. In R. C. Gupta (Ed.), *Nutraceuticals: Efficacy, safety and toxicity* (pp. 811−822). Academic Press & Elsevier.

Malik, S. S., Saeed, A., Baig, M., Asif, N., Masood, N., & Yasmin, A. (2018). Anticarcinogenecity of microbiota and probiotics in breast cancer. *International Journal of Food Properties, 21*, 655−666.

Mantzourani, I., Chondrou, P., Bontsidis, C., Karolidou, K., Terpou, A., Alexopoulos, A., Bezirtzoglou, E., Galanis, A., & Plessas, S. (2019). Assessment of the probiotic potential of lactic acid bacteria isolated from kefir grains: Evaluation of adhesion and antiproliferative properties in in vitro experimental systems. *Annals of Microbiology, 69*, 751−763.

Marinelli, L., Tenore, G. C., & Novellino, E. (2017). Probiotic species in the modulation of the anticancer immune response. *Seminars in Cancer Biology, 46*, 182−190.

Markowiak, P., & Śliżewska, K. (2017). Effects of probiotics, prebiotics, and synbiotics on human health. *Nutrients, 9*, 1021.

Matsuya-Ogawa, M., Shibata, T., Itoh, H., Murakami, H., Yaguchi, C., Sugihara, K., & Kanayama, N. (2019). Oncoprotective effects of short-chain fatty acids on uterine cervical neoplasia. *Nutrition and Cancer, 71*, 312−319.

Meegan, M. J., & O'Boyle, N. M. (2019). Special issue "anticancer drugs.". *Pharmaceuticals, 12*, 134.

Mendes, M. C. S., Paulino, D. S. M., Brambilla, S. R., Camargo, J. A., Persinoti, G. F., & Carvalheira, J. B. C. (2018). Microbiota modification by probiotic supplementation reduces colitis associated colon cancer in mice. *World Journal of Gastroenterology., 24*, 1995−2008.

Mendoza, L. (2019). Potential effect of probiotics in the treatment of breast cancer. *Oncology Reviews, 13*, 134−138.

MFMER (2020a). Mayo Foundation for Medical Education and Research—Breast cancer. Retrieved from: https://www.mayoclinic.org/diseases-conditions/breast-cancer/symptoms-causes/syc-20352470. Accessed September 3, 2020.

MFMER (2020b). Mayo Foundation for Medical Education and Research—Cervical cancer. Retrieved from: https://www.mayoclinic.org/diseases-conditions/cervical-cancer/symptoms-causes/syc-20352501. Accessed September 3, 2020.

MFMER (2020c). Mayo Foundation for Medical Education and Research—Colon cancer. Retrieved from: https://www.mayoclinic.org/diseases-conditions/colon-cancer/symptoms-causes/syc-20353669. Accessed September 3, 2020.

Mima, K., Nishihara, R., Qian, Z. R., Cao, Y., Sukawa, Y., Nowak, J. A., Yang, J. H., Dou, R. X., Masugi, Y., Song, M. Y., et al. (2016). Fusobacterium nucleatum in colorectal carcinoma tissue and patient prognosis. *Gut, 65*, 1973−1980.

Mirhadi, E., Nassirli, H., & Malaekeh-Nikouei, B. (2020). An updated review on therapeutic effects of nanoparticle-based formulations of saffron components (safranal, crocin, and crocetin). *Journal of Pharmaceutical Investigation, 50*, 47−58.

Mnich, E., Ibran, J., & Chmiela, M. (2018). Treatment of Helicobacter pylori infections in the light of the increase of antibiotic resistance. *Postepy Higieny i Medycyny Doswiadczlnej, 72*, 143−158.

Monshikarimi, A., Ostadrahimi, A., Jafarabadi, M. A., EivaziZiaei, J., Barzeghari, A., Esfahani, A., Payahoo, L., Aamazadeh, F., & Farrin, N. (2019). Does combination of Lactobacillus rhamnosus Heriz I and beta glucan improve quality of life in women with breast cancer receiving chemotherapy? A randomized double-blind placebo-controlled clinical trial. *Nutrition & Food Science, 50*, 569–578.

Motevaseli, E., Shirzad, M., Raoofian, R., Hasheminasab, S. M., Hatami, M., Dianatpour, M., & Modarressi, M. H. (2013). Differences in vaginal lactobacilli composition of Iranian healthy and bacterial vaginosis infected women: A comparative analysis of their cytotoxic effects with commercial vaginal probiotics. *Iranian Red Crescent Medical Journal, 15*, 199–206.

Motevaseli, E., Shirzad, M., Akrami, S. M., Mousavi, A. S., Mirsalehian, A., & Modarressi, M. H. (2013). Normal and tumour cervical cells respond differently to vaginal lactobacilli, independent of pH and lactate. *Journal of Medical Microbiology, 62*, 1065–1072.

Mrozek-Wilczkiewicz, A., Kalinowski, D., Musioł, R., Finster, J., Szurko, A., Serafin, K., Knas, M., Kamalapuram, S. K., Kovacevic, Z., Jampílek, J., Ratuszna, A., Rzeszowska-Wolny, J., Richardson, D. R., & Polański, J. (2010). Investigating anti-proliferative activity of styrylazanaphthalenes and azanaphthalenediones. *Bioorganic & Medicinal Chemistry, 18*, 2664–2671.

Mukaisho, K., Nakayama, T., Hagiwara, T., Hattori, T., & Sugihara, H. (2015). Two distinct etiologies of gastric cardia adenocarcinoma: Interactions among pH, Helicobacter pylori, and bile acids. *Frontiers in Microbiology, 6*, 412.

Mushtaq, M., Gani, A., & Masoodi, F. A. (2019). Himalayan cheese (Kalari/Kradi) fermented with different probiotic strains: In vitro investigation of nutraceutical properties. *LWT—Food Science and Technolgy, 104*, 5360.

Nair, M. R. B., Chouhan, D., Sen Gupta, S., & Chattopadhyay, S. (2016). Fermented foods: Are they tasty medicines for Helicobacter pylori associated peptic ulcer and gastric cancer? *Frontiers in Microbiology, 7*, UNSP 1148.

Nami, Y., Abdullah, N., Haghshenas, B., Radiah, D., Rosli, R., & Khosroushahi, A. Y. (2014). Assessment of probiotic potential and anticancer activity of newly isolated vaginal bacterium Lactobacillus plantarum 5BL. *Microbiology and Immunology, 58*, 492–502.

Nasiri, Z., Montazeri, H., Akbari, N., Mirfazli, S. S., & Tarighi, P. (2021). Synergistic cytotoxic and apoptotic effects of local probiotic Lactobacillus brevis isolated from regional dairy products in combination with Tamoxifen. *Nutrition and Cancer, 73*(2), 290–299.

National Breast Cancer Foundation, 2019. https://www.nationalbreastcancer.org/what-is-breast-cancer/. Accessed September 11, 2020.

Navaei, M., Haghighat, S., Janani, L., Vafa, S., Totmaj, A. S., Lahiji, M. R., Emamat, H., Salehi, Z., Amirinejad, A., Izad, M., & Yarrati, M. (2020). The effects of synbiotic supplementation on antioxidant capacity and arm volumes in survivors of breast cancer-related lymphedema. *Nutrition and Cancer, 72*, 6273.

Nazir, Y., Hussain, S. A., Hamid, A. A., & Song, Y. (2018). Probiotics and their potential preventive and therapeutic role for cancer, high serum cholesterol, and allergic and HIV diseases. *BioMed Research International, 2018*, 3428437.

Newton, J., Palladino, E. N. D., Weigel, C., Maceyka, M., Gräler, M. H., Senkal, C. E., Enriz, R. D., Marvanová, P., Jampílek, J., Lima, S., Milstien, S., & Spiegel, S. (2020). Targeting defective sphingosine kinase 1 in Niemann-Pick type C disease: Discovery of a SphK1 activator that mitigates cholesterol accumulation. *Journal of Biological Chemistry, 295*(27), 9121–9133.

NHS. (2018a). Overview—Cervical cancer. Retrieved from: https://www.nhs.uk/conditions/cervical-cancer/. Accessed September 11, 2020.

NHS. (2018b). Probiotics. Retrieved from: https://www.nhs.uk/conditions/probiotics/. Accessed September 3, 2020.

NHS. (2019). Overview—Breast cancer in women. Retrieved from: https://www.nhs.uk/conditions/breast-cancer/. Accessed September 3, 2020.

NIH. (2019). Probiotics: What you need to know. Retrieved from: https://www.nccih.nih.gov/health/probiotics-what-you-need-to-know. Accessed September 3, 2020.

Norouzi, Z., Salimi, A., Halabian, R., & Fahimi, H. (2018). Nisin, a potent bacteriocin and anti-bacterial peptide, attenuates expression of metastatic genes in colorectal cancer cell lines. *Microbial Pathogenesis., 123*, 18389.

Nouri, Z., Karami, F., Neyazi, N., Modarressi, M. H., Karimi, R., Khorramizadeh, M. R., Taheri, B., & Motevaseli, E. (2016). Dual anti-metastatic and anti-proliferative activity assessment of two probiotics on HeLa and HT-29 cell lines. *Cell Journal, 18*, 127–134.

Nowak, A., Kuberski, S., & Libudzisz, Z. (2014). Probiotic lactic acid bacteria detoxify N-nitrosodimethylamine. *Food Additives & Contaminants: Part A: Chemistry, Analysis, Control, Exposure and Risk Assessment, 31*, 1678–1687.

Nowak, A., Paliwoda, A., & Blasiak, J. (2019). Anti-proliferative, pro-apoptotic and anti-oxidative activity of Lactobacillus and Bifidobacterium strains: A review of mechanisms and therapeutic perspectives. *Critical Reviews in Food Science and Nutrition, 59*, 3456–3467.

Nozari, S., Faridvand, Y., Etesami, A., Beiki, M. A. K., Mazrakhondi, S. A. M., & Abdolalizadeh, J. (2019). Potential anticancer effects of cell wall protein fractions from Lactobacillus paracasei on human intestinal Caco-2 cell line. *Letters in Applies Microbiology, 69*, 148–154.

Ortiz, A. L. A., Vega, F. J., & Vargas, M. S. (2013). Dietary supplements as a treatment for cervical cancer; A systemic review. *Nutricion Hospitalaria, 28*, 1770–1780.

Pan, M. F., Wan, C. X., Xie, Q., Huang, R. H., Tao, X. Y., Shah, N. P., & Wei, H. (2016). Changes in gastric microbiota induced by Helicobacter pylori infection and preventive effects of Lactobacillus plantarum ZDY 2013 against such infection. *Journal of Dairy Science, 99*, 970–981.

Pandey, K. R., Naik, S. R., & Vakil, B. V. (2015). Probiotics, prebiotics and synbiotics—A review. *Journal of Food Science and Technology, 52*, 7577–7587.

Parida, S., & Sharma, D. (2020). Microbial alterations and risk factors of breast cancer: Connections and mechanistic insights. *Cells, 9*, 1091.

Parisa, A., Roya, G., Mahdi, R., Shabnam, R., Maryam, E., & Malihe, T. (2020). Anti-cancer effects of Bifidobacterium species in colon cancer cells and a mouse model of carcinogenesis. *PLoS One, 15*, e0232930.

Park, J. M., Jeong, M., Kim, E. H., Han, Y. M., Kwon, S. H., & Hahm, K. B. (2015). Omega-3 polyunsaturated fatty acids intake to regulate Helicobacter pylori-associated gastric diseases as nonantimicrobial dietary approach. *BioMed Research International, 2015*, 712363.

Pellegrini, M., Ippolito, M., Monge, T., Violi, R., Cappello, P., Ferrocino, I., Cocolin, L. S., De Francesco, A., Bo, S., & Finocchiaro, C. (2020). Gut microbiota composition after diet and probiotics in overweight breast cancer survivors: A randomized open-label pilot intervention trial. *Nutrition, 74*, UNSP 110749.

Pentak, D., Kozik, V., Bąk, A., Dybał, P., Sochanik, A., & Jampílek, J. (2016). Methotrexate and cytarabine-loaded nanocarriers for multidrug cancer therapy. Spectroscopic study. *Molecules, 21*, 1689.

Pineiro, M., Asp, N. G., Reid, G., Macfarlane, S., Morelli, L., Brunser, O., & Tuohy, K. L. (2008). FAO technical meeting on prebiotics. *Journal of Clinical Gastroenterology, 42*, S156–S159.

Plachá, D., & Jampílek, J. (2019). Graphenic materials for biomedical applications. *Nanomaterials, 9*, 1758.

Plummer, M., Franceschi, S., Vignat, J., Forman, D., & de Martel, C. (2015). Global burden of gastric cancer attributable to Helicobacter pylori. *International Journal of Cancer, 136*, 487–490.

Poonia, A. (2017). Potential of milk proteins as nanoencapsulation materials in food industry. In S. Ranjanm, N. Dasgupta, & N. Lichtfouse (Eds.), *Nanoscience in food and agriculture 5. Book series: Sustainable agriculture reviews 26*. Springer, Cham, Switzerland, 139–168.

Pourmollaei, S., Barzegari, A., Farshbaf-Khalili, A., Nouri, M., Fattahi, A., Shahnazi, M., & Dittrich, R. (2020). Anticancer effect of bacteria on cervical cancer: Molecular aspects and therapeutic implications. *Life Sciences, 246*, 117413.

Puccetti, M., Xiroudaki, S., Ricci, M., & Giovagnoli, S. (2020). Postbiotic-enabled targeting of the host-microbiota-pathogen interface: Hints of antibiotic decline? *Pharmaceutics, 12*, 624.

Qiu, G. J., Yu, Y., Wang, Y. P., & Wang, X. Y. (2019). The significance of probiotics in preventing radiotherapy-induced diarrhea in patients with cervical cancer: A systematic review and *meta*-analysis. *International Journal of Surgery, 65*, 61–69.

Ragul, K., Kandasamy, S., Devi, P. B., & Shetty, P. H. (2020). Evaluation of functional properties of potential probiotic isolates from fermented brine pickle. *Food Chemistry, 311*, 126057.

Rajoka, M. S. R., Mehwish, H. M., Fang, H. Y., Padhiar, A. A., Zeng, X. R., Khurshid, M., He, Z. D., & Zhao, L. Q. (2019). Characterization and anti-tumor activity of exopolysaccharide produced by Lactobacillus kefiri isolated from Chinese kefir grains. *Journal of Functional Foods, 63*, 103588.

Ranjbar, S., Seyednejad, S. A., Azimi, H., Rezaeizadeh, H., & Rahimi, R. (2019). Emerging roles of probiotics in prevention and treatment of breast cancer: A comprehensive review of their therapeutic potential. *Nutrition and Cancer, 71*, 112.

Ranji, P., Agah, S., Heydari, Z., Rahmati-Yamchi, M., & Alizadeh, A. M. (2019). Effects of Lactobacillus acidophilus and Bifidobacterium bifidum probiotics on the serum biochemical parameters, and the vitamin D and leptin receptor genes on mice colon cancer. *Iranian Journal of Basic Medical Sciences, 22*, 631–636.

Ren, Q., Yang, B., Zhu, G. Z., Wang, S. Y., Fu, C. L., Zhang, H., Ross, R. P., Stanton, C., Chen, H. Q., & Chen, W. (2020). Antiproliferation activity and mechanism of c9, t11, c15-CLNA and t9, t11, c15-CLNA from Lactobacillus plantarum ZS2058 on colon cancer cells. *Molecules, 25*, 1225.

Richards, J. L., Yap, Y. A., McLeod, K. H., Mackay, C. R., & Marino, E. (2016). Dietary metabolites and the gut microbiota: An alternative approach to control inflammatory and autoimmune diseases. *Clinical & Translational Immunology, 5*, UNSP e82.

Russo, F., Linsalata, M., & Orlando, A. (2014). Probiotics against neoplastic transformation of gastric mucosa: Effects on cell proliferation and polyamine metabolism. *World Journal of Gastroenterology., 20*, 13258–13272.

Saadat, Y. R., Khosroushahi, A. Y., Movassaghpour, A. A., Talebi, M., & Gargari, B. P. (2020). Modulatory role of exopolysaccharides of Kluyveromyces marxianus and Pichia kudriavzevii as probiotic yeasts from dairy products in human colon cancer cells. *Journal of Functional Foods, 64*, 103675.

Seifert, A., Freilich, S., Kashi, Y., & Livney, Y. D. (2019). Protein-oligosaccharide conjugates as novel prebiotics. *Polymers for Advanced Technologies, 30*, 2577–2585.

Settanni, C. R., Quaranta, G., Bibbo, S., Gasbarrini, A., Cammarota, G., & Ianiro, G. (2020). Oral supplementation with lactobacilli to prevent colorectal cancer in preclinical models. *Minerva Gastroenterologica e Dietologica, 66*, 4869.

Shah, B. R., Li, B., Al Sabbah, H., Xu, W., & Mráz, J. (2020). Effects of prebiotic dietary fibers and probiotics on human health: With special focus on recent advancement in their encapsulated formulations. *Trends in Food Science & Technology, 102*, 178–192.

Shamekhi, S., Abdolalizadeh, J., Ostadrahimi, A., Mohammadi, S. A., Barzegari, A., Lotfi, H., Bonabi, E., & Zarghami, N. (2020). Apoptotic effect of Saccharomyces cerevisiae on human colon cancer SW480 cells by regulation of Akt/NF-& x138;B signaling pathway. *Probiotics and Antimicrobial Proteins, 12*, 311–319.

Sharifi, M., Moridnia, A., Mortazavi, D., Salehi, M., Bagheri, M., & Sheikhi, A. (2017). Kefir: A powerful probiotics with anticancer properties. *Medical Oncology, 34*, 183.

Sharma, M., Chandel, D., & Shukla, G. (2020). Antigenotoxicity and cytotoxic potentials of metabiotics extracted from isolated probiotic, Lactobacillus rhamnosus MD 14 on Caco-2 and HT-29 human colon cancer cells. *Nutrition and Cancer, 72*, 110–119.

Shi, L. H., Balakrishnan, K., Thiagarajah, K., Mohd Ismail, N. I., & Yin, O. S. (2016). Beneficial properties of probiotics. *Tropical Life Sciences Research, 27*, 73–90.

Shibahara-Sone, H., Gomi, A., Iino, T., Kano, M., Nonaka, C., Watanabe, O., Miyazaki, K., & Ohkusa, T. (2016). Living cells of probiotic Bifidobacterium bifidum YIT 10347 detected on gastric mucosa in humans. *Beneficial Microbes, 7*, 319–326.

Shimizu, Y. (2018). Gut microbiota in common elderly diseases affecting activities of daily living. *World Journal of Gastroenterology, 24*, 4750–4758.

Sivamaruthi, B. S., Kesika, P., & Chaiyasut, C. (2020). The role of probiotics in colorectal cancer management. *Evidence-Based Complementary an Alternative Medicine, 2020*, 3535982.

Sivieri, K., Morales, M. L. V., Adorno, M. A. T., Sakamoto, I. K., Saad, S. M. I., & Rossi, E. A. (2013). Lactobacillus acidophilus CRL 1014 improved "gut health" in the SHIME (R) reactor. *BMC Gastroenterology, 13*, 100.

Song, H., Wang, W. Y., Shen, B., Jia, H., Hou, Z. Y., Chen, P., & Sun, Y. W. (2018). Pretreatment with probiotic Bifico ameliorates colitis-associated cancer in mice: Transcriptome and gut flora profiling. *Cancer Science, 109*, 666–677.

Spaczyńska, E., Mrozek-Wilczkiewicz, A., Malarz, K., Kos, J., Goněc, T., Oravec, M., Gawecki, R., Bąk, A., Doháňošová, J., Kapustíková, I., Liptaj, T., Jampílek, J., & Musioł, R. (2019). Design and synthesis of anticancer 1-hydroxynaphthalene-2-carboxanilides with p53 independent mechanism of action. *Scientific Reports, 9*, 6387.

Strumylaite, L., Zickute, J., Dudzevicius, J., & Dregval, L. (2006). Salt-preserved foods and risk of gastric cancer. *Medicina (Kaunas), 42*, 164–170.

Sungur, T., Aslim, B., Karaaslan, C., & Aktas, B. (2017). Impact of exopolysaccharides (EPSs) of Lactobacillus gasseri strains isolated from human vagina on cervical tumor cells (HeLa). *Anaerobe, 47*, 137–144.

Swanson, K. S., Gibson, G. R., Hutkins, R., Reimer, R. A., Reid, G., Verbeke, K., Scott, K. P., Holscher, H. D., Azad, M. B., Delzenne, N. M., & Sanders, M. E. (2020). The International Scientific Association for Probiotics and Prebiotics (ISAPP) consensus statement on the definition and scope of synbiotics. *Nature Reviews Gastroenterology & Hepatology, 17*(11), 687–701.

Takagi, A., Kano, M., & Kaga, C. (2015). Possibility of breast cancer prevention: Use of soy isoflavones and fermented soy beverage produced using probiotics. *International Journal of Molecular Sciences, 16*, 10907–10920.

Takeda, S., Takeshita, M., Matsusaki, T., Kikuchi, Y., Tsend-ayush, C., Oyunsuren, T., Miyata, M., Maeda, K., Yasuda, S., Aiba, Y., Koga, Y., & Igoshi, K. (2015). In vitro and in vivo anti-Helicobacter pylori activity of probiotics isolated from Mongolian dairy products. *Food Science and Technology Research, 21*, 399–406.

The Nobel Prize. (2020). Ilya Mechnikov Biographical. Retreived from: https://www.nobelprize.org/prizes/medicine/1908/mechnikov/biographical/. Accessed July 29, 2020.

Tiptiri-Kourpeti, A., Spyridopoulou, K., Santarmaki, V., Aindelis, G., Tompoulidou, E., Lamprianidou, E. E., Saxami, G., Ypsilantis, P., Lampri, E. S., Simopoulos, C., Kotsianidis, I., Galanis, A., Kourkoutas, Y., Dimitrellou, D., & Chlichlia, K. (2016). Lactobacillus casei exerts antiproliferative effects accompanied by apoptotic cell death and up-regulation of TRAIL in colon carcinoma cells. *PLoS One, 11*, e0147960.

Tomas, L. (2009). Best breastfeeding and formulas. *Journal of Complementary Medicine, 8*, 3240.

Tomasik, P., & Tomasik, P. (2020). Probiotics, non-dairy prebiotics and postbiotics in nutrition. *Applied Sciences, 10*, 1470.

Utz, V. E. M., Perdigon, G., & de LeBlanca, A. D. (2019). Oral administration of milk fermented by Lactobacillus casei CRL431 was able to decrease metastasis from breast cancer in a murine model by modulating immune response locally in the lungs. *Journal of Functional Foods, 54*, 263–270.

Vafa, S., Haghighat, S., Janani, L., Totmaj, A. S., Navaei, M., Amirinejad, A., Emamat, H., Salehi, Z., & Zarrati, M. (2020). The effects of synbiotic supplementation on serum inflammatory markers and edema volume in breast cancer with lymphedema. *EXCLI Journal, 19*, 115.

Verhoeven, V., Renard, N., Makar, A., Van Royen, P., Bogers, J. P., Lardon, F., Peeters, M., & Baay, M. (2013). Probiotics enhance the clearance of human papillomavirus-related cervical lesions: A prospective controlled pilot study. *European Journal of Cancer Prevention, 22*, 4651.

Vettorazzi, M., Angelina, E., Lima, S., Goněc, T., Otevřel, J., Marvanová, P., Padrtová, T., Mokrý, P., Bobáľ, P., Acosta, L. M., Palma, A., Cobo, J., Bobáľová, J., Csöllei, J., Malík, I., Alvarez, S., Spiegel, S., Jampílek, J., & Enriz, R. D. (2017). Search of new structural scaffolds for sphingosine kinase 1 inhibitors. *European Journal of Medicinal Chemistry, 139*, 461–481.

Vettorazzi, M., Lima, S., Acosta, L., Yépes, F., Palma, A., Cobo, J., Tengler, J., Malík, I., Alvarez, S., Spiegel, S., Cabedo, N., Cortes, D. M., Sanz, J. M., Jampílek, J., & Enriz, R. D. (2019). Design, synthesis, and biological evaluation of sphingosine kinase 2 inhibitors with anti-inflammatory activity. *Archiv der Pharmazie, 352*, 1800298.

Wang, Z. Q., Wang, Q. X., Wang, X., Zhu, L., Chen, J., Zhang, B. L., Chen, Y., & Yuan, Z. Y. (2019). Gut microbial dysbiosis is associated with development and progression of radiation enteritis during pelvic radiotherapy. *Journal of Cellular and Molecular Medicine, 23*, 3747–3756.

Wei, H. Y., Chen, L. K., Lian, G. H., Yang, J. W., Li, F. J., Zou, Y. Y., Lu, F., & Yin, Y. (2018). Antitumor mechanisms of bifidobacteria. *Oncology Letters, 16*, 38.

Wei, Y. L., Li, F., Li, L., Huang, L. L., & Li, Q. H. (2019). Genetic and biochemical characterization of an exopolysaccharide with in vitro antitumoral activity produced by Lactobacillus fermentum YL-11. *Frontiers in Microbiology, 10*, 2898.

Westerik, N., Reid, G., Sybesma, W., & Kort, R. (2018). The probiotic Lactobacillus rhamnosus for alleviation of Helicobacter pylori-associated gastric pathology in East Africa. *Frontiers in Microbiology, 9*, 1873.

Westmeier, D., Posselt, G., Hahlbrock, A., Bartfeld, S., Vallet, C., Abfalter, C., Docter, D., Knauer, S. K., Wessler, S., & Stauber, R. H. (2018). Nanoparticle binding attenuates the pathobiology of gastric cancer-associated Helicobacter pylori. *Nanoscale, 10*, 1453–1463.

Wilson, A. S., Koller, K. R., Ramaboli, M. C., Nesengani, L. T., Ocvirk, S., Chen, C. X., Flanagan, C. A., Sapp, F. R., Merritt, Z. T., Bhatti, F., Thomas, T. K., & O'Keefe, S. D. J. (2020). Diet and the human gut microbiome: An international review. *Digestive Diseases and Sciences, 65*, 723–740.

Yang, P., Zhou, Y., Chen, B., Wan, H. W., Jia, G. Q., Bai, H. L., & Wu, X. T. (2009). Overweight, obesity and gastric cancer risk: Results from a meta-analysis of cohort studies. *European Journal of Cancer, 45*, 2867–2873.

Yeo, S. K., & Liong, M. T. (2010). Angiotensin I-converting enzyme inhibitory activity and bioconversion of isoflavones by probiotics in soymilk supplemented with prebiotics. *International Journal of Food Sciences and Nutrition, 61*, 161–181.

Zamberi, N. R., Abu, N., Mohamed, N. E., Nordin, N., Keong, Y. S., Beh, B. K., Zakaria, Z. A., Rahman, N. M. A. N. A., & Alitheen, N. B. (2016). The antimetastatic and antiangiogenesis effects of kefir water on murine breast cancer cells. *Integrative Cancer Therapies., 15*, NP53–NP66.

Zandu, S. K., Sharma, A., Garg, K., Bakshi, H., & Singh, I. (2020). Probiotics for treating disorders: Microencapsulation a boon to potentiate their therapeutic applications. *Biointerface Research in Applied Chemistry, 10*, 5068–5075.

Zhang, M., & Zhang, J. (2020). PEG3 mutation is associated with elevated tumor mutation burden and poor prognosis in breast cancer. *Bioscience Reports, 40*, BSR20201648.

Zhang, T., Pan, D. D., Yang, Y. J., Jiang, X. X., Zhang, J. X., Zeng, X. Q., Wu, Z., Sun, Y. Y., & Guo, Y. X. (2020). Effect of Lactobacillus acidophilus CICC 6074 S-layer protein on colon cancer HT-29 cell proliferation and apoptosis. *Journal of Agricutural and Food Chemistry, 68*, 2639–2647.

Zhang, Y. (2019). Probiotic effects of Lactobacillus casei Zhang: From single strain omics to metagenomics. *Chinese Science Bulletin, 64*, 307–314.

Zheng, C. H., Chen, T. T., Wang, Y. Q., Gao, Y., Kong, Y., Liu, Z. X., & Deng, X. R. (2019). A randomised trial of probiotics to reduce severity of physiological and microbial disorders induced by partial gastrectomy for patients with gastric cancer. *Journal of Cancer, 10*, 568–576.

Żółkiewicz, J., Marzec, A., Ruszczyński, M., & Feleszko, W. (2020). Postbiotics—A step beyond pre- and probiotics. *Nutrients, 12*, 2189.

Žuntar, I., Petric, Z., Bursać-Kovačević, D., & Putnik, P. (2020). Safety of probiotics: Functional fruit beverages and nutraceuticals. *Foods, 9*, 947.

Chapter 14

Probiotics in mitigation of food allergies and lactose intolerance

Bhuvan Shankar Vadala[1], Prasant Kumar[2] and Mitesh Kumar Dwivedi[3]

[1]Sri Venkateswara University, Tirupati, India, [2]Ingress Bio-Solutions Pvt Ltd, Ahmedabad, India, [3]C.G. Bhakta Institute of Biotechnology, Uka Tarsadia University, Maliba Campus, Bardoli, India

14.1 Introduction of probiotics and the gut microbiome

The probiotic word is a combination of two words—pro and bios—pro is a Latin word which means "good," bios is a Greek word which means "for life"; probiotics full meaning is "good for life." The original observation of the positive role played by certain bacteria was first introduced by Russian scientist Eile Mechinikoff, who at the beginning of the 20th century suggested that it would be possible to modify the gut flora and to replace harmful microbes with useful microbes. German scientist Warner Kollath used the word for the first time in 1950. Fujji and Cook gave details of probiotics as compounds in 1970; Parker defined probiotics as a live organism in 1990. In 2001, FAO/WHO (Food and Agriculture Organization & World Health Organization), on behalf of international scientists who worked on probiotics, defined them as live organisms with health benefits for the host (Schepper et al., 2017).

Probiotics are live microbes that are beneficial and bring health benefits when consumed through yogurt, milk, curd, and other dairy products. They are helpful in sustaining a healthy digestive tract by maintaining a healthy community of microflora like *Lactobacillus acidophilus, Lactobacillus rhamnosus* GG, *Saccharomyces boulardii, Bifidobacterium bifidum*, and *Bacillus coagulans*; these gut microbiota acts as a friendly bacterium and play a major role in immune system regulation (Kapse & Chandekar, 2020).

Probiotics consumption will boost our immune system by maintaining healthy gut microflora. Probiotics is naturally available in dairy products, dietary supplements, and foods; they can also be used as complementary and alternative medicine. Probiotics build a symbiotic relationship between microbiota and humans (La Fata et al., 2018), while the usage of antibiotics will disturb our gut microbiota and raise the risk of allergic diseases, particularly in children and elderly people. The gut microbiome is useful to human metabolism as gut bacteria break down indigestible compounds from the diet, biosynthesize amino acids and vitamins (Magnúsdóttir & Thiele, 2018; Shivaji, 2017). The gut microbiome has three types of microbes (1) pathogenic (harmful bacteria), (2) commensal (host, no use bacteria), (3) symbiotic (useful bacteria) (Ho & Bunyavanich, 2018). Every human being contains trillions of microbes in the gut. These microbes play an important role in our health and diseases. Good microbes called probiotics help to maintain and boost our gut system and prevent or protect it from pathogens and allergies.

14.2 Food allergies and lactose intolerance

Hygiene is most important in the early age of life and throughout adulthood. Food allergy is an abnormal response to a food triggered by the body's immune system. Our immune system responds to a harmless food as if it's a threat. Food allergies are being considered as pediatric diseases nowadays, and being observed with other diseases like cardiovascular (Evans et al., 2019), diabetes (Ierodiakonou et al., 2016), neurodegenerative (Sarkar & Banerjee, n.d.), and cancers (Smyth et al., 2020). These food allergies are gradually increasing, including an increased report in elders. These food allergy root causes are pleomorphic, and many factors are involved such as abnormal immune response, hampered gut barrier function, age-related factors, malnutrition or abnormality in nutrition, vitamin-D deficiency (VDD), and hormonal imbalance; all those things affect our immune system and lead to food allergies (Massimo et al., 2019). The food allergy symptoms include stomach upset like gas, bloating, constipation, diarrhea, and heartburn. An unhealthy ecosystem of the gut has various symptoms including sleep disturbances, skin irritation, food intolerances, and unintentional weight changes (Caffarelli et al., 2011; Lee et al., 2020; Massimo et al., 2019).

Among all food allergies, diarrhea is most commonly observed. The rotavirus is the main and common pathogen in diarrhea (Cameron et al., 2017). Diarrhea types include nosocomial diarrhea (ND), antibiotic-associated diarrhea (AAD), *Clostridium difficile* diarrhea (CDD), travelers' diarrhea (TD), and radiation diarrhea (Harald, 2019). Vitamin-D plays the significant role in immune response and its impacts in the function of macrophages, epithelial cells, B cells, T cells, and dendritic cells. VDD is an effective food allergy. It mainly causes disequilibrium at the intestinal level that damages immune tolerance, injuries to the epithelial barrier, and an increase in susceptibility to infections, VDD is noneffective tight junctions in the skin this effect on skin allergy sensitization eczema (Giannetti et al., 2020).

Cow milk allergy (CMA) is the common food allergy observed in infants and young children. IgE mediated CMA's is one of the most common food allergies in infants and young children. CMA can result in anaphylactic reactions, and has long term implications on growth and nutrition. CMA symptoms are eczema and gastrointestinal functional disorders in children around 2 years of age, and other reported IgE-mediated food allergies include egg allergy, peanut allergy, soy allergy, fish allergy, tree nuts allergy, and wheat allergy (Du et al., 2017; Ferraro et al., 2019). Dysbiosis disrupts the ecosystem of the gut, resulting in various symptoms such as indigestion, constipation, and diarrhea. Gut microbiome imbalance is the cause of dysbiosis (Ho & Bunyavanich, 2018).

14.3 Lactose intolerance

Lactose intolerance (LI) is another common gastrointestinal condition that arises due to the inability of lactose digestion and of essential dietary lactose required for normal function. Lactose is usually absorbed through hydrolysis catalyzed by lactase enzymes into D-glucose and D-galactose; more than 70% of people around the world are suffering from LI (Heine et al., 2017). LI results after acute diarrhea due to milk consumption. The LI patient needs to avoid a diet which contains lactose such as dairy products (milk, cheese, etc.) (Deng et al., 2015). Milk acts as nutrient-rich food and takes the place of a major part of a healthful diet (Horner et al., 2011). If we avoid milk and other dairy products in our daily intake, it would lead to low bone density. Those who avoid milk due to LI consume significantly less calcium and have poorer bone health including a probable higher risk of osteoporosis (Leis et al., 2020).

Primary LI symptoms in young children are mild gastrointestinal symptoms including abdominal pain, flatulence, diarrhea, vomiting, nausea, and bowel sounds. Secondary LI symptoms in young children's gastrointestinal functional disease include viral gastroenteritis, giardiasis, nonIgE-mediated cow's milk enteropathy, and celiac disease.

With LI inflammatory bowel disease, hydrogen breath tests (HBTs) are commonly used to identify LI (Garg & Gibson, 2011). This LI causes nutrition diseases, rickets, osteoporosis, osteomalacia, and calcium deficiency. The main reason for LI is that so many people avoid milk products in the daily and early stages of life (Martínez Vázquez et al., 2020). Several methods are there to measure lactose digestion in humans: (1) HBT, (2) lactose tolerance test (LTT), (3) determination of fecal pH test, (4) plasma glucose test (PGT), and (5) genotyping test (GT) (Gayathri & Vasudha, 2018).

14.4 Role of probiotics in mitigation of food allergies and lactose intolerance

Nowadays, probiotics are the best remedy for food allergies and LI treatment. The major advantage of probiotics treatment is a lower-cost development and their natural availability. Food allergy is considered a type-1 hypersensitivity reaction mediated by protein antigens present in different food sources, indicated by the hyper levels of IgE antibodies which can lead to severe clinical reactions.

Food allergens are specific components of food recognized by the individual's immune system that result in characteristic allergic symptoms. The most serious and potentially fatal allergic reaction is anaphylaxis. Anaphylaxis is a life-threatening type of allergic reaction due to allergens. A few of the other allergic symptoms include vomiting, feeding disorders, reflux, abdominal pain, dysphagia, diarrhea, growth failure, and bloody stools. Several studies show promising results by using probiotics in treatment successfully, but the evidence is still conflicting and inconclusive. Most systematic trials and experiments performed on probiotics and food allergy focused on the role of probiotics in preventing food allergy (Tan-Lim & Esteban-Ipac, 2018).

The gut microbiome is known as a friendly and beneficial bacteria, playing a major role in regulating physiological, immunological, and structural changes in the gut region. These beneficial bacteria were helpful in the modulation of immune responses by targeting Th-1, Th-2, Th-17, and regulatory T cells known as Treg cells, and B cells. For treating food allergies, present strategies employed are allergen-specific immunotherapy; it is a specific and targeted treatment procedure to induce tolerance in individuals against specific food allergens.

The presence of huge and active commensal microbiota in our intestine since childhood will be helpful in the process of developing regulatory T cells and tolerance. Breast milk from the mother contains oligosaccharides which promote *Bifidobacteria* growth and activity, and also *Lactobacilli*. There is an association between developing allergic diseases and the presence of commensal microbiota during infant times. The common and useful microbiota with specific biological activities includes the following microflora—*Lactobacilli*, *Bifidobacteria*, and *Streptococci* strains—which are the most common microflora present in healthy human beings and on dairy products. These probiotics show a direct impact on the immune system when taken in adequate quantities and change the intestinal microflora of the host (Erkki et al., 2009).

In the pathogenesis of intestinal inflammation of ulcer colitis, the T-cell activation plays a major role. *Clostridium butyricum* is a probiotic and has been employed in the treatment of immune diseases (Rao & Samak, 2013).

14.4.1 Mechanism of action of probiotics

The mechanism by which probiotics exert its effects are schematically represented in Fig. 14.1.

14.4.2 Role of probiotics mitigation in lactose intolerance

Lactose is a disaccharide consisting of D-galactose and D-glucose. Biochemically, it has two aldohexoses classified as O-β-D-galactopyranosyl-(1—4)-β-glucose. Lactose denotes the major carbohydrate of mammalian milk and very few other sources of this carbohydrate occur in nature. Even the blood glucose tests use lactose maldigestion as an indicator for failure to raise blood glucose levels which are above 1.1—1.4 mmol/L. These two tests have many discrepancies for different reasons (Lan et al., 2016).

To mitigate LI, people started using cultured bacteria as probiotics to overcome problems associated with lactose digestion. Irritable bowel syndrome (IBS) is one of the most common gut functional diseases and one of the most common diseases in gastrointestinal clinical practice. It is defined classically as a chronic disorder characterized by abdominal pain/discomfort and disturbed defecation not explained by structural and biochemical abnormalities. IBS symptoms overlap with those of coeliac disease, LI, food allergies, and bile salt malabsorption (Andrew & Norma, 2018). Researchers hypothesized that intake of probiotics and vitamin B6 may be useful to improve symptoms in LI patients through a positive modulation of gut microbial composition and relative metabolism (Vitellio et al., 2019). They started using some of the selected probiotic strains to improve the gut microbiota of the patient. This approach represented a valid therapeutic way to treat functional gastrointestinal disorders (FGIDs), even with concomitant LI.

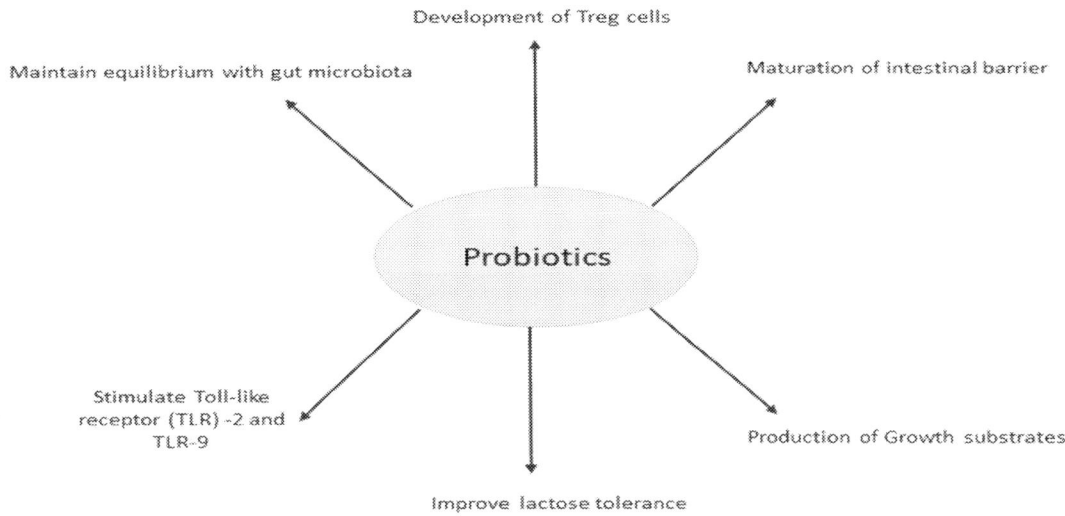

FIGURE 14.1 Mechanism by which probiotics protect our health.

This way of probiotic supplementation. with specific strains useful in maintaining the balance of essential intestinal microflora, can be altered by several factors which include (lifestyle, diet type, stressful life, anxiety, excessive antibiotic usage, and so on). Hence, probiotics are known to have a role in the mitigation of LI, for treatment of FGIDs, as well as carbohydrate malabsorption (De Giorgio et al., 2004). Other symptoms associated with LI are diarrhea. Several studies were performed on AAD and acute diarrhea to check the effect of probiotics on those two symptoms. AAD occurs in 4%–30% of antibiotic-treated patients and is caused by a disturbance of the intestinal microbiota, direct tissue damage, or modulation of the immune system.

The meta-analyses were then repeated, stratifying the probiotic strains used: *S. boulardii*, *L. GG* and probiotic mixtures, which significantly reduced the development of AAD; only *S. boulardii* was effective for *C. difficile*-associated diarrhea. The majorities of the studies (total 97) were focused on acute diarrhea using rota-virus-associated diarrhea in children (Vitellio et al., 2019).

14.5 Dietary management strategies

Since the advancement of technology and knowledge gained, people started focusing on well-being and disease prevention strategies. This was also initiated by increasing the immunity power through healthy diets, daily exercise, yoga, and intake of additional dietary supplements (Jonkers & Stockbrügger, 2007). To increase the function of the gastrointestinal tract as the main target. In particular, carbohydrates digestion and absorption were one of the main concerned areas which were shed more light in the past few years. Digestion of carbohydrates in the small intestine takes place by absorbing the hydrolysis disaccharides, oligosaccharides, and polysaccharides into respective monomers, but in certain cases physiological or pathological conditions, like as in case of LI—these carbohydrates hardly got hydrolyzed and absorbed, and fermented by intestinal microbiota, once they reach the gut lumen (Prochaska & Piekutowski, 1994). Research-based studies showed that consumption of commercial probiotics increased specific intestinal microbiota, but it is not reflected in the total microflora present in the intestine (Corgneau et al., 2017).

The majority of reported research cases state that specific bacteria do not increase unless the person starts to consume very high doses of probiotics in the form of supplements and not in naturally available food products (Vitellio et al., 2019). Several studies have been shown that microorganisms, with the ability to modulate the intestinal and systemic immune response, could be used in bacterial and viral respiratory infections to improve their outcomes (Brown & Valiere, 2004; Clua et al., 2017; de Vrese et al., 2005, 2006; Eguchi et al., 2019; Hao et al., 2015; Winkler et al., 2005).

14.6 Therapeutic applications

Probiotics are live microorganisms; their consumption will help us stay healthy by maintaining the equilibrium and physiological functions of our intestine microflora. Very recently, probiotics were defined as "live microorganisms" which transit the gastrointestinal tract and help keep our health stable, with positive benefits. Probiotics have been reported in many studies that they are having a major role as therapeutic agents by increasing immunity, decreasing the levels of cholesterol, improving intolerance of lactose, and helpful in preventing a few types of cancers, such as colon cancer, and so on. At present, there has been a trend of using probiotic-based health products in the form of either fermented dairy products or nutritional supplements, and statistics showed that market demand is also very high and is growing forward worldwide because of their various benefits. Almost 80% of these fermented dairy products contain "Bifidus" and "Acidophilus."

Probiotics have several health benefits for both humans and animals: helpful in LI indication, increases the capacity of bioavailability of nutrients, confirms lactose digestion, sustains the git microbiota and many more. Probiotics have antagonistic effects related to intestinal and foodborne pathogens like *Esherichia coli, Staphylococcus aureus*, and many more (Holzapfel et al., 1998).

14.7 Intake of probiotics

In general, probiotics are identified by the strains of bacteria they belong to, both species and subspecies (World Gastroenterology Organisation, 2017). Tables 14.1 and 14.2 shows the strain ID and local names of common genera of microbial strains and their forms that are most frequently used in probiotic products.

TABLE 14.1 List of commercially used strains as probiotics.

Genus	Species	Subspecies	Strain ID	References
Lactobacillus	rhamnosus	None	GG/PL60/PL62	World Gastroenterology Organisation (2017)
Bifidobacterium	animalis	Lactis	DN-173000	World Gastroenterology Organisation (2017)
Bifidobacterium	Longum	Longum	35624	World Gastroenterology Organisation (2017)

TABLE 14.2 Probiotics in various forms.

Type of probiotic	Biological important	Microflora
Yogurt	Biological impacts are there but very palatable and few are colonisable gut bacteria very palatable.	Lactobacillus delbrueckii var bulgaricus, Streptococcus salivarius var thermophilus
Milk, fruits, drinks	Very palatable	Lactobacillus casei, Lactobacillus plantarum, Lactobacillus reuteri
Additional supplements (capsules, tablets, powders)	Long shell life, with some proven benefits	Lactobacillus acidophilus, Bifidobacteria

TABLE 14.3 Animals studies and clinical trials of probiotics and its biological effects as a treatment of food allergic disorders.

Probiotic strain	Biological effects of probiotics	References
Lactobacilli and Bifidobacteria	Gut barriers maturations	Rao and Samak (2013), Wosinska L et al. (2019)
Bifidobacterium breve	Immunomodulation: suppression of IgE production	Ren et al. (2018)
Genetically modified Lactococcus lactis	Interleukin-10 production	de Moreno de Leblanc et al. (2011)
Lactobacillus paracasei I 1688, Lactobacillus salivarius I 1794	Increase in Th-1 immune response, increase level of IL-12 and IL-10 cytokine production	Castellazzi et al. (2007), Kimoto et al. (2004)
Lactobacillus casei, Lactobacillus rhamnousus, Lactobacillus acidophilus, and Lactobacillus delbrueckii subsp. Bulgaricus, Bifidobacterium longum, Bifidobacterium breve, and Streptococcus salivarius subsp. thermophilus	Reduce the level of IL-6, antiinflammatory and protective effects	Plaza-Díaz et al. (2017), Kaci et al. (2014)
Lactobacillus rhamnosus GG (ATCC 53103) & Bifidobacterium lactis (Bb-12)	Immune system regulation: Increased FOXP3$^+$ Tregs and & TGF-3 production	Dwivedi et al. (2016)

14.8 Future prospective of probiotic in food allergies

In the current scenario, food allergies are increasing worldwide due to globalization, and people are very concerned about hygienic food habits and the consumption of different types of food in daily routines. Research activities currently focus on understanding the mechanism of an allergy and the possibility to reduce the food allergic problems. Various animal models and clinical trial studies unveiled the potential of probiotics in the treatment of allergic diseases (Tables 14.3 and 14.4). However, selection of the most beneficial probiotic strain for specific types of allergic problems, the dose, and the timing of supplementation, still need to be determined.

TABLE 14.4 Probiotics used in food allergy.

Probiotic strains	Clinical evidence showing Positives effects against food allergic disorders	References
Lactobacillus GG *(LGG)* and *L. gasseri*	Treatment of allergic rhinitis	Kawase et al. (2009)
Lactobacillus GG	Reduction of asthma and eczema	Kalliomäki et al. (2001)
Lactobacillus salivarius and Fructo-oligosaccharide (FOS)	Treatment of atopic dermatitis	Wu et al. (2012)
Lactobacillus rhamnosus GG (ATCC 53103) & *Bifidobacterium lactis* (Bb-12)	Suppression of allergic sensitization and airway inflammation	Feleszko et al. (2007)
Lactobacillus rhamnosus GG	Reduction in cow milk allergy	Taylor et al. (2007), Tan-Lim & Esteban-Ipac (2018)
LGG, *Lactobacillus acidophilus* La-5, and *Bifidobacterium animalis*	Atopic eczema	Özdemir (2018)
Lactobacillus rhamnosus CGMCC 1.3724	Peanut allergy	Hsiao Chih et al. (2017)
Lactobacillus, Bifidobacterium	Atopy and food hypersensitivity	Zhang et al. (2016)

14.9 Conclusions

Probiotic organisms are beneficial for human beings and confer normal health. The probiotic microbiome is known as friendly bacteria to the consumer when provided externally in a diet for maintaining a healthy status in present-day scenarios. Growing evidence shows extensive usage of probiotics due to their nutrition and health benefits have negligible side effects.

From reported studies, it has been proven that gut microbiota composition is vulnerable to disruptions starting after birth and are were associated with the changes in host-microbiota homeostasis which leads to the development of food allergies. All these reported studies supported that gut microbiota are playing a major role in the manifestation of food allergies. But further studies are required to validate the particular role of the gut microbiota in the mitigation of food allergies. To conclude this chapter, the emerging evidence suggests that therapeutic strategies in modifying gut microbiota composition are useful in preventing, managing, and treating food allergies and will help pave the way for prophylactic and therapeutic routes for mitigating food allergies.

References

Andrew, S., & Norma, I. (2018). Lactose intolerance, dairy avoidance, and treatment options. *Nutrients*, *1994*. Available from https://doi.org/10.3390/nu10121994.

Brown, A. C., & Valiere, A. (2004). Probiotics and medical nutrition therapy. *Nutrition in Clinical Care: An Official Publication of Tufts University*, *7*(2), 56–68.

Caffarelli, C., Coscia, A., Ridolo, E., Povesi Dascola, C., Gelmett, C., Raggi, V., Volta, E., Vanell, M., & Dall'Aglio, P. P. (2011). Parents' estimate of food allergy prevalence and management in Italian school-aged children. *Pediatrics International*, *53*(4), 505–510. Available from https://doi.org/10.1111/j.1442-200X.2010.03294.x.

Cameron, D., Hock, Q. S., Kadim, M., Mohan, N., Ryoo, E., Sandhu, B., Yamashiro, Y., Jie, C., Hoekstra, H., & Guarino, A. (2017). Probiotics for gastrointestinal disorders: Proposed recommendations for children of the Asia-Pacific region. *World Journal of Gastroenterology*, *23*(45), 7952–7964. Available from https://doi.org/10.3748/wjg.v23.i45.7952.

Castellazzi, A. M., Valsecchi, C., Montagna, L., Malfa, P., Ciprandi, G., Avanzini, M. A., & Marseglia, G. L. (2007). *In vitro* activation of mononuclear cells by two probiotics: *Lactobacillus paracasei* I 1688, *Lactobacillus salivarius* I 1794, and their Mixture (PSMIX). *Immunological Investigations*, *36*(4), 413–421.

Clua, P., Kanmani, P., Zelaya, H., Tada, A., Humayun Kober, A. K. M., Salva, S., Alvarez, S., Kitazawa, H., & Villena, J. (2017). Peptidoglycan from immunobiotic lactobacillus rhamnosus improves resistance of infant Mice to respiratory syncytial viral infection and secondary pneumococcal pneumonia. *Frontiers in Immunology*, *8*. Available from https://doi.org/10.3389/fimmu.2017.00948.

Corgneau, M., Scher, J., Ritie-Pertusa, L., Le, D. T. L., Petit, J., Nikolova, Y., Banon, S., & Gaiani, C. (2017). Recent advances on lactose intolerance: Tolerance thresholds and currently available answers. *Critical Reviews in Food Science and Nutrition*, *57*(15), 3344–3356. Available from https://doi.org/10.1080/10408398.2015.1123671.

De Giorgio, R., Barbara, G., Stanghellini, V., Cremon, C., Salvioli, B., De Ponti, F., & Corinaldesi, R. (2004). Diagnosis and therapy of irritable bowel syndrome. *Alimentary Pharmacology and Therapeutics*, 20(2), 10–22. Available from https://doi.org/10.1111/j.1365-2036.2004.02038.x.

de Moreno de Leblanc, A., Del Carmen, S., Zurita-Turk, M., Santos Rocha, C., van de Guchte, M., Azevedo, V., Miyoshi, A., & Leblanc, J. G. (2011). Importance of IL-10 modulation by probiotic microorganisms in gastrointestinal inflammatory diseases. *ISRN Gastroenterology*, 892971. Available from https://doi.org/10.5402/2011/892971, Epub 2011 Feb 8. PMID: 21991534; PMCID: PMC3168568.

de Vrese, M., Winkler, P., Rautenberg, P., Harder, T., Noah, C., Laue, C., Ott, S., Hampe, J., Schreiber, S., Heller, K., & Schrezenmeir, J. (2005). Effect of *Lactobacillus gasseri* PA 16/8, *Bifidobacterium longum* SP 07/3, *B. bifidum* MF 20/5 on common cold episodes: A double blind, randomized, controlled trial. *Clinical Nutrition*, 24(4), 481–491. Available from https://doi.org/10.1016/j.clnu.2005.02.006.

de Vrese, M., Winkler, P., Rautenberg, P., Harder, T., Noah, C., Laue, C., Ott, S., Hampe, J., Schreiber, S., Heller, K., & Schrezenmeir, J. (2006). Probiotic bacteria reduced duration and severity but not the incidence of common cold episodes in a double blind, randomized, controlled trial. *Vaccine*, 24(44–46), 6670–6674. Available from https://doi.org/10.1016/j.vaccine.2006.05.048.

Deng, Y., Misselwitz, B., Dai, N., & Fox, M. (2015). Lactose intolerance in adults: Biological mechanism and dietary management. *Nutrients*, 7(9), 8020–8035. Available from https://doi.org/10.3390/nu7095380.

Du, T., Foong, G., & Lack, R. X. (2017). Prevention of food allergy—Early dietary interventions. *Allergology International: Official Journal of the Japanese Society of Allergology*, 66(1).

Dwivedi, M., Kumar, P., Laddha, N. C., & Kemp, E. H. (2016). Induction of regulatory T cells: A role for probiotics and prebiotics to suppress autoimmunity. *Autoimmunity Reviews*, 15(4), 379–392. Available from https://doi.org/10.1016/j.autrev.2016.01.002, Epub 2016 Jan 7. PMID: 26774011.

Eguchi, K., Fujitani, N., Nakagawa, H., & Miyazaki, T. (2019). Prevention of respiratory syncytial virus infection with probiotic lactic acid bacterium *Lactobacillus gasseri* SBT2055. *Scientific Reports*, 9(1). Available from https://doi.org/10.1038/s41598-019-39602-7.

Erkki, S., Kaarina, K., & Mikael, K. (2009). Probiotics in the treatment and prevention of allergy in children. *World Allergy Organization Journal*, 69–76. Available from https://doi.org/10.1097/wox.0b013e3181a45ee5.

Evans, M. A., Sano, S., & Walsh, K. (2019). Cardiovascular disease, aging, and clonal hematopoiesis. *Annual Review of Pathology*, 24.

Feleszko, W., Jaworska, J., Rha, R. D., Steinhausen, S., Avagyan, A., Jaudszus, A., Ahrens, B., Groneberg, D. A., Wahn, U., & Hamelmann, E. (2007). Probiotic-induced suppression of allergic sensitization and airway inflammation is associated with an increase of T regulatory-dependent mechanisms in a murine model of asthma. *Clinical & Experimental Allergy*, 37(4), 498–505. Available from https://doi.org/10.1111/j.1365-2222.2006.02629.x, PMID: 17430345.

Ferraro, V., Zanconato, S., & Carraro, S. (2019). Timing of food introduction and the risk of food allergy. *Nutrients*, 11(5). Available from https://doi.org/10.3390/nu11051131.

Garg, M., & Gibson, P. R. (2011). Lactose intolerance in inflammatory bowel disease. *Alimentary Pharmacology and Therapeutics*, 34(9), 1140–1141. Available from https://doi.org/10.1111/j.1365-2036.2011.04836.x.

Gayathri, D., & Vasudha, M. (2018). Lactose intolerance with special emphasis on probiotics for management. *EC Nutrition*, 13, 325–332.

Giannetti, A., Bernardini, L., Cangemi, J., Gallucci, M., Masetti, R., & Ricci, G. (2020). Role of vitamin D in prevention of food allergy in infants. *Frontiers in Pediatrics*, 8. Available from https://doi.org/10.3389/fped.2020.00447.

Hao, Q., Dong, B. R., & Wu, T. (2015). Probiotics for preventing acute upper respiratory tract infections. *Cochrane Database of Systematic Reviews*, 2015(2). Available from https://doi.org/10.1002/14651858.CD006895.pub3.

Harald, B. (2019). Probiotics and prebiotics in clinical tests: An update. *F1000Research*, 1157. Available from https://doi.org/10.12688/f1000research.19043.1.

Heine, R. G., Alrefaee, F., Bachina, P., De Leon, J. C., Geng, L., Gong, S., Madrazo, J. A., Ngamphaiboon, J., Ong, C., & Rogacion, J. M. (2017). Lactose intolerance and gastrointestinal cow's milk allergy in infants and children—Common misconceptions revisited. *World Allergy Organization Journal*, 10(1). Available from https://doi.org/10.1186/s40413-017-0173-0.

Ho, H. E., & Bunyavanich, S. (2018). Role of the microbiome in food allergy. *Current Allergy and Asthma Reports*, 18(4). Available from https://doi.org/10.1007/s11882-018-0780-z.

Holzapfel, W. H., Haberer, P., Snel, J., Schillinger, U., & Huis In'T Veld, J. H. J. (1998). Overview of gut flora and probiotics. *International Journal of Food Microbiology*, 41(2), 85–101. Available from https://doi.org/10.1016/S0168-1605(98)00044-0.

Horner, T. W., Dunn, M. L., Eggett, D. L., & Ogden, L. V. (2011). β-Galactosidase activity of commercial lactase samples in raw and pasteurized milk at refrigerated temperatures. *Journal of Dairy Science*, 94(7), 3242–3249. Available from https://doi.org/10.3168/jds.2010-3742.

Hsiao, K. C., Ponsonby, A. L., Axelrad, C., Pitkin, S., & Tang, M. L. K. (2017). PPOIT Study Team. Long-term clinical and immunological effects of probiotic and peanut oral immunotherapy after treatment cessation: 4-year follow-up of a randomised, double-blind, placebo-controlled trial. *The Lancet Child Adolescent Health*, 1(2), 97–105. Available from https://doi.org/10.1016/S2352-4642(17)30041-X, Epub 2017 Aug 15. Erratum in: Lancet Child Adolesc Health. 2017 Nov;1(3):e2. PMID: 30169215.

Ierodiakonou, D., Garcia-Larsen, V., Logan, A., Groome, A., Cunha, S., Chivinge, J., Robinson, Z., Geoghegan, N., Jarrold, K., Reeves, T., Tagiyeva-Milne, N., Nurmatov, U., Trivella, M., Leonardi-Bee, J., & Boyle, R. J. (2016). Timing of allergenic food introduction to the infant diet and risk of allergic or autoimmune disease a systematic review and meta-analysis. *JAMA—Journal of the American Medical Association*, 316(11), 1181–1192. Available from https://doi.org/10.1001/jama.2016.12623.

Jonkers, D., & Stockbrügger, R. (2007). Review article: Probiotics in gastrointestinal and liver diseases. *Alimentary Pharmacology and Therapeutics*, 26(2), 133–148. Available from https://doi.org/10.1111/j.1365-2036.2007.03480.x.

Kaci, G., Goudercourt, D., Dennin, V., Pot, B., Doré, J., Ehrlich, S. D., Renault, P., Blottière, H. M., Daniel, C., & Delorme, C. (2014). Anti-inflammatory properties of Streptococcus salivarius, a commensal bacterium of the oral cavity and digestive tract. *Applied and Environmental Microbiology*, *80*(3), 928–934. Available from https://doi.org/10.1128/AEM.03133-13, Epub 2013 Nov 22. PMID: 24271166; PMCID: PMC3911234.

Kalliomäki, M., Salminen, S., Arvilommi, H., Kero, P., Koskinen, P., & Isolauri, E. (2001). Probiotics in primary prevention of atopic disease: A randomised placebo-controlled trial. *The Lancet*, *357*(9262), 1076–1079. Available from https://doi.org/10.1016/S0140-6736(00)04259-8, PMID: 11297958.

Kapse, A. N., & Chandekar, C. J. (2020). Probiotic assessment of bacteria isolated from milk of domestic animals in prevention of enteric bacterial infections. *World Journal of Pharmacy and Pharmaceutical Sciences*, *9*(10), 2247–2256.

Kawase, M., He, F., Kubota, A., Hiramatsu, M., Saito, H., Ishii, T., Yasueda, H., & Akiyama, K. (2009). Effect of fermented milk prepared with two probiotic strains on Japanese cedar pollinosis in a double-blind placebo-controlled clinical study. *International Journal of Food Microbiology*, *128*(3), 429–434. Available from https://doi.org/10.1016/j.ijfoodmicro.2008.09.017, Epub 2008 Oct 7. PMID: 18977549.

Kimoto, H., Mizumachi, K., Okamoto, T., & Kurisaki, J. (2004). New Lactococcus strain with immunomodulatory activity: Enhancement of Th1-type immune response. *Microbiology and Immunology*, *48*(2), 75–82. Available from https://doi.org/10.1111/j.1348-0421.2004.tb03490.x, PMID: 14978331.

La Fata, G., Weber, P., & Mohajeri, M. H. (2018). Probiotics and the gut immune system: Indirect regulation. *Probiotics and Antimicrobial Proteins*, *10*(1), 11–21. Available from https://doi.org/10.1007/s12602-017-9322-6.

Lan, B., Yang, F., Lu, D., & Lin, Z. (2016). Specific immunotherapy plus *Clostridium butyricum* alleviates ulcerative colitis in patients with food allergy. *Scientific Reports*, *6*. Available from https://doi.org/10.1038/srep25587.

Lee, K. H., Song, Y., Wu, W., Yu, K., & Zhang, G. (2020). The gut microbiota, environmental factors, and links to the development of food allergy. *Clinical and Molecular Allergy*, *18*(1). Available from https://doi.org/10.1186/s12948-020-00120-x.

Leis, R., de Castro, M. J., de Lamas, C., Picáns, R., & Couce, M. L. (2020). Effects of prebiotic and probiotic supplementation on lactase deficiency and lactose intolerance: A systematic review of controlled trials. *Nutrients*, *12*(5). Available from https://doi.org/10.3390/nu12051487.

Magnúsdóttir, S., & Thiele, I. (2018). Modeling metabolism of the human gut microbiome. *Current Opinion in Biotechnology*, *51*, 90–96. Available from https://doi.org/10.1016/j.copbio.2017.12.005.

Martínez Vázquez, S. E., Nogueira de Rojas, J. R., Remes Troche, J. M., Coss Adame, E., Rivas Ruíz, R., & Uscanga Domínguez, L. F. (2020). Importancia de la intolerancia a la lactosa en individuos con síntomas gastrointestinales. *Revista de Gastroenterologia de Mexico*, *85*(3), 321–331. Available from https://doi.org/10.1016/j.rgmx.2020.03.002.

Massimo, D. M., Maddalena, S. M., Angelo, V., & Lia, G. (2019). Food allergies and ageing. *International Journal of Molecular Sciences*, 5580. Available from https://doi.org/10.3390/ijms20225580.

Özdemir, O. (2018). Role and use of probiotics in allergic diseases: Review of the literature. *İstanbul Medical Journal*, *19*, 95–104. Available from https://doi.org/10.5152/imj.2018.09735.

Plaza-Díaz, J., Ruiz-Ojeda, F. J., Vilchez-Padial, L. M., & Gil, A. (2017). Evidence of the anti-inflammatory effects of probiotics and synbiotics in intestinal chronic diseases. *Nutrients*, *9*(6), 555. Available from https://doi.org/10.3390/nu9060555, PMID: 28555037; PMCID: PMC549053.

Prochaska, L. J., & Piekutowski, W. V. (1994). On the synergistic effects of enzymes in food with enzymes in the human body. A literature survey and analytical report. *Medical Hypotheses*, *42*(6), 355–362. Available from https://doi.org/10.1016/0306-9877(94)90152-X.

Rao, R. K., & Samak, G. (2013). Protection and restitution of gut barrier by probiotics: Nutritional and clinical implications. *Current Nutrition and Food Science*, *9*(2), 99–107. Available from https://doi.org/10.2174/15734013113090200004.

Ren, J., Zhao, Y., Huang, S., Lv, D., Yang, F., Lou, L., Zheng, Y., Zhang, J., Liu, S., Zhang, N., & Bachert, C. (2018). Immunomodulatory effect of Bifidobacterium breve on experimental allergic rhinitis in BALB/c mice. *Experimental and Therapeutic Medicine*, *16*(5), 3996–4004.

Sarkar, R., & Banerjee, S. (n.d.). Gut microbiota in neurodegenerative disorders. *Journal of Neuroimmunology*, 15. https://doi.org/10.1016/j.jneuroim.2019.01.004. Epub.

Schepper, J. D., Irwin, R., Kang, J., Dagenais, K., Lemon, T., Shinouskis, A., Parameswaran, N., & McCabe, L. R. (2017). Probiotics in gut-bone signaling. *Advances in experimental medicine and biology* (Vol. 1033, pp. 225–247). New York LLC: Springer. Available from https://doi.org/10.1007/978-3-319-66653-2_11.

Shivaji, S. (2017). We are not alone: A case for the human microbiome in extra intestinal diseases. *Gut Pathogens*, *9*(1). Available from https://doi.org/10.1186/s13099-017-0163-3.

Smyth, E. C., Nilsson, M., Grabsch, H. I., van Grieken, N. C., & Lordick, F. (2020). Gastric cancer. *The Lancet*, *396*(10251), 635–648. Available from https://doi.org/10.1016/S0140-6736(20)31288-5.

Tan-Lim, C. S. C., & Esteban-Ipac, N. A. R. (2018). Probiotics as treatment for food allergies among pediatric patients: A meta-analysis. *World Allergy Organization Journal*, *11*(1). Available from https://doi.org/10.1186/s40413-018-0204-5.

Taylor, A. L., Dunstan, J. A., & Prescott, S. L. (2007). Probiotic supplementation for the first 6 months of life fails to reduce the risk of atopic dermatitis and increases the risk of allergen sensitization in high-risk children: A randomized controlled trial. *The Journal of Allergy and Clinical Immunology*, *119*(1), 184–191. Available from https://doi.org/10.1016/j.jaci.2006.08.036, Epub 2006 Oct 13. PMID: 17208600.

Vitellio, P., Celano, G., Bonfrate, L., Gobbetti, M., Portincasa, P., & De Angelis, M. (2019). Effects of bifidobacterium longum and lactobacillus rhamnosus on gut microbiota in patients with lactose intolerance and persisting functional gastrointestinal symptoms: A randomised, double-blind, cross-over study. *Nutrients*, *11*(4). Available from https://doi.org/10.3390/nu11040886.

Winkler, P., de Vrese, M., Laue, C., & Schrezenmeir, J. (2005). Effect of a dietary supplement containing probiotic bacteria plus vitamins and minerals on common cold infections and cellular immune parameters. *International Journal of Clinical Pharmacology and Therapeutics*, *43*(7), 318–326. Available from https://doi.org/10.5414/CPP43318.

Wosinska, L., Cotter, P. D., O'Sullivan, O., & Guinane, C. (2019). The potential impact of probiotics on the gut microbiome of athletes. *Nutrients*, *11*(10), 2270. Available from https://doi.org/10.3390/nu11102270.

World Gastroenterology Organisation. (2017). Global guidelines probiotics and prebiotics.

Wu, K. G., Li, T. H., & Peng, H. J. (2012). Lactobacillus salivarius plus fructo-oligosaccharide is superior to fructo-oligosaccharide alone for treating children with moderate to severe atopic dermatitis: A double-blind, randomized, clinical trial of efficacy and safety. *British Journal of Dermatology*, *166*(1), 129–136. Available from https://doi.org/10.1111/j.1365-2133.2011.10596.x, Epub 2011 Dec 6. PMID: 21895621.

Zhang, G. Q., Hu, H. J., Liu, C. Y., Zhang, Q., Shakya, S., & Li, Z. Y. (2016). Probiotics for prevention of atopy and food hypersensitivity in early childhood: A PRISMA-compliant systematic review and meta-analysis of randomized controlled trials. *Medicine (Baltimore)*, *95*(8), e2562. Available from https://doi.org/10.1097/MD.0000000000002562, PMID: 26937896; PMCID: PMC4778993.

Chapter 15

Probiotics in the prevention and treatment of nosocomial infections

Julie Kalabalik-Hoganson, Malgorzata Slugocki and Elif Özdener-Poyraz

School of Pharmacy and Health Sciences, Fairleigh Dickinson University, Florham Park, NJ, United States

15.1 Introduction

Nosocomial infections, also known as healthcare-associated infections, are defined as infections that are obtained during the process of providing health care to a patient and were not present at the time of admission. Nosocomial infections may develop in hospitals or other healthcare settings, such as long-term care facilities or ambulatory settings or even following discharge. Nosocomial infections may be associated with invasive procedures, indwelling medical devices, or prosthetic devices, and the type of infection is based on the source and type of pathogen (Sikora & Zahra, 2020). This chapter focuses on the use of probiotics for the prevention and treatment of three major nosocomial infections in adults and pediatrics: hospital-acquired pneumonia (HAP), ventilator-associated pneumonia (VAP), and *Clostridium difficile* infection (CDI).

15.1.1 Description of probiotics

The World Health Organization defines probiotics as live microorganisms that offer health benefits to a host when provided in adequate amounts (Alexandre et al., 2014). A microbiome is a collection of microbial genomes of a host, including bacteria, viruses, fungi, protozoa, and archae (Akrami & Sweeney, 2018). The health benefits of fermented milk products date back to the 1800s. The first genera of probiotic species used to treat disease were *Bifidobacterium* and *Lactobacillus acidophilus*. Those microorganisms were used to treat conditions, such as constipation, diarrhea, and eczema. In the 1930s *Lactobacillus bulgaricus* and *Streptococcus thermophilus* were tested as health-promoting bacteria, in the form of yogurt starters. They were found incapable of colonizing the human intestine, leading to questioning yogurt as delivery vehicle. It was around this time that *L. acidophilus* was discovered to also colonize the human colon (McFarland, 2015).

Probiotics are thought to provide a protective effect against pathogenic bacteria via three biological mechanisms: (1) direct antimicrobial activity, (2) epithelium barrier function reinforcement, and (3) immunomodulation (Alexandre et al., 2014). Probiotics may stimulate production of mucins, stabilize cell junctions, and decrease permeability. Their antimicrobial effects may be due to decreased luminal pH, production of bactericidal toxins, and competition for nutrition and adhesion (Bailey & Yeung, 2011). Since mucus is the first layer of defense in the intestines and the mucus layer may thin due to inflammation and allow penetration of bacteria, the ability of probiotics to increase mucin production and block pathogenic infiltration would be helpful in this setting. In addition, probiotic bacteria produce antimicrobial chemicals including organic acids (lactic, acetic, formic, propionic, and butyric), ethanol, hydrogen peroxide, bacteriocins, and short-chain fatty acids (Karacaer et al., 2017). Immunomodulatory effects may be due to the stimulation of phagocytes, cytokines, immunoglobulins, and increased epithelial recovery and apoptosis prevention (Bailey & Yeung, 2011). Probiotics are labeled based on genus, species, and strain. Each strain of probiotic may exert different health effects (Hill et al., 2014). Probiotic research suggests that the beneficial effects of probiotics can only be attributed to a specific strain or strains tested, and not to species (Guarner et al., 2012). Ideally, a probiotic candidate should satisfy five broad requirements: survival to the target, interaction with host systems, antipathogenic actions, safety, and manufacturing concerns. This has a number of implications, such as results reporting or documentation of dose-specific effects (Guarner et al., 2012).

Probiotics are available in various forms: foods, pharmaceuticals, dietary supplements, capsules, tablets, beverages, and powders (Bailey & Yeung, 2011). There is a significant amount of heterogeneity in probiotic species, doses, and routes of administration in the probiotic-published literature, making clear recommendations for their use complex (Blot et al., 2016; Virk & Wiersinga, 2019). Probiotics contain various microorganisms; most formulations are combinations of *Lactobacillus*, *Bifidobacterium*, and *Saccharomyces* species. Ingested probiotics must survive passage through the gastrointestinal tract, resisting gastric acid, bile salts, and digestive enzymes and successfully adhere to intestinal epithelium to exert pharmacological effect. In the United States, many probiotics are classified as dietary supplements, which means they do not require the approval of the US Food and Drug Administration (FDA) to be marketed and are available without a prescription (U.S. Department of Health and Human Services, 2020). An ongoing issue in this therapeutic category is the lack of validity of probiotic contents in commercial products (Sanders, 2008). The FDA uses their own terms for regulatory purposes; however, its authority over probiotic products is not meaningful and makes it difficult for consumers to select properly formulated and labeled products. The lack of a meaningful oversight also prevents probiotics from being included on hospital formularies or insurance reimbursement (Simpson et al., 2019).

With regard to safety, probiotics are considered overall safe on the basis of the assumption that some species, like *Lactobacilli* and *Bifidobacteria*, are normal residents of the human digestive system, and as such do not pose toxicity or infectivity risk (Guarner et al., 2012). Probiotics have been reported to carry the risk of causing systemic infection via bacterial translocation due to intestinal barrier defects. Risk factors for severe infection due to probiotics seem to be underlying immunodeficiency, debilitation, or chronic disease. In addition, it has been suggested relative contraindications to probiotic use are immunosuppression, central venous catheterization, and cardiac valvular disease, specifically for *Lactobacillus* species (Urben et al., 2014). Although not well studied, the risk of transferring antimicrobial resistance from antibiotic-resistance genes in probiotic isolates has been suggested (Bailey & Yeung, 2011). Critically ill patients are at higher risk for adverse effects of probiotics, which include sepsis, fungemia, and gastrointestinal ischemia. Although probiotics are generally safe for use, risks should be weighed against benefits before use in specific patient populations (Didari et al., 2014).

15.2 Hospital-acquired pneumonia and ventilator-associated pneumonia

15.2.1 Epidemiology, pathophysiology, and clinical presentation

Hospital-acquired pneumonia is defined as "pneumonia not incubating at the time of hospital admission and occurring 48 hours or more after admission." Ventilator-associated pneumonia is defined as "pneumonia occurring greater than 48 hours after endotracheal intubation." HAP refers to episodes of pneumonia not associated with mechanical ventilation (Kalil et al., 2016). The clinical presentation of HAP involves new lung infiltrate with clinical evidence of infectious origin and new-onset fever, sputum that is purulent, leukocytosis, and a decrease in oxygenation. The rate of HAP is 5–10 per 1000 hospital admissions (Nosocomial Infections—StatPearls—NCBI Bookshelf, n.d.). VAP presents similarly to HAP but in patients who have undergone endotracheal intubation. VAP is estimated to affect 10%–20% of patients receiving mechanical ventilation for greater than 48 hours (Nosocomial Infections—StatPearls—NCBI Bookshelf, n.d.). Microaspiration of pathogens around the endotracheal tube cuff in the trachea or build-up of biofilm on the endotracheal tube internal lumen and movement of pathogens toward distal airways contributes to the development of VAP (Coppadoro et al., 2019). Approximately half of HAP patients will develop serious complications including empyema, septic shock, and renal failure. VAP is associated with increased use of hospital resources and increased hospital length of stay. Some studies suggest VAP increases length of mechanical ventilation by up to 11.5 days and increases hospitalization by up to 13.1 days compared to patients without VAP. The cost associated with providing care for a VAP patient is approximately $40,000 per patient. Crude mortality rates associated with VAP range from 20% to 50% (Kalil et al., 2016; Shio-Shin et al., 2020). HAP and VAP antimicrobial treatment regimens target the organisms most implicated in these infections: *Staphylococcus aureus*, *Pseudomonas*, *Acinetobacter*, *Escherichia coli*, and *Klebsiella* species (Shio-Shin et al., 2020). In the setting of growing antimicrobial resistance and multidrug-resistant organisms, preventative strategies for nosocomial infections have been explored, including use of probiotics.

Bacterial communities, similar to those found in upper respiratory tracts, have been identified in alveoli and bronchioles, suggesting that microinhalation may lead to the colonization of lower airways. Ventilator-associated pneumonia involves respiratory and digestive tract pathogenic colonization, biofilms, and microaspirations of bacteria-contaminated secretions. The utility of probiotics in ventilator-associated pneumonia is based on two hypotheses:

competitive reduction in pathogenic bacteria in oropharyngeal and gastric environments in mechanically ventilated patients and immune system modulation (Alexandre et al., 2014).

The Society for Healthcare Epidemiology of America and Infectious Diseases Society of America released practice recommendations for preventing ventilator-associated pneumonia in acute care hospitals in 2014. The guideline recommended avoiding intubation if possible, minimizing sedation, minimizing patient transport while ventilated, using weaning protocols, improving physical conditioning, reducing secretion pooling above the endotracheal tube cuff, head of bed elevation, and maintaining ventilator circuits. The guidelines also note the potential role of selective oral or digestive decontamination, oral care with chlorhexidine, ultrathin polyurethane endotracheal tube cuffs, automated control of endotracheal tube cuff pressure, saline instillation before tracheal suctioning, and mechanical tooth brushing, although there is insufficient evidence to support these practices. Prophylactic probiotics are discussed in the guidelines as an option to possibly lower VAP rates in adults, although the authors state there is insufficient data on the impact of probiotics on mechanical ventilation duration, length of stay, and mortality (Klompas et al., 2014). Probiotics are not included in the 2016 clinical practice guidelines by the Infectious Diseases Society of America and the American Thoracic Society (Kalil et al., 2016).

15.2.2 Dysbiosis in critically ill patients

Critical illness affects composition and diversity of the microbiome, leading to dysbiosis. The microbiome of critically ill patients lacks microbial diversity and demonstrates a single taxon and loss of microbial site specificity. Studies support the fact that there is a shift in gut microbiota in critically ill patients compared to healthy controls, with an increase in bacterial genera that cause invasive disease and antimicrobial resistance. Critical care dysbiosis leads gut barrier dysfunction, cellular apoptosis, and translocation of pathogenic bacteria, potentially contributing to multiorgan dysfunction (Haak et al., 2017). Several factors affect the gut microbiome of critically ill patients including the use of opioids, vasoactive drugs, antibiotics, gastrointestinal prophylaxis agents, and nutrient deprivation. Although the duration and impact of critical illness dysbiosis is not yet known, it is predictive of clinical outcomes and mortality in critically ill patients (Akrami & Sweeney, 2018).

15.2.3 Probiotics in the prevention and treatment of ventilator-associated pneumonia in adults

The majority of literature available on nosocomial pneumonia and probiotics focuses on VAP and suggests that probiotics are associated with a reduced incidence of VAP. The studies are varied in the strains and species of probiotics studied and fail to demonstrate a reduction in mortality or length of stay. A Cochrane review of 8 studies with 1083 participants between the years of 2006 and 2011 provided evidence that probiotics reduce VAP incidence but do not affect other outcomes, such as mortality, ICU length of stay, or mechanical ventilation duration. The subgroup analysis failed to identify one superior strain of probiotic. Generalizability of the review findings was limited by differences in participants, types of probiotics used in the included studies, small sample sizes, and clinical and statistical heterogeneity (Bo et al., 2014). A randomized trial by Zeng et al. (2016) failed to demonstrate a benefit from a probiotic capsule containing *Bacillus subtilis* and *Enterococcus faecalis* in intubated patients in terms of the incidence of clinically suspected VAP, mechanical ventilation duration, hospital length of stay, or mortality. In a double-blind, concealed randomized, placebo-controlled trial of adult ICU patients mechanically ventilated for more than 48 hours, there was no difference in 28-day mortality rates, ICU mortality rates, or mortality at 90 days between the enterally administered probiotic (*Ergyphilus*, 2×10^{10} lactic acid bacteria, mostly *Lactobacillus rhamnosus* GG) once a day group and the placebo group. A reduction of 28-day mortality was observed in a prespecified subgroup analysis of severe sepsis patients; however, a higher mortality rate was associated with probiotics in nonsevere sepsis patients (Barraud et al., 2010). Morrow et al. evaluated the oropharyngeal and gastric administration of *L. rhamnosus GG* and VAP incidence in 146 mechanically ventilated patients. Patients who received *L. rhamnosus GG* were significantly less likely to develop VAP compared to placebo and less likely to develop *C. difficile*-associated diarrhea. Patients in the probiotic group also had shorter duration of VAP-indicated antibiotics. Adverse events associated with probiotics were not identified in this study (Morrow et al., 2010). A prospective, randomized, open-label controlled trial of 150 adult hospitalized patients expected to receive mechanical ventilation for 72 hours or longer evaluated the probiotic *Lactobacillus casei* compared to the control group. There was no difference in rates of VAP, length of hospital or ICU stay, mortality, or diarrhea in this study (Rongrungruang et al., 2015). In a prospective, double-blind, randomized trial of 100 adult critically ill patients who were mechanically ventilated for more than 48 hours, patients who received a probiotic preparation of *Lactobacillus*, *Bifidobacterium*, and *Streptococcus* species daily for 14 days had a lower incidence of microbiologically confirmed VAP, shorter duration of ICU stay, shorter duration of hospital stay, and less gastric residuals compared to the placebo group. Similar to other studies, there was no difference in ICU mortality and duration of mechanical ventilation between groups (Mahmoodpoor et al., 2019).

Another group of dietary substances that confer beneficial health effects on the host are prebiotics. Prebiotics are selectively fermented ingredients (usually nondigestible polysaccharides and oligosaccharides) that result in specific changes in the composition and/or activity of the gastrointestinal microbiota. Prebiotics affect intestinal bacteria by increasing the numbers of beneficial anaerobic bacteria and decreasing the population of potentially pathogenic microorganisms (Guarner et al., 2012). When a prebiotic is administered with a specific probiotic to enhance the engraftment and growth of that microbe, the combination is termed "synbiotic" (Mills et al., 2018). A randomized controlled trial evaluating daily *Bifidobacterium breve* strain Yakult, *L. casei* strain Shirota, and galactooligosaccharides versus no synbiotics in 72 mechanically ventilated ICU patients identified a lower incidence of VAP in the synbiotic group, with no difference in mortality between groups. The amount of *Bifidobacterium*, *Lactobacillus*, and organic acids was greater in the synbiotic group according to the fecal analysis (Shimizu et al., 2018). Of note, this study had several methodological limitations (Reisinger & Stadlbauer, 2019).

Chlorhexidine is an antiseptic that has been used to reduce the incidence of VAP as part of oral care in intubated patients. Chlorhexidine has been associated with bacterial resistance and hypersensitivity. Klarin et al. investigated the use of *Lactobacillus plantarum 299*, a probiotic bacterium that adheres to gastrointestinal mucosa and blocks pathogenic microorganisms, and how it compares to chlorhexidine for oral care in mechanically ventilated ICU patients. *L. plantarum 299* was as effective as chlorhexidine with regard to inhibiting the incidence of emerging pathogenic bacteria, and there were no adverse events reported with use of *L. plantarum 299*. VAP incidence was similar in both groups, although this study was not powered to detect a difference in this area (Klarin et al., 2018).

Several meta-analyses have been conducted on this topic and overall support a reduction in VAP incidence with probiotic use. Although there was no reduction in mortality, a meta-analysis by Gu et al. (2012) in 2013 revealed an association between probiotics and a reduction in incidence of nosocomial infections, VAP, and length of ICU stay among trauma patients. A systematic review and meta-analysis by Liu et al. in 2012 found probiotics significantly reduced nosocomial pneumonia rates [odds ratio (OR) = 0.75, 95% confidence interval (CI) 0.57–0.97, $P = .03$, $I^2 = 46\%$]. However, there was no significant difference for in-hospital mortality, ICU mortality, duration of hospital stay, or duration of ICU stay (Liu et al., 2012). A letter to the editor as a follow-up to this meta-analysis found no significant effect of probiotics on nosocomial pneumonia when a random-effects model was applied to the data, rather than a fixed-effects model as originally used by Liu and colleagues (Silvestri et al., 2012). A meta-analysis of five randomized controlled trials from 2013 did not find a significant decrease in the incidence of VAP due to probiotics [risk ratio (RR) 0.94, 95% CI 0.85–1.04, $P = .22$], although probiotics were associated with a decreased risk of VAP due to *Pseudomonas aeruginosa* (RR 0.30, 95% CI 0.11–0.91, $P = .03$) (Wang et al., 2013). A meta-analysis of 30 trials that included 2972 patients published in 2016 identified a significant decrease in infections with use of probiotics in critically ill patients (RR 0.80, 95% CI 0.68–0.95, $P = .009$, $I^2 = 36\%$), including VAP incidence (RR 0.74, 95% CI 0.61–0.90, $P = .002$, $I^2 = 19\%$). No differences in mortality, length of stay, or diarrhea were noted (Manzanares et al., 2016). With regard to specific strains of probiotics for VAP, a network meta-analysis of 14 parallel randomized controlled trials from 2006 to 2016 including 2036 patients demonstrated the combination of *Bifidobacterium longum*, *L. bulgaricus*, and *Streptococcus thermophiles* is more efficacious than *Ergyphilus* for preventing VAP. *L. rhamnosus* was found to be more effective than placebo. The most efficacious probiotic for reducing hospital and ICU mortality was Synbiotic 2000FORTE®. The authors found the most efficacious probiotic for preventing VAP is the combination of *B. longum*, *L. bulgaricus*, and *S. thermophiles*. This network meta-analysis shed light on the selection of probiotic strains for use in ICU, although significant heterogeneity among study protocols existed (Fan et al., 2019). The most recent meta-analysis conducted by Su and colleagues in 2020 included 14 studies involving 1975 subjects comparing probiotics with controls for VAP prevention. Probiotics were associated with decreased VAP incidence (OR 0.62, 95% CI 0.45–0.85, $P = .003$, $I^2 = 43\%$) among 13 studies in the meta-analysis; however, the finding was no longer significant when only including 6 double-blinded studies (OR 0.72, 95% CI 0.44–1.19, $P = .20$, $I^2 = 55\%$). Patients who received probiotics, based on two studies, received a significantly shorter duration of antibiotics for VAP (mean difference −1.44, 95% CI −2.88 to −0.01, $P = .048$, $I^2 = 30\%$). There were no significant differences in ICU mortality, ICU stay, duration of mechanical ventilation, or diarrhea occurrence (Su et al., 2020).

15.2.4 Probiotics in the prevention and treatment of ventilator-associated pneumonia in pediatrics

Infants are born with sterile gastrointestinal tracts but are quickly exposed to microorganisms starting with labor when the offspring ingests bacteria belonging to the mother (Manzoni et al., 2013). Bacterial colonization occurs rapidly and seems to be dependent on diet, gestational age, and mode of delivery (Armstrong, 2011). Babies that are born prematurely, or through cesarean section, or given antibiotics early on in life may have disturbances in the natural bacterial colonization process (Manzoni et al., 2013). A study by Gronlund et al. (2000) show that infants with health gut colonization with *Bacteroides* spp. have increased number of gut cells that produce IgA, IgG, and IgM in the first months of life. The mechanism for which probiotics prevent pneumonia is by reducing bacterial translocation into the lungs thereby decreasing bacterial load that causes infection Currently there are no guidelines regarding how and for what indication to use probiotics in pediatric patients (May & So, 2014).

The incidence of nosocomial infections in pediatric patients varies from 5% to 10%, most of them being gastrointestinal or respiratory infections (World Health Organization Report on the Burden of Endemic Health Care-Associated Infection Worldwide, 2011). Pediatric mortality attributed to nosocomial infections is estimated to be 11% (Richards et al., 1999). Probiotic use in pediatric patients has been studied for a wide variety of indications including acute gastroenteritis, prevention of antibiotic-associated diarrhea, prevention of nosocomial diarrhea, and respiratory tract infections in day care centers (Hojsak, 2017). There is a limited amount of studies that investigate the use of probiotics for HAP and VAP in the pediatric patient population (May & So, 2014).

Wang et al. (2014) investigated the utilization of probiotics in full-term infants who are critically ill. In this randomized study, 50 critically ill infants were given probiotics containing *L. casei*, *L. acidophilus*, *B. subtilis*, and *E. faecalis* three times a day for 8 days and 50 critically ill infants were given placebo. The dose of the probiotic was not mentioned. They found that patients that received probiotics had less cases of nosocomial pneumonia [8 (16%) vs 18 (36%); $P = .023$] and a shorter hospital stays (13 ± 3.5 vs 15.8 ± 5.3; $P = 0.03$) (Wang et al., 2014). The effects of *Lactobacillus* GG (LGG) at a dose of 10^9 colony-forming units (CFU) in 100 mL of a fermented milk product was studied in preventing nosocomial respiratory tract infections in pediatric patients in a randomized, double-blinded, placebo-controlled trial. There were 376 patients enrolled in the LGG arm and 366 patients enrolled in the placebo arm. There were less patients that developed respiratory tract infections in the probiotic arm [8/376 (2.1%) vs 20/366 (5.5%)]. The risk of respiratory tract infections were less in the probiotic arm compared to the placebo arm [RR: 0.38 (95% CI 0.18–0.85); NNT: 30 (95% CI 16–159)]. Patients in the placebo arm were found to be 3.17 times more likely to develop respiratory infections than the arm receiving probiotics (OR: 3.17, 95% CI 1.35–7.43). There was no difference between the arms regarding the duration of hospital stay (Hojsak et al., 2010).

An open-label randomized controlled study based in India by Banupriya et al. showed that prophylactic probiotic use can reduce the risk of VAP in sick children being treated in the pediatric intensive care unit. There were 150 children with a mean age of 2.9 years who were randomized into the probiotic group or the control group. Patients in the probiotic arm received capsules containing 700 million CFU of *L. acidophilus*, 400 million CFU of *L. rhamnosus*, 300 million CFU of *Lactobacillus plantaris*, 300 million CFU of *L. casei*, 300 million CFU of *L. bulgaricus*, 300 million CFU of *Bifidobacterium infantis*, 300 million CFU of *B. breve*, 400 million CFU of *B. longum*, and 300 million CFU of *S. thermophilus* equaling a total of 3.3 billion CFU of probiotics. Study subjects received probiotics twice daily for 7 days or until discharge, whichever was earlier. Results showed that the incidence of VAP in children in the probiotic arm was less than the control arm [12 (17.1%) vs 35 (48.6%); $P < 0.001$]. The mean duration of ICU stay and hospital stay were also lower in the probiotic arm (7.7 ± 4.60 vs 12.54 ± 9.91; $P < 0.001$), (13.13 ± 7.71 vs 19.17 ± 13.51; $P = 0.001$). The mean mechanical ventilation duration was 6.24 ± 3.24 in the probiotic group and 10.35 ± 8.87 in the control arm ($P = 0.001$). There were no probiotic-related adverse effects reported (Banupriya et al., 2015).

A study by Li et al. investigated neonates undergoing mechanical ventilation and pathogenic bacteria colonization in oropharynx and lower respiratory tract and the time it takes to develop VAP. Subjects were randomized to either the probiotic or control arm. Those in the probiotic arm received *Bifidobacterium*, *Lactobacillus*, and *S. thermophiles* at a total dose of 0.33 g/day. Subjects in the probiotic arm had less bacterial colonization of the oropharynx and lower respiratory tract (35% vs. 51%, $P < .05$). The time to VAP development was also delayed in those that received probiotics ($P < .05$). There were no adverse effects reported in patients receiving probiotics (Li et al., 2012).

The limited data that are available make it difficult to make a recommendation in favor of probiotic use for HAP or VAP in pediatric patients. The size of available studies is generally small and single-centered. A variety of probiotic species at differing doses and frequencies of administration are used in the trials. In addition, although all the study subjects are considered pediatric, there is a large age range among them making it difficult to make any targeted recommendations. More effort needs to be placed in investigating the use of probiotics for nosocomial respiratory infections in the pediatric patient population.

15.3 *Clostridium difficile* infection

15.3.1 Epidemiology, pathophysiology, and clinical presentation

C. difficile is recognized as the most common cause of infectious diarrhea in the healthcare setting. In 2010, the incidence of CDI has plateaued at about 500,000 cases annually in the United States, after a 10-year period of steady increase (Roecker & Bates, 2020). Although historically recognized as a nosocomial infection, it has become more prevalent in the community setting with an estimated number of 28% of cases being identified as acquired in the community (Roecker & Bates, 2020). A multicenter cohort study has reviewed records of 2,025,678 patients from a network of community hospitals between 2013 and 2017. The findings suggest a decreasing trend in healthcare facility-associated CDI, and an increasing proportion of cases classified as community acquired (Turner et al., 2019). The increased community prevalence of CDI has also been accompanied by an increase in morbidity and mortality associated with CDI. This development has coincided with the emergence of a previously rare strain of *C. difficile*, known as polymerase chain reaction ribotype 027, North American Pulse-field type 1, commonly referred to in literature as ribotype 027. This strain is characterized by causing more severe CDI outbreaks with an increased severity, refractory to traditional therapy, and a greater risk for relapse (Depestel & Aronoff, 2013).

Reports indicate that the incidence of CDI has also been increasing among hospitalized children across United States. A retrospective cohort study of hospitalized children evaluated CDI at 22 freestanding children's hospitals in the United States from 2001 to 2006. The annual incidence increased over the study period from 2.6 to 4.0 cases per 1000 admissions (Depestel & Aronoff, 2013). Data suggest that 26% of children hospitalized with CDI were infants younger than 1 year, and 5% were neonates. However, it is not certain whether these rates of hospitalization represent true disease or asymptomatic carriage. Asymptomatic carriage of *C. difficile* has been reported to be around 33% for patients aged 0–34 months (Schutze & Willoughby, 2013). It is generally more common in infants through the first year of age, and diminishes with age as lower intestinal microbiota becomes established (Sammons et al., 2013).

C. difficile is a gram-positive, anaerobic, spore-forming bacillus, which causes disease via toxin release. *C. difficile* colonization follows the disruption of normal colonic flora by antibiotics. Once colonization of *C. difficile* occurs, two toxins, A and B, are released to mediate diarrhea and colitis. The production and adhesion of toxins is essential for the disease to manifest. The major contributor to the pathogenicity of CDI is toxin A, an enterotoxin, that causes intestinal fluid secretion and injury to the intestinal mucosa. This injury is mediated via an inflammatory process that involves disaggregation of actin, intracellular calcium release, and damage to neurons. Toxin B is a nonenterotoxic cytotoxin that causes a stronger damage to the colonic mucosa than toxin A, through depolymerization of filamentous actin (Roecker & Bates, 2020). This process causes an endothelial damage in early stages of the disease, with small areas of necrosis in the surface epithelium. The secretion of neutrophils, nuclear debris, and other inflammatory elements leads to formation of pseudomembranes, white, and yellowish plaques that can become inflamed. Pseudomembranous plaques can be up to two centimeters in diameter and are initially scattered and dispersed around the areas of normal mucosa (Farooq et al., 2015). With progression of the disease, pseudomembranous plaques grow in size and can cover the entirety of the mucosa (Roecker & Bates, 2020).

Rates of disease are much higher among elderly and patients exposed to antibiotic agents (Roecker & Bates, 2020). Furthermore, due to an increase in the severity of CDI, many cases result in colectomies and death. In addition to ribotype 027, other genotypes have been reported to be associated with a more complicated disease outcome. Those include ribotypes 078/126, 056, and 018. Microbial factors attributed to increased virulence of these strains include mutations in the regulatory gene *tcdC* causing hyperproduction of toxins A and B, production of a binary toxin, antibiotic resistance, improved toxin binding to target cells, and mutations in surface layer proteins that increase *C. difficile*'s adherence to intestinal epithelium (Depestel & Aronoff, 2013).

Several patient risk factors have been identified as posing increased risk of acquiring CDI. Those include recent healthcare exposure, chemotherapy, patients undergoing gastrointestinal surgery or receiving tube feedings, impaired immune response, and presence of underlying chronic comorbidities. Another postulated risk factor for the acquisition of CDI has been acid suppressive medication therapy. This association still needs confirmation via prospective, randomized trials. All antibiotics have been implicated in CDI, but the most likely ones are fluoroquinolones, clindamycin, carbapenems, and third/fourth generations of cephalosporins. The most common onset for CDI is during or shortly after the completion of antimicrobial therapy; however, onset can be delayed for ≥ 3 months (Roecker & Bates, 2020).

An ongoing challenge in the management of CDI is recurrence of symptoms. This can occur as a consequence of relapse of the original infection, or reinfection with a new strain from an outside source. It has been reported that 12%–24% of patients experience at least one recurrence, and the risk of further recurrences increases from 50% to 65% if a patient has had more than two prior episodes. The cause for CDI recurrence is not completely understood;

however, it does not appear to be a result of *C. difficile*'s resistance to standard antimicrobial regimen that is used to treat it. Several mechanisms have been postulated, including new or continued disturbances in gut microbiota, with subsequent loss of colonization resistance; persistence of *C. difficile* spores in the gastrointestinal tract; a defective host immune response to *C. difficile* and/or its toxins; or reinfection with a new strain (Depestel & Aronoff, 2013).

Risk factors for community-acquired CDI have not been fully assessed. Studies suggest a greater risk in smokers and those >50 years of age. *C. difficile* has been isolated from the environment in outpatient healthcare areas and day care centers, possibly serving as a reservoir for transmission. This suggests a possibility for an even greater transmission of *C. difficile* in the community as compared to hospital setting. Furthermore, exposure to household contacts with CDI and children less than 2 years of age could also serve as a reservoir for transmission, as these groups are known to be highly colonized with *C. difficile* (Depestel & Aronoff, 2013).

Pediatric and neonatal patient risk factors include increased length of stay and antibiotic treatment, formula feeding as opposed to breastfeeding, as well as vaginal birth due to possible vaginal colonization with *C. difficile* (Lees et al., 2016). It is worth noting that while the rates of CDI have increased in pediatric patients, the severity of the disease (e.g., colectomy and in-hospital deaths) has not increased as much as it has in adults (Antonara & Leber, 2016).

CDI presents with a scale of symptoms ranging from asymptomatic carriage to severe clinical disease. Most commonly, CDI manifests as mild or moderate diarrhea, rarely with blood or mucous. Additional symptoms include fever, abdominal cramps, as well as peripheral leukocytosis (Sammons et al., 2013). Severe colitis may result in paralytic ileus or toxic megacolon, which in effect may present with minimal or no diarrhea. Complications of severe colitis include dehydration, electrolyte disturbances, bowel perforation, hypotension, renal failure, sepsis, and death. Reports suggest that although severe CDI can occur among children, complications related to CDI are uncommon, occurring at a rate of 0%−12%. Recurrent episodes are associated with increased morbidity and mortality and rates of recurrence are similar among adults and children (Sammons et al., 2013).

In addition to intestinal manifestations of CDI, rare symptoms occurring outside of the intestines have been reported as well. Those include bacteremia, peritonitis, perianal abscess, surgical site infections, and musculoskeletal infections, including septic arthritis, osteomyelitis, reactive arthritis, and acute flexor tenosynovitis. In children, rare extraintestinal manifestations include rectal prolapse and hemolytic uremic syndrome (Sammons et al., 2013).

15.3.2 Probiotics in the prevention and treatment of *C. difficile* infection in adults

There are multiple mechanisms by which probiotics could affect the onset and course of CDI: consumption of vegetative *C. difficile* by probiotics, which has an inhibitory effect; counteracting germination of *C. difficile* spores; secretion of inhibitory compounds by probiotics, which counteract the activity of toxins A and B; or secretion of bacteroicins, microbial peptides secreted by probiotics. Other effects of probiotics that can inhibit *C. difficile* include altering pH, increasing mucosal IgA levels, and increasing mucin production. In addition to the genus and species of a probiotic, the particular strain is important as well as health benefits can be strain specific (Mills et al., 2018).

The use of probiotics has been studied for the prevention and treatment of CDI with conflicting results (Cho et al., 2020). The pace of research into probiotics has accelerated in recent years: in 2001−2005, more than four times as many human clinical trials on probiotics were published as in 1996−2000 (Guarner et al., 2012). It is important to note that meta-analyses performed before it was discovered that efficacy of probiotics was strain specific, were often flawed due to pooling of different probiotic strains or pooling different indications together (McFarland, 2015). A systematic review and meta-analysis of 31 randomized controlled trials including 8672 patients, have found probiotics to be effective for the prevention of *C. difficile*-associated diarrhea. The results suggest that the risk of *C. difficile*-associated diarrhea is reduced by 60% when probiotics are given with antibiotics. Trials enrolling participants at high risk for *C. difficile*-associated diarrhea saw an even higher benefit, with risk reduction of 70% (Goldenberg et al., 2018). Shen et al. conducted a meta-analysis of probiotic use for CDI prevention in hospitalized adults receiving oral or intravenous antibiotic therapy. In this study, four probiotic genera were evaluated, in various dosage forms: *Lactobacillus*, *Saccharomyces*, *Bifidobacterium*, and *Streptococcus*. Of the *Lactobacillus* genus, *L. acidophilus*, *L. rhamnosus*, and *L. casei* species were studied in a capsule and a drink formulation (Shen et al., 2017). *Lactobacillus* was also evaluated in combination with *Bifidobacterium* and *Streptococcus* genera. Daily doses of *Saccharomyces*, *Lactobacillus*, and *Lactobacillus* in combination with other species were 20 billion, 50 billion, and 30 billion CFU, respectively. Duration of therapy with probiotics varied from 14 to 21 days. In the studied trials, the timing of administration of probiotics ranged from 1 to 7 days after the first antibiotic dose. This meta-analysis demonstrated efficacy of probiotics in the study population, along with timely probiotic administration. This was demonstrated in other systematic reviews as well, but probiotic use has not been incorporated into the standard of care when prescribing antibiotics to hospitalized adults (Shen et al., 2017). The most likely reason is that the largest high-quality trial (PLACIDE) that evaluated the use of two probiotic genera in older adults has concluded that there is no evidence that probiotics were effective in preventing CDI (Allen et al., 2013).

Although evidence is limited, treatment of CDI with probiotics to improve symptoms and prevent recurrence has been observed to have a potentially beneficial effect. A meta-analysis of 31 randomized controlled trials showed that adjunct probiotics in patients with antibiotic-associated diarrhea reduced occurrences of severe diarrhea. Another, more stringent meta-analysis that included six randomized controlled trials has shown a reduced risk for recurrent CDI, but efficacy was only observed in two of the six trials. Thus there is a paucity of evidence supporting a role for probiotics in treating CDI and preventing recurrences as most studies have focused on prevention, subsequently excluding such patients (Ollech et al., 2016).

Supplementation with specific probiotics has been effective in preventing various negative outcomes, including antibiotic-associated diarrhea and CDI. Evidence seems to be most abundant on the combination of *L. acidophilus* CL1285, *L. casei* LBC80R, *L. rhamnosus* CLR2, Bio-K + , especially on its effectiveness in preventing CDI in healthcare settings (McFarland et al., 2018). The evidence on the effectiveness of *Lactobacillus*-containing preparations comes from randomized controlled trials as well as facility level interventions (Allen et al., 2013; Barker et al., 2017; Dudzicz et al., 2018; Hudson et al., 2019; Lahtinen et al., 2012; Łukasik & Szajewska, 2018; Nagata et al., 2016; Trick et al., 2018; Wong et al., 2014).

Bio-K + formulation acts to reduce the effects of CDI thanks to a number of properties: effective delivery to target organ, ability to survive in the gastrointestinal tract, good compatibility with antibiotics that are given to treat CDI, and effective mechanism of action (direct inhibition of *C. difficile* growth and *C. difficile* toxin neutralization). The formulation has been shown to have high survival rates in a simulated gastric fluid medium, as well as a higher concentration in the host stool (a surrogate for presence within the intestine). *L. casei* and *L. rhamnosus* also seem to be more resistant to vancomycin, while *L. acidophilus* is more susceptible. This is beneficial since antibiotics can significantly affect the viability of probiotics (McFarland et al., 2018).

Species of *Lactobacillus* and *Bifidobacterium* are also commonly used as probiotics, as are yeast *Saccharomyces cerevisiae* and some *E. coli* and *Bacillus* species. Those species are known to have a beneficial effect on the host and as such fulfill the scientific definition of a probiotic. Lactic acid bacteria, including *Lactobacillus* species, have a dual function because they can also serve as fermentation agents, conferring additional benefits on the host. Fermentation is a process by which a microorganism transforms food into other products, usually through the production of lactic acid, ethanol, and other metabolic end-products (Guarner et al., 2012).

TABLE 15.1 Probiotics for pediatric CDI and antibiotic-associated diarrhea.

Probiotics strain	Recommended pediatric dose	Specific indication
Single-strain probiotics		
Lactobacillus rhamnosus GG	$10^{10}-10^{11}$ CFU, twice daily	Treatment of acute infectious diarrhea
Saccharomyces boulardii, strain of *Saccharomyces cerevisiae*	200 mg, three times daily	Treatment of acute infectious diarrhea
Indian Dahi containing *Lactococcus lactis*, *Lactococcus lactis cremoris*, and *Leuconostoc mesenteroides cremoris*	10^{10} CFU of each strain, 2 or 3 times per day	Treatment of acute infectious diarrhea
S. boulardii, strain of *S. cerevisiae*	250 mg, twice daily	Prevention of antibiotic-associated diarrhea
L. rhamnosus GG	10^{10} CFU, once or twice daily	Prevention of antibiotic-associated diarrhea
Bifidobacterium lactis Bb12 + *Streptococcus thermophilus*	$10^7 + 10^6$ CFU/g of formula	Prevention of antibiotic-associated diarrhea
L. rhamnosus (strains E/N, Oxy and Pen)	2×10^{10}, twice daily	Prevention of antibiotic-associated diarrhea
L. rhamnosus GG	$10^{10}-10^{11}$ CFU, twice daily	Prevention of nosocomial pneumonia
B. lactis Bb12 + *S. thermophilus*	$10^8 + 10^7$ CFU/g of formula	Prevention of nosocomial pneumonia
Probiotic combinations		
Lactobacillus helveticus R0052 (CNCM I-1722) + *L. rhamnosus* R0011 (CNCM I-1720) in capsules or sachets	2×10^9 to 4×10^{10} CFU/day	CDI pediatric, adult

A study that assessed the ability of *L. plantarum* Inducia and the prebiotic xylitol has found this combination to inhibit the germination of *C. difficile* spores. Another study assessed the ability of four different *Bifidobacterium* strains to inhibit in vitro *C. difficile* growth when cocultured with various prebiotics. Researchers observed a reduction in toxicity when *B. longum* and *B. breve* were cultured in a cell line exposed to *C. difficile*, using oligofructosaccharides as prebiotics (Mills et al., 2018). Fermentation of oligofructose in the colon results in a number of physiologic effects, including increased number of bifidobacteria in the colon, increased absorption of calcium, and increased fecal weight (Guarner et al., 2012).

15.3.3 Probiotics in the prevention and treatment of *Clostridium difficile* infection in pediatrics

In the treatment of acute diarrhea in children, *L. reuteri* ATCC 55730, *L. rhamnosus* GG, *L. casei* DN-114 001, and *Saccharomyces boulardii* have been shown to reduce the severity and duration of diarrheal illness by one day. In the prevention of adult and childhood diarrhea, there is only suggestive evidence that LGG, *L. casei* DN-114 001, and *S. boulardii* are effective. In antibiotic-associated diarrhea, there is strong evidence of efficacy for *S. boulardii* or *L. rhamnosus* GG in adults or children who are receiving antibiotic therapy. One study indicated that *L. casei* DN-114 001 is effective in hospitalized adult patients for preventing antibiotic-associated diarrhea and *C. difficile* diarrhea (Guarner et al., 2012). Tables 15.1 and 15.2 present the specific probiotic strains, formulations, and doses used for the prevention and treatment of pediatric and adult CDI or antibiotic-associated diarrhea.

TABLE 15.2 Probiotics for adult CDI and antibiotic-associated diarrhea.

Probiotic strain	Recommended adult dose	Specific indication
Single-strain probiotics		
Enterococcus faecium LAB SF68	10^8 CFU, three times daily	Treatment of acute diarrhea
Lactobacillus paracasei B 21060 or *Lactobacillus rhamnosus* GG	10^9 CFU, twice daily	Treatment of acute diarrhea
Saccharomyces boulardii, strain of *Saccharomyces cerevisiae*	10^9 CFU per capsule of 250 mg, 2–6 capsules per day	Treatment of acute diarrhea
E. faecium SF68 in powder or sachets	10^8 CFU, three times daily	Prevention of antibiotic-associated diarrhea
S. boulardii, strain of *S. cerevisiae*	1 g or 4×10^9 CFU/day	Prevention of antibiotic-associated diarrhea
L. rhamnosus GG	10^{10}–10^{11} CFU, twice daily	Prevention of antibiotic-associated diarrhea
Lactobacillus casei DN-114001 in fermented milk	10^{10} CFU, twice daily	Prevention of antibiotic-associated diarrhea
Bacillus clausii (Enterogermina strains)	2×10^9 spores, three times daily	Prevention of antibiotic-associated diarrhea
Lactobacillus acidophilus CL1285 + *L. casei* LBC80R	5×10^{10} CFU, once or twice daily	Prevention of antibiotic-associated diarrhea
L. casei DN-114001 in fermented milk	10^{10} CFU, twice daily	Prevention of *C. difficile* diarrhea
L. acidophilus + *Bifidobacterium bifidum* (Cultech strains)	2×10^{10} CFU each strain, once daily	Prevention of *C. difficile* diarrhea
Oligofructose	4 g, three times per day	Prevention of *C. difficile* diarrhea
Probiotic combinations		
L. rhamnosus HN001 + *L. acidophilus* NCFM	10^9 CFU each, once daily	Prevention of *C. difficile* diarrhea
L. acidophilus CL1285 + *L. casei* LBC80R	5×10^9 CFU, once or twice daily	Prevention of *C. difficile* diarrhea
S. boulardii, strain of *S. cerevisiae*	2–3×10^9 for 28 days, followed for another 4 weeks	Prevention of *C. difficile* diarrhea
Lactobacillus helveticus R0052 (CNCM I-1722) + *L. rhamnosus* R0011 (CNCM I-1720) in capsules or sachets	2×10^9 to 4×10^{10} CFU/day	Prevention of *C. difficile* diarrhea
L. acidophilus CL1285 + *L. casei* Lbc80r + *L. rhamnosus* CLR2 in fermented drink or capsules (Bio-K +)	1×10^{11} CFU/day	CDI, antibiotic-associated diarrhea

15.4 Conclusion

The available literature highlights the volume of research that has been conducted in the area of probiotic use for the prevention and treatment of nosocomial infections. Most of the available evidence points to a definite benefit of probiotics for preventing CDI. Data from studies for HAP or VAP are conflicting but suggest a potential benefit for preventing VAP in adults. Challenges with interpreting and applying probiotic literature are the variability in VAP diagnosis definitions, lack of quality control of probiotic products used, and a large variety in probiotic species and strains, doses, combinations, and routes of administration studied. Although the current evidence available demonstrates a potential benefit of probiotics for VAP and CDIs, a general consensus on the optimal strain, dose, timing, and duration of therapy is less clear. More studies are needed to clarify the optimal dose, duration, and combination of strains according to the indication and patient population.

References

Akrami, K., & Sweeney, D. A. (2018). The microbiome of the critically ill patient. *Current Opinion in Critical Care*, *24*(1), 49–54. Available from https://doi.org/10.1097/MCC.0000000000000469.

Alexandre, Y., Le Blay, G., Boisramé-Gastrin, S., Le Gall, F., Héry-Arnaud, G., Gouriou, S., Vallet, S., & Le Berre, R. (2014). Probiotics: A new way to fight bacterial pulmonary infections? *Medecine et Maladies Infectieuses*, *44*(1), 9–17. Available from https://doi.org/10.1016/j.medmal.2013.05.001.

Allen, S. J., Wareham, K., Wang, D., Bradley, C., Hutchings, H., Harris, W., Dhar, A., Brown, H., Foden, A., Gravenor, M. B., & Mack, D. (2013). Lactobacilli and bifidobacteria in the prevention of antibiotic-associated diarrhoea and Clostridium difficile diarrhoea in older inpatients (PLACIDE): A randomised, double-blind, placebo-controlled, multicentre trial. *The Lancet*, *382*(9900), 1249–1257. Available from https://doi.org/10.1016/S0140-6736(13)61218-0.

Antonara, S., & Leber, A. L. (2016). Diagnosis of Clostridium difficile infections in children. *Journal of Clinical Microbiology*, *54*(6), 1425–1433. Available from https://doi.org/10.1128/JCM.03014-15.

Armstrong, C. (2011). AAP reports on use of probiotics and prebiotics in children. *American Family Physician*, *83*(7), 849–852. Available from http://www.aafp.org/afp/2011/0401/p839.pdf.

Bailey, J. L., & Yeung, S. Y. (2011). Probióticos para la Prevención de Enfermedades: Un Enfoque en la Neumonía Asociada a Ventilación Mecánica. *Annals of Pharmacotherapy*, *45*(11), 1425–1432. Available from https://doi.org/10.1345/aph.1Q241.

Banupriya, B., Biswal, N., Srinivasaraghavan, R., Narayanan, P., & Mandal, J. (2015). Probiotic prophylaxis to prevent ventilator associated pneumonia (VAP) in children on mechanical ventilation: An open-label randomized controlled trial. *Intensive Care Medicine*, *41*(4), 677–685. Available from https://doi.org/10.1007/s00134-015-3694-4.

Barker, A. K., Duster, M., Valentine, S., Hess, T., Archbald-Pannone, L., Guerrant, R., & Safdar, N. (2017). A randomized controlled trial of probiotics for Clostridium difficile infection in adults (PICO). *Journal of Antimicrobial Chemotherapy*, *72*(11), 3177–3180. Available from https://doi.org/10.1093/jac/dkx254.

Barraud, D., Blard, C., Hein, F., Marçon, O., Cravoisy, A., Nace, L., Alla, F., Bollaert, P. E., & Gibot, S. (2010). Probiotics in the critically ill patient: A double blind, randomized, placebo-controlled trial. *Intensive Care Medicine*, *36*(9), 1540–1547. Available from https://doi.org/10.1007/s00134-010-1927-0.

Blot, S., Torres, A., & Francois, B. (2016). Evidence in the eye of the beholder: About probiotics and VAP prevention. *Intensive Care Medicine*, *42*(7), 1182–1184. Available from https://doi.org/10.1007/s00134-016-4353-0.

Bo, L., Li, J., Tao, T., Bai, Y., Ye, X., Hotchkiss, R. S., Kollef, M. H., Crooks, N. H., & Deng, X. (2014). Probiotics for preventing ventilator-associated pneumonia. *Cochrane Database of Systematic Reviews*, *2014*(10). Available from https://doi.org/10.1002/14651858.CD009066.pub2.

Cho, J. M., Pardi, D. S., & Khanna, S. (2020). Update on treatment of Clostridioides difficile infection. *Mayo Clinic Proceedings*, *95*(4), 758–769. Available from https://doi.org/10.1016/j.mayocp.2019.08.006.

Coppadoro, A., Bellani, G., & Foti, G. (2019). Non-pharmacological interventions to prevent ventilator-associated pneumonia: A literature review. *Respiratory Care*, *64*(12), 1586–1595. Available from https://doi.org/10.4187/respcare.07127.

Depestel, D. D., & Aronoff, D. M. (2013). Epidemiology of Clostridium difficile infection. *Journal of Pharmacy Practice*, *26*(5), 464–475. Available from https://doi.org/10.1177/0897190013499521.

Didari, T., Solki, S., Mozaffari, S., Nikfar, S., & Abdollahi, M. (2014). A systematic review of the safety of probiotics. *Expert Opinion on Drug Safety*, *13*(2), 227–239. Available from https://doi.org/10.1517/14740338.2014.872627.

Dudzicz, S., Kujawa-Szewieczek, A., Kwiecień, K., Więcek, A., & Adamczak, M. (2018). Lactobacillus plantarum 299v reduces the incidence of clostridium difficile infection in nephrology and transplantation ward—Results of one year extended study. *Nutrients*, *10*(11). Available from https://doi.org/10.3390/nu10111574.

Fan, Q. L., Yu, X. M., Liu, Q. X., Yang, W., Chang, Q., & Zhang, Y. P. (2019). Synbiotics for prevention of ventilator-associated pneumonia: A probiotics strain-specific network meta-analysis. *Journal of International Medical Research*, *47*(11), 5349–5374. Available from https://doi.org/10.1177/0300060519876753.

Farooq, P. D., Urrunaga, N. H., Tang, D. M., & von Rosenvinge, E. C. (2015). Pseudomembranous colitis. *Disease-a-Month*, *61*(5), 181−206. Available from https://doi.org/10.1016/j.disamonth.2015.01.006.

Goldenberg, J. Z., Mertz, D., & Johnston, B. C. (2018). Probiotics to prevent Clostridium difficile infection in patients receiving antibiotics. *JAMA—Journal of the American Medical Association*, *320*(5), 499−500. Available from https://doi.org/10.1001/jama.2018.9064.

Gronlund, M. M., Arvilommi, H., Kero, P., Lehtonen, O. P., & Isolauri, E. (2000). Importance of intestinal colonisation in the maturation of humoral immunity in early infancy: A prospective follow up study of healthy infants aged 0−6 months. *Archives of Disease in Childhood: Fetal and Neonatal Edition*, *83*(3), F186−F192. Available from https://doi.org/10.1136/fn.83.3.f186.

Gu, W. J., Wei, C. Y., & Yin, R. X. (2012). Lack of efficacy of probiotics in preventing ventilator-associated pneumonia: A systematic review and meta-analysis of randomized controlled trials. *Chest*, *142*(4), 859−868. Available from https://doi.org/10.1378/chest.12-0679.

Guarner, F., Khan, A. G., Garisch, J., Eliakim, R., Gangl, A., Thomson, A., Krabshuis, J., Lemair, T., Kaufmann, P., De Paula, J. A., Fedorak, R., Shanahan, F., Sanders, M. E., Szajewska, H., Ramakrishna, B. S., Karakan, T., & Kim, N. (2012). World gastroenterology organisation global guidelines: Probiotics and prebiotics october 2011. *Journal of Clinical Gastroenterology*, *46*(6), 468−481. Available from https://doi.org/10.1097/MCG.0b013e3182549092.

Haak, B. W., Levi, M., & Wiersinga, W. J. (2017). Microbiota-targeted therapies on the intensive care unit. *Current Opinion in Critical Care*, *23*(2), 167−174. Available from https://doi.org/10.1097/MCC.0000000000000389.

Hill, C., Guarner, F., Reid, G., Gibson, G. R., Merenstein, D. J., Pot, B., Morelli, L., Canani, R. B., Flint, H. J., Salminen, S., Calder, P. C., & Sanders, M. E. (2014). Expert consensus document: The international scientific association for probiotics and prebiotics consensus statement on the scope and appropriate use of the term probiotic. *Nature Reviews Gastroenterology and Hepatology*, *11*(8), 506−514. Available from https://doi.org/10.1038/nrgastro.2014.66.

Hojsak, I. (2017). Probiotics in children: What is the evidence? *Pediatric Gastroenterology, Hepatology and Nutrition*, *20*(3). Available from https://doi.org/10.5223/pghn.2017.20.3.139.

Hojsak, I., Abdović, S., Szajewska, H., Milošević, M., Krznarić, Z., & Kolaček, S. (2010). Lactobacillus GG in the prevention of nosocomial gastrointestinal and respiratory tract infections. *Pediatrics*, *125*(5), e1171−e1177. Available from https://doi.org/10.1542/peds.2009-2568.

Hudson, S. L., Arnoczy, G., Gibson, H., Thurber, C., Lee, J., & Kessell, A. (2019). Probiotic use as prophylaxis for Clostridium difficile-associated diarrhea in a community hospital. *American Journal of Infection Control*, *47*(8), 1028−1029. Available from https://doi.org/10.1016/j.ajic.2018.12.018.

Kalil, A. C., Metersky, M. L., Klompas, M., Muscedere, J., Sweeney, D. A., Palmer, L. B., Napolitano, L. M., O'Grady, N. P., Bartlett, J. G., Carratalà, J., El Solh, A. A., Ewig, S., Fey, P. D., File, T. M., Restrepo, M. I., Roberts, J. A., Waterer, G. W., Cruse, P., Knight, S. L., & Brozek, J. L. (2016). Management of adults with hospital-acquired and ventilator-associated pneumonia: 2016 clinical practice guidelines by the Infectious Diseases Society of America and the American Thoracic Society. *Clinical Infectious Diseases*, *63*(5), e61−e111. Available from https://doi.org/10.1093/cid/ciw353.

Karacaer, F., Hamed, I., Özogul, F., Glew, R. H., & Özcengiz, D. (2017). The function of probiotics on the treatment of ventilator-associated pneumonia (VAP): Facts and gaps. *Journal of Medical Microbiology*, *66*(9), 1275−1285. Available from https://doi.org/10.1099/jmm.0.000579.

Klarin, B., Adolfsson, A., Torstensson, A., & Larsson, A. (2018). Can probiotics be an alternative to chlorhexidine for oral care in the mechanically ventilated patient? A multicentre, prospective, randomised controlled open trial. *Critical Care*, *22*(1). Available from https://doi.org/10.1186/s13054-018-2209-4.

Klompas, M., Branson, R., Eichenwald, E. C., Greene, L. R., Howell, M. D., Lee, G., Magill, S. S., Maragakis, L. L., Priebe, G. P., Speck, K., Yokoe, D. S., & Berenholtz, S. M. (2014). Strategies to prevent ventilator-associated pneumonia in acute care hospitals: 2014 update. *Infection Control and Hospital Epidemiology*, *35*(8), 915−936. Available from https://doi.org/10.1086/677144.

Lahtinen, S. J., Forssten, S., Aakko, J., Granlund, L., Rautonen, N., Salminen, S., Viitanen, M., & Ouwehand, A. C. (2012). Probiotic cheese containing Lactobacillus rhamnosus HN001 and Lactobacillus acidophilus NCFM® modifies subpopulations of fecal lactobacilli and Clostridium difficile in the elderly. *Age (Melbourne, Vic.)*, *34*(1), 133−143. Available from https://doi.org/10.1007/s11357-011-9208-6.

Lees, E. A., Miyajima, F., Pirmohamed, M., & Carrol, E. D. (2016). The role of Clostridium difficile in the paediatric and neonatal gut—A narrative review. *European Journal of Clinical Microbiology and Infectious Diseases*, *35*(7), 1047−1057. Available from https://doi.org/10.1007/s10096-016-2639-3.

Li, X. C., Wang, J. Z., & Liu, Y. H. (2012). Effect of probiotics on respiratory tract pathogen colonization in neonates undergoing mechanical ventilation. *Chinese Journal of Contemporary Pediatrics*, *14*(6), 406−408. Available from http://www.cjcp.org/EN/article/downloadArticleFile.do?attachType = PDF&id = 12832.

Liu, K. X., Zhu, Y. G., Zhang, J., Tao, L. L., Lee, J. W., Wang, X. D., & Qu, J. M. (2012). Probiotics' effects on the incidence of nosocomial pneumonia in critically ill patients: A systematic review and meta-analysis. *Critical Care*, *16*(3). Available from https://doi.org/10.1186/cc11398.

Łukasik, J., & Szajewska, H. (2018). Effect of a multispecies probiotic on reducing the incidence of antibiotic-associated diarrhoea in children: A protocol for a randomised controlled trial. *BMJ Open*, *8*(5). Available from https://doi.org/10.1136/bmjopen-2017-021214.

Mahmoodpoor, A., Hamishehkar, H., Asghari, R., Abri, R., Shadvar, K., & Sanaie, S. (2019). Effect of a probiotic preparation on ventilator-associated pneumonia in critically ill patients admitted to the intensive care unit: A prospective double-blind randomized controlled trial. *Nutrition in Clinical Practice*, *34*(1), 156−162. Available from https://doi.org/10.1002/ncp.10191.

Manzanares, W., Lemieux, M., Langlois, P. L., & Wischmeyer, P. E. (2016). Probiotic and synbiotic therapy in critical illness: A systematic review and meta-analysis. *Critical Care*, *20*(1). Available from https://doi.org/10.1186/s13054-016-1434-y.

Manzoni, P., De Luca, D., Stronati, M., Jacqz-Aigrain, E., Ruffinazzi, G., Luparia, M., Tavella, E., Boano, E., Castagnola, E., Mostert, M., & Farina, D. (2013). Prevention of nosocomial infections in neonatal intensive care units. *American Journal of Perinatology*, *30*(2), 81−88. Available from https://doi.org/10.1055/s-0032-1333131.

May, M. E., & So, T. Y. (2014). Overview of probiotics use in the pediatric population. *Clinical Pediatrics*, *53*(13), 1231−1238. Available from https://doi.org/10.1177/0009922813518427.

McFarland, L. V. (2015). From yaks to yogurt: The history, development, and current use of probiotics. *Clinical Infectious Diseases*, S85−S90. Available from https://doi.org/10.1093/cid/civ054.

McFarland, L. V., Ship, N., Auclair, J., & Millette, M. (2018). Primary prevention of Clostridium difficile infections with a specific probiotic combining Lactobacillus acidophilus, L. casei, and L. rhamnosus strains: Assessing the evidence. *Journal of Hospital Infection*, *99*(4), 443−452. Available from https://doi.org/10.1016/j.jhin.2018.04.017.

Mills, J. P., Rao, K., & Young, V. B. (2018). Probiotics for prevention of Clostridium difficile infection. *Current Opinion in Gastroenterology*, *34*(1), 3−10. Available from https://doi.org/10.1097/MOG.0000000000000410.

Morrow, L. E., Kollef, M. H., & Casale, T. B. (2010). Probiotic prophylaxis of ventilator-associated pneumonia: A blinded, randomized, controlled trial. *American Journal of Respiratory and Critical Care Medicine*, *182*(8), 1058−1064. Available from https://doi.org/10.1164/rccm.200912-1853OC.

Nagata, S., Asahara, T., Wang, C., Suyama, Y., Chonan, O., Takano, K., Daibou, M., Takahashi, T., Nomoto, K., & Yamashiro, Y. (2016). The effectiveness of Lactobacillus beverages in controlling infections among the residents of an aged care facility: A randomized placebo-controlled double-blind trial. *Annals of Nutrition and Metabolism*, *68*(1), 51−59. Available from https://doi.org/10.1159/000442305.

Nosocomial Infections—StatPearls—NCBI Bookshelf. (n.d.). Retrieved (2020).

Ollech, J. E., Shen, N. T., Crawford, C. V., & Ringel, Y. (2016). Use of probiotics in prevention and treatment of patients with Clostridium difficile infection. *Best Practice and Research: Clinical Gastroenterology*, *30*(1), 111−118. Available from https://doi.org/10.1016/j.bpg.2016.01.002.

Reisinger, A., & Stadlbauer, V. (2019). Letter on \synbiotics modulate gut microbiota and reduce enteritis and ventilator-associated pneumonia in patients with sepsis: A randomized controlled trial\. *Critical Care*, *23*(1). Available from https://doi.org/10.1186/s13054-019-2319-7.

Richards, M. J., Edwards, J. R., Culver, D. H., & Gaynes, R. P. (1999). Nosocomial infections in pediatric intensive care units in the United States. *Pediatrics*, e39. Available from https://doi.org/10.1542/peds.103.4.e39.

Roecker, A., & Bates, B. (2020). Gastrointestinal infections and enterotoxigenic poisonings. In J. Dipiro, G. Yee, L. Posey, & S. Haines (Eds.), *Pharmacotherapy: A pathophysiologic approach* (11th ed.). McGraw-Hill. Available from http://accesspharmacy.mhmedical.com/content.aspx?aid = 1174444671.

Rongrungruang, Y., Krajangwittaya, D., Pholtawornkulchai, K., Tiengrim, S., & Thamlikitkul, V. (2015). Randomized controlled study of probiotics containing Lactobacillus casei (Shirota strain) for prevention of ventilator-associated pneumonia. *Journal of the Medical Association of Thailand*, *98*(3), 253−259. Available from http://www.jmatonline.com/index.php/jmat/article/viewfile/6041/5739.

Sammons, J. S., Toltzis, P., & Zaoutis, T. E. (2013). Clostridium difficile infection in children. *JAMA Pediatrics*, *167*(6), 567−573. Available from https://doi.org/10.1001/jamapediatrics.2013.441.

Sanders, M. E. (2008). Probiotics: Definition, sources, selection, and uses. *Clinical Infectious Diseases*, *46*(2), S58−S61. Available from https://doi.org/10.1086/523341.

Schutze, G. E., & Willoughby, R. E. (2013). Clostridium difficile infection in infants and children. *Pediatrics*, *131*(1), 196−200. Available from https://doi.org/10.1542/peds.2012-2992.

Shen, N. T., Maw, A., Tmanova, L. L., Pino, A., Ancy, K., Crawford, C. V., Simon, M. S., & Evans, A. T. (2017). Timely use of probiotics in hospitalized adults prevents Clostridium difficile infection: A systematic review with meta-regression analysis. *Gastroenterology*, *152*(8), 1889−1900. e9. Available from https://doi.org/10.1053/j.gastro.2017.02.003.

Shimizu, K., Yamada, T., Ogura, H., Mohri, T., Kiguchi, T., Fujimi, S., Asahara, T., Yamada, T., Ojima, M., Ikeda, M., & Shimazu, T. (2018). Synbiotics modulate gut microbiota and reduce enteritis and ventilator-associated pneumonia in patients with sepsis: A randomized controlled trial. *Critical Care*, *22*(1). Available from https://doi.org/10.1186/s13054-018-2167-x.

Shio-Shin, J., Yin-Chun, C., Wei-Cheng, L., Wen-Sen, L., Po-Ren, H., & Chin-Wan, H. (2020). Epidemiology, treatment, and prevention of nosocomial bacterial pneumonia. *Journal of Clinical Medicine*, 275. Available from https://doi.org/10.3390/jcm9010275.

Sikora, A., & Zahra, F. (2020). Nosocomial infections. [Updated 2021 Feb 10]. In: StatPearls [Internet]. Treasure Island (FL): StatPearls Publishing; 2021 Jan. Available from: https://www.ncbi.nlm.nih.gov/books/NBK559312/.

Silvestri, L., van Saene, H. K. F., & Gregori, D. (2012). Probiotics do not significantly reduce nosocomial pneumonia. *Critical Care*, *16*(6). Available from https://doi.org/10.1186/cc11654.

Simpson, M., Lyon, C., & Jarrett, J. B. (2019). Do probiotics reduce C diff risk in hospitalized patients. *Journal of Family Practice*.

Su, M., Jia, Y., Li, Y., Zhou, D., & Jia, J. (2020). Probiotics for the prevention of ventilator-associated pneumonia: A meta-analysis of randomized controlled trials. *Respiratory Care*, *65*(5), 673−685. Available from https://doi.org/10.4187/respcare.07097.

Trick, W. E., Sokalski, S. J., Johnson, S., Bunnell, K. L., Levato, J., Ray, M. J., & Weinstein, R. A. (2018). Effectiveness of probiotic for primary prevention of Clostridium difficile infection: A single-center before-and-after quality improvement intervention at a tertiary-care medical center. *Infection Control and Hospital Epidemiology*, *39*(7), 765−770. Available from https://doi.org/10.1017/ice.2018.76.

Turner, N. A., Grambow, S. C., Woods, C. W., Fowler, V. G., Moehring, R. W., Anderson, D. J., & Lewis, S. S. (2019). Epidemiologic trends in Clostridioides difficile infections in a regional community hospital network. *JAMA Network Open*, *2*(10), e1914149. Available from https://doi.org/10.1001/jamanetworkopen.2019.14149.

U.S. Department of Health and Human Services. (2020). Probiotics: What you need to know. National Center for Complementary and Integrative Health. Retrieved from https://www.nccih.nih.gov/health/probiotics-what-you-need-to-know.

Urben, L. M., Wiedmar, J., Boettcher, E., Cavallazzi, R., Martindale, R. G., & McClave, S. A. (2014). Bugs or drugs: Are probiotics safe for use in the critically ill? *Current Gastroenterology Reports*, *16*(7). Available from https://doi.org/10.1007/s11894-014-0388-y.

Virk, H. S., & Wiersinga, W. J. (2019). Current place of probiotics for VAP. *Critical Care*, *23*(1). Available from https://doi.org/10.1186/s13054-019-2325-9.

Wang, Y., Gao, L., Zhang, Y. H., Shi, C. S., & Ren, C. M. (2014). Efficacy of probiotic therapy in full-term infants with critical illness. *Asia Pacific Journal of Clinical Nutrition*, *23*(4), 575–580. Available from https://doi.org/10.6133/apjcn.2014.23.4.14.

Wang, J., Liu, K. X., Ariani, F., Tao, L. L., Zhang, J., & Qu, J. M. (2013). Probiotics for preventing ventilator-associated pneumonia: A systematic review and meta-analysis of high-quality randomized controlled trials. *PLoS One*, *8*(12). Available from https://doi.org/10.1371/journal.pone.0083934.

Wong, S., Jamous, A., O'Driscoll, J., Sekhar, R., Weldon, M., Yau, C. Y., Hirani, S. P., Grimble, G., & Forbes, A. (2014). A Lactobacillus casei Shirota probiotic drink reduces antibiotic-associated diarrhoea in patients with spinal cord injuries: A randomised controlled trial. *British Journal of Nutrition*, *111*(4), 672–678. Available from https://doi.org/10.1017/S0007114513002973.

World Health Organization. (2011). *Report on the burden of endemic health care-associated infection worldwide*. World Health Organization. Available from https://apps.who.int/iris/bitstream/handle/10665/80135/9789241501507_eng.pdf.

Zeng, J., Wang, C. T., Zhang, F. S., Qi, F., Wang, S. F., Ma, S., Wu, T. J., Tian, H., Tian, Z. T., Zhang, S. L., Qu, Y., Liu, L. Y., Li, Y. Z., Cui, S., Zhao, H. L., Du, Q. S., Ma, Z., Li, C. H., Li, Y., ... Wang, Y. P. (2016). Effect of probiotics on the incidence of ventilator-associated pneumonia in critically ill patients: A randomized controlled multicenter trial. *Intensive Care Medicine*, *42*(6), 1018–1028. Available from https://doi.org/10.1007/s00134-016-4303-x.

Chapter 16

Role of probiotics in urological health

Santosh S. Waigankar
Kokilaben Dhirubhai Ambani Hospital, Mumbai, India

16.1 Introduction

Even in this modern era of highly effective antibiotics and medical advances, urogenital infections are still among the most common reasons for a woman to consult a gynecologist or a urologist (Waigankar & Patel, 2011). An estimated one billion women around the world suffer from infections, such as bacterial vaginosis (BV), urinary tract infection (UTI), and yeast vaginitis (Reid & Bruce, 2003). The well-known association between abnormal vaginal microbial flora and its formidable risk in the increased incidence of UTI underscores the importance of understanding the microbial flora and its efforts to maintain it for ensuring urogenital health. The medical fraternity takes surprisingly urogenital infections less seriously. The increasing awareness among people regarding the entity and the available newer advanced treatment options has brought them into the limelight. The importance of restoring these depleting commensals with "probiotics" has resurfaced in a big way (Waigankar & Patel, 2011). In our daily practice as private practitioners, specialists, and super specialists, we come across many instances where the patients complain of loose motions after or during a course of antibiotics. We prescribe "Sporolac," which alleviates the symptoms. Once again, the Lactobacillus does the trick. Even the food industry has begun exploiting this "bug" through a variety of their products, for example, Probiotic-curd/yogurt, which is nothing but usual dahi fortified with the "probiotic bug" (Waigankar & Patel, 2011). Probiotics can be considered a promising alternative to antibiotics capable of displacing harmful bacteria through various mechanisms (Bustamante et al., 2020). This chapter focuses on probiotics for the prevention and treatment of infectious diseases occurring in the urogenital tract.

16.2 Vaginal microbiota

The microbial species inhabiting the vaginal tract play an essential role in maintaining health and preventing infection. These amount to 50 compared to the 800 species inhabiting the gut. Despite the proximity of the vagina to the anus, the different microbes present in the vagina are much lower than in the gut. The reason is still unclear. The present species in the vaginal mucosa vary between premenopausal women and those who have gone through menopause. The *Lactobacillus* species generally dominate microbial flora of a healthy premenopausal woman, the most common of which are *L. iners*, *L. crispatus*, *L. gasseri*, and *L. jenesenii*, followed by *L. acidophilus*, *L. fermentum*, *L. plantarum*, *L. brevis*, *L. casei*, *L. vaginalis*, *L. delbrueckii*, *L. salivarius*, *L. reuteri*, and *L. rhamnosus*. Various factors, such as hormonal changes (particularly estrogen), vaginal pH, and glycogen content, affect the *Lactobacilli* colonization in the vagina. The menstrual cycle can also cause hormonal changes (Antonio et al., 1999; Bertuccini et al., 2017; Burton & Reid, 2002; Cribby et al., 2008; Vasquez et al., 2002; Waigankar & Patel, 2011; Yoshimura & Okamura, 2001).

16.3 Commensal microbial flora and preventing UTI

The defensive role of *Lactobacillus* depends on multiple factors (Donders et al., 2000; Klebanoff et al., 1999; Reid & Bruce, 2001; Reid, 1999; Waigankar & Patel, 2011), namely: (1) Symbiotic relation with potential pathogenic organisms. (2) Capacity to produce antibacterial materials, such as H_2O_2, to restrict the growth of pathogens. (3) Producing biosurfactants that stop pathogen adherence. (4) Priming the macrophages, leukocytes, cytokines, and other host defenses3.

16.4 Scope of the problem

The number of women affected annually is high, and hence urogenital infections constitute a significant health problem. These being common in women are because the urethra is reasonably short and straight, making it easier for germs to spread into the bladder (Bustamante et al., 2020). The nonsexually transmitted urogenital infections include BV, UTIs, and yeast vaginitis (Reid & Bruce, 2003).

16.5 Urinary tract infection

Annually several hundred million women suffer from UTIs all around the world. The incidence of uncomplicated UTI in women is 0.5 episodes/person/year, with a recurrence rate of between 27% and 48%. The annual cost of healthcare services is staggering, reaching $2 billion in the United States alone and over $6 billion worldwide. Multiple risk factors predisposed to UTI include sexual intercourse with numerous partners and spermicidal agents' exposure (Foxman et al., 2000; Gupta et al., 2000; Hooton et al., 1996; Scholes, 2000; Waigankar & Patel, 2011). Spermicides lead to *Lactobacilli* loss and an increase in pH, which stimulates gram-negative organisms' growth and subsequent UTI (Waigankar & Patel, 2011). McGroarty demonstrated the impact of nonoxynol-9 on the development and adherence of urogenital bacteria and Candida. Additional risk factors found in postmenopausal women include a history of previous genitourinary surgery, altered bladder function, and estrogen loss (McGroarty et al., 1990). Stamm and Hooton reported *Escherichia coli* as the agent responsible in most cases (up to 85%), followed by *Staphylococcus saprophyticus* Enterococci (Desforges et al., 1993; Hooton et al., 1996). The incidence of asymptomatic bacteriuria increases with age. Krieger et al. found that 1%–2% of school-aged girls are afflicted, compared to 2%–5% of premenopausal women and 10%–15% of postmenopausal women (Krieger, 1986). The development of multidrug resistance has led to the emergence of milder prophylactic therapies to minimize the high cost of therapies (Akgül & Karakan, 2018). The effects of probiotics on UTIs remain controversial (Akgül & Karakan, 2018; Grin et al., 2013; Schwenger et al., 2015). Some evidence states that there is no benefit from probiotics administration (Schwenger et al., 2015). Other evidence shows a shortening of the average duration of illness and a considerable reduction of the infection rate (Akgül & Karakan, 2018; Borchert et al., 2008).

16.6 Bacterial vaginosis

BV is nothing but a vaginal inflammation caused by an imbalance of the vaginal flora with overgrowth of several bacterial species and decreased *Lactobacilli*. Women at reproductive age develop vaginosis more frequently. Falagas et al. (2007) and Fredricks et al. (2005) found that it manifests as an overgrowth of anaerobic or Gram-negative organisms, predominantly *Gardnerella vaginalis*, *Atopobium vaginae*, *Megasphaera* species, *Mycoplasma hominis*, *Mobiluncus* species, *Ureaplasma urealyticum*, *Prevotella*, and *Peptostreptococcus* species. The common symptoms, which the women present with, were malodorous vaginal discharge and sometimes vulvovaginal irritation (Livengood et al., 1990). It is known that *Lactobacillus* spp. produces lactic acid protecting the vagina from colonization by pathogens. When this balance is disturbed, *Lactobacillus* start decreasing or missing, and vaginosis occurs. Few investigators have tried to restore this imbalance of the vaginal flora by oral or vaginal administration of *Lactobacilli* and *L. acidophilus* seems to positively affect the prevention and treatment of BV (Falagas et al., 2007; Homayouni et al., 2014; Rosenstein et al., 1997). The mechanism of action of *Lactobacillus* remains unknown. Few in vitro studies highlighted reducing H_2O_2 and bacteriocins by specific *Lactobacillus* against pathogens involved in BV (Alvarez-Olmos et al., 2004) (Rosenstein et al., 1997). It is treated using different antibiotics, such as metronidazole, clindamycin, tinidazole, and secnidazole, administered orally or intra-vaginally (Menard, 2011). Administration of *L. acidophilus* and *L. fermentum* RC-14 for an extended period of 2 months is also found to be beneficial (Falagas et al., 2007; Homayouni et al., 2014). Study results have been encouraging for probiotics' effectiveness in preventing and treating vaginal imbalance in BV. But to understand the effect on preventing and treating vaginosis and by which strains, more robust studies or evidence is needed (Stavropoulou & Bezirtzoglou, 2020). Probiotics are found to be effective in preventing and treating vaginal imbalance in BV. Recent studies undertaken are certainly encouraging, but more research and clinical studies are necessary to prove the efficiency of preventing and treating vaginosis.

16.7 Yeast vaginitis

Yeast vaginitis is a prevalent problem. It is estimated to affect around 1:5 black American women and close to 1:10 white women (Foxman et al., 2000). The etiologies of this entity have been well studied. As with BV and UTI, the intestine is the primary source of the infecting fungal organisms. Disruption of the normal flora due to antibiotic abuse can lead to overgrowth in the vagina (Reid & Bruce, 2003). Symptomatology includes developing a white vaginal discharge characterized by its malodorous, nonhomogeneous caseous appearance, accompanied by vaginal and introital itch and irritation. Abbott showed that only 34% of patients with these classic symptoms had positive cultures, and hence there is a risk of over diagnosis (Abbott, 1995). This is also the most "self-diagnosed" condition by women leading to self-therapy and over-the-counter medications. Thus many women find themselves taking cyclical treatment. It is known that *Candida albicans* is the primary cause of infections (around 85%). Other yeasts, such as *Candida glabrata*, *Candida krusei*, and *Candida tropicalis*, also infect the host (Reid & Bruce, 2003).

16.8 Modes of administration of probiotics

There are three modes of administering probiotics in literature (Bustamante et al., 2020): (1) topical; (2) oral; (3) intravaginal; and (4) combination.

16.8.1 Topical application of probiotics or prebiotics

Investigators have done significant research in the topical mode of administration of probiotics. Zeng et al. (2010) compared the efficacy of a nonantibiotic sucrose gel with an antibiotic metronidazole gel to treat BV. In the 560 subjects evaluated, researchers concluded that sucrose gel could restore the normal vaginal flora and be used as a novel treatment for BV. Sucrose gel and metronidazole gel exhibited different mechanisms of action in treating BV. Sucrose gel causes a shift of vaginal bacterial flora, thereby promoting lactobacilli growth, which generates lactic acid that reduces the vaginal pH and secrete antibacterial substances, inhibiting the adhesion and replication of the pathogenic anaerobic bacteria. Metronidazole gel inhibits the growth of both the pathogenic bacteria and the beneficial lactobacilli. However, it is also believed that once the metronidazole gel treatment is complete, *Lactobacillus* will recover faster than the pathogenic bacteria because *Lactobacillus* is more resistant to metronidazole than anaerobic bacteria. Another triple-blind clinical trial (Khazaeian et al., 2018) showed that sucrose vaginal gel might be considered a possible alternative to metronidazole vaginal gel to treat BV. Hemmerling et al. (2010) evaluated the colonization efficiency, safety, tolerability, and acceptability of *L. crispatus* CTV-05 (Latin-V) administered by a vaginal applicator. The results showed that *L. crispatus* CTV-05 colonized 11 test group women at day 10 or day 28. The endogenous *Lactobacillus* flora at baseline line did not influence colonization. The product was well tolerated and accepted.

16.8.2 Oral administration of probiotics

Authors also researched traditional ways of taking medicines as a route of administering (Vujic et al., 2013), in a randomized, double-blind, multicentric, placebo-controlled trial, evaluated the efficacy of orally administered probiotics (*L. rhamnosus* GR-1 and *L. reuteri* RC-1) in 544 women older than 18 years of age diagnosed with vaginal infection. They concluded that Oral probiotics could be an alternative, side-effect-free treatment for one of the most common gynecology indications, combining the good aspects of both metronidazole and vaginal capsules. Petricevic et al. (2008) provide evidence for an alternative modality to restore the normal vaginal flora using specific probiotic strains administered orally. Heczko et al. (2015) showed that oral probiotics lengthened remission in patients with recurrent BV/AV and improved clinical and microbiological parameters. van de Wijgert & Verwijs (2020) evaluated the impact of vaginal probiotics on BV and vulvovaginal candidiasis (VVC) cure and recurrence, as well as vaginal microbiota composition and vaginal detection of probiotic strains. They found *Lactobacilli*-containing vaginal probiotics hold promise for BV cure and prevention, but not for VVC.

16.8.3 Intravaginal administration of probiotics

Pericolini et al. (2017) demonstrated that vaginal administration of probiotic *Saccharomyces cerevisiae* live yeast and, in part, inactivated whole yeast *S. cerevisiae*, used as postchallenge therapeutics, was able to positively influence the course of vaginal candidiasis by accelerating the clearance of the fungus. Their data showed for the first time that *S. cerevisiae*-based ingredients, particularly the living cells, can exert beneficial therapeutic effects on a widespread vaginal mucosal infection. De Gregorio et al. (2020) conducted a double-blind, randomized clinical trial to assess the safety of vaginal *Lactobacilli*-gelatine capsules vaginally administered to healthy, sexually active women. They found that subjects well-tolerated vaginal *Lactobacilli*-gelatine capsules so they could be proposed as an adequate alternative to restore vaginal *Lactobacilli* in sexually active women.

16.8.4 Combination therapies

Probiotics can also be administered in more than one route of administration. Their series concluded combining the recommended first-line therapies of oral metronidazole and vaginal clindamycin, or oral metronidazole with an extended-course of a commercially available vaginal-*L. acidophilus* probiotic does not reduce BV recurrence.

16.9 What does the evidence say?

In 2017 the Cochrane review (Braga et al., 2017) summarized that despite the marketing and the benefits associated with probiotics, there is little scientific evidence supporting the use of probiotics. The reviews did not provide any high-quality evidence for the prevention of illnesses through the use of probiotics. They further suggested more trials to understand probiotics better and confirm when their use is beneficial and cost-effective. Things have certainly changed since then, with more trials and meta-analysis done to look into probiotics' efficacy as an effective alternative treatment to prevent and treat urogenital infections in females. de Vrese et al. (2019) showed in their meta-analysis that oral intake of a probiotic product containing *Lactobacillus* strains either as yogurt or in capsule form might improve the microbial pattern in different forms of vaginal dysbiosis.

16.10 Conclusion

The current literature is inconclusive yet promising regarding probiotics for preventing UTIs since no large clinical trials have been performed. The existing clinical trial designs do not focus on precautions or clinical scenarios on using probiotics in severe UTI episodes warranting additional treatment. It is worth mentioning that until further research is completed, *Lactobacillus* probiotic strains, formulated as suppositories, may be considered but not definitively recommended. These probiotic suppositories could be regarded as a safe alternative to antimicrobials for UTI prophylaxis in high-risk women when antimicrobial resistance is the issue. Future RCTs should study these strains for a more extended period.

References

Abbott, J. (1995). Clinical and microscopic diagnosis of vaginal yeast infection: A prospective analysis. *Annals of Emergency Medicine*, 25(5), 587–591. Available from https://doi.org/10.1016/S0196-0644(95)70168-0.

Akgül, T., & Karakan, T. (2018). The role of probiotics in women with recurrent urinary tract infections. *Turkish Journal of Urology*, 44(5), 377–383. Available from https://doi.org/10.5152/tud.2018.48742.

Alvarez-Olmos, M. I., Barousse, M. M., Rajan, L., Van Der Pol, B. J., Fortenberry, D., Orr, D., & Fidel, P. L. (2004). Vaginal lactobacilli in adolescents: Presence and relationship to local and systemic immunity, and to bacterial vaginosis. *Sexually Transmitted Diseases*, 31(7), 393–400. Available from https://doi.org/10.1097/01.OLQ.0000130454.83883.E9.

Antonio, M. A. D., Hawes, S. E., & Hillier, S. L. (1999). The identification of vaginal Lactobacillus species and the demographic and microbiologic characteristics of women colonized by these species. *Journal of Infectious Diseases*, 180(6), 1950–1956. Available from https://doi.org/10.1086/315109.

Bertuccini, L., Russo, R., Iosi, F., & Superti, F. (2017). Effects of Lactobacillus rhamnosus and Lactobacillus acidophilus on bacterial vaginal pathogens. *International Journal of Immunopathology and Pharmacology*, 30(2), 163–167. Available from https://doi.org/10.1177/0394632017697987.

Borchert, D., Sheridan, L., Papatsoris, A., Faruquz, Z., Barua, J. M., Junaid, I., Pati, Y., Chinegwundoh, F., & Buchholz, N. (2008). Prevention and treatment of urinary tract infection with probiotics: Review and research perspective. *Indian Journal of Urology*, 24(2), 139–144. Available from https://doi.org/10.4103/0970-1591.40604.

Braga, V. L., Rocha, L. P. d S., Bernardo, D. D., Cruz, C. d O., & Riera, R. (2017). What do cochrane systematic reviews say about probiotics as preventive interventions? *Sao Paulo Medical Journal*, 135(6), 578–586. Available from https://doi.org/10.1590/1516-3180.2017.0310241017.

Burton, J. P., & Reid, G. (2002). Evaluation of the bacterial vaginal flora of 20 postmenopausal women by direct (Nugent score) and molecular (polymerase chain reaction and denaturing gradient gel electrophoresis) techniques. *Journal of Infectious Diseases*, 186(12), 1770–1780. Available from https://doi.org/10.1086/345761.

Bustamante, M., Oomah, B. D., Oliveira, W. P., Burgos-Díaz, C., Rubilar, M., & Shene, C. (2020). Probiotics and prebiotics potential for the care of skin, female urogenital tract, and respiratory tract. *Folia Microbiologica*, 65(2), 245–264. Available from https://doi.org/10.1007/s12223-019-00759-3.

Cribby, S., Taylor, M., & Reid, G. (2008). Vaginal microbiota and the use of probiotics. *Interdisciplinary Perspectives on Infectious Diseases*, 1–9. Available from https://doi.org/10.1155/2008/256490.

De Gregorio, P. R., Maldonado, N. C., Pingitore, E. V., Terraf, M. C. L., Tomás, M. S. J., de Ruiz, C. S., Santos, V., Wiese, B., Bru, E., Paiz, M. C., Reina, M. F., Schujman, D. E., & Nader-Macías, M. E. F. (2020). Intravaginal administration of gelatine capsules containing freeze-dried autochthonous lactobacilli: A double-blind, randomised clinical trial of safety. *Beneficial Microbes*, *11*(1), 5–17. Available from https://doi.org/10.3920/BM2019.0081.

de Vrese, M., Laue, C., Papazova, E., Petricevic, L., & Schrezenmeir, J. (2019). Impact of oral administration of four lactobacillus strains on nugent score—Systematic review and meta-analysis. *Beneficial Microbes*, *10*(5), 483–496. Available from https://doi.org/10.3920/BM2018.0129.

Desforges, J. F., Stamm, W. E., & Hooton, T. M. (1993). Management of urinary tract infections in adults. *New England Journal of Medicine*, *329*(18), 1328–1334. Available from https://doi.org/10.1056/NEJM199310283291808.

Donders, G. G. G., Bosmans, E., Dekeersmaecker, A., Vereecken, A., Van Bulck, B., & Spitz, B. (2000). Pathogenesis of abnormal vaginal bacterial flora. *American Journal of Obstetrics and Gynecology*, *182*(4), 872–878. Available from https://doi.org/10.1016/S0002-9378(00)70338-3.

Falagas, M. E., Betsi, G. I., & Athanasiou, S. (2007). Probiotics for the treatment of women with bacterial vaginosis. *Clinical Microbiology and Infection*, *13*(7), 657–664. Available from https://doi.org/10.1111/j.1469-0691.2007.01688.x.

Foxman, B., Barlow, R., D'Arcy, H., Gillespie, B., & Sobel, J. D. (2000). Candida vaginitis: Self-reported incidence and associated costs. *Sexually Transmitted Diseases*, *27*(4), 230–235. Available from https://doi.org/10.1097/00007435-200004000-00009.

Fredricks, D. N., Fiedler, T. L., & Marrazzo, J. M. (2005). Molecular identification of bacteria associated with bacterial vaginosis. *New England Journal of Medicine*, *353*(18), 1899–1911. Available from https://doi.org/10.1056/NEJMoa043802.

Grin, P. M., Kowalewska, P. M., Alhazzani, W., & Fox-Robichaud, A. E. (2013). Lactobacillus for preventing recurrent urinary tract infections in women: Meta-analysis. *Canadian Journal of Urology*, *20*(1), 6607–6614. Available from http://www.canjurol.com/html/subscriber/Spdf/V20I01/V20I1_05_DrGrin.pdf.

Gupta, K., Hillier, S. L., Hooton, T. M., Roberts, P. L., & Stamm, W. E. (2000). Effects of contraceptive method on the vaginal microbial flora: A prospective evaluation. *Journal of Infectious Diseases*, *181*(2), 595–601. Available from https://doi.org/10.1086/315267.

Heczko, P. B., Tomusiak, A., Adamski, P., Jakimiuk, A. J., Stefanski, G., Mikolajczyk-Cichonska, A., Suda-Szczurek, M., & Strus, M. (2015). Supplementation of standard antibiotic therapy with oral probiotics for bacterial vaginosis and aerobic vaginitis: A randomised, double-blind, placebocontrolled trial. *BMC Women's Health*, *15*(1). Available from https://doi.org/10.1186/s12905-015-0246-6.

Hemmerling, A., Harrison, W., Schroeder, A., Park, J., Korn, A., Shiboski, S., Foster-Rosales, A., & Cohen, C. R. (2010). Phase 2a study assessing colonization efficiency, safety, and acceptability of lactobacillus crispatus CTV-05 in women with bacterial vaginosis. *Sexually Transmitted Diseases*, *37*(12), 745–750. Available from https://doi.org/10.1097/OLQ.0b013e3181e50026.

Homayouni, A., Bastani, P., Ziyadi, S., Mohammad-Alizadeh-Charandabi, S., Ghalibaf, M., Mortazavian, A. M., & Mehrabany, E. V. (2014). Effects of probiotics on the recurrence of bacterial vaginosis: A review. *Journal of Lower Genital Tract Disease*, *18*(1), 79–86. Available from https://doi.org/10.1097/LGT.0b013e31829156ec.

Hooton, T. M., Scholes, D., Hughes, J. P., Winter, C., Roberts, P. L., Stapleton, A. E., Stergachis, A., & Stamm, W. E. (1996). A prospective study of risk factors for symptomatic urinary tract infection in young women. *New England Journal of Medicine*, *335*(7), 468–474. Available from https://doi.org/10.1056/NEJM199608153350703.

Khazaeian, S., Navidian, A., Navabi-Rigi, S., Araban, M., Mojab, F., & Khazaeian, S. (2018). Comparing the effect of sucrose gel and metronidazole gel in treatment of clinical symptoms of bacterial vaginosis: A randomized controlled trial. *Trials*, *19*, 585. Available from https://doi.org/10.1186/s13063-018-2905-z.

Klebanoff, S. J., Watts, D. H., Mehlin, C., & Headley, C. M. (1999). Lactobacilli and vaginal host defense: Activation of the human immunodeficiency virus type 1 long terminal repeat, cytokine production, and NF-κB. *Journal of Infectious Diseases*, *179*(3), 653–660. Available from https://doi.org/10.1086/314644.

Krieger, J. N. (1986). Complications and treatment of urinary tract infections during pregnancy. *Urologic Clinics of North America*, *13*(4), 685–693.

Livengood, C. H., Thomason, J. L., & Hill, G. B. (1990). Bacterial vaginosis: Diagnostic and pathogenetic findings during topical clindamycin therapy. *American Journal of Obstetrics and Gynecology*, *163*(2), 515–520. Available from https://doi.org/10.1016/0002-9378(90)91187-H.

McGroarty, J. A., Soboh, F., Bruce, A. W., & Reid, G. (1990). The spermicidal compound nonoxynol-9 increases adhesion of Candida species to human epithelial cells in vitro. *Infection and Immunity*, *58*. Available from https://doi.org/10.1128/IAI.58.6.

Menard, J. P. (2011). Antibacterial treatment of bacterial vaginosis: Current and emerging therapies. *International Journal of Women's Health*, *3*(1), 295–305. Available from https://doi.org/10.2147/ijwh.s23814.

Pericolini, E., Gabrielli, E., Ballet, N., Sabbatini, S., Roselletti, E., CayzeeleDecherf, A., Pélerin, F., Luciano, E., Perito, S., Jüsten, P., & Vecchiarelli, A. (2017). Therapeutic activity of a Saccharomyces cerevisiae-based probiotic and inactivated whole yeast on vaginal candidiasis. *Virulence*, *8*(1), 74–90. Available from https://doi.org/10.1080/21505594.2016.1213937.

Petricevic, L., Unger, F. M., Viernstein, H., & Kiss, H. (2008). Randomized, double-blind, placebo-controlled study of oral lactobacilli to improve the vaginal flora of postmenopausal women. *European Journal of Obstetrics and Gynecology and Reproductive Biology*, *141*(1), 54–57. Available from https://doi.org/10.1016/j.ejogrb.2008.06.003.

Reid, G. (1999). The scientific basis for probiotic strains of Lactobacillus. *Applied and Environmental Microbiology*, *65*(9), 3763–3766. Available from https://doi.org/10.1128/aem.65.9.3763-3766.1999.

Reid, G., & Bruce, A. W. (2001). Selection of Lactobacillus strains for urogenital probiotic applications. *Journal of Infectious Diseases*, *183*, S77–S80. Available from https://doi.org/10.1086/318841.

Reid, G., & Bruce, A. W. (2003). Urogenital infections in women: Can probiotics help? *Postgraduate Medical Journal, 79*(934), 428–432. Available from https://doi.org/10.1136/pmj.79.934.428.

Rosenstein, I. J., Fontaine, E. A., Morgan, D. J., Sheehan, M., Lamont, R. F., & Taylor-Robinson, D. (1997). Relationship between hydrogen peroxide-producing strains of lactobacilli and vaginosis-associated bacterial species in pregnant women. *European Journal of Clinical Microbiology & Infectious Diseases, 16*, 517–522. Available from https://doi.org/10.1007/bf01708235.

Scholes, D. (2000). Risk factors for recurrent urinary tract infection in young women. *Journal of Infectious Diseases, 182*(4), 1177–1182. Available from https://doi.org/10.1086/315827.

Schwenger, E. M., Tejani, A. M., & Loewen, P. S. (2015). Probiotics for preventing urinary tract infections in adults and children. *Cochrane Database of Systematic Reviews, 2015*(12). Available from https://doi.org/10.1002/14651858.CD008772.pub2.

Stavropoulou, E., & Bezirtzoglou, E. (2020). Probiotics in medicine: A long debate. *Frontiers in Immunology, 11*. Available from https://doi.org/10.3389/fimmu.2020.02192.

van de Wijgert, J. H. H. M., & Verwijs, M. C. (2020). Lactobacilli-containing vaginal probiotics to cure or prevent bacterial or fungal vaginal dysbiosis: A systematic review and recommendations for future trial designs. *BJOG: An International Journal of Obstetrics and Gynaecology, 127*(2), 287–299. Available from https://doi.org/10.1111/1471-0528.15870.

Vasquez, A., Jakobsson, T., Ahrne, S., Forsum, U., & Molin, G. (2002). Vaginal Lactobacillus flora of healthy Swedish women. *Journal of Clinical Microbiology, 40*(8), 2746–2749. Available from https://doi.org/10.1128/JCM.40.8.2746-2749.2002.

Vujic, G., Jajac Knez, A., Despot Stefanovic, V., & Kuzmic Vrbanovic, V. (2013). Efficacy of orally applied probiotic capsules for bacterial vaginosis and other vaginal infections: A double-blind, randomized, placebo-controlled study. *European Journal of Obstetrics and Gynecology and Reproductive Biology, 168*(1), 75–79. Available from https://doi.org/10.1016/j.ejogrb.2012.12.031.

Waigankar, S., & Patel, V. (2011). Role of probiotics in urogenital healthcare. *Journal of Mid-Life Health, 2*(0), 5–10. Available from https://doi.org/10.4103/0976-7800.83253.

Yoshimura, T., & Okamura, H. (2001). Short term oral estriol treatment restores normal premenopausal vaginal flora to elderly women. *Maturitas, 39*(3), 253–257. Available from https://doi.org/10.1016/S0378-5122(01)00212-2.

Zeng, Z. M., Liao, Q. P., Yao, C., Geng, L., Feng, L. H., Shi, H. R., Xin, X. Y., Li, P., Wang, H. L., Pang, Y. C., Liu, S. W., & Jiang, S. B. (2010). Directed shift of vaginal flora after topical application of sucrose gel in a phase III clinical trial: A novel treatment for bacterial vaginosis. *Chinese Medical Journal, 123*(15), 2051–2057. Available from https://doi.org/10.3760/cma.j.issn.0366-6999.2010.15.018.

Chapter 17

Role of probiotics in prevention and treatment of Candida vaginitis and Bacterial vaginosis

Adekemi Titilayo Adesulu-Dahunsi

Food Science and Technology Programme, College of Agriculture, Engineering and Science, Bowen University, Iwo, Nigeria

17.1 Introduction

Lactic acid bacteria (LAB) are known to colonize diverse environments and habitats. They have also been reported as part of the normal microflora that is found in the human mucosal surfaces such as the gastrointestinal tract (GIT), vagina, and oral cavity (Aureli et al., 2011; Pfeiler & Klaenhammer, 2007). The predominant LAB found in the human vagina are the *Lactobacillus* species; they are found to colonize the vagina of women of reproductive ages. *Lactobacillus* species exist as part of human microbiota where they help to fight off disease, thereby boosting the host immune system (Holzapfel et al., 2001). The lowering of pH in the GIT in humans is considered helpful in maintaining general health. Similarly, the broad spectrum of antimicrobial activity observed among LAB species, especially in the *Lactobacillus* species, has been reported; therefore, the antibacterial activity exhibited by these LAB species may be useful to control the undesirable microbiota in the GIT (Lavilla-Lerma et al., 2013; Patel et al., 2014). LAB strains produce different types of compounds; vitamins, bioactive peptides, and antibacterial compounds (LeBlanc et al., 2013; Li et al., 2014). Antimicrobial compounds produced by probiotic LAB are lactic acid, hydrogen peroxide, and bacteriocin thus causes pH reduction (Dortu & Thonart, 2009). The existence of beneficial LAB in the vagina has caused a reduction in the occurrence of sexually transmitted diseases (Reid et al., 2001). Research studies have shown that *Lactobacillus rhamnosus* and *Lactobacillus reuteri* that were isolated from some fermented foods reduces the risk of urinary tract infections in women by colonizing the vagina (Reid et al., 2001). LAB when consumed improves the GIT health, enhances the immune system and bioavailability of nutrients, reduces lactose intolerance symptoms in allergic patients, and reduces the risk of having cancer (Parvez et al., 2006; Saikali et al., 2004). There are several benefits that accompany the consumption of probiotics, as probiotics improve the intestinal health by the regulation of microbiota, development of the immune system, synthesizing and enhancing the bioavailability of nutrients, reducing symptoms of lactose intolerance, and reducing the risk of certain other diseases (Arshad et al., 2018; Castro-González et al., 2019; Forestier et al., 2001; Nagpal et al., 2012).

The Centers for Disease Control and Prevention estimated that the statistics of women in the world suffering from nonsexually transmitted vaginal infections such as Candida vaginitis (CV), Bacterial vaginosis (BV), and other yeast related infections around the globe is more than one billion (Kerry et al., 2018; Waigankar & Patel, 2011). And the commonly associated species with BV are *Gardnerella vaginalis*, *Ureaplasma urealyticum*, and *Mycoplasma hominis* (Hanson et al., 2016; Waigankar & Patel, 2011). An increase in the incidence of BV and CV or any form of UTI could be attributed to abnormal or unhealthy vaginal microflora. Antonio et al. (1999) assessed *Lactobacillus* species, colonizing the vagina of 300 women with the aid of vaginal swabs and inoculating in the appropriate medium, several strains of *Lactobacillus* (*Lactobacillus crispatus*, *Lactobacillus jensenii*, *Lactobacillus gasseri*, *Lactobacillus fermentum*, *Lactobacillus oris*, *L. reuteri*, *Lactobacillus ruminis*, *Lactobacillus vaginalis*) were isolated and identified from sexually active women using whole-chromosomal DNA probes to 20 American Type Culture Collection *Lactobacillus* strains. All the *Lactobacillus* species were qualitatively tested for hydrogen peroxide production on tetramethylbenzidine agar to know the potential benefits of these *Lactobacillus* species in women's vaginas and the species specificity of lactobacilli were also determined; more than 94 % of *L. crispatus* and *L. jensenii* isolates were found to produce H_2O_2, *L. crispatus* and *L. jensenii* were reported as the predominant vaginal lactobacilli. From their study, cases of women lacking H_2O_2-producing vaginal lactobacilli were reported to develop BV than the vagina colonized by these strains of *Lactobacillus*, thus they deduced that *L. crispatus* and *L. jensenii* has the potential to protect women from developing BV by inhibiting the growth of potential microbes that can result in this type of infection. Probiotic *Lactobacillus* has been extensively reported to be used in the effective treatment of BV. This chapter assesses the positive roles and evidence of the protective functions of probiotic *Lactobacillus*, and in the treatment of CV and BV.

17.2 Healthy vaginal microflora and probiotic lactobacilli

Probiotic lactobacilli are bacteria that are found in the human genital system without causing any harm to the host disease. Probiotics play a crucial role in the maintenance of vaginal health and the prevention of infections. Lactobacilli exist as abundance vaginal bacteria in women, by inhibiting the binding of other microbes to the epithelial cells through the production of lactic acid which kills or inhibits the growth of other bacteria that may be present around the vagina. The vaginal flora is the bacteria that live inside the vagina. The normal vaginal flora of humans is mainly dominated by *Lactobacillus* species. The antagonism feature displayed by probiotic lactobacilli has a protective influence on the vaginal mucosae. Several species of *Lactobacillus* have been reported to colonize women's vagina, these include; *Lactobacillus brevis, Lactobacillus casei, L. vaginalis, Lactobacillus delbrueckii, Lactobacillus salivarius, L. reuteri*, and *L. rhamnosus* (Kerry et al., 2018). Genus *Lactobacillus* is the largest group of family Lactobacteriaceae, they are nonspore forming, Gram-positive rods (Collins et al., 1991; Hammes & Vogel, 1995). Several *Lactobacillus* species have been isolated from different sources where they serve as probiotics (Adesulu-Dahunsi et al., 2018; Bautista-Gallego et al., 2013; Tham et al., 2012). *Lactobacillus* produces acid, hydrogen peroxide, and bacteriocins, and the species are among the most frequent microorganisms used as probiotic and may alter the microbiota of host by colonizing the GIT, various researchers have reported the beneficial effect of *Lactobacillus* on the health and wellbeing of humans (Castro-González et al., 2019; Ducrotté et al., 2012; Hempel et al., 2012; Wang et al., 2010).

Lactobacillus species perform the function of regulating and creating a healthy vaginal microenvironment, by creating an ambient temperature for the survival of beneficial microorganisms, once there is an alteration in the microbial composition of the vagina, the vaginal health will be compromised and may result in CV or BV. It has been recommended that the populations and numbers of the *Lactobacillus* species in human can be balanced by administering supplements from probiotics (Kerry et al., 2018; Waigankar & Patel, 2011). The presence of *Lactobacillus* species in the vagina performs important roles in the maintenance of a healthy vagina pH of around 4, this slight acidic environment helps protect against infection and invasion of any unwanted microorganisms and ensuring a healthy vaginal ecosystem (Miller et al., 2016). Clinical studies have revealed that the predominant microbe in human vagina is *Lactobacillus* species, and research has shown that the presence of H_2O_2-producing strains of *Lactobacillus* in the vagina has resulted in a decrease in the occurrence of gonorrhea, CV, BV, and other related infections (Cohen et al., 1995; Hawes et al., 1996; Royce et al., 1999; Sewankambo et al., 1997; Taha et al., 1999). Probiotic lactobacilli restore the natural balance of vaginal health. They alsoperform excellent roles in the maintenance of the natural balance of microflora in the vagina and are recognized as safe microorganisms without causing any harm to the host (Heravi et al., 2011).

17.3 Vaginitis (vaginal infection)

Vaginitis imply is a vaginal infection that results in inflammation of the vagina due to an imbalance in the vaginal microbial flora, this sometimes is accompanied by smell caused by bacteria, yeast, or viruses. The commonest examples of vaginitis/inflammation due to the overgrowth of bacteria or fungus are *Bacteria vaginosis* and *C. vaginitis*, these two types of vaginitis may not be because of sexually transmitted infection. Other types of sexually transmitted vaginitis include; *Chlamydia, Gonorrhea, Trichomoniasis*, and *Viral vaginitis*. Symptoms of vaginitis may include a change in the color of vaginal discharge with a very noticeable odor, burning feeling after urinating, swelling, soreness, or itching in the vagina. *C. vaginitis* and *BV* are the two most common causes of vaginitis which are related to the microorganisms that live in the woman's vagina. These two can have very similar symptoms. *C. vaginitis* is yeast infections caused by the overgrowth of the yeast in the body, while BV occurs when there is imbalance in the number of bacteria (Lactobacilli) (Miller et al., 2016). The vaginal microbiota of BV infected humans would have a reduced number of lactobacilli as compared with a healthy person.

BV results from the changes in the normal balance of the vaginal flora, and sometimes the symptoms in women are not pronounced, some of the symptoms include; burning sensation when urinating, a fishy smell that gets stronger after having sex, itching in the vagina, and thin discharges from the vagina which may be in different colors. *Lactobacillus* species can keep the vagina slightly acidic, by so inhibiting the growth of the bad bacteria, so, therefore, lactobacilli levels in the vagina must be maintained. Studies have reported the synergism between *G. vaginalis* with other bacteria in causing BV, some of these bacteria include; *Prevotella, Mobiluncus, Bacteroides, Peptostreptococcus, Fusobacterium, Veillonella, Eubacterium*. Other types of bacteria that have been reportedly associated with BV are; *M. hominis, U. urealyticum, Streptococcus viridans*, and *Atopobium vaginae* (Mulu et al., 2015). Several behaviors that can upset the natural balance of *Lactobacillus* species in women's vagina includes; douching, use of scented soaps/detergents, bubble baths, use of vaginal deodorants, sitting on public toilets, swimming pools, oral or anal sex, and having multiple sex partners, all these activities predisposes women to have BV and CV by altering the vagina pH/acidity level.

17.4 Probiotic roles in the prevention and treatment of vaginal infection

The predominance of lactobacilli in the human vaginal microbiota has been reported since the 1800s, as the pH of the vagina is 4 which makes it inhibitory to other pathogenic microorganisms that may be associated with vaginal microflora (Martin et al., 2008). Parvez et al. (2006) described the application of probiotics in the prevention and treatment of GIT infections (Parvez et al., 2006). Some LAB strains have found their applications as probiotic, as they confer health-promoting effects on humans. Health-promoting effects of probiotics include: antagonism, pathogen interference, anticarcinogenic and antimutagenic activities, modulations of the immune system, reduction in lactose intolerance and cholesterol levels, reduction in the incidence of diarrhea, and prevention of urinary tract infections (Bansal et al., 2016; Vidhyalakshmi et al., 2016). Since the healthy microbial flora of women's vaginas is predominated by *Lactobacillus* species, the use of probiotics to preserve vaginal health and treat any form of genital infection is essential. Recently, research has shown that microbes causing vaginal infections are becoming resistant to antibiotics and conventional drugs; thus, there is a need for the development of dietary supplements using nonpathogenic microbes, especially probiotics that will act against the pathogens and serve as an alternative to antibiotics, which have side effects. There are many functional attributes displayed by probiotics that make them desirable to serve as supplements for medicines and any type of antibiotics.

Probiotics are viable microorganisms that confer a beneficial effect on the host when adequate quantities are consumed (WHO, 2010). The roles and positive impact probiotics perform in the preservation of vaginal health is enormous. *Lactobacillus* species are found to primarily colonize women's vaginas, thereby preventing any form of bacterial or fungal genital infection in women (Ventolini, 2013; Ventolini & Sawyer, 2015). The contribution of probiotics in the prevention and treatment of urinary tract infections and other associated diseases is a rapid and evolving area of research in the past decades. Probiotics are effective agents for the treatment and prevention of vaginitis. The therapeutic effect of probiotic lactobacilli has been investigated in women having vaginal and urinary tract infections (Arshad et al., 2018; Parvez et al., 2006). It has been reported that the absence of vaginal lactobacilli in adult women would result in the development of BV. The inhibitory substances produced by vaginal lactobacilli serves as protection against infections because they can inhibit the growth of *G. vaginalis* in the vaginal epithelium.

Some probiotic lactobacilli are reported to be effective when administered orally or intra-vaginally, where they have been found to colonize the vagina and cure women with vaginitis, thus preventing re-occurrences. Several studies have reported the use of probiotic *Lactobacillus* for protection against CV and BV (Ventolini & Sawyer, 2015). In the treatment of CV, BV, and other forms of yeast infections, sometimes the bacterial populations return to normal proportions after treatment and sometimes, they do not. The potential use of required doses of probiotic *Lactobacillus* strains in the prevention and treatment of CV and BV has been widely reported (De Seta et al., 2014; Ehrstrom et al., 2010; Vicariotto et al., 2012). To be able to prescribe the appropriate dosage of probiotics for the treatment of any form of vaginal infection, the relationship among the vaginal microbiome must be well researched and understood (Ventolini & Sawyer, 2015). Mendling (2015) also reported the effectiveness of using an appropriate amount of probiotic LAB in the treatment of vaginal infection. Hawes et al. (1996) researched the production of inhibitory substances such as hydrogen peroxide by vaginal lactobacilli and the effectiveness of this *Lactobacillus* strain against BV, but not against CV. The effectiveness of the vaginal lactobacilli in the prevention and treatment of BV was also carried out by Abad and Safdar (2009).

Ventolini and Sawyer (2015) made some recommendations on the protective functions of probiotic vaginal lactobacilli against yeast infections; some of their recommendations are as follows: (1) the innate immune function of the vaginal epithelium is supported by the vaginal microflora; (2) the protective functions of the probiotic lactobacilli are species/strain specific as detected in *L. rhamnosus GR-1* and *L. reuteri RC-14*; (3) in the effective treatment of CV and

BV, the activities of the probiotic lactobacilli are synergistic; and (4) the use of probiotic lactobacilli in the treatment of BV can be achieved singly, while it may not be achieved when used to treat CV.

The in vivo assessment of resistance to intraperitoneal infection by *Candida albicans* was performed to examine the effect of a diet supplemented with probiotic *L. casei* and was administered to malnourished mice. The result of the study showed the mice that were fed with the supplemented feed had a high resistance to yeast infection, and they deduced that malnutrition decreases the production of several interleukins that were sensitive to infection, and the treatments given normalized the immune response to *C. albicans* (Villena et al., 2011). In the prevention and treatment of CV and BV, researchers have also recommended the usage of probiotics as an adjuvant (Morelli & Capurso, 2012; Petrova et al., 2015). Dietary probiotic supplementation of fermented foods, especially dairy food products, has been widely explored for use as probiotics in humans (Adesulu-Dahunsi et al., 2018, 2021). The clinical and nutritional evaluations have greatly helped the scientists in understanding specific roles performed by strains of probiotics. Some of these roles include regulation of energy in catabolic and anabolic processes, tolerance to acid and bile, adherence to the gut epithelial cells, ability to inhibit pathogenic microbes, safety-evaluations, and serviceability as beneficial supplements for human health. Extensive research studies in biomedicals and microbiology are being carried out to evaluate new strains of probiotics and these strains are being explored for improving human health, though some limitations and side effects that could result from their use are also being researched. The research studies conducted by Saleki et al. (2018) compared the use of clotrimazole alone and the administration of clotrimazole with probiotics in the treatment of CV and BV. The result of the treatments showed that clotrimazole, when used singly or with probiotics, are effective in the treatment of these diseases. The safety evaluation of using probiotics as adjuvant therapy in the treatment of vaginal infection in non-pregnant females was carried out, and it was deduced that probiotics lactobacilli can be effectively used to improve the short term clinical cure and mycological cure (Xie et al., 2017). BV can be effectively treated with probiotic *Lactobacillus* (Ventolini & Sawyer, 2015). The potential use of probiotics in the treatment of CV have been reported by researchers (De Seta et al., 2014; Ehrstrom et al., 2010; Vicariotto et al., 2012) *Lactobacillus* strains showing probiotic properties have also been recommended in the prevention and treatment of vaginal infection (Mendling, 2015). Probiotic lactobacilli can be used to stimulate the development of the good/ beneficial microorganisms, thereby ameliorating the effects of the pathogens which may cause infection in the vagina (Dunne, 2001; Gismondo et al., 1999). The use of probiotic *Lactobacillus* strains is effective in the prevention and treatment of any form of vaginal infections.

Well-characterized strains of *Lactobacillus* have been reportedly used to treat and reduce the risk of gastrointestinal infections in humans (Salminen et al., 2005). *Lactobacillus* from different sources, especially those from food origins have been successfully characterized to strain levels using different molecular biological tools (Adesulu-Dahunsi et al., 2017a, 2017b). Different vaginal *Lactobacillus* species have also been identified, using the polyphasic approaches; the predominant lactobacilli includes *Lactobacillus acidophilus, L. fermentum, Lactobacillus plantarum, L. brevis, L. jensenii, L. casei, Lactobacillus cellobiosus, Lactobacillus leichmanii, L. delbrueckii, L. gasseri, L. crispatus*, and *L. salivarius* (Levison et al., 1977; Nagy et al., 1991; Rogosa & Sharpe, 1960). *L. acidophilus* has not been isolated from various vaginal microflora studies up till date. Martinez et al. (2008) used culture-dependent and -independent approaches to examine vaginal Lactobacilli from healthy women and those infected with CV, the result of the analysis showed the presence of *L. crispatus*.

Vitali et al. (2007) studied the structure and dynamics of vaginal microflora in healthy women and those who had CV infection, using PCR-denaturing gradient gel electrophoresis (PCR-DGGE), real-time PCR universal *Eubacteriam* primers, and *Lactobacillus* genus-specific primers, their reports showed the dominance of *Lactobacillus* species in the healthy vaginal flora. In an in vitro analysis, *L. reuteri* and *L. rhamnosus* were found to inhibit yeast growth, the presence of the *Lactobacillus* species could play an essential role in vivo (Martinez et al., 2009a). Martinez et al. (2009b) performed a randomized, double-blind, placebo-controlled trial of the treatment of vaginitis using fluconazole with or without a 4-week treatment of probiotic *Lactobacillus*. After 4 weeks of treatment, the ones that were administered probiotics had less vaginal discharge with less associated symptoms, which suggested that probiotic augmentation in the treatments of vaginitis can improve associated symptoms.

17.5 Conclusion

The development and use of probiotics for the treatment of vaginitis are emerging rapidly because of the development of resistance towards the conventional drugs/antibiotics by the pathogenic microbes, which may have an adverse effect on the protective flora and even result in exposure to infection. Probiotics are tailored to confer health benefits when consumed; therefore, the ability of these probiotics to inhabit and maintain the normal vaginal microbiota has engineered them with the ability to resist any form of invader(s) that may likely penetrate the vagina. Several reports have documented the use of probiotic lactobacilli in the treatment of vaginitis. Vaginal infections occur as a result of an imbalance in the normal vaginal microbiota, which is characterized by a decrease in the number of lactobacilli present in the vagina and a concomitant overgrowth of the *Candida* species, though, several treatments using antifungal drugs such as clindamycin and metronidazole has been administered for the treatment and clinal cure of CV and BV, but due to the increase in the resistance to these conventional drugs and usual reoccurrence of vaginitis, probiotic has been successfully employed in the treatment and prevention of any form of GIT infections as the probiotic pills have no side effect whatsoever and have shown to possess some exceptional properties. Vaginitis can be prevented by maintaining good personal hygiene and keeping the vagina clean and dry. Consumption of fermented foods and dairy products such as cheese and yogurt with active cultures will also be recommended to keep and maintain a healthy vagina.

References

Abad, C. L., & Safdar, N. (2009). The role of *Lactobacillus probiotics* in the treatment or prevention of urogenital infections—A systematic review. *Journal of Chemotherapy, 21*(3), 243—252.

Adesulu-Dahunsi, A. T., Jeyaram, K., & Sanni, A. I. (2018). Probiotic and technological properties of exopolysaccharide producing lactic acid bacteria isolated from some cereal-based Nigerian indigenous fermented food products. *Food Control, 92*, 225—231.

Adesulu-Dahunsi, A. T., Sanni, A. I., & Jeyaram, K. (2017a). Rapid differentiation among Lactobacillus, Pediococcus and Weissella species from some Nigerian indigenous fermented foods. *LWT Food Science and Technology, 77*, 39—44.

Adesulu-Dahunsi, A. T., Sanni, A. I., & Jeyaram, K. (2021). Diversity and technological characterization of *Pediococcus pentosaceus* strains isolated from Nigerian traditional fermented foods. *LWT Food Science and Technology, 140*, 110697.

Adesulu-Dahunsi, A. T., Sanni, A. I., Jeyaram, K., & Banwo, K. (2017b). Genetic diversity of *Lactobacillus plantarum* strains from selected indigenous fermented foods in Nigeria. *LWT Food Science and Technology, 82*, 199—206.

Antonio, A. D., Hawes, S. E., & Hillier, S. L. (1999). The identification of vaginal Lactobacillus species and the demographic and microbiologic characteristics of women colonized by these species. *Journal of Infectious Diseases, 180*, 1950—1956.

Arshad, F., Mehmood, R., Rubina, K., Hussain, S., Khan, A., & Farooq, O. (2018). Lactobacilli as probiotics and their isolation from different sources. *British Journal of Research, 5*(3), 43.

Aureli, P., Capurso, L., Castellazzi, A. M., Clerici, M., Giovannini, M., Morelli, L., & Zuccotti, G. V. (2011). Probiotics and health: An evidence-based review. *Pharmaceutical Research, 63*, 366—376.

Bansal, S., Mangal, M., Sharma, S. K., Yadav, D. N., & Gupta, R. K. (2016). Optimization of process conditions for developing yoghurt like probiotic product from peanut. *LWT Food Science and Technology, 73*, 6—12.

Bautista-Gallego, J., Arroyo-Lopez, F. N., Rantsiou, K., Jimenez-Dıaz, R., Garrido-Fernandez, A., & Cocolin, L. (2013). Screening of lactic acid bacteria isolated from fermented table olives with probiotic potential. *Food Research International, 50*, 135—142.

Castro-González, J. M., Castro, P., Sandoval, H., & Castro-Sandoval, D. (2019). Probiotic lactobacilli precautions. *Frontiers in Microbiology, 10*, 375.

Cohen, C. R., Duerr, A., Pruithinithada, H., et al. (1995). Bacterial vaginosis and HIV seroprevalence among female commercial sex workers in Chiang Mai, Thailand. *AIDS (London, England), 9*, 1093—1097.

Collins, M. D., Rodrigues, U., Aguirre, M., Farrow, J. A., Martinez- Murcia, A., Philips, B. A., Williams, A. M., & Wallbanks, S. (1991). Phylogeneticanalysis of the genus Lactobacillus and related lactic acid bacteria as determined by reverse transcriptase sequencing of 16S rRNA. *FEMS Microbiology Letters, 77*, 5—12.

De Seta, F., Parazzini, F., De Leo, R., Banco, R., Maso, G. P., De Santo, D., et al. (2014). Lactobacillus plantarum P17630 for preventing *Candida vaginitis* recurrence: A retrospective comparative study. *European Journal of Obstetrics & Gynecology and Reproductive Biology, 182*, 136—139.

Dortu, C., & Thonart, P. H. (2009). Les bactériocines des bactéries lactiques: Caractéristiques et interest pour la bi-conversation des produits alimentaires. *Biotechnology, Agronomy and Society and Environment, 13*, 143—154.

Ducrotté, P., Sawant, P., & Jayanthi, V. (2012). Clinical trial: *Lactobacillus plantarum* 299v (DSM 9843) improves symptoms of irritable bowel syndrome. *World Journal of Gastroenterology: WJG, 18*, 4012—4018.

Dunne, R. (2001). Adaptation of bacteria to the intestinal niche: Probiotics and gut disorder. *Inflammatory Bowel Diseases, 7*, 136—145.

Ehrstrom, S., Daroczy, K., Rylander, E., Samuelsson, C., Johannesson, U., Anzén, B., et al. (2010). Lactic acid bacteria colonization and clinical outcome after probiotic supplementation in conventionally treated bacterial vaginosis and vulvovaginal candidiasis. *Microbes and Infection/Institut Pasteur, 12*, 691—699.

Forestier, C., De Champs, C., Vatoux, C., & Joly, B. (2001). Probiotic activities of *Lactobacillus casei* rhamnosus: In-vitro adherence to intestinal cells and antimicrobial properties. *Research in Microbiology, 152*, 167—173.

Gismondo, M. R., Drago, L., & Lombardi, A. (1999). Review of probiotics available to modify gastrointestinal flora. *International Journal of Antimicrobial Agents, 12*, 287—292.

Hammes, W. P., & Vogel, R. F. (1995). The genus Lactobacillus. In B. J. B. Wood, & W. H. Holzapfel (Eds.), *The genera of lactic acid bacteria. The lactic acid bacteria* (Vol. 2, pp. 19—52). Glasgow, United Kingdom: Chapman and Hall.

Hanson, L., Vusse, L. V., Jerme, M., Abad, C. L., & Safdar, N. (2016). Probiotics for treatment and prevention of urogenital infections in women: A systematic review. *Journal of Midwifery & Women's Health, 61*, 339—355.

Hawes, S. E., Hillier, S. L., Benedetti, J., Stevens, C. E., Koutsky, L. A., Welncr-Hanssen, P., et al. (1996). Hydrogen peroxide-producing lactobacilli and acquisition of vaginal infections. *The Journal of Infectious Diseases, 174*, 1058–1063.

Hempel, S., Newberry, S. J., Maher, A. R., Wang, Z., Miles, J. N. V., Shanman, R., & Shekelle, P. G. (2012). Probiotics for the prevention and treatment of antibiotic associated diarrhea: A systematic review and meta-analysis. *Journal of the American Medical Association, 307*, 1959–1969.

Heravi, R. M., Kermanshahi, M., Sankian, M., Nassiri, M. R., Moussavi, A. H., et al. (2011). Screening of lactobacilli bacteria isolated from gastrointestinal tract of broiler chickens for their use as probiotic. *African Journal of Microbiology Research, 5*, 1858–1868.

Holzapfel, W. H., Haberer, P., Geisen, R., Björkroth, J., & Schillinger, U. (2001). Taxonomy and important features of probiotic microorganisms in food and nutrition. *American Journal of Clinical Nutrition, 73*, 365–373.

Kerry, R. G., Patra, J. K., Gouda, S., Park, Y., Shin, H., & Das, G. (2018). Benefaction of probiotics for human health: A review. *Journal of Food and Drug Analysis, 26*, 927–939.

Lavilla-Lerma, L., Perez-Pulido, R., Martınez-Bueno, M., Maqueda, M., & Valdivia, E. (2013). Characterization of functional, safety, and gut survival related characteristics of Lactobacillus strains isolated from farmhouse goat's milk cheeses. *International Journal of Food Microbiology, 163*, 136–145.

LeBlanc, J. G., Milani, C., deGiori, G. S., Sesma, F., VanSinderen, D., & Ventura, M. (2013). Bacteria as it amin suppliers to their host: A gut microbiota perspective. *Current Opinion in Biotechnology, 24*, 160–168.

Levison, M. E., Corman, L. C., Carrington, E. R., & Kaye, D. (1977). Quantitative microflora of the vagina. *American Journal of Obstetrics and Gynecology, 127*, 80–85.

Li, W., Ji, J., Rui, X., Yu, J., Tang, W., Chen, X., et al. (2014). Production of exopolysaccharides by *Lactobacillus helveticus* MB2-1 and its functional characteristics in vitro. *LWT Food Science and Technology, 59*, 732–739.

Martin, R., Soberon, N., Vaneechoutte, M., Florez, A. B., Vazquez, F., et al. (2008). Characterization of indigenous vaginal lactobacilli from healthy women as probiotic candidates. *International Microbiology: The Official Journal of the Spanish Society for Microbiology, 11*, 261–266.

Martinez, R. C., Franceschini, S. A., Patta, M. C., et al. (2009b). Improved cure of bacterial vaginosis with single dose of tinidazole (2 g), *Lactobacillus rhamnosus* GR-1, and *Lactobacillus reuteri* RC-14: A randomized, double-blind, placebo-controlled trial. *Canadian Journal of Microbiology, 55*, 133–138.

Martinez, R. C., Franceschini, S. A., Patta, M. C., Quintana, S. M., Candido, R. C., Ferreira, E. C., et al. (2009a). Improved treatment of vulvovaginal candidiasis with fluconazole plus probiotic *Lactobacillus rhamnosus* GR-1 and Lactobacillus reuteri RC- 14. *Letters in Applied Microbiology, 48*, 269–274.

Martinez, R. C., Franceschini, S. A., Patta, M. C., Quintana, S. M., Nunes, A. C., Moreira, J. L., et al. (2008). Analysis of Vaginal lactobacilli from Healthy and Infected Brazilian Women. *Applied and Environmental Microbiology, 74*, 4539–4542.

Mendling, W. (2015). Guideline: *Vulvovaginal candidasis* (AWMF 015/072), S2k (excluding chronic mucocutaneous candidosis). *Mycos, 58*, 1–15.

Miller, E. A., Beasley, D. E., Dunn, R. R., & Archie, E. A. (2016). Lactobacilli dominance and vaginal pH: Why is the human vaginal microbiome unique? *Frontiers in Microbiology, 7*, 1936.

Morelli, L., & Capurso, L. (2012). FAO/WHO guidelines on probiotics: 10 years later. *Journal of Clinical Gastroenterology, 46*, S1–S2.

Mulu, W., Yimer, M., Zenebe, Y., & Abera, B. (2015). *Common causes of vaginal infections and antibiotic susceptibility of aerobic bacterial isolates in women of reproductive age attending at Felegehiwot referral Hospital, Ethiopia: A cross sectional study*. BMC Women's Health (15, p. 42).

Nagpal, R., Kumar, A., Kumar, M., Behare, P. V., Jain, S., & Yadav, H. (2012). Probiotics, their health benefits and applications for developing healthier foods: A review. *FEMS Microbiology Letters, 334*, 1–15.

Nagy, E., Petterson, M., & Mardh, P. A. (1991). Antibiosis between bacteria isolated from the vagina of women with and without signs of Bacterial vaginosis. *APMIS: Acta Pathologica, Microbiologica, et Immunologica Scandinavica, 99*, 739–744.

Parvez, S., Malik, K. A., Ah Kang, S., & Kim, H. Y. (2006). Probiotics and their fermented food products are beneficial for health. *Journal of Applied Microbiology, 100*, 1171–1185.

Patel, A., Prajapatia, J. B., Holst, O., & Ljungh, A. (2014). Determining probiotic potential of exopolysaccharide producing lactic acid bacteria isolated from vegetables and traditional Indian fermented food products. *Food Bioscience, 5*, 27–33.

Petrova, M. I., Lievens, E., Malik, S., Imholz, N., & Lebeer, S. (2015). Lactobacillus species as biomarkers and agents that can promote various aspects of vaginal health. *Frontiers in Physiology, 6*, 81.

Pfeiler, E. A., & Klaenhammer, T. R. (2007). The genomics of lactic acid bacteria. *Trends in Microbiology, 15*, 546–553.

Reid, G., Bruce, A. W., Fraser, N., Heinemann, C., Owen, J., & Henning, B. (2001). Oral probiotics can resolve urogenital infections. *FEMS Immunology & Medical Microbiology Letters, 30*, 49–52.

Rogosa, M., & Sharpe, M. E. (1960). Species differentiation of human vaginal lactobacilli. *Journal of General Microbiology, 23*, 197–201.

Royce, R. A., Thorp, J., Granados, J. L., & Savitz, D. A. (1999). Bacterial vaginosis associated with HIV infection in pregnant women from North Carolina. *Journal of Acquired Immune Deficiency Syndromes and Human Retrovirology, 20*, 382–386.

Saikali, J., Picard, C., & Freitas, M. (2004). Fermented milks, probiotic cultures and colon cancer. *Nutrition and Cancer, 49*, 14–24.

Saleki, S., Farid, M., Azizi, L., Amiri, M., & Afrakhteh, M. (2018). Probiotics and treatment of vulvovaginal candidiasis. *Journal of Enteric Pathogens, 6*(1), 22–26.

Salminen, S. J., Gueimonde, M., & Isolauri, E. (2005). Probiotics that modify disease risk. *The Journal of Nutrition, 135*, 1294–1298.

Sewankambo, N., Gray, R. H., Wawer, M. J., et al. (1997). HIV-1 infection associated with abnormal vaginal flora morphology and bacterial vaginosis. *Lancet, 350*, 546–550.

Taha, E. T., Gray, R. H., Kumwenda, N. I., et al. (1999). HIV infection and disturbances of vaginal flora during pregnancy. *Journal of Acquired Immune Deficiency Syndromes and Human Retrovirology, 20*, 52–59.

Tham, C. S., Peh, K. K., Bhat, R., & Liong, M. T. (2012). Probiotic properties of bifidobacteria and lactobacilli isolated from local dairy products. *Annals of Microbiology, 62*, 1079–1087.

Ventolini, G. (2013). New insides on vaginal immunity and recurrent infections. *Journal of Genital System & Disorders, 2*, 1.

Ventolini, G., & Sawyer, C. (2015). Probiotic vaginal lactobacilli: Are they protecting against fungal infections? *Journal of Bacteriology & Mycology, 2*(1), 2015.

Vicariotto, F., Del, P. M., Mogna, L., & Mogna, G. (2012). Effectiveness of the association of 2 probiotic strains formulated in a slow release vaginal product in women affected by vulvovaginal candidiasis: A pilot study. *Journal of Clinical Gastroenterology, 46*, S73–S80.

Vidhyalakshmi, R., Valli, N. C., Narendra, K. G., & Sunkar, S. (2016). Bacillus circulans exopolysaccharide: Production, characterization and bioactivities. *International Journal of Biological Macromolecules, 87*, 405–414.

Villena, J., Salva, S., Agüero, G., & Alvarez, S. (2011). Immunomodulatory and protective effect of probiotic *Lactobacillus casei* against *Candida albicans* infection in malnourished mice. *Microbiology and Immunology, 55*, 434–445.

Vitali, B., Pugliese, C., Biagi, E., Candela, M., Turroni, S., Bellen, G., et al. (2007). Dynamics of vaginal bacterial communities in women developing bacterial vaginosis, candidiasis, or no infection, analyzed by PCR-denaturing gradient gel electrophoresis and real-time PCR. *Applied and Environmental Microbiology, 73*, 5731–5741.

Waigankar, S. S., & Patel, V. (2011). Role of probiotics in urogenital healthcare. *Journal of Mid-Life Health, 2*, 5–10.

Wang, Y., Li, C., Liu, P., Ahmed, Z., Xiao, P., & Bai, X. (2010). Physical characterization of exopolysaccharide produced by *Lactobacillus plantarum* KF5 isolated from Tibet Kefir. *Carbohydrate Polymers, 82*, 895–903.

WHO. (2010). http://www.who.int/foodsafety/fs_management/en/probiotic_guidelines.pdf.

Xie, H. Y., Feng, D., Wei, D. M., Mei, L., Chen, H., Wang, X., & Fang, F. (2017). Probiotics for vulvovaginal candidiasis in non-pregnant women. *Cochrane Database of Systematic Reviews* (11), Art. No.: CD010496.

Chapter 18

Role of probiotics in the prevention and treatment of oral diseases

Devang Bharatkumar Khambholja[1], Prasant Kumar[2], Rushikesh G. Joshi[3] and Hiteshkumar V. Patel[4]

[1]*P.G. Department of Medical Technology, B.N. Patel Institute of Paramedical and Science (Paramedical Division), Anand, India,* [2]*Ingress Bio-Solutions Pvt. Ltd., Ahmedabad, India,* [3]*Department of Biochemistry and Forensic Science, University School of Sciences, Gujarat University, Ahmedabad, India,* [4]*Department of Biochemistry, Shri A.N. Patel PG Institute of Science and Research, Anand, India*

18.1 Introduction

Our oral cavity is a home for a wide verities of microorganisms, which are directly or indirectly linked with good health and disease states. Among microorganisms, bacteria are the major colonizer of the oral cavity. The diversity of oral microbiota depends on oral hygiene practice, nature of colonized surfaces, nutritional status, age and health status of host, and other environmental factors (Dewhirst et al., 2010; Sivamaruthi et al., 2020). The disturbance in the homeostatic equilibrium of the microflora has consequences in the development and progression of oral diseases, such as periodontal diseases (gingivitis and periodontitis), dental caries, and halitosis (oral malodor) (Sivamaruthi et al., 2020).

Oral diseases, particularly dental caries, are the most predominant of human diseases globally. It affects people of all age groups and is independent of gender and race. Basically, dental caries is a multifactorial chronic disease, mainly initiated by the production of certain organic acids (methanoic acid, formic acid, propionic acid, lactic acid, acetic acid) by oral microbes. These organic acids lower down the oral pH, which ultimately causes teeth demineralization and produces cavities on teeth surfaces. However, teeth demineralization can be corrected by the use of certain chemical agents such as fluorides, but an imbalance in oral microbiota may provoke cavitation by the release of certain bacterial enzymes such as glucansucrases (Selwitz et al., 2007).

Another predominant oral disease in humans is periodontal disease, which mainly includes gingivitis and periodontitis. According to the World Health Organization, the majority of children have signs of gingivitis, and among the adults, the initial stages of periodontal disease, are highly prevalent (WHO). Gingivitis and periodontitis are a continuum of the same inflammatory disease. However, not all patients with gingivitis will develop to periodontitis. The management of gingivitis is both a primary prevention strategy for periodontitis and a secondary prevention strategy for recurrent periodontitis (Chapple et al., 2015). Generally, gingivitis is considered as a nondestructive type of periodontal disease, but untreated, it can progress to periodontitis. Periodontitis is a chronic infectious disease-causing inflammation of teeth-supporting tissues such as gingival, periodontal ligament, cementum, and alveolar bone leading to tissue destruction and tooth loss (Khambholja & Mehta, 2019). It is mainly caused by diverse subgingival microbiota, which are in a dysbiosis state. Major putative pathogens of periodontal diseases are *Porphyromonas gingivalis*, *Aggregatibacter actinomycetemcomitans*, *Actinobacillus actinomycetemcomitans*, *Prevotella intermedia*, *Streptococcus mutans*, *Treponema denticola*, and *Bacteroides forsythus* (Carranza et al., 2006; Chahbouni et al., 2013; Dzink et al., 1988; Faveri et al., 2009; Hung et al., 2002; Ishikawa et al., 2002; Miura et al., 2005). Along with infection causing pathogens, it is also depending on host inflammatory immune response that inflicts the irreversible damage on the periodontium and teeth loss (Hajishengallis et al., 2012).

Halitosis, or oral malodor, is a condition which significantly impedes a person's social and interpersonal life, and hampers self-esteem (Shringeri et al., 2019). Oral malodor may be a cosymptom of common oral diseases, such as dental caries or periodontal diseases (Georgiou et al., 2018). Also, it seems that it is primarily attributed to coating of the tongue dorsum (43.4%) and periodontal diseases (11.2%) (Quirynen et al., 2009). Oral malodor is the result of degradation of both endogenous and exogenous organic compounds present in the oral cavity by some oral anaerobic microorganisms. This degradation process leads to the formation of highly volatile sulfur compounds (VSCs) (methyl mercaptan, hydrogen sulfide, and dimethyl sulfide), that give the unpleasant odor (Georgiou et al., 2018).

Globally, oral diseases, especially dental caries and periodontal infections, are common and can pose unwanted health complications. Some of these problems demand for the usage of antibiotics, which may cause gastrointestinal (GI) side effects, severe allergic reactions, and the emergence of antibiotic resistance (Agarwal et al., 2011; Babaji et al., 2012). Thus there is an urgent need for alternative therapy that can address these problems. Some alternatives and efficient therapeutic strategies are now employed to treat oral disease. Probiotics therapy is one such alternative that has increased recognition by the modern healthcare system over the past decades (Teughels et al., 2008). Probiotics can be characterized as living organisms that valuably impact the well-being of the host when utilized in adequate quantities (Ali Hassan et al., 2020). Currently available probiotic products include a wide range of bacterial and fungal species that are consumed in a variety of preparations (Hasslöf & Stecksén-Blicks, 2020). Initially, probiotics have been used for the prevention and treatment of GI diseases. In the past two decades, there has been an increased interest in the possible use of probiotics in oral healthcare. Several studies have been reported that certain probiotic bacteria strains like *Lactobacillus reuteri* (Keller et al., 2012; Krasse et al., 2006), *Lactobacillus rhamnosus* (Nase et al., 2001), *Bifidobacterium* spp. (Grudianov et al., 2002), and *Lactobacillus plantarum* have positive effects on tooth adhesion and their action against oral diseases (Morales et al., 2017). Presently, probiotics are broadly used in the prevention and treatment of many dental disorders. Large numbers of clinical trials have shown that use of probiotics improves the clinical parameters such as plaque index, bleeding index, pocket depth, and gingival index (Benic et al., 2019; Invernici et al., 2018; Vivekananda et al., 2010). Also, it can control plaque formation and prevent the breakdown of oral microbial homeostasis. The present chapter explores the therapeutic values of various probiotics for maintaining oral health.

18.2 Role of probiotics in prevention and treatment of dental caries

Dental caries are the most recorded common diseases worldwide in this era, and developing countries are the most affected by this major human disease (Petersen, 2004). Globally, it is estimated that 2.3 billion people suffer from caries of permanent teeth and more than 530 million children suffer from caries of primary teeth. It was projected that about US$544.41 billion was used for treating dental diseases in 2015 worldwide, and the cost of dental treatment varies based on the treatment procedures and interventions (Righolt et al., 2018). Dental caries are a multifactorial chronic disease where the hard tissues of the teeth are infected by cariogenic bacteria resulting in demolition and demineralization of the teeth. Dental caries are a major public health problem globally and is the most widespread noncommunicable disease, ultimately it will generate inequity between tooth minerals and oral microbial biofilms. Many aspects have been studied that relate to this common human disease (Featherstone et al., 2003; Hassell & Harris, 1995; Krol, 2003; Selwitz et al., 2007). The living microbes in the oral cavity produces organic acids through the carbohydrate metabolism, which decreases the pH and causes the demineralization in teeth. Constant demineralization ultimately causes a cavity on tooth surfaces. Additionally, long-term exposure of organic acids will produce dental caries. Though, the most effective methods to prevent caries are by promoting remineralization and slowing down demineralization. This can be achieved with fluoride treatments. It is extensively accepted that the regular use of fluoride, such as in dentifrice and drinking water, is very effective at preventing dental caries. Fluoride has effects on the microorganism by creating an imbalance in oral microbial population (Selwitz et al., 2007).

Many another possible and effective therapeutic strategies, other than antimicrobials, are now developed to treat oral diseases. Many microbial enzymes like glucanase (dextranase and mutanase), deoxyribonucleases (DNases), and ionic detergents are leading in use to destroy plaque biofilms in oral cavity. The use of microbial protease inhibitors and the antimicrobial photodynamic therapy are feasible ways of treating oral infection (Allaker & Ian Douglas, 2015). In the same way, probiotics are also predictable as a potent therapeutic agent for dental diseases. Probiotics are live microorganisms which, when administered in suitable amounts, confer a health benefit to the host.

Generally lactic acid-producing bacteria are present naturally in human normal flora, human milk, and cow's milk (Martín et al., 2003; Tulini et al., 2016). For hundreds of years these bacteria have been used to ferment cow's milk into yogurt, which helps to extend the durability of the milk. Fermentation of milk into yogurt helps to improve digestion (Scott et al., 2015). The consumption of probiotic milk supplemented *L. rhamnosus* GG reduces (6%) the growth of dental caries and the concentration of *S. mutans* in children. Another study determined that the short-term consumption of cheese containing two probiotic strains (*L. rhamnosus* GG ATCC 53103 and *L. rhamnosus* LC 705) might reduce the oral cariogenic microbial flora in young adults (Ahola et al., 2002).

The scientific evidence to support the beneficial effect on the efficacy and safety of probiotics is still not clear. However, probiotic effects are strain specific; therefore each individual bacterial strain must be checked respectively.

The mechanism of the probiotic action must be demonstrated via both in vitro and in vivo studies, to allow prediction of the applicable scope and potential side effects (Busscher et al., 1997; Rodrigues et al., 2004; Schwandt et al., 2005).

The ionic concentration, insoluble extracellular polymeric substance, and degree of mineral loss, were analyzed from isolated dental biofilm. The results indicated that daily administration of the beverages decreased the pH value of dental biofilm and reduced enamel demineralization. Many research groups have been working on this aspect; for example, Lin et al. (2004) has isolated *Lactobacillus paracasei* subsp. *paracasei* NTU 101 (NTU 101; DSMZ 28047) from an infant and has shown several functional properties over the past decade. It has been used to prevent metabolic syndrome based on its hypocholesterolemia by using it in yogurt and probiotic products with demonstrated safety and health benefits (Chiu et al., 2006). It also demonstrated antiatherosclerotic (Tsai et al., 2009), antihypertensive (Liu et al., 2011), and antifat accumulation effects (Cheng et al., 2015). It has also been used for the prevention of gastric mucosal lesions (Liu et al., 2009) and shown to have antiosteoporotic (Chiang et al., 2012), anticariogenic (Lin et al., 2004), and immunomodulating effects (Tsai et al., 2008, 2010).

It has been reported that the consumption of probiotic milk containing *L. rhamnosus* GG ($5-10 \times 10^5$ CFU/mL) for 7 months (5 days/wk) significantly reduced the occurrence of dental caries in children. Especially, probiotic milk intervention reduced *S. mutans* count and cumulative caries score in 3- to 4-year-old children compared with the placebo control. This study claimed that probiotic milk could be considered a health supplement to improve the oral health of daycare children (Nase et al., 2001). The protective effect was linked to the effective transfer of *L. reuteri* from mothers to children (Stensson et al., 2014).

Over a century ago, Elie Metchnikoff described the beneficial effects of fermented dairy products to changes the microbial balance in the gut; he believed that harmful effects of toxins produced by intestinal bacteria could be replaced by beneficial effects of lactic acid bacteria. Many beneficial effects on health have been attributed to probiotics. Traditionally, probiotic bacteria have been used for the prevention and treatment of GI infections or other related diseases (De Vrese & Schrezenmeir, 2008; Saxelin et al., 2005). The strongest evidence available on the beneficial effects of probiotics *Lactobacilli* and *Bifidobacteria* is related to the prevention or treatment of infections in the lower part of the GI tract. In addition, probiotics are better than placebo for preventing acute infections of the upper respiratory tract and reducing the use of antibiotics in both children and adults. The use of probiotics to combat biofilm-mediated oral diseases, dental caries, and gingivitis/periodontitis has been studied during the past 20 years (Busscher et al., 1997; Rodrigues et al., 2004; Schwandt et al., 2005).

It has been reported that regular use of probiotics can help to control halitosis. A patient infected with the *Fusobacterium nucleatum* organism will produce volatile sulfide components, but after taking *Weissella cibaria*, it will be reduced (Kang et al., 2006). *Streptococcus salivarius* also suppress volatile sulfide effects by competing for colonization areas with volatile sulfide-producing species (Burton et al., 2005).

In concluding the content, dental caries arise, owing to bacterial infection that causes demineralization and destruction of the tooth. Tooth decay is a slow process in which the action of primarily acidogenic bacteria in the bacteria-laden biofilm and accumulation of food debris on the tooth surface lead to tooth damage, tooth loss, and infection (Chen & Wang, 2010). Dental caries result from the environmental changes in the oral cavity. It has adverse effects on oral health due to acid production from fermentable carbohydrates. *S. mutans* has the ability to form dental plaque on tooth surfaces; this is dependent on the expression of surface proteins involved in the synthesis of the extracellular glucan matrix. Among these proteins, glucosyltransferases (GtfB, GtfC, and GtfD) synthesize glucan from sucrose; other surface proteins, such as glucan-binding proteins (Gbps), contribute to biofilm growth through the bacterial interaction with extracellular glucan (Banas & Vickerman, 2003; Duque et al., 2011; Lynch et al., 2007).

18.3 Role of probiotics in the prevention and treatment of periodontal diseases

Periodontal diseases (gingivitis and periodontitis) are infectious diseases, causing inflammation of teeth-supporting tissues such as gingival, periodontal ligament, cementum, and alveolar bone, leading to tissue destruction and teeth loss (Damor et al., 2020; Khambholja & Mehta, 2019). Large-scale population studies have shown that periodontal diseases are mostly associated with poor oral hygiene. Some of the oral bacterial species organize in biofilm and trigger the local destructive inflammation of teeth-supporting tissues. The formation of bacterial biofilm around the teeth often causes the gingival inflammation called plaque-induced gingivitis (Mariotti, 1999; Morales et al., 2017). It is the most common form of periodontal disease across the globe. Gingivitis and periodontitis are regarded as a continuum of the same inflammatory process (Morales et al., 2017). Usually, it is considered that periodontitis is the advancement of gingivitis. However, it is also important to highlight that not all cases of gingivitis progress into the periodontitis (Kinane & Attstrom, 2005; Smith et al., 2000). The extent of biofilm formation, the virulence of the biofilm bacteria, and the host immune responses to the biofilm are the major factors that determine the progress of the periodontal diseases (Botero et al., 2015). The culprit bacteria associated with periodontal diseases include *P. gingivalis*, *A. actinomycetemcomitans*, *A. actinomycetemcomitans*, *Prevotella melaninogenica*, *T. denticola*, and *Tannerella forsythia* (Carranza et al., 2006; Chahbouni et al., 2013; Dzink et al., 1988; Faveri et al., 2009; Hung et al., 2002; Ishikawa et al., 2002; Miura et al., 2005).

The conventional approach of periodontal treatment is mostly comprised of mechanical debridement, the disruption of the biofilm, and the restoration of damage tissues (Vives-Soler & Chimenos-Küstner, 2020). Use of antibiotics, antimicrobial products in the form of mouthwashes or dentifrices, have been tested for their adjunctive efficacy in reducing bacterial biofilm and periodontal diseases. However, antibiotics are not innocuous drugs, since they are accompanied by side effects and the potential emergence of antibiotic-resistant bacterial strains (Nguyen et al., 2019). Therefore there is an urgent need of alternative therapy that can modulate the composition of oral biofilms, prevent colonization of pathogenic organisms, and obstruct the development of colonized pathogens. Probiotic therapy is one alternative that has gained recognition by the contemporary healthcare system over the past decade (Teughels et al., 2008). Many experimental studies and clinical trials have proven that certain GI bacteria have the capacity to restrict the growth of oral pathogens (Meurman, 2005). Certain GI bacteria, such as *Bifidobacterium* spp. and *Lactobacillus*, have the potential to restrict the growth of carcinogenic streptococci (Meurman, 2005). The probable mechanisms of probiotic action in oral cavity could be identical to that suggested in the GI tract (Fig. 18.1). In the GI track, a combination of probiotics (viable bacteria and yeasts) and prebiotics (inulin, fructose oligosaccharides and others) increases the abundance of short-chain fatty acids, such as butyric acid, which modulates histone acetylation and mucin production. Another short-chain fatty acid, propionic acid, regulates the action of lipogenic enzymes in the liver (Den Besten et al., 2013; Nagpal et al., 2018). Reports also suggest that probiotics along with prebiotics, increases phagocytic activity of macrophages, controls inflammation, and restores the normal microbial balance in the GI tract (Mishra et al., 2020). Similar action can also be expected from the use of oral probiotics and prebiotics in the periodontal diseases.

The probiotic approach represents a breakthrough technique to maintain oral health by using natural beneficial bacteria normally found in healthy mouths to provide a natural protection against the bacteria believed to be harmful to teeth-supporting tissues (Morales et al., 2017). Earlier studies on various species of probiotics have revealed mixed effects on oral pathogens. In a double-blind, randomized, placebo-controlled clinical trial, the effectiveness of the probiotic strain in the treatment of gingivitis was tested (Krasse et al., 2006). Fifty-nine patients with moderate to severe gingivitis were included and given one of two different formulation of *L. reuteri* (LR-1 or LR-2) or a corresponding placebo. At day 0 (baseline) and day 14 (after completion of treatment) plaque index and gingival index were measured. Saliva samples were also collected to determine total *Lactobacilli* count. Gingival index reduced significantly in all study groups ($P < .0001$). Moreover, compared to placebo, significant reductions were observed in plaque index in the both study groups. Also, at 14 days, 65% and 95% patient's saliva samples were colonized with *L. reuteri* in LR-1 and LR-2, respectively, suggesting the probiotic organism was efficacious in reducing both plaque and gingivitis (Krasse et al., 2006). Another study on *L. reuteri*, 30 systemically healthy, chronic periodontitis (mean age 41 years) was included. The study period was 42 days. "Split-mouth" design was used for the scaling and root planning (SRP), which

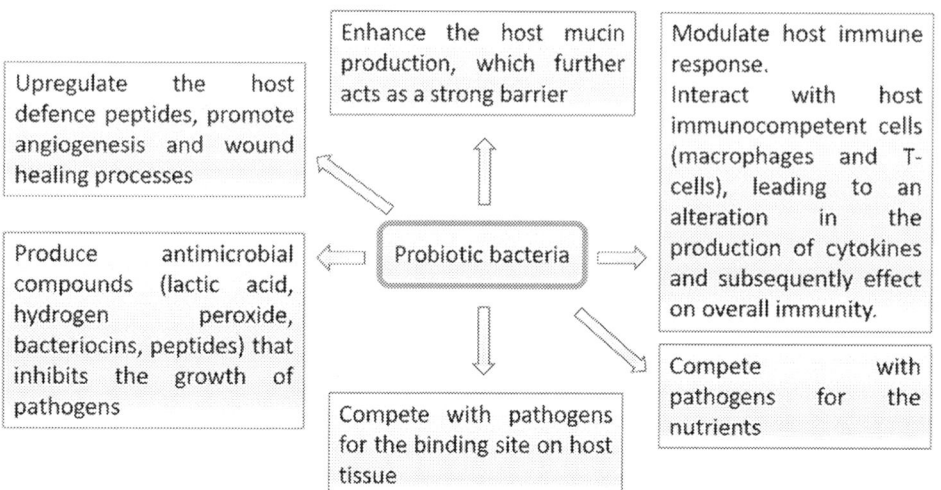

FIGURE 18.1 Mechanism of probiotic action.

was performed on day 0; two quadrants (either right or left) were treated with SRP, whereas the remaining two quadrants were left untreated. *L. reuteri* Prodentis lozenges, or the corresponding placebo lozenges, were taken twice daily from day 21 to day 42. Assessment of clinical parameters and level oral pathogens were made on day 0 before SRP treatment, on day 21 before administration of the lozenges, and on day 42. At day 42, the plaque index, gingival index, and gingival bleeding index were significantly reduced by all treatment modalities. Compared to SRP + placebo and placebo alone, the treatment with SRP + probiotics and probiotics alone were capable to significantly reduce all clinical parameters as well as concentration of selected oral pathogens (Vivekananda et al., 2010). Clinical studies that evaluated various probiotic strains for the prevention and treatment of periodontal diseases are summarized in Table 18.1.

In the field of tissue regeneration, mesenchymal stem cells (MSC) have potential roles as therapeutic agents. The oral cavity possesses several MSC-like cells with regeneration properties that can be explored for therapeutic applications (Nagpal et al., 2018). Studies propose that if the correct balance can be maintained in the oral microbiota, the regenerative cells present in the oral cavity can be activated, leading to an improvement in the wound healing process (Mishra et al., 2020). Recently in a Chinese study, the effects of balanced pathogenic bacteria *P. gingivalis* and probiotics *L. reuteri* extracts on gingival MSCs were tested (Han et al., 2020). The results suggest that the balance between pathogenic bacteria and probiotics enhanced the migration, osteogenic differentiation, and cell proliferation of MSCs. Moreover, local inoculation of the mixture of *L. reuteri* and *P. gingivalis* also promoted the wound healing process. The study also suggests that reuterin from *L. reuteri* neutralizes the action of the lipopolysachharides of *P. gingivalis*, reducing the inflammation and promoting wound healing (Han et al., 2020). The probiotic chewing gum containing *L. reuteri* also decreased levels of proinflammatory cytokines in gingival crevicular fluid (Twetman et al., 2009). However, several studies have found that probiotics did not show any significant improvement compared to the placebo. In a human experimental gingivitis study with *L. brevis* CD2 lozenge use, no marked differences in the gingival crevicular fluid levels of cytokines were reported compared to the placebo (Lee et al., 2015).

Contrary, a study on rat models, observed that oral administration of probiotic mixture (*L. paracasei* LPC-37, *Bifidobacterium lactis* HN0019, *L. rhamnosus* HN001, *Lactobacillus acidophilus* NCFM) was able to promote even gut-skin-healing process (Tagliari et al., 2019).

18.4 Role of probiotics in the prevention and treatment of halitosis

Oral halitosis or oral malodor is common problem affecting people of all ages. When severe and longstanding, it may reduce social interactions and self-confidence (Porter & Scully, 2006). Severe oral malodor is mostly caused by oral, or occasionally nasopharyngeal, disease. Reports now agree that about 90% of halitosis originates within the oral cavity. The most common cause is oral bacterial plaque, particularly on the dorsum of the tongue and teeth. Poor oral hygiene and infection and inflammation of gingival and periodontal tissues are considerable factors in oral malodor (Porter & Scully, 2006). Putrefactive activities of tongue microbiota contribute a significant role in generating volatile malodorous compounds (Allaker & Stephen, 2017). Malodorous compounds such as VSC, hydrogen sulfide, methyl mercaptan, organic acids, ammonia, skatole, and cadaverine are claimed to be the major contributors to oral halitosis (Allaker & Stephen, 2017; Tangerman & Winkel, 2010). Bacteria responsible for halitosis include mainly *Porphyromonas gingivitis*, *F. nucleatum*, *T. denticola*, *P. intermedia*, and *T. forsythia* (Aung et al., 2015; De Boever & Loesche, 1995; Iwamoto et al., 2010; Persson et al., 1990; Suzuki et al., 2014; Takahashi, 2015).

The treatment modality for halitosis is generally elimination or growth retardation of responsible pathogenic organisms. Conventionally, chemotherapeutic agents such as chlorhexidine, cetylpyridinium, triclosan, essential oils, chlorine dioxide, and sodium bicarbonate have usually been effective, but only for a short period of time. Also, disturbance of oral cavity homeostasis is a substantial negative side effect of such agents (Fedorowicz et al., 2008; Scully & Greenman, 2012; Van Steenberghe et al., 2001). Novel approaches such as probiotics are spotlighted to replace these side effects and to provide an inhibitory effect on oral halitosis (Table 18.2). *Streptococcus salivarus*, a common oral bacterium, is often present in oral surfaces and represents the predominant organism in the tongue microbiota of healthy individuals (Kazor et al., 2003). Several studies on its strains suggest potential applications of this organism, as it reduces the production of VSCs (Bustamante et al., 2020). In an in vitro study, *S. salivarus* strain K12 has been reported to inhibit the growth of several oral halitosis-associated bacterial species (Masdea et al., 2012). Anti-VSC activities have also been reported in certain strains of probiotic bacteria *W. cibaria* (Lee et al., 2020; Jang et al., 2016; Kang et al., 2006), *Enterococcus faecium* (Suzuki et al., 2016) and *Streptococcus thermophilus* (Lee & Baek, 2014). Generally, this anti-VSC effect of such probiotic organisms could be due to the production of hydrogen peroxide and/or by competing for the colonization area with VSC-producing species (Flichy-Fernández et al., 2010). *S. salivarius* strain

TABLE 18.1 Potential role of probiotics in the prevention and treatment of periodontal diseases.

Probiotic strain/product	Mode of delivery	Sample size (age)	Study outcomes/therapeutic properties	Reference
Probiotic milk drink "Yakult"	Milk drink	28 (20–33 years)	PI increased significantly in probiotic group at the end of the probiotic intake. Significantly less BOP and lower GCF volume in probiotic group compared with placebo. Daily consumption of a probiotic milk drink reduces the effects of plaque-induced gingival inflammation.	Slawik et al. (2011)
Lactobacillus reuteri	Tablets	40 (20–24 years)	No significant change in clinical parameters between the groups after probiotic intake Total anaerobic counts and counts of Prevotella intermedia reduced significantly in saliva after 4 and 8 weeks respectively. Subgingival Porphyromonas gingivalis counts reduced significantly after 4 weeks.	Iniesta et al. (2012)
Lactobacillus salivarius WB21	Oil drops	42	Oil drops containing L. salivarius WB21 improved BOP and inhibited the reproduction of total and VSC-producing periodontopathic bacteria compared with the placebo group.	Suzuki et al. (2012)
Lactobacillus rhamnosus GG (LGG) + Bifidobacterium animalis BB-12	Lozenges	77 (Test group: 24.6 year; control group: 24 years)	Both PI and GI decrease significantly compared to control. In saliva, no probiotic-induced changes were found in the microbial compositions. The probiotic lozenge improved the periodontal status without affecting the oral microbiota.	Toiviainen et al. (2014)
Lactobacillus brevis CD2	Lozenges	34 (Test group: 22.1 year; control group: 21.6 years)	No significant change in clinical parameters between the groups after probiotic intake Microscopically, prostaglandin E2 levels reduced significantly in the test group even though matrix metalloproteinase-8 and nitric oxide levels did not show any difference.	Lee et al. (2015)
L. rhamnosus SP1	Sachets	28 (Test group: 52.7 ± 7.3 years; control group: 46.9 ± 10.3 years)	Clinical parameters were equally improved compared to scaling and root planning. Both test and control groups showed improvements in clinical parameters. The test group, however, showed greater reductions in PPD than the control. Also, at initial visits and after 1-year follow-up, the test group showed a statistically significant reduction in number of participants with PPD ≥ 6 mm.	Morales et al. (2016)
Lactobacillus plantarum L-137 (heat killed)	Capsules	39 (Mean age: 66.2 years)	Daily heat killed L-137 intake can decrease the depth of periodontal pockets in patients undergoing supportive periodontal therapy.	Iwasaki et al. (2016)

(Continued)

TABLE 18.1 (Continued)

Probiotic strain/product	Mode of delivery	Sample size (age)	Study outcomes/therapeutic properties	Reference
Bacillus subtilis, Bacillus megaterium, and Bacillus pumulus spore	Toothpaste, mouthrinse, and toothbrush cleaner	30 (18–31 years)	No significant differences were observed between a placebo and a bacilli-containing toothpaste, mouthrinse, and toothbrush cleaner on gingivitis parameters.	Alkaya et al. (2016)
L. salivarius + L. reuteri	Capsule/direct	32 (25–49 years)	Significant improvement in PI, MGI, and BI noticed in test group. PPD reduction and CAG revealed no statistical significance. Microbial assessment using N-benzoyl-DL-arginine-naphthylamide and halitosis assessment using organoleptic scores showed reduction in test group compared to control group.	Penala et al. (2016)
Bifidobacterium animalis sp. lactis DN-173010	Yogurt	51 (16–26 years)	All parameters (PI, GI, BOP, GCF volume and interlukin-13 total) were significantly improved in test group (probiotics) compared to control group.	Kuru et al. (2017)
L. plantuarum + L. brevis + Pediococcus acidilactici	Tablets	59 (Test group: 30.9 ± 12.2 years; control group: 32.5 ± 13.6 years)	No significant improvements were observed in clinical index and GI. However, significant reduction was noticed in the growth of pathogenic organism "Tannerella forsythia."	Montero et al. (2017)
L. rhamnosus GG + B. lactis BB-12	Lozenges	101 (13–15 years)	Short-term daily consumption of strains GG and BB-12 probiotic lozenges improved the gingival health in adolescents and decreased the microbial counts of Actinobacillus actinomycetemcomitans, and P. gingivalis.	Alanzi et al. (2018)
Bifidobacterium animalis ssp. lactis HN019	Lozenges	30	Significant improvement in all clinical and immunological parameter were observed in test (probiotics) group compared to control. HN019 reduced the adhesion of P. gingivalis to BEC and showed antimicrobial potential against periodontopathogen.	Invernici et al. (2020)
L. rhamnosus SP1	Sachets group I: placebo, group II: probiotics, group III: antibiotic azithromycin	47 (>35 years)	Both probiotics or antibiotic as an adjunct to SRP failed to provide additional benefits in the treatment of stage III periodontitis.	Morales et al. (2021)

BI, Bleeding index; *BOP*, Bleeding on probing; *CAG*, Clinical attachment gain; *CFU*, Colony-forming units; *GCF*, Gingival crevicular fluid; *GI*, Gingival index; *MGI*, Modified gingival index; *PI*, Plaque index; *PPD*, Probing pocket depth; *VSC*, Volatile sulphur compound.

K12 produces two antibiotic bacteriocins, salivaricin A and salivaricin B. Both the bacteriocins have an inhibitory effect against several species of Gram-positive bacteria responsible for oral malodor (Teughels et al., 2008).

A prospective, double-blind, placebo-controlled, randomized study was conducted on 25 healthy young adults with mean age of 22 years to evaluate the efficacy of a probiotic chewing gum containing *L. reuteri* (Keller et al., 2012). The organoleptic score suggesting the beneficial effect of probiotic chewing gum; however, no effect was noticed on the levels of measured VSCs which could explain this reduction. In a prospective, triple-blind, placebo-controlled, randomized study, contradict observations were noticed. The study was conducted on probiotic group ($n = 32$) and placebo group ($n = 32$). The probiotic group consumed two lozenges containing *S. salivarius* M18 (3.6×10^9 CFU/lozenge) per

TABLE 18.2 Potential role of probiotics in the prevention and treatment of oral halitosis.

Probiotic strain	Mode of delivery (product name)	Study outcomes/therapeutic properties	Reference
Lactobacillus salivarius G60	Chewing gum	Significant reduction in halitosis was observed in probiotic + inulin combination study group.	Mousquer et al. (2020)
Lactobacillus reuteri	Chewing gum	No significance difference noticed in organoleptic score and in cysteine rinse evaluation compared to placebo group.	Keller et al. (2012)
Lactobacillus brevis CD2	Lozenges	No improvement in organoleptic score and VSC concentration.	Marchetti et al. (2015)
Lactobacillus paracasei	Toothpaste (hyperbiotics, activated charcoal probiotic spearmint)	Supports heathy teeth and freshness breath.	Mishra et al. (2020)
Lactobacillus sp.	Mouthwash (Cuchupe mouthwash, fresh mint stick L-8020 10 mL)	Prevents cavity formation and fight bad breath.	Mishra et al. (2020)
L. salivarius, L. paracasei, L. reuteri, Lactobacillus sakei, and Streptococcus salivarius M18	Chewable tablets (hyperbiotics prodental: probiotics)	Dissolve biofilms, combats halitosis, controls dysbiosis, and restores microbial balance.	Mishra et al. (2020)
L. salivarius and L. reuteri	Mouthrinse	Microbiological and clinical parameters were significantly reduced. Significant reductions were observed in pocket depth and halitosis.	Penala et al. (2016)
L. salivarius WB21	Chewable tablet	Reduction in halitosis and pathogenic bacteria.	Suzuki et al. (2014)
S. salivarius M18	Lozenges	Plaque index and gingival index scores were not significantly. Significant reduction in VSCs were observed.	Benic et al. (2019)
L. reuteri	Chewing gum	Organoleptic scores reduction. No reduction in VSCs concentration.	Keller et al. (2012)
S. salivarus strain K12	In vitro study	Growth inhibition of several bacterial pathogens associated with oral malodor.	Masdea et al. (2012)
S. salivarus BLIS K12	Lozenges (E.N.T. Biotic)	Promotes healthy oral bacteria and freshen breath.	Mishra et al. (2021)
S. salivarus BLIS strain K12 and M18	Lozenges (Thera Breath Oral care Probiotics)	Improve oral malodor.	Mishra et al. (2021)
L. salivarius WB21 + xylitol	Tablet	Improvement was observed in oral halitosis and also showed beneficial effects on bleeding on probing from the periodontal pocket.	Iwamoto et al. (2010)
S. salivarius K12	Lozenges	Reduction was observed in breath levels of VSCs.	Burton et al. (2005)
Weissella cibaria CMU	Tablet	Significant reduction in organoleptic score and VSC concentration.	Lee et al. (2020)

day for 1 month. Assessments were carried out at baseline, at the end of the intervention, and at a 3-month follow-up (Benic et al., 2019). Plaque index and gingival index scores were not significantly influenced by the probiotic intervention; however, the level of VSCs reduced significantly. Also, in 3-month follow-up, the VSC levels in the placebo group returned to baseline levels whereas those in the probiotic group decreased further (Benic et al., 2019).

In another study, a probiotic tablet containing *Lactobacillus salivarius* WB21 was investigated for its effect on oral malodor in a 14-day, double-blind, placebo-controlled, randomized crossover trial (Suzuki et al., 2014). Organoleptic test scores significantly reduced in both the probiotic and placebo periods compared with the respective baseline scores. In contrast, the average probing pocket depth and the level of measured VSCs decreased significantly in the probiotic period compared with the placebo period. Bacterial quantitative analysis found significant reduction in pathogenic organisms during probiotic intervention period.

In a double-blind, randomized, placebo-controlled trial study, the effectiveness of the local use of probiotics was assessed as an adjunct to SRP in the treatment of patient with chronic periodontitis and halitosis. The trial involving 32 systemically healthy chronic periodontitis patients. After SRP, the patients were randomly assigned into the test and control groups. The test group used probiotic mouthwash for 15 days after SRP and received subgingival delivery of probiotic solution at baseline (immediately after SRP), 1 week, 2 weeks, and 4 weeks. The control group received placebo mouthwash and subgingival delivery of placebo. A mixture of two probiotic organisms, *L. salivarius* and *L. reuteri* per capsule was used in the study. Each capsule contains both organisms at 2×10^9 CFU. The patient was given 2 capsules a day and asked to empty the capsule in 10-mL distilled water and rinse for 1 minutes daily twice for 14 days. All the microbiological and clinical parameters were significantly reduced in both groups at the end of the 3-month study. Furthermore, the study also showed that the adjunctive use of probiotics offers clinical benefit in terms of pocket depth and halitosis reduction (Penala et al., 2016).

Contradictory, studies on *L. reuteri* (Keller et al., 2012) and *L. brevis* CD2 (Marchetti et al., 2015) consumption were not found to reduced organoleptic scores and volatile sulfur concentration. Intake of *Lactobacillus casei* also did not show considerable changes in the organoleptic scores or volatile sulfur concentration, even though presence of the *L. casei* in the tongue plaque during the treatment (Sutula et al., 2013). However, a recent study on same genus *Lactobacillus*, suggesting strong deleterious activity of this organism against oral pathogens. *Lactobacillus gasseri* HHuMIN D culture supernatant inhibited halitosis producing anaerobic microorganisms 88.8% and strong antimicrobial activity against deleterious oral bacteria (Mann et al., 2021). A probiotic gum containing *L. salivarius* G60 (LS) and inulin was investigated for its effect on oral halitosis in double-blind, phase II clinical trial (Mousquer et al., 2020). Forty-four patients (mean age 35 ± 15 years) completed the trial. The patients were randomly assigned into the LS (1 billion CFU) + inulin (1 g), LS (1 billion CFU) and placebo groups. Patients treated with LS + inulin showed statistically significant reduction in oral halitosis compared to LS and placebo groups. Suggesting, the combination of prebiotics and probiotics can be a promising approach for patients with oral halitosis (Mousquer et al., 2020).

18.5 Conclusions

In conclusion, probiotics can correct microbiological and clinical outcomes in the prevention and treatment of oral diseases. Several studies and clinical trials have been reported that the use of probiotics helps to prevent dental caries and minimizes the risk of caries progression in children and adults. Also, consumption of probiotics can improve organoleptic score in halitosis and recovers the treatment outcomes of chronic periodontitis and gingivitis with or without the application of nonsurgical periodontal therapy. However, certain studies and clinical trials have some deficiencies such as limited information and inconclusive evidence, due to the wide variety of probiotics that have been included in studies, making it hard to identify effectiveness of each probiotic strain. Moreover, the efficacy of probiotics to modulate host immune response, the efficiency of different probiotic species and administration protocols, and fluctuations in long-term microbiome composition, merit further investigation.

References

Agarwal, E., Bajaj, P., Guruprasad, C. N., Naik, S., & Pradeep, A. R. (2011). Probiotics: A novel step towards oral health. *Archives of Oral Sciences & Research*, 1(2), 108–115.

Ahola, A. J., Yli-Knuuttila, H., Suomalainen, T., Poussa, T., Ahlström, A., Meurman, J. H., & Korpela, R. (2002). Short-term consumption of probiotic-containing cheese and its effect on dental caries risk factors. *Archives of Oral Biology*, 47(11), 799–804. Available from https://doi.org/10.1016/S0003-9969(02)00112-7.

Alanzi, A., Honkala, S., Honkala, E., Varghese, A., Tolvanen, M., & Söderling, E. (2018). Effect of *Lactobacillus rhamnosus* and *Bifidobacterium lactis* on gingival health, dental plaque, and periodontopathogens in adolescents: a randomised placebo-controlled clinical trial. *Beneficial Microbes*, 9(4), 593–602.

Ali Hassan, S., Bhateja, S., Arora, G., & Francis, P. (2020). Use of probiotics in dental. *IP International Journal of Periodontology and Implantology*, 5(3), 101–103. Available from https://doi.org/10.18231/j.ijpi.2020.023.

Alkaya, B., Laleman, I., Keceli, S., Ozcelik, O., Cenk Haytac, M., & Teughels, W. (2016). Clinical effects of probiotics containing Bacillus species on gingivitis: a pilot randomized controlled trial. *Journal of Periodontal Research*, 52(3), 497–504.

Allaker, R. P., & Ian Douglas, C. W. (2015). Non-conventional therapeutics for oral infections. *Virulence*, *6*(3), 196−207. Available from https://doi.org/10.4161/21505594.2014.983783.

Allaker, R. P., & Stephen, A. S. (2017). Use of probiotics and oral health. *Current Oral Health Reports*, *4*(4), 309−318. Available from https://doi.org/10.1007/s40496-017-0159-6.

Aung, E. E., Ueno, M., Zaitsu, T., Furukawa, S., & Kawaguchi, Y. (2015). Effectiveness of three oral hygiene regimens on oral malodor reduction: A randomized clinical trial. *Trials*, *16*(1). Available from https://doi.org/10.1186/s13063-015-0549-9.

Babaji, P., Keswani, K., Lau, H., Lau, M., Punga, R., & Sharma, N. (2012). Role of probiotics in oral health: A review of the literature. *Journal of Education and Ethics in Dentistry*, *2*(2), 52−55. Available from https://doi.org/10.4103/0974-7761.121256.

Banas, J. A., & Vickerman, M. M. (2003). Glucan-binding proteins of the oral streptococci. *Critical Reviews in Oral Biology and Medicine*, *14*(2), 89−99. Available from https://doi.org/10.1177/154411130301400203.

Benic, G. Z., Farella, M., Morgan, X. C., Viswam, J., Heng, N. C., Cannon, R. D., & Mei, L. (2019). Oral probiotics reduce halitosis in patients wearing orthodontic braces: A randomized, triple-blind, placebo-controlled trial. *Journal of Breath Research*, *13*(3). Available from https://doi.org/10.1088/1752-7163/ab1c81.

Botero, J. E., Rösing, C. K., Duque, A., Jaramillo, A., & Contreras, A. (2015). Periodontal disease in children and adolescents of Latin America. *Periodontology*, *67*(1), 34−57. Available from https://doi.org/10.1111/prd.12072, 2000.

Burton, J. P., Chilcott, C. N., & Tagg, J. R. (2005). The rationale and potential for the reduction of oral malodour using *Streptococcus salivarius* probiotics. *Oral diseases*, *11*(1), 29−31. Available from https://doi.org/10.1111/j.1601-0825.2005.01084.x.

Busscher, H. J., Van Hoogmoed, C. G., Geertsema-Doornbusch, G. I., Van Der Kuijl-Booij, M., & Van Der Mei, H. C. (1997). *Streptococcus thermophilus* and its biosurfactants inhibit adhesion by *Candida* spp. on silicone rubber. *Applied and Environmental Microbiology*, *63*(10), 3810−3817. Available from https://doi.org/10.1128/aem.63.10.3810-3817.1997.

Bustamante, M., Oomah, B. D., Mosi-Roa, Y., Rubilar, M., & Burgos-Díaz, C. (2020). Probiotics as an adjunct therapy for the treatment of halitosis, dental caries and periodontitis. *Probiotics and Antimicrobial Proteins*, *12*(2), 325−334. Available from https://doi.org/10.1007/s12602-019-9521-4.

Carranza, F. A., Newman, M. G., Takei, H. H., & Klokkevold, P. R. (2006). *Carranza's clinical periodontology*.

Chahbouni, H., Maltouf, A. F., & Ennibi, O. (2013). Aggregatibacter actinomycetemcomitans et Porphyromonas gingivalis dans les parodontites agressives au Maroc-Etude preliminaire. *Odonto-Stomatologie Tropicale = Tropical Dental Journal*, *36*(143), 5−10.

Chapple, I. L., Van der Weijden, F., Doerfer, C., Herrera, D., Shapira, L., Polak, D., Madianos, P., Louropoulou, A., Machtei, E., Donos, N., Greenwell, H., Van Winkelhoff Ari, J., Eren Kuru, B., Arweiler, N., Teughels, W., Aimetti, M., Molina, A., Montero, E., & Graziani, F. (2015). Primary prevention of periodontitis: Managing gingivitis. *Journal of Clinical Periodontology*, *42*(16), S71−S76. Available from https://doi.org/10.1111/jcpe.12366.

Chen, F., & Wang, D. (2010). Novel technologies for the prevention and treatment of dental caries: A patent survey. *Expert Opinion on Therapeutic Patents*, *20*(5), 681−694. Available from https://doi.org/10.1517/13543771003720491.

Cheng, M. C., Tsai, T. Y., & Pan, T. M. (2015). Anti-obesity activity of the water extract of *Lactobacillus paracasei* subsp. paracasei NTU 101 fermented soy milk products. *Food and Function*, *6*(11), 3522−3530. Available from https://doi.org/10.1039/c5fo00531k.

Chiang, S. S., Liao, J. W., & Pan, T. M. (2012). Effect of bioactive compounds in lactobacilli-fermented soy skim milk on femoral bone microstructure of aging mice. *Journal of the Science of Food and Agriculture*, *92*(2), 328−335. Available from https://doi.org/10.1002/jsfa.4579.

Chiu, C. H., Lu, T. Y., Tseng, Y. Y., & Pan, T. M. (2006). The effects of Lactobacillus-fermented milk on lipid metabolism in hamsters fed on high-cholesterol diet. *Applied Microbiology and Biotechnology*, *71*(2), 238−245. Available from https://doi.org/10.1007/s00253-005-0145-0.

Damor, C. R., Patel, D. D., Chauhan, R. M., Pithadiya, R. S., & Khambholja, D. B. (2020). Efficacy of *Azadirachta indica* (neem) extract embedded onto guided tissue regeneration membrane against *Neisseria* sp. CDK-10 and *Micrococcus* sp. CDK-23 isolated from periodontal plaque. *Journal of Advanced Scientific Research*, *11*(4), 56−61.

De Boever, E. H., & Loesche, W. J. (1995). Assessing the contribution of anaerobic microflora of the tongue to oral malodor. *Journal of the American Dental Association (1939)*, *126*(10), 1384−1393. Available from https://doi.org/10.14219/jada.archive.1995.0049.

De Vrese, M., & Schrezenmeir, J. (2008). Probiotics, prebiotics, and synbiotics. *Advances in Biochemical Engineering/Biotechnology*, *111*, 1−66. Available from https://doi.org/10.1007/10_2008_097.

Den Besten, G., Van Eunen, K., Groen, A. K., Venema, K., Reijngoud, D. J., & Bakker, B. M. (2013). The role of short-chain fatty acids in the interplay between diet, gut microbiota, and host energy metabolism. *Journal of Lipid Research*, *54*(9), 2325−2340. Available from https://doi.org/10.1194/jlr.R036012.

Dewhirst, F. E., Chen, T., Izard, J., Paster, B. J., Tanner, A. C. R., Yu, W. H., Lakshmanan, A., & Wade, W. G. (2010). The human oral microbiome. *Journal of Bacteriology*, *192*(19), 5002−5017. Available from https://doi.org/10.1128/JB.00542-10.

Duque, C., Stipp, R. N., Wang, B., Smith, D. J., Höfling, J. F., Kuramitsu, H. K., Duncan, M. J., & Mattos-Graner, R. O. (2011). Downregulation of GbpB, a component of the VicRK regulon, affects biofilm formation and cell surface characteristics of *Streptococcus mutans*. *Infection and Immunity*, *79*(2), 786−796. Available from https://doi.org/10.1128/IAI.00725-10.

Dzink, J. L., Socransky, S. S., & Haffajee, A. D. (1988). The predominant cultivable microbiota of active and inactive lesions of destructive periodontal diseases. *Journal of Clinical Periodontology*, *15*(5), 316−323. Available from https://doi.org/10.1111/j.1600-051X.1988.tb01590.x.

Faveri, M., Figueiredo, L. C., Duarte, P. M., Mestnik, M. J., Mayer, M. P. A., & Feres, M. (2009). Microbiological profile of untreated subjects with localized aggressive periodontitis. *Journal of Clinical Periodontology*, *36*(9), 739−749. Available from https://doi.org/10.1111/j.1600-051X.2009.01449.x.

Featherstone, J. D. B., Adair, S. M., Anderson, M. H., Berkowitz, R. J., Bird, W. F., Crall, J. J., Den Besten, P. K., Donly, K. J., Glassman, P., Milgrom, P., Roth, J. R., Snow, R., & Stewart, R. E. (2003). Caries management by risk assessment: consensus statement, April 2002. *Journal of the California Dental Association*, *31*(3), 257−269.

Fedorowicz, Z., Aljufairi, H., Nasser, M., Outhouse Trent, L., & Pedrazzi, V. (2008). *Mouthrinses for the treatment of halitosis*. Wiley. Available from https://doi.org/10.1002/14651858.cd006701.pub2.

Flichy-Fernández, A. J., Alegre-Domingo, T., Peñarrocha-Oltra, D., & Peñarrocha-Diago, M. (2010). Probiotic treatment in the oral cavity: An update. *Medicina Oral, Patologia Oral y Cirugia Bucal*, 15(5), e677–e680. Available from https://doi.org/10.4317/medoral.15.e677.

Georgiou, A. C., Laine, M. L., Deng, D. M., Brandt, B. W., Van Loveren, C., & Dereka, X. (2018). Efficacy of probiotics: Clinical and microbial parameters of halitosis. *Journal of Breath Research*, 12(4). Available from https://doi.org/10.1088/1752-7163/aacf49.

Grudianov, A. I., Dmitrieva, N. A., & Fomenko, E. V. (2002). Primenenie tabletirovannykh form probiotikov Bifidumbakterina i Atsilakta v kompleksnom lechenii vospalitel'nykh zabolevanii parodonta. *Stomatologiya*, 81(1), 39–43.

Hajishengallis, G., Darveau, R. P., & Curtis, M. A. (2012). The keystone-pathogen hypothesis. *Nature Reviews Microbiology*, 10(10), 717–725. Available from https://doi.org/10.1038/nrmicro2873.

Han, N., Jia, L., Guo, L., Su, Y., Luo, Z., Du, J., Mei, S., & Liu, Y. (2020). Balanced oral pathogenic bacteria and probiotics promoted wound healing via maintaining mesenchymal stem cell homeostasis. *Stem Cell Research and Therapy*, 11(1). Available from https://doi.org/10.1186/s13287-020-1569-2.

Hassell, T. M., & Harris, E. L. (1995). Genetic influences in caries and periodontal diseases. *Critical Reviews in Oral Biology and Medicine*, 6(4), 319–342. Available from https://doi.org/10.1177/10454411950060040401.

Hasslöf, P., & Stecksén-Blicks, C. (2020). The impact of nutrition and diet on oral health. *Monographs in Oral Science, Basel, Karger*, 28, 99–107.

Hung, S. L., Lin, Y. W., Wang, Y. H., Chen, Y. T., Su, C. Y., & Ling, L. J. (2002). Permeability of *Streptococcus mutans* and *Actinobacillus actinomycetemcomitans* through guided tissue regeneration membranes and their effects on attachment of periodontal ligament cells. *Journal of Periodontology*, 73(8), 843–851. Available from https://doi.org/10.1902/jop.2002.73.8.843.

Iniesta, M., Herrera, D., Montero, E., Zurbriggen, M., Matos, A. R., Marín, M. J., Beltran, S., Llama-Palacio, A., & Sanz, M. (2012). Probiotic effects of orally administered *Lactobacillus reuteri*-containing tablets on the subgingival and salivary microbiota in patients with gingivitis. A randomized clinical trial. *Journal of Clinical Periodontology*, 39(8), 736–744.

Invernici, M. M., Furlaneto, F. A. C., Salvador, S. L., Ouwehand, A. C., Salminen, S., Mantziari, A., Vinderola, G., Ervolino, E., Santana, S., Felix Silva, P. H., & Messora, M. R. (2020). *Bifidobacterium animalis* subsp *lactis* HN019 presents antimicrobial potential against periodontopathogens and modulates the immunological response of oral mucosa in periodontitis patients. *PLOS ONE*, 15(9), 1–20.

Invernici, M. M., Salvador, S. L., Silva, P. H. F., Soares, M. S. M., Casarin, R., Palioto, D. B., Souza, S. L. S., Taba, M., Novaes, A. B., Furlaneto, F. A. C., & Messora, M. R. (2018). Effects of Bifidobacterium probiotic on the treatment of chronic periodontitis: A randomized clinical trial. *Journal of Clinical Periodontology*, 45(10), 1198–1210. Available from https://doi.org/10.1111/jcpe.12995.

Ishikawa, I., Kawashima, Y., Oda, S., Iwata, T., & Arakawa, S. (2002). Three case reports of aggressive periodontitis associated with *Porphyromonas gingivalis* in younger patients. *Journal of Periodontal Research*, 37(5), 324–332. Available from https://doi.org/10.1034/j.1600-0765.2002.01613.x.

Iwamoto, T., Suzuki, N., Tanabe, K., Takeshita, T., & Hirofuji, T. (2010). Effects of probiotic *Lactobacillus salivarius* WB21 on halitosis and oral health: An open-label pilot trial. *Oral Surgery, Oral Medicine, Oral Pathology, Oral Radiology and Endodontology*, 110(2), 201–208. Available from https://doi.org/10.1016/j.tripleo.2010.03.032.

Iwasaki, K., Maeda, K., Hidaka, K., Nemoto, K., Hirose, Y., & Deguchi, S. (2016). Daily Intake of Heat-killed *Lactobacillus plantarum* L-137 Decreases the Probing Depth in Patients Undergoing Supportive Periodontal Therapy. *Oral Health and Preventive Dentistry*, 14(3), 207–214.

Jang, H. J., Kang, M. S., Yi, S. H., Hong, J. Y., & Hong, S. P. (2016). Comparative study on the characteristics of *Weissella cibaria* CMU and probiotic strains for oral care. *Molecules (Basel, Switzerland)*, 21(12). Available from https://doi.org/10.3390/molecules21121752.

Kang, M. S., Chung, J., Kim, S. M., Yang, K. H., & Oh, J. S. (2006). Effect of *Weissella cibaria* isolates on the formation of *Streptococcus mutans* biofilm. *Caries Research*, 40(5), 418–425. Available from https://doi.org/10.1159/000094288.

Kang, M. S., Kim, B. G., Chung, J., Lee, H. C., & Oh, J. S. (2006). Inhibitory effect of *Weissella cibaria* isolates on the production of volatile sulphur compounds. *Journal of Clinical Periodontology*, 33(3), 226–232. Available from https://doi.org/10.1111/j.1600-051X.2006.00893.x.

Kazor, C. E., Mitchell, P. M., Lee, A. M., Stokes, L. N., Loesche, W. J., Dewhirst, F. E., & Paster, B. J. (2003). Diversity of bacterial populations on the tongue dorsa of patients with halitosis and healthy patients. *Journal of Clinical Microbiology*, 41(2), 558–563. Available from https://doi.org/10.1128/JCM.41.2.558-563.2003.

Keller, M. K., Hasslöf, P., Dahlén, G., Stecksén-Blicks, C., & Twetman, S. (2012). Probiotic supplements (*Lactobacillus reuteri* DSM 17938 and ATCC PTA 5289) do not affect regrowth of mutans streptococci after full-mouth disinfection with chlorhexidine: A randomized controlled multicenter trial. *Caries Research*, 46(2), 140–146. Available from https://doi.org/10.1159/000337098.

Khambholja, D. B., & Mehta, K. B. (2019). Efficacy of tulsi (*Ocimum sanctum*) extract incorporated onto guided tissue regeneration (GTR) membrane against periodontal pathogens. *International Journal of Health Sciences and Research*, 9(2), 68–76.

Kinane, D. F., & Attstrom, R. (2005). Advances in the pathogenesis of periodontitiss. Group B consensus report of the fifth European workshop in periodontology. *Journal of Clinical Periodontology*, 32(s6), 130–131. Available from https://doi.org/10.1111/j.1600-051x.2005.00823.x.

Krasse, P., Carlsson, B., Dahl, C., Paulsson, A., Nilsson, A., & Sinkiewicz, G. (2006). Decreased gum bleeding and reduced gingivitis by the probiotic *Lactobacillus reuteri*. *Swedish Dental Journal*, 30(2), 55–60.

Krol, D. M. (2003). Dental caries, oral health, and pediatricians. *Current Problems in Pediatric and Adolescent Health Care*, 33(8), 253–270. Available from https://doi.org/10.1016/S1538-5442(03)00093-2.

Kuru, B. E., Laleman, I., Yalnızoğlu, T., Kuru, L., & Teughels, W. (2017). The Influence of a *Bifidobacterium animalis* Probiotic on Gingival Health: A Randomized Controlled Clinical Trial. *Journal of Periodontology*, 88(11), 1115–1123.

Lee, D. S., Lee, S. A., Kim, M., Nam, S. H., & Kang, M. S. (2020). Reduction of halitosis by a tablet containing *Weissella cibaria* CMU: A randomized, double-blind, placebo-controlled study. *Journal of Medicinal Food*, 23(6), 649–657. Available from https://doi.org/10.1089/jmf.2019.4603.

Lee, J. K., Kim, S. J., Ko, S. H., Ouwehand, A. C., & Ma, D. S. (2015). Modulation of the host response by probiotic *Lactobacillus brevis* CD2 in experimental gingivitis. *Oral Diseases*, 21(6), 705–712. Available from https://doi.org/10.1111/odi.12332.

Lee, S. H., & Baek, D. H. (2014). Effects of *Streptococcus thermophilus* on volatile sulfur compounds produced by *Porphyromonas gingivalis*. *Archives of Oral Biology*, 59(11), 1205–1210. Available from https://doi.org/10.1016/j.archoralbio.2014.07.006.

Lin, F. M., Chiu, C. H., & Pan, T. M. (2004). Fermentation of a milk-soymilk and Lycium chinense Miller mixture using a new isolate of *Lactobacillus paracasei* subsp. paracasei NTU101 and *Bifidobacterium longum*. *Journal of Industrial Microbiology and Biotechnology*, 31(12), 559–564. Available from https://doi.org/10.1007/s10295-004-0184-z.

Liu, C. F., Hu, C. L., Chiang, S. S., Tseng, K. C., Yu, R. C., & Pan, T. M. (2009). Beneficial preventive effects of gastric mucosal lesion for soy-skim milk fermented by lactic acid bacteria. *Journal of Agricultural and Food Chemistry*, 57(10), 4433–4438. Available from https://doi.org/10.1021/jf900465c.

Liu, C. F., Tung, Y. T., Wu, C. L., Lee, B. H., Hsu, W. H., & Pan, T. M. (2011). Antihypertensive effects of Lactobacillus-fermented milk orally administered to spontaneously hypertensive rats. *Journal of Agricultural and Food Chemistry*, 59(9), 4537–4543. Available from https://doi.org/10.1021/jf104985v.

Lynch, D. J., Fountain, T. L., Mazurkiewicz, J. E., & Banas, J. A. (2007). Glucan-binding proteins are essential for shaping *Streptococcus mutans* biofilm architecture. *FEMS Microbiology Letters*, 268(2), 158–165. Available from https://doi.org/10.1111/j.1574-6968.2006.00576.x.

Mann, S., Park, M. S., Johnston, T. V., Ji, G. E., Hwang, K. T., & Ku, S. (2021). Oral probiotic activities and biosafety of *Lactobacillus gasseri* HHuMIN D. *Microbial Cell Factories*, 20(1), 75. Available from https://doi.org/10.1186/s12934-021-01563-w.

Marchetti, E., Tecco, S., Santonico, M., Vernile, C., Ciciarelli, D., Tarantino, E., Marzo, G., & Pennazza, G. (2015). Multi-sensor approach for the monitoring of halitosis treatment via *Lactobacillus brevis* (CD2)—containing lozenges—a randomized, double-blind placebo-controlled clinical trial. *Sensors (Switzerland)*, 15(8), 19583–19596. Available from https://doi.org/10.3390/s150819583.

Mariotti, A. (1999). Dental plaque-induced gingival diseases. *Annals of periodontology/the American Academy of Periodontology*, 4(1), 7–19. Available from https://doi.org/10.1902/annals.1999.4.1.7.

Martín, R., Langa, S., Reviriego, C., Jiménez, E., Marín, M. L., Xaus, J., Fernández, L., & Rodríguez, J. M. (2003). Human milk is a source of lactic acid bacteria for the infant gut. *Journal of Pediatrics*, 143(6), 754–758. Available from https://doi.org/10.1016/j.jpeds.2003.09.028.

Masdea, L., Kulik, E. M., Hauser-Gerspach, I., Ramseier, A. M., Filippi, A., & Waltimo, T. (2012). Antimicrobial activity of *Streptococcus salivarius* K12 on bacteria involved in oral malodour. *Archives of Oral Biology*, 57(8), 1041–1047. Available from https://doi.org/10.1016/j.archoralbio.2012.02.011.

Meurman, J. H. (2005). Probiotics: Do they have a role in oral medicine and dentistry? *European Journal of Oral Sciences*, 113(3), 188–196. Available from https://doi.org/10.1111/j.1600-0722.2005.00191.x.

Mishra, S., Rath, S., & Mohanty, N. (2020). Probiotics—A complete oral healthcare package. *Journal of Integrative Medicine*, 18(6), 462–469. Available from https://doi.org/10.1016/j.joim.2020.08.005.

Miura, M., Hamachi, T., Fujise, O., & Maeda, K. (2005). The prevalence and pathogenic differences of *Porphyromonas gingivalis* fimA genotypes in patients with aggressive periodontitis. *Journal of Periodontal Research*, 40(2), 147–152. Available from https://doi.org/10.1111/j.1600-0765.2005.00779.x.

Montero, E., Iniesta, M., Rodrigo, M., Marín, M. J., Figuero, E., Herrera, D., & Sanz, M. (2017). Clinical and microbiological effects of the adjunctive use of probiotics in the treatment of gingivitis: A randomized controlled clinical trial. *Journal of Clinical Periodontology*, 44(7), 708–716.

Morales, A., Bravo-bown, J., Bedoya, J., & Gamonal, J. (2017). Probiotics and periodontal diseases. In J. F. Manakil (Ed.), *Insights into various aspects of oral health* (pp. 73–96). IntechOpen. Available from https://doi.org/10.5772/intechopen.68814.

Morales, A., Carvajal, P., Silva, N., Hernandez, M., Godoy, C., Rodriguez, G., Cabello, R., Garcia-Sesnich, J., Hoare, A., Diaz, P. I., & Gamonal, J. (2016). Clinical Effects of *Lactobacillus rhamnosus* in Non-Surgical Treatment of Chronic Periodontitis: A Randomized Placebo-Controlled Trial With 1-Year Follow-Up. *Journal of Periodontology*, 87(8), 944–952.

Morales, A., Contador, R., Bravo, J., Carvajal, P., Silva, N., Strauss, F. J., & Gamonal, J. (2021). Clinical effects of probiotic or azithromycin as an adjunct to scaling and root planning in the treatment of stage III periodontitis: a pilot randomized controlled clinical trial. *BMC Oral Health*, 21(12), 1–15.

Mousquer, C., Della Bona, A., Milani, D., Callegari-Jacques, S., Ishikawa, K., Mayer, M., Rösing, C., & Fornari, F. (2020). Are *Lactobacillus salivarius* G60 and inulin more efficacious to treat patients with oral halitosis and tongue coating than the probiotic alone and placebo? A randomized clinical trial. *The Journal of Periodontology*, 91(6), 775–783. Available from https://doi.org/10.1002/JPER.19-0089.

Nagpal, R., Wang, S., Ahmadi, S., Hayes, J., Gagliano, J., Subashchandrabose, S., Dalane, W. K., Becton, T., Read, R., & Yadav, H. (2018). Human-origin probiotic cocktail increases short-chain fatty acid production via modulation of mice and human gut microbiome. *Scientific Reports*, 8, 12649. Available from https://doi.org/10.1038/s41598-018-30114-4.

Nase, L., Hatakka, K., Savilahti, E., Saxelin, M., Pönkä, A., Poussa, T., Korpela, R., & Meurman, J. H. (2001). Effect of long-term consumption of a probiotic bacterium, *Lactobacillus rhamnosus* GG, in milk on dental caries and caries risk in children. *Caries Research*, 35(6), 412–420. Available from https://doi.org/10.1159/000047484.

Nguyen, C. C., Hugie, C. N., Kile, M. L., & Navab-Daneshmand, T. (2019). Association between heavy metals and antibiotic-resistant human pathogens in environmental reservoirs: A review. *Frontiers of Environmental Science and Engineering*, 13(3). Available from https://doi.org/10.1007/s11783-019-1129-0.

Penala, S., Butchibabu, K., Pathakota, K. R., Avula, J., Koppolu, P., Lakshmi, B. V., Pandey, R., & Mishra, A. (2016). Efficacy of local use of probiotics as an adjunct to scaling and root planing in chronic periodontitis and halitosis: A randomized controlled trial. *Journal of Research in Pharmacy Practice*, 5(2), 86–93. Available from https://doi.org/10.4103/2279-042X.179568.

Persson, S., Edlund, M., Claesson, R., & Carlsson, J. (1990). The formation of hydrogen sulfide and methyl mercaptan by oral bacteria. *Oral Microbiology and Immunology*, 5(4), 195–201. Available from https://doi.org/10.1111/j.1399-302X.1990.tb00645.x.

Petersen, P. E. (2004). Challenges to improvement of oral health in the 21st century—The approach of the WHO Global Oral Health Programme. *International Dental Journal*, 54(6), 329–343. Available from https://doi.org/10.1111/j.1875-595x.2004.tb00009.x, FDI World Dental Press Ltd.

Porter, S. R., & Scully, C. (2006). Oral malodour (halitosis). *BMJ (Clinical Research ed.)*, 333(7569), 632–635. Available from https://doi.org/10.1136/bmj.38954.631968.AE.

Quirynen, M., Dadamio, J., Van Den Velde, S., De Smit, M., Dekeyser, C., Van Tornout, M., & Vandekerckhove, B. (2009). Characteristics of 2000 patients who visited a halitosis clinic. *Journal of Clinical Periodontology*, 36(11), 970–975. Available from https://doi.org/10.1111/j.1600-051X.2009.01478.x.

Righolt, A. J., Jevdjevic, M., Marcenes, W., & Listl, S. (2018). Global-, regional-, and country-level economic impacts of dental diseases in 2015. *Journal of Dental Research*, 97(5), 501–507. Available from https://doi.org/10.1177/0022034517750572.

Rodrigues, L., Van Der Mei, H., Teixeira, J. A., & Oliveira, R. (2004). Biosurfactant from *Lactococcus lactis* 53 inhibits microbial adhesion on silicone rubber. *Applied Microbiology and Biotechnology*, 66(3), 306–311. Available from https://doi.org/10.1007/s00253-004-1674-7.

Saxelin, M., Tynkkynen, S., Mattila-Sandholm, T., & De Vos, W. M. (2005). Probiotic and other functional microbes: From markets to mechanisms. *Current Opinion in Biotechnology*, 16(2), 204–211. Available from https://doi.org/10.1016/j.copbio.2005.02.003.

Schwandt, L. Q., Van Weissenbruch, R., Van Der Mei, H. C., Busscher, H. J., & Albers, F. W. J. (2005). Effect of dairy products on the lifetime of provox2 voice prostheses in vitro and in vivo. *Head and Neck*, 27(6), 471–477. Available from https://doi.org/10.1002/hed.20180.

Scott, K. P., Antoine, J.-M., Midtvedt, T., & van Hemert, S. (2015). Manipulating the gut microbiota to maintain health and treat disease. *Microbial Ecology in Health & Disease*, 26, 25877. Available from https://doi.org/10.3402/mehd.v26.25877.

Scully, C., & Greenman, J. (2012). Halitology (breath odour: Aetiopathogenesis and management). *Oral Diseases*, 18(4), 333–345. Available from https://doi.org/10.1111/j.1601-0825.2011.01890.x.

Selwitz, R. H., Ismail, A. I., & Pitts, N. B. (2007). Dental caries. *Lancet*, 369(9555), 51–59. Available from https://doi.org/10.1016/S0140-6736(07)60031-2.

Shringeri, P. I., Fareed, N., Battur, H., & Khanagar, S. (2019). Role of probiotics in the treatment and prevention of oral malodor/halitosis: A systematic review. *Journal of Indian Association of Public Health Dentistry*, 17(2), 90–96. Available from https://doi.org/10.4103/jiaphd.jiaphd_171_18.

Sivamaruthi, B. S., Kesika, P., & Chaiyasut, C. (2020). A review of the role of probiotic supplementation in dental caries. *Probiotics and Antimicrobial Proteins*, 12(4), 1300–1309. Available from https://doi.org/10.1007/s12602-020-09652-9.

Slawik, S., Staufenbiel, I., Schilke, R., Nicksch, S., Weinspach, K., Stiesch, M., & Eberhard, J. (2011). Probiotics affect the clinical inflammatory parameters of experimental gingivitis in humans. *European Journal of Clinical Nutrition*, 65(7), 857–863.

Smith, M., Seymour, G., & Cullinan, M. (2000). Histopathological features of chronic and aggressive periodontitis. *Periodontology*, 53, 45–54. Available from https://doi.org/10.1111/j.1600-0757.2010.00354.x.

Stensson, M., Koch, G., Coric, S., Abrahamsson, T. R., Jenmalm, M. C., Birkhed, D., & Wendt, L. K. (2014). Oral administration of *Lactobacillus reuteri* during the first year of life reduces caries prevalence in the primary dentition at 9 years of age. *Caries Research*, 48(2), 111–117. Available from https://doi.org/10.1159/000354412.

Sutula, J., Coulthwaite, L. A., Thomos, L. V., & Verran, J. (2013). The effect of a commercial probiotic drink containing *Lactobacillus casei* strain Shirota on oral health in healthy dentate people. *Microbial Ecology in Health and Disease*, 24, 1–12.

Suzuki, N., Higuchi, T., Nakajima, M., Fujimoto, A., Morita, H., Yoneda, M., Hanioka, T., & Hirofuji, T. (2016). Inhibitory effect of *Enterococcus faecium* WB2000 on volatile sulfur compound production by *Porphyromonas gingivalis*. *International Journal of Dentistry*, 2016. Available from https://doi.org/10.1155/2016/8241681.

Suzuki, N., Tanabe, K., Takeshita, T., Yoneda, M., Iwamoto, T., Oshiro, S., Yamashita, Y., & Hirofuji, T. (2012). Effects of oil drops containing *Lactobacillus salivarius* WB21 on periodontal health and oral microbiota producing volatile sulfur compounds. *Journal of Breath. Research*, 6(1), 017106.

Suzuki, N., Yoneda, M., Tanabe, K., Fujimoto, A., Iha, K., Seno, K., Yamada, K., Iwamoto, T., Masuo, Y., & Hirofuji, T. (2014). *Lactobacillus salivarius* WB21-containing tablets for the treatment of oral malodor: A double-blind, randomized, placebo-controlled crossover trial. *Oral Surgery, Oral Medicine, Oral Pathology and Oral Radiology*, 117(4), 462–470. Available from https://doi.org/10.1016/j.oooo.2013.12.400.

Tagliari, E., Campos, L. F., Campos, A. C., Costa-Casagrande, T. A., & de Noronha, L. (2019). Effect of probiotic oral administration on skin wound healing in rats. *Arquivos Brasileiros de Cirurgia Digestiva*, 32(3). Available from https://doi.org/10.1590/0102-672020190001e1457.

Takahashi, N. (2015). Oral microbiome metabolism: From \who are they?\to\what are they doing?\. *Journal of Dental Research*, 94(12), 1628–1637. Available from https://doi.org/10.1177/0022034515606045.

Tangerman, A., & Winkel, E. G. (2010). Extra-oral halitosis: An overview. *Journal of Breath Research*, 4(1). Available from https://doi.org/10.1088/1752-7155/4/1/017003.

Teughels, W., Van Essche, M., Sliepen, I., & Quirynen, M. (2008). Probiotics and oral healthcare. *Periodontology 2000*, 48(1), 111–147. Available from https://doi.org/10.1111/j.1600-0757.2008.00254.x.

Toiviainen, A., Jalasvuori, H., Lahti, E., Gursoy, U., Salminen, S., Fontana, M., Flannagan, S., Eckert, G., Kokaras, A., Paster, B., & Söderling, E. (2014). Impact of orally administered lozenges with *Lactobacillus rhamnosus* GG and *Bifidobacterium animalis* subsp. *lactis* BB-12 on the number of salivary mutans streptococci, amount of plaque, gingival inflammation and the oral microbiome in healthy adults. *Clinical Oral Investigations*, *19*(1), 77–83.

Tsai, Y. T., Cheng, P. C., Fan, C. K., & Pan, T. M. (2008). Time-dependent persistence of enhanced immune response by a potential probiotic strain *Lactobacillus paracasei* subsp. paracasei NTU 101. *International Journal of Food Microbiology*, *128*(2), 219–225. Available from https://doi.org/10.1016/j.ijfoodmicro.2008.08.009.

Tsai, T. Y., Chu, L. H., Lee, C. L., & Pan, T. M. (2009). Atherosclerosis-preventing activity of lactic acid bacteria-fermented milk-soymilk supplemented with momordica charantia. *Journal of Agricultural and Food Chemistry*, *57*(5), 2065–2071. Available from https://doi.org/10.1021/jf802936c.

Tsai, Y. T., Cheng, P. C., & Pan, T. M. (2010). Immunomodulating activity of *Lactobacillus paracasei* subsp. paracasei NTU 101 in enterohemorrhagic *Escherichia coli* O157H7-infected mice. *Journal of Agricultural and Food Chemistry*, *58*(21), 11265–11272. Available from https://doi.org/10.1021/jf103011z.

Tulini, F. L., Hymery, N., Haertlé, T., Le Blay, G., & De Martinis, E. C. P. (2016). Screening for antimicrobial and proteolytic activities of lactic acid bacteria isolated from cow, buffalo and goat milk and cheeses marketed in the southeast region of Brazil. *Journal of Dairy Research*, *83*(1), 115–124. Available from https://doi.org/10.1017/S0022029915000606.

Twetman, S., Derawi, B., Keller, M., Ekstrand, K., Yucel-Lindberg, T., & Stecksén-Blicks, C. (2009). Short-term effect of chewing gums containing probiotic *Lactobacillus reuteri* on the levels of inflammatory mediators in gingival crevicular fluid. *Acta Odontologica Scandinavica*, *67*(1), 19–24. Available from https://doi.org/10.1080/00016350802516170.

Van Steenberghe, D., Avontroodt, P., Peeters, W., Pauwels, M., Coucke, W., Lijnen, A., & Quirynen, M. (2001). Effect of different mouthrinses on morning breath. *Journal of Periodontology*, *72*(9), 1183–1191. Available from https://doi.org/10.1902/jop.2000.72.9.1183.

Vivekananda, M. R., Vandana, K. L., & Bhat, K. G. (2010). Effect of the probiotic *Lactobacilli reuteri* (prodentis) in the management of periodontal disease: A preliminary randomized clinical trial. *Journal of Oral Microbiology*, *2*(2010). Available from https://doi.org/10.3402/jom.v2i0.5344.

Vives-Soler, A., & Chimenos-Küstner, E. (2020). Effect of probiotics as a complement to non-surgical periodontal therapy in chronic periodontitis: A systematic review. *Medicina Oral, Patologia Oral y Cirugia Bucal*, *25*(2), e161–e167. Available from https://doi.org/10.4317/medoral.23147.

Chapter 19

Role of probiotics in infections with multidrug-resistant organisms

Basavaprabhu Haranahalli Nataraj and Rashmi Hogarehalli Mallappa

Molecular Biology Unit, Dairy Microbiology Division, ICAR-National Dairy Research Institute, Karnal, India

19.1 Introduction

Though antimicrobial resistance is an enduring threat that evolved over the years, the magnitude of microbial proficiency has been recently amplified with newer dimensions, thereby making antimicrobial resistance (AMR) a topmost health threat. Escalating microbial resistance to last-resort antibiotics apprize a cautionary tale that might jeopardize the existence of humankind in the near future. The global annual deaths due to AMR were reported to be nearly 700,000, and it has been anticipated that the death curve may show an uptick hike to 10 million by 2050 (Ghosh et al., 2019). Albeit resistance among all microbial communities is of paramount public health concern in one way or another, the broadened resistance pattern among the clinically relevant pathogens is highly worrying since it has a direct and immediate impact on the success of empiric antibiotic therapy in the human clinical sector. However, care should be taken on growing AMR in all the sectors (human medicine, agriculture, and animal husbandry) since resistance from bacteria of humans, animals, or the environmental origin may spread among each other, and from one country to another without geographical boundaries. Worldwide easy accessibility to antibiotics and their subsequent abuse by consumers, medical practitioners, or veterinarians/paraveterinarians has injured the harmony and coherence of the microbial ecosystem with the emergence of difficult-to-treat infection-causing bugs. It has been suggested that suboptimal exposure of bacterial cells to drugs harnesses bacterial evolutionary processes to surpass the selective antibiotic pressures, which over time might certainly stretch the resistance dose to higher concentrations (Ching et al., 2019). Bacterial demonstrate antibiotic resistance by exhibiting intrinsic and extrinsic features. As intrinsic/innate resistance, bacteria display one or more sophisticated mechanisms such as remodeling the outer membrane permeability toward antibiotics, production of inactivating enzymes, modification in the drug target site, fostering antibiotic efflux pumps, or the resistance may be due to chromosomal mutations that alter the resistance phenotype. Though intrinsic resistance dramatically limits the therapeutic options, it is not laterally transferable among the environmental bacteria as these phenotypes are the outcome of core and fixed genetic makeup. On other hand, the acquired resistance is a major public health concern as the antibiotic-resistant genes are localized on the mobile genetic elements (mobilome), such as plasmids or flanked between insertion sequence elements. Unfortunately, microbes with acquired resistance can disseminate the AMR genes (ARGs) in the environmental or commensal microbes via horizontal gene transfer (transduction, transformation, or conjugation) (Peterson & Kaur, 2018). As an outcome, several clinically relevant antibiotic-resistant bacteria have emerged with a knack to resist a diverse group of existing antimicrobials. To enlist such superbugs, the World Health Organization (WHO) has made collective efforts to categorize such superbugs on a priority basis for the discovery of innovative drugs using contemporary approaches. At the critical importance, the most Gram-negative pathogens, such as *Acinetobacter baumannii* (carbapenem resistant), *Pseudomonas aeruginosa* (carbapenem resistant), and Enterobacteriaceae (carbapenem resistant and 3rd-generation cephalosporin resistant), have been listed. In the current scenario, these are the topmost priority pathogens against which modern researchers are currently focusing to develop complementary drugs. Under the second priority (high), the organisms, such as *Enterococcus faecium*, vancomycin-resistant *Staphylococcus aureus* (methicillin resistant and *vancomycin* intermediate and resistant), *Helicobacter pylori* (clarithromycin resistant), *Campylobacter* (fluoroquinolone resistant), *Salmonella* spp. (fluoroquinolone resistant), and *Neisseria gonorrhoeae* (3rd-generation cephalosporin resistant and fluoroquinolone resistant), have been listed.

Likewise, *Streptococcus pneumoniae*, penicillin-nonsusceptible *Haemophilus influenzae*, ampicillin-resistant *Shigella* spp., and fluoroquinolone resistant have been identified under third priority (medium) (Shrivastava et al., 2018).

To address the enduring threat of AMR, the holistic approach of "One Health" is imperative, which necessitates the active involvement of multidisciplinary professionals with a goal to protect all living organisms in the environment. This involves restricting the abuse/overprescribing of antibiotics, strict regulatory restrictions, improved antibiotic stewardship, sanitation, continued active surveillance, and protecting the effectiveness of currently existing antibiotics. More importantly, the timely discovery of novel antimicrobials or alternatives to antibiotics is indispensable when the preexisting drug is no longer effective (McEwen & Collignon, 2018). Developing novel therapeutic avenues to fight against resistant infections, especially those caused by ESKAPE bugs (*Enterococcus faecium*, *S. aureus*, *Klebsiella pneumoniae*, *A. baumannii*, *P. aeruginosa*, and *Enterobacter* spp.), is indeed the need of the hour. Having said this, several alternatives to antibiotics are now well studied for their efficacy and effectiveness against ESKAPE pathogens. Among, the bacteriophages, endolysins, antimicrobial peptides, antibodies, stem cell therapy, liposomes, photodynamic light therapy, silver nanoparticles, Faecal Microbial Transplantation (FMT), and probiotics are some of the portfolios of alternatives approach (Czaplewski et al., 2016; Ghosh et al., 2019; Rello et al., 2019). However, their effective dosage and mode of action vary among the therapies depending upon the mode and site of application. Henceforth, a careful therapeutic selection is essential to derive maximum response based on the target applications. Amid the several alternatives, the probiotic arena is a strenuous protagonist among alternatives to antibiotics that is widely studied and applied in both human and animal disease control. With this goal, the present chapter aims to recapitulate the role of probiotics in combating multidrug-resistant organisms vis-à-vis their infections by focusing on their mode of antagonistic actions lucidly and understandably.

19.2 Probiotics

The microbiome is an integral part of human life that is inoculated right from birth. The microbial eubiosis in several organs of the human system confers a balanced and healthy condition. On the contrary, microbial dysbiosis is a most serious conundrum that is now well correlated to the onset of several lifestyle diseases (Brüssow, 2020). To overcome such disturbances, fermented milk products have been long recommended as both therapeutics and prophylactics without solid scientific evidences. Such beneficial properties of fermented milk products were scrutinized by Russian Nobel Laureate Elie Metchnikoff and 27-year-old Bulgarian physician Stamen Grigorov, who noticed the longevity of Bulgarian people after consumption of fermented milk products like yogurt or sour milk. However, the scientific hypothesis of Metchnikoff was further strengthened by coining the term probiotics by German scientist Werner Kollath in 1953, and in 1992 by Fuller who defined probiotics as "a live microbial feed supplement which beneficially affects the host animal by improving its intestinal microbial balance" (Gasbarrini et al., 2016). Since then several amendments have been made to define probiotics by FAO/WHO. Nevertheless, an internationally agreed definition of probiotics is now defined as "live microorganisms that, when administered in adequate amounts, confer a health benefit on the host" (Martín & Langella, 2019). Although several genera among lactic acid bacteria (LAB) and non-LAB are studied as potential probiotics, the European Food Safety Authority panel accorded the Qualified Presumption of Safety for selected species under *Lactobacillus* and *Bifidobacterium* based on their safe footing. Though probiotics intervention was traditionally confined to overrule the gastrointestinal complications, they are now being used as an adjunct therapeutic avenue in ameliorating allergies, neurodegenerative diseases, cancers, and management of lifestyle diseases, such as hypertension, type-2 diabetes, metabolic syndrome, and nonalcoholic fatty liver (Asher et al., 2020; Koutnikova et al., 2019).

While addressing the growing threat of AMR, the use of probiotics instead of antibiotics for treating infectious diseases is a well-accepted and noteworthy approach. Briefly, the idea of this concept is that instead of using antibiotics to curb pathogenic microbes, the use of probiotics would aid to establish beneficial microbes successfully in the target niche and thus may hinder the growth and implantation of disease-causing microbes. Limiting the frequency of antibiotics usage coupled with the subsequent complementary use of probiotics may also curtail the microbial exposure to antibiotics and therefore may help to decrease the rate of development of resulting antibiotic-resistant strains. The same is currently being practiced to overcome the recurrent infection of drug-resistant *Clostridium difficile* during antibiotic-associated diarrhea (AAD). To avoid AAD, remedial probiotic therapy is generally prescribed to restore the intestinal microbiota and to exclude the pathogens that dwell under antibiotic selective pressure (*Clostridium difficile*). However, the concern of modern researchers is to completely avoid the antibiotic applications during such infection and to replace them with probiotics (Kerna & Brown, 2018).

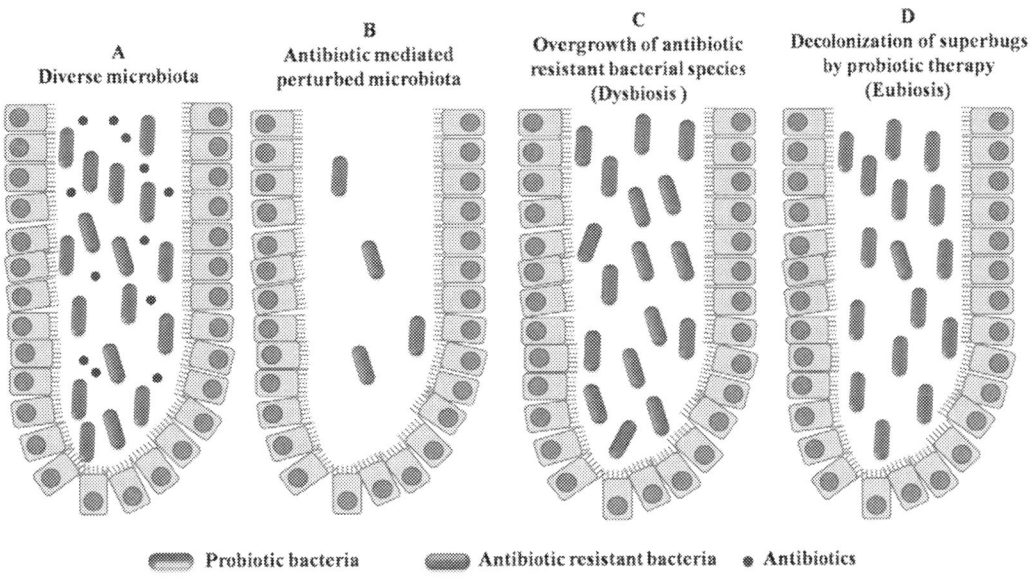

FIGURE 19.1 Pictorial representation of antibiotics induced gut microbial perturbation (A and B), overgrowth of drug-resistant bugs/dysbiosis (C), and subsequent gut microbial replenishment by probiotic therapy (D).

Human gut is considered as an epicenter of bacterial resistance since the colonization of the multidrug-resistant (MDR) superbugs has the propensity to spread the ARGs to other commensal and pathogenic organisms in the gut (Maharjan et al., 2018). Hence, comprehending the consequences of gut exposure to antibiotics is vital to prevent the spread of antibiotic resistance. Equilibrium in the microflora residing in the gut econiche is paramount to maintain a balanced state of health since microbial perturbation is believed to be relevant in causing disease mechanisms. However, the use of antibiotics to subside the symptoms of gut dysbiosis will provide an environment favorable to the colonization of antibiotic-resistant strains, which demonstrate a hike in the frequency of treatment failure, and finally leads to poor therapeutic outcomes (Guk et al., 2020). Henceforth, the use of microbial therapies, such as FMT or probiotics, as live biotherapeutics to treat the enteric resistant infections is a better complementary option to decolonize resistant bugs from the intestinal milieu as illustrated in Fig. 19.1. Although probiotics intervention is mainly targeted to confront gut-mediated infections, the therapeutic horizon is now expanded beyond the gut, such as treatment of resistant urogenital infections, skin/wound infections, vaginal infections, respiratory/pulmonary infections via direct gastrointestinal, topical, intravaginal, and intranasal administrations (Argenta et al., 2016; Forsythe, 2011; Lopes et al., 2017; Naderi et al., n.d.; van de Wijgert & Verwijs, 2020). The various probiotic delivery vehicles in different routes include lyophilized tablets/powders, nonlyophilized tablets/powders, and fermented beverages and yogurt (Newman & Arshad, 2020). In this regard, we hereby highlight the general and disease-organ-specific mechanisms of actions of probiotics while ruining the MDR infections.

19.3 General mechanisms of actions of probiotics against MDR bacteria

19.3.1 Antibacterial action

Antimicrobial action is an important attribute that should be demonstrated by all probiotic strains. This helps the bacteria to inhibit the growth and establishment of the competitive microflora in a particular niche. The antibacterial activity of probiotic strains is majorly attributed to the production of several metabolites extracellularly in culture supernatant or its vicinity. LAB are the natural cell factory of multifarious compounds, such as organic acids (lactic and acetic acid), hydrogen peroxide, free fatty acids, ethanol, diacetyl, mevalonolactone, δ-dodecalactone, acetaldehyde, acetoin, hydroxyl fatty acids, phenyllactic acid, cyclic dipeptides, carbon dioxide, reuterin, surfactants, siderophores, exopolysaccharides, reutericyclin, and bacteriocins (Kanmani et al., 2013; Šušković et al., 2010). However, each of these compounds exhibits different modes of action on the bacterial cells as presented in Fig. 19.2. It is important to mention here that temporal secretion of several antimicrobial compounds by probiotics at a given time may act synergistically would aid in demonstrating multiple inhibitory actions against pathogenic microflora. This perhaps helps to overcome the development of AMR by target pathogen against all the compounds at a given time since cellular modifications to

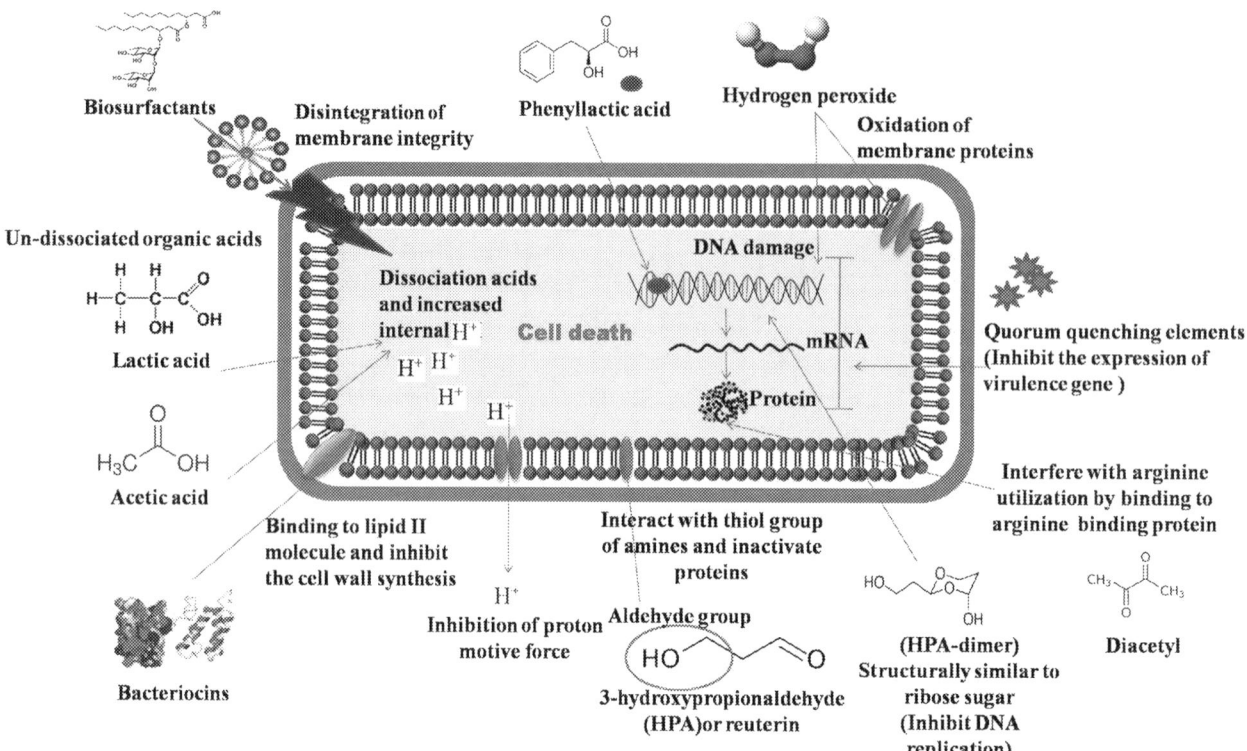

FIGURE 19.2 Mode of action of probiotic derived metabolites on bacterial cell.

resistant multiple stresses is indeed too energetic and an unfavorable process for any biological system thereof. On the other hand, the synergistic use of cell-free supernatant (CFS) (source of antimicrobial agents) and antibiotics to kill the target pathogens might minimize the lethal antibiotic dose that otherwise demands a higher concentration. In a study, synergistic use of CFS (*Lactobacillus rhamnosus* and *Lactobacillus casei*) and gentamicin had reduced the antibiotic requirement (minimum inhibitory concentration and minimum bactericidal concentration) to kill the *P. aeruginosa* (Aminnezhad et al., 2015).

19.3.2 Antibiofilm action

Microbial biofilm of single-species or polymicrobial communities arranged in a three-dimensional structure on both biotic and abiotic surfaces is a significant threat to the therapeutic world since bacteria in the biofilms behave 10–1000 times resistant to antimicrobials and other stress including overcoming the host immune system compared to the planktonic state (Shivaprasad et al., 2020). Microbes in the biofilms display multifactorial actions by hampering the penetration of antibiotics inside the biofilm structure that ultimately fails the functioning of antibiotic therapy. The failure of antibiotics to disrupt the multidrug-resistant bacterial biofilms necessitated alternative and more intense natural antibiofilm agents. Interestingly, probiotic LAB are the natural hub of several and most effective biodetergents. The CFS or outer membrane contains extracellularly synthesized biosurfactants of protein–carbohydrate complexes, lipids, or fatty acids. Few representatives of probiotic lactobacilli-derived biosurfactants are surfactin, glycoprotein, protein-like, etc. (Hajfarajollah et al., 2018). Being amphiphilic compounds, they reduce the interfacial tension between the contact surface and bacterial surface and thus aid in halting the biofilm formation. At the molecular level, the biosurfactants from probiotic lactobacilli have been shown to downregulate the expression of biofilm-related genes. In this context, the purified biosurfactants extracted from the *Lactobacillus reuteri* have significantly downregulated the expression of *glucosyltransferases* (*gtfs*) and *fructosyltransferase* (*ftf*) genes that play a critical role in the initial adhesion of *Streptococcus mutans* (Salehi et al., 2020). Besides demonstrating antibiofilm actions, they exhibit lethal actions on the target pathogens by inducing the ultrastructural membrane details like membrane pore formation (fatty acid moieties of biosurfactants inserting into the cell membrane and smaller acyl tails of the biosurfactant into the plasma membrane triggering disruptions of the plasma membrane) (Deepansh et al., 2016). Production of biosurfactants by probiotic strains has been reported inhibiting the adhesion of resistant pathogenic microflora in the human gastrointestinal tract and vaginal econiche (Nelson et al., 2020). Therefore probiotic-derived biosurfactants may have valuable applications as antiadhesive or antibiofilm agents in combating the multidrug-resistant bacterial biofilms on the hospital settings and biomedical surfaces.

19.3.3 Antiquorum sensing

Quorum sensing is an interbacterial communication of the bacteria belonging to the same community via synthesis of signaling molecules like autoinducers (AIs) at a particular population density/ threshold where bacteria sense the AIs and regulate the expression of several downstream regulatory proteins and virulent genes (bacterial motility, biofilm formation, plasmid conjugation, and production of other virulence factors to invade host) (Kiymaci et al., 2018). Both Gram-positive and Gram-negative bacteria produce AIs. Examples for AIs are autoinducing peptides produced by Gram-positive bacteria, acylatedhomoserine lactone (AHL) produced by Gram-negative bacteria, pseudomonas quinolone signal, autoinducer-2 (AI-2) for intra- and interspecies communication regardless of whether they are Gram-negative or Gram-positive bacteria, autoinducer-3 (AI-3) (Deng et al., 2020; Zhang & Li, 2016). It is interesting to note that the probiotic bacteria extracellularly synthesize several soluble proteins, exopolysaccharides, and organic acids that show proven efficacy to attenuate the quorum sensing and their subsequent virulence expression. The lactic acid produced by *Pediococcus acidilactici* M7 significantly attenuated the virulence phenotypes of *P. aeruginosa*, such as swimming-swarming-twitching motility, protease activity, elastase activity, pyocyanin production, and biofilm formation (Kiymaci et al., 2018). Similarly, the acidified supernatant of *Lactococcus lactis*, *Lactobacillus rhamnosus*, and *Lactobacillus fermentum* had a quorum quenching mechanism by significantly reducing the AHL level and thus reducing the elastase activity. Moreover, the supernatant could diminish the expression of lasI and rhlI genes (AHL synthase) of *P. aeruginosa* (Rana et al., 2020). Since antibiotics and related peptides target the growth-related process of pathogens, it imparts antibiotic selection pressure. Therefore harnessing the antiquorum sensing knack of probiotics may be a promising alternative that could potentially impede microbial pathogenesis.

19.3.4 Antivirulence property

Bacterial virulence is the collective regulation and expression of several virulence determinates, such as toxins and adhesins, and cell surface adhesion molecules, such as pili, adhesins, chaperons, and sortase (Alekshun & Levy, 2004). In this regard, the biosurfactants from probiotic *Lactobacillus helveticus* strains have shown in vitro antibiofilm and antiinvasion ability against *S. aureus* (Jiang et al., 2019). Moreover, the release of exopolysaccharides from *Lactobacillus acidophilus* A4 was shown to abrogate the biofilm formation by *Escherichia coli* by downregulating the expression of curli production genes (*crl*, *csgA*, and *csgB*) and chemotaxis gene (*cheY*) (Kim et al., 2009). Phenyllactic acid, another antimicrobial compound produced by probiotic lactobacilli, has been shown to inhibit enterococcal biofilm formation, cellular motility, and exopolysaccharide production by downregulating the expression of Ebppili (*ebpABC*) and Epa polysaccharide genes (*epaABE*) (Liu et al., 2020). The CFS of *Lactobacillus acidophilus* GP1B displayed *in vivo* antivirulence potential against *C. difficile* by decreasing the transcriptomic response of *luxS*, *tcdA*, *tcdB*, and *txeR* genes (Yun et al., 2014). On the other hand, probiotics attenuate the mucoadhesion of pathogenic microbes by lowering the expression of host MUC-related genes (Mack et al., 1999). These dynamic antivirulence mechanisms of probiotics with clear molecular mechanisms further recommend the exploitation of probiotics as safe biotherapy to counteract the devastating diseases.

19.3.5 Antitoxic property

Microbial toxins pose a significant threat to public health since they are carcinogenic, genotoxic, cytotoxic, teratogenic, allergenic, and dermato-, nephro-, and hepatotoxic (Hathout & Aly, 2014). Hence, probiotics could be a powerful biological strategy to counteract the effects of microbial toxins. Although underlying mechanisms of antitoxic effects of probiotics have been poorly understood, researchers proposed three pertinent mechanisms. These include neutralization or degradation of toxins by secretion of protease, surface binding of toxins by probiotic cells, and blocking the production of toxins (Corbo et al., 2018). For example, *L. acidophilus* and *L. fermentum* decreased the production of α-toxin from *C. perfringens* without influencing cell biomass. More importantly, probiotic strains even degraded the established α-toxin (Guo et al., 2017). Similarly, an engineered probiotic *Lactobacillus paracasei* BL23 expressing antitoxin antibody on the cell surface neutralized the toxin B (TcdB) produced by *C. difficile* (Andersen et al., 2016). On the other hand, *L. acidophilus* exhibited the inhibitory action against the cholera toxin and Shiga-toxin produced by *Vibrio cholera* and *Shigella dysenteriae* by hindering the expression of *CTX-B* and *Stx1* expression (Alamdary & Bakhshi, 2020). The serine protease secreted in the CFS of probiotic *Bacillus clausii* strain O/C inactivated cytotoxins of *Clostridium difficile* and *Bacillus cereus* (Ripert et al., 2016). The antidiarrheal knack of probiotics is mainly attributed to the antitoxic effects of probiotics since several of them have protective actions against verotoxin producing *E. coli* (EHEC) and Shiga toxin-producing *E. coli* O157:H7 (Asahara et al., 2004). Indirectly, probiotics modulate the host immune response to protect against bacterial toxins (Surendran Nair et al., 2017). Besides bacterial toxins, several probiotic lactobacilli have been shown to detoxify or bind and reduce the bioavailability or transepithelial transport of mycotoxins such as aflatoxin B_1, deoxynivalenol, fumonisins, ochratoxin A, and patulin (Chlebicz & Śliżewska, 2020; Fuchs et al., 2008).

19.3.6 Antiinvasion actions

Cell surface-mediated bacterial adhesion and subsequent invasion of bacteria into host tissues are the two pragmatic phenomena while inducing pathogenicity. The binding specificity of pathogens to the host epithelial cells will be conferred by various cell surface-anchored components, such as pilus, surface proteins, and bacterial capsule. Once attached, the cells undergo internalization into the nonprofessional phagocytes to facilitate cell invasion either by zipper or trigger mechanisms via actin filament reorganization. In Zipper mode of bacterial invasion, the host-associated E-cadherin and hepatocyte growth factor receptor "Met" serve as the receptors for internalins that facilitate the pathogen internalization. In trigger mode, pathogenic bacteria activate the host Rho GTPase-mediated signal transduction mechanisms to form cup-like protrusion (ruffles) via cytoskeleton rearrangement (Ribet & Cossart, 2015). However, several probiotic strains and their CFS have shown the protective efficacy against enteropathogenic invading pathogens in various cell culture models through three different invasion inhibition assays, that is, protective, competitive, and displacement mode (Khodaii et al., 2017). Besides, several probiotic LAB have been shown to inhibit the invasion of urinary tract pathogens (Lai et al., 2020). Though antiinvasion mechanisms are poorly understood, the target pathogen shedding and strengthening the intestinal barriers via expression of adherence (claudin, occludin, ZO-1) and tight junction and adherence (E-cadherin and β-catenin) junction protein expression (Moroni et al., 2006; Yu et al., 2012) are the two proposed antiinvasion mechanisms of probiotics. However, further studies are necessary to comprehend this particular mechanistic action of probiotics.

19.3.7 Intrabacterial and interbacterial aggregation

Several bacteria in the environment exhibit the process of autoaggregation/autoagglutination/flocculation by which bacteria among the same community can form clumps or aggregate that eventually settles down. Autoaggregation is one among the cell surface properties wherein the process is mediated by self-recognizing of the cell surface patterns or autoagglutinins, such as surface proteins, exopolysaccharides, teichoic acids, pilus, fimbriae, M-proteins, and MSCRAMMs (microbial surface components recognizing adhesive matrix molecules). However, these autoagglutinins vary widely among the pathogenic and beneficial bacteria. For example, *A. baumannii*, an opportunistic pathogen, exhibits AtaA factor. Whereas probiotic lactobacilli display LysM-containing serine/threonine-rich protein as an agglutinin factor (Trunk et al., 2018). Though the process of autoaggregation among pathogenic bacteria is unseemly since numerous studies correlate the autoaggregation with biofilm formation (Chenia & Duma, 2017), the same may be desirable among probiotics bacteria. Several studies have established that probiotic bacteria exhibiting superior autoaggregation portray better biofilm formation, intestinal adhesion, and subsequent establishment (Leccese Terraf et al., 2014). Besides, an autoaggregation phenotype also protects the bacterial cells from physical or chemical stress. This perhaps helps to overcome gastrointestinal stress that a probiotic strain undergoes upon oral administration for successful colonization in the intestine and thereby indirectly prevent the adhesion of pathogenic bacteria in the gut or other econiche. On the contrary, interspecies cell-to-cell coaggregation is a desirable property of the probiotics that indirectly aid in the pathogen elimination from the host tissue by preventing the pathogenic bacterial adhesion via blocking the adhesion sites (cell surface patterns) (Dlamini et al., 2019).

19.3.8 Bacterial colonization interference

Bacterial adhesion is a crucial step in the colonization of both probiotic and pathogenic bacteria. The effective colonization of pathogens is a way to cause several infections by triggering several signal transduction mechanisms and subsequent invasion. To counteract this, probiotics exhibits decolonization capability via protective (exclusion), competitive,

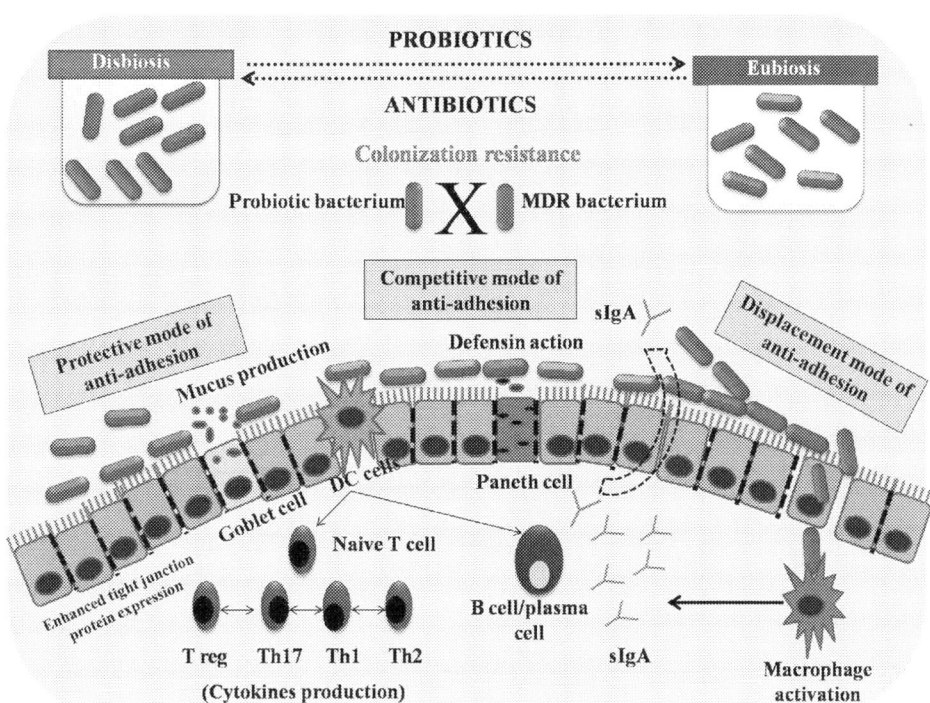

FIGURE 19.3 Colonization resistance mechanisms of probiotic bacteria against multidrug-resistant superbugs.

and displacement modes (Fig. 19.3) (Candela et al., 2008). In protective mode, an effective adhesion of probiotic bacterium to the host tissue will avoid the adhesion of pathogens since the adhesion receptors on the host tissues are preoccupied with probiotics. Whereas probiotics compete directly or indirectly with the tropic limiting nutrients or physically for the adhesion sites either by creating active competition to binding sites or passively by out-competing with pathogenic bacteria by killing of targets microbes through the production of antimicrobial substances. For example, competition for nutrients like monomeric glucose, N-acetyl-glucosamine, and sialic acid in the intestinal niche has been reviewed to favor the elimination of *C. difficile* from the gut (Surendran Nair et al., 2017). Although pathogen displacement by probiotics is unclear, several studies suggest that probiotics can also displace the previously adhered pathogens from the tissue surface (Collado et al., 2007). This is perhaps due to the in vivo production of certain antimicrobials and biosurfactants that may unfasten the adhered pathogens from the host tissue. These manifestations of probiotics suggest both therapeutic and prophylaxis roles in abating microbial adhesion mediated pathogenesis.

19.3.9 Immunomodulation

Several researchers have noted the improvement in the immunocompetence of the human subjects upon the probiotics intervention by modulating both mucosal innate and adaptive immune systems via microbe-associated molecular pattern—pattern recognition receptor interactions. Probiotics associated cell surface appendages or their metabolites like short-chain fatty acids interact with the toll-like receptor on the gut enterocytes or dendritic cells (DCs) (located in lamina propria) and thus modulates/inhibits the signal transduction mechanisms, such as nuclear factor-κB and mitogen-activated protein kinases, that are earlier triggered by pathogens leading to altered cytokines production in the host (Yousefi et al., 2019). While certain probiotic *Lactobacillus* strains have also been reported to induce heme-oxygenase in DCs to produce T-regulatory cells. On the other hand, the probiotics mediated a balance between T lymphocytes expressing CD-4 surface molecule (T-helper cells) by the suppression of Th1 response (proinflammatory response-TNF-alpha, IL-6, interferon) and stimulation of Th2 response stimulates the host-associated antiinflammatory cytokines (IL-4, IL-10, TGF-beta) production and subsequent activation of humoral response, B-cell proliferation and antibody production (sIgA) (Forsythe & Bienenstock, 2010). Besides regulating a balance between Th1 and Th2 cells, a balance between pathogenic (proinflammatory) and nonpathogenic (antiinflammatory) Th17 cells was also observed by probiotics since Th17 differentiation into nonpathogenic Th17 is influenced by surrounding antiinflammatory cytokines. The antiinflammatory effect of probiotics is linked to the downregulation of proinflammatory IL-17 cytokine production, upstream Th-17-secreted cytokines (IL-23, TGF-β), and downstream Th-17-secreted cytokines (IL-1β, IL-6, TNF-α,

IFNγ, IL-12) (Owaga et al., 2015; Wu et al., 2018). On the other side, several strains of probiotics have enhanced epithelial mucus production by goblet cells by increasing the expression of MUC genes (an innate immune system) (Plaza-Diaz et al., 2014). Interestingly, the supplementation of soluble protein factor (p40) from *L. rhamnosus* GG triggers epidermal growth factor (Yan et al., 2013) and thus suggested the resuscitation ability of probiotics in the inflammation-mediated injured tissues in colitis. Probiotics also trigger the induction of paneth cells to produce broad-spectrum host-associated eukaryotic antimicrobial peptides like β-defensin-2 (hBD-2), which protects against invading pathogens in the lumen (Cazorla et al., 2018). Similarly, the lipid component of probiotic cells has been documented to increase the NK-cell activity (Yahfoufi et al., 2018).

19.3.10 Antidrug resistance property

Typical phenotypes, such as the antibiotic efflux pumps, drug inactivating enzymes, and modification of drug action, are the important mechanisms by which bacteria show resistance to different antibiotics. Very interestingly, probiotics could reverse the antibiotic resistance exhibited by MDR superbugs by lowering the expression of resistance genes. Recently, the CFS from few gut microbes and probiotic species, such as *Bacteroides fragilis*, *Bifidobacterium longum*, *Clostridium butyricum*, *Clostridioides difficile*, *Clostridium perfringens*, *Enterococcus faecium*, *Lactobacillus plantarum*, and probiotic strain of *C. butyricum* MIYAIRI 588, has shown to suppress the transcription of *bla* $_{CTX-M}$ gene during the growth phase of ESBL *E. coli* coupled with reduced transmissibility of antibiotic-resistant *bla* gene to gut microbiota/probiotics (Kunishima et al., 2019). Similarly in another study, coculturing of commensal and probiotic bacteria with MDR bacteria (*Klebsiella pneumonia* and *A. baumannii*) has resulted in differential expression of several genes that are responsible for the biology of antibiotic resistance. These shreds of evidence suggest that probiotics may certainly hamper the development and spread of AMR of community bacteria while living together in a specific ecosystem (Chan et al., 2018). However, further studies are warranted to comprehend such mechanisms in other antibiotic-resistant genes of various superbugs.

19.4 Probiotics in organ-specific resistant infections

19.4.1 Role of probiotics in urogenital infections

Urogenital infections are among the most frequently observed microbial infections that are causing a significant global economic loss in society. In fact, compared to men, women significantly suffer from urogenital infections as reported in the United States (Smelov et al., 2016). Amid the several classifications of urogenital infections, microbe-associated infections are of great interest as they contribute to AMR. Several microbes, such as uropathogenic *E. coli*, *Candida* spp., *Enterococcus* spp., *P. aeruginosa*, *Klebsiella* spp., *Enterobacter* spp., *Proteus* spp., coagulase-negative staphylococci, *Morganella* spp., *Acinetobacter* spp., and *Citrobacter* (Zaid, 2014). Very importantly, the rampant antibiotic usage in the clinical sectors has pushed these microbes to dwell under antibiotic selective pressure and few are now resistant to last-line antibiotics. These microbes initially form biofilms/establish in the organs of the lower urogenital tract and then may also lead to sepsis by ascending traffic to the upper genital tract. Therefore while developing the empiric therapies against such pathogens, the factors, such as bacterial biofilm production, intracellular bacterial colonization, and the quality of the host immune, response (antiadhesion chemokine production, state of glycosaminoglycans, and proinflammatory cytokine production), should be considered for effective mitigation of infections. In this regard, probiotics and their bioactive metabolites have been considered as a panacea in treating urogenital infections and thus have been incorporated into gender foods to overcome microbial infections (Patrignani et al., 2019; Waigankar & Patel, 2011). Several metabolites produced by probiotics limit the growth of microbes, the biosurfactant produced by probiotics hamper/disrupt the biofilm formation, and they also prime the macrophages, leukocytes, cytokines, and other host defenses (Waigankar & Patel, 2011). The ex vivo and in vitro assays have suggested the bio-competency (bacteriostatic, antiinflammatory, antibiofilm, and pathogen exclusion) of probiotics or probiotic-based formulations against urogenital pathogens (*E. coli*, *K. pneumoniae*, and *Proteus mirabilis*) (Defne et al., 2020; Nicklas et al., 2019). More importantly, the probiotic isolates viz. *L. casei* and *L. reuteri* have shown antibiofilm and antiadherence activities against MDR *P. mirabilis* (Shaaban et al., 2020).

On the other hand, bacterial vaginosis (BV) is the most commonly observed gynecological threat characterized by perturbed vaginal lactobacilli and overgrowth of anaerobic and putrefying microbes (Basavaprabhu et al., 2020). Nevertheless, excessive use of antibiotics to treat BV has witnessed the emergence of antibiotic-resistant episodes in the BV pathogens (Beigi et al., 2004). Hence, the alternative use of probiotics either orally or intravaginal route to reestablish the microbial homeostasis in the vaginal econiche is widely accepted and applied (Bohbot et al., 2018). Among the several species of probiotic *Lactobacillus*, *Lactobacillus crispatus* and *Lactobacillus gasseri* have been commonly recommended as vaginal probiotics due to their native/autochthonous status. The mechanism of actions of probiotics against BV pathogens includes antimicrobial, antibiofilm, coaggregation, competitive exclusion, host immunomodulation, and reepithelialization (Basavaprabhu et al., 2020; Mitchell et al., 2015). It is important to note that few multicentre, randomized, double-blind, placebo-controlled trials also underscore equal potency of probiotics to combat the recurrent BV infections similar to the group treated with metronidazole antibiotics (van de Wijgert & Verwijs, 2020; Ya et al., 2010).

19.4.2 Role of probiotics in the resistant skin and wound infections

Skin is considered to be the largest organ of the integumentary system that covers the human body. A loss in skin integrity by cut or break may lead to entry, colonization, and invasion of exogenous microorganisms of the environment. These microbes may adversely trigger the host immune response leading to inflammation in the surface that alters the wound healing properties. Microorganisms, such as *Staphylococcus*, *Corynebacterium*, *Clostridium*, and *Pseudomonas*, have been isolated from skin or wound infections that adversely affect the wound healing properties (Frank et al., 2009). With the growing concern of AMR while treating cutaneous and systemic infections, alternative therapeutic agents have been evaluated to investigate their ability to accelerate wound healing and decrease the incidence of chronic wounds. Probiotics administration in wound management is a new strategy and is found to regulate both in direct and indirect modes (Fijan et al., 2019). Indirect mode suggested by the literature suggests that the orally administered probiotics improve the wound healing process, such as tissue oxygenation levels, blood pressure, inflammation, and the immune response. Whereas the topical applications of probiotics could directly overcome the local infections by ameliorating the local inflammation, direct antagonism with pathogens, and improved tissue healing by reepithelialization, more specifically by the increase in the expression levels of collagen type 1 and transcription growth factor-beta 1 (TGF-beta 1) (Tsiouris & Tsiouri, 2017). The metabolites in the CFS of probiotic lactobacilli have also been shown to inhibit *Propionibacterium acnes* and *S. aureus* and thus they seem to be an interesting alternative to combat acne lesions (Mottin & Suyenaga, 2018). On the other hand, biofilm-forming superbugs associated wound infections (*S. aureus*, *P. aeruginosa*, *Enterococcus faecalis*, *A. baumannii*, *E. coli*, *K. pneumoniae*, *Enterobacter* spp., *Peptostreptococcus* spp., etc.) are more common and are sometimes difficult-to-treat with antibiotics in the immunocompromised individuals since it may cause sepsis/may enter the bloodstream. There is also corroborative evidence on the translocation of gut colonized MRSA to the wound site (Krezalek et al., 2018). Hence, it is important to keep both wound infection sites and gut free from such resistant bugs. Nevertheless, numerous studies have demonstrated the antagonistic ability of several probiotics strains against MRSA isolates either direct competitive exclusion (adhesion and internalization inhibition) and indirectly by host immune stimulation (Hafez et al., 2013). Despite excluding the pathogens by bacterial interferences modes, probiotics have also been reported to confer anticytotoxic effect/protective against drug-resistant *S. aureus*- and *P. aeruginosa*-infected epidermal keratinocytes and also on Vero cells (Hafez et al., 2013; Prince et al., 2012). Alternatively, probiotics intervention has also resulted in improved tight junction function and expression of claudin 1, ZO-1, and occludin in keratinocytes infected with *S. aureus* and thus may prevent the pathogen invasion. Besides displaying the protective effects at in vitro experiments, the topical applications of probiotics have also impeded the adhesion of *P. aeruginosa*, *S. aureus*, and *S. epidermidis* both upon animal and human experimentation and improved wound healing by reducing the inflammation (Lukic et al., 2017).

19.4.3 Probiotics in gut-mediated resistant infections

Human gut insights through metagenomic approaches have underscored the presence of an extraordinarily complex and dynamic microbial community that can vary dramatically with several factors (Schloissnig et al., 2013). The healthy gut microbiota is relatively stable and therefore ingested pathogens can be eliminated through a large number of residing commensal microbes. By contrast, the antibiotic intervention drastically disturbs the gut microbiome by killing the antibiotic susceptible individuals. Depending upon the antibiotics been used in the therapy, the collateral enrichment or selection of antibiotic-resistant bugs, such as *Clostridium difficile*, ESBL-secreting *E. coli*, *Pseudomonas*, *Enterococci*, and *Acinetobacter* spp. predominates in the niche. This perhaps damages the gut barrier property and allows bacterial/their lipopolysaccharides (LPS) translocation into the bloodstream which leads to healthcare-associated infections such as bacteremia/sepsis/endotoxemia (Melzer & Petersen, 2007). Moreover, this process may trigger the horizontal transfer of resistant genes from resistant bugs to commensal bugs. Moreover, gut-mediated resistance may facilitate easy and widespread dissemination of resistant genes in the environment via defecation. Therefore a technique like selective digestive decontamination (SDD) and use of probiotics to reestablish balanced gut microflora or prophylactic use of probiotics to create colonization resistance against antibiotic-resistant bugs have been overlooked to decolonize resistant bugs. In fact, studies could not differentiate the noninferiority of probiotics compared with SDD in resistant digestive tract infection prevention (Oudhuis et al., 2011). Probiotics have proven efficacy to overcome AAD. Several in vitro and in vivo studies have shown that probiotics directly compete to the adhesion sites and other nutrients with superbugs and thus obstruct the colonization of multidrug resistant bugs via protective, competitive, and displacement mode of exclusion in the intestinal milieu (Cunha et al., 2017; Jayashree et al., 2018; Quigley et al., 2019; Ren et al., 2012). On the other hand, probiotics indirectly eliminate the pathogens by altering the host immune modulation such as stimulation of secretory immunoglobulins and antimicrobial human β-defensin (Möndel et al., 2009) while also strengthening the intestinal epithelial by enhancing the expression of tight junction and adherence junction proteins.

19.4.4 Role of probiotics in resistant pulmonary infections

With the efforts of the human microbiome project, it now well established that microbes have coevolved with humans and each organ systems have their unique microbial profile. Homeostasis in the microbial community in an organ system is crucial to maintain overall health and wellness (Salehi et al., 2020). Likewise, our respiratory tract harbors niche-specific numerous microbes, such as *Staphylococcus* spp., *Propionibacterium* spp., *Corynebacterium* spp., *Moraxella* spp., *Streptococcus* spp., *Dolosigranulum* spp., *Haemophilus* spp., *Rothia* spp., *Leptotrichia* spp., *Prevotella*spp., *Veillonella* spp., and *Tropheryma whipplei* (Man et al., 2017). Their alterations and dysbiosis have also been linked to the onset of several inflammatory lung diseases. Such microbial imbalance in the respiratory tract has also been observed in pneumonia patients (De Steenhuijsen Piters et al., 2016). Albeit the antibiotics were essential to control the upper and lower respiratory tract infections, the reduced antibiotic susceptibility by respiratory pathogens *S. pneumoniae*, *H. influenzae*, *P. aeruginosa*, and *Mycobacterium tuberculosis* has pushed the clinicians to unravel alternatives therapies to combat difficult-to-treat-infections (Guitor & Wright, 2018). Although the application of probiotics was traditionally limited to the gastrointestinal site, the advances in probiotic research have paved the way to exploit the therapeutic proficiency of probiotics in curbing disease in different organs. In this regard, the role of probiotics in respiratory infections is now becoming fairly apparent. Studies inferred that their mode of action remains largely the same in curbing the infectious disease irrespective of organs/tissue. Though the preventive mechanisms of probiotics in pulmonary associated infections are less intuitive, it has been postulated that probiotics may protect the host by displaying direct antimicrobial activity against respiratory pathogens, competitive exclusion of pathogens, reinforcement of the epithelial barrier function (enhancing the expression of tight junction proteins), enhanced production of host antimicrobial proteins, such as defensins-2, increased mucus production, and immunomodulation (enhancing the humoral and cell-mediated immunity) (Alexandre et al., 2014; Robinson, 2017). Regarding the route of probiotic administration in respiratory infections, both oral and intranasal applications of probiotics have been overlooked with sufficient availability of commercially viable technologies to produce probiotic-based formulation modalities (Katarina et al., 2020). Importantly, the intranasal application of probiotics has been reported to have more potency to trigger the immune functioning of the lungs more easily and can easily decolonize the adhered drug-resistant bugs than the intragastric route (Park et al., 2011; Pellaton et al., 2012). On the contrary, there is also sufficient evidence displaying the increased expression of antiinflammatory IL-10 cytokine and suppression of proinflammatory cytokines in lungs upon oral administration probiotics in the *S. aureus* and *P. aeruginosa* induced pulmonary infectious murine model (Shoaib et al., 2019; Vieira et al., 2016). Moreover, probiotic consumption appears to be a feasible way to decrease the incidence of respiratory infections in randomized, double-blind, placebo-controlled clinical trials (Chong et al., 2019; Fujita et al., 2013; Hor et al., 2018; Wang et al., 2016).

19.5 Conclusion

It has been well documented in various experimental settings that probiotics from various sources exhibit inhibitory actions against MDR superbugs. The bactericidal and bacteriostatic effect of probiotics was conferred by the extracellular secretion of various metabolites, such as bacteriocins, organic acids, and hydrogen peroxides. Irrespective of their administration in organs/tissue, the probiotic-mediated MDR bacterial clearance is attributed by the collection of both direct antagonistic actions (antimicrobial, antibiofilm, antivirulence, coaggregation, and bacterial interferences) and indirect modes (enhancing the humoral and cell-mediated immunity of the host to fight against MDR infections, enhancing the expression of tight and adherent junction proteins, triggering the production of broad-spectrum host-associated antimicrobial peptides, and enhancing the mucus expression across the mucus lining). While the in vivo and multicentric studies underscore that intervention with specific strains of probiotics to ameliorate the MDR bacterial infections may be effective. However, randomized trials with large population size without the limitation of geographical boundaries are further needed to validate statistically and to infer more confidently.

References

Alamdary, S. Z., & Bakhshi, B. (2020). Lactobacillus acidophilus attenuates toxin production by Vibrio cholerae and shigella dysenteriae following intestinal epithelial cells infection. *Microbial Pathogenesis*, 149. Available from https://doi.org/10.1016/j.micpath.2020.104543.

Alekshun, M. N., & Levy, S. B. (2004). Targeting virulence to prevent infection: To kill or not to kill? *Drug Discovery Today: Therapeutic Strategies*, 1(4), 483–489. Available from https://doi.org/10.1016/j.ddstr.2004.10.006.

Alexandre, Y., Le Blay, G., Boisramé-Gastrin, S., Le Gall, F., Héry-Arnaud, G., Gouriou, S., Vallet, S., & Le Berre, R. (2014). Probiotics: A new way to fight bacterial pulmonary infections? *Medecine et Maladies Infectieuses*, 44(1), 9–17. Available from https://doi.org/10.1016/j.medmal.2013.05.001.

Aminnezhad, S., Kermanshahi, R. K., & Ranjbar, R. (2015). Evaluation of synergistic interactions between cell-free supernatant of Lactobacillus strains and Amikacin and genetamicin against Pseudomonas aeruginosa. *Jundishapur Journal of Microbiology*, 8(4). Available from https://doi.org/10.5812/jjm.8(4)2015.16592.

Andersen, K. K., Strokappe, N. M., Hultberg, A., Truusalu, K., Smidt, I., Mikelsaar, R. H., Mikelsaar, M., Verrips, T., Hammarström, L., & Marcotte, H. (2016). Neutralization of Clostridium difficile toxin B mediated by engineered lactobacilli that produce single-domain antibodies. *Infection and Immunity*, 84(2), 395–406. Available from https://doi.org/10.1128/IAI.00870-15.

Argenta, A., Satish, L., Gallo, P., Liu, F., & Kathju, S. (2016). Local application of probiotic bacteria prophylaxes against sepsis and death resulting from burn wound infection. *PLoS One*, 11(10). Available from https://doi.org/10.1371/journal.pone.0165294.

Asahara, T., Shimizu, K., Nomoto, K., Hamabata, T., Ozawa, A., & Takeda, Y. (2004). Probiotic bifidobacteria protect mice from lethal infection with shiga toxin-producing Escherichia coli O157:H7. *Infection and Immunity*, 72(4), 2240–2247. Available from https://doi.org/10.1128/IAI.72.4.2240-2247.2004.

Asher, D., Kai, R., Amanda, Y., Michael, Q., Hayden, R., Don, W., Tynan, C., Dylan, R., Cheng, C., & Jing, S. (2020). Efficacy of probiotics in patients of cardiovascular disease risk: A systematic review and meta-analysis. *Current Hypertension Reports*. Available from https://doi.org/10.1007/s11906-020-01080-y.

Basavaprabhu, H. N., Sonu, K. S., & Prabha, R. (2020). Mechanistic insights into the action of probiotics against bacterial vaginosis and its mediated preterm birth: An overview. *Microbial Pathogenesis*, 141. Available from https://doi.org/10.1016/j.micpath.2020.104029.

Beigi, R. H., Austin, M. N., Meyn, L. A., Krohn, M. A., & Hillier, S. L. (2004). Antimicrobial resistance associated with the treatment of bacterial vaginosis. *American Journal of Obstetrics and Gynecology*, 191(4), 1124–1129. Available from https://doi.org/10.1016/j.ajog.2004.05.033.

Bohbot, J. M., Daraï, E., Bretelle, F., Brami, G., Daniel, C., & Cardot, J. M. (2018). Efficacy and safety of vaginally administered lyophilized Lactobacillus crispatus IP 174178 in the prevention of bacterial vaginosis recurrence. *Journal of Gynecology Obstetrics and Human Reproduction*, 47(2), 81–86. Available from https://doi.org/10.1016/j.jogoh.2017.11.005.

Brüssow, H. (2020). Problems with the concept of gut microbiota dysbiosis. *Microbial Biotechnology*, 13(2), 423–434. Available from https://doi.org/10.1111/1751-7915.13479.

Candela, M., Perna, F., Carnevali, P., Vitali, B., Ciati, R., Gionchetti, P., Rizzello, F., Campieri, M., & Brigidi, P. (2008). Interaction of probiotic Lactobacillus and Bifidobacterium strains with human intestinal epithelial cells: Adhesion properties, competition against enteropathogens and modulation of IL-8 production. *International Journal of Food Microbiology*, 125(3), 286–292. Available from https://doi.org/10.1016/j.ijfoodmicro.2008.04.012.

Cazorla, S. I., Maldonado-Galdeano, C., Weill, R., De Paula, J., & Perdigón, G. D. V. (2018). Oral administration of probiotics increases Paneth cells and intestinal antimicrobial activity. *Frontiers in Microbiology*, 9. Available from https://doi.org/10.3389/fmicb.2018.00736.

Chan, A. P., Choi, Y., Brinkac, L. M., Krishnakumar, R., DePew, J., Kim, M., Hinkle, M. K., Lesho, E. P., & Fouts, D. E. (2018). Multidrug resistant pathogens respond differently to the presence of co-pathogen, commensal, probiotic and host cells. *Scientific Reports*, 8(1). Available from https://doi.org/10.1038/s41598-018-26738-1.

Chenia, H. Y., & Duma, S. (2017). Characterization of virulence, cell surface characteristics and biofilm-forming ability of Aeromonas spp. isolates from fish and sea water. *Journal of Fish Diseases*, 40(3), 339–350. Available from https://doi.org/10.1111/jfd.12516.

Ching, C., Orubu, E. S. F., Wirtz, V. J., & Zaman, M. H. (2019). Bacterial antibiotic resistance development and mutagenesis following exposure to subminimal inhibitory concentrations of fluoroquinolones in vitro: A systematic literature review protocol. *BMJ Open*, 9(10). Available from https://doi.org/10.1136/bmjopen-2019-030747.

Chlebicz, A., & Śliżewska, K. (2020). In vitro detoxification of aflatoxin B1, deoxynivalenol, fumonisins, T-2 toxin and zearalenone by probiotic bacteria from genus Lactobacillus and Saccharomyces cerevisiae yeast. *Probiotics and Antimicrobial Proteins*, 12(1), 289–301. Available from https://doi.org/10.1007/s12602-018-9512-x.

Chong, H. X., Yusoff, N. A. A., Hor, Y. Y., Lew, L. C., Jaafar, M. H., Choi, S. B., Yusoff, M. S. B., Wahid, N., Abdullah, M. F. I. L., Zakaria, N., Ong, K. L., Park, Y. H., & Liong, M. T. (2019). Lactobacillus plantarum DR7 improved upper respiratory tract infections via enhancing immune and inflammatory parameters: A randomized, double-blind, placebo-controlled study. *Journal of Dairy Science*, 102(6), 4783–4797. Available from https://doi.org/10.3168/jds.2018-16103.

Collado, M. C., Meriluoto, J., & Salminen, S. (2007). In vitro analysis of probiotic strain combinations to inhibit pathogen adhesion to human intestinal mucus. *Food Research International*, *40*(5), 629–636. Available from https://doi.org/10.1016/j.foodres.2006.11.007.

Corbo, M. R., Campaniello, D., Speranza, B., Altieri, C., Sinigaglia, M., & Bevilacqua, A. (2018). Neutralisation of toxins by probiotics during the transit into the gut: Challenges and perspectives. *International Journal of Food Science and Technology*, *53*(6), 1339–1351. Available from https://doi.org/10.1111/ijfs.13745.

Cunha, S., Mendes., Rego, D., Meireles, D., Fernandes, R., Carvalho, A., & Martins da Costa, P. (2017). Effect of competitive exclusion in rabbits using an autochthonous probiotic. *World Rabbit Science*, *25*(2), 123–134. Available from https://doi.org/10.4995/wrs.2017.4533.

Czaplewski, L., Bax, R., Clokie, M., Dawson, M., Fairhead, H., Fischetti, V. A., Foster, S., Gilmore, B. F., Hancock, R. E. W., Harper, D., Henderson, I. R., Hilpert, K., Jones, B. V., Kadioglu, A., Knowles, D., Ólafsdóttir, S., Payne, D., Projan, S., Shaunak, S., & Rex, J. H. (2016). Alternatives to antibiotics—A pipeline portfolio review. *The Lancet Infectious Diseases*, *16*(2), 239–251. Available from https://doi.org/10.1016/s1473-3099(15)00466-1.

De Steenhuijsen Piters, W. A. A., Huijskens, E. G. W., Wyllie, A. L., Biesbroek, G., Van Den Bergh, M. R., Veenhoven, R. H., Wang, X., Trzcinski, K., Bonten, M. J., Rossen, J. W. A., Sanders, E. A. M., & Bogaert, D. (2016). Dysbiosis of upper respiratory tract microbiota in elderly pneumonia patients. *ISME Journal*, *10*(1), 97–108. Available from https://doi.org/10.1038/ismej.2015.99.

Deepansh, S., Singh, S. B., & Shailly, K. (2016). *Biosurfactants of Probiotic Lactic Acid Bacteria* (pp. 17–29). Springer Science and Business Media LLC. Available from https://doi.org/10.1007/978-3-319-26215-4_2.

Defne, G., Kalayci, Y. F., Merve, B., Deniz, C. F., & Anğ, K. M. (2020). In vitro effects of various probiotic products on growth and biofilm formation of clinical UPEC strains. *Acta Biologica Marisiensis*, 5–14. Available from https://doi.org/10.2478/abmj-2020-0001.

Deng, Z., Luo, X. M., Liu, J., & Wang, H. (2020). Quorum sensing, biofilm, and intestinal mucosal barrier: Involvement the role of probiotic. *Frontiers in Cellular and Infection Microbiology*, 10. Available from https://doi.org/10.3389/fcimb.2020.538077.

Dlamini, Z. C., Langa, R. L. S., Aiyegoro, O. A., & Okoh, A. I. (2019). Safety evaluation and colonisation abilities of four lactic acid bacteria as future probiotics. *Probiotics and Antimicrobial Proteins*, *11*(2), 397–402. Available from https://doi.org/10.1007/s12602-018-9430-y.

Fijan, S., Frauwallner, A., Langerholc, T., Krebs, B., Ter Haar, J. A., Heschl, A., Mičetić Turk, D., & Rogelj, I. (2019). Efficacy of using probiotics with antagonistic activity against pathogens of wound infections: An integrative review of literature. *BioMed Research International*, *2019*. Available from https://doi.org/10.1155/2019/7585486.

Forsythe, P. (2011). Probiotics and lung diseases. *Chest*, *139*(4), 901–908. Available from https://doi.org/10.1378/chest.10-1861.

Forsythe, P., & Bienenstock, J. (2010). Immunomodulation by commensal and probiotic bacteria. *Immunological Investigations*, *39*(4–5), 429–448. Available from https://doi.org/10.3109/08820131003667978.

Frank, D. N., Wysocki, A., Specht-Glick, D. D., Rooney, A., Feldman, R. A., St., Amand, A. L., Pace, N. R., & Trent, J. D. (2009). Microbial diversity in chronic open wounds. *Wound Repair and Regeneration*, *17*(2), 163–172. Available from https://doi.org/10.1111/j.1524-475X.2009.00472.x.

Fuchs, S., Sontag, G., Stidl, R., Ehrlich, V., Kundi, M., & Knasmüller, S. (2008). Detoxification of patulin and ochratoxin A, two abundant mycotoxins, by lactic acid bacteria. *Food and Chemical Toxicology*, *46*(4), 1398–1407. Available from https://doi.org/10.1016/j.fct.2007.10.008.

Fujita, R., Iimuro, S., Shinozaki, T., Sakamaki, K., Uemura, Y., Takeuchi, A., Matsuyama, Y., & Ohashi, Y. (2013). Decreased duration of acute upper respiratory tract infections with daily intake of fermented milk: A multicenter, double-blinded, randomized comparative study in users of day care facilities for the elderly population. *American Journal of Infection Control*, *41*(12), 1231–1235. Available from https://doi.org/10.1016/j.ajic.2013.04.005.

Gasbarrini, G., Bonvicini, F., & Gramenzi, A. (2016). Probiotics history. *Journal of Clinical Gastroenterology*, *50*, S116–S119. Available from https://doi.org/10.1097/MCG.0000000000000697.

Ghosh, C., Sarkar, P., Issa, R., & Haldar, J. (2019). Alternatives to conventional antibiotics in the era of antimicrobial resistance. *Trends in Microbiology*, *27*(4), 323–338. Available from https://doi.org/10.1016/j.tim.2018.12.010.

Guitor, A. K., & Wright, G. D. (2018). Antimicrobial resistance and respiratory infections. *Chest*, *154*(5), 1202–1212. Available from https://doi.org/10.1016/j.chest.2018.06.019.

Guk, J., Guedj, J., Burdet, C., Andremont, A., de Gunzburg, J., Ducher, A., & Mentré, F. (2020). Modeling the effect of DAV132, a novel colon-targeted adsorbent, on fecal concentrations of moxifloxacin and gut microbiota diversity in healthy volunteers. *Clinical Pharmacology and Therapeutics*. Available from https://doi.org/10.1002/cpt.1977.

Guo, S., Liu, D., Zhang, B., Li, Z., Li, Y., Ding, B., et al. (2017). Two Lactobacillus species inhibit the growth and α-toxin production of Clostridium perfringens and induced proinflammatory factors in chicken intestinal epithelial cells in vitro. *Frontiers in Microbiology*, 8.

Hafez, M. M., Maghrabi, I. A., & Zaki, N. M. (2013). Toward an alternative therapeutic approach for skin infections: Antagonistic activity of lactobacilli against antibiotic-resistant Staphylococcus aureus and Pseudomonas aeruginosa. *Probiotics and Antimicrobial Proteins*, *5*(3), 216–226. Available from https://doi.org/10.1007/s12602-013-9137-z.

Hajfarajollah, H., Eslami, P., Mokhtarani, B., & Akbari Noghabi, K. (2018). *Biosurfactants from probiotic bacteria: A review. Biotechnology and applied biochemistry*. Wiley-Blackwell Publishing Ltd. Available from https://doi.org/10.1002/bab.1686.

Hathout, A. S., & Aly, S. E. (2014). Biological detoxification of mycotoxins: A review. *Annals of Microbiology*, *64*(3), 905–919. Available from https://doi.org/10.1007/s13213-014-0899-7.

Hor, Y. Y., Lew, L. C., Lau, A. S. Y., Ong, J. S., Chuah, L. O., Lee, Y. Y., Choi, S. B., Rashid, F., Wahid, N., Sun, Z., Kwok, L. Y., Zhang, H., & Liong, M. T. (2018). Probiotic Lactobacillus casei Zhang (LCZ) alleviates respiratory, gastrointestinal & RBC abnormality via immuno-modulatory, anti-inflammatory & anti-oxidative actions. *Journal of Functional Foods*, *44*, 235–245. Available from https://doi.org/10.1016/j.jff.2018.03.017.

Jayashree, S., Karthikeyan, R., Nithyalakshmi, S., Ranjani, J., Gunasekaran, P., & Rajendhran, J. (2018). Anti-adhesion property of the potential probiotic strain Lactobacillus fermentum 8711 against methicillin-resistant Staphylococcus aureus (MRSA). *Frontiers in Microbiology*, 9. Available from https://doi.org/10.3389/fmicb.2018.00411.

Jiang, X., Yan, X., Gu, S., Yang, Y., Zhao, L., He, X., Chen, H., Ge, J., & Liu, D. (2019). Biosurfactants of Lactobacillus helveticus for biodiversity inhibit the biofilm formation of Staphylococcus aureus and cell invasion. *Future Microbiology*, *14*(13), 1133–1146. Available from https://doi.org/10.2217/fmb-2018-0354.

Kanmani, P., Satish Kumar, R., Yuvaraj, N., Paari, K. A., Pattukumar, V., & Arul, V. (2013). Probiotics and its functionally valuable products—A review. *Critical Reviews in Food Science and Nutrition*, *53*(6), 641–658. Available from https://doi.org/10.1080/10408398.2011.553752.

Katarina, J., Shari, K., Eline, B., Ilke, D. B., Eline, C., Sarah, L., & Filip, K. (2020). Probiotic nasal spray development by spray drying. *European Journal of Pharmaceutics and Biopharmaceutics*. Available from https://doi.org/10.1016/j.ejpb.2020.11.008.

Kerna, N., & Brown, T. (2018). A complementary medicine approach to augmenting antibiotic therapy: Current practices in the use of probiotics during antibiotic therapy. *Int J Complement Alt Med*, *11*, 62–66.

Khodaii, Z., Ghaderian, S. M. H., & Natanzi, M. M. (2017). Probiotic bacteria and their supernatants protect enterocyte cell lines from enteroinvasive Escherichia coli (EIEC) invasion. *International Journal of Molecular and Cellular Medicine*, *6*(3), 183–189. Available from http://ijmcmed.org/article-1-722-en.pdf.

Kim, Y., oh, S., & Kim, S. H. (2009). Released exopolysaccharide (r-EPS) produced from probiotic bacteria reduce biofilm formation of enterohemorrhagic Escherichia coli O157:H7. *Biochemical and Biophysical Research Communications*, *379*(2), 324–329. Available from https://doi.org/10.1016/j.bbrc.2008.12.053.

Kiymaci, M. E., Altanlar, N., Gumustas, M., Ozkan, S. A., & Akin, A. (2018). Quorum sensing signals and related virulence inhibition of Pseudomonas aeruginosa by a potential probiotic strain's organic acid. *Microbial Pathogenesis*, *121*, 190–197. Available from https://doi.org/10.1016/j.micpath.2018.05.042.

Koutnikova, H., Genser, B., Monteiro-Sepulveda, M., Faurie, J. M., Rizkalla, S., Schrezenmeir, J., & Clement, K. (2019). Impact of bacterial probiotics on obesity, diabetes and non-alcoholic fatty liver disease related variables: A systematic review and meta-analysis of randomised controlled trials. *BMJ Open*, *9*(3). Available from https://doi.org/10.1136/bmjopen-2017-017995.

Krezalek, M. A., Hyoju, S., Zaborin, A., Okafor, E., Chandrasekar, L., Bindokas, V., Guyton, K., Montgomery, C. P., Daum, R. S., Zaborina, O., Boyle-Vavra, S., & Alverdy, J. C. (2018). Can methicillin-resistant Staphylococcus aureus silently travel from the gut to the wound and cause postoperative infection? Modeling the "Trojan Horse Hypothesis". *Annals of Surgery*, *267*(4), 749–758. Available from https://doi.org/10.1097/SLA.0000000000002173.

Kunishima, H., Ishibashi, N., Wada, K., Oka, K., Takahashi, M., Yamasaki, Y., Aoyagi, T., Takemura, H., Kitagawa, M., & Kaku, M. (2019). The effect of gut microbiota and probiotic organisms on the properties of extended spectrum beta-lactamase producing and carbapenem resistant Enterobacteriaceae including growth, beta-lactamase activity and gene transmissibility. *Journal of Infection and Chemotherapy*, *25*(11), 894–900. Available from https://doi.org/10.1016/j.jiac.2019.04.021.

Lai, T. M., Lin, P. P., Hsieh, Y. M., & Tsai, C. C. (2020). Evaluation of inhibitory activity of domestic probiotics for against invasion and infection by Proteus mirabilis in the urinary tract. *Journal of Infection in Developing Countries*, *14*(4), 366–372. Available from https://doi.org/10.3855/JIDC.12203.

Leccese Terraf, M. C., Mendoza, L. M., Juárez Tomás, M. S., Silva, C., & Nader-Macías, M. E. F. (2014). Phenotypic surface properties (aggregation, adhesion and biofilm formation) and presence of related genes in beneficial vaginal lactobacilli. *Journal of Applied Microbiology*, *117*(6), 1761–1772. Available from https://doi.org/10.1111/jam.12642.

Liu, F., Sun, Z., Wang, F., Liu, Y., Zhu, Y., Du, L., Wang, D., & Xu, W. (2020). Inhibition of biofilm formation and exopolysaccharide synthesis of Enterococcus faecalis by phenyllactic acid. *Food Microbiology*, 86. Available from https://doi.org/10.1016/j.fm.2019.103344.

Lopes, E. G., Moreira, D. A., Gullón, P., Gullón, B., Cardelle-Cobas, A., & Tavaria, F. K. (2017). Topical application of probiotics in skin: Adhesion, antimicrobial and antibiofilm in vitro assays. *Journal of Applied Microbiology*, *122*(2), 450–461. Available from https://doi.org/10.1111/jam.13349.

Lukic, J., Chen, V., Strahinic, I., Begovic, J., Lev-Tov, H., Davis, S. C., Tomic-Canic, M., & Pastar, I. (2017). Probiotics or pro-healers: The role of beneficial bacteria in tissue repair. *Wound Repair and Regeneration*, *25*(6), 912–922. Available from https://doi.org/10.1111/wrr.12607.

Mack, D. R., Michail, S., Wei, S., Mcdougall, L., & Hollingsworth, M. A. (1999). Probiotics inhibit enteropathogenic E. coli adherence in vitro by inducing intestinal mucin gene expression. *American Journal of Physiology-Gastrointestinal and Liver Physiology*, 276.

Maharjan, A., Bhetwal, A., Shakya, S., Satyal, D., Shah, S., Joshi, G., Khanal, P. R., & Parajuli, N. P. (2018). Ugly bugs in healthy guts! Carriage of multidrug-resistant and ESBL-producing commensal enterobacteriaceae in the intestine of healthy nepalese adults. *Infection and Drug Resistance*, *11*, 547–554. Available from https://doi.org/10.2147/IDR.S156593.

Man, W. H., De Steenhuijsen Piters, W. A. A., & Bogaert, D. (2017). The microbiota of the respiratory tract: Gatekeeper to respiratory health. *Nature Reviews. Microbiology*, *15*(5), 259–270. Available from https://doi.org/10.1038/nrmicro.2017.14.

Martín, R., & Langella, P. (2019). Emerging health concepts in the probiotics field: Streamlining the definitions. *Frontiers in Microbiology*, *10*, 1047.

McEwen, S. A., & Collignon, P. J. (2018). Antimicrobial resistance: A one health perspective. *American Society for Microbiology*. Available from https://doi.org/10.1128/9781555819804.ch25.

Melzer, M., & Petersen, I. (2007). Mortality following bacteraemic infection caused by extended spectrum beta-lactamase (ESBL) producing E. coli compared to non-ESBL producing E. coli. *Journal of Infection*, *55*(3), 254–259. Available from https://doi.org/10.1016/j.jinf.2007.04.007.

Mitchell, C., Fredricks, D., Agnew, K., & Hitti, J. (2015). Hydrogen-peroxide producing lactobacilli are associated with lower levels of vaginal IL13, independent of bacterial vaginosis. *Sexually Transmitted Diseases*, 42.

Möndel, M., Schroeder, B. O., Zimmermann, K., Huber, H., Nuding, S., Beisner, J., Fellermann, K., Stange, E. F., & Wehkamp, J. (2009). Probiotic E. coli treatment mediates antimicrobial human β-defensin synthesis and fecal excretion in humans. *Mucosal Immunology*, 2(2), 166–172. Available from https://doi.org/10.1038/mi.2008.77.

Moroni, O., Kheadr, E., Boutin, Y., Lacroix, C., & Fliss, I. (2006). Inactivation of adhesion and invasion of food-borne Listeria monocytogenes by bacteriocin-producing Bifidobacterium strains of human origin. *Applied and Environmental Microbiology*, 72(11), 6894–6901. Available from https://doi.org/10.1128/AEM.00928-06.

Mottin, V. H. M., & Suyenaga, E. S. (2018). An approach on the potential use of probiotics in the treatment of skin conditions: Acne and atopic dermatitis. *International Journal of Dermatology*, 57(12), 1425–1432. Available from https://doi.org/10.1111/ijd.13972.

Naderi, A., Kasra-Kermanshahi, R., Gharavi, S., Fooladi, A. A. I., Alitappeh, M. A., & Saffarian, P. (2014). Study of antagonistic effects of Lactobacillus strains as probiotics on multi drug resistant (MDR) bacteria isolated from urinary tract infections (UTIs). *Iranian Journal of Basic Medical Sciences*, 17(3), 201.

Nelson, J., El-Gendy, A. O., Mansy, M. S., Ramadan, M. A., & Aziz, R. K. (2020). The biosurfactants iturin, lichenysin and surfactin, from vaginally isolated lactobacilli, prevent biofilm formation by pathogenic Candida. *FEMS Microbiology Letters*, 367(15). Available from https://doi.org/10.1093/femsle/fnaa126.

Newman, A. M., & Arshad, M. (2020). The role of probiotics, prebiotics and synbiotics in combating multidrug-resistant organisms. *Clinical Therapeutics*, 42(9), 1637–1648. Available from https://doi.org/10.1016/j.clinthera.2020.06.011.

Nicklas, D., Finnegan, P., Siler, Z., Peterson, M., & Sarangapani, S. (2019). 1447. Ex vivo human bladder tissue model to evaluate lactobacillus-containing formulations as preventative treatment against common urogenital pathogens. *Open Forum Infectious Diseases*.

Oudhuis, G. J., Bergmans, D. C., Dormans, T., Zwaveling, J. H., Kessels, A., Prins, M. H., Stobberingh, E. E., & Verbon, A. (2011). Probiotics vs antibiotic decontamination of the digestive tract: Infection and mortality. *Intensive Care Medicine*, 37(1), 110–117. Available from https://doi.org/10.1007/s00134-010-2002-6.

Owaga, E., Hsieh, R.-H., Mugendi, B., Masuku, S., Shih, C.-K., & Chang, J.-S. (2015). Th17 cells as potential probiotic therapeutic targets in inflammatory bowel diseases. *International Journal of Molecular Sciences*, 16(9), 20841–20858. Available from https://doi.org/10.3390/ijms160920841.

Park, B., Iwase, T., & Liu, G. Y. (2011). Intranasal application of S. epidermidis prevents colonization by methicillin-resistant Staphylococcus aureus in mice. *PLoS One*, 6(10). Available from https://doi.org/10.1371/journal.pone.0025880.

Patrignani, F., Siroli, L., Parolin, C., Serrazanetti, D. I., Vitali, B., & Lanciotti, R. (2019). Use of Lactobacillus crispatus to produce a probiotic cheese as potential gender food for preventing gynaecological infections. *PLoS One*, 14(1). Available from https://doi.org/10.1371/journal.pone.0208906.

Pellaton, C., Nutten, S., Thierry, A. C., Boudousquié, C., Barbier, N., Blanchard, C., Corthésy, B., Mercenier, A., & Spertini, F. (2012). Intragastric and intranasal administration of Lactobacillus paracasei NCC2461 modulates allergic airway inflammation in mice. *International Journal of Inflammation*, 2012. Available from https://doi.org/10.1155/2012/686739.

Peterson, E., & Kaur, P. (2018). Antibiotic resistance mechanisms in bacteria: relationships between resistance determinants of antibiotic producers, environmental bacteria, and clinical pathogens. *Frontiers in Microbiology*, 9, 2928.

Plaza-Diaz, J., Gomez-Llorente, C., Fontana, L., & Gil, A. (2014). Modulation of immunity and inflammatory gene expression in the gut, in inflammatory diseases of the gut and in the liver by probiotics. *World Journal of Gastroenterology*, 20(42), 15632–15649. Available from https://doi.org/10.3748/wjg.v20.i42.15632.

Prince, T., McBain, A. J., & O'Neill, C. A. (2012). Lactobacillus reuteri protects epidermal keratinocytes from Staphylococcus aureus-induced cell death by competitive exclusion. *Applied and Environmental Microbiology*, 78(15), 5119–5126. Available from https://doi.org/10.1128/AEM.00595-12.

Quigley, L., Coakley, M., Alemayehu, D., Rea, M. C., Casey, P. G., O'Sullivan, Ó., Murphy, E., Kiely, B., Cotter, P. D., Hill, C., & Ross, R. P. (2019). Lactobacillus gasseri APC 678 reduces shedding of the pathogen Clostridium difficile in a murine Model. *Frontiers in Microbiology*, 10. Available from https://doi.org/10.3389/fmicb.2019.00273.

Rana, S., Bhawal, S., Kumari, A., Kapila, S., & Kapila, R. (2020). pH-dependent inhibition of AHL-mediated quorum sensing by cell-free supernatant of lactic acid bacteria in Pseudomonas aeruginosa PAO1. *Microbial Pathogenesis*, 142. Available from https://doi.org/10.1016/j.micpath.2020.104105.

Rello, J., Parisella, F. R., & Perez, A. (2019). Alternatives to antibiotics in an era of difficult-to-treat resistance: New insights. *Expert Review of Clinical Pharmacology*, 12(7), 635–642. Available from https://doi.org/10.1080/17512433.2019.1619454.

Ren, D., Li, C., Qin, Y., Yin, R., Li, X., Tian, M., Du, S., Guo, H., Liu, C., Zhu, N., Sun, D., Li, Y., & Jin, N. (2012). Inhibition of Staphylococcus aureus adherence to Caco-2 cells by lactobacilli and cell surface properties that influence attachment. *Anaerobe*, 18(5), 508–515. Available from https://doi.org/10.1016/j.anaerobe.2012.08.001.

Ribet, D., & Cossart, P. (2015). How bacterial pathogens colonize their hosts and invade deeper tissues. *Microbes and Infection*, 17(3), 173–183. Available from https://doi.org/10.1016/j.micinf.2015.01.004.

Ripert, G., Racedo, S. M., Elie, A. M., Jacquot, C., Bressollier, P., & Urdaci, M. C. (2016). Secreted compounds of the probiotic Bacillus clausii strain O/C inhibit the cytotoxic effects induced by Clostridium difficile and Bacillus cereus toxins. *Antimicrobial Agents and Chemotherapy*, 60(6), 3445–3454. Available from https://doi.org/10.1128/AAC.02815-15.

Robinson, J. L. (2017). Probiotics for modification of the incidence or severity of respiratory tract infections. *Pediatric Infectious Disease Journal*, 36(11), 1093–1095. Available from https://doi.org/10.1097/INF.0000000000001714.

Salehi, B., Dimitrijević, M., Aleksić, A., Neffe-Skocińska, K., Zielińska, D., Kołożyn-Krajewska, D., Sharifi-Rad, J., Stojanović-Radić, Z., Prabu, S. M., Rodrigues, C. F., & Martins, N. (2020). Human microbiome and homeostasis: Insights into the key role of prebiotics, probiotics, and symbiotics. *Critical Reviews in Food Science and Nutrition*. Available from https://doi.org/10.1080/10408398.2020.1760202.

Schloissnig, S., Arumugam, M., Sunagawa, S., Mitreva, M., Tap, J., Zhu, A., Waller, A., Mende, D. R., Kultima, J. R., Martin, J., Kota, K., Sunyaev, S. R., Weinstock, G. M., & Bork, P. (2013). Genomic variation landscape of the human gut microbiome. *Nature*, *493*(7430), 45–50. Available from https://doi.org/10.1038/nature11711.

Shaaban, M., El-Rahman, O. A. A., Al-Qaidi, B., & Ashour, H. M. (2020). Antimicrobial and antibiofilm activities of probiotic lactobacilli on antibiotic-resistant proteus mirabilis. *Microorganisms*, *8*(6), 1–13. Available from https://doi.org/10.3390/microorganisms8060960.

Shivaprasad, D., Taneja, N. K., Lakra, A., & Sachdev, D. (2020). In vitro and in situ abrogation of biofilm formation in E. coli by vitamin C through ROS generation, disruption of quorum sensing and exopolysaccharide production. *Food Chemistry*.

Shoaib, A., Xin, L., & Xin, Y. (2019). Oral administration of Lactobacillus acidophilus alleviates exacerbations in Pseudomonas aeruginosa and Staphylococcus aureus pulmonary infections. *Pakistan Journal of Pharmaceutical Sciences*, *32*(4), 1621–1630. Available from http://www.pjps.pk/wp-content/uploads/pdfs/32/4/Paper-21.pdf.

Shrivastava, S. R., Shrivastava, P. S., & Ramasamy, J. (2018). World health organization releases global priority list of antibiotic-resistant bacteria to guide research, discovery, and development of new antibiotics. *JMS—Journal of Medical Society*, *32*(1), 76–77. Available from https://doi.org/10.4103/jms.jms_25_17.

Smelov, V., Naber, K., & Bjerklund Johansen, T. E. (2016). Improved classification of urinary tract infection: Future considerations. *European Urology, Supplements*, *15*(4), 71–80. Available from https://doi.org/10.1016/j.eursup.2016.04.002.

Surendran Nair, M., Amalaradjou, M. A., & Venkitanarayanan, K. (2017). Antivirulence properties of probiotics in combating microbial pathogenesis. *Advances in Applied Microbiology*, *98*, 1–29. Available from https://doi.org/10.1016/bs.aambs.2016.12.001.

Šušković, J., Kos, B., Beganović, J., Pavunc, A. L., Habjanič, K., & Matoć, S. (2010). Antimicrobial activity—The most important property of probiotic and starter lactic acid bacteria. *Food Technology and Biotechnology*, *48*(3), 296–307. Available from http://www.ftb.com.hr/48/48-296.pdf.

Trunk, T., Khalil, H. S., & Leo, J. C. (2018). Bacterial autoaggregation. *AIMS Microbiology*, 4.

Tsiouris, C. G., & Tsiouri, M. G. (2017). Human microflora, probiotics and wound healing. *Wound Medicine*, *19*, 33–38. Available from https://doi.org/10.1016/j.wndm.2017.09.006.

van de Wijgert, J. H. H. M., & Verwijs, M. C. (2020). Lactobacilli-containing vaginal probiotics to cure or prevent bacterial or fungal vaginal dysbiosis: A systematic review and recommendations for future trial designs. *BJOG: An International Journal of Obstetrics and Gynaecology*, *127*(2), 287–299. Available from https://doi.org/10.1111/1471-0528.15870.

Vieira, A. T., Rocha, V. M., Tavares, L., Garcia, C. C., Teixeira, M. M., Oliveira, S. C., Cassali, G. D., Gamba, C., Martins, F. S., & Nicoli, J. R. (2016). Control of Klebsiella pneumoniae pulmonary infection and immunomodulation by oral treatment with the commensal probiotic Bifidobacterium longum 51A. *Microbes and Infection*, *18*(3), 180–189. Available from https://doi.org/10.1016/j.micinf.2015.10.008.

Waigankar, S. S., & Patel, V. (2011). Role of probiotics in urogenital healthcare. *Journal of Mid-Life Health*, 5. Available from https://doi.org/10.4103/0976-7800.83253.

Wang, Y., Li, X., Ge, T., Xiao, Y., Liao, Y., Cui, Y., Zhang, Y., Ho, W., Yu, G., & Zhang, T. (2016). Probiotics for prevention and treatment of respiratory tract infections in children: A systematic review and meta-analysis of randomized controlled trials. *Medicine (United States)*, *95*(31). Available from https://doi.org/10.1097/MD.0000000000004509.

Wu, X., Tian, J., & Wang, S. (2018). Insight into non-pathogenic Th17 cells in autoimmune diseases. *Frontiers in Immunology*, *9*(MAY). Available from https://doi.org/10.3389/fimmu.2018.01112.

Ya, W., Reifer, C., & Miller, L. E. (2010). Efficacy of vaginal probiotic capsules for recurrent bacterial vaginosis: A double-blind, randomized, placebo-controlled study. *American Journal of Obstetrics and Gynecology*, *203*(2), 120.e1–120.e6. Available from https://doi.org/10.1016/j.ajog.2010.05.023.

Yahfoufi, N., Mallet, J. F., Graham, E., & Matar, C. (2018). Role of probiotics and prebiotics in immunomodulation. *Current Opinion in Food Science*, *20*, 82–91. Available from https://doi.org/10.1016/j.cofs.2018.04.006.

Yan, F., Liu, L., Dempsey, P. J., Tsai, Y. H., Raines, E. W., Wilson, C. L., Cao, H., Cao, Z., Liu, L., & Polk, D. B. (2013). A Lactobacillus rhamnosus GG-derived soluble protein, p40, stimulates ligand release from intestinal epithelial cells to transactivate epidermal growth factor receptor. *Journal of Biological Chemistry*, *288*(42), 30742–30751. Available from https://doi.org/10.1074/jbc.M113.492397.

Yousefi, B., Eslami, M., Ghasemian, A., Kokhaei, P., Salek Farrokhi, A., & Darabi, N. (2019). Probiotics importance and their immunomodulatory properties. *Journal of Cellular Physiology*, *234*(6), 8008–8018. Available from https://doi.org/10.1002/jcp.27559.

Yu, Q., Zhu, L., Wang, Z., Li, P., & Yang, Q. (2012). Lactobacillus delbrueckii ssp. lactis R4 prevents Salmonella typhimurium SL1344-induced damage to tight junctions and adherens junctions. *Journal of Microbiology*, *50*(4), 613–617. Available from https://doi.org/10.1007/s12275-012-1596-5.

Yun, B., Oh, S., & Griffiths, M. W. (2014). Lactobacillus acidophilus modulates the virulence of Clostridium difficile. *Journal of Dairy Science*, *97*(8), 4745–4758. Available from https://doi.org/10.3168/jds.2014-7921.

Zaid, A. M. (2014). Distribution of bacterial uropathogens and their susceptibility patterns over twelve years (2001–2013) in Palestine. *The International Arabic Journal of Antimicrobial Agents*.

Zhang, W., & Li, C. (2016). Exploiting quorum sensing interfering strategies in gram-negative bacteria for the enhancement of environmental applications. *Frontiers in Microbiology*, 6. Available from https://doi.org/10.3389/fmicb.2015.01535.

Chapter 20

Probiotics in the prevention and treatment of infections with *Helicobacter pylori*, Enterohemorrhagic *Escherichia coli*, and *Rotavirus*

Nilanjana Das[1], Mangala Lakshmi Ragavan[1] and Sanjeeb Kumar Mandal[2]

[1]*Department of Biomedical Sciences, School of Bio Sciences and Technology, Vellore, India,* [2]*Sri Shakthi Institute of Engineering and Technology, Coimbatore, India*

20.1 Introduction

Probiotics are known living microorganisms having a positive effect on intestinal microecology and improved health conditions (Yousefi et al., 2019). Most of the reported probiotics are bacteria especially *Lactobacillus* strains, which produce lactic acid (Ghasemian et al., 2018). However, recently different species of bacteria belonging to the genera viz. *Bifidobacterium* spp. and *Bacillus* spp. and yeast genus *Saccharomyces* spp. are also being used as probiotics. The potential application of probiotics includes prevention and treatment of gastrointestinal (GI) infections, inflammatory bowel disease, lactose intolerance, allergies, urogenital infections, cystic fibrosis, various cancers, reduction of antibiotic side effects, oral health, such as prevention of dental caries, periodontal diseases, and oral malodour (Singh et al., 2013). Probiotics have been used for the treatment of many GI diseases, such as antibiotic-associated diarrhea, acute diarrhea, functional digestive disorders, and inflammatory bowel diseases (Yousefi et al., 2019).

The beneficial aspects of probiotics have made them as a best replacement of antibiotics to combat complex disorders, such as GI, digestive system, and nervous system (Roobab et al., 2020). Hence, application of probiotics is considered as a promising remedial treatment for GI diseases to improve overall good health by preventing establishment of pathogens (Judkins et al., 2020). Probiotic microorganisms can execute their antipathogenic activity by several mechanisms, such as production of antimicrobial compounds, competition for nutrient substrates, competitive exclusion, enhancement of intestinal barrier function, maintaining intestinal epithelial integrity, enhancing immunomodulatory effects, increasing mucin production, and secretion from goblet cells (Zhang et al., 2018). Thus probiotics are recommended as alternative biotherapeutic agents for intestinal pathogenic infections. Probiotic strains *Lactobacillus acidophilus*, *Bifidobacterium lactis*, and *Streptococcus thermophilus* are showing antagonistic activity against pathogenic infections (Saracino et al., 2020).

GI hemorrhage is potentially life threatening and remains a significant health problem in humans. In western countries, 10%–20% of adults below 40 years are having peptic ulcer disease. The peptic ulcer is well known upper GI disease caused by *Helicobacter pylori* (den Hoed & Kuipers, 2020). It is a gram-negative bacteria observed on the surface of gastric epithelial cells and gastric mucus, which cause gastric cancer (GC) in humans. Hence, *H. pylori* is classified as a biological carcinogen by WHO (Lambert & Hull, 1996). *H. pylori* gastroenteritis treated by many probiotics viz., *Lactobacillus acidophilus*, *L. casei* strain Shirota, and *Lactobacillus fermentum* are demonstrated in clinical studies (Misra et al., 2019).

Foodborne diseases are one of the most significant health problems during the last decades. It can be caused by bacteria, virus, parasites, and their toxins. The host tolerance level to microbial infections greatly varies among the same species or different species. For example, most of the *E. coli* types are harmless and keeps our gut system healthy.

However, some of the *E. coli* strains can cause diarrhea from contaminated foods or drinks (Meng et al., 2013). Infections caused by enterohemorrhagic *Escherichia coli* (EHEC) start from mild diarrhea to hemolytic uremic syndrome (HUS). Thus it causes renal failure among the children's in many countries. The severity of this disease usually occurred due to the release of Shiga toxins (Stx). The use of antibiotics to treat EHEC infections is generally avoided as it can result in increased stx expression (Mühlen et al., 2020). Probiotics can be used for the treatment of biofilm forming pathogens, such as *E. coli* and other pathogens in humans. *Lactobacillus* and *Bifidobacterium* are helpful to treat many GI diseases including EHEC. The extracellular activity of probiotic bacteria prevents biofilm formation of pathogenic *E. coli* (Fang et al., 2018).

In case of the viruses, most of the gastroenteritis is caused by rotavirus (RV). It is highly contagious among infants and children under 5 years in worldwide (Sen et al., 2020). Especially, different viral strains with several stages frequently cause gastroenteritis in the first year of life (Gómez-Rial et al., 2020). Vaccines are available to prevent the disease, but it has only limited strategies for challenging diarrhea caused by RV infection (Fernandez-Duarte et al., 2018). Probiotics can be used for the treatment of viral gastroenteritis effectively in humans. It is a promising approach for modulating GI tract (GIT) microbiota to control the colonization of enteric pathogens in the GIT (Khaneghah et al., 2020). This chapter will be focused on prevention and treatment of GI diseases using probiotics.

20.2 Probiotics and their health implications

GI system is a resident flora of various microorganisms, referred as microflora or microbiota. These are present in varying concentrations throughout the gut. They include species of bacteria, Eukarya, and viruses (Rahmani et al., 2019). Essential metabolites with dietary and therapeutic characteristics are provided by probiotics which confer numerous health benefits and proper maintenance of the gut health. The probiotics enter into the body through food and exist naturally or being infused in food. It is necessary to understand the mechanism of action of the probiotic strains, their interaction with the gut microflora, and their clinical significance (Misra et al., 2019). The colonization of the microbes in the digestive tract is initiated from birth by *Bifidobacterium*, Enterobacteriaceae, *Staphylococcus*, and *Streptococcus*. These are transmitted from vagina, skin, and breast milk in infants whereas, in adults, diet plays a crucial role in the maintenance of this microbiota. Disruption in the microbiome results in various kinds of GI disorders (Bozzi Cionci et al., 2018).

Probiotics exert antagonistic activity on host system by competing with pathogens for their adhesion site, growth nutrients, and producing antimicrobial compounds, such as lactic acid and acetic acid. The competitive exclusion activity of probiotics depends on their administration in the GIT to prevent the colonization of pathogens/selectively reducing populations of pathogenic bacteria (Sharma et al., 2019). Some of the probiotic strains *S. faecalis*, *C. butyricum*, and *B. mesentericus* promote the growth of bifidobaterium, which selectively inhibits the growth of pathogenic bacteria. It also produces glutamine to maintain mucosal integrity and enhances the protection of mucosal barrier (Singh et al., 2013). Probiotics are resistant to bile juice and stomach acid and adhere to the epithelial lining of the gut. They have the ability to fight against and prevent GI infections by modulating innate and cell-mediated immunity (Rahmani et al., 2019). *Lactobacillus* probiotic strains inhibit gastroenteric and foodborne pathogens as well as food spoilage fungi, as they can resist or survive under simulated GI transit conditions and adhere to the mucin layer and form biofilms.

Acute diarrheal disease considered as one of the most common GI diseases affecting all age of people in worldwide. This kind of GI disease can be treated by probiotics due to their therapeutic properties (Mantegazza et al., 2018). Most of the gastroenterologists believed that probiotics are useful in treating GI diseases, and nutritionists use probiotics to prevent disease or maintain good health. Recent studies showed the antisclerosis activity of *B. subtilis* and *B. coagulans* (Mohammadsadeghi et al., 2019), antiulcerogenic activity of yeast strain (*S. cerevisiae*) (Banik et al., 2019), and antimicrobial activity (against *Salmonella enterica* and *Clostridium difficile*) of *Lactobacillus* spp. (Moens et al., 2019; Mohanty et al., 2019). Synbiotics also play a significant role in combating against pathogen colonization and infection with enteric pathogens. The promising effects of synbiotics are generally derived from prebiotics and probiotics, due to their combinational effectiveness (Peng et al., 2019).

The effects of probiotics/synbiotic on various inflammatory and antiinflammatory markers in various disease conditions have also been investigated (Kazemi et al., 2019). Moreover, this intervention helped to decrease inflammation in case of inflammatory bowel disease, arthritis, fatty liver, and other diseases. The antiinflammatory activity of bifidobacterium (Devi et al., 2018), *L. plantarum*, and *Kluyveromyces marxianus* against inflammatory bowel disease (Chopade et al., 2019), anticholestrolamic activity of *L. kunkeei* (Mo et al., 2019; Sakandar et al., 2019), and cholesterol-lowering capabilities of *L. plantarum* YS5 (Nami et al., 2019) has also been reported. Moreover, the daily consumption of probiotic yogurt containing *L. acidophilus* and *B. lactis* is associated with the reduction in blood sugar, improved endothelial function, and reduced cardiovascular risk (Rezazadeh et al., 2019).

Probiotics have a potential to be used for food allergies treatment in pediatric patients (Tan-Lim & Esteban-Ipac, 2018). The use of probiotics (*L. rhamnosus*) can alleviate the symptoms of milk allergy in children. Ma et al. (2019) provides molecular insights into the application of probiotic mixtures to reduce food allergies and even intestinal immune homeostasis. The use of probiotics (*Lactobacillus* and *Bifidobacteria*) was considered as an effective treatment strategy for treatment of human food allergies (Yang et al., 2018). Particular attention should be given to the common prescription of antibiotics and probiotics to ensure that probiotic strains are not susceptible to infection. However, some yeast strain, such as *S. boulardii*, is resistant to most prescribed antibiotics (Neut et al., 2017). A combination of prebiotic polymer nanoparticles and probiotics (*Pediococcus acidilactici*) has been suggested as an alternative to antibiotics, providing a potential strategy for addressing bacterial resistance (Kim et al., 2019). However, probiotics are origin specific strain which could deliver the effectiveness on particular disease for the prevention and treatment.

20.3 Infections caused by *Helicobacter pylori*, enterohemorrhagic *Escherichia coli*, and *rotavirus*

H. pylori is one of the most common pathogens causing GI diseases, such as peptic ulcer, gastritis, and lymphoma [mucosa-associated lymphoid tissue (MALT), lymphoma] in half of the world's population, particularly in children (Rahmani et al., 2019). The prevalence of *H. pylori* infection is associated with hygiene levels among the population. In developing countries, the prevalence remains high due to their socioeconomic status and hygiene level. Thus improvement in sanitation and methods of eradication has changed the epidemiology of *H. pylori* infection (Hooi et al., 2017). The colonization of *H. pylori* causes GC in humans. The interaction between human cells, virulence factors from microbes, and their environment is considered as a complex structure, which is responsible for the prevalence and mortality of GC worldwide (Amieva & Peek, 2016). Acid tolerance, flagella-mediated motility toward epithelium cells, interaction with adhesion receptors, and release of toxic substances are critical steps for *H. pylori* to establish successful colonization, persistent infection, and disease pathogenesis (Kao et al., 2016).

H. pylori infection can be diagnosed by two methods viz. noninvasive and invasive. Noninvasive method is more reliable diagnostic tool for *H. pylori infection*, such as urea breath tests, serum IgG antibody tests, and fecal antigen tests. Invasive tests viz. culture, histology, and rapid urease tests are only applicable for an upper GI endoscopy. The infection caused by *H. pylori* can be treated with a combination of antimicrobials and acid-suppressive drugs (den Hoed & Kuipers, 2020). Clarithromycin, amoxicillin, metronidazole, and proton-pump inhibitors (PPIs) including triple therapy (two antibiotics and a PPI) are prescribed as a first-line eradication therapy for *H. pylori* infection. Despite the applications of different treatments, the infection rate is still increasing both in developed and developing states. The challenge of treatment failure is caused due to the resistance of *H. pylori* to antibiotics and its side effects.

Potential of probiotics to cure *H. pylori* infection is well-documented. Probiotics combined with conventional treatment regime appear to have great potential in eradicating *H. pylori* infection. Therefore probiotics provide an excellent alternative approach to manage *H. pylori* load and its threatening disease outcome (Qureshi et al., 2019). It is noted that anti-*H. pylori* activity of probiotics is strain specific. Therefore establishing standard guidelines regarding the dose and formulation of individual strain is inevitable. However, use of probiotics as a supplement will increase eradication and reduce side effects associated with treatment (Eslami et al., 2019).

EHEC, a foodborne pathogen causes human diseases starting from diarrhea to life-threatening complications. Potential sources for EHEC infections are ruminants, cattle and foods, such as undercooked beef products, unpasteurized milk, and contaminated vegetables, and water. These bacteria create a severe bloody diarrhea and some high-risk diseases, such as HUS, hemorrhagic colitis, and thrombotic thrombocytopenic purpura (TTP). EHEC disease occurred at very low infectious dose around 50–100 bacteria, even though it is considered as a very serious pathogen. There are 400 serotypes in EHEC, but O157:H7 is the most often associated with severe diseases in worldwide (Jubelin et al., 2018). *E. coli* O157:H7, a prototype of EHEC, has also been known as one of the pathogens that is transferred from food. It is one of the natural intestinal flora of animals, including cow, goat, and sheep. Accordingly, contaminated dairy products, such as nonpasteurized milk, meat products, and undone hamburger, are other important ways of transmission of these bacteria (Dimidi et al., 2017).

The dynamic in vitro models of human gut provide new insights into EHEC pathogenesis for elucidating spatial and temporal modulation of EHEC survival and virulence along the GIT (Jubelin et al., 2018). The colonization of EHEC achieved through the formation of lesions on the intestine for attaching and effacing of bacteria, when there is a loss of microvilli in humans (Stevens & Frankel, 2014). The virulence factors of EHEC allow bacteria to colonize in the intestine to deliver toxic substances, such as Stx to the host cells. This Stx is mainly responsible for HUS disease (Bergan et al., 2012).

HUS is a rare disease associated with Stx-producing *E. coli* (STEC). The leading cause of typical HUS in children can cause major outbreaks. Dini et al. (2016) demonstrated the in vitro activity of a microbial mixture of five probiotic strains isolated from kefir grains for reducing the cytotoxic effect on STEC infected epithelial Hep-2 cells. A study by Bian et al. (2016) demonstrated the antimicrobial potential of *Lactobacillus helveticus* KLDS against STEC. Many antibiotics failed to treat EHEC infections, especially antibiotics belonging to quinolone family induce the bacterial SOS response, which instigate the production and release of phages from the bacteria. Thus treatment of STEC infections with antibiotics is generally not advised (Kakoullis et al., 2019). Despite major progresses in the understanding of STEC-HUS mechanisms, no specific treatment is currently available. However, some of the therapeutic approaches and promising strategies viz. antibody therapy, vaccinations, antimicrobial agents, such as probiotics, and phages are outlined by Mühlen and Dersch (2020).

RV is recognized as the single most important agent for causing diarrhea in infants, which occur worldwide. Most symptomatic infections occur in children between 3 months and 2 years of age. In temperate countries, RV infections show winter seasonality, whereas infections occur year-round in most tropical countries. RV spreads via the fecal–oral route, primarily through person-to-person transmission. Only a few virus particles are required to infect the susceptible host (Iturriza-Gómara & Cunliffe, 2020). Initially virus infects enterocytes that induce diarrhea due to the destruction of absorptive enterocytes and it stimulates intestinal secretion by RV nonstructural protein 4 for activation of the enteric nervous system. The severe infection of RV can lead to acute gastroenteritis and viraemia. Also, RV able to replicate in systemic sites, but it is limited. Reinfection of RV is common throughout life, but the severity of disease decreased with repeated infections (Crawford et al., 2017). RV infection has broad spectrum of targets apart from the intestine, such as nervous system, liver, and pancreas. In addition, it triggers the development of autoimmune diseases, such as celiac disease and type 1 diabetes (Gomez-Rial et al., 2019).

Better understanding on mechanism of interactions between virus, host, and microbiota could provide new approach for vaccine development. For example, NoV or RV vaccine are designed based on the specific interactions between viral strains and the host, which target specific viral groups. This could enhance the host defense system (Lee & Ko, 2016). Although vaccines have proven effective in decreasing the strength of RV-induced diarrhea, researchers are searching continuously for alternative ways to prevent this disease. Probiotics have the capacity to prevent and improve health conditions against RV (Salas-Cárdenas et al., 2018).

This chapter is a compilation of research updates on the potential role of probiotics toward the prevention and treatment of diseases caused by the three pathogens viz. *H. pylori*, *EHEC*, and RV. The role of probiotics in the prevention of GI diseases is illustrated in Fig. 20.1. Normal gut microbiota is unable to block/prevent pathogen colonization and

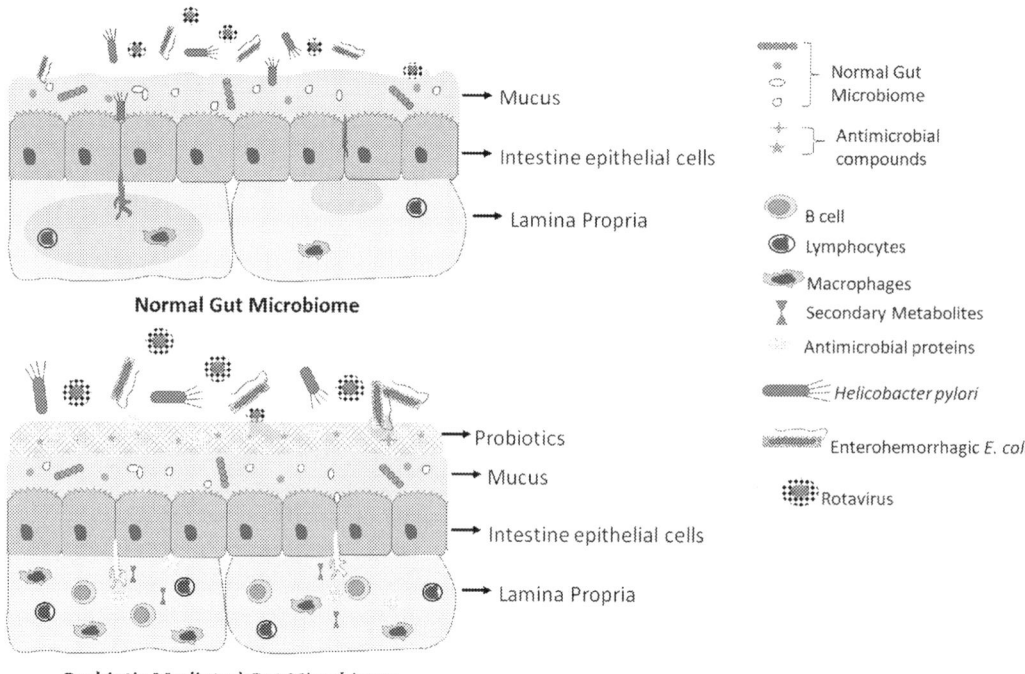

FIGURE 20.1 Normal and probiotic mediated gut microbiome.

release of their toxins in the host intestine. In case of probiotic-mediated gut microbiome, the colonization of pathogens was inhibited by probiotics through production of secondary *meta*bolites, antimicrobial compounds and improved host immunity. Research prospects discussed in this chapter will encourage future researchers to focus on new attempts toward the development of advanced protocol for the control of *H. pylori*, EHEC, and RV.

20.4 Helicobacter pylori

H. pylori is a Gram-negative bacillus, helical, flagellated, and microaerophillic organisms present in the gastric mucosa causing diseases of the upper GIT and GC (Dunne et al., 2014). It is the bacterium linked with gastric malignancy, estimated to be the cause of 60% of GC cases (Parkin, 2006). They are highly pathogenic when bound to gastric epithelial cells. It is a common pathogen reported by Warren and Marshall in Australia in the year 1983 (Wroblewski et al., 2010). The infection with this bacterium occurs all over the world though the epidemiology of *H. pylori* infection is not yet clear. Difference was noted in the prevalence of infection within and between countries, such as Sweden 11%, Canada and the United States 30%, Spain 60.3%, and China 83.4% (Eusebi et al., 2014). High prevalence about 80% or more have been documented in parts of China and some South American and Eastern European states (Roberts et al., 2016). *H. pylori* infection in childhood may persist throughout life if not treated properly (Arslan et al., 2017). Giemsa staining and rapid urease test are more reliable and used to detect *H. pylori* infection as preliminary examination (Fan et al., 2020). Further examination done by upper endoscopy or EGD, breath test, and stool culture. Those who have noncardia gastric problems (atrophic gastritis, GI metaplasia, and dysplasia), weak metabolic control, and poor glycemic conditions (type 2 diabetes) are highly susceptible to *H. pylori* infection compared to gastric cardia cancer (Hassan et al., 2020).

For the last two decades, the recommended treatment for *H. pylori* eradication is the standard triple therapy (Papastergiou et al., 2014a,b), using a PPI/ranitidine bismuth citrate, combined with clarithromycin and amoxicillin or metronidazole. Sometimes the failure of *H. pylori* eradication occurs and the factors involved include poor diet, poor patient compliance, a high bacterial load of the gastric, internalization of bacteria, gastric acidity, gene polymorphisms, antimicrobial washout, and most importantly, and antibiotic resistance. However, the increase in the prevalence of macrolide resistance, mainly clarithromycin, has decreased the efficacy of these therapies in most parts of the world, resulting the necessity of studying other possible therapies (bismuth quadruple, sequential, and hybrid therapies) to eradicate the pathogen. Due to the rapid development of quinolone resistance, levofloxacin-based regimens should be reserved as a second-line treatment option. Due to the fact that it is difficult to treat *H. pylori* infection mainly because of acquired resistance to commonly used antibiotics, there is a growing interest to use probiotics in conjunction with antibiotic regimens to eradicate *H. pylori* (Goderska et al., 2018).

Eradication of *H. pylori* infection has been reported as an effective strategy for the treatment of peptic ulcers and lymphoma associated with gastric mucus as well as the prevention of GC (Moss, 2017). The eradication of *H. pylori* was an essential factor to the prevention of GC was confirmed based on the agreement of Maastricht v/Florence, the Kyoto global agreement and the Toronto agreement (Fischbach & Malfertheiner, 2018). The eradication of *H. pylori* was significantly lower in GC patients, especially elders. In some cases, eradiation of *H. pylori* with antibiotics are affecting the gut microbiota among children. Thus further studies are needed to eradicate this infection without affecting the gut microbiota in children. In order to eradicate *H. pylori* infection, new therapeutic strategies viz. probiotic supplementation, berberine supplementation, and dual therapy were introduced with reduced adverse effects (Peng et al., 2019). In recent years antibiotic resistance to clarithromycin has been increased rapidly in many countries (Afsahi et al., 2018). Antibacterial drugs are improved using natural ingredients viz. probiotic, green tea, honey, and olive oil to treat *H. pylori* infection (Hassan et al., 2020). Probiotics have been proven to be useful in the treatment of several GI diseases. Among them, the anti-*H. pylori* activity has also been studied (Aiba et al., 2015).

20.4.1 How probiotics act against *H. pylori* infection?

Many probiotic bacteria and yeasts viz. *Bacillus* spp., *Enterobacter cloacae*, *Enterococcus faecium*, *Lactobacillus acidophilus*, *Lactobacillus paracasei*, *Lactobacillus fermentum*, *Lactobacillus pentosus*, *Lactobacillus plantarum*, *Lactococcus lactis*, *Leuconostoc citreum*, *Leuconostoc lactis*, *Staphylococcus auricularis*, *Staphylococcus epidermidis*, *Stenotrophomonas maltophilia*, *Weissella confusa*, and *Saccharomyces cerevisiaeare* reported to have significant effects on *H. pylori* infection (Lin et al., 2009; Lopez-Brea et al., 2008; Techo et al., 2019). Probiotic supplementation therapy is an emerging therapy for *H. pylori* treatment (Chey et al., 2017). It is a feasible way to treat *H. pylori* infection. Probiotic therapy can enhance the therapeutic effects of antibiotics as well as maintenance of host GI microbiota.

Moreover, probiotics along with antibiotics could improve the eradication rate and reduce the side effects (Song et al., 2019). Probiotics act on *H. pylori* infection through the following mechanisms: (1) mucus barrier enhancement, (2) adhesion inhibition, (3) antibacterial substances secretion, and (4) immunity modulation (Ji & Yang, 2020). The mechanism of probiotics on *H. pylori* infection was illustrated in Fig. 20.1.

H. pylori damages the gastric mucosa using its virulence factors, such as CagA and VacA (Backert et al., 2016). It causes gastritis due to decrease in mucus secretion on a damaged epithelium (Lesbros-Pantoflickova et al., 2007). Probiotics can positively affect the epithelial barrier function, which is strain specific (Karczewski et al., 2010). Probiotics can protect the mucosal barrier from damage by different mechanisms including modification of the expression of mucus and epithelial junction proteins and releasing the bioactive molecules to stabilize the barrier which prevents its disruption by the pathogens (Sakarya & Gunay, 2014). SabA and VacA are important virulence factors of *H. pylori*, inhibition of their expression is critically important to regulate inflammation and prevent tumor formation (Qureshi et al., 2019). A reduction in SabA gene expression mediated by an unknown effect or molecule was reported. The authors suggested the effect or molecule to be either an antimicrobial substance or a bacterial surface molecule released into the conditioned medium. Reuterin from *L. reuteri* inhibited the growth of *H. pylori* and downregulated the virulence gene expression of vacA and flaA (Urrutia-Beca et al., 2018). These studies indicate that probiotics on repairing the gastric mucosal barrier can effectively prevent the initial infection and reinfection of the *H. pylori*.

The regulation of intestinal epithelium by probiotics achieved by their surface compounds, such as surface layer proteins, flagella, pili, and capsular polysaccharides, for specific constitution of microbial-associated molecular patterns to select and bind respective receptors on the host. This regulation enhances the gut epithelium barrier function by triggering signaling pathways to produce cytokines/inhibit apoptosis to reduce inflammation in the intestine. The metabolites of probiotics viz. secreted proteins, organic acids, indole, extracellular vesicles, and bacteriocins on host receptors also regulate gut epithelial barrier function (Liu et al., 2020).

Several experiments have been conducted to propose various possible probiotic's antagonistic effect on *H. pylori* (Karczewski et al., 2010). Adhesion of *H. pylori* to gastric epithelial cells was inhibited by *Clostridium butyricum*, *Lactobacillus salivarius*, and *L. plantarum* (Kabir et al., 1997; Takahashi et al., 2000; Zhao et al., 2018). It was also noted that culture supernatants of *B. subtilis*, *L. plantarum*, *C. butyricum*, and *W. confuse* inhibited the growth and morphology of *H. pylori* (Nam et al., 2002; Pinchuk et al., 2001; Takahashi et al., 2000; Zhao et al., 2018). In vitro coaggregation of probiotics, such as *L. gasseri* and *L. reuteri* DSM17648, significantly prevent/reduce *H. pylori* colonization in the host intestine (Chen et al., 2010; Holz et al., 2015). There was a report on affinity of *Saccharomyces boulardii* to sialic acid receptor followed by the inhibition of *H. pylori* from binding (Sakarya & Gunay, 2014).

The antiadherence effects of probiotics occurred by bacterial competition for nutrients and binding sites on epithelial cells. Inhibitory effects of LAB prevent infection in an early stage of *H. pylori* colonization. Also, *Lactobacillus* strains can reduce the growth of *H. pylori* and inhibit its urease activity, which reduces *H. pylori* adhesion to intestinal cell line. Thus lactic acid bacteria can play an important role in preventing the colonization of *H. pylori* infection. Many *Lactobacillus* strains and their cell-free supernatant inhibit the urease activity of *H. pylori*, which significantly reduce *H. pylori* infection in humans (Rezaee et al., 2019). These reports indicate that probiotics are having potentiality for the destruction/prevention of *H. pylori* biofilm formation, which may improve the effect of the antibiotics for the treatment of *H. pylori* infection (Ji & Yang, 2020).

Probiotics inhibits pathogen colonization by producing antibacterial substances, such as lactic acid, short-chain fatty acids (SCFAs), hydrogen peroxide, and bacteriocin (Homan & Orel, 2015). Lactic acid secreted by probiotic lowers down the surrounding pH making it unfavorable for the growth of *H. Pylori* (Aiba et al., 1998; Sgouras et al., 2004). Direct action of *L. gasseri* Kx110A1 and *L. brevis* ATCC14869 on *H. pylori* was demonstrated by de Klerk et al. (2016). In addition to organic acids, hydrogen peroxide produced by probiotics could cause oxidative damage to pathogenic proteins, membrane lipids and DNA by forming peroxygen ions, thus injuring the *H. pylori* cell (Batdorj et al., 2007). SCFAs are showing strong antibacterial activity due to their incomplete ionization. It also acts as a proton carrier, which induce acidification in the cytoplasm and accumulation of toxin anions to damage *H. pylori* cells (Poppi et al., 2015). Bacteriocin production by probiotics has been considered as one of the most essential properties (Dobson et al., 2011). Bacteriocin-mediated inhibition of *H. pylori* has been reported by *Bacillus subtilis* (Pinchuk et al., 2001) and *W. confusa* (Nam et al., 2002). The bacteriocin from *L. plantarum* and *L. acidophilus* can also inhibit or reduce the urease activity, which reduces *H. pylori* infection (Rezaee et al., 2019).

In vivo effects of probiotics on *H. pylori* were studied using animal models (Johnson-Henry et al., 2004; Kabir et al., 1997; Lesbros-Pantoflickova et al., 2007). It was reported that the number of *H. pylori* was decreased using *L. salivarius* WB1004 strain to the level of less than one-hundredth in the gastric mucosa by using germfree mice.

(Kabir et al., 1997). Similar experiment was carried out to decrease the number of *H. pylori* colonized in gastric mucosa to the level of less than one-hundredth using germfree mice model (Takahashi et al., 2000). Oral administration of *Lactobacillus casei* Shirota strain for 9 months decreased the number of *H. pylori* colonized in the gastric mucosa of C57BL/6 mice and inflammation score of the gastric mucosa was also found to be decreased (Sgouras et al., 2004).

H. pylori was eradicated by the treatment with *Lactobacillus rhamnosus* R0001 strain and *L. acidophilus* R0052 strain, and the inflammation score was decreased in 5 out of 7 mice (Johnson-Henry et al., 2004). It was evident from various animal studies that probiotics were significantly effective to reduce the degree of inflammation caused by *H. pylori*. The studies conducted during the period 2010 and 2014, *Lactobacillus* and *Bifidobacterium* species showed high inhibitory effect on *H. pylori* and reduced inflammatory responses. Bifidobacterium showed high inhibitory effect along with *Lactococcus*, *Enterococcus*, and *Pediococcus*, could inhibit the growth of *H. pylori*, and the use of *Pediococcus* alone led to the elimination of *H. pylori* infection. The studies conducted after 2014, all of them were conducted using *Lactobacillus* and *Bifidobacteria* sp. on the C57Bl/6 mouse model. All of the investigated probiotics showed an inhibitory effect on the growth of *H. pylori* and inhibited inflammatory responses in epithelial cells. Some of the probiotic strains reduced the release of inflammatory factors on gastric mucosa. *H. pylori* gastritis is associated with interleukin (IL)-8, which can be discovered in early stage of infection. This chemotactic compound activates neutrophils, which induced the degeneration and necrosis of gastric mucosa cell, also stimulated mucosal monocytes and dendritic cells to produce tumor necrosis factor, IL-1, and IL-6 (Fu, 2014).

In human studies, *Lactobacillus reuteri* and *Lactobacillus gasseri* alone with PPIs showed a high eradication effect on *H. pylori* infections, which suggested the use of probiotics as the future therapeutic protocols in human. In relation to the treatment process, probiotics should not be used as a single treatment for the eradication of *H. pylori*. However, their use in standard treatment as a supplement will increase eradication and reduce side effects associated with treatment. It is widely believed that probiotics can improve the eradication of *H. pylori* and reduce side effects during standard treatment, but some probiotic bacterial species could help with drug therapy. The diversity of gut microbiota was altered shortly after *H. pylori* eradication. However, it was restored after 2 months in patients treated with triple therapy (O'Connor et al., 2019). Many clinical studies have been reported to examine the effect of probiotics on *H. pylori* infection (Goderska et al., 2018). Probiotics alone can reduce *H. pylori* load in the stomach, but it cannot be cured. However, the mixed strains of probiotics showed increased antimicrobial activity on *H. pylori* infection, which reduce the delta value of UBT, and alleviate gastric mucosal inflammation (Song et al., 2019). The effect of single treatment with probiotics, combined effects of probiotics with other drugs, combined effects of probiotics with eradication therapy using PPI, and antimicrobial drugs are useful in *H. pylori* treatment. Role of probiotics for the treatment of *H. pylori* infection is shown in Table 20.1. Therefore probiotics are having significant impact on the treatment or prevention of *H. pylori* infection (Kamiya et al., 2019).

20.4.2 Efficacy of probiotics as vaccine delivery system for *H. pylori* infection

In 1984 the vaccine against *H. pylori* was discovered by Marshall and Warren (1984). *H. pylori* was reported as the third GC causing notorious agent throughout the world. So, there was a need for searching a potential vaccine for the control of *H. pylori* infection (International Agency for Research on Cancer, 2013). The severe antimicrobial resistance and therapy-related side effects still remain as an obstacle to eradicate *H. pylori* bacteria. *Lactobacillus* supplementation along with triple therapy can increase *H. pylori* eradication rates and reduce the incidence of therapy-related diarrhea in children (Fang et al., 2019). The efficacy of these triple regimens has decreased lately to rates lower than 70%, due to *H. pylori* resistance to key antibiotics, mainly clarithromycin, followed by metronidazole and levofloxacin (Goderska et al., 2018). Probiotics, such as *L. acidophilus*, *L. gasseri* OLL2716, and *B. infantis*, along with antibiotic-PPI could improve the eradication rate in adjuvant therapy. However, there was no report on the adverse symptoms. Probiotic yeast *S. boulardii* has been deemed to have a therapeutic potential for many GI and extraintestinal diseases in recent years. *L. reuteri* and *S. boulardii* have the ability to increase eradication rate and reduce adverse effects. There was no significant decrease in the eradication rate with the mixture of *L. reuteri* strains. Therefore the effects of multistrain probiotics on the treatment of *H. pylori* mainly depends on specific combination and not all of them were valid in eradicating *H. pylori* infection (Zhang et al., 2017).

Lactococci was suggested as an ideal recombinant vaccine vehicle due to their potentiality to induce both acquired and innate immunity in the host. Production of recombinant *H. pylori* antigens, such as UreB, CagA, and NapA, were widely demonstrated in *L. lactis* followed by their efficacy in preclinical studies (Gu, Song, et al., 2009; Kim et al., 2009). To study surface display expression of *H. pylori* antigens in probiotics, recombinant UreBE-SpaxX (Ure B fragment E and fragment Spax of *Staphylococcus aureus*) was constructed (Song & Gu, 2009). SpaxX is a cell wall anchor

TABLE 20.1 Probiotics for the treatment of *Helicobacter pylori* infection.

Probiotics	Effects against *H. pylori* infection	References
L. acidophilus, *L. plantarum*, and *L. rhamnosus*	Reduction of inflammation in mice	Asgari et al. (2020)
L. plantarum	Induce apoptosis in gastric cancer cells	Maleki-Kakelar et al. (2020)
L. casei, *L. paracasei*, *L. acidophilus*, *B. lactis*, and *S. thermophilus* strains	Bacteriostatic and bactericidal activity	Saracino et al. (2020)
LAB isolates: 19, 4, 8, 11, 12, 13, 15, 16, and 17	Antagonistic effects through bacteriocins and organic acids	Mabeku et al. (2020)
L. fermentum UCO-979C	Modulation of gastric innate immunity by exopolysaccharides	Garcia-Castillo et al. (2020)
Lactobacillus spp.	Reduce inflammation in mice	Chen et al. (2019)
Lactic acid bacteria	Inhibits urease activity and adhesion on epithelial cell line	Rezaee et al. (2019)
L. plantarum ZDY2013	Antiinflammatory effects and antiadhesion	Zhao et al. (2018)
L. rhamnosus	Reduce gastric pathology	Westerik et al. (2018)
Enterococcus faecium L-3	Antimicrobial activity by enterococcal bacteriocins	Baryshnikova et al. (2017)
L. paracasei strain 06TCa19	Prevent gastric inflammation	Takeda et al. (2017)
L. fermentum UCO-979C	Biofilm formation prevents infection	Salas-Jara et al. (2016)
L. reuteri DSM17648	Specific binding antagonist to *H. pylori*	Holz et al. (2015)
L. reuteri	Antibactericidal activity	Delgado et al. (2015)
L. casei	Antagonistic activity including antibiotic resistant strains	Enany and Abdalla (2015)
	Inhibits *H. pylori* motility	Isobe et al. (2012)

of *S. aureus* and its fusion with Ure BE provided enhanced adjuvant activity. Western blotting of the recombinant *L. lactis* cell wall extract with polyclonal chicken antiserum confirmed its efficacy. Zhou et al. (2015) used the spores of *Bacillus subtilis* to deliver recombinant urease B antigen, and *H. pylori* load was found to be reduced significantly (84%) in mice. Recently Peng, Zhang, et al. (2018) reported a vaccine containing recombinant NapA *L. lactis* which demonstrated production of protective antibodies in orally administered mice and reduction in *H. pylori* colonization was noted. Despite a large number of researches in vaccine development, the progress is still lacking.

20.5 Enterohemorrhagic *Escherichia coli*

E. coli isolates are considered as endogenous microbiota of the human gut, causing significant diarrheal and extraintestinal diseases in humans. The bacteria are commonly transmitted through ingestion of contaminated food, such as undercooked meat, particularly beef products, cross-contaminated raw vegetables, sprouts, and seeds (Tozzoli et al., 2014). Pathogenic *E. coli* associated with GI illness have been categorized into eight pathotypes based on their virulence profiles: EHEC; enterotoxigenic *E. coli*; enteropathogenic *E. coli*; enteroinvasive *E. coli*; enteroaggregative *E. coli*; diffusely adherent *E. coli*; adherent invasive *E. coli*; and STEC (Roussel et al., 2017). EHEC O157:H7 is one of the main human pathogens found in contaminated food and water. Development of infection by this bacterium in human manifests itself as diarrhea without bleeding and in severe cases as severe intestinal inflammation along with bleeding (Sahshorpour et al., 2014).

20.5.1 Origin, definition, and characteristics

The EHEC O157:H7, a *E. coli* prototype, Gram-negative *bacillus* was identified in 1982 and recognized as an important organism related to public health in North America and European countries based on clinical, epidemiological, and laboratory investigations (Riley et al., 1983). *E. coli* serotypes showing similar pathogenic potentiality was termed as EHEC (Levine & Edelman, 1984). EHEC is associated with hemorrhagic colitis outbreaks and represent the main trigger of HUS throughout the world was reported by Johnson and Taylor (2008). In particular, O157:H7 is the main serotype associated with hemorrhagic colitis and HUS outbreaks (Karmali et al., 2010; Masana et al., 2010). HUS affects mostly children under age 10 and was characterized by the production of acute renal failure, thrombocytopenia and microangiopathic hemolytic anemia, with a mortality rate of 1%–4% (Spinale et al., 2013).

Hemolytic uremic syndrome, previously termed as a mysterious disease, was recognized as a complication caused by *E. coli* O157:H7 in developed countries. TTP having a prodrome of diarrhea or abdominal pain also caused by *E. coli* O157:H7 (Griffin & Tauxe, 1991). Other complications of *E. coli* O157:H7 infection include gross anal dilatation (Vickers et al., 1988), which cause death. EHEC, including *E. coli* O157:H7, causes severe illness in humans due to the production of Stx (Nawrocki et al., 2020).

The primary EHEC virulence factor is the Stx, targets cells expressing the glycolipid globotriaosylceramide, disrupts host protein synthesis, and causes apoptotic cell death (Dallman et al., 2015). It is also called as SETC infection. Management of STEC-mediated diseases including HUS by probiotics has also recently been reported in many studies. The administration of certain probiotics, such as *Lactobacillus* strains (*L. rhamnosus* LR04, LR06, *L. delbrueckii*, *L. pentosus*, *L. fermentum*, *L. crispatus*, *L. plantarum*, *L. lactis*, *L. kefir*, *L. gasseri* CCDM215, *L. accidophila* CCDM149, *L. helveticus* KLDS, *L. casei*, *L. paracasei* NZU101), *E. coli* Nissle, *Enterococcus faecium* YF5, *Enterococcus faecalis* (Symbioflor), and *Bifidobacterium longum*, reduces colonization and carriage of STEC into humans or reservoir animals, which will prevent and/or reduce the risk of infection and transmission of the pathogenic bacteria (Mühlen & Dersch, 2020). Endothelial dysfunction has been recognized as the trigger event in the development of microangiopathic process, which causes podocyte injury in HUS patients. Glomerular endothelial cells are the primary target of the toxic effects of Stx, which triggers a cascade of signaling events resulting in the loss of endothelial antiadhesive, antiinflammatory, and thromboresistant properties (Zoja et al., 2019). Stx directly induces complement activation through alternative pathway on the surface of endothelial cells by increasing C3 deposition and thrombus formation on microvascular endothelial cells after perfusion with human serum. The over activation of complement system on renal and blood cells contributes abnormal vascular function and prothrombotic processes in Stx-HUS patients (Morigi et al., 2011).

EHEC interacts with the follicle-associated epithelium (Peyer's patches) in distal ileum and translocate across the intestinal epithelium by M cells and induces apoptosis in infected macrophages, which release toxin to *lamina propria*. This toxin entered into bloodstream to reach target organs in humans (Etienne-Mesmin et al., 2011). Long polar fimbriae in Payer's patches play a significant role in EHEC pathogenesis. The significant association was observed between the presence of *lpf* operons and EHEC pathogenicity (Cordonnier et al., 2017). Therefore the terminal ileum and colon are considered to be the main sites of EHEC colonization in humans (Lewis et al., 2015). EHEC infection also mediated by outer membrane protein A (OmpA), which located at periplasmic space in the bacterial membrane. OmpAper plays multiple roles in EHEC pathogenesis. OmpA contains two terminuses, such as N-terminus (OmpA), which forms a transmembrane domain, and C-terminus (OmpAper), which forms a dimer and binds to peptidoglycan layer. The OmpAper is responsible for acid tolerance and high osmotic pressure during pathogenesis (Wang et al., 2016).

Children are more susceptible to EHEC infection due to their microbiome metabolites, which induce species-specific enhancement of EHEC pathogenesis. The four specific metabolites viz. 4-methyl benzoic acid, 3,4-dimethylbenzoic acid, hexanoic acid, and heptanoic acid from human microbiome could induce the expression of flagellin, a bacterial protein associated with the motility of EHEC, and increased epithelial injury. The possible release of Stx from dead and dying bacteria and the risk of resistance development have restricted the usage of antibiotics against EHEC (Cheng et al., 2017). Furthermore, in-depth investigation of EHEC infection within the GI tract is highly needed to predict human intestinal pathophysiology (Tovaglieri et al., 2019).

20.5.2 Treatment of EHEC infection

The Centers for Disease Control and Prevention reported that foodborne *E. coli* O157:H7 is responsible for over 63,000 illnesses every year in the United States. In general, the prevention of foodborne diseases must be based on good hygienic practices and control of the contamination of foods by biological and chemical hazards (Jenssen et al., 2016). Also, there was a trend of reducing the usage of antibiotics in order to control the antibiotics resistant pathogens. Other alternative treatments included application of antibodies to endotoxins, vaccines, and microorganisms producing antimicrobial agents, which have been tried by many researchers (Fernebro, 2011; Gu, Liu, et al., 2009; Rahal et al., 2012).

According to Rabanal et al. (2015), antibiotics are generally required to treat EHEC-associated intestinal disease. However, the increasing issue of antibiotic resistance is a global threat to the public health. In addition, lysis of EHEC O157:H7 cells following antibiotic treatment can result in the release of virulence factors, such as endotoxin, Stx, and cytosine-phosphate-guanine (CpG)-containing oligonucleotides, all of which trigger the immune system, resulting in an exacerbated inflammatory response.

EHEC O157:H7 vaccine was developed by inserting the bivalent antigen espA-Tir-M (ET), which is composed of espA and the Tir central domain (Tir-M) and was inserted into *Lactobacillus acidophilus*. Specific immune responses were evaluated in mice and protection against EHEC O157:H7 both in vitro and in vivo (Lin et al., 2017). It was demonstrated that LA-ET induced both humoral and cellular immune responses in mice and was considered as a promising vaccine against EHEC O157:H7 infection. Haiwen et al. (2019) reported that Lactoferricin B, derived from lactoferrin in whey could efficiently attenuate O157:H7-induced epithelial barrier damage and dysregulation of inflammation status, while maintaining microbiota homeostasis in the intestine.

The neutralization of toxin has been considered as one of the strategies to reduce its effect. Antibodies cαStx1 and cαStx2 have been directly engineered against the B subunit of Stx1 and A subunit of Stx2, respectively (Bitzan et al., 2009). Camelid single antibodies against Stx2 have been tested for their protective characteristics. The antisingle-chain antibodies (VHH) were obtained with two copies of anti-Stx2B VHH and one antiserum albumin VHH. The antitoxin effect of VHH may serve as an alternative for the treatment of HUS (Mejias et al., 2016). The suitability of an adjuvant is important in vaccine development to enhance the immunogenicity and reactivity of the antigens in the host immune system. The intranasal immunization of dams and later passive immunization of their offspring with either recombinant EspB or γ-intimin C280 plus MALP2 as adjuvant significantly reduced the intestinal colonization of bacteria and uremia level in serum which was demonstrated in the infant mice (Rabinovitz et al., 2016).

The recombinant nanovaccine candidate could induce the strong humoral and mucosal immune responses and protect the mice from live EHEC O157:H7 challenge. The effective techniques to prevent/control EHEC infection include vaccination against extremely immunogenic part of attachment factors. A chimeric trivalent recombinant protein rEIT (EspA, Intimin, Tir) has been reported for their significant immunogenicity against *E. coli* O157:H7. The recombinant proteins are then encapsulated with chitosan nanoparticle as a nanovaccine. Prevention of EHEC infection by chitosan nanostructure coupled with synthetic recombinant antigen has been reported by Khanifar et al. (2019). The use of oral injection combined vaccination routes achieved higher humoral and mucosal immunogenicity levels compared to other methods.

Phages play a major role in controlling bacterial densities in the biosphere, including humans, which is the basis of sustainable phage therapy. Phages could be used therapeutically, as an additional tool or in combination with antibiotics to treat bacterial infections that do not respond to conventional antibiotics. Moreover, they can be chosen to be harmless to the commensal bacteria, such as those of the gut microflora. The oral application of phages to humans is very safe and is commercially available for the decontamination of foods (Merabishvili et al., 2012). The phage therapy proved to be efficient toward the biocontrol of pathogenic *E. coli* (Alam et al., 2011; Chibani-Chennoufi et al., 2004; Tanji et al., 2005). Recently probiotic lactic acid bacterium *Lactococcus lactis* also considered a safe vaccine vehicle for EHEC infection (Sreerohini et al., 2019).

20.5.3 Role of probiotics on EHEC infection

Probiotics promote the GIT homeostasis and stimulate the growth of indigenous beneficial gut microbiota by inhibiting the growth of pathogenic microbes. Therefore probiotics are recommended as alternative biotherapeutic agents for intestinal pathogenic infections (Misra et al., 2019). Inhibition of EHEC infection through application of probiotic bacteria is of crucial importance. Zhao Zhao et al. (1998) showed that probiotic bacteria were found to be capable of decreasing *E. coli* O157:H7 in animals. Ota (1999) reported that consumption of yogurt caused more lactobacilli to be colonized in the intestine, which could prevent colonization of EHEC. In the study by Shu and Gill (2002), *Bifidobacterium lactis* HN019 reduced the infection *E. coli* O157:H7 and suggested that this reduction might be associated with enhanced immune protection conferred by the probiotic. Other researchers also reported that probiotics showed the potentiality for the control of *E. coli* O157:H7 infections (Medellin-Pena & Griffiths, 2009; Ogawa et al., 2001; Shu & Gill, 2002).

In the study by Brashears et al. (2003), 686 colonies isolated from goat stool were investigated for identification of *Lactobacilli*. Following identification of the tolerance of acidic and alkaline conditions, 15 genera had the ability to inhibit *E. coli*, where *Lactobacillus crispatus* was found to be the most competent strain. The probiotic *Lactobacillus plantarum* strain CIDCA 83114 isolated from kefir grains was also successfully assayed against EHEC pathogenesis in vitro (Hugo et al., 2008). There was a report that podophage CA933P proved to be a potential candidate for the biocontrol of EHEC CA933P, which was found to be capable of infecting certain strains of serotypes O145:H25, ONT: H12, and O13:H6 of STEC, and could also infect enteroinvasive *E. coli*, *Shigella flexneri* 2, *Sh. flexneri* 3, and *Pseudomonas aeruginosa* (Dini & De Urraza, 2013).

It has been suggested that probiotics are effective in preventing adhesion and invasion of enteric pathogens (Dini et al., 2016). Probiotics may reduce intestinal infections by competing with pathogens for binding sites on the intestinal wall as well as for nutrients, and also by producing antibacterial compounds and lactic acid, or via immunomodulation. Lin et al. (2017) reported that *L. acidophilus* (LA) and recombinant *L. acidophilus* (LA-ET) were both effective to exclude EHEC O157 from LoVo cells in exclusion and competition assays. This highlighted the important role of probiotics in interrupting progressive infection with EHEC O157:H7. Hesari et al. (2017) reported the antagonistic activity of probiotic bacteria viz. *L. plantarum* and *L. fermentum* isolated from traditional dairy products against *E. coli* O157:H7. The metabolites produced by the investigated bacteria inhibited the growth of *E. coli* O157:H7, which can be considered as an important solution for the prevention and treatment of *E. coli* O157:H7 infection and improve human health.

Jin-Cheng et al. (2017) reported the antagonistic activity of *Lactobacillus acidophilus* KLDS1.0901, KLDS1.0902, KLDS1.1003, and NCFM against *E. coli* O157:H7. The probiotic potential of *L. acidophilus* strains was investigated based on adhesion assay to Caco-2 cells and antiinflammatory effects by IL-8 produced in Caco-2 cells. The adhesion ability and antiinflammatory effects of *L. acidophilus* strains showed a strain-dependent manner. In general, *L. acidophilus* KLDS1.0901 and NCFM showed better probiotic potential compared to KLDS1.0902 and KLDS1.1003. Therefore the use of *L. acidophilus* KLDS1.0901 and NCFM was suggested to prevent or treat the diseases associated with *E. coli* O157:H7.

In 2007 a systematic review suggested that the probiotic combination *L. acidophilus* NP51 and *P. freudenreichii* was effective in increasing animal resistance to STEC (Sargeant et al., 2007). Furthermore, it was reported that probiotics could significantly reduce fecal STEC dismissal in ruminant animals, reservoirs of the pathogenic bacteria (Callaway et al., 2009). In 2012 Mogna et al. demonstrated a significant in vitro inhibitory effect against the growth of STEC by five probiotic strains (*L. rhamnosus* LR04, *L. rhamnosus* LR06, *L. delbrueckii* subsp. *Delbrueckii* LDD01, *L. pentosus* LPS01, and *B. breve* BR03). In 2013 Rund et al. tested the probiotic *E. coli* strain Nissle 1917 (EcN) for antagonistic effects on three different STEC strain. Results showed that the probiotic EcN had very efficient antagonistic activity on the STEC strains tested. Tan et al. (2013) reported that the probiotic strain *Enterococcus faecium* YF5, when cocultured with an STEC strain, inhibited the pathogen's replication. In the same year it was demonstrated that *Lactobacillus plantarum* and *Lactobacillus fermentum* strains could negatively influence the adhesion of STEC (Arena et al., 2014; Likotrafiti et al., 2013). In the last decade different in vitro studies have assessed the antimicrobial potential of different probiotic strains against STEC and probiotic supplementation for the prevention and treatment of pediatric GI diseases has been employed (Baldassarre et al., 2016, 2018). Probiotics are known to be effective in the management of acute gastroenteritis in children as an adjunct to rehydration therapy. Recent reports of probiotics for the treatment of EHEC infection is given in Table 20.2.

The results of the studies open the possibility for probiotic modulation to antagonize STEC specifically. No specific treatment is currently available despite major progresses in understanding the STEC-HUS mechanisms. The data obtained in vitro and in vivo studies cannot be extrapolated to humans. Only clinical trials in humans will determine the effective probiotic strains and doses. In conclusion, it is important to investigate the promising role of probiotics, which can modify the intestinal microbiota of patients with STEC strain infection and to confirm the real efficacy of probiotics at least to reduce the severity of HUS.

20.6 Rotavirus

RV belonging to the family of Reoviridae is found to be present in various foods and transmitted via fecal—oral route (Cui et al., 2018). RV is considered as a major cause of infectious gastroenteritis and mortality in infants and young children all over the world, especially under age of 5 years (Bwogi et al., 2016; Mizukoshi et al., 2014). RV is the main cause of diarrheal health among children <5 years worldwide, accounting for 146,000 deaths in 2015. The RV infection was prevalent in both developing and developed countries. In fact, almost every child was found to be infected below the age 5, and probably more than once, because reinfections occurred frequently (Azagra-Boronat et al., 2020; Crawford et al., 2017). This causes serious problems in the developing and low-income countries, such as South Asian and African countries (Pant et al., 2007). In 2016 there was a report that RV was responsible for causing 29.5% of diarrhea deaths in the age group of below 5 years, and 202,300 deaths among all the age groups occurred throughout the world (Khalil, 2017). In China, more than 33% of acute gastroenteritis caused due to RV, and children were more

TABLE 20.2 Probiotics for the treatment of Enterohemorrhagic *E. coli* (EHEC) infection.

Probiotic strains	Mode of action against EHEC	References
L. acidophilus	The length of intestinal villi and goblet cells was increased to promote antiinflammatory effects	Mirabdollah Elahi et al. (2020)
Lactobacillus casei LC2W	Down regulation of proinflammatory cytokines to protect intestinal barrier function	Wang et al. (2020)
Lactobacillus helveticus ASCC 511	Intestinal epithelial cell integrity was improved to exert antiinflammatory effects	Ho et al. (2020)
L. plantarum CCMA 0743 and *L. paracasei* CCMA 0505	Antagonistic activity by inhibition of pathogen colonization	Fonseca et al. (2021)
Lactobacillus fermentum (LF: MTCC-5898)	Modulation of tight junction to repair intestinal barrier function	Bhat et al. (2020)
Lactococcus lactis	Production of Stx neutralizing antibodies (EspB)	Sreerohini et al. (2019)
phage-resistant *Lactobacillus plantarum* (LP + PR) mutant	Inhibition of adhesion and invasion abilities	Nagarajan et al. (2019)
Saccharomyces boulardii CNCM I-745	Maintaining the integrity of tight junctions to enhance the antiinflammatory activity	Czerucka and Rampal (2019)
Bioengineered *Lactobacillus casei*	Production of metabolites (conjugated linoleic acid) for antimicrobial activity	Tabashsum et al. (2019)
E. coli Nissle 1917	Secretes DegP, a bifunctional protein with protease and chaperone activity to prevents biofilm formation	Fang et al. (2018)
Bioengineered *Lactobacillus* along with cocoa/peanut	Production of bioactive metabolites (conjugated linoleic acids) to prevent colonization and induce antiinflammatory activity	Peng (2018)
Lactobacillus casei	Production of conjugated linoleic acids for their antagonistic and antiinflammatory activities	Peng, Tabashsum, et al. (2018), Peng, Zhang, et al. (2018)
Recombinant *L. acidophilus* (LA-ET) ATCC4356	Immunomodulation thorough inhibition of A/E lesions	Lin et al. (2017)
Lactobacillus casei NA-2	Production of exopolysaccharides to exert antibiofilm activity	Xu et al. (2020)
Lactobacillus curvatus TUCO-5E	Growth of pathogen was inhibited by their antagonistic activity	Quilodrán-Vega et al. (2016)
Lactobacillus lactis VB94 and *L. lactis* VB69	Production of bacteriocin could prevent colonization of pathogen	Gómez et al. (2016)

susceptible under the age group of 24 months (Dian et al., 2017). In addition, RV infections caused anxieties on parents and economic loss to households and the societies. In the United Kingdom, an estimated cost was reported as £25 million (based on 2008–2009 prices) annually to patients and the health services (Tam & O'Brien, 2016).

RV is a naked double-strand RNA virus. It has shorter (<3 days) incubation period and transmitted via person to person by the fecal–oral route or contaminated infected surfaces. This virus is highly resistant at room temperature and can survive in stools for months. RV primarily infects enterocytes, which results severe diarrhea in children. It infects the villi of small intestinal epithelial cells (IECs), where it can replicate to cause clinical sign and symptoms of the disease (Bouseettine et al., 2020; Chaudhary et al., 2019). Innate immune responses are the first line defenses critical to battle RV infection (Holloway & Coulson, 2013). The mucosal tissues in the GI tract are considering as a main portal entry of RV, which cause severe acute intestinal infection in children's and livestock animals. The main symptoms of RVs gastroenteritis are nausea, low-grade fever, vomit, and acute watery diarrhea. However, it can spread systematically to cause viremia and infect multiple organs. The pathogenesis of RV has been studied already via IECs and immune cells' interactions, where it triggers innate immune response to increase detrimental effects in the host (Villena et al., 2016).

20.6.1 Treatment of rotavirus infection

Treatment of RV diarrhea mainly depends on the supply of oral rehydration solutions for the replacement of fluid loss. However, this strategy is not effective to reduce the severity and shorten the duration of the disease (Telmesani, 2010). There is no specific medicine for the treatment of RV infections. Administration of a variety of liquids, nonspecific antiviral medicines, as well as nursing to relieve symptoms are commonly used as clinical treatments for RV infections (Nan et al., 2014). Parents would be more concerned with safety and side effects of clinical treatments considering the physiological immaturity of infants and young children as well as their susceptibility to various adverse factors. To prevent the RV infection, vaccines are available but they are not globally implemented due to the high cost and requirements of cold storage. RV vaccines offer low protection in developing countries as a consequence of malnutrition, micronutrient deficiencies, and suboptimal breastfeeding (Kandasamy et al., 2016; Rigo-Adrover et al., 2017). Two RV vaccines viz. RotaTeq (Merck, USA) and Rotarix (GlaxoSmithKline, Belgium) are being used worldwide to reduce the number of outbreaks in many countries and were proven safe. Both vaccines are live attenuated and are highly ($>90\%$) effective in preventing severe RV disease in high-income countries (Payne et al., 2015; Yeung et al., 2016), but efficacy is reduced in low-income countries to $\approx 50\%-60\%$. The impact of RV vaccination is greater in low-income countries, saving more infant lives due to the higher RV diarrhea burden in these countries. Other live-attenuated RV vaccines are in use in some countries, and various others are in development, including a nonreplicating parenteral vaccine. Current data suggest that live attenuated vaccines, regardless of strain composition, have similar efficacy and effectiveness and confer comparable levels of cross-protection against a variety of RV genotypes (Iturriza-Gómara & Cunliffe, 2020).

The ability of immunoregulatory probiotic microorganisms (immunobiotics) is useful to prevent/control intestinal infections caused by RVs and the effects have been studied for these important groups of beneficial microbes. The modulation of intestinal antiviral innate immunity by immunobiotics and their beneficial impact on RV infection have been reported by Villena et al. (2016). The effects of probiotics on alleviating RV infections in infants and young children are controversial in clinical studies. These controversies happened because of diversities (such as varying patient profiles and probiotic strains) of these studies (Cui et al., 2016; Park et al., 2017).

Meta-analysis is considered as an effective tool to address a broad range of research questions in the field of food microbiology (Gonzales-Barron et al., 2013). It generates reliable and precise estimation of a particular intervention by integrating and synthesizing data from a large number of studies independently, which is unlikely to be obtained through only a single study. Previous studies on meta-analysis to test the effects of probiotics on RV infections were mainly focused on duration of diarrhea (Ahmadi et al., 2015; Wanke & Szajewska, 2014). In 2019 Yang et al. aimed to explore the effects of probiotics on RV infections in infants and young children with large numbers of clinical studies conducted in China adopting a meta-analysis approach. They investigated various factors influencing the effects of probiotics with regard to various symptoms. Findings of this study gave support to recommend probiotics for preventing or treatment of childhood RV infections (Rigo-Adrover et al., 2017).

According to a systematic review and meta-analysis of RV-1 and RV-5, the hospitalization and emergency visit were reduced by 85% and 90% respectively, in Latin America. However, more randomized control studies and meta-analysis are required in future to support the benefit of vaccination against RV especially at low income health care facilities (Velázquez et al., 2017). Moreover, most studies only measured partial vaccine coverage, yet full dose coverage is necessary for accurate protection against RV (Rosettie et al., 2018). The introduction of RV vaccine is partly responsible for the significant reduction in the burden of RV-associated diarrhea in sub-Saharan Africa. Therefore there is a need to encourage the remaining countries to introduce the vaccine to their routine national immunization programs (Godfrey et al., 2020).

20.6.2 Efficacy of probiotics

Probiotics are regarded as alternatives for treatment of infectious diseases, including gastroenteritis caused by RV infections (Kandasamy et al., 2016; Kawahara et al., 2017). Probiotics are members of the normal microbiota in humans or animals and generally regarded as safe. Application of probiotics, alone or combined with other treatment procedures, has attracted attention to food microbiologists and pediatricians. Commonly used probiotics for the treatment of RV infections in infants and young children include, *L. lactis*, *L. paracasei*, *L. rhamnosus*, *B. longum*, *B. infantis*, and *Enterococcus faecalis*. The efficacy of a commercially available probiotic product containing two probiotic cell types, such as *Bifidobacterium longum* BORI and *Lactobacillus acidophilus* AD031, was tested in infants and/or toddlers with RV-associated symptoms. The results showed that a probiotic formula containing *B. longum* BORI and *L. acidophilus*

AD031 could reduce the duration of RV diarrhea in young Korean children (Park et al., 2017). Because of their potential benefits in enhancing gut barrier functions and innate immunity of recipients, as well as being generally regarded as safe, probiotics were recommended as effective alternatives to prevent or treat childhood RV infections (Fernandez-Duarte et al., 2018; Kawahara et al., 2017).

NSP4 protein is a viral toxin that triggers various cellular responses, which leads to RV associated diarrhea. This protein has been associated with interferon production inhibition by inducing the degradation of interferon regulatory factors IRF3, IRF5, and IRF7 in RV pathogenesis process. Some of the probiotics from *Bifidobacterium* and *Lactobacillus* species along with prebiotics (inulin, HMO, scGOS, lcFOS) showed improved antiviral response by decreased expression of NSP4 and increased levels of specific anti-RV IgAs. Moreover, these probiotics and prebiotics are useful for the prevention of RV infection and reduced incidence of reinfections (Gonzalez-Ochoa et al., 2017).

In 2020 Ignasi Azagra-Boronat et al. reported beneficial effects of probiotic (*Lactobacilli* and *Bifidobacteria*) supplementation with different strains in infectious diarrhea caused by RV in young children. Preclinical models of RV infection were adopted as a good strategy to screen for the efficacy of new probiotic strains or to test their comparative efficacy. Neonatal Lewis rats were supplemented with *B. breve* M-16V, *L. acidophilus* NCFM, *L. helveticus* R0052, or *L. salivarius* PS2 from days 2 to 14 of life. All probiotics viz. *L. acidophilus* NCFM, *B. breve* M-16V, and *L. helveticus* R0052 caused a reduction of several clinical variables of severity and incidence of diarrhea except *L. salivarius* PS2. RV infection of MA104 cells was decreased using probiotic extract binding to Hsc70 and ß3 integrin receptors. Probiotic extracts significantly exerted their antiviral activity by interfering with RV adhesion on MA104 cell receptors, with proteins in probiotic extracts competitively interacting with cell surface receptors necessary to reduce RV infection (Salas-Cárdenas et al., 2018).

20.6.3 Role of probiotics on RV infection

RV gastroenteritis seems to be modulated by nutritional interventions, such as bioactive components of breast milk, probiotics, or prebiotics (Rigo-Adrover et al., 2017). Probiotics, such as *Lactobacillus* and *Bifidobacterium* species, and *Saccharomyces boulardii* have been associated with the prevention of RV infection, to shorter duration and severity of RV diarrhea, to reduced incidence of reinfections and to the modulation of the immune response and viral shedding (Gonzalez-Ochoa et al., 2017). Moreover, *Lactobacillus* and *Bifidobacterium* species have been associated to the stimulation of production of cytokines IL25, IL33, and TGF by intestinal cells; IL22 by innate immune cells; and IL12, IL25, IL10, and TGF, by antigen- presenting cells, resulting in improved intestinal barrier function, reduced effector, and increased regulatory immune responses (Vlasova et al., 2016).

Probiotics have been reported for their beneficial effects by several mechanisms, such as alleviation of oxidative stress, protective modulation of gut microbiota and associated metabolic profiles, enhancement of T-cell differentiation, ileal cytokine production, and serum IgG Ab levels. *Lactobacilli* and *bifidobacteria* provide significant health benefits to host by improving feed conversion and growth performance, modulating immune responses and intestinal crypt dynamics, and ultimately protecting the host from pathogens including RV. The strongest evidence of *Lactobacilli/Bifidobacteria*-mediated protection against RV diarrhea and infection was observed in pediatric patients by human clinical trials (Vlasova et al., 2016). Effects of probiotics against RV infection are shown in Table 20.3.

In vitro and in vivo studies revealed some more mechanisms of probiotics against RV infection, which includes production of antimicrobial substances (lactic acid, nitric oxide, H_2O_2, and bacteriocins), stimulation of antimicrobial peptides, mucin production by epithelial cells, stimulation of local adaptive (specific IgA response), and innate immune responses (Gonzalez-Ochoa et al., 2017). The modulation of RV immune response by probiotics and prebiotics has been associated with a generalized antiviral response via pattern recognition receptor signaling and through promoting type I IFNs, which are key regulators of IFN signaling pathway (Ishizuka et al., 2016; Kang et al., 2015).

The use of immunobiotics to beneficially modulate IFN and inflammatory signaling pathways in IECs and immune cells is an attractive target for preventive or therapeutic intervention against RVs infection. Furthermore, the advances in the knowledge of the molecular crosstalk between immunobiotics and the gut innate immune system have provided light into the microorganism-sensing signals that allow these beneficial microorganisms to improve intestinal immune responses. Activation of receptors by RV induces secretion of proinflammatory mediators that can lead to increase local tissue damage and immunopathology. Therefore activation of receptors plays a significant role to reduce the risk of RV infection by modulating deregulation of intestinal immune responses (Villena et al., 2016). This new molecular information might be helpful to improve the development of functional foods and/or pharmabiotics using immunobiotics aimed to reduce mortality and severity of RVs disease.

TABLE 20.3 Effects of probiotics on rotavirus infection.

Probiotics	Effects against RV	References
L. acidophilus NCFM, B. breve M-16V, and L. helveticus R0052	Specific anti-RV humoral response to prevent RV infection	Azagra-Boronat et al. (2020)
B. longum BORI cell extract	Stimulates antiviral activity to prevent RV colonization	Han et al. (2019)
Antimicrobial protein from L. casei (Lafti L26-DSL) and B. adolescentis (DSM 20083)	Blocks RV entry by a direct effect on the viral particle	Fernandez-Duarte et al. (2018)
Bifidobacterium breve M-16V along with short-chain galactooligosaccharide/long-chain fructooligosaccharide	Enhances early immune response against reinfection of RV	Rigo-Adrover et al. (2018)
Probiotics along with rice bran L. rhamnosus GG (LGG) and E. coli Nissle (EcN)	The prophylactic efficacy of synbiotic combination prevents human RV diarrhea in neonatal gnotobiotic pigs	Nealon et al. (2017), Yang et al. (2015)
B. longum BORI and L. acidophilus AD031	Reduced the duration of rotavirus diarrhea in young Korean children	Park et al. (2017)
Metabolites from Lactobacillus and Bifidobacetrium species	Probiotic metabolites controlled NSP4 protein to prevent cell damage and electrolyte loss	Olaya Galán et al. (2016)
B. thermophilum RBL67	Stimulates specific humoral response (IgA) to inhibit RV	Gagnon et al. (2016)
L. rhamnosus strain GG and E. coli Nissle	Immunomodulatory effects (B cell response) against RV infection	Kandasamy et al. (2016)
B. longum and L. acidophilus	Decrease the duration of diarrhea in RV-affected patients	Lee et al. (2015)
Lactobacillus strains isolated from human intestine	Antimicrobial effects against RV	Liévin-Le Moal and Servin (2014)
L. plantarum NCIMB8826	Human interferon-β (huIFN-β) significantly reduces microbial colitis and inflammatory activity	Wang et al. (2012)
L. lactis NZ9000	Induce the formation of anti-VP8 antibodies with an increased mucosal IgA against RV spike protein	Marelli et al. (2011)

20.7 Conclusion and future perspectives

The role of probiotics on various GI infections (H. pylori, EHEC, and RV) has been identified by numerous in vitro, in vivo, and clinical studies. The mechanism or action of probiotics on GI infections includes immunomodulation, competition for adhesion, secretion of antimicrobial substances, strengthening the mucosal barrier, coaggregation. Antibiotic resistance is the biggest challenge for the current eradication treatment options. The efficacy of probiotics as a tool to deliver anti-H. pylori vaccines should be taken into consideration despite the limitation of scarcity in preclinical and clinical trials. Probiotics could significantly improve the antibiotic therapy of H. pylori infection and also reduce the side effects of the treatment. In human studies, L. reuteri and L. gasseri alone with PPIs have a high eradication effect on H. pylori infections, which is suggested as the use of probiotics as the future therapeutic protocols in patients.

Moreover, the reviewed studies opened new perspectives for probiotic modulation specifically antagonizing EHEC. The relationship between probiotics and the immune system have been reported in many studies for defending the host against the colonization of pathogenic E. coli. However, probiotics produce many potential compounds, such as peroxides, fatty acids, and bacteriocins, which are highly specific to kill pathogenic bacteria, including E. coli O157:H7. Eradication of EHEC by probiotics has been reported in several in vitro studies. It also demonstrates the possible roles of probiotic in modifying the biofilms microbial ecology against EHEC through secretion of extracellular antibiofilm factors, metabolic activity, growth inhibition, and coaggregation. It has also been revealed that the impacts of probiotics are strain-specific. Therefore an ideal strain of probiotic for interfering and competing with pathogenic biofilms should be screened and identified at the molecular level for specific pathophysiological states.

Due to the potential benefits in enhancing gut barrier functions and innate immunity of recipients, as well as being generally regarded as safe, probiotics were recommended as effective alternatives to prevent or treat childhood RV infections. Although multiple probiotic microorganisms could be utilized in RV treatments, some studies have not identified any significant therapeutic effects. The beneficial activity of probiotics and prebiotics is associated with the healthy intestinal microbiota balance, intestinal epithelial barrier, and the interactions with viral particles to prevent RV cell entry. This could increase generalized antiviral response and levels of specific anti-RVs IgAs and reduce the expression of viral enterotoxins NSP4 and NSP1. More evidence is needed to support the beneficial effects and the mechanisms of prebiotics and probiotics against RV gastroenteritis.

A number of researches and clinical trials are conducted to examine the therapeutic effects of probiotics in pediatric patients. However, the use of probiotics needs to be controlled and clinical recommendations need to be followed. Therefore the underlying mechanisms of the therapeutic effects of probiotics in humans still remain unclear. To discover new probiotics, it is suggested to report complete profile of probiotic tested describing its genus species, dose, formulation, and molecular mechanism involved to provide appropriate data for further analysis, which may help to propose future guidelines for strain specific and evidence-based therapy.

References

Afsahi, A., Mahmoudi, H., Ebrahimi, A., Aeini, Z., & Esmaeili, D. (2018). Evaluation of the effect of *Lactobacillus planetarium* probiotics produced from broad bean seed in prevention of *Helicobacter pylori* in stomach tissue of C57BL/6 mice. *Journal of Cancer Science and Therapy, 10*(4), 85–89.

Ahmadi, E., Alizadeh-Navaei, R., & Rezai, M. S. (2015). Efficacy of probiotic use in acute rotavirus diarrhea in children: A systematic review and meta-analysis. *Caspian Journal of Internal Medicine, 6*(4), 187–195.

Aiba, Y., Nakano, Y., Koga, Y., Takahashi, K., & Komatsu, Y. (2015). A highly acid-resistant novel strain of *Lactobacillus johnsonii* No. 1088 has antibacterial activity, including that against *Helicobacter pylori*, and inhibits gastrin-mediated acid production in mice. *Microbiologyopen, 4*(3), 465–474.

Aiba, Y., Suzuki, N., Kabir, A. M., Takagi, A., & Koga, Y. (1998). Lactic acid mediated suppression of *Helicobacter pylori* by the oral administration of *Lactobacillus salivariusas* a probiotic in a gnotobioticmurine model. *The American Journal of Gastroenterology, 93*(11), 2097–2101.

Alam, M., Akhter, M. Z., Yasmin, M., Ahsan, C. R., & Nessa, J. (2011). Local bacteriophage isolates showed anti-*Escherichia coli* O157:H7 potency in an experimental ligated rabbit ileal loop model. *Canadian Journal of Microbiology, 57*, 408–415.

Amieva, M., & Peek, R. M., Jr (2016). Pathobiology of Helicobacter pylori–induced gastric cancer. *Gastroenterology, 150*(1), 64–78.

Arena, M. P., Russo, P., Capozzi, V., López, P., Fiocco, D., & Spano, G. (2014). Probiotic abilities of riboflavin-overproducing *Lactobacillus* strains: a novel promising application of probiotics. *Applied Microbiology and Biotechnology, 98*(17), 7569–7581.

Arslan, N., Yılmaz, O., & Demiray-Gürbüz, E. (2017). Importance of antimicrobial susceptibility testing for the management of eradication in *Helicobacter pylori* infection. *World Journal of Gastroenterology: WJG, 23*(16), 2854–2869.

Asgari, B., Kermanian, F., Yaghoobi, M. H., Vaezi, A., Soleimanifar, F., & Yaslianifard, S. (2020). The anti-Helicobacter pylori effects of *Lactobacillus acidophilus*, *L. plantarum*, and *L. rhamnosus* in stomach tissue of C57BL/6 mice. *Visceral Medicine, 36*(2), 137–143.

Azagra-Boronat, I., Massot-Cladera, M., Knipping, K., Garssen, J., Ben Amor, K., Knol, J., Franch, À., Castell, M., Rodríguez-Lagunas, M. J., & Pérez-Cano, F. J. (2020). Strain-specific probiotic properties of *bifidobacteria* and *lactobacilli* for the prevention of diarrhea caused by rotavirus in a preclinical model. *Nutrients, 12*(2), 498.

Backert, S., Neddermann, M., Maubach, G., & Naumann, M. (2016). Pathogenesis of *Helicobacter pylori* infection. *Helicobacter, 21*(Suppl. 1), 19–25.

Baldassarre, M. E., Di Mauro, A., Mastromarino, P., Fanelli, M., Martinelli, D., Urbano, F., Capobianco, D., & Laforgia, N. (2016). Administration of a multi-strain probiotic product to women in the perinatal period differentially affects the breast milk cytokine profile and may have beneficial effects on neonatal gastrointestinal functional symptoms, A randomized clinical trial. *Nutrients, 8*(11), 677.

Baldassarre, M. E., Palladino, V., Amoruso, A., Pindinelli, S., Mastromarino, P., Fanelli, M., Di Mauro, A., & Laforgia, N. (2018). Rationale of probiotic supplementation during pregnancy and neonatal period. *Nutrients, 10*(11), 1693.

Banik, A., Mondal, J., Rakshit, S., Ghosh, K., Sha, S. P., Halder, S. K., Ghosh, C., & Mondal, K. C. (2019). Amelioration of cold-induced gastric injury by a yeast probiotic isolated from traditional fermented foods. *Journal of Functional Foods, 59*, 164–173.

Baryshnikova, N., Ermolenko, E., Svarval, A., Alechina, G., Ferman, R., Roshina, N., Colobov, A., Uspenskiy, Y., Haertlé, T., & Suvorov, A. (2017). *Enterococcus faecium* L-3 in eradication of *Helicobacter pylori*: In-vivo and in-vitro. *International Journal of Clinical & Medical Microbiology, 2*(2), 123.

Batdorj, B., Trinetta, V., Dalgalarrondo, M., Prevost, H., Dousset, X., Ivanova, I., Haertle, T., & Chobert, J. M. (2007). Isolation, taxonomic identification and hydrogen peroxide production by *Lactobacillys delbrueckii* subsp. *lactis* T31, isolated from Mongolian yoghurt: Inhibitory activity on food-borne pathogens fool-borne pathogens. *Journal of Applied Microbiology, 103*(3), 584–593.

Bergan, J., Lingelem, A. B. D., Simm, R., Skotland, T., & Sandvig, K. (2012). Shiga toxins. *Toxicon, 60*(6), 1085–1107. Available from https://doi.org/10.1016/j.toxicon.2012.07.016.

Bhat, M. I., Kapila, S., & Kapila, R. (2020). *Lactobacillus fermentum* (MTCC-5898) supplementation renders prophylactic action against *Escherichia coli* impaired intestinal barrier function through tight junction modulation. *LWT, 123*, 109118.

Bian, X., Wang, T. T., Xu, M., Evivie, S. E., Luo, G. W., Liang, H. Z., Yu, S. F., & Huo, G. C. (2016). Effect of *Lactobacillus* strains on intestinal microflora and mucosa immunity in *Escherichia coli* O157: H7-induced diarrhea in mice. *Current Microbiology, 73*(1), 65–70.

Bitzan, M., Poole, R., Mehran, M., Sicard, E., Brockus, C., Thuning-Roberson, C., & Rivière, M. (2009). Safety and pharmacokinetics of chimeric anti-Shiga toxin 1 and anti-Shiga toxin 2 monoclonal antibodies in healthy volunteers. *Antimicrobial Agents and Chemotherapy, 53*(7), 3081.

Bozzi Cionci, N., Baffoni, L., Gaggìa, F., & Di Gioia, D. (2018). Therapeutic microbiology: The Role of Bifidobacterium breve as food supplement for the prevention/treatment of paediatric diseases. *Nutrients, 10*(11), 1723.

Bouseettine, R., Hassou, N., Hatib, A., Berradi, B., Bessi, H., & Ennaji, M. M. (2020). Worldwide emerging and reemerging rotavirus genotypes: genetic variability and interspecies transmission in health and environment, In. *Emerging and Reemerging Viral Pathogens*, 1017–1040.

Brashears, M. M., Galyean, M. L., Loneragan, G. H., Mann, J. E., & Killinger-Mann, K. (2003). Prevalence of *Escherichia coli* O157: H7 and performance by beef feedlot cattle given *Lactobacillus* direct-fed microbials. *Journal of Food Protection, 66*(5), 748–754.

Bwogi, J., Malamba, S., Kigozi, B., Namuwulya, P., Tushabe, P., Kiguli, S., Byarugaba, D. K., Desselberger, U., Iturriza-Gomara, M., & Karamagi, C. (2016). The epidemiology of rotavirus disease in under-five-year-old children hospitalized with acute diarrhea in central Uganda, 2012–2013. *Archives of Virology, 161*(4), 999–1003.

Callaway, T. R., Carr, M. A., Edrington, T. S., Anderson, R. C., & Nisbet, D. J. (2009). Diet, *Escherichia coli* O157: H7, and cattle: a review after 10 years. *Current Issues in Molecular Biology, 11*(2), 67–80.

Chaudhary V., Anand V. and Singh P., Rotavirus: A correlation of animals and human, 2019.

Chen, X., Tian, F., Liu, X., Zhao, J., Zhang, H. P., Zhang, H., & Chen, W. (2010). In vitro screening of *Lactobacilli* with antagonistic activity against *Helicobacter pylori* from traditionally fermented foods. *Journal of Dairy Science, 93*(12), 5627–5634.

Chen, Y. H., Tsai, W. H., Wu, H. Y., Chen, C. Y., Yeh, W. L., Chen, Y. H., Hsu, H. Y., Chen, W. W., Chen, Y. W., Chang, W. W., & Lin, T. L. (2019). Probiotic *Lactobacillus spp.* act against *Helicobacter pylori*-induced inflammation. *Journal of Clinical Medicine, 8*(1), 90.

Cheng, C., Balasubramanian, S., Fekete, A., Krischke, M., Mueller, M. J., Hentschel, U., Oelschlaeger, T. A., & Abdelmohsen, U. R. (2017). Inhibitory potential of streptphonium A against Shiga toxin production in enterohemorrhagic *Escherichia coli* (EHEC) strain EDL933. *Natural Product Research, 31*(23), 2818–2823.

Chey, W. D., Leontiadis, G. I., Howden, C. W., & Moss, S. F. (2017). ACG Clinical Guideline: Treatment of *Helicobacter pylori* Infection. *The American Journal of Gastroenterology, 112*(2), 212–239.

Chibani-Chennoufi, S., Sidoti, J., Bruttin, A., Kutter, E., Sarker, S., & Brüssow, H. (2004). In vitro and in vivo bacteriolytic activities of *Escherichia coli* phages: Implications for phage therapy. *Antimicrobial Agents and Chemotherapy, 48*(7), 2558.

Chopade, L. R., Paradeshi, J. S., Amrutkar, K. P., & Chaudhari, B. L. (2019). Finding out potent probiotic cultures from ayurvedic formulation *Takrarishta* through *in-vitro* probiotic characterization and principal component analysis. *LWT, 100*, 205–212.

Cordonnier, C., Etienne-Mesmin, L., Thévenot, J., Rougeron, A., Rénier, S., Chassaing, B., Darfeuille-Michaud, A., Barnich, N., Blanquet-Diot, S., & Livrelli, V. (2017). Enterohemorrhagic *Escherichia coli* pathogenesis: Role of Long polar fimbriae in Peyer's patches interactions. *Scientific Reports, 7*(1), 1–14.

Crawford, S., Ramani, S., Tate, J., Tate, J. E., Parashar, U. D., Svensson, L., Hagbom, M., Franco, M. A., Greenberg, H. B., O'Ryan, M., Kang, G., Desselberger, U., & Estes, M. K. (2017). Rotavirus infection. *Nature Reviews Disease Primers, 3*, 17083.

Cui, Q., Fu, Q., Zhao, X., Song, X., Yu, J., Yang, Y., Sun, K., Bai, L., Tian, Y., Chen, S., & Jia, R. (2018). Protective effects and immunomodulation on piglets infected with rotavirus following resveratrol supplementation. *PLoS One, 13*(2), e0192692.

Cui, Y., Ye, P., Zhao, Y., Xu, H., Dong, J., Luo, J., & Fu, Y. (2016). Effect of *Bifidobacterium tetravaccine* tablets-assisted therapy on T lymphocyte subpopulation of children with rotavirus enteritis. *International Journal of Clinical and Experimental Medicine, 9*(8), 15804–15811.

Czerucka, D., & Rampal, P. (2019). Diversity of *Saccharomyces boulardii* CNCM I-745 mechanisms of action against intestinal infections. *World Journal of Gastroenterology, 25*(18), 2188.

Dallman, T. J., Ashton, P. M., Byrne, L., Perry, N. T., Petrovska, L., Ellis, R., Allison, L., Hanson, M., Holmes, A., Gunn, G. J., & Chase-Topping, M. E. (2015). Applying phylogenomics to understand the emergence of Shiga-toxin-producing *Escherichia coli* O157:H7 strains causing severe human disease in the UK. *Microbial Genomics, 1*(3).

de Klerk, N., Maudsdotter, L., Gebreegziabher, H., Saroj, S. D., Eriksson, B., Eriksson, O. S., Roos, S., Lindén, S., Sjölinder, H., & Jonsson, A. B. (2016). *Lactobacilli* reduce *Helicobacter pylori* attachment to host gastric epithelial cells by inhibiting adhesion gene expression. *Infection and Immunity, 84*(5), 1526–1535.

Delgado, S., Leite, A. M., Ruas-Madiedo, P., & Mayo, B. (2015). Probiotic and technological properties of *Lactobacillus spp.* strains from the human stomach in the search for potential candidates against gastric microbial dysbiosis. *Frontiers in Microbiology, 5*, 766.

den Hoed, C. M., & Kuipers, E. J. (2020). Helicobacter pylori *infection*. Hunter's Tropical medicine and emerging infectious diseases (pp. 476–480).

Devi, S. M., Kurrey, N. K., & Halami, P. M. (2018). In vitro anti-inflammatory activity among probiotic *Lactobacillus* species isolated from fermented foods. *Journal of Functional Foods, 47*, 19–27.

Dian, Z., Fan, M., Wang, B., Feng, Y., Ji, H., Dong, S., Zhang, A. M., Liu, L., Niu, H., & Xia, X. (2017). The prevalence and genotype distribution of rotavirus A infection among children with acute gastroenteritis in Kunming, China. *Archives of Virology, 162*(1), 281–285.

Dimidi, E., Christodoulides, S., Scott, S. M., & Whelan, K. (2017). Mechanisms of action of probiotics and the gastrointestinal microbiota on gut motility and constipation. *Advances in Nutrition, 8*(3), 484–494.

Dini, C., & De Urraza, P. J. (2013). Effect of buffer systems and disaccharides concentration on *Podoviridae coliphage* stability during freeze drying and storage. *Cryobiology, 66*(3), 339–342.

Dini, C., Bolla, P. A., & de Urraza, P. J. (2016). Treatment of in vitro enterohemorrhagic *Escherichia coli* infection using phage and probiotics. *Journal of Applied Microbiology, 121*(1), 78–88.

Dobson, A., Cotter, P. D., Ross, R. P., & Hill, C. (2011). Bacteriocin production: A probiotic trait? *Applied and Environmental Microbiology, 78*(1), 1–6.

Dunne, C., Dolan, B., & Clyne, M. (2014). Factors that mediate colonization of the human stomach by *Helicobacter pylori*. *World Journal of Gastroenterology: WJG, 20*(19), 5610–5624.

Enany, S., & Abdalla, S. (2015). In vitro antagonistic activity of *Lactobacillus casei* against *Helicobacter pylori*. *Brazilian Journal of Microbiology, 46*(4), 1201–1206.

Eslami, M., Yousefi, B., Kokhaei, P., Moghadas, A. J., Moghadam, B. S., Arabkarid, V., & Niazie, Z. (2019). Are probiotics useful for therapy of *Helicobacter pylori* diseases. *Comparative Immunology, Microbiology and Infectious Diseases, 64*, 99–108.

Etienne-Mesmin, L., Chassaing, B., Sauvanet, P., Denizot, J., Blanquet-Diot, S., Darfeuille-Michaud, A., Pradel, N., & Livrelli, V. (2011). Interactions with M cells and macrophages as key steps in the pathogenesis of enterohemorragic *Escherichia coli* infections. *PLoS One, 6*(8), e23594.

Eusebi, L. H., Zagari, R. M., & Bazzoli, F. (2014). Epidemiology of *Helicobacter pylori* infection. *Helicobacter, 19*(Suppl. 1), 1–5.

Fan, C. C., Chen, C. H., Chou, C., Kao, T. Y., Cheng, A. N., Lee, A. Y. L., & Kuo, C. L. (2020). A time-saving—modified Giemsa stain is a better diagnostic method of *Helicobacter pylori* infection compared with the rapid urease test. *Journal of Clinical Laboratory Analysis, 34*(4), e23110. Available from https://doi.org/10.1002/jcla.23110.

Fang, K., Jin, X., & Hong, S. H. (2018). Probiotic Escherichia coli inhibits biofilm formation of pathogenic *E. coli* via extracellular activity of DegP. *Scientific Reports, 8*(1), 4939.

Fang, H. R., Zhang, G. Q., Cheng, J. Y., & Li, Z. Y. (2019). Efficacy of *Lactobacillus*-supplemented triple therapy for *Helicobacter pylori* infection in children: a meta-analysis of randomized controlled trials. *European Journal of Pediatrics, 178*(1), 7–16.

Fernandez-Duarte, K. P., Olaya-Galán, N. N., Salas-Cárdenas, S. P., Lopez-Rozo, J., & Gutierrez-Fernandez, M. F. (2018). *Bifidobacterium adolescentis* (DSM 20083) and *lactobacillus casei* (Lafti L26-DSL): Probiotics able to block the in vitro adherence of rotavirus in MA104 cells. *Probiotics Antimicrob Proteins, 10*(1), 56–63.

Fernebro, J. (2011). Fighting bacterial infections—Future treatment options. *Drug Resistance Updates: Reviews and Commentaries in Antimicrobial and Anticancer Chemotherapy, 14*, 125–139.

Fischbach, W., & Malfertheiner, P. (2018). *Helicobacter pylori* infection: When to eradicate, how to diagnose and treat. *Deutsches Ärzteblatt International, 115*(25), 429–436.

Fonseca, H. C., de Sousa Melo, D., Ramos, C. L., Dias, D. R., & Schwan, R. F. (2021). Probiotic properties of *Lactobacilli* and their ability to inhibit the adhesion of enteropathogenic bacteria to caco-2 and ht-29 cells. *Probiotics and Antimicrobial Proteins, 13*, 102–112.

Fu, H. W. (2014). *Helicobacter pylori* neutrophil-activating protein: From molecular pathogenesis to clinical applications. *World Journal of Gastroenterology: WJG, 20*(18), 5294–5301.

Gagnon, M., Vimont, A., Darveau, A., Fliss, I., & Jean, J. (2016). Study of the ability of *Bifidobacteria* of human origin to prevent and treat rotavirus infection using colonic cell and mouse models. *PLoS One, 11*(10), e0164512.

Garcia-Castillo, V., Marcial, G., Albarracín, L., Tomokiyo, M., Clua, P., Takahashi, H., Kitazawa, H., Garcia-Cancino, A., & Villena, J. (2020). The Exopolysaccharide of *Lactobacillus fermentum* UCO-979C Is Partially Involved in Its Immunomodulatory Effect and Its Ability to Improve the Resistance against Helicobacter pylori Infection. *Microorganisms, 8*(4), 479.

Ghasemian, A., Eslami, M., Shafiei, M., Najafipour, S., & Rajabi, A. (2018). Probiotics and their increasing importance in human health and infection control. *Reviews in Medical Microbiology, 29*(4), 153–158. Available from https://doi.org/10.1097/MRM.0000000000000147.

Goderska, K., Pena, S. A., & Alarcon, T. (2018). *Helicobacter pylori* treatment: Antibiotics or probiotics. *Applied Microbiology and Biotechnology, 102*(1), 1–7.

Godfrey, O., Zhang, W., Amponsem-Boateng, C., Bonney Oppong, T., Zhao, Q., & Li, D. (2020). Evidence of rotavirus vaccine impact in sub-Saharan Africa: Systematic review and meta-analysis. *PLoS One, 15*(4), e0232113.

Gómez, N. C., Ramiro, J. M., Quecan, B. X., & de Melo Franco, B. D. (2016). Use of potential probiotic lactic acid bacteria (LAB) biofilms for the control of *Listeria monocytogenes, Salmonella Typhimurium*, and *Escherichia coli* O157:H7 biofilms formation. *Frontiers in Microbiology, 7*, 863.

Gómez-Rial, J., Rivero-Calle, I., Salas, A., & Martinón-Torres, F. (2020). Rotavirus and autoimmunity. *Journal of Infection, 81*(2), 183–189.

Gonzales-Barron, U., Cadavez, V., Sheridan, J. J., & Butler, F. (2013). Modelling the effect of chilling on the occurrence of *Salmonella* on pig carcasses at study, abattoir and batch levels by meta-analysis. *International Journal of Food Microbiology, 163*(2–3), 101–113.

Gonzalez-Ochoa, G., Flores-Mendoza, L. K., Icedo-Garcia, R., Gomez-Flores, R., & Tamez-Guerra, P. (2017). Modulation of rotavirus severe gastroenteritis by the combination of probiotics and prebiotics. *Archives of Microbiology, 199*(7), 953–961.

Griffin, P. M., & Tauxe, R. V. (1991). The epidemiology of infections caused by *Escherichia coli* O157:H7, other enterohemorrhagic *E. coli*, and the associated hemolytic uremic syndrome. *Epidemiologic Reviews, 13*(1), 60–98.

Gu, J., Liu, Y., Yu, S., Wang, H., Wang, Q., Yi, Y., Zhu, F., Yu, X. J., et al. (2009). Enterohemorrhagic Escherichia coli trivalent recombinant vaccine containing EspA, intimin and Stx2 induces strong humoral immune response and confers protection in mice. *Microbes and Infection/Institut Pasteur, 11*, 835–841.

Gu, Q., Song, D., & Zhu, M. (2009). Oral vaccination of mice against *Helicobacter pylori* with recombinant *Lactococcus lactis* expressing urease subunit B. *FEMS Immunology and Medical Microbiology*, 56(3), 197−203.

Haiwen, Z., Rui, H., Bingxi, Z., Qingfeng, G., Jifeng, Z., Xuemei, W., & Beibei, W. (2019). Oral administration of bovine lactoferrin-derived lactoferricin (Lfcin) B could attenuate enterohemorrhagic *Escherichia coli* O157:H7 induced intestinal disease through improving intestinal barrier function and microbiota. *Journal of Agricultural and Food Chemistry*, 67(14), 3932−3945.

Han, Y. O., Jeong, Y., You, H. J., Ku, S., Ji, G. E., & Park, M. S. (2019). The anti-rotaviral activity of low molecular weight and non-proteinaceous substance from *Bifidobacterium longum* BORI cell extract. *Microorganisms*, 7(4), 108.

Hassan, M. N., Arif, A., Shahzad, M. S., Ibrahim, M., Rahman, H. A., Razaq, M. A., & Ahmed, R. (2020). Global prevalence of *Helicobacter pylori* and its effect on human health. *Pure and Applied Biology*, 9(1), 936−948.

Hesari, M. R., Darsanaki, R. K., & Salehzadeh, A. (2017). Antagonistic activity of probiotic bacteria isolated from traditional dairy products against *E. coli* O157: H7. *Journal of Medical Bacteriology*, 6(3-4), 23−30.

Ho, S. W., El-Nezami, H., & Shah, N. P. (2020). The protective effects of enriched citrulline fermented milk with *Lactobacillus helveticus* on the intestinal epithelium integrity against *Escherichia coli* infection. *Scientific Reports*, 10(1), 1−15.

Holloway, G., & Coulson, B. S. (2013). Innate cellular responses to rotavirus infection. *Journal of General Virology*, 94(6), 1151−1160.

Holz, C., Busjahn, A., Mehling, H., Arya, S., Boettner, M., Habibi, H., & Lang, C. (2015). Significant reduction in *Helicobacter pylori* load in humans with non-viable *Lactobacillus reuteri* DSM17648: A pilot study. *Probiotics and Antimicrobial Proteins*, 7(2), 91−100.

Homan, M., & Orel, R. (2015). Are probiotics useful in *Helicobacter pylori* eradication? *World Journal of Gastroenterology: WJG*, 21(37), 10644−10653.

Hooi, J. K., Lai, W. Y., Ng, W. K., Suen, M. M., Underwood, F. E., Tanyingoh, D., Malfertheiner, P., Graham, D. Y., Wong, V. W. S., Wu, J. C., Chan, F. K. L., Sung, J. J. Y., Kaplan, G. G., & Ng, S. C. (2017). Global prevalence of *Helicobacter pylori* infection: Systematic review and meta-analysis. *Gastroenterology*, 153(2), 420−429.

Hugo, A. A., Kakisu, E., De Antoni, G. L., & Pérez, P. F. (2008). *Lactobacilli* antagonize biological effects of enterohaemorrhagic *Escherichia coli* in vitro. *Letters in Applied Microbiology*, 46(6), 613−619.

International Agency for Research on Cancer GLOBOCAN. (2013). *Estimated cancer incidence, mortality and prevalence worldwide in 2012*. World Health Organisation.

Ishizuka, T., Kanmani, P., Kobayashi, H., Miyazaki, A., Soma, J., Suda, Y., Aso, H., Nochi, T., Iwabuchi, N., Xiao, J. Z., & Saito, T. (2016). Immunobiotic *Bifidobacteria* strains modulate rotavirus immune response in porcine intestinal epitheliocytes via pattern recognition receptor signaling. *PLoS One*, 11(3), e0152416.

Isobe, H., Nishiyama, A., Takano, T., Higuchi, W., Nakagawa, S., Taneike, I., Fukushima, Y., & Yamamoto, T. (2012). Reduction of overall *Helicobacter pylori* colonization levels in the stomach of Mongolian gerbil by *Lactobacillus johnsonii* La1 (LC1) and its in vitro activities against *H. pylori* motility and adherence. *Bioscience, Biotechnology, and Biochemistry*, 76(4), 850−852.

Iturriza-Gómara, M., & Cunliffe, N. A. (2020). Viral gastroenteritis. *Hunter's Tropical Medicine and Emerging Infectious Diseases*, 289−307.

Jenssen, G. R., Vold, L., Hovland, E., Bangstad, H. J., Nygård, K., & Bjerre, A. (2016). Clinical features, therapeutic interventions and long-term aspects of hemolytic-uremic syndrome in Norwegian children: A nationwide retrospective study from 1999−2008. *BMC Infectious Diseases*, 16(1), 1−10.

Ji, J., & Yang, H. (2020). Using probiotics as supplementation for *Helicobacter pylori* antibiotic therapy. *International Journal of Molecular Sciences*, 21(3), 1136. Available from https://doi.org/10.3390/ijms21031136.

Jin-cheng, D., Fei, L., Bai-liang, L., Xin, B., Evivie, S. E., Min, X., Xiu-yun, D., & Gui-cheng, H. (2017). In vitro assessment of probiotic potential of *Lactobacillus acidophilus* and antagonistic activity against *Escherichia coli* O157: H7. *Journal of Northeast Agricultural University (English Edition)*, 24(1), 59−69.

Johnson, S., & Taylor, C. M. (2008). What's new in haemolytic uraemic syndrome? *European Journal of Pediatrics*, 167, 965−971.

Johnson-Henry, K. C., Mitchell, D. J., Avitzur, Y., Galindo-Mata, E., Jones, N. L., & Sherman, P. M. (2004). Probiotics reduce bacterial colonization and gastric inflammation in *H. pylori*-infected mice. *Digestive Diseases and Sciences*, 49(7−8), 1095−1102.

Jubelin, G., Desvaux, M., Schüller, S., Etienne-Mesmin, L., Muniesa, M., & Blanquet-Diot, S. (2018). Modulation of enterohaemorrhagic *Escherichia coli* survival and virulence in the human gastrointestinal tract. *Microorganisms*, 6(4), 115. Available from https://doi.org/10.3390/microorganisms6040115.

Judkins, T. C., Archer, D. L., Kramer, D. C., & Solch, R. J. (2020). Probiotics, Nutrition, and the Small Intestine. *Current Gastroenterology Reports*, 22(1), 2.

Kabir, A. M., Aiba, Y., Takagi, A., Kamiya, S., Miwa, T., & Koga, Y. (1997). Prevention of *Helicobacter pylori* by *Lactobacilli* in a gnotobiotic murine model. *Gut*, 41(1), 49−55.

Kakoullis, L., Papachristodoulou, E., Chra, P., & Panos, G. (2019). Shiga toxin-induced haemolytic uraemic syndrome and the role of antibiotics: A global overview. *The Journal of Infection*, 79, 75−94.

Kamiya, S., Yonezawa, H., & Osaki, T. (2019). Role of Probiotics in eradication therapy for *Helicobacter pylori* Infection. *Advances in Experimental Medicine and Biology*, 1149, 243−255.

Kandasamy, S., Vlasova, A. N., Fischer, D., Kumar, A., Chattha, K. S., Rauf, A., Shao, L., Langel, S. N., Rajashekara, G., & Saif, L. J. (2016). Differential effects of *Escherichia coli* Nissle and *Lactobacillus rhamnosus* strain GG on human rotavirus binding, infection, and B cell immunity. *The Journal of Immunology*, 196(4), 1780−1789.

Kang, J. Y., Lee, D. K., Ha, N. J., & Shin, H. S. (2015). Antiviral effects of *Lactobacillus ruminis* SPM0211 and *Bifidobacterium longum* SPM1205 and SPM1206 on rotavirus-infected Caco-2 cells and a neonatal mouse model. *Journal of Microbiology*, 53(11), 796−803.

Kao, C. Y., Sheu, B. S., & Wu, J. J. (2016). *Helicobacter pylori* infection: An overview of bacterial virulence factors and pathogenesis. *Biomedical Journal*, *39*(1), 14−23.

Karczewski, J., Troost, F. J., Konings, I., Dekker, J., Kleerebezem, M., Brummer, R. J. M., & Wells, J. M. (2010). Regulation of human epithelial tight junction proteins by *Lactobacillus plantarum* in vivo and protective effects on the epithelial barrier. *American Journal of Physiology. Gastrointestinal and Liver Physiology*, *298*(6), G851−G859.

Karmali, M. A., Gannon, V., & Sargeant, J. M. (2010). Verocytotoxin-producing *Escherichia coli* (VTEC). *Veterinary Microbiology*, *140*, 360−370.

Kawahara, T., Makizaki, Y., Oikawa, Y., Tanaka, Y., Maeda, A., Shimakawa, M., Komoto, S., Moriguchi, K., Ohno, H., & Taniguchi, K. (2017). Oral administration of *Bifidobacterium bifidum* G9−1 alleviates rotavirus gastroenteritis through regulation of intestinal homeostasis by inducing mucosal protective factors. *PLoS One*, *12*(3), e0173979.

Kazemi, A., Soltani, S., Ghorabi, S., Keshtkar, A., Daneshzad, E., Nasri, F., & Mazloomi, S. M. (2019). Effect of probiotic and synbiotic supplementation on inflammatory markers in health and disease status: A systematic review and meta-analysis of clinical trials. *Clinical Nutrition (Edinburgh, Scotland)*, *39*(3), 789−819.

Khalil, I. A. M. (2017). The global burden of rotavirus diarrheal diseases: Results from the Global Burden of Diseases Study 2016. *Open Forum Infectious Diseases*, *4*(Suppl. 1), S363.

Khaneghah, A. M., Abhari, K., Eş, I., Soares, M. B., Oliveira, R. B. A., Hosseini, H., Rezaei, M., Balthazar, C. F., Silva, R., Cruz, A. G., Ranadheera, C. S., & Sant'Ana, A. S. (2020). Interactions between probiotics and pathogenic microorganisms in hosts and foods: A review. *Trends in Food Science & Technology*, *95*, 205−218.

Khanifar, J., Hosseini, R. H., Kazemi, R., Ramandi, M. F., Amani, J., & Salmanian, A. H. (2019). Prevention of EHEC infection by chitosan nanostructure coupled with synthetic recombinant antigen. *Journal of Microbiological Methods*, *157*, 100−107.

Kim, S. J., Lee, J. Y., Jun, D. Y., Song, J. Y., Lee, W. K., Cho, M. J., & Kim, Y. H. (2009). Oral administration of *Lactococcus lactis* expressing *Helicobacter pylori* Cag7-ct383 protein induces systemic anti-Cag7 immune response in mice. *FEMS Immunology and Medical Microbiology*, *57*(3), 257−268.

Kim, W. S., Han, G. G., Hong, L., Kang, S. K., Shokouhimehr, M., Choi, Y. J., & Cho, C. S. (2019). Novel production of natural bacteriocin via internalization of dextran nanoparticles into probiotics. *Biomaterials*, *218*, 119360.

Lambert, J., & Hull, R. (1996). Upper gastrointestinal tract disease and probiotics. *Asia Pacific Journal of Clinical Nutrition*, *5*(1), 31−35.

Lee, D. K., Park, J. E., Kim, M. J., Seo, J. G., Lee, J. H., & Ha, N. J. (2015). Probiotic bacteria, *B. longum* and *L. acidophilus* inhibit infection by rotavirus in vitro and decrease the duration of diarrhea in pediatric patients. *Clinics and Research in Hepatology and Gastroenterology*, *39*(2), 237−244.

Lee, H., & Ko, G. P. (2016). Antiviral effect of vitamin A on norovirus infection via modulation of the gut microbiome. *Scientific Reports*, *6*, 25835. Available from https://doi.org/10.1038/srep25835.

Lesbros-Pantoflickova, D., Corthe'Sy-Theulaz, I., & Blum, A. L. (2007). *Helicobacter pylori* and probiotics. *The Journal of Nutrition*, *137*(3 Suppl. 2), 812S−818S.

Levine, M. M., & Edelman, R. (1984). Enteropathogenic *Escherichia coli* of classic serotypes associated with infant diarrhea: Epidemiology and pathogenesis. *Epidemiologic Reviews*, *6*, 31−51.

Lewis, S. B., Cook, V., Tighe, R., & Schüller, S. (2015). Enterohemorrhagic *Escherichia coli* colonization of human colonic epithelium in vitro and ex vivo. *Infection and Immunity*, *83*, 942−949.

Liévin-Le Moal, V., & Servin, A. L. (2014). Anti-infective activities of *Lactobacillus* strains in the human intestinal microbiota: From probiotics to gastrointestinal anti-infectious biotherapeutic agents. *Clinical Microbiology Reviews*, *27*(2), 167.

Likotrafiti, E., Tuohy, K. M., Gibson, G. R., & Rastall, R. A. (2013). Development of antimicrobial synbiotics using potentially-probiotic faecal isolates of *Lactobacillus fermentum* and *Bifidobacterium longum*. *Anaerobe*, *20*, 5−13.

Lin, R., Zhang, Y., Long, B., Li, Y., Wu, Y., Duan, S., Zhu, B., Wu, X., & Fan, H. (2017). Oral immunization with recombinant *Lactobacillus acidophilus* expressing espA-Tir-M confers protection against enterohemorrhagic Escherichia coli O157:H7 challenge in mice. *Frontiers in Microbiology*, *8*, 417.

Lin, W. H., Lin, C. K., Sheu, S. J., Hwang, C. F., Ye, W. T., Hwang, W. Z., & Tsen, H. Y. (2009). Antagonistic activity of spent culture supernatants of lactic acid bacteria against *Helicobacter pylori* growth and infection in human gastric epithelial AGS cells. *Journal of Food Science*, *74*(6), 225−230.

Liu, Q., Yu, Z., Tian, F., Zhao, J., Zhang, H., Zhai, Q., & Chen, W. (2020). Surface components and metabolites of probiotics for regulation of intestinal epithelial barrier. *Microbial Cell Factories*, *19*(1), 23. Available from https://doi.org/10.1186/s12934-020-1289-4.

Lopez-Brea, M., Alarcon, T., Domingo, D., & Diaz-Reganon, J. (2008). Inhibitory effect of gram-negative and gram positive microorganisms against *Helicobacter pylori*. *The Journal of Antimicrobial Chemotherapy*, *61*(1), 139−142.

Ma, J., Zhang, J., Li, Q., Shi, Z., Wu, H., Zhang, H., Tang, L., Yi, R., Su, H., & Sun, X. (2019). Oral administration of a mixture of probiotics protects against food allergy via induction of CD103$^+$ dendritic cells and modulates the intestinal microbiota. *Journal of Functional Foods*, *55*, 65−75.

Mabeku, L. B. K., Ngue, S., Nguemo, I. B., & Leundji, H. (2020). Potential of selected lactic acid bacteria from Theobroma cacao fermented fruit juice and cell-free supernatants from cultures as inhibitors of *Helicobacter pylori* and as good probiotic. *BMC Research Notes*, *13*(1), 64.

Maleki-Kakelar, H., Dehghani, J., Barzegari, A., Barar, J., Shirmohamadi, M., Sadeghi, J., & Omidi, Y. (2020). *Lactobacillus plantarum* induces apoptosis in gastric cancer cells via modulation of signaling pathways in *Helicobacter pylori*. *BioImpacts: BI*, *10*(2), 65.

Mantegazza, C., Molinari, P., D'Auria, E., Sonnino, M., Morelli, L., & Zuccotti, G. V. (2018). Probiotics and antibiotic-associated diarrhea in children: A review and new evidence on *Lactobacillus rhamnosus* GG during and after antibiotic treatment. *Pharmacological Research: The Official Journal of the Italian Pharmacological Society*, *128*, 63−72.

Marelli, B., Perez, A. R., Banchio, C., de Mendoza, D., & Magni, C. (2011). Oral immunization with live *Lactococcus lactis* expressing rotavirus VP8* subunit induces specific immune response in mice. *Journal of Virological Methods, 175*(1), 28–37.

Marshall, B. J., & Warren, R. M. (1984). Unidentified curved *Bacilli* in the stomach of patients with gastritis and peptic ulceration. *The Lancet, 1* (8390), 1311–1315.

Masana, M. O., Leotta, G. A., Del Castillo, L. L., D'Astek, B. A., Palladino, P. M., Galli, L., Vilacoba, E., Carbonari, C., et al. (2010). Prevalence, characterization, and genotypic analysis of *Escherichia coli* O157:H7/NM from selected beef exporting abattoirs of Argentina. *Journal of Food Protection, 73*, 649–656.

Medellin-Pena, M. J., & Griffiths, M. W. (2009). Effect of molecules secreted by *Lactobacillus acidophilus* strain La-5 on *Escherichia coli* O157:H7 colonization. *Applied and Environmental Microbiology, 75*(4), 1165.

Mejias, M. P., Hiriart, Y., Lauche, C., Fernandez-Brando, R. J., Pardo, R., Bruballa, A., et al. (2016). Development of camelid single chain antibodies against Shiga toxin type 2 (Stx2) with therapeutic potential against Hemolytic Uremic Syndrome (HUS). *Scientific Reports, 6*, 24913.

Meng, J., LeJeune, J. T., Zhao, T., & Doyle, M. P. (2013). *Enterohemorrhagic* Escherichia coli. *Food microbiology* (pp. 287–309). American Society of Microbiology, Chpater 12.

Merabishvili, M., De Vos, D., Verbeken, G., Kropinski, A. M., Vandenheuvel, D., Lavigne, R., Wattiau, P., Mast, J., Ragimbeau, C., Mossong, J., & Scheres, J. (2012). Selection and characterization of a candidate therapeutic bacteriophage that lyses the *Escherichia coli* O104:H4 strain from the 2011 outbreak in Germany. *PLoS One, 7*(12), e52709.

Mirabdollah Elahi, S. S., Mirnejad, R., Kazempoor, R., & Sotoodehnejadnematalahi, F. (2020). Study of the Histopathologic Effects of Probiotic *Lactobacillus acidophilus* in Exposure to E. coli O157:H7 in Zebrafish Intestine. *Iranian Red Crescent Medical Journal, 22*(4).

Misra, S., Mohanty, D., & Mohapatra, S. (2019). Applications of probiotics as a functional ingredient in food and gut health. *Journal of Food and Nutrition Research, 7*(3), 213–223.

Mizukoshi, F., Kuroda, M., Tsukagoshi, H., Sekizuka, T., Funatogawa, K., Morita, Y., Noda, M., Katayama, K., & Kimura, H. (2014). A food-borne outbreak of gastroenteritis due to genotype G1P [8] rotavirus among adolescents in Japan. *Microbiology and Immunology, 58*(9), 536–539.

Mo, R., Zhang, X., & Yang, Y. (2019). Effect of probiotics on lipid profiles in hypercholesterolaemic adults: A meta-analysis of randomized controlled trials. *Medicina Clínica (English Edition), 152*(12), 473–481.

Moens, F., den Abbeele, P. V., Basit, A. W., Dodoo, C., Chatterjee, R., Smith, B., & Gaisford, S. (2019). A four-strain probiotic exerts positive immunomodulatory effects by enhancing colonic butyrate production in vitro. *International Journal of Pharmaceutics, 555*, 1–10.

Mohammadsadeghi, F., Afsharmanesh, M., & Ebrahimnejad, H. (2019). The substitution of humic material complex with mineral premix in diet and interaction of that with probiotic on performance, intestinal morphology and microflora of chickens. *Livestock Science, 228*, 1–4.

Mohanty, D., Panda, S., Kumar, S., & Ray, P. (2019). In vitro evaluation of adherence and anti-infective property of probiotic *Lactobacillus plantarum* DM 69 against *Salmonella enterica*. *Microbial Pathogenesis, 126*, 212–217.

Morigi, M., Galbusera, M., Gastoldi, S., Locatelli, M., Buelli, S., Pezzotta, A., Pagani, C., Noris, M., Gobbi, M., Stravalaci, M., & Rottoli, D. (2011). Alternative pathway activation of complement by Shiga toxin promotes exuberant C3a formation that triggers microvascular thrombosis. *The Journal of Immunology, 187*(1), 172–180.

Moss, S. F. (2017). The clinical evidence linking *Helicobacter pylori* to gastric cancer. *Cellular and Molecular Gastroenterology and Hepatology, 3* (2), 183–191.

Mühlen, S., & Dersch, P. (2020). Treatment strategies for infections with Shiga toxin-producing *Escherichia coli*. *Frontiers in Cellular and Infection Microbiology, 10*, 169.

Mühlen, S., Ramming, I., Pils, M. C., Koeppel, M., Glaser, J., Leong, J., Flieger, A., Stecher, B., & Dersch, P. (2020). Identification of antibiotics that diminish disease in a murine model of enterohemorrhagic *Escherichia coli* infection. *Antimicrobial Agents and Chemotherapy, 64*(4), e02159–19.

Nagarajan, V., Peng, M., Tabashsum, Z., Salaheen, S., Padilla, J., & Biswas, D. (2019). Antimicrobial effect and probiotic potential of phage resistant *Lactobacillus plantarum* and its interactions with zoonotic bacterial pathogens. *Foods, 8*(6), 194.

Nam, H., Ha, M., Bae, O., & Lee, Y. (2002). Effect of *Weissella confusa* strain PL9001 on the adherence and growth of *Helicobacter pylori*. *Applied and Environmental Microbiology, 68*(9), 4642–4645.

Nami, Y., Bakhshayesh, R. V., Manafi, M., & Hejazi, M. A. (2019). Hypocholesterolaemic activity of a novel autochthonous potential probiotic *Lactobacillus plantarum* YS5 isolated from yogurt. *LWT, 111*, 876–882.

Nan, X., Jinyuan, W., Yan, Z., Maosheng, S., & Hongjun, L. (2014). Epidemiological and clinical studies of rotavirus-induced diarrhea in China from1994–2013. *Human Vaccines & Immunotherapeutics, 10*(12), 3672–3680.

Nawrocki, E. M., Mosso, H. M., & Dudley, E. G. (2020). A toxic environment: A growing understanding of how microbial communities affect *Escherichia coli* O157:H7 Shiga toxin expression. *Applied and Environmental Microbiology, 86*(24).

Nealon, N. J., Yuan, L., Yang, X., & Ryan, E. P. (2017). Rice bran and probiotics alter the porcine large intestine and serum metabolomes for protection against human rotavirus diarrhea. *Frontiers in Microbiology, 8*, 653.

Neut, C., Mahieux, S., & Dubreuil, L. J. (2017). Antibiotic susceptibility of probiotic strains: Is it reasonable to combine probiotics with antibiotics? *Medecine et Maladies Infectieuses, 47*(7), 477–483.

O'Connor, A., Liou, J. M., Gisbert, J. P., & O'Morain, C. (2019). Review: Treatment of *Helicobacter pylori* infection 2019. *Helicobacter, 24*(Suppl. 1), e12640. Available from https://doi.org/10.1111/hel.12640.

Ogawa, M., Shimizu, K., Nomoto, K., Takahashi, M., Watanuki, M., Tanaka, R., Tanaka, T., Hamabata, T., et al. (2001). Protective effect of *Lactobacillus casei* strain Shirota on Shiga toxin-producing *Escherichia coli* O157:H7 infection in infant rabbits. *Infection and Immunity, 69*, 1101–1108.

Olaya Galán, N. N., Ulloa Rubiano, J. C., Velez Reyes, F. A., Fernandez Duarte, K. P., Salas Cardenas, S. P., & Gutierrez Fernandez, M. F. (2016). In vitro antiviral activity of *Lactobacillus casei* and *Bifidobacterium adolescentis* against rotavirus infection monitored by NSP 4 protein production. *Journal of Applied Microbiology, 120*(4), 1041−1051.

Ota, A. (1999). Protection against an infectious disease by enterohaemorrhagic *E. coli* 0-157. *Medical Hypotheses, 53*(1), 87−88.

Pant, N., Marcotte, H., Brüssow, H., Svensson, L., & Hammarström, L. (2007). Effective prophylaxis against rotavirus diarrhea using a combination of *Lactobacillus rhamnosus* GG and antibodies. *BMC Microbiology, 7*(1), 1−9.

Papastergiou, V., Georgopoulos, S. D., & Karatapanis, S. (2014a). Treatment of *Helicobacter pylori* infection: Meeting the challenge of antimicrobial resistance. *World Journal of Gastroenterology: WJG, 20*(29), 9898−9911.

Papastergiou, V., Georgopoulos, S. D., & Karatapanis, S. (2014b). Treatment of *Helicobacter pylori* infection: Past, present and future. *World Journal of Gastrointestinal Pathophysiology, 5*(4), 392−399.

Park, M. S., Kwon, B., Ku, S., & Ji, G. E. (2017). The efficacy of *Bifidobacterium longum* BORI and *Lactobacillus acidophilus* AD031 probiotic treatment in infants with rotavirus infection. *Nutrients, 9*(887). Available from https://doi.org/10.3390/nu9080887.

Parkin, D. M. (2006). The global health burden of infection-associated cancers in the year 2002. *International Journal of Cancer. Journal International du Cancer, 118*(12), 3030−3044.

Payne, D. C., Selvarangan, R., Azimi, P. H., Boom, J. A., Englund, J. A., Staat, M. A., Halasa, N. B., Weinberg, G. A., Szilagyi, P. G., Chappell, J., & McNeal, M. (2015). Long-term consistency in rotavirus vaccine protection: RV5 and RV1 vaccine effectiveness in United States children, 2012−2013. *Clinical Infectious Diseases, 61*(12), 1792−1799.

Peng, M. (2018). *Stimulation of growth and metabolites production of Lactobacillus in control of enteric bacterial pathogen infection and improving gut health* (Doctoral dissertation).

Peng, C., Hu, Y., Ge, Z. M., Zou, Q. M., & Lyu, N. H. (2019). Diagnosis and treatment of *Helicobacter pylori* infections in children and elderly populations. *Chronic Diseases and Translational Medicine, 5*(4), 243−251.

Peng, M., Tabashsum, Z., Patel, P., Bernhardt, C., & Biswas, D. (2018). Linoleic acids overproducing Lactobacillus casei limits growth, survival, and virulence of *Salmonella* Typhimurium and enterohaemorrhagic *Escherichia coli*. *Frontiers in Microbiology, 9*, 2663.

Peng, X., Zhang, R., Duan, G., Wang, C., Sun, N., Zhang, L., Chen, S., Fan, Q., & Xi, Y. (2018). Production and delivery of *Helicobacter pylori* NapA in *Lactococcus lactis* and its protective efficacy and immune modulatory activity. *Scientific Reports, 8*(1), 6435. Available from https://doi.org/10.1038/s41598-018-24879-x.

Pinchuk, I. V., Bressollier, P., Verneuil, B., Fenet, B., Sorokulova, I. B., Megraud, F., & Urdaci, M. C. (2001). In vitro anti-*Helicobacter pylori* activity of the probiotic strain *Bacillus subtilis* 3 is due to secretion of antibiotics. *Antimicrobial Agents and Chemotherapy, 45*(11), 3156−3161.

Poppi, L. B., Rivaldi, J. D., Coutinho, T. S., Astolfi-Ferreira, C. S., Ferreira, A. J. P., & Mancilha, I. M. (2015). Effect of *Lactobacillus* sp isolates supernatant on *Escherichia coli* O157:H7 enhances the role of organic acids production as a factor for pathogen control. *Pesquisa Veterinaria Brasileira, 35*(4), 353−359.

Quilodrán-Vega, S. R., Villena, J., Valdebenito, J., Salas, M. J., Parra, C., Ruiz, A., Kitazawa, H., & García, A. (2016). Isolation of lactic acid bacteria from swine milk and characterization of potential probiotic strains with antagonistic effects against swine-associated astrointestinal pathogens. *Canadian Journal of Microbiology, 62*(6), 514−524.

Qureshi, N., Li, P., & Gu, Q. (2019). Probiotic therapy in *Helicobacter pylori* infection: A potential strategy against a serious pathogen. *Applied Microbiology and Biotechnology, 103*(4), 1573−1588.

Rabanal, F., Grau-Campistany, A., Vila-Farrés, X., Gonzalez-Linares, J., Borràs, M., Vila, J., Manresa, A., & Cajal, Y. (2015). A bioinspired peptide scaffold with high antibiotic activity and low in vivo toxicity. *Scientific Reports, 5*(1), 1−11.

Rabinovitz, B. C., Larzábal, M., Vilte, D. A., Cataldi, A., & Mercado, E. C. (2016). The intranasal vaccination of pregnant dams with Intimin and EspB confers protection in neonatal mice from *Escherichia coli* (EHEC) O157:H7 infection. *Vaccine, 34*, 2793−2797.

Rahal, E. A., Kazzi, N., Nassar, F. J., & Matar, G. M. (2012). *Escherichia coli* O157:H7—Clinical aspects and novel treatment approaches. *Frontiers in Cellular and Infection Microbiology, 2*, 138.

Rahmani, P., Moradzadeh, A., & Farahmand, F. (2019). Giving probiotics to your children for gastrointestinal problems: In the light of scientific findings. *PharmaNutrition, 10*, 100164. Available from https://doi.org/10.1016/j.phanu.2019.100164.

Rezaee, P., Kermanshahi, R. K., & Falsafi, T. (2019). Antibacterial activity of *lactobacilli* probiotics on clinical strains of *Helicobacter pylori*. *Iran. Journal of Basic Medical Sciences, 22*(10), 1118−1124.

Rezazadeh, L., Gargari, B. P., Jafarabadi, M. A., & Alipour, B. (2019). Effects of probiotic yogurt on glycemic indexes and endothelial dysfunction markers in patients with metabolic syndrome. *Nutrition (Burbank, Los Angeles County, Calif.), 62*, 162−168.

Rigo-Adrover, M., Saldaña-Ruíz, S., Van Limpt, K., Knipping, K., Garssen, J., Knol, J., Franch, A., Castell, M., & Pérez-Cano, F. J. (2017). A combination of scGOS/lcFOS with *Bifidobacterium breve* M-16V protects suckling rats from rotavirus gastroenteritis. *European Journal of Nutrition, 56*(4), 1657−1670.

Rigo-Adrover, M. D. M., VanLimpt, K., Knipping, K., Garssen, J., Knol, J., Costabile, A., Franch, À., Castell, M., & Pérez-Cano, F. J. (2018). Preventive effect of a synbiotic combination of galacto-and fructooligosaccharides mixture with *Bifidobacterium breve* M-16V in a model of multiple rotavirus infections. *Frontiers in Immunology, 9*, 1318.

Riley, L. W., Remis, R. S., Helgerson, S. D., McGee, H. B., Wells, J. G., Davis, B. R., Hebert, R. J., Olcott, E. S., Johnson, L. M., Hargrett, N. T., & Blake, P. A. (1983). *Hemorrhagic colitis* associated with a rare *Escherichia coli* serotype. *New England Journal of Medicine, 308*(12), 681−685.

Roberts, S. E., Morrison-Rees, S., Samuel, D. G., Thorne, K., Akbari, A., & Williams, J. G. (2016). Review article: The prevalence of *Helicobacter pylori* and the incidence of gastric cancer across Europe. *Alimentary Pharmacology & Therapeutics, 43*(3), 334−345.

Roobab, U., Batool, Z., Manzoor, M. F., Shabbir, M. A., Khan, M. R., & Aadil, R. M. (2020). Sources, formulations, advanced delivery and health benefits of probiotics. *Current Opinion in Food Science, 32*, 17–28.

Rosettie, K. L., Vos, T., Mokdad, A. H., Flaxman, A. D., Khalil, I., Troeger, C., & Weaver, M. R. (2018). Indirect rotavirus vaccine effectiveness for the prevention of rotavirus hospitalization: A systematic review and meta-analysis. *The American Journal of Tropical Medicine and Hygiene, 98*(4), 1197–1201.

Roussel, C., Sivignon, A., de Wiele, T. V., & Blanquet-Diot, S. (2017). Foodborne enterotoxigenic *Escherichia coli*: From gut pathogenesis to new preventive strategies involving probiotics. *Future Microbiology, 12*(1), 73–93.

Sahshorpour, M., Amani, J., Jafari, M., & Salmanian, A. H. (2014). Expression of recombinant chimeric EspA-intimin protein in *Nicotiana tobaccum* for oral vaccine development. *Journal of Plant Genetic Researches, 1*(1), 77–94.

Sakandar, H. A., Kubow, S., & Sadiq, F. A. (2019). Isolation and *in-vitro* probiotic characterization of fructophilic lactic acid bacteria from Chinese fruits and flowers. *LWT, 104*, 70–75.

Sakarya, S., & Gunay, N. (2014). *Saccharomyces boulardii* expresses neuraminidase activity selective for α-2, 3-linked sialic acid that decreases *Helicobacter pylori* adhesion to host cells. *APMIS: Acta Pathologica, Microbiologica, et Immunologica Scandinavica, 122*(10), 941–950.

Salas-Cárdenas, S. P., Olaya-Galán, N. N., Fernández, K., Velez, F., Guerrero, C. A., & Gutiérrez, M. F. (2018). Decreased rotavirus infection of MA104 cells via probiotic extract binding to Hsc70 and ß3 integrin receptors. *Universitas Scientiarum, 23*(2), 219–239.

Salas-Jara, M. J., Sanhueza, E. A., Retamal-Díaz, A., González, C., Urrutia, H., & García, A. (2016). Probiotic *Lactobacillus fermentum* UCO-979C biofilm formation on AGS and Caco-2 cells and *Helicobacter pylori* inhibition. *Biofouling, 32*(10), 1245–1257.

Saracino, I. M., Pavoni, M., Saccomanno, L., Fiorini, G., Pesci, V., Foschi, C., Piccirilli, G., Bernardini, G., Holton, J., Figura, N., Lazzarotto, T., Borghi, C., & Vaira, B. (2020). Antimicrobial efficacy of five probiotic strains against *Helicobacter pylori*. *Antibiotics, 9*(5), 244.

Sargeant, J. M., Amezcua, M. R., Rajic, A., & Waddell, L. (2007). Pre-harvest interventions to reduce the shedding of *E. coli* O157 in the faeces of weaned domestic ruminants: a systematic review. *Zoonoses and Public Health, 54*(6-7), 260–277.

Sen, A., Ding, S., & Greenberg, H. B. (2020). *The role of innate immunity in regulating rotavirus replication, pathogenesis, and host range restriction and the implications for live rotaviral vaccine development*. Mucosal vaccines (pp. 683–697). Academic Press, Chapter 40.

Sgouras, D., Maragkoudakis, P., Petraki, K., Martinez-Gonzalez, B., Eriotou, E., Michopoulos, S., Kalantzopoulos, G., Tsakalidou, E., & Mentis, A. (2004). In vitro and in vivo inhibition of *Helicobacter pylori* by *Lactobacillus casei* Shirota. *Applied and Environmental Microbiology, 70*(1), 518–526.

Sharma, K., Pooranachithra, M., Balamurugan, K., & Goel, G. (2019). Probiotic mediated colonization resistance against *E. coli* infection in experimentally challenged *Caenorhabditis elegans*. *Microbial Pathogenesis, 127*, 39–47.

Shu, Q., & Gill, H. S. (2001). A dietary probiotic (*Bifidobacterium lactis* HN019) reduces the severity of *Escherichia coli* O157:H7 infection in mice. *Medical Microbiology and Immunology, 189*(3), 147–152.

Shu, Q., & Gill, H. S. (2002). Immune protection mediated by the probiotic *Lactobacillus rhamnosus* HN001 (DR20™) against *Escherichia coli* O157:H7 infection in mice. *FEMS Immunology & Medical Microbiology, 34*(1), 59–64.

Singh, V. P., Sharma, J., Babu, S., Rizwanulla., & Singla, A. (2013). Role of probiotics in health and disease: A review. *Journal of the Pakistan Medical Association, 63*(2), 253–257.

Song, D., & Gu, Q. (2009). Surface expression of *Helicobacter pylori* urease subunit B gene E fragment on *Lactococcus lactis* by means of the cell wall anchor of *Staphylococcus aureus* protein A. *Biotechnology Letters, 31*(7), 985–989.

Song, H., Zhou, L., Liu, D., Ge, L., & Li, Y. (2019). Probiotic effect on *Helicobacter pylori* attachment and inhibition of inflammation in human gastric epithelial cells. *Experimental and Therapeutic Medicine, 18*(3), 1151–1562.

Spinale, J., Ruebner, R., Copelovitch, L., & Kaplan, B. (2013). Long-term outcomes of Shiga toxin hemolytic uremic syndrome. *Pediatric Nephrology (Berlin, Germany), 28*, 2097–2105.

Sreerohini, S., Balakrishna, K., & Parida, M. (2019). Oral immunization of mice with *Lactococcus lactis* expressing Shiga toxin truncate confers enhanced protection against Shiga toxins of *Escherichia coli* O157:H7 and Shigella dysenteriae. *APMIS: Acta Pathologica, Microbiologica, et Immunologica Scandinavica, 127*(10), 671–680.

Stevens, M. P., & Frankel, G. M. (2014). The locus of enterocyte effacement and associated virulence factors of enterohemorrhagic *Escherichia coli*. *Microbiology Spectrum, 2*(4).

Tabashsum, Z., Peng, M., Bernhardt, C., Patel, P., Carrion, M., & Biswas, D. (2019). Synbiotic-like effect of linoleic acid overproducing *Lactobacillus casei* with berry phenolic extracts against pathogenesis of enterohemorrhagic *Escherichia coli*. *Gut Pathogens, 11*(1), 1–11.

Takahashi, M., Taguchi, H., Yamaguchi, H., Osaki, T., & Kamiya, S. (2000). Studies of the effect of *Clostridium butyricum* on *Helicobacter pylori* in several test models including gnotobiotic mice. *Journal of Medical Microbiology, 49*(7), 635–642.

Takeda, S., Igoshi, K., Tsend-Ayush, C., Oyunsuren, T., Sakata, R., Koga, Y., Arima, Y., & Takeshita, M. (2017). *Lactobacillus paracasei* strain 06TCa19 suppresses inflammatory chemokine induced by *Helicobacter pylori* in human gastric epithelial cells. *Human Cell, 30*(4), 258–266.

Tam, C. C., & O'Brien, S. J. (2016). Economic cost of *campylobacter, norovirus* and rotavirus disease in the United Kingdom. *PLoS One, 11*(2).

Tan, Q., Xu, H., Xu, F., Aguilar, Z. P., Yang, Y., Dong, S., Chen, T., & Wei, H. (2013). Survival, distribution, and translocation of Enterococcus faecalis and implications for pregnant mice. *FEMS Microbiology Letters, 349*(1), 32–39.

Tanji, Y., Shimada, T., Fukudomi, H., K., Miyanaga, Nakai, Y., & Unno, H. (2005). Therapeutic use of phage cocktail for controlling *Escherichia coli* O157: H7 in gastrointestinal tract of mice. *Journal of Bioscience and Bioengineering, 100*(3), 280–287.

Tan-Lim, C. S. C., & Esteban-Ipac, N. A. R. (2018). Probiotics as treatment for food allergies among pediatric patients: A meta-analysis. *World Allergy Organization Journal*, *11*(1), 25.

Techo, S., Visseanguan, W., Vilaichone, R. K., & Tanasupawat, S. (2019). Characterization and antibacterial activity against *Helicobacter pylori* of lactic acid bacteria isolated from Thai fermented rice noodle. *Probiotics and Antimicrobial Proteins*, *11*(1), 92−102.

Telmesani, A. M. (2010). Oral rehydration salts, zinc supplement and rota virus vaccine in the management of childhood acute diarrhea. *Journal of Family and Community Medicine*, *17*(2), 79.

Tovaglieri, A., Sontheimer-Phelps, A., Geirnaert, A., Prantil-Baun, R., Camacho, D. M., Chou, D. B., Jalili-Firoozinezhad, S., de Wouters, T., Kasendra, M., Super, M., & Cartwright, M. J. (2019). Species-specific enhancement of enterohemorrhagic *E. coli* pathogenesis mediated by microbiome metabolites. *Microbiome*, *7*(1), 1−21.

Tozzoli, R., Grande, L., Michelacci, V., Ranieri, P., Maugliani, A., Caprioli, A., & Morabito, S. (2014). Shiga toxin-converting phages and the emergence of new pathogenic *Escherichia coli*: a world in motion. *Frontiers in Cellular and Infection Microbiology*, *4*, 80.

Urrutia-Beca, V. H., Escamilla-Garcia, E., de la Garza-Ramos, M. A., Tamez-Guerra, P., Gomez-Flores, R., & Urbina-Rios, C. S. (2018). In vitro antimicrobial activity and downregulation of virulence gene expression on *Helicobacter pylori* by reuterin. *Probiotics and Antimicrobial Proteins*, *10*(2), 168−175.

Velázquez, R. F., Linhares, A. C., Muñoz, S., Seron, P., Lorca, P., DeAntonio, R., & Ortega-Barria, E. (2017). Efficacy, safety and effectiveness of licensed rotavirus vaccines: A systematic review and meta-analysis for Latin America and the Caribbean. *BMC Pediatrics*, *17*(1), 1−12.

Vickers, D., Morris, K., Coulthard, M., & Eastham, E. (1988). Anal Signs in haemolytic uraemic syndrome. *The Lancet*, *331*(8592), 998.

Villena, J., Vizoso-Pinto, M. G., & Kitazawa, H. (2016). Intestinal innate antiviral immunity and immunobiotics: Beneficial effects against rotavirus infection. *Frontiers in Immunology*, *7*, 563.

Vlasova, A. N., Kandasamy, S., Chattha, K. S., Rajashekara, G., & Saif, L. J. (2016). Comparison of probiotic *Lactobacilli* and *bifidobacteria* effects, immune responses and rotavirus vaccines and infection in different host species. *Veterinary Immunology and Immunopathology*, *172*, 72−84.

Wang, G., Tang, H., Zhang, Y., Xiao, X., Xia, Y., & Ai, L. (2020). The intervention effects of *Lactobacillus casei* LC2W on *Escherichia coli* O157:H7-induced mouse colitis. *Food Science and Human Wellness*, *9*(3), 289−294.

Wang, H., Li, Q., Fang, Y., Yu, S., Tang, B., Na, L., Yu, B., Zou, Q., Mao, X., & Gu, J. (2016). Biochemical and functional characterization of the periplasmic domain of the outer membrane protein A from enterohemorrhagic *Escherichia coli*. *Microbiological Research*, *182*, 109−115.

Wang, Z., Yu, Q., Gao, J., & Yang, Q. (2012). Mucosal and systemic immune responses induced by recombinant Lactobacillus spp. expressing the hemagglutinin of the avian influenza virus H5N1. *Clinical and Vaccine Immunology: CVI*, *19*(2), 174.

Wanke, M., & Szajewska, H. (2014). Probiotics for preventing healthcare-associated diarrhea in children: A meta-analysis of randomized controlled trials. *Pediatria Polska*, *89*(1), 8−16.

Westerik, N., Reid, G., Sybesma, W., & Kort, R. (2018). The probiotic Lactobacillus rhamnosus for alleviation of helicobacter pylori-associated gastric pathology in East Africa. *Frontiers in Microbiology*, *9*, 1873.

Wroblewski, L. E., Peek, R. M., Jr, & Wilson, K. T. (2010). *Helicobacter pylori* and gastric cancer: Factors that modulate disease risk. *Clinical Microbiology Reviews*, *23*(4), 713−739.

Xu, X., Peng, Q., Zhang, Y., Tian, D., Zhang, P., Huang, Y., Ma, L., Dia, V. P., Qiao, Y., & Shi, B. (2020). Antibacterial potential of a novel *Lactobacillus casei* strain isolated from Chinese northeast sauerkraut and the antibiofilm activity of its exopolysaccharides. *Food & Function*, *11*(5), 4697−4706.

Yang, B., Luo, Y., Liu, Z., Yang, P., & Gui, Y. (2018). Probiotics SOD inhibited food allergy via downregulation of STAT6-TIM4 signaling on DCs. *Molecular Immunology*, *103*, 71−77.

Yang, X., Twitchell, E., Li, G., Wen, K., Weiss, M., Kocher, J., Lei, S., Ramesh, A., Ryan, E. P., & Yuan, L. (2015). High protective efficacy of rice bran against human rotavirus diarrhea via enhancing probiotic growth, gut barrier function and innate immunity. *Scientific Reports*, *5*(1), 1−12.

Yeung, K. H. T., Tate, J. E., Chan, C. C., Chan, M. C., Chan, P. K., Poon, K. H., Siu, S. L. Y., Fung, G. P. G., Ng, K. L., Chan, I. M. C., & Yu, P. T. (2016). Rotavirus vaccine effectiveness in Hong Kong children. *Vaccine*, *34*(41), 4935−4942.

Yousefi, B., Eslami, M., Ghasemian, A., Kokhaei, P., Farrokhi, A. S., & Darabi, N. (2019). Probiotics importance and their immunomodulatory properties. *Journal of Cellular Physiology*, *234*(6), 8008−8018. Available from https://doi.org/10.1002/jcp.27559.

Zhang, S. Y., Guo, J. Q., & Liu, L. (2017). Treating bacteria with bacteria: The role of probiotics in the eradication of *Helicobacter pylori*. *International Journal of Clinical and Experimental Medicine*, *10*(3), 4330−4341.

Zhang, Z., Lv, J., Pan, L., & Zhang, Y. (2018). Roles and applications of probiotic *Lactobacillus* strains. *Applied Microbiology and Biotechnology*, *102*(19), 8135−8143.

Zhao Zhao, T., Doyle, M. P., Harmon, B. G., Brown, C. A., Mueller, P. E., & Parks, A. H. (1998). Reduction of carriage of enterohemorrhagic *Escherichia coli* O157:H7 in cattle by inoculation with probiotic bacteria. *Journal of Clinical Microbiology*, *36*(3), 641.

Zhao, K., Xie, Q., Xu, D., Guo, Y., Tao, X., Wei, H., & Wan, C. (2018). Antagonistics of *Lactobacillus plantarum* ZDY2013 against *Helicobacter pylori* SS1 and its infection in vitro in human gastric epithelial AGS cells. *Journal of Bioscience and Bioengineering*, *126*(4), 458−463.

Zhou, Z., Gong, S., Li, X. M., Yang, Y., Guan, R., Zhou, S., Yao, S., Xie, Y., Ou, Z., Zhao, J., & Liu, Z. (2015). Expression of *Helicobacter pylori* urease B on the surface of *Bacillus subtilis* spores. *Journal of Medical Microbiology*, *64*(Pt 1), 104−110.

Zoja, C., Buelli, S., & Morigi, M. (2019). Shiga toxin triggers endothelial and podocyte injury: The role of complement activation. *Pediatric Nephrology*, *34*(3), 379−388.

Chapter 21

Role of probiotics in the management of fungal infections

Archana Chaudhari[1], Ankit Bharti[2] and Mitesh Kumar Dwivedi[3]

[1]*Vyara Clinical Laboratory Pvt Ltd., Tapi, India,* [2]*Aura Skin and Dental Clinic, Tapi, India,* [3]*C.G. Bhakta Institute of Biotechnology, Faculty of Science, Uka Tarsadia University, Maliba Campus, Bardoli, India*

21.1 Introduction

Fungal pathogens have a major impact upon human health globally. It is estimated that, at any given time, over a quarter of the world's population have a fungal infection of the skin among which dermatophytes affect between 20% and 25% (Wu et al., 2011) of people worldwide. Over a million people die each year from an invasive fungal infection and additionally, 75% of women suffer at least one episode of vulvovaginal candidiasis (VVC) during their lifetime (Brown et al., 2012). *Candida* is the most isolated microorganism (40%–70%) from clinical specimens (Pfaller et al., 2006). In fact, in US hospital, the leading cause of healthcare-associated bloodstream infections is *Candida* (Magill et al., 2014). Mortality rates for those suffering systemic fungal infections are unacceptably high, reaching 50% in many cases. This is because fungal infections are often difficult to diagnose and are particularly challenging to treat (Brown et al., 2012; Köhler et al., 2015; Perlroth et al., 2007). The leading cause of invasive mold infection (*Aspergillus*) is estimated to cause 300,000 infections every year worldwide (Brown et al., 2012). In addition, it is estimated that about 12% of *Aspergillus* infections are resistant to antifungal medications (Rivero-Menendez et al., 2016).

There is a dire need for new antifungal treatment considering that fungal infections have tremendously escalated in clinical field along with the emergence of antifungal resistant fungal pathogens while there are few antifungal drugs to treat the diseased. There is an urgent medical need for more precise diagnostics along with safer and more effective antifungal drugs and host directed therapies. The search for antifungal drug targets is suppressed by the fact that, as eukaryotes, fungi share fundamental mechanisms of cell growth and division with humans. The search for diagnostic markers that can differentiate fungal commensalism from infection is particularly difficult. As a result, the advancement of effective new clinical tools is determined upon a thorough understanding of fungal pathogenicity and antifungal immunity. Probiotics have been proved to have antifungal activity against *Candida glabrata* (Chew et al., 2015a,b), *Candida albicans* (Chew et al., 2015a,b; Song & Lee, 2017; Zhao et al., 2016), *Aspergillus* spp. (Crowley et al., 2013), and dermatophytes (Guo et al., 2011, 2012) and thus probiotics are promising antifungal agents.

21.2 Probiotics

Probiotics are living microorganisms that confer health benefit to the host when administered in adequate amount (Suez et al., 2019). Probiotics have been described to play a beneficial role through their diverse mode of action that include lowering pH, antagonism by producing antimicrobial compounds; compete with the pathogen for binding sites and receptors sites, nutrients, and growth factors; stimulate immunomodulatory cells; improve barrier function of intestinal mucosa; modulate inflammatory responses; and produce hydrogen peroxide (H_2O_2) and organic acids (Amara & Shibl, 2015; Deidda et al., 2016; Guo et al., 2011, 2012; Matsubara, Bandara, Ishikawa, et al., 2016; Matsubara, Bandara, Mayer, et al., 2016; Matsubara, Wang, et al., 2016; Shehata et al., 2016).

21.3 Probiotics in fungal diseases

Potential probiotic microorganisms and probiotics have proved an amazing antagonistic activity toward a wide range of clinical pathogens. *Lactobacillus acidophilus* ATCC 4495, *Lactobacillus plantarum* NRRL B-4496 have shown significant antifungal activity (Cortés-Zavaleta et al., 2014). *L. acidophilus*, *Bifidobacterium lactis*, *Bifidobacterium longum*, and *Bifidobacterium bifidum* probiotic strains have the potential to reduce enteral fungal colonization and decrease invasive fungal sepsis rates in low−birth-weight neonates (Roy et al., 2014). *L. acidophilus* ATCC 4356 have been proved to produce substances with anti-*Candida* activity that inhibited its growth by 45.1% (Vilela et al., 2015). *Lactobacillus buchneri* showed antagonistic potential against *C. albicans* (Shokryazdan et al., 2017). Several in vitro investigations have been performed on the antifungal effects of probiotics as shown in Table 21.1.

Clinical studies suggest that probiotics administered in many cases together with conventional antifungal drugs lead to faster healing, synergy of the drug and half dose of conventional drug needed (Lau et al., 2016; Rishi et al., 2011; Russo et al., 2019; Shah et al., 2013). *L. acidophilus* GLA-14 and *Lactobacillus rhamnosus* HN001 used along with Clotrimazole reduced symptoms and recurrence of the disease in case of VVC (Russo et al., 2019). Probiotic *L. rhamnosus* GR-1 and *Lactobacillus reuteri* RC-14 along with fluconazole increased the effectiveness of an antifungal pharmaceutical agent in curing VVC disease (Fu et al., 2017). Usage of Probiotic Inersan along with doxycycline decreased plaque index and gingivial index within a period of 2 months in case of aggressive peritonitis (Degnan, 2012). *L. acidophilus*, *B. longum*, and *B. bifidum* along with fluconazole showed significant reduction in VVC disease recurrence (Denkova et al., 2013).

Probiotics have been tested clinically for the management of fungal pathogens of oral (Keller & Kragelund, 2018; Matsubara, Bandara, Ishikawa, et al., 2016; Matsubara, Bandara, Mayer, et al., 2016; Matsubara, Wang, et al., 2016; Mishra et al., 2016; Santos et al., 2009; Shah et al., 2013), gastrointestinal systems (Zuo & Ng, 2018), and urogenital infections (Davar et al., 2016; Fu et al., 2017; Russo et al., 2019) with promising results, thus supporting some probiotics as potential antifungal agents (Table 21.2).

21.3.1 Probiotics in oral fungal infections

The humans' oral cavity has a dynamic ecosystem. Oral mucosa that is in continuous contact with the external environment is easily colonized by microbes. The microflora that resides in oral cavity is diverse with varied atmospheric, nutritional, and physiochemical traits. Temperature, pH, nutrient availability, saliva, and gingival crevicular fluid are other factors that mainly have effects on the oral cavity (Gaidhane et al., 2018; Kogade et al., 2019; Puri et al., 2017; Thow et al., 2017; Uddin et al., 2017). Even a slight disturbance in this physiological activity may lead to endogenous and exogenous infections, debility, and illnesses and allow few selected species to survive (Balwani et al., 2019; Mittal et al., 2018). Oral health conditions usually associated with decreased levels of beneficial bacteria include gingivitis, thrush, cold sores, etc. With the growth in the complexity of microbes, there is a need to revolutionize alternative solution to block pathogenesis of oral infections and consequently decrease them. Probiotics have demonstrated to be efficient in treating diseases associated to the gut. Dental diseases stem from digestive problems. Recent studies have investigated novel antifungal treatment alternatives to treat oral diseases. The most significant is the consumption of probiotics that has been claimed as a substitute for prophylaxis and therapy of oral candidiasis. Probiotics can be administered in several forms, such as lozenges, mouth rinses, and capsules.

Lactobacillus fermentum, *L. rhamnosus*, *Lactobacillus salivarius*, *Lactobacillus casei*, *L. acidophilus*, and *L. plantarum* can be normally found in human saliva or dental plaque, even though only accounting for 1% of cultivable microbes. Majority of the probiotic agents may act as a protective shield to keep the harmful microflora away and reside in space that might then be colonized by them. When administered probiotics show beneficial effects by inhibiting pathogens in dental biofilm, antimicrobial substance production, and nutrient and adhesion sites' competition with oral pathogens. Some of the indirect probiotic action includes immunomodulation of the host's response, improvement in mucosal permeability, effect on nonimmunological defense mechanisms, regulation of mucosal penetrability, and prevention of plaque development by neutralizing the free electrons. The decrease in oral pathogens can be attained both by decrease in pH and the production of antimicrobial products like bacteriocins by probiotic *L. reuteri* (Charalampopoulos, 2009; Lahtinen et al., 2011).

The pathological proliferation of *C. albicans* is called candidiasis, and it is the most common form of fungal oral infection in humans. The infection may also arise due to the immunocompromised state of the host, triggered by radiotherapy and chemotherapy. Patients receiving cytotoxic drugs are highly susceptible to fungal infections that not only cause pain and discomfort but can also extent to the esophagus, leading to disseminated candidiasis (Lashof et al.,

TABLE 21.1 In vitro investigations on antifungal effects of probiotics.

Reference	Probiotics	Pathogen	Results	Comments
Hasslöf et al. (2010)	L. plantarum 299v, L. plantarum 931, L. rhamnosus GG ATCC 53103, L. rhamnosus LB21, and Lactobacillus paracasei	Ms: • Reference strains: S. mutans NCTC 10449, S. mutans Ingbritt, and Streptococcus sobrinus OMZ176 • Clinical isolates: S. mutans P1:27 and S. mutans P2:29	C. albicans: • 10^9–10^5 CFU/mL: all lactobacilli strains inhibited the growth of the Ms strains completely (except L. acidophilus La5) • 10^3 CFU/mL: only L. plantarum 299v and L. plantarum 931 displayed a total growth inhibition for all Ms. L. rhamnosus GG ATCC 53103 inhibited the growth slightly for 3 Ms	L. acidophilus La5: weaker inhibition capacity in comparison with the other probiotic strains ($P < .05$). All the tested Lactobacillus strains reduced Candida growth, but the effect was generally weaker than for Ms
		C. albicans: • Reference strains: C. albicans ATCC 28366 and C. albicans ATCC 10231 • Clinical isolates: C. albicans 1957, C. albicans 3339, and C. albicans GDM8	C. albicans: • 10^9 and 10^7 CFU/mL: all lactobacilli except L. acidophilus La5 and Lactobacillus reuteri PTA 5289 inhibited all Candida strains completely • 10^5 CFU/mL: L. rhamnosus strains, L. paracasei, and L. reuteri PTA 5289 displayed a slight inhibition. L. acidophilus La5 showed no inhibition. L. plantarum and L. reuteri ATCC 55730 executed a total inhibition • 10^3 CFU/mL: No inhibition was recorded except for the L plantarum strains	
Murzyn et al. (2010)	Saccharomyces boulardii	C. albicans SC5314	• Active compounds of probiotic yeast reduced Candida virulence factors (hyphae formation, cell adhesion, and biofilm formation) • Yeast extract and capric acid reduced the expression of HWP1, INO1, and CSH1 genes in C. albicans cells	Capric acid was the main compound affecting hyphae formation, Candida adhesion, and biofilm formation
Ishijima et al. (2012)	Streptococcus salivarius K12	C. albicans (clinical isolate)	• S. salivarius reduced adherence of mycelial form to plastic substratum, increased the number of planktonic Candida cells in culture medium, but did not inhibit C. albicans strain • Probiotic bacteria preferentially bound to hyphae	S. salivarius K12 was not directly fungicidal but appeared to inhibit Candida adhesion to the substratum

(Continued)

TABLE 21.1 (Continued)

Köhler et al. (2012)	*L. rhamnosus* GR-1 and *L. reuteri* RC-14, *Lactobacillus johnsonii* PV016, and *Staphylococcus aureus* ATCC 25923 (controls)	*C. albicans* SC5314	• 48 h: *Lactobacillus* GR-1 and RC-1 showed visible zones of fungal growth inhibition around them • *L. johnsonii*: very weak inhibition zone • *S. aureus*: no inhibition zones • *C. albicans* growth was suppressed at low pH by the *Lactobacillus* culture supernatants • Probiotic-inhibited genes associated with biofilm formation	Lactic acid at low pH environment: major role in fungal growth inhibition. Glucose or other nutrient exhaustion was not a likely cause for fungal inhibition. H_2O_2 production may be an anti-*Candida* factor
Coman et al. (2014)	*L. rhamnosus* IMC 501	• Gram-positive, gram-negative bacteria • *C. albicans*, *Candida glabrata*, *Candida krusei*, *Candida parapsilosis*, and *Candida tropicalis*	*L. rhamnosus*: Inhibitory activity against both gram-positive and gram-negative bacteria, and against two *C. albicans* strains (ATCC 10261 and ISS7)	
	L. paracasei IMC 502		*L. paracasei*: Inhibitory effect on gram-positive and gram-negative bacteria, especially *S. aureus* and *Proteus mirabilis*. All *Candida* spp. were inhibited except *C. glabrata* and *C. tropicalis*	*L. paracasei* IMC 502: higher activity toward all the pathogens, especially *Candida* strains; strong inhibition registered for SYNBIO
	Combination of both (SYNBIO)		SYNBIO: Inhibitory activity against most of the bacteria and fungi strains, especially *C. albicans* and *C. krusei*	
Verdenelli et al. (2014)	*L. paracasei* subsp. *paracasei*, *L. plantarum*, *L. fermentum*, *L. rhamnosus* IMC 501, and *L. paracasei* IMC 502	*C. albicans*, *C. glabrata*, *C. krusei*, *C. parapsilosis*, and *C. tropicalis* (clinical isolates)	• Well diffusion assay: no inhibition against *Candida* spp. • Radial method: All lactobacilli had the capacity to inhibit *Candida* in different degrees	Inhibition and coaggregation ability vary according to the *Lactobacillus* strain and the pathogen involved
Kheradmand et al. (2014)	*L. plantarum* (ATCC 8014) and *L. johnsonii* (clinical isolate) enriched or not with SeNPs	*C. albicans* (ATCC 14053)	Conventional hole-plate diffusion: • *L. plantarum* and *L. johnsonii* supernatant grown with selenium dioxide showed potent anti-*Candida* activity • No antifungal effect was observed with supernatant without selenium time-kill assay • No viable *C. albicans* was present after 4 h incubation with culture supernatants grown with selenium dioxide • Viable *C. albicans* cells were present even after 24 h incubation with culture supernatants grown without selenium dioxide	Direct antifungal effect was observed when selenium-enriched *Lactobacillus* spp were cocultured with *C. albicans*. The strong inhibition of *C. albicans* by supernatant of selenium-enriched *Lactobacillus* spp. indicated the release of potent exometabolites

			After 0.5 h, Lactobacillus strains without SeNPs decreased the viability of C. albicans by approximately 10-fold. SeNP-enriched species decreased 1000-fold	
Ujaoney et al. (2014)	L. acidophilus, L. rhamnosus, L. salivarius, Bifidobacterium bifidum, Streptococcus thermophilus, Bifidobacterium infantis, Lactobacillus GG, and Bacillus coagulans BC30	C. albicans 10341	Probiotics supernatant provided a stronger and significant inhibitory effect on biofilm formation than their bacterial counterparts	Depletion of nutrients in the culture media by overgrowth of the probiotic bacteria may inhibit fungal growth
Vilela et al. (2015)	L. acidophilus ATCC 4356	C. albicans ATCC 18804	• L. acidophilus culture filtrate reduced the growth of C. albicans cells by 45.1% • Less hyphae formation in the presence of L. acidophilus cells or culture filtrate	L. acidophilus produced substances with anti-Candida activity, presenting an indirect effect on Candida
Chew et al. (2015a, 2015b)	L. rhamnosus GR-1 and L. reuteri RC-14	C. glabrata ATCC 2001 and clinical isolates	• Probiotic strains exhibit growth inhibitory activities (bacterial cells and supernatant) and candidicidal activity against C. glabrata • Both probiotic strains exhibited strong autoaggregation and coaggregation in the presence of Candida	Lactobacilli may prevent C. glabrata colonization through the formation of aggregates. Reduction of pH plays role on the antifungal effect of probiotic, but not H_2O_2. Other inhibitory mechanisms or pathways may be involved

CFU, Colony-forming units; H_2O_2, hydrogen peroxide; MATH, microbial adhesion to hydrocarbons; Ms, mutants Streptococci; SeNPs, selenium dioxide nanoparticles; XTT, tetrazolium salt (Matsubara, Bandara, Ishikawa, et al., 2016; Matsubara, Bandara, Mayer, et al., 2016; Matsubara, Wang, et al. 2016.

TABLE 21.2 Clinical investigations on the antifungal effects of probiotics in the oral cavity, urogenital tract, and gastrointestinal tract of humans.

Reference	Site of action	Probiotic	Pathogen	Results	Comments
Romeo et al. (2011)	Gastrointestinal tract	L. reuteri (ATCC 55730) and L. rhamnosus (ATCC 53103)	Candida spp.	• Probiotic reduced significantly Candida stool colonization • L. reuteri group had a significant higher reduction in gastrointestinal symptoms than the L. rhamnosus and control groups • Probiotics reduced the incidence of abnormal neurological outcome	Probiotics may prevent gastrointestinal colonization by Candida, protect from late-onset sepsis, and reduce abnormal neurological outcomes in preterms
Mendonça et al. (2012)	Oral cavity	Lactobacillus casei and Bifidobacterium breve	C. albicans, C. tropicalis, Candida guilliermondii, C. glabrata, Candida lipolytica, C. krusei, Candida kefyr, and Candida parapsilosis	• Reduction of Candida prevalence from 92.9% to 85.7% • Increase of anti-Candida IgA levels	C. albicans was the most frequently species isolated before and after probiotic consumption
Sutula et al. (2012)	Oral cavity	L. casei Shirota	Candida spp., Streptococcus mutans, and gram-negative anaerobic species	• No effect of probiotic on occurrence and viability of Candida • No significant change in the viability of Streptococcus mutans and gram-negative anaerobes	Small sample group (n = 7) completed the study protocol
Vicariotto et al. (2012)	Urogenital tract	Lactobacillus fermentum LF10 and L. acidophilus LA02 (arabinogalactan and fructooligosaccharides as prebiotics)	Candida spp.	• Probiotic significantly solved Candida yeast symptoms in 86.6% of patients after 28 days • At the end of the second month, recurrences were recorded in 11.5% of patients	Probiotic may establish and maintain a protective barrier effect against vaginal Candida
Demirel et al. (2013)	Gastrointestinal tract	Saccharomyces boulardii	Candida spp.	• Candida colonization of the skin and stool were similar between probiotic and nystatin groups • Clinical sepsis and number of sepsis attacks were significantly lower in the probiotic group	Prophylactic S. boulardii and nystatin were equally effective in reducing candidal colonization and invasive fungal infection
Hu et al. (2013)	Urogenital tract and oral cavity	Bifidobacterium and Lactobacillus (DanActive or YoPlus yogurt)	Candida spp.	• Less fungal colonization among women was observed after probiotic consumption • HIV-infected women had significantly lower vaginal fungal colonization after DanActive yogurt consumption	Reduced oral fungal colonization was observed in HIV-infected women consuming probiotic yogurts, but not statistically significant

Study	Site	Probiotic	Target	Findings	Conclusion
Kumar et al. (2013)	Gastrointestinal tract	L. acidophillus, L. rhamnosus, B. longum, B. bifidum, S. boulardii, and Saccharomyces thermophilus	Candida spp.	• Probiotic therapy avoided a significant increase in the number of patients colonized by Candida spp. • Probiotic significantly reduced the presence of Candida in the urine, but not in the blood	Probiotics may be an alternative strategy to reduce Candida infection in GI tract and urine in children receiving broad-spectrum antibiotics
Sutula et al. (2013)	Oral cavity	L. casei Shirota	• Candida spp. • Gram-negative anaerobic species	• Lactobacillus level in saliva was increased during probiotic consumption period • Candida and anaerobic species levels were unaffected by the therapy • Morning breath scores measured were not significantly affected	Confirmation of the temporary and intake-dependent presence of Lactobacillus
Li et al. (2014)	Oral cavity	Lactobacillus bulgaricus, Bifidobacterium longum, and Streptococcus thermophilus	Candida spp.	Detection rate of Candida spp. was reduced in the probiotic group; significant relief of clinical signs and symptoms after probiotic administration	No adverse events were observed
Roy et al. (2014)	Gastrointestinal tract	L. acidophilus, Bifidobacterium lactis, B. longum, and B. bifidum	Candida spp.	• Probiotic therapy reduced the duration of hospitalization and stool fungal colonization • Fungal infection was significant less in the probiotic group • Full feed establishment was earlier in probiotic group	Probiotics may reduce enteral fungal colonization and reduce invasive fungal sepsis in low-birth-weight neonates
Ishikawa et al. (2015)	Oral cavity	L. rhamnosus HS111, Lactobacillus acidophillus HS101, and Bifidobacterium bifidum	Candida spp.	• Significant reduction of Candida infection after probiotic administration • C. albicans was the most prevalent species before and after the probiotic therapy	Reduction of Candida infection was independent of initial Candida level, colonizing species, or age of denture
Kovachev et al. (2015)	Urogenital tract	L. acidophilus, L. rhamnosus, and L. delbrueckii subsp. bulgaricus, and S. thermophiles	C. albicans	• Probiotic reduced clinical complaints • Probiotic therapy improved the investigated parameters: vaginal fluorine, vaginal tissue changes, and pH	Local application of probiotics may improve the efficacy of conventional antifungals and prevent relapse
Kraft-Bodi et al. (2015)	Oral cavity	Lactobacillus reuteri DSM 17938 and L. reuteri ATCC PTA 5289	Candida spp.	• Significant reduction of Candida cells in saliva and plaque after probiotic administration • No differences in the levels of supragingival plaque or bleeding on probing were observed	"Strong taste" of the tablets and gastric upset were compliances reported in both control and experimental groups

CFU, Colony-forming units; ELISA, enzyme-linked immunosorbent assay; GI, gastrointestinal; HIV, human immunodeficiency virus; IgA, immunoglobulin A; RCT, randomized controlled trial; VVC, vulvovaginal candidiasis (Matsubara, Bandara, Ishikawa, et al. 2016; Matsubara, Bandara, Mayer, et al., 2016; Matsubara, Wang, et al. 2016).

2004). As for the efficiency of probiotics in the treatment of yeast infections, it is measured in comparison with the one already achieved by antifungal medications. Probiotics have the added benefit on not causing microbial resistance and being generally less aggressive to the host's organism. (Elahi et al., 2005) tested the pattern of colonization of *L. fermentum* and *L. acidophilus* in mice on the intake of probiotic strains and observed a sudden decline in *C. albicans* count. Continuous consumption of probiotics considerably reduced the amount of fungal infection in the oral cavity, therefore preserving the protective effect for a persistent period after the termination of application (Meurman & Stamatova, 2007). Li et al. (2014) proved that adding a probiotic to nystatin increases the reduction in *C. albicans* colonization versus the nystatin monotherapy. An investigation tested *L. acidophulus* and *L. rhamnosus* in their capabilities to reduce *Candida* spp. infections, and both were effective (Ishikawa et al., 2015; Miyazima et al., 2017). Another study tested the antifungal capabilities of *L. rhamnosus* and *L. casei* on resin surface dentures. Both strains were effective at reducing yeast proliferation and did not affect the roughness of the resin, an added benefit for patients who use removable oral prosthetics (Song & Lee, 2017). *L. rhamnosus* has been shown to reduce *C. albicans*' counts in saliva (Hatakka et al., 2007). *L. reuteri* has also been proved to reduce *C. albicans* counts in saliva and dentures (Kraft-Bodi et al., 2015).

A recent double-blinded, placebo-controlled, randomized trial demonstrated that probiotic capsules containing *Lactobacillus bulgaricus*, *Streptococcus thermophilus*, *L. acidophilus*, and *B. bifidum* significantly reduced candidal loads in patients with Sjogren syndrome (Kamal et al., 2020). This study was the first to administer probiotics systemically by using capsules. Previous studies found that probiotics effectively reduce *Candida* levels in older denture wearers and children receiving broad-spectrum antibiotics (Ishikawa et al., 2015; Kumar et al., 2013; Mendonça et al., 2012). In complete denture wearers, daily consumption of cheese supplemented with probiotics also reduced *Candida* loads (Miyazima et al., 2017). Probiotics have been studied in combination with nystatin, showing an increase in the reduction of *Candida* associated stomatitis compared with conventional therapy (Li et al., 2014). A significant increase in anti-*Candida* immunoglobulin A levels has also been demonstrated after consuming the probiotics *L. casei* and *Bifidobacterium breve* (Mendonça et al., 2012). An additional study concluded that epithelial cells acquire improved defense functions after the intake of probiotics (Boirivant & Strober, 2007). Further research is required to understand the species that are therapeutically efficacious in the prophylaxis and treatment of oral candidiasis.

21.3.2 Probiotics therapy for dermal infections

In the human body, there are bacteria, viruses, and microbial eukaryotic communities that are specific to each anatomical part of the human body, for example, the gastrointestinal tract, the skin, the vagina, and the mouth (Slattery et al., 2016). The human microbiota consists of approximately 100 trillion microorganisms. Each body region carries its own characteristic microbial communities (Bennett et al., 2014). Skin is one of the largest organs of the human body that harbors 10^6 microflora and acts as a barrier protecting the inner part of the body (Grice & Segre, 2011; Scharschmidt & Fischbach, 2013). Skin microbiota is linked to some serious skin diseases and wound infections, as well as contributing to the defense system of the skin. Dysbiosis occurring in the skin microbiota might be instrumental in inflammatory skin diseases, such as psoriasis, atopic dermatitis, and acne vulgaris (Zeeuwen et al., 2013). Probiotics and prebiotics are extensively employed in dermatology. Investigating the application of probiotics in treating atopic dermatitis, acne, eczema, allergies, skin aging, bacterial and fungal infections, and chronic diabetic foot ulcers has yielded promising results (Fuchs-Tarlovsky et al., 2016).

Dermatophytosis is an infection caused by a dermatophyte mainly on hair, skin, and nails, usually of the genus *Trichophyton*, *Microsporum*, and few *Epidermophyton* genera. *Tinea capitis*, *Tinea pedis*, and *Onychomycosis* are common dermal infections. They are distributed within the entire world, particularly tropical and subtropical hot and wet countries. Dermatophytes infect human skin cells that are rich in keratin protein. Skin, hair and nail are the foremost necessary parts of body that are enriched with keratin. Therefore dermatophytosis that are caused by dermatophytes are restricted solely to these keratinous tissues.

There are three main sources for dermatophytosis. Some of the anthropophilic form of dermatophyte's spreads from one person to another by direct contact with infected person or by contact to infected macerated skin cells. The geophilic form of dermatophytes that resides in keratinous materials of soil as saprophytes is transmitted to individuals by contact through contaminated soil. The zoophilic form of dermatophytes spreads from animals that are mostly domestic and a few wild animals (AlokKumar & Rahul, 2016).

Oral and topical antifungal agents are used as treatment for fungus infections caused by dermatophytes. Generally, it involves the usage of antifungal agents of the allylamine category (mainly terbinafine) and of azoles, such as ketoconazole, miconazole, and oxiconazole. Most fungal infections are often managed with topical medical care alone. The major clinical form of dermatophyte infection is onychomycosis that is followed by *Tinea corporis*, *T. pedis*, and *T. capitis*. There is a preference for treatments that combine topical and systemic drugs, and the most widely used drugs are ciclopirox olamine (topical) and fluconazole (systemic). Itraconazole, fluconazole, and terbinafine are efficient in the treatment of onychomycosis and have a good safety report. Terbinafine produces the best results for the dermatophyte pathogen. For *Candida* and nondermatophyte infections, the azoles are mostly the recommended therapy. Topical medical care with the fungicidal allylamine antifungals has slightly more cure rates than with fungistatic azoles. Topical terbinafine, ciclopirox olamine is the best agent against dermatophytosis. The toxicity and limited spectrum of currently available antifungals and the steady development of resistance to the available drugs are a topic of concern; as a result, alternative therapies are urgently needed.

The use of probiotic bacteria against microbial infections has emerged as an alternative therapeutic technique for fungal infections in view to the limitations of the currently available antimicrobials. Probiotics and prebiotics are extensively employed in dermatology. Investigating the application of probiotics in treating atopic dermatitis, acne, eczema, allergies, skin aging, bacterial and fungal infections, and chronic diabetic foot ulcers has yielded promising results (Fuchs-Tarlovsky et al., 2016).

L. reuteri has been shown to inhibit the growth of *Trichophyton tonsurans* (Guo et al., 2011). Apart from this, another study also showed antifungal activity of *Lactobacillus* against *Microsporum canis*, *Microsporum gypseum*, and *Epidermophyton floccosum* (Guo et al., 2012). *L. plantarum* have been shown to produce antifungal activity against *Aspergillus fumigatus* (Crowley et al., 2013). *L. casei* have been used to show antidermatophytosis effect against *Trichophyton rubrum*, *T. verocosum*, *M. canis*, and *M. gypseum* in the formulation development of topical gel (Mehdi-Alamdarloo et al., 2016). *L. acidophilus* bacterial secretions show strong effect against *C. albicans* and *T. rubrum* fungi adopted in this study (Alwan et al., 2020).

21.3.3 Probiotics in vaginal fungal infections

Candida spp. though being a commensal fungi of the vaginal mucosa may cause symptoms when the balance among the fungus, mucosa, and host defense mechanisms is disturbed, leading to the development of candidiasis (Cassone & Cauda, 2012; Costa et al., 2013; Hebecker et al., 2014; Matsubara, Bandara, Ishikawa, et al., 2016; Salvatori et al., 2016; Thompson et al., 2010).

VVC is a very common infection that affects both immunocompromised and immunocompetent women, presenting indications of vulval and vaginal inflammation caused by several *Candida* species, mainly *C. albicans* (Dovnik et al., 2015; Makanjuola et al., 2018). It is well seen that most women suffer from one or more episodes of VVC in the course of their life. This infection affects women's mental health, quality of life along with sexual activity due to its severe symptoms: excoriation, vulvar erythema, pruritus, and a vaginal discharge along with a change in vaginal odor (Blostein et al., 2017). VVC can be treated by the use of systemic or topical antifungals, depending on the extent of infection. Nevertheless, high rates of antifungal resistance have been reported (Khan et al., 2018; Wang et al., 2016). Due to the increase in antifungal resistance and various studies that proved that certain probiotic strains inhibit *Candida* species (Matsubara, Bandara, Ishikawa, et al., 2016; Matsubara, Bandara, Mayer, et al., 2016; Matsubara, Wang, et al., 2016; Mishra et al., 2016; Santos et al., 2009; Shah et al., 2013), studies have been performed to evaluate the clinical application of *Lactobacillus* for the VVC treatment (Buggio et al., 2019; Xie et al., 2017). (Pendharkar et al., 2015) evaluated that the antifungal efficacy of EcoVag, a commercially available probiotic product composed of *L. rhamnosus* (DSM 14870) and *Lactobacillus gasseri* (DSM 14869) combined with fluconazole for the treatment of VVC where results showed that the group treated with the antifungal plus EcoVag had a 100% cure rate. However, after the end of treatment, there was a relapse in 33% of the women treated with fluconazole alone, requiring afresh treatment, while there was no relapse of in any case in group treated with the combination regimen. In a similar study, Davar et al. (2016) investigated the effect of Pro-Digest that contains *L. acidophilus*, *B. bifidum*, and *B. longum* along with fluconazole for the treatment of recurrent VVC. The authors found that the recurrence rate of the group treated with fluconazole was 35.5% compared with 7.2% for the group treated with fluconazole plus Pro-Digest. These studies suggest that probiotics may enhance the effect of fluconazole and provide a sustainable and protective solution at the end of antifungal therapy.

21.3.4 Probiotics in systemic fungal infections

Systemic invasive fungal infections are growing public health problem and cause severe invasive injuries, with symptoms, such as organ dysfunction along with hematogenous infection in the host (Bongomin et al., 2017; Huseyin et al., 2017). The most commonly isolated common filamentous fungi and yeast during clinical practices are *C. albicans*,

Cryptococcus neoformans, and *A. fumigatus*. Invasive fungi will infect throughout the body in people with low immunity (Kamei & Watanabe, 2005; Paul & Kannan, 2019; Szalewski et al., 2018), causing a variety of fungal diseases (Abdulkareem et al., 2015; Chrétien et al., 2002; Kato et al., 2018; Mayer & Kronstad, 2019; van de Veerdonk et al., 2017) having high relapse rate and mortalities (Bays & Thompson, 2019; Bongomin et al., 2017; Fairlamb et al., 2016; Paul & Kannan, 2019; Perlin et al., 2017; Robbins et al., 2017). In addition, the increase in the use of antifungal drugs in clinical practice has led to the increase in the rate of fungal resistance (Fairlamb et al., 2016; Robbins et al., 2017). Because multidrug-resistant *Candida auris* was first reported in Japan in 2009, the incidence of multiple drug resistant fungi makes the control of invasive fungi more serious (Larkin et al., 2017; Sherry et al., 2017). Thus new strategies regarding antifungal therapy on these drug-resistant invasive fungi are necessary. Invasive fungi and bacteria can distribute in the oral cavity, skin, intestinal tract and other parts of the human body (Mason et al., 2012; Prieto et al., 2016). There is a symbiotic relationship between invasive fungi and bacteria in the host (Limon et al., 2017), which forms a delicate microecological dynamic balance and plays an important role in maintaining human health (Diaz et al., 2014; Kumamoto, 2016; Manrique et al., 2017; Sam et al., 2017).

Bacillus is a common Gram-positive bacterium, distributed in soil, water, animal intestines, and other natural environments. Some *bacilli* are probiotics for the human body and play an important role in maintaining microbial balance. Symparasitism of *Bacillus* and *C. albicans* in the human intestinal tract inhibits invasion by *C. albicans*. A lipopeptide secreted from *Bacillus* spp. leads to the inhibition of fungal biofilm formation through its surfactant properties and reduction in the expression of specific biofilm formation genes (Rautela et al., 2014). *Enterococcus faecalis* is a Gram-positive bacterium abundant in the intestinal tract of the human body. It belongs to the normal flora of the body. Some strains of *E. faecalis* have been developed as probiotics for body regulation. Therefore this species plays an important role in maintaining the stability of the flora in the intestinal tract (Cuív et al., 2018). It has been proved that *E. faecalis* has particular inhibitory effects on intestinal colonization and invasion during *C. albicans* infection (Garsin & Lorenz, 2013).

Lactobacilli serve as excellent probiotics in the human body. They live in large numbers in human intestines and vaginas and maintain the dynamic balance among microorganisms. They are also closely related to the intestinal colonization of fungi. Production of lactic acid and other substances during the growth process reduces the pH of the environment. However, it has been demonstrated that the antifungal effect of *Lactobacillus* is not related to the reduced pH (Matsubara, Bandara, Mayer, et al., 2016) and different species of *Lactobacillus* have different mechanisms of the inhibiting fungal growth. For instance, the development of fungi is inhibited by *L. rhamnosus* by competing with fungi for adhesion sites (do Carmo et al., 2016). *Lactobacillus* inhibits the transformation of *C. albicans* from yeast to mycelium phase through the short chain fatty acids and lactic acid secretion (Er et al., 2019; Liang et al., 2016). *Lactobacilli* species produce butyrate that not only inhibits filamentation growth of *C. albicans* but also inhibit melanin and capsule formation in *C. neoformans* along with enhancing the effector functions of macrophages (Nguyen et al., 2011). *L. plantarum* strain produces a substance that halts the hyphae and germ tube growth as well as influences the *A. fumigatus* cell metabolism (Crowley et al., 2013; Kim, 2005).

In brief, several *Lactobacilli* species have various inhibitory effects on *C. neoformans*, *C. albicans*, and *A. fumigatus* mycelium formation, growth, bud tube germination, virulence, and biofilm formation. Hence, probiotics *Lactobacilli* can be used as therapy adjuvants for intestinal tract, oral cavity, and vaginal candidiasis to enhance antitumor effect and improve antifungal effects (Azevedo et al., 2020; Shively et al., 2018).

21.4 Future perspectives

With the increase in the number of immunocompromised persons, an increase in the number of cases with fungal infections has occurred. Probiotics offer an alternative means of treatment. Nevertheless, there is a need for detailed convincing research on in vitro, in vivo, and clinical trials from probiotic administration, which clearly proves the benefits and side effects of each. More importance needs to be given to the selection of probiotic used along with the methods and experimental setup. Further research on probiotics used in dentistry may help and assist in providing localized passive immunization against dental caries. The synergism between conventional drugs and probiotic microorganisms also needs to be defined. Further studies on combinations of prebiotics and probiotics and development of synbiotics can prove to be advantageous for skin-related diseases and can be used as a cotherapy in treatment.

21.5 Conclusions

As probiotics have a limited success in treating immune-mediated diseases, prebiotics can be used along with probiotics or as a supplement for them. Studies demonstrate that the biotherapeutic formulas comprising both suitable microbial strains along with synergistic prebiotics may lead to the improvement of the probiotic effect in the small intestine and the colon. These "enhanced" probiotic products may prove to be even better in their protective and stimulatory effect and may be even more superior to their components administered separately (Bomba et al., 2002; Markowiak & Ślizewska, 2017). However, the use of probiotics needs more standardization and validation, thereby providing an insight to newer therapeutic targets for infection.

Acknowledgment

We are grateful to Uka Tarsadia University, Maliba Campus, Tarsadi, Gujarat, India, for providing the facilities needed for the preparation of this chapter.

References

Abdulkareem, A. F., Lee, H. H., Ahmadi, M., & Martinez, L. R. (2015). Fungal serotype-specific differences in bacterial-yeast interactions. *Virulence*, 6(6), 652–657. Available from https://doi.org/10.1080/21505594.2015.1066962.

AlokKumar, S., & Rahul, M. (2016). Management of Tinea corporis, Tinea cruris, and Tinea pedis: A comprehensive review. *Indian Dermatology Online Journal*, 77. Available from https://doi.org/10.4103/2229-5178.178099.

Alwan, A. H., Abdulkareem, A. F., & Alwan, B. H. (2020). Antifungal effect of Lactobacillus acidophilus crude extract. *PalArch's Journal of Archaeology of Egypt/Egyptology*, 17(7), 7616–7622.

Amara, A. A., & Shibl, A. (2015). Role of Probiotics in health improvement, infection control and disease treatment and management. *Saudi Pharmaceutical Journal*, 23(2), 107–114. Available from https://doi.org/10.1016/j.jsps.2013.07.001.

Azevedo, M. J., de Lurdes Pereira, M., Araujo, R., Ramalho, C., Zaura, E., & Sampaio-Maia, B. (2020). Influence of delivery and feeding mode in oral fungi colonization—A systematic review. *Microbial Cell*, 7(2), 36–45. Available from https://doi.org/10.15698/mic2020.02.706.

Balwani, M., CharulataP, B., Prakash, K., & Amit, P. (2019). Awareness about kidney and its related function/dysfunction in school going children: A survey from the Central India. *Saudi Journal of Kidney Diseases and Transplantation*, 202. Available from https://doi.org/10.4103/1319-2442.252911.

Bays, D. J., & Thompson, G. R. (2019). Fungal infections of the stem cell transplant recipient and hematologic malignancy patients. *Infectious Disease Clinics of North America*, 33(2), 545–566. Available from https://doi.org/10.1016/j.idc.2019.02.006.

Bennett, J. E., Dolin, R., & Blaser, M. J. (2014). *Mandell, douglas, and bennett's principles and practice of infectious diseases: 2-volume set* (Vol. 2). Elsevier Health Sciences.

Blostein, F., Levin-Sparenberg, E., Wagner, J., & Foxman, B. (2017). Recurrent vulvovaginal candidiasis. *Annals of Epidemiology*, 27(9), 575–582.e3. Available from https://doi.org/10.1016/j.annepidem.2017.08.010.

Boirivant, M., & Strober, W. (2007). The mechanism of action of probiotics. *Current Opinion in Gastroenterology*, 23(6), 679–692. Available from https://doi.org/10.1097/MOG.0b013e3282f0cffc.

Bomba, A., Nemcová, R., Mudroňová, D., & Guba, P. (2002). The possibilities of potentiating the efficacy of probiotics. *Trends in Food Science and Technology*, 13(4), 121–126. Available from https://doi.org/10.1016/S0924-2244(02)00129-2.

Bongomin, F., Sara, G., Rita, O., & David, D. (2017). Global and multi-national prevalence of fungal diseases—Estimate precision. *Journal of Fungi*, 57. Available from https://doi.org/10.3390/jof3040057.

Brown, D. G., Denning, D. W., Gow, N. A. R., Levitz, S. M., Netea, M. G., & White, T. C. (2012). Hidden killers: Human fungal infections. *Science Translational Medicine*. Available from https://doi.org/10.1126/scitranslmed.3004404, 165rv13.

Buggio, L., Somigliana, E., Borghi, A., & Vercellini, P. (2019). Probiotics and vaginal microecology: Fact or fancy? *BMC Women's Health*, 19(1). Available from https://doi.org/10.1186/s12905-019-0723-4.

Cassone, A., & Cauda, R. (2012). Candida and candidiasis in HIV-infected patients: Where commensalism, opportunistic behavior and frank pathogenicity lose their borders. *AIDS (London, England)*, 26(12), 1457–1472. Available from https://doi.org/10.1097/QAD.0b013e3283536ba8.

Charalampopoulos, D. (2009). *Prebiotics and probiotics science and technology* (Vol. 1). Springer Science & Business Media.

Chew, S. Y., Cheah, Y. K., Seow, H. F., Sandai, D., & Than, L. T. L. (2015a). In vitro modulation of probiotic bacteria on the biofilm of Candida glabrata. *Anaerobe*, 34, 132–138. Available from https://doi.org/10.1016/j.anaerobe.2015.05.009.

Chew, S. Y., Cheah, Y. K., Seow, H. F., Sandai, D., & Than, L. T. L. (2015b). Probiotic Lactobacillus rhamnosus GR-1 and Lactobacillus reuteri RC-14 exhibit strong antifungal effects against vulvovaginal candidiasis-causing Candida glabrata isolates. *Journal of Applied Microbiology*, 118(5), 1180–1190. Available from https://doi.org/10.1111/jam.12772.

Chrétien, F., Lortholary, O., Kansau, I., Neuville, S., Gray, F., & Dromer, F. (2002). Pathogenesis of cerebral Cryptococcus neoformans infection after fungemia. *Journal of Infectious Diseases*, 186(4), 522–530. Available from https://doi.org/10.1086/341564.

Coman, M. M., Verdenelli, M. C., Cecchini, C., Silvi, S., Orpianesi, C., Boyko, N., & Cresci, A. (2014). In vitro evaluation of antimicrobial activity of Lactobacillus rhamnosus IMC 501®, Lactobacillus paracasei IMC 502® and SYNBIO® against pathogens. *Journal of Applied Microbiology*, 117(2), 518–527.

Cortés-Zavaleta, O., López-Malo, A., Hernández-Mendoza, A., & García, H. S. (2014). Antifungal activity of lactobacilli and its relationship with 3-phenyllactic acid production. *International Journal of Food Microbiology*, 173, 30–35. Available from https://doi.org/10.1016/j.ijfoodmicro.2013.12.016.

Costa, A. C. B. P., Pereira, C. A., Junqueira, J. C., & Jorge, A. O. C. (2013). Recent mouse and rat methods for the study of experimental oral candidiasis. *Virulence*, *4*(5), 391–399. Available from https://doi.org/10.4161/viru.25199.

Crowley, S., Mahony, J., Morrissey, J. P., & van Sinderen, D. (2013). Transcriptomic and morphological profiling of Aspergillus fumigatus Af293 in response to antifungal activity produced by Lactobacillus plantarum 16. *Microbiology (United Kingdom)*, *159*(10), 2014–2024. Available from https://doi.org/10.1099/mic.0.068742-0.

Cuív, P., Giri, R., Hoedt, E. C., McGuckin, M. A., Begun, J., & Morrison, M. (2018). Enterococcus faecalis AHG0090 is a genetically tractable bacterium and produces a secreted peptidic bioactive that suppresses nuclear factor kappa B activation in human gut epithelial cells. *Frontiers in Immunology*, *9*. Available from https://doi.org/10.3389/fimmu.2018.00790.

Davar, R., Nokhostin, F., Eftekhar, M., Sekhavat, L., Bashiri Zadeh, M., & Shamsi, F. (2016). Comparing the recurrence of vulvovaginal candidiasis in patients undergoing prophylactic treatment with probiotic and placebo during the 6 months. *Probiotics and Antimicrobial Proteins*, *8*(3), 130–133. Available from https://doi.org/10.1007/s12602-016-9218-x.

Degnan, F. H. (2012). Clinical studies involving probiotics: When FDA's investigational new drug rubric applies-and when it may not. *Gut Microbes*, *3*(6), 485–489. Available from https://doi.org/10.4161/gmic.22158.

Deidda, F., Angela, A., Serena, A., Marco, P., Teresa, G., Mario, D. P., & Luca, M. (2016). In vitro activity of Lactobacillus fermentum LF5 against different Candida species and Gardnerella vaginalis. *Journal of Clinical Gastroenterology*, *50*(Suppl. 2), S168–S170. Available from https://doi.org/10.1097/mcg.0000000000000692.

Demirel, G., Celik, I. H., Erdeve, O., Saygan, S., Dilmen, U., & Canpolat, F. E. (2013). Prophylactic Saccharomyces boulardii versus nystatin for the prevention of fungal colonization and invasive fungal infection in premature infants. *European Journal of Pediatrics*, *172*(10), 1321–1326.

Denkova, R., Yanakieva, V., Denkova, Z., Nikolova, V., & Radeva, V. (2013). In vitro inhibitory activity of Bifidobacterium and Lactobacillus strains against Candida albicans. *Bulgarian Journal of Veterinary Medicine*, *16*(3).

Diaz, P. I., Strausbaugh, L. D., & Dongari-Bagtzoglou, A. (2014). Fungal-bacterial interactions and their relevance to oral health: Linking the clinic and the bench. *Frontiers in Cellular and Infection Microbiology*, *4*. Available from https://doi.org/10.3389/fcimb.2014.00101.

do Carmo, M. S., Noronha, F. M. F., Arruda, M. O., da Silva Costa, Ê. P., Bomfim, M. R. Q., Monteiro, A. S., Ferro, T. A. F., Fernandes, E. S., Girón, J. A., & Monteiro-Neto, V. (2016). Lactobacillus fermentum ATCC 23271 displays in vitro inhibitory activities against Candida spp. *Frontiers in Microbiology*, *7*. Available from https://doi.org/10.3389/fmicb.2016.01722.

Dovnik, A., Golle, A., Novak, D., Arko, D., & Takač, I. (2015). Treatment of vulvovaginal candidiasis: A review of the literature. *Acta Dermatovenerologica Alpina, Pannonica et Adriatica*, *24*(1), 5–7. Available from https://doi.org/10.15570/actaapa.2015.2.

Elahi, S., Pang, G., Ashman, R., & Clancy, R. (2005). Enhanced clearance of Candida albicans from the oral cavities of mice following oral administration of Lactobacillus acidophilus. *Clinical and Experimental Immunology*, *141*(1), 29–36. Available from https://doi.org/10.1111/j.1365-2249.2005.02811.x.

Er, S., İstanbullu Tosun, A., Arik, G., & Kivanç, M. (2019). Anticandidal activities of lactic acid bacteria isolated from the vagina. *Turkish Journal of Medical Sciences*, *49*(1), 375–383. Available from https://doi.org/10.3906/sag-1709-143.

Fairlamb, A. H., Gow, N. A. R., Matthews, K. R., & Waters, A. P. (2016). Drug resistance in eukaryotic microorganisms. *Nature Microbiology*, *1*(7). Available from https://doi.org/10.1038/nmicrobiol.2016.92.

Fu, J., Ding, Y., Wei, B., Wang, L., Xu, S., Qin, P., Wei, L., & Jiang, L. (2017). Epidemiology of Candida albicans and non-C.albicans of neonatal candidemia at a tertiary care hospital in Western China. *BMC Infectious Diseases*, *17*(1). Available from https://doi.org/10.1186/s12879-017-2423-8.

Fuchs-Tarlovsky, V., Marquez-Barba, M. F., & Sriram, K. (2016). Probiotics in dermatologic practice. *Nutrition (Burbank, Los Angeles County, Calif.)*, *32*(3), 289–295. Available from https://doi.org/10.1016/j.nut.2015.09.001.

Gaidhane, A., Sinha, A., Khatib, M., Simkhada, P., Behere, P., Saxena, D., Unnikrishnan, B., Khatib, M., Ahmed, M., & Zahiruddin, Q. S. (2018). A systematic review on effect of electronic media on diet, exercise, and sexual activity among adolescents. *Indian Journal of Community Medicine*, *43*(5), S56–S65. Available from https://doi.org/10.4103/ijcm.IJCM_143_18.

Garsin, D. A., & Lorenz, M. C. (2013). Candida albicans and Enterococcus faecalis in the gut: Synergy in commensalism? *Gut Microbes*, *4*(5). Available from https://doi.org/10.4161/gmic.26040.

Grice, E. A., & Segre, J. A. (2011). The skin microbiome. *Nature Reviews. Microbiology*, *9*(4), 244–253. Available from https://doi.org/10.1038/nrmicro2537.

Guo, J., Brosnan, B., Furey, A., Arendt, E. K., Murphy, P., & Coffey, A. (2012). Antifungal activity of Lactobacillus against Microsporum canis, Microsporum gypseum and Epidermophyton floccosum. *Bioengineered Bugs*, *3*(2), 104–113. Available from https://doi.org/10.4161/bbug.19624.

Guo, J., Mauch, A., Galle, S., Murphy, P., Arendt, E. K., & Coffey, A. (2011). Inhibition of growth of Trichophyton tonsurans by Lactobacillus reuteri. *Journal of Applied Microbiology*, *111*(2), 474–483. Available from https://doi.org/10.1111/j.1365-2672.2011.05032.x.

Hasslöf, P., Hedberg, M., Twetman, S., & Stecksén-Blicks, C. (2010). Growth inhibition of oral mutans streptococci and candida by commercial probiotic lactobacilli-an in vitro study. *BMC Oral Health*, *10*(1), 1–6.

Hatakka, K., Ahola, A. J., Yli-Knuuttila, H., Richardson, M., Poussa, T., Meurman, J. H., & Korpela, R. (2007). Probiotics reduce the prevalence of oral Candida in the elderly a randomized controlled trial. *Journal of Dental Research*, *86*(2), 125–130. Available from https://doi.org/10.1177/154405910708600204.

Hebecker, B., Naglik, J. R., Hube, B., & Jacobsen, I. D. (2014). Pathogenicity mechanisms and host response during oral Candida albicans infections. *Expert Review of Anti-Infective Therapy*, *12*(7), 867–879. Available from https://doi.org/10.1586/14787210.2014.916210.

Hu, H., Merenstein, D. J., Wang, C., Hamilton, P. R., Blackmon, M. L., Chen, H., Calderone, R. A., & Li, D. (2013). Impact of eating probiotic yogurt on colonization by Candida species of the oral and vaginal mucosa in HIV-infected and HIV-uninfected women. *Mycopathologia*, *176*(3-4), 175−181.

Huseyin, C. E., O'Toole, P. W., Cotter, P. D., & Scanlan, P. D. (2017). Forgotten fungi—The gut mycobiome in human health and disease. *FEMS Microbiology Reviews*, *41*(4), 479−511. Available from https://doi.org/10.1093/femsre/fuw047.

Ishijima, S. A., Hayama, K., Burton, J. P., Reid, G., Okada, M., Matsushita, Y., & Abe, S. (2012). Effect of Streptococcus salivarius K12 on the in vitro growth of Candida albicans and its protective effect in an oral candidiasis model. *Applied and Environmental Microbiology*, *78*(7), 2190−2199.

Ishikawa, K. H., Mayer, M. P. A., Miyazima, T. Y., Matsubara, V. H., Silva, E. G., Paula, C. R., Campos, T. T., & Nakamae, A. E. M. (2015). A multispecies probiotic reduces oral candida colonization in denture wearers. *Journal of Prosthodontics*, *24*(3), 194−199. Available from https://doi.org/10.1111/jopr.12198.

Kamal, Y., Kandil, M., Eissa, M., Yousef, R., & Elsaadany, B. (2020). Probiotics as a prophylaxis to prevent oral candidiasis in patients with Sjogren's syndrome: A double-blinded, placebo-controlled, randomized trial. *Rheumatology International*, *40*(6), 873−879. Available from https://doi.org/10.1007/s00296-020-04558-9.

Kamei, K., & Watanabe, A. (2005). Aspergillus mycotoxins and their effect on the host. *Medical Mycology*, *43*(1), S95−S99. Available from https://doi.org/10.1080/13693780500051547.

Kato, H., Yoshimura, Y., Suido, Y., Ide, K., Sugiyama, Y., Matsuno, K., & Nakajima, H. (2018). Prevalence of, and risk factors for, hematogenous fungal endophthalmitis in patients with Candida bloodstream infection. *Infection*, *46*(5), 635−640. Available from https://doi.org/10.1007/s15010-018-1163-z.

Keller, M. K., & Kragelund, C. (2018). Randomized pilot study on probiotic effects on recurrent candidiasis in oral lichen planus patients. *Oral Diseases*, *24*(6), 1107−1114. Available from https://doi.org/10.1111/odi.12858.

Khan, M., Ahmed, J., Gul, A., Ikram, A., & Lalani, F. K. (2018). Antifungal susceptibility testing of vulvovaginal Candida species among women attending antenatal clinic in tertiary care hospitals of Peshawar. *Infection and Drug Resistance*, *11*, 447−456. Available from https://doi.org/10.2147/IDR.S153116.

Kheradmand, E., Rafii, F., Yazdi, M. H., Sepahi, A. A., Shahverdi, A. R., & Oveisi, M. R. (2014). The antimicrobial effects of selenium nanoparticle-enriched probiotics and their fermented broth against Candida albicans. *DARU Journal of Pharmaceutical Sciences*, *22*(1), 1−6.

Kim, J. D. (2005). Antifungal activity of lactic acid bacteria isolated from Kimchi against Aspergillus fumigatus. *Mycobiology*, *33*(4), 210−214.

Kogade., Gaidhane, A., Choudhari, S., Khatib, M. N., Kawalkar, U., Gaidhane, S., & Zahiruddin, Q. S. (2019). Socio-cultural determinants of infant and young child feeding practices in rural India. *Medical Science*, *23*(100), 1015−1022.

Köhler, G. A., Assefa, S., & Reid, G. (2012). Probiotic interference of Lactobacillus rhamnosus GR-1 and Lactobacillus reuteri RC-14 with the opportunistic fungal pathogen Candida albicans. *Infectious diseases in obstetrics and gynecology*, 2012.

Köhler, J. R., Casadevall, A., & Perfect, J. (2015). The spectrum of fungi that infects humans. *Cold Spring Harbor Perspectives in Medicine*, *5*(1). Available from https://doi.org/10.1101/cshperspect.a019273.

Kovachev, S. M., & Vatcheva-Dobrevska, R. S. (2015). Local probiotic therapy for vaginal Candida albicans infections. *Probiotics and Antimicrobial Proteins*, *7*(1), 38−44.

Kraft-Bodi, E., Jørgensen, M. R., Keller, M. K., Kragelund, C., & Twetman, S. (2015). Effect of probiotic bacteria on oral Candida in frail elderly. *Journal of Dental Research*, *94*, 181−186. Available from https://doi.org/10.1177/0022034515595950.

Kumamoto, C. A. (2016). The fungal mycobiota: Small numbers, large impacts. *Cell Host and Microbe*, *19*(6), 750−751. Available from https://doi.org/10.1016/j.chom.2016.05.018.

Kumar, S., Bansal, A., Chakrabarti, A., & Singhi, S. (2013). Evaluation of efficacy of probiotics in prevention of Candida colonization in a PICU—A randomized controlled trial. *Critical Care Medicine*, *41*(2), 565−572. Available from https://doi.org/10.1097/CCM.0b013e31826a409c.

Lahtinen, S., Ouwehand, A. C., Salminen, S., & von Wright, A. (2011). *Lactic acid bacteria: Microbiological and functional aspects. Lactic acid bacteria: Microbiological and functional aspects* (fourth edition, pp. 1−761). CRC Press. Available from https://www.taylorfrancis.com/books/e/9781439836781.

Larkin, E., Hager, C., Chandra, J., Mukherjee, P. K., Retuerto, M., Salem, I., Long, L., Isham, N., Kovanda, L., Borroto-Esoda, K., Wring, S., Angulo, D., & Ghannoum, M. (2017). The emerging pathogen Candida auris: Growth phenotype, virulence factors, activity of antifungals, and effect of SCY-078, a novel glucan synthesis inhibitor, on growth morphology and biofilm formation. *Antimicrobial Agents and Chemotherapy*, *61*(5). Available from https://doi.org/10.1128/AAC.02396-16.

Lashof, A. M. L. O., De Boc, R., Herbrecht, R., de Pauwa, B. E., Krcmery, V., Aoun, M., Akova, M., Cohen, J., Siffnerová, H., Egyed, M., Ellis, M., Marinus, A., Sylvester, R., & Kullberg, B. J. (2004). An open multicentre comparative study of the efficacy, safety and tolerance of fluconazole and itraconazole in the treatment of cancer patients with oropharyngeal candidiasis. *European Journal of Cancer*, 1314−1319. Available from https://doi.org/10.1016/j.ejca.2004.03.003.

Lau, C. S. M., Ward, A., & Chamberlain, R. S. (2016). Probiotics improve the efficacy of standard triple therapy in the eradication of Helicobacter pylori: A *meta*-analysis. *Infection and Drug Resistance*, *9*, 275−289. Available from https://doi.org/10.2147/IDR.S117886.

Li, D., Li, Q., Liu, C., Lin, M., Li, X., Xiao, X., Zhu, Z., Gong, Q., & Zhou, H. (2014). Efficacy and safety of probiotics in the treatment of Candida-associated stomatitis. *Mycoses*, *57*(3), 141−146. Available from https://doi.org/10.1111/myc.12116.

Liang, W., Guan, G., Dai, Y., Cao, C., Tao, L., Du, H., Nobile, C. J., Zhong, J., & Huang, G. (2016). Lactic acid bacteria differentially regulate filamentation in two heritable cell types of the human fungal pathogen Candida albicans. *Molecular Microbiology*, *102*(3), 506−519. Available from https://doi.org/10.1111/mmi.13475.

Limon, J. J., Skalski, J. H., & Underhill, D. M. (2017). Commensal fungi in health and disease. *Cell Host and Microbe*, *22*(2), 156−165. Available from https://doi.org/10.1016/j.chom.2017.07.002.

Magill, S. S., Edwards, J. R., Bamberg, W., Beldavs, Z. G., Dumyati, G., Kainer, M. A., Lynfield, R., Maloney, M., McAllister-Hollod, L., Nadle, J., Ray, S. M., Thompson, D. L., Wilson, L. E., & Fridkin, S. K. (2014). Multistate point-prevalence survey of health care-associated infections. *New England Journal of Medicine*, *370*(13), 1198−1208. Available from https://doi.org/10.1056/NEJMoa1306801.

Makanjuola, O., Bongomin, F., & Fayemiwo, S. A. (2018). An update on the roles of non-albicans candida species in vulvovaginitis. *Journal of Fungi*, *4*(4). Available from https://doi.org/10.3390/jof4040121.

Manrique, P., Dills, M., & Young, M. J. (2017). The human gut phage community and its implications for health and disease. *Viruses*, *9*(6). Available from https://doi.org/10.3390/v9060141.

Markowiak, P., & Śliżewska, K. (2017). Effects of probiotics, prebiotics, and synbiotics on human health. *Nutrients*, *9*(9). Available from https://doi.org/10.3390/nu9091021.

Mason, K. L., Downward, J. R. E., Mason, K. D., Falkowski, N. R., Eaton, K. A., Kao, J. Y., Young, V. B., & Huffnaglea, G. B. (2012). Candida albicans and bacterial microbiota interactions in the cecum during recolonization following broad-spectrum antibiotic therapy. *Infection and Immunity*, *80*(10), 3371−3380. Available from https://doi.org/10.1128/IAI.00449-12.

Matsubara, V. H., Bandara, H. M. H. N., Ishikawa, K. H., Mayer, M. P. A., & Samaranayake, L. P. (2016). The role of probiotic bacteria in managing periodontal disease: A systematic review. *Expert Review of Anti-Infective Therapy*, *14*(7), 643−655. Available from https://doi.org/10.1080/14787210.2016.1194198.

Matsubara, V. H., Bandara, H. M. H. N., Mayer, M. P. A., & Samaranayake, L. P. (2016). Probiotics as antifungals in mucosal candidiasis. *Clinical Infectious Diseases*, *62*(9), 1143−1153. Available from https://doi.org/10.1093/cid/ciw038.

Matsubara, V. H., Wang, Y., Bandara, H. M. H. N., Mayer, M. P. A., & Samaranayake, L. P. (2016). Probiotic lactobacilli inhibit early stages of Candida albicans biofilm development by reducing their growth, cell adhesion, and filamentation. *Applied Microbiology and Biotechnology*, *100*(14), 6415−6426. Available from https://doi.org/10.1007/s00253-016-7527-3.

Mayer, F. L., & Kronstad, J. (2019). The spectrum of interactions between cryptococcus neoformans and bacteria. *Journal of Fungi*, *5*(2). Available from https://doi.org/10.3390/jof5020031.

Mehdi-Alamdarloo, S., Ameri, A., Moghimipour, E., Gholipour, S., & Saadatzadeh, A. (2016). Formulation development of a topical probiotic gel for antidermatophytosis effect. *Jundishapur Journal of Natural Pharmaceutical Products*, *11*(3). Available from https://doi.org/10.17795/jjnpp-35893.

Mendonça, F. H. B. P., dos Santos, S. S. F., de Faria, I. D. S., Gonçalves e Silva, C. R., Jorge, A. O. C., & Leão, M. V. P. (2012). Effects of probiotic bacteria on Candida presence and IgA anti-Candida in the oral cavity of elderly. *Brazilian Dental Journal*, *23*(5), 534−538. Available from https://doi.org/10.1590/S0103-64402012000500011.

Meurman, J. H., & Stamatova, I. (2007). Probiotics: Contributions to oral health. *Oral Diseases*, *13*(5), 443−451. Available from https://doi.org/10.1111/j.1601-0825.2007.01386.x.

Mishra, R., Shobha, T., Monika, R., & Molay, B. (2016). Antimicrobial efficacy of probiotic and herbal oral rinses against Candida albicans in children: A randomized clinical trial. *International Journal of Clinical Pediatric Dentistry*, *9*(1), 25−30. Available from https://doi.org/10.5005/jp-journals-10005-1328.

Mittal, V., Jagzape, T., & Sachdeva, P. (2018). Care seeking behaviour of families for their sick infants and factors impeding to their early care seeking in rural part of central India. *Journal of Clinical and Diagnostic Research*, *12*(4), SC08−SC12. Available from https://doi.org/10.7860/JCDR/2018/28130.11401.

Miyazima, T. Y., Ishikawa, K. H., Mayer, M. P. A., Saad, S. M. I., & Nakamae, A. E. M. (2017). Cheese supplemented with probiotics reduced the Candida levels in denture wearers—RCT. *Oral Diseases*, *23*(7), 919−925. Available from https://doi.org/10.1111/odi.12669.

Murzyn, A., Krasowska, A., Stefanowicz, P., Dziadkowiec, D., & Łukaszewicz, M. (2010). Capric acid secreted by *S. boulardii* inhibits *C. albicans* filamentous growth, adhesion and biofilm formation. *Plos one*, *5*(8), e12050.

Nguyen, L. N., Lopes, L. C. L., Cordero, R. J. B., & Nosanchuk, J. D. (2011). Sodium butyrate inhibits pathogenic yeast growth and enhances the functions of macrophages. *Journal of Antimicrobial Chemotherapy*, *66*(11), 2573−2580. Available from https://doi.org/10.1093/jac/dkr358.

Paul, S., & Kannan, I. (2019). Molecular identification and antifungal susceptibility pattern of Candida species isolated from HIV infected patients with candisiasis. *Current Medical Mycology*, *5*(1), 21−26. Available from https://doi.org/10.18502/cmm.5.1.533.

Pendharkar, S., Brandsborg, E., Hammarström, L., Marcotte, H., & Larsson, P. G. (2015). Vaginal colonisation by probiotic lactobacilli and clinical outcome in women conventionally treated for bacterial vaginosis and yeast infection. *BMC Infectious Diseases*, *15*(1). Available from https://doi.org/10.1186/s12879-015-0971-3.

Perlin, D. S., Rautemaa-Richardson, R., & Alastruey-Izquierdo, A. (2017). The global problem of antifungal resistance: Prevalence, mechanisms, and management. *The Lancet Infectious Diseases*, *17*.

Perlroth, J., Choi, B., & Spellberg, B. (2007). Nosocomial fungal infections: Epidemiology, diagnosis, and treatment. *Medical Mycology*, *45*(4), 321−346. Available from https://doi.org/10.1080/13693780701218689.

Pfaller, M. A., Pappas, P. G., & Wingard, J. R. (2006). Invasive fungal pathogens: Current epidemiological trends. *Clinical Infectious Diseases*, *43*(1), S3−S14. Available from https://doi.org/10.1086/504490.

Prieto, D., Correia, I., Pla, J., & Román, E. (2016). Adaptation of Candida albicans to commensalism in the gut. *Future Microbiology*, *11*(4), 567−583. Available from https://doi.org/10.2217/fmb.16.1.

Puri, S., Fernandez, S., Puranik, A., Anand, D., Gaidhane, A., Quazi Syed, Z., Patel, A., Uddin, S., & Thow, A. M. (2017). Policy content and stakeholder network analysis for infant and young child feeding in India. *BMC Public Health*, *17*. Available from https://doi.org/10.1186/s12889-017-4339-z.

Rautela, R., Singh, A. K., Shukla, A., & Cameotra, S. S. (2014). Lipopeptides from Bacillus strain AR2 inhibits biofilm formation by Candida albicans. *Antonie van Leeuwenhoek, International Journal of General and Molecular Microbiology, 105*(5), 809–821. Available from https://doi.org/10.1007/s10482-014-0135-2.

Rishi, P., Preet, S., & Kaur, P. (2011). Effect of L. plantarum cell-free extract and co-trimoxazole against Salmonella Typhimurium: A possible adjunct therapy. *Annals of Clinical Microbiology and Antimicrobials, 10*. Available from https://doi.org/10.1186/1476-0711-10-9.

Rivero-Menendez, O., Alastruey-Izquierdo, A., Mellado, E., & Cuenca-Estrella, M. (2016). Triazole resistance in Aspergillus spp.: A worldwide problem? *Journal of Fungi, 2*(3). Available from https://doi.org/10.3390/jof2030021.

Robbins, N., Caplan, T., & Cowen, L. E. (2017). Molecular evolution of antifungal drug resistance. *Annual Review of Microbiology, 71*, 753–775. Available from https://doi.org/10.1146/annurev-micro-030117-020345.

Romeo, M. G., Romeo, D. M., Trovato, L., Oliveri, S., Palermo, F., Cota, F., & Betta, P. (2011). Role of probiotics in the prevention of the enteric colonization by Candida in preterm newborns: incidence of late-onset sepsis and neurological outcome. *Journal of Perinatology, 31*(1), 63–69.

Roy, A., Chaudhuri, J., Sarkar, D., Ghosh, P., & Chakraborty, S. (2014). Role of enteric supplementation of Probiotics on late-onset sepsis by Candida species in preterm low birth weight neonates: A randomized, double blind, placebo-controlled trial. *North American Journal of Medical Sciences, 6*(1), 50–57. Available from https://doi.org/10.4103/1947-2714.125870.

Russo, R., Superti, F., Karadja, E., & De Seta, F. (2019). Randomised clinical trial in women with Recurrent Vulvovaginal Candidiasis: Efficacy of probiotics and lactoferrin as maintenance treatment. *Mycoses*. Available from https://doi.org/10.1111/myc.12883.

Salvatori, O., Puri, S., Tati, S., & Edgerton, M. (2016). Innate immunity and saliva in Candida albicans-mediated oral diseases. *Journal of Dental Research, 95*(4), 365–371. Available from https://doi.org/10.1177/0022034515625222.

Sam, Q. H., Chang, M. W., & Chai, L. Y. A. (2017). The fungal mycobiome and its interaction with gut bacteria in the host. *International Journal of Molecular Sciences, 18*(2). Available from https://doi.org/10.3390/ijms18020330.

Santos, A. L., Jorge, A. O. C., dos Santos, S. S. F., e Silva, C. R. G., & Leão, M. V. P. (2009). Influence of probiotics on Candida presence and IgA anti-Candida in the oral cavity. *Brazilian Journal of Microbiology, 40*(4), 960–964. Available from https://doi.org/10.1590/s1517-83822009000400030.

Scharschmidt, T. C., & Fischbach, M. A. (2013). What lives on our skin: Ecology, genomics and therapeutic opportunities of the skin microbiome. *Drug Discovery Today: Disease Mechanisms, 10*(3–4), e83–e89. Available from https://doi.org/10.1016/j.ddmec.2012.12.003.

Shah, M. P., Gujjari, S. K., & Chandrasekhar, V. S. (2013). Evaluation of the effect of probiotic (Inersan R) alone, combination of probiotic with doxycycline and doxycycline alone on aggressive periodontitis—A clinical and microbiological study. *Journal of Clinical and Diagnostic Research, 7*(3), 595–600. Available from https://doi.org/10.7860/JCDR/2013/5225.2834.

Shehata, M. G., El Sohaimy, S. A., El-Sahn, M. A., & Youssef, M. M. (2016). Screening of isolated potential probiotic lactic acid bacteria for cholesterol lowering property and bile salt hydrolase activity. *Annals of Agricultural Sciences, 61*(1), 65–75. Available from https://doi.org/10.1016/j.aoas.2016.03.001.

Sherry, L., Ramage, G., Kean, R., Borman, A., Johnson, E. M., Richardson, M. D., & Rautemaa-Richardson, R. (2017). Biofilm-forming capability of highly virulent, multidrug-resistant Candida auris. *Emerging Infectious Diseases, 23*(2), 328–331. Available from https://doi.org/10.3201/eid2302.161320.

Shively, C. A., Register, T. C., Appt, S. E., Clarkson, T. B., Uberseder, B., Clear, K. Y. J., Wilson, A. S., Chiba, A., Tooze, J. A., & Cook, K. L. (2018). Consumption of mediterranean vs western diet leads to distinct mammary gland microbiome populations. *Cell Reports, 25*(1), 47–56.e3. Available from https://doi.org/10.1016/j.celrep.2018.08.078.

Shokryazdan, P., Faseleh Jahromi, M., Liang, J. B., & Ho, Y. W. (2017). Probiotics: From isolation to application. *Journal of the American College of Nutrition, 36*(8), 666–676. Available from https://doi.org/10.1080/07315724.2017.1337529.

Slattery, J., MacFabe, D. F., & Frye, R. E. (2016). The significance of the enteric microbiome on the development of childhood disease: A review of prebiotic and probiotic therapies in disorders of childhood. *Clinical Medicine Insights: Pediatrics, 10*. Available from https://doi.org/10.4137/cmped.s38338.

Song, Y. G., & Lee, S. H. (2017). Inhibitory effects of *Lactobacillus rhamnosus* and *Lactobacillus casei* on Candida biofilm of denture surface. *Archives of Oral Biology, 76*, 1–6. Available from https://doi.org/10.1016/j.archoralbio.2016.12.014.

Suez, J., Zmora, N., Segal, E., & Elinav, E. (2019). The pros, cons, and many unknowns of probiotics. *Nature Medicine, 25*(5), 716–729. Available from https://doi.org/10.1038/s41591-019-0439-x.

Sutula, J., Coulthwaite, L., Thomas, L., & Verran, J. (2012). The effect of a commercial probiotic drink on oral microbiota in healthy complete denture wearers. *Microbial Ecology in Health and Disease, 23*(1), 18404.

Sutula, J., Coulthwaite, L. A., Thomas, L. V., & Verran, J. (2013). The effect of a commercial probiotic drink containing *Lactobacillus casei* strain Shirota on oral health in healthy dentate people. *Microbial Ecology in Health and Disease, 24*(1), 21003.

Szalewski, D. A., Hinrichs, V. S., Zinniel, D. K., & Barletta, R. G. (2018). The pathogenicity of Aspergillus fumigatus, drug resistance, and nanoparticle delivery. *Canadian Journal of Microbiology, 64*(7), 439–453. Available from https://doi.org/10.1139/cjm-2017-0749.

Thompson, G. R., Patel, P. K., Kirkpatrick, W. R., Westbrook, S. D., Berg, D., Erlandsen, J., Redding, S. W., & Patterson, T. F. (2010). Oropharyngeal candidiasis in the era of antiretroviral therapy. *Oral Surgery, Oral Medicine, Oral Pathology, Oral Radiology and Endodontology, 109*(4), 488–495. Available from https://doi.org/10.1016/j.tripleo.2009.11.026.

Thow, A. M., Karn, S., Devkota, M. D., Rasheed, S., Roy, S., Suleman, Y., Hazir, T., Patel, A., Gaidhane, A., Puri, S., Godakandage, S., Senarath, U., & Dibley, M. J. (2017). Opportunities for strengthening infant and young child feeding policies in South Asia: Insights from the SAIFRN policy analysis project. *BMC Public Health, 17*. Available from https://doi.org/10.1186/s12889-017-4336-2.

Uddin, S., Mahmood, H., Senarath, U., Zahiruddin, Q., Karn, S., Rasheed, S., & Dibley, M. (2017). Analysis of stakeholders networks of infant and young child nutrition programmes in Sri Lanka, India, Nepal, Bangladesh and Pakistan. *BMC Public Health, 17*. Available from https://doi.org/10.1186/s12889-017-4337-1.

Ujaoney, S., Chandra, J., Faddoul, F., Chane, M., Wang, J., Taifour, L., Mamtani, M. R., Thakre, T. P., Kulkarni, H., Mukherjee, P., & Ghannoum, M. A. (2014). In vitro effect of over-the-counter probiotics on the ability of Candida albicans to form biofilm on denture strips. *American Dental Hygienists' Association, 88*(3), 183–189.

van de Veerdonk, F. L., Gresnigt, M. S., Luigina, R., Netea, M. G., & Jean-Paul, L. (2017). Aspergillus fumigatus morphology and dynamic host interactions. *Nature Reviews. Microbiology*, 661–674. Available from https://doi.org/10.1038/nrmicro.2017.90.

Verdenelli, M. C., Coman, M. M., Cecchini, C., Silvi, S., Orpianesi, C., & Cresci, A. (2014). Evaluation of antipathogenic activity and adherence properties of human *Lactobacillus* strains for vaginal formulations. *Journal of Applied Microbiology, 116*(5), 1297–1307.

Vicariotto, F., Del Piano, M., Mogna, L., & Mogna, G. (2012). Effectiveness of the association of 2 probiotic strains formulated in a slow release vaginal product, in women affected by vulvovaginal candidiasis: a pilot study. *Journal of Clinical Gastroenterology, 46*, S73–S80.

Vilela, S. F. G., Barbosa, J. O., Rossoni, R. D., Santos, J. D., Prata, M. C. A., Anbinder, A. L., Jorge, A. O. C., & Junqueira, J. C. (2015). Lactobacillus acidophilus ATCC 4356 inhibits biofilm formation by C. albicans and attenuates the experimental candidiasis in Galleria mellonella. *Virulence, 6*(1), 29–39. Available from https://doi.org/10.4161/21505594.2014.981486.

Wang, F. J., Zhang, D., Liu, Z. H., Wu, W. X., Bai, H. H., & Dong, H. Y. (2016). Species distribution and in vitro antifungal susceptibility of vulvovaginal Candida isolates in China. *Chinese Medical Journal, 129*(10), 1161–1165. Available from https://doi.org/10.4103/0366-6999.181964.

Wu, S. X., Guo, N. R., Li, X. F., Liao, W. Q., Chen, M., Zhang, Q. Q., Li, C. Y., Li, R. Y., Bulmer, G. S., Li, D. M., & Xi, L. Y. (2011). Human pathogenic fungi in China—Emerging trends from ongoing national survey for 1986, 1996, and 2006. *Mycopathologia, 171*(6).

Xie, H. Y., Feng, D., Wei, D. M., Mei, L., Chen, H., Wang, X., & Fang, F. (2017). Probiotics for vulvovaginal candidiasis in non-pregnant women. *Cochrane Database of Systematic Reviews, 2017*(11). Available from https://doi.org/10.1002/14651858.CD010496.pub2.

Zeeuwen, P. L. J. M., Kleerebezem, M., Timmerman, H. M., & Schalkwijk, J. (2013). Microbiome and skin diseases. *Current Opinion in Allergy and Clinical Immunology, 13*(5), 514–520. Available from https://doi.org/10.1097/ACI.0b013e328364ebeb.

Zhao, C., Lv, X., Fu, J., He, C., Hua, H., & Yan, Z. (2016). In vitro inhibitory activity of probiotic products against oral Candida species. *Journal of Applied Microbiology, 121*(1), 254–262. Available from https://doi.org/10.1111/jam.13138.

Zuo, T., & Ng, S. C. (2018). The gut microbiota in the pathogenesis and therapeutics of inflammatory bowel disease. *Frontiers in Microbiology, 9*. Available from https://doi.org/10.3389/fmicb.2018.02247.

Chapter 22

Role of probiotics in the prevention and management of diabetes and obesity

Rashmi Hogarehalli Mallappa[1], Chandrasekhar Balasubramaniam[1], Monica Rose Amarlapudi[1], Shweta Kelkar[1], Gbenga Adedeji Adewumi[2], Saurabh Kadyan[1], Diwas Pradhan[1] and Sunita Grover[1]

[1]Molecular Biology Unit, Dairy Microbiology Division, ICAR-National Dairy Research Institute, Karnal, India, [2]Department of Microbiology, Faculty of Science, University of Lagos, Lagos, Nigeria

22.1 Introduction

Diabetes and obesity emerged as dual or combined epidemic (diabesity) and are of important public health issue worldwide (Bhupathiraju & Hu, 2016; Ng et al., 2021). By 2030, the global prevalence of diabetes is projected to increase by 10.1%, and the higher prevalence of diabetes was identified in association with obesity (IDF data). Diabetes is a chronic metabolic disease, characterized by elevated levels of blood glucose (blood sugar), which is either a result of the incompetence of the pancreas to produce enough insulin [type 1 diabetes (T1D)], or failure of the body to effectively use the insulin it produces [type 2 diabetes (T2D)] (American Diabetes Association). The increased blood glucose as a result of T1D or T2D, and over time, can cause serious complications to the body (physical component, mental component, cogitative component, psychological and social components), such as diabetic retinopathy, neuropathy, nephropathy, hypertension, foot ulceration, and congestive heart failure (Aikaterini et al., 2017). Moreover, many of these complications significantly deteriorate the quality, productivity, and expectancy of patient's life (Papatheodorou et al., 2017).

The increasing prevalence of diabetes was found in association with obesity, which not only increases the risk of developing diabetes particularly T2D but also compounds its health risks and complicates the management. Although T1D has been largely precipitated by immune destruction of insulin and perseveres in lean individuals, recent reports showed that their obesity rate surpassed that of the general population (Mottalib et al., 2017). This close relationship between diabetes and obesity led to the connotation "diabesity," suggesting a causal pathophysiological link between both phenomena (Ng et al., 2021). However, the molecular mechanisms underlying these complications are complex to understand and three main hypotheses have been developed in recent years to bridge the gap between epidemiology and pathobiochemistry of diabesity: (1) the "inflammation hypothesis," where obesity represents a state of chronic low-grade systemic inflammation in which inflammatory molecules produced by infiltrating macrophages in adipose tissue exert pathological changes in β-cells and insulin-sensitive tissues; (2) the "lipid overflow hypothesis," when the storage capacity of adipose tissue is exceeded with surplus lipids, accumulation of lipids in organs (steatosis) including the pancreas, results in insulin resistance; and (3) the "adipokine hypothesis," where expanding volume of adipose tissue during obesity raises circulating levels of these inflammatory markers, is therefore thought to contribute to insulin resistance (Chadt et al., 2018).

Various genetic and environmental/lifestyle factors are considered responsible for the pathogenesis of diabetes and obesity and the number of patients is increasing rapidly in recent decades reflecting lifestyle changes as a major contributor toward higher prevalence of diabesity globally (Kolb & Martin, 2017). Advances in the understanding of the pathogenesis of diabetes and obesity have revealed the role of gut microbiota dysbiosis as a driving factor of these diseases, besides suggesting therapeutic strategies to restore healthy host–microbiota relationship (gut symbiosis/eubiosis) in the management of T2D and obesity (Gurung et al., 2020).

The amelioration of gut dysbiosis using specific group of probiotics, prebiotics, and synbiotics has been found beneficial in the prevention and treatment of different disease disorders, including diabetes and obesity, as they are well-known ingredients of functional foods and nutraceuticals and may provide beneficial health effects, by influencing intestinal microbial ecology and immunity (Panwar et al., 2013; Sunita et al., 2012). Accumulating evidence highlighted the role of probiotics as prophylactics or therapeutics in the management of diabetes and obesity as probiotics−gut microbiota, and host interaction directs and contributes to a plethora of essential physiological functions, such as energy metabolism, metabolic signaling in glucose metabolism and secretion of hormones (insulin and gut hormones), formation of the immune system, regulation of integrity, and mobility of the gut barrier (Ahmad et al., 2019). Hence, this chapter is dedicated to discuss the pathophysiology of diabetes mellitus (DM) and obesity, and the role of probiotics as gut microbiota modulators, prophylactics in the prevention, and therapeutics in the management of DM and obesity.

22.2 Pathophysiology and risk factors of diabetes mellitus and obesity

DM is a complex metabolic disorder associated with an increased risk of microvascular and macrovascular disease. The last century has been characterized by remarkable leads in our understanding of the pathophysiological mechanisms leading to DM and obesity. Further advancements in understanding the role of human microbial ecosystem in relation to health and disease have provided substantial evidence on the role of gut microbiota in metabolic diseases including DM and obesity.

22.2.1 Pathophysiology and risk factors of T1D

T1D is a chronic autoimmune disorder, caused by insulin deficiency that eventually leads to hyperglycemia. Over the past three decades, knowledge of T1D has grown substantially on many aspects of the disease, including its heterogeneity, pancreatic pathology, and epidemiology.

T1DM results from the autoimmune destruction of β cells in the pancreas leading to insulin deficiency. Pathogenesis of T1DM is different from that of T2DM, where both insulin resistance and reduced secretion of insulin by the β cells play a synergistic role. Various factors, such as genetic (major histocompatibility complex region often called HLA (human leukocyte antigen), environmental (rubella, coxsackievirus B or enteroviruses), toxins, nutrients (cow's milk, cereals), and immunological (islet cell-specific antibodies or other organ-specific antibodies and antibodies against certain treatment therapies) are involved in the destruction of β cells of the endocrine pancreas and lead to insulin deficiency. The application of genome-wide association studies (GWASs) has robustly revealed several genetic contributors or loci that act on the immune system in the pathogenesis of T1D. These observations strongly strengthened the concept of a stronger autoimmune component of T1D in younger children. However, genetic susceptibility cannot explain the increased incidence of T1D in the older age category, which is very likely attributed to the growing impact of environmental factors. There is substantial evidence of gut microbiota influencing genes (directly or indirectly) associated with immune responses to pathogens and commensals and it is likely that autoimmunity would be affected directly or indirectly as well. Although results often vary between studies, the gut microbial composition and diversity patterns have considerably varied between T1D and healthy subject in most of the longitudinal and cross-sectional human studies (Vaarala, 2012; Zheng et al., 2018).

22.2.2 Gut microbiota in T1D

Several studies have revealed that human gut microbiome can influence the pathogenesis of immune diseases, predominantly autoimmune diseases including T1D. The origin of T1D was speculated to be gut microbiota dysbiosis (i.e., bacterial imbalance in composition and function), associated with compromised gut permeability and a major vulnerability of the immune system. Gut microbial composition and function are *dynamic* in infancy and several studies emphasized the role of the intestinal microbiota in the maturation and development of immune functions. However, at the same time, it can be affected by multiple factors during course of development. During childbirth, gut microbiome of infants is largely influenced by delivery mode. However, the gut microbiome of vaginally delivered infants was found closer to the mother's vaginal microbiome (Dunn et al., 2017; Mitchell et al., 2020). Later, during child development, gut microbiome is largely affected by diet, antibiotics usage, medicine, life style, and other socio economic and geographic factors. For example, high-fat and high-sugar diet affected the incidence of diabetes by causing dysbiosis of gut microbiota, particularly the decreased *Bifidobacterium* spp., which affects GI tract metabolism and immune homeostasis (Brown et al., 2012). Besides, use of antibiotics or antiinfective medications early in childhood may increase the risk of T1D by affecting the development of gut-microbial-mediated immunity (Langdon et al., 2016; Vangay et al., 2015). In addition, socio-demographic and behavioral factors influenced the gut microbial composition and function and showed varied results in T1D onset (Traversi et al., 2020).

Various studies have established significant differences in the microbial composition (microbiome) and function (metabolome) between subjects with T1D or islet autoimmunity and healthy control (Siljander et al., 2019; Vaarala, 2012). Though most of the findings originated from cross-sectional studies, they could not establish a direct link between gut microbiota and T1D, and the interplay between host and microbes in the development of T1D; however, these studies are important steps in the direction of assessing the role of gut microbiota in the pathogenesis of T1D (Dedrick et al., 2020).

Along with the diverse microbiota, the presence of specific gut microflora has crucial role in development of nascent immune system. The disturbed homeostasis of gut microbiome accelerates the progression of hyperglycemia or T1D. In the human gut ecosystem, *Firmicutes* and *Bacteroidetes* are the dominant phyla accounting for almost 90% of the total microbial population, which without any surprise alterations in their composition affect the gut immune system (Shen et al., 2018). Hence, *Firmicutes/Bacteroidetes* (F/B) *ratio* has been widely accepted to have an important influence in maintaining normal *gut homeostasis and immune system* (Belkaid & Hand, 2014). Increased or decreased F/B *ratio* is regarded as dysbiosis. Compared with healthy control group, the *Firmicutes/Bacteroides* (F/B) ratio was found significantly reduced in T1D patients (Bibbò et al., 2017). A reduction in F/B ratio was also seen in other studies of different geographic origin. However, contradictory data with regard to F/B ratio in T1D individuals have also been published (Zhou et al., 2020). These differences may be attributed to different sample sizes, sequencing and data analysis approaches, and geographical location. Another common gut microbiome shift associated with the T1D is the decreased microbial diversity, which has been widely reported both in T1D children. In intestinal bacterial taxonomic studies, significant reduction in the abundance of butyrate producers, such as *Clostridium* clusters IV and XIVa, and mucin-degrading bacteria, such as *Prevotella* and *Akkermansia*, was were reported in T1D patients (Fig. 22.1). A significant decrease in *Bifidobacterium* was also reported in T1D subjects by several studies, which used several techniques including analysis of microbial culturome, transcriptome and proteome besides 16S ribosomal RNA (rRNA) gene sequencing. In addition, the colonization of intestinal *Candida albicans* was also reported to be positively linked to T1D development (Zhou et al., 2020).

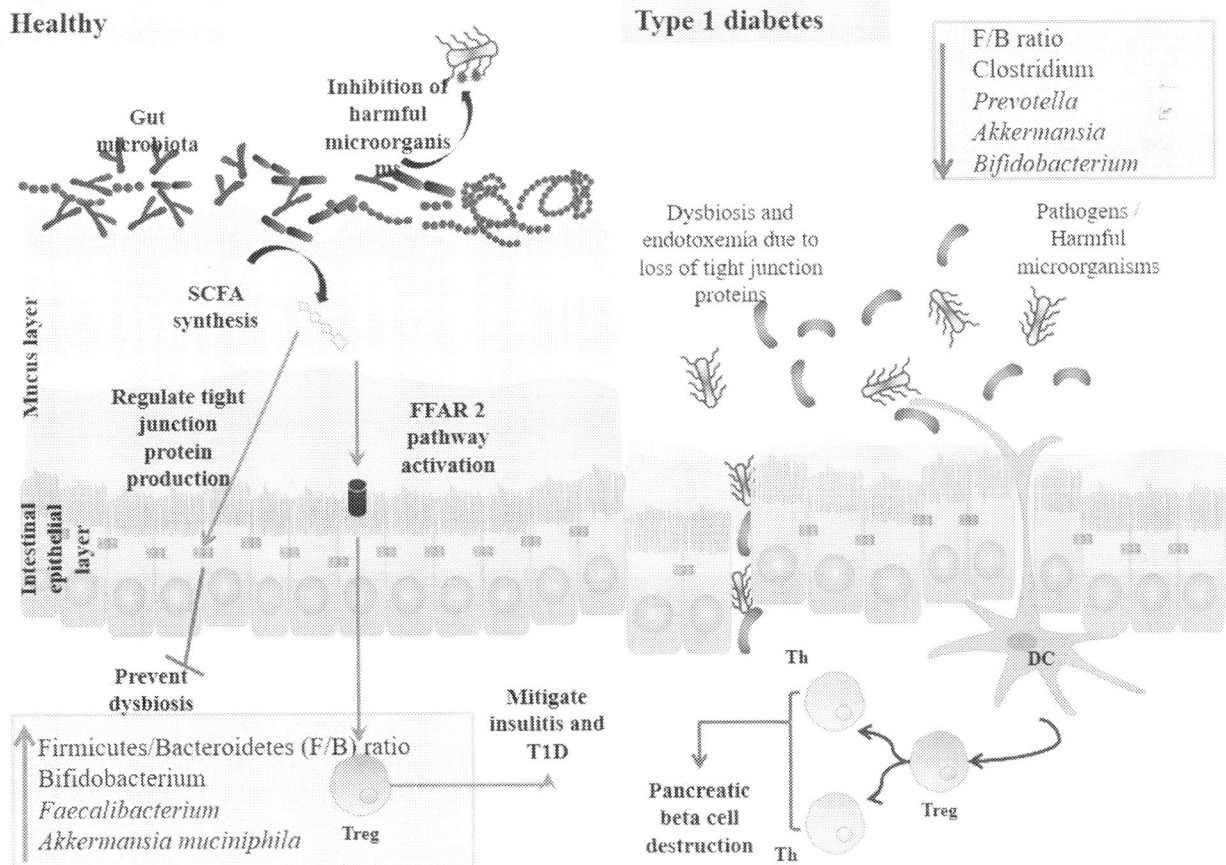

FIGURE 22.1 Gut microbiome in healthy and type 1 diabetic conditions.

The microbiome in the human gut ecosystem interacts with host epithelial cells in two major pathways mainly through "toll-like receptors (TLRs)" and "free fatty acid receptors—2/3." As mentioned earlier, lipopolysacharide (LPS) is one of the factors that interact with host cells via TLRs. Other than the cell surface compounds like LPS, gut microorganisms *Faecalibacterium prausnitzii* and *Clostridium leptum* of Firmicutes phylum play key role in the production of short-chain fatty acids (SCFAs) (for their own benefit). For certain gut microorganisms, SCFAs are the readily accessible energy source. Among them butyrate is the dominant SCFA that aids in the production of tight junction proteins preventing the translocation of certain pathobionts and inflammatory compounds (LPS). Several studies reported that the SCFA, especially butyrate, has the ability to trigger the regulation of T cell [differentiation and proliferation of T regulatory cells (Tregs)] via FFAR 2 pathway and thereby reduce the progression of insulitis and diabetes. Meanwhile, the SCFAs, such as acetate and propionate, help in the migration of the T cells, which are regulated by butyrate. Studies prove that the development of T1D is inversely proportional to the butyrate concentration (in blood and feces during medical diagnosis) (Mishra et al., 2019; Wen & Wong, 2017).

Like microbiome, metabolome plays a key role in gut homeostasis. Branched chain amino acids (leucine, isoleucine, and valine) are also equally important in maintaining the gut homeostasis. They trigger the stimulation of S6K1 (kinase that phosphorylates IRS-1) and m-TOR (kinase complex). Regulation of S6K1 increases the insulin sensitivity and thereby reduces insulin resistance (Barlow et al., 2015; Mishra et al., 2019; Sikalidis & Maykish, 2020). Therefore depending on the type of metabolites produced by gut microbiota the mode of action changes, that is, they can act either as triggering factors or as ameliorating factors in the progression of T1D.

Recent studies found that gut microbiome also have direct impact on the wellness of pancreas (due to anatomic relation of pancreas and gut). Long back pancreas was considered as a sterile organ, but the recent studies show that the pancreas is having its own hub of microorganisms which can modulate the gut immune system (gut—pancreas axis) (Dedrick et al., 2020; Thomas & Jobin, 2020). SCFA (butyrate) produced by gut microbiota triggers the regulation of cathelicidins and related antimicrobial peptide (CRAMP) by islet cells of pancreas during T1D.

22.2.3 Pathophysiology and risk factors of T2D

T2D is a complex, polygenic disease with heterogenous pathophysiology, characterized by impairment in the metabolism of carbohydrates, lipids, and proteins. It has a multifactorial etiology, comprising complex interactions among factors, such as genetic predisposition, lifestyle, diet and environmental elements, and epigenetic changes (Kolb & Martin, 2017), that affect β-cell function and tissue (muscle, liver, adipose tissue, and pancreas) insulin sensitivity (Fig. 22.2). Hyperglycemia (high blood sugar levels) results when insulin secretion from β cells is unable to compensate for insulin

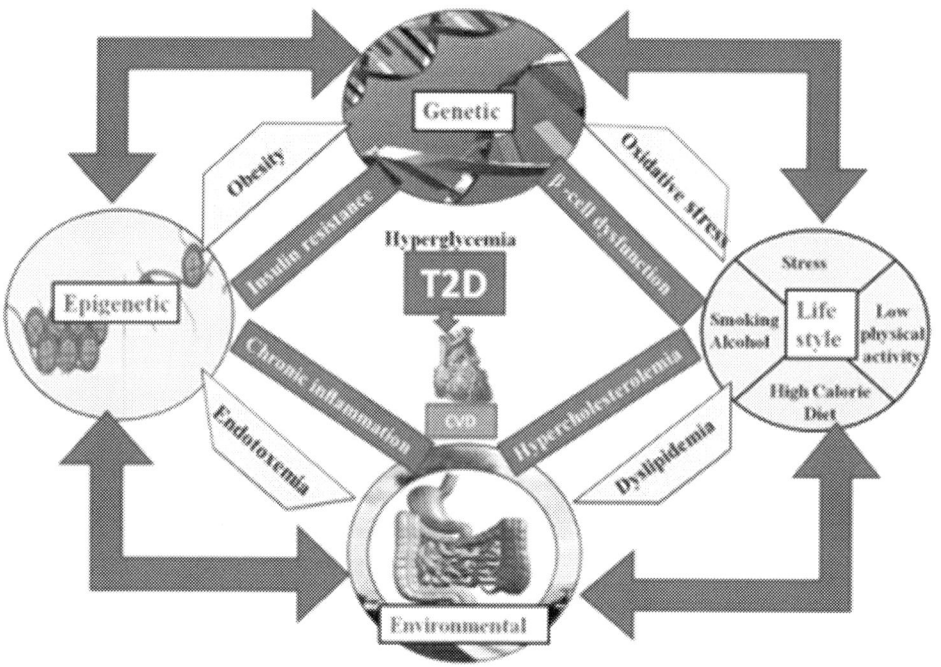

FIGURE 22.2 Pathophysiology of type 2 diabetes.

resistance (Cerf, 2013; Zaccardi et al., 2016). The progressive decline in the β-cell function and mass over time with hyperglycemia marks the development of T2D (Dendup et al., 2018; Kahn et al., 2014).

Obesity is the leading risk factor for T2D. Ectopic fat in the liver, muscles, and pancreas from surplus calories and physical inactivity contributes to β-cell dysfunction and insulin resistance (Zaccardi et al., 2016). Besides, inflammation induced by specific proinflammatory cytokines, oxidative and endoplasmic-reticulum (ER) stress, raised lipid levels, and amyloid accumulation also triggers β-cell dysfunction (Hasnain et al., 2016; Phillips et al., 2014). Group of gastrointestinal hormones are the largest endocrine organ of the body and nervous system including the brain also acts on β cells in response to nutrient signals (insulinotropic effect/incretin effect) (Nauck et al., 1986) and the diminished incretin effect was reported with the occurrence of T2D (Boer & Holst, 2020). The pathophysiology of T2D is now a 90-year-old perspective (Zaccardi et al., 2016). The advanced cellular and molecular understanding of diabetes in the last decades have shifted the traditional "glucocentric" view of diabetes to broader and more inclusive pathophysiological changes that resulted in a better patient phenotyping and therapeutic approach. The most important pathophysiological shifts observed in the last decade is the gut microbial shift (alteration in the gut microbial composition), which today are the important pathophysiological target of T2D (Blandino et al., 2016). The role of gut microbiota in T2D diabetes has been well established with several preclinical animal models of T2D and in clinical trials. The results of these studies found potential application in the use of gut microbiota in clinical applications for understanding its role in pathophysiology of T2D and management of T2D with gut microbiota-directed dietary strategies using probiotics, prebiotics, and synbiotics.

22.2.4 Role of gut microbiota in T2D

Dysbiosis in the composition and function of the gut microbiota has been associated with the pathophysiology of most chronic diseases ranging from common intestinal diseases and metabolic diseases to respiratory, urinary, neurological, cardiovascular, and respiratory *illness* (Durack & Lynch, 2019). exception in this aspect. Indeed, there is a substantial body of literature on the role of gut microbiota on glucose metabolism generated with well-designed preclinical animal and clinical human studies on T2D. An increasing number of data obtained during the last decade have indicated changes in gut bacterial composition or function in T2D patients. Analysis of this gut microbial "dysbiosis" using metagenomic approaches has enabled the detection of alterations in specific bacteria, clusters of bacteria, or bacterial functions associated with the occurrence or development of T2D (Delzenne et al., 2015; Woldeamlak et al., 2019). Though these studies yielded substantial results to corroborate the role of gut microbiota in T2D, concerns have been raised about the variability of the results. Considerable differences in the diversity of microbiota, *Bacteroides/Firmicutes* ratio, and different taxa have been reported in association with T2D in different studies. Recently a large study observed that different microbes were found associated with the same metabolic outcomes in different geographical areas (He et al., 2018). Though it appeared challenging to derive conclusive results with respect to a definite group of bacterial taxa associated with T2D, it is important to note that differences between results and interpretations are common features of gut microbial studies since gut microbial composition is highly influenced by host genetic factors, health, diet, and geography as discussed in several studies. However, the major contributors of gut microbial dysbiosis (pathobionts) have been found to be associated with low-grade inflammation, endotoxemia, and increased intestinal permeability in T2D (Delzenne et al., 2015) and disparities regarding the association of particular taxonomic groups of gut bacteria with the disease. A recent systematic review summarized the evidence of 42 human clinical studies, which reported microbial associations with T2D. Among the commonly reported findings, the bacterial genera of *Bifidobacterium*, *Bacteroides*, *Faecalibacterium*, *Akkermansia*, and *Roseburia* were negatively associated with the development of T2D, while the genera of *Ruminococcus*, *Fusobacterium*, and *Blautia* were positively associated with T2D. The *Lactobacillus* genus, which is among the most studied probiotic genera presented a complex case with conflicting results when considering its association to T2D. But, an association of this genera tends to be species specific or even strain specific, which clearly explained the inconsistency associated with establishing its role in the development of T2D (Gurung et al., 2020). On the other hand, other commensal beneficial gut microbial organisms (probionts including bifidobacteria and lactobacilli) have been found to play a key role in the management of T2D by improving gut inflammation, endotoxemia, and gut barrier function (Cani & Delzenne, 2009). Currently, the use of pro-, pre-, and synbiotics and other new strategies, such as gut microbiota transplant, or even antibiotic therapy, has been proposed to be useful tools to modulate the development of obesity and insulin resistance through the diet (Muñoz-Garach et al., 2016).

22.2.5 Pathophysiology and risk factors of obesity

Obesity, a trivial metabolic disorder in its infancy, has reached pandemic proportions. It is generally defined as possessing excess body weight (BW) with respect to a given height (Gadde et al., 2018). Obesity is the most common abnormality that contributes to a constellation of symptoms generally leading to a metabolic syndrome. It is widely associated with numerous other chronic diseases, such as hypertension, T2D, and cardiovascular diseases. Its global presence is accentuated by an obesogenic environment characterized by easy access to low-cost calorie dense food, evolving technologies that obviate physical activity coupled with cheap nonphysical entertainment. In addition, excessive intake of carbohydrates and sugars furthered by an increasing emphasis on consumption of a low-fat diet is also a potential contributor to the obesogenic environment. The simple causative factors favoring the obesogenic environment have aided in the rampant spread of the disorder and making obesity one among the prime health concerns across the globe in current times. Obesity is a multifactorial disorder with a complex pathogenesis involving genetic, medical, socio-cultural, physiological, epigenetic, and a multitude of other factors contributing to causation and its persistence (Oussaada et al., 2019). At the most basic level, obesity is simply believed to be caused due to an abnormal energy homeostasis characterized by increased calorie intake, exceeding the ongoing energy expenditure (Emilio, 2013). Like diabetes, gene—environmental interaction has been found associated with the development of obesity (Sheikh et al., 2017). GWASs have discovered associations of numerous SNPs and genes with obesity (Schlauch et al., 2020).

The neurological connection to obesity is also being gradually established. The obesity genes are found to have considerable influence on the central nervous system. The suppression of appetite and energy expenditure is augmented by leptin-melanocortin pathway (Izquierdo et al., 2019). Ghrelin is secreted in abundance in the stomach when the body is in the restriction of food, hence inducing satiety. It is a peptide hormone that binds to its cognate receptors and enhances the expression of neuropeptide Y (NPY) and agouti-related protein (AgRP) in the orexigenic neurons. The melanocortin-4 receptor (MC4R) in the hypothalamus binds AgRP showing antagonistic activity, NPY binds to its respective receptor, increasing appetite and decreasing energy expenditure. The Leptin hormone regulates hunger by binding to orexigenic neurons located within the hypothalamus and leads to pathway inhibition through the production of AgRP/NPY. Furthermore, the binding of leptin to anorexigenic neurons leads to the expression of proopiomelanocortin (POMC) and cocaine- and amphetamine-related transcript (CART), which in turn stimulates this pathway. Both POMC and CART induce the expression of MC4R in the PVN, decreasing the appetite and increasing energy expenditure (Oussaada et al., 2019).

In addition, other related genes expressed in hypothalamus, having role in energy balance and appetite includes brain-derived neurotrophic factor (*BDNF*) and fat mass and obesity-associated (*FTO*) genes. *BDNF* plays a significant role in developmental stages where it is involved in modulating energy metabolism through neuronal survival, maturation, and differentiation during hypothalamic development. Enzyme coded by *FTO* has demethylation ability and plays a crucial role in the regulation of food intake and energy expenditure in both mice and humans (Oussaada et al., 2019).

Although genetic factors exclusively cannot be accounted for the rapid increase in obesity prevalence during the past 40 years, it is possible that the interplay between genetic factors and environmental influences binate the risk of obesity by favoring a positive energy balance (higher calorie intake, less physical activity, or both) and/or result in the biological defense of increased fat mass. The long list of potentially relevant environmental factors includes changes in diet composition and lifestyle, environmental toxins, infections, changes in the microbiome, and many others as well.

The coevolved human microbiota is having complex and diverse role in human health. The gut microbiota has cohabited humans and have become an essential part, earning the sobriquet of a "hidden organ" with many important and indispensable functions. The dysbiosis in gut microbiota (quantitative and/or qualitative deficiency of the gut microbiota) probably is a basis of many disorders, including obesity. The plethora of scientific studies including preclinical, clinical, and *meta*-analysis clearly revealed the direct role of gut microbiota in the obesity as it directly affects the food digestion, absorption, and metabolism besides controlling appetite and energy balance. On the other hand, lifestyle and food regimen affect the diversity of the gut microbiota and the ensuing dysbiosis.

22.2.6 Gut microbiota and obesity

As already stated, obesity is a consequence of a multitude of factors. It is strongly believed that the gut microbiome is one of the leading contributors to the disease pathogenesis. The consortia of microbes in the gut not only aids in digestion and absorption of nutrients but also plays a crucial role in the homeostatic maintenance of metabolism, immunity, and gut barrier integrity (Francine et al., 2021). The alterations in gut microbiota composition and function together modulate the host energy metabolism. As an increasing body of literature hint at the involvement of GM in regulating metabolism and immune homeostasis, a putative GM imbalance (dysbiosis) can be a probable trigger for both metabolic and autoimmune disorder. Lately, many studies have shown that a correlation between BW maintenance and GM is extremely likely and have also demonstrated that gut microbiome changes decrease BW and fat mass and ameliorate insulin sensitivity (Francine et al., 2021; Lee et al., 2020).

Ley et al. (2006) devised a genetic model of obesity, wherein he revealed that gnotobiotic mice upon colonization with the microbiota from a genetically obese (ob/ob) mice resulted in an elevated fat mass and BW. Furthermore, alterations in gut microbiota composition in obese individuals have resulted in an increased energy harvest from food and also assisted in the development of adiposity.

The scientific investigations have encountered a 50% reduction in *Bacteroidetes and a proportional increase of abundance of Firmicutes on* comparing the GM composition in genetically obese mice to their lean counterparts. In addition, the findings revealed an increase in number of Gram-negative species in GM as a consequence of consuming high-fat diets, promoting greater intestinal absorption of lipopolysaccharides, the increase of which is defined as "metabolic endotoxemia." Few studies have also highlighted that endotoxemia leads to fasted hyperglycemia and hyperinsulinemia, BW gain, similar to the one found in high-fat-fed mice. In addition, high-fat diets have been shown to promote the growth of pathobionts, triggering an innate immune-mediated inflammatory response, that culminate with proinflammatory cytokinesor toxic compounds' production. Fat storage is also influenced by other pathways including production of choline leading to the synthesis of very low-density lipoproteins and stimulation of bile acid farnesoid X receptor, which ultimately induces an increase in adiposity (Francine et al., 2021).

Several studies also illustrated the possible mechanisms used by the gut microbiota to modulate inflammation. Systemic inflammation is a type of inflammation triggered by the translocation of lipopolysaccharides LPSs, embedded in the outer membrane of Gram-negative bacteria. This was aided by an impaired intestinal barrier functioning of obese individuals conferring a higher permeability compared with that of lean individuals. Second, metabolites like SCFA of gut bacteria were found to influence the host immune system. They were responsible for the activation of regulatory T cells with antiinflammatory capacity through stimulating expression of the transforming growth factor (TGFβ) from human intestinal epithelial cells. Besides, SCFA supplementation modulated insulin resistance and improved obesity. In other animal studies, *F. prausnitzii*, a prolific butyrate producer has shown to alleviate insulin resistance through induction of GLP-1 hormone secretion from the colonic L cells by signaling through the fatty acid receptor FFAR2. Another mechanism through which butyrate and propionate may influence host glucose metabolism is the activation of intestinal gluconeogenesis via complementary mechanisms.

In humans, several studies have illustrated that specific alterations in GM structure led to a proportional increase in *Firmicutes* and to a decrease in *Bacteroidetes* phylum. Also, studies have shown that subjects with low bacterial richness have higher titers of C-reactive protein and leptins, dyslipidemia, and insulin resistance, gain more weight, and have higher adiposity and inflammatory phenotype compared to that with high bacterial gene counts.

On comprehensive analysis, studies have revealed that obese individuals have a GM featured by a decrease in antiinflammatory bacteria and a global rise in pathogens. Such changes trigger a pronounced decrease in SCFAs' production, which ultimately impair intestinal barrier integrity and increase mucus degradation potential.

22.3 Probiotics for the management of diabetes and obesity

Consumers are increasingly interested in health management through diet and dietary supplements. The use of evidence-based approaches to improve diets and lifestyles is a trend that continues to grow among health-conscious consumers (Binda et al., 2020). A plethora of scientific evidence supports the claims related to the health benefits of probiotics. Among, major health benefits are improvement of nutritional and intestinal health of host, development, enhancement and maintenance of the immune health, and improvement in the metabolic health through their antioxidative, anticholesterol, antiobesity, and antidiabetic properties.

Most of these health benefits are strain specific and are imparted by an adequate number of probiotic bacteria in a dose-dependent manner. Some of the health benefits of these probiotic strains are well established with adequate scientific documentation while others, such as their impact on respiratory, reproductive, and neurological health and use in immune-compromised hosts, require additional scientific studies to be established.

The antidiabetic and antiobesity effects of probiotics are well studied with several preclinical and clinical studies, systematically reviewed, and assessed for potential application in them through *meta*-analysis studies.

22.3.1 Probiotics for the management of T1D

Probiotics are "symbionts of human gut microflora", have the ability to ameliorate host health by modulating immune system, protecting the gut membrane integrity by regulating certain gut microbial metabolic activities (production of SCFAs and secretion of gut hormones), and managing the bowel mechanisms, competitive pathogen exclusion, inhibitory action on certain harmful microorganisms (antimicrobial activity), and reduction of endotoxemia, and most

TABLE 22.1 Antidiabetic efficacy of probiotics against T1D.

Probiotic	Study model	Study design	Study outcome	References
Lactobacillus johnsonii N6.2	Bio-breeding diabetes-prone (BBDP) rat	Administered 10^8 CFU by oral gavage	Enhanced mucin production and upregulated Cox-2 gene. Decreased reactive oxygen species in the ileum	Valladares et al. (2010)
Lactobacillus johnsonii strain N6.2	BBDP rats	Administered 10^8 CFU daily for 21 days	Elevated Th17 cell differentiation and proliferation	Lau et al. (2011)
VSL#3	Four-week-old NOD mice	Administration of 3×10^{11}/g of viable lyophilized bacteria	Inhibits IL-1β and enhanced indoleamine 2,3-dioxygenase and IL-33 expression. Reduced differentiation/expansion of Th1 and Th17 cells in the intestinal mucosa cells	Dolpady et al. (2016)
Clostridium butyricum CGMCC0313.1	Three-week-old female NOD mice	Supplementation of *Clostridium butyricum* CGMCC0313.1 in powder form	Increased $\alpha 4\beta 7^+$ (the gut homing receptor) and Treg migration to pancreas. Enhanced the *Firmicutes/Bacteroidetes* ratio and butyrate-producing bacteria subgroups	Jia et al. (2017)

importantly help in maintaining the gut homeostasis. The mechanism of action of probiotic in the gut system is entirely strain specific. Several studies reported that specific strains of probiotics regulated both antiinflammatory (increased IL-10 levels) and proinflammatory cascades depending on the host health. All these above-mentioned properties of probiotics attenuate the progression of T1D- and diabetes-related health issues (obesity, cardiovascular disease, and hypertension) (Bermudez-Brito et al., 2012; Panwar et al., 2013).

The metabolites like SCFAs activate FFAR-2/3 pathways that regulate the proliferation and differentiation of Tregs (Table 22.1). Furthermore, FFAR 2 pathway enhanced the production of GLP-1 from the host intestinal cells. In some studies, GLP-1 was reported to elevate the beta cell (pancreatic beta cell) production which in essence increased the insulin secretion and reduced blood sugar levels (called as incretin effect). In this aspect, two potential probiotics *Lactobacillus kefiranofaciens* M and *Lactobacillus kefiri* K administration were reported to elevate the secretion of GLP-1 and antiinflammatory cytokine IL-10 (Wei et al., 2015).

Some studies reported that probiotic administration could modulate immune system by reducing certain inflammatory cytokines (IL-1, IL-6, IL-8, interferon-gamma, and TNF-α), high sensitivity C-reactive protein and by suppressing NF-kB pathway (systemic low-grade inflammation). This immunomodulation along with antioxidative property of probiotics has direct effect on reducing both insulin resistance and hyperglycemia condition. Besides, probiotics attenuated the circulation of endotoxin, which eventually affects glucose metabolism (Ruan et al., 2015; Shah & Swami, 2017).

22.3.2 Probiotics for the management of T2D

The gut microbial dysbiosis has been *described* to be *associated* with the development of T2D in several studies (Wei-Zheng et al., 2020). Hence, gut microbial-directed or -derived dietary strategies are promising avenue for the *management of* glycemic disorders including T2D. *Probiotics* have enormous *potential* for modifying *the gut* microbiota, achieving gut homeostasis besides conferring antidiabetic potential with the secretion of incretin hormones, production of SCFAs, and improvement of gut barrier function and inflammation (Panwar et al., 2013; Sunita et al., 2012; Wang et al., 2017).

Production of SCFAs (butyrate and propionate) by probionts proved to be involved in triggering/inducing the secretion of GLP-1, which is an important gut hormone with insulinotropic and satietogenic effects (Lin et al., 2012). The teratogenic effect of SCFA in the endogenous secretion of GLP-1 demonstrated via activation of SCFA receptors (ffar3 and ffar2), which clearly concluded the involvement of colonic epithelial receptors (G protein-coupled receptors) in the detection of luminal contents particularly bacterial metabolites (SCFA) in the host's energy metabolism via GLP-1 release, as well as the gut barrier and mucosal defense functions (Silva et al., 2020).

Several in vitro cell line models have demonstrated the antidiabetic effect of probiotics through their insulinotropic and satietogenic, hypoglycemic, antiinflammatory, and antioxidative effects (Fig. 22.3). The multistrain probiotic VSL#3 stimulated the GLP-1 secretion with increased expression of proglucagon and proprotein convertase/prohormone convertase (PC1/3) genes responsible for GLP-1 synthesis, which is a key insulinotropic and satietogenic hormone.

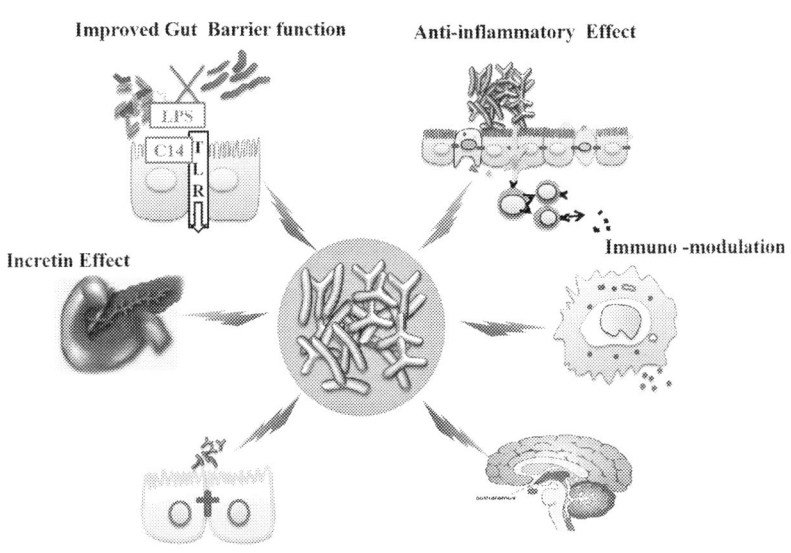

FIGURE 22.3 Mechanism of action of probiotics in type 2 diabetes.

TABLE 22.2 Antidiabetic efficacy of probiotic interventions against T2D in preclinical animal models.

Probiotic	Animal model	Result	References
Shubat (probiotic fermented Camel Milk)	Streptozotocin induced type-1 diabetes in male Wistar rats	Promotes production of GLP-1 improves function of β cells	Manaer et al. (2015)
Clostridium butyricum CGMCC0313.1 (CB0313.1)	Leptin db/db mice	(1) Decreased blood lipids and inflammation; (2) reversed hypohepatias and reduced glucose output; (3) decreased ratio of Firmicutes to Bacteroidetes; and (4) increased butyrate-producing bacteria	Jia et al. (2017)
Lactobacillus rhamnosus MTCC:5957, Lactobacillus rhamnosus MTCC:5897, and Lactobacillus fermentum MTCC:5898	Streptozotocin-induced type-1 diabetes in male Wistar rats	Improved glucose metabolism. Downregulated genes involved in regulating gluconeogenesis pathway	Yadav et al. (2018)
Composite	Db/db Mice	Enhanced intestinal barrier function. Upregulation of GLP-1 production	Wang et al. (2020)

Interestingly, the increased expression of Free Fatty Acid Receptor -3 (FFAR3) gene was also reported both in VSL#3-treated and butyrate-treated NCI-H716 cells (Enteroendocrine L cells) with concomitant increase in GLP-1 secretion (Tolhurst et al., 2012; Yadav et al., 2018). Besides, many probiotic administrations (Lactobacillus rhamnosus GG and Bifidobacterium adolescentis) demonstrated the enhancement in glycemic regulations and reduction in the glycated hemoglobin (HbA1c), with the inhibition of proinflammatory cytokines, α-amylase, and α-glucosidase (Sanborn et al., 2020; Tundis et al., 2010). The inhibition action of above-mentioned enzymes successfully imparted the antidiabetic effect with reduced hyperglycemia in diabetic subjects (Grom et al., 2020). Furthermore, it was reported that oxidative stress that imposed damage to insulin-secreting ß cells was prevented by the metabolites of Lactobacillus plantarum 2142 (Paszti-Gere et al., 2013).

Several preclinical and clinical studies have also proved the efficacy of probiotics against T2D. Oral administration of probiotics in preclinical studies using different animal models unanimously proved the antidiabetic potential of probiotics (Table 22.2) by addressing the role of probiotics in the improvement of glucose metabolism with decreased gluconeogenesis, GLP-1 production with improved function of β cells, enhancement of intestinal barrier function with decreased inflammation and gut homeostatis with decreased ratio of Firmicutes to Bacteroidetes and increased butyrate-producing bacteria (Balakumar et al., 2018).

TABLE 22.3 Antidiabetic efficacy of probiotic interventions against T2D in human clinical trials.

Probiotics	Model	Study design	Study outcome	References
L. acidophilus, L. casei, and B. bifidum	Clinical trial of 60 pregnant women	2×10^9 CFU/g of each probiotic strain for 6 weeks	Positive impact on controllic triglycerides and glycemic index	Karamali et al. (2016)
S. thermophilus, L. casei, L. acidophilus, and B. lactis	Clinical trial involving 60 individuals	Kefir (600 mL/day for 8 weeks)	Enhanced insulin resistance and decreased serum level	Alihosseini et al. (2017)
L. rhamnosus CGMCC1.3724	Clinical trial including 105 obese people	2 capsules/day of 10 mg/capsule of probiotic	Enhanced weight loss, satiety and decreased depression	Sanchez et al. (2017)
L. acidophilus La-5 and B. lactis BB-12	Clinical trial with 50 people	120 g/day of fermented milk with 10^9 CFU of each probiotic for 6 weeks	Increased glycemic control and decrease TNF-α	Tonucci et al. (2017)
B. pseudocatenulatum CECT 7765	Animal (mice)	1 capsule/day (10^9 CFU of the probiotic) for 13 weeks	Reduced obesity and depressive behavior	Agusti et al. (2018)
L. casei 01	In vitro and clinical trials	Prato cheese (50 g), Minas Frescal cheese (50 g), and whey beverage (300 mL). Postprandial study for 2 h	Observed great inhibiton of α-amylase and α-glucosidase	Grom et al. (2020)
L. rhamnosus GG	Human (200 people of age 55–75 years)	2 capsules/day (1012 CFUs/capsule) for 3 months	Controlled glycemic index and stabilized HbA1c levels	Sanborn et al. (2020)

Besides, human clinical studies have conveyed the antidiabetic efficacy of several probiotic strains, such as *Bifidobacterium animalis* subsp. *lactis* BB-12 and *Lactobacillus acidophilus* La-5, which inhibited TNF-α, a proinflammatory cytokine, and controlled the glycemic index (Karamali et al., 2016; Sanborn et al., 2020) whereas the probiotic strain *L. casei* 01 offered greater inhibition of α-amylase and α-glucosidase toward antihyperglycemic properties. Another antidiabetic action of potential probiotics was attributed to the production of bioactive peptides during milk fermentations (Ahtesh et al., 2018; Chaudhari et al., 2017). Thus diary fermented products were found to be a helpful supplement to treat diabetes. Interestingly, *Bifidobacterium pseudocatenulatum* CECT 7765 has positively impacted in significantly reducing depressive behavioral attributes associated with T2D (Agusti et al., 2018) (Table 22.3). Hence, the administration of potential probiotics has proven to be the most beneficial and convenient way to effectively prevent and manage the T2D or DM.

22.3.3 Probiotics for the management of obesity

Obesity is one of the most common kinds of lifestyle-associated disease that causes irreversible health conditions. It also causes great economic loss and weakens the society financially due to the prolonged treatments involved in its cure. Obesity is also a cause of several other comorbidities, such as cardiovascular diseases, various metabolic disorders including diabetes and disorders of respiratory, and muscle-skeletal dieseases. However, fortunately obesity disease can be prevented by adopting the fundamentals of balance diet and dietary supplements including probiotics that provides a greater number of beneficial bacteria to combat gut bacterial dysbiosis-associated obesity. The science of probiotics has rapidly evolved since last few decades as it confers many technological and health promoting attributes. The use of probiotics can successfully offer a wide range of effective as well as sustainable methodology for addressing most common public health issues even in many developing nations. Probiotics generally possess some crucial antiobesity properties that is linked with various mechanisms and functions namely improvement in lipid profile and insulin sensitivity, cytokine regulation (IL-10, IL-17, IL-22), controlling the signals of leptin hormone, and lowering the proinflammatory genes; all these properties resulted from studies performed in human and animal models. Due to all these major antiobesity properties observed along with other related beneficial functions of probiotics, that is, adjusting the gut dysbiosis that ultimately recreates the natural balance in the intestinal microbiota. Much of the emphasis is given toward the identification of these beneficial and live microorganisms in the management of metabolic syndrome and obesity. Therefore consumption of probiotics as an antiobesity and antiobesogenic agent plays a significant role in the prevention and management of obesity. Many of the studies have recommended *Lactobacillus* and *Bifidobacterium* to be the most important genera for the appropriate management of obesity and other related health consequences. Few human studies have also demonstrated the reduction of total cholesterol including low-density lipoprotein (LDL) cholesterol, while showing a significant rise in high-density lipoprotein (HDL) cholesterol after the consumption of probiotics by various individuals. Some of the animal studies involving the DIO mice administered with known beneficial probiotic microorganisms, such as *Lactobacillus rhamnosus*, *Bifidobacterium bifidum*, and *Lactobacillus acidophilus* showed possible enhancements and modulation of gut microbiota. Few probiotic microorganisms, namely *Lactobacillus* (*L. casei* strain Shirota, *L. gasseri*, *L. rhamnosus*, *L. plantarum*), along with *Bifidobacterium* (*B. breve* B3, *B. longum*, *B. Infantis*) supported most studies by exhibiting the antiobesity characteristics during 4–6 weeks of consumption. Probiotic strain mainly *L. rhamnosus* CGMCC1.3724 proved to be the most functional and beneficial strain for the efficient prevention and management of obesity-related issues and exhibited extraordinary antiobesity characteristics (Daniali et al., 2020).

Tomé-Castro et al. (2021) evaluated the efficacy of probiotics as a therapeutic agent against obesity issues wherein they performed 23 randomized controlled trials to demonstrate positive effect of probiotics in the management of obesity along with the reduction of BMI values. Some studies have also shown that some of the specific probiotic strains, namely *Lactobacillus bulgaricus*, *Lactobacillus acidophilus*, and *Streptococcus thermophilus*, along with others have presented a vital strategy in preventing obesity and overweight in terms of altering different parameters along with important biomarkers, such as cholesterol, LDL, and triglycerides level, in addition to few others when multiple strains were used in combination Table 22.4. These above-mentioned probiotics not only showed a significant reduction in the BMI values but also decreased the hip circumference of probiotic administered individuals. Thus probiotics could play a very significant role in the prevention and management of obesity and other metabolic syndromes.

TABLE 22.4 Antiobesity effect of probiotics established in preclinical and clinical studies.

Probiotic	Model	Study design	Study outcome	References
Lactobacillus gasseri SBT2055 (LG2055)	Human	To check the regulation of abdominal adiposity by probiotics (*Lactobacillus gasseri* SBT2055) in adults with obese tendencies in an RCT	Probiotic LG2055 ↓ abdominal adiposity and ↓ body weight	Kadooka et al. (2010)
Lactobacillus casei strain Shirota (LcS)	Human	To check the effects of the *Lactobacillus casei* strain on obesity in children: a pilot study	Reduced fecal concentrations of *Bifidobacterium* as well as *Bacteroides fragilis*, *Atopobium* cluster, and *Lactobacillus gasseri*. There was a significant drop in body weight and an increase in HDL cholesterol	Karimi et al. (2015) and Nagata et al. (2017)
Lactobacillus reuteri (*L. reuteri*) V340	Human and animal (mice)	To evaluate the influence on biomarkers, such as inflammation and insulin resistance, cardiovascular and hepatic issues	Lowered the cholesterol absorption, inflammation, and insulin resistance	Tenorio-Jiménez et al. (2018)
Bifidobacterium animalis subsp. *lactis* CECT 8145 (Ba8145)	Clinical study	Influence of daily consumption on human body measurement-related biomarkers	Enhanced the anthropometric biomarkers, largely in women. Also increased *Akkermansia* genus in the gut	Pedret et al. (2019)
Lactobacillus genera	Animal	Imbalance of normal gut microflora	Probiotics delivered during lactation period	Sotoudegan et al. (2019)
Lactobacillus rhamnosus GG	Animal model	Effect on gut microflora, leptin resistance	Enhanced the gut microflora, improved leptin resistance, and decreased amount of proteobacteria	Cheng et al. (2020)
Lactobacillus rhamnosus GG, *L. paracasei* HII01 (with xylooligosaccharide), *Bacillus amyloliquefaciens* SC06, and *Sachharomyces boulardii*	Human and animal (mice and rats)	Effect on *Firmicutes*/*Bacteroidetes* during the treatment of obesity	Exhibited a low level of ratio, reduction of LDL cholesterol, which prevented the obesity and ultimately reduced body weight	Stojanov et al. (2020)

22.4 Conclusions

In the era of life style diseases, diabetes and obesity (diabesity) have gained prominence over other diseases owing to the commonality in their pathophysiology. In the current scenario, these lifestyle diseases stand as slow poison to humans that can silently deteriorate the quality, productivity, and expectancy of patient's life. Various genetic and environmental/lifestyle factors are responsible in the pathogenesis of diabesity. Lately, the gut microbiota has also been increasingly linked with the causation of diabetes and obesity. In this regard, several studies have shown promising results with respect to probiotics, which can aid in the retrieval and restoration of a healthy gut microbiota, thereby achieving immune and energy homeostasis in gut as "symbionts of human gut microflora." The mechanism of action of probiotic in the gut system is entirely strain specific. Mostly, probiotics modulate the gut system by triggering the regulation of certain pro- and antiinflammatory cascades. Collaterally metabolites like SCFAs can activate FFAR-2/3 pathways that regulate the proliferation and differentiation of Tregs as well as GLP-1 enhancement, decreased gluconeogenesis, increased butyrate-producing bacteria, and improved function of Beta cells. Above all, *Bifidobacterium animalis* subsp. *lactis* BB-12 and *Lactobacillus acidophilus* La-5 are regarded as antidiabetic strains based on the clinical trials. The antidiabetic potential of probiotics is also attributed toward the production of bioactive peptides bearing antioxidative and antidiabetic potential. Thus fermented dairy products were found to be a potential supplement to treat diabetes. Antidiabetic potential also ameliorates the obesity by improving lipid profile and regulating leptin hormone. Many of the studies have recommended *Lactobacillus* and *Bifidobacterium* to be the most important genera for the appropriate management of obesity and other related health consequences. Thus probiotics could play a very significant role in the prevention and management of obesity and other metabolic syndromes.

References

Agusti, A., Moya-Pérez, A., Campillo, I., Montserrat-de la Paz, S., Cerrudo, V., Perez-Villalba, A., & Sanz, Y. (2018). Bifidobacterium pseudocatenulatum CECT 7765 ameliorates neuroendocrine alterations associated with an exaggerated stress response and anhedonia in obese mice. *Molecular Neurobiology*, 55(6), 5337–5352. Available from https://doi.org/10.1007/s12035-017-0768-z.

Ahmad, A., Yang, W., Chen, G., Shafiq, M., Javed, S., Zaidi, S. S. A., Shahid, R., Liu, C., & Bokhari, H. (2019). Analysis of gut microbiota of obese individuals with type 2 diabetes and healthy individuals. *PLoS One*, 14(12). Available from https://doi.org/10.1371/journal.pone.0226372.

Ahtesh, F. B., Stojanovska, L., & Apostolopoulos, V. (2018). Anti-hypertensive peptides released from milk proteins by probiotics. *Maturitas*, 115, 103–109. Available from https://doi.org/10.1016/j.maturitas.2018.06.016.

Aikaterini, T., Athanasia, K. P., & Andreas, M. (2017). Type 2 diabetes and quality of life. *World Journal of Diabetes*, 120. Available from https://doi.org/10.4239/wjd.v8.i4.120.

Alihosseini, N., Moahboob, S. A., Farrin, N., Mobasseri, M., Taghizadeh, A., & Ostadrahimi, A. R. (2017). Effect of probiotic fermented milk (kefir) on serum level of insulin and homocysteine in type 2 diabetes patients. *Acta Endocrinologica (Bucharest)*, 13(4), 431.

Balakumar, M., Prabhu, D., Sathishkumar, C., Prabu, P., Rokana, N., Kumar, R., Raghavan, S., Soundarajan, A., Grover, S., Batish, V. K., Mohan, V., & Balasubramanyam, M. (2018). Improvement in glucose tolerance and insulin sensitivity by probiotic strains of Indian gut origin in high-fat diet-fed C57BL/6J mice. *European Journal of Nutrition*, 57(1), 279–295. Available from https://doi.org/10.1007/s00394-016-1317-7.

Barlow, G. M., Yu, A., & Mathur, R. (2015). Role of the gut microbiome in obesity and diabetes mellitus. *Nutrition in Clinical Practice*, 30(6), 787–797. Available from https://doi.org/10.1177/0884533615609896.

Belkaid, Y., & Hand, T. W. (2014). Role of the microbiota in immunity and inflammation. *Cell*, 157(1), 121–141. Available from https://doi.org/10.1016/j.cell.2014.03.011.

Bermudez-Brito, M., Plaza-Díaz, J., Muñoz-Quezada, S., Gómez-Llorente, C., & Gil, A. (2012). Probiotic mechanisms of action. *Annals of Nutrition and Metabolism*, 61(2), 160–174. Available from https://doi.org/10.1159/000342079.

Bhupathiraju, S. N., & Hu, F. B. (2016). Epidemiology of obesity and diabetes and their cardiovascular complications. *Circulation Research*, 118(11), 1723–1735. Available from https://doi.org/10.1161/CIRCRESAHA.115.306825.

Bibbò, S., Dore, M. P., Pes, G. M., Delitala, G., & Delitala, A. P. (2017). Is there a role for gut microbiota in type 1 diabetes pathogenesis? *Annals of Medicine*, 49(1), 11–22. Available from https://doi.org/10.1080/07853890.2016.1222449.

Binda, S., Hill, C., Johansen, E., Obis, D., Pot, B., Sanders, M. E., Tremblay, A., & Ouwehand, A. C. (2020). Criteria to qualify microorganisms as "probiotic" in foods and dietary supplements. *Frontiers in Microbiology*, 11. Available from https://doi.org/10.3389/fmicb.2020.01662.

Blandino, G., Inturri, R., Lazzara, F., Di Rosa, M., & Malaguarnera, L. (2016). Impact of gut microbiota on diabetes mellitus. *Diabetes & Metabolism*, 303–315. Available from https://doi.org/10.1016/j.diabet.2016.04.004.

Boer, G. A., & Holst, J. J. (2020). Incretin hormones and type 2 diabetes—Mechanistic insights and therapeutic approaches. *Biology*, 9(12), 1–20. Available from https://doi.org/10.3390/biology9120473.

Brown, K., DeCoffe, D., Molcan, E., & Gibson, D. L. (2012). Diet-induced dysbiosis of the intestinal microbiota and the effects on immunity and disease. *Nutrients*, 4(8), 1095–1119. Available from https://doi.org/10.3390/nu4081095.

Cani, P. D., & Delzenne, N. M. (2009). The role of the gut microbiota in energy metabolism and metabolic disease. *Current Pharmaceutical Design*, *15*(13), 1546–1558. Available from https://doi.org/10.2174/138161209788168164.

Cerf, M. E. (2013). Beta cell dysfunction and insulin resistance. *Frontiers in Endocrinology*, *4*. Available from https://doi.org/10.3389/fendo.2013.00037.

Chadt, A., Scherneck, S., Joost, H. G., & Hasani, H. (2018). Molecular links between obesity and diabetes:"diabesity.". *Endotext*.

Chaudhari, D. D., Singh, R., Mallappa, R. H., Rokana, N., Kaushik, J. K., Bajaj, R., Batish, V. K., & Grover, S. (2017). Evaluation of casein & whey protein hydrolysates as well as milk fermentates from lactobacillus helveticus for expression of gut hormones. *Indian Journal of Medical Research*, *146*(September), 409–419. Available from https://doi.org/10.4103/ijmr.IJMR_802_15.

Cheng, Y. C., & Liu, J. R. (2020). Effect of Lactobacillus rhamnosus GG on energy metabolism, leptin resistance, and gut microbiota in mice with diet-induced obesity. *Nutrients*, *12*(9), 2557.

Daniali, M., Nikfar, S., & Abdollahi, M. (2020). A brief overview on the use of probiotics to treat overweight and obese patients. *Expert Review of Endocrinology and Metabolism*, *15*(1), 1–4. Available from https://doi.org/10.1080/17446651.2020.1719068.

Dedrick, S., Sundaresh, B., Huang, Q., Brady, C., Yoo, T., Cronin, C., Rudnicki, C., Flood, M., Momeni, B., Ludvigsson, J., & Altindis, E. (2020). The role of gut microbiota and environmental factors in type 1 diabetes pathogenesis. *Frontiers in Endocrinology*, *11*. Available from https://doi.org/10.3389/fendo.2020.00078.

Delzenne, N. M., Cani, P. D., Everard, A., Neyrinck, A. M., & Bindels, L. B. (2015). Gut microorganisms as promising targets for the management of type 2 diabetes. *Diabetologia*, *58*(10), 2206–2217. Available from https://doi.org/10.1007/s00125-015-3712-7.

Dendup, T., Feng, X., Clingan, S., & Astell-Burt, T. (2018). Environmental risk factors for developing type 2 diabetes mellitus: A systematic review. *International Journal of Environmental Research and Public Health*, *15*(1). Available from https://doi.org/10.3390/ijerph15010078.

Dolpady, J., Sorini, C., Di Pietro, C., Cosorich, I., Ferrarese, R., Saita, D., Clementi, M., Canducci, F., & Falcone, M. (2016). Oral probiotic VSL# 3 prevents autoimmune diabetes by modulating microbiota and promoting indoleamine 2, 3-dioxygenase-enriched tolerogenic intestinal environment. *Journal of Diabetes Research*, *2016*.

Dunn, A. B., Jordan, S., Baker, B. J., & Carlson, N. S. (2017). The maternal infant microbiome: Considerations for labor and birth. *MCN: The American Journal of Maternal/Child Nursing*, *42*(6), 318–325. Available from https://doi.org/10.1097/NMC.0000000000000373.

Durack, J., & Lynch, S. V. (2019). The gut microbiome: Relationships with disease and opportunities for therapy. *Journal of Experimental Medicine*, *216*(1), 20–40. Available from https://doi.org/10.1084/jem.20180448.

Emilio, G. J. (2013). Obesidad: Análisis etiopatogénico y fisiopatológico. *Endocrinología y Nutrición*, 17–24. Available from https://doi.org/10.1016/j.endonu.2012.03.006.

Francine, S., Margarida, F.-B., Pedro, B., & Natália, C.-M. (2021). Obesity and gut microbiome: Review of potential role of probiotics. *Porto Biomedical Journal*, *6*(1), e111. Available from https://doi.org/10.1097/j.pbj.0000000000000111.

Gadde, K. M., Martin, C. K., Berthoud, H. R., & Heymsfield, S. B. (2018). Obesity: Pathophysiology and management. *Journal of the American College of Cardiology*, *71*(1), 69–84. Available from https://doi.org/10.1016/j.jacc.2017.11.011.

Grom, L. C., Coutinho, N. M., Guimarães, J. T., Balthazar, C. F., Silva, R., Rocha, R. S., Freitas, M. Q., Duarte, M. C. K. H., Pimentel, T. C., Esmerino, E. A., Silva, M. C., & Cruz, A. G. (2020). Probiotic dairy foods and postprandial glycemia: A mini-review. *Trends in Food Science and Technology*, *101*, 165–171. Available from https://doi.org/10.1016/j.tifs.2020.05.012.

Gurung, M., Li, Z., You, H., Rodrigues, R., Jump, D. B., Morgun, A., & Shulzhenko, N. (2020). Role of gut microbiota in type 2 diabetes pathophysiology. *EBioMedicine*, *51*. Available from https://doi.org/10.1016/j.ebiom.2019.11.051.

Hasnain, S. Z., Prins, J. B., & McGuckin, M. A. (2016). Oxidative and endoplasmic reticulum stress in β-cell dysfunction in diabetes. *Journal of Molecular Endocrinology*, *56*(2), R33–R54. Available from https://doi.org/10.1530/JME-15-0232.

He, Y., Wu, W., Zheng, H. M., Li, P., McDonald, D., Sheng, H. F., Chen, M. X., Chen, Z. H., Ji, G. Y., Zheng, Z. D. X., Mujagond, P., Chen, X. J., Rong, Z. H., Chen, P., Lyu, L. Y., Wang, X., Wu, C. B., Yu, N., Xu, Y. J., ... Zhou, H. W. (2018). Regional variation limits applications of healthy gut microbiome reference ranges and disease models. *Nature Medicine*, *24*(10), 1532–1535. Available from https://doi.org/10.1038/s41591-018-0164-x.

Izquierdo, A. G., Crujeiras, A. B., Casanueva, F. F., & Carreira, M. C. (2019). Leptin, obesity, and leptin resistance: Where are we 25 years later? *Nutrients*, *11*(11). Available from https://doi.org/10.3390/nu11112704.

Jia, L., Li, D., Feng, N., Shamoon, M., Sun, Z., Ding, L., & Chen, Y. Q. (2017). Anti-diabetic effects of Clostridium butyricum CGMCC0313. 1 through promoting the growth of gut butyrate-producing bacteria in type 2 diabetic mice. *Scientific reports*, *7*(1), 1–15.

Jia, L., Shan, K., Pan, L. L., Feng, N., Lv, Z., Sun, Y., Li, J., Wu, C., Zhang, H., Chen, W., & Diana, J. (2017). Clostridium butyricum CGMCC0313. 1 protects against autoimmune diabetes by modulating intestinal immune homeostasis and inducing pancreatic regulatory T cells. *Frontiers in immunology*, *8*, 1345.

Kadooka, Y., Sato, M., Imaizumi, K., Ogawa, A., Ikuyama, K., Akai, Y., Okano, M., Kagoshima, M., & Tsuchida, T. (2010). Regulation of abdominal adiposity by probiotics (Lactobacillus gasseri SBT2055) in adults with obese tendencies in a randomized controlled trial. *Eur J Clin Nutr.*, *64*(6), 636–643. Available from https://doi.org/10.1038/ejcn.2010.19, Epub 2010 Mar 10. PMID: 20216555.

Kahn, S. E., Cooper, M. E., & Del Prato, S. (2014). Pathophysiology and treatment of type 2 diabetes: Perspectives on the past, present, and future. *The Lancet*, *383*(9922), 1068–1083. Available from https://doi.org/10.1016/S0140-6736(13)62154-6.

Karamali, M., Dadkhah, F., Sadrkhanlou, M., Jamilian, M., Ahmadi, S., Tajabadi-Ebrahimi, M., Jafari, P., & Asemi, Z. (2016). Effects of probiotic supplementation on glycaemic control and lipid profiles in gestational diabetes: A randomized, double-blind, placebo-controlled trial. *Diabetes & Metabolism*, 234–241. Available from https://doi.org/10.1016/j.diabet.2016.04.009.

Karimi, G., Sabran, M. R., Jamaluddin, R., Parvaneh, K., Mohtarrudin, N., Ahmad, Z., Khazaai, H., & Khodavandi, A. (2015). The anti-obesity effects of Lactobacillus casei strain Shirota versus Orlistat on high fat diet-induced obese rats. *Food & Nutrition Research*, 59, 29273. Available from https://doi.org/10.3402/fnr.v59.29273.

Kolb, H., & Martin, S. (2017). Environmental/lifestyle factors in the pathogenesis and prevention of type 2 diabetes. *BMC Medicine*, 15(1). Available from https://doi.org/10.1186/s12916-017-0901-x.

Langdon, A., Crook, N., & Dantas, G. (2016). The effects of antibiotics on the microbiome throughout development and alternative approaches for therapeutic modulation. *Genome Medicine*, 8(1). Available from https://doi.org/10.1186/s13073-016-0294-z.

Lau, K., Benitez, P., Ardissone, A., Wilson, T. D., Collins, E. L., Lorca, G., Li, N., Sankar, D., Wasserfall, C., Neu, J., & Atkinson, M. A. (2011). Inhibition of type 1 diabetes correlated to a Lactobacillus johnsonii N6. 2-mediated Th17 bias. *The Journal of Immunology*, 186(6), 3538–3546.

Lee, C. J., Sears, C. L., & Maruthur, N. (2020). Gut microbiome and its role in obesity and insulin resistance. *Annals of the New York Academy of Sciences*, 1461(1), 37–52. Available from https://doi.org/10.1111/nyas.14107.

Ley, R. E., Turnbaugh, P. J., Klein, S., & Gordon, J. I. (2006). Human gut microbes associated with obesity. *Nature*, 1022–1023. Available from https://doi.org/10.1038/4441022a.

Lin, H. V., Frassetto, A., Kowalik, E. J., Nawrocki, A. R., Lu, M. M., Kosinski, J. R., Hubert, J. A., Szeto, D., Yao, X., Forrest, G., & Marsh, D. J. (2012). Butyrate and propionate protect against diet-induced obesity and regulate gut hormones via free fatty acid receptor 3-independent mechanisms. *PLoS One*, 7(4). Available from https://doi.org/10.1371/journal.pone.0035240.

Manaer, T., Yu, L., Zhang, Y., Xiao, X. J., & Nabi, X. H. (2015). Anti-diabetic effects of shubat in type 2 diabetic rats induced by combination of high-glucose-fat diet and low-dose streptozotocin. *Journal of Ethnopharmacology*, 169, 269–274.

Mishra, S., Wang, S., Nagpal, R., Miller, B., Singh, R., Taraphder, S., & Yadav, H. (2019). Probiotics and prebiotics for the amelioration of type 1 diabetes: Present and future perspectives. *Microorganisms*, 7(3). Available from https://doi.org/10.3390/microorganisms7030067.

Mitchell, C. M., Mazzoni, C., Hogstrom, L., Bryant, A., Bergerat, A., Cher, A., Pochan, S., Herman, P., Carrigan, M., Sharp, K., Huttenhower, C., Lander, E. S., Vlamakis, H., Xavier, R. J., & Yassour, M. (2020). Delivery mode affects stability of early infant gut microbiota. *Cell Reports Medicine*, 1(9). Available from https://doi.org/10.1016/j.xcrm.2020.100156.

Mottalib, A., Kasetty, M., Mar, J. Y., Elseaidy, T., Ashrafzadeh, S., & Hamdy, O. (2017). Weight management in patients with type 1 diabetes and obesity. *Current Diabetes Reports*, 17(10). Available from https://doi.org/10.1007/s11892-017-0918-8.

Muñoz-Garach, A., Diaz-Perdigones, C., & Tinahones, F. J. (2016). Microbiota y diabetes mellitus tipo 2. *Endocrinologia y Nutricion*, 63(10), 560–568. Available from https://doi.org/10.1016/j.endonu.2016.07.008.

Nagata, S., Chiba, Y., Wang, C., & Yamashiro, Y. (2017). The effects of the Lactobacillus casei strain on obesity in children: a pilot study. *Benef Microbes*, 8(4), 535–543. Available from https://doi.org/10.3920/BM2016.0170, Epub 2017 Jun 16. PMID: 28618860.

Nauck, M., Stöckmann, F., Ebert, R., & Creutzfeldt, W. (1986). Reduced incretin effect in Type 2 (non-insulin-dependent) diabetes. *Diabetologia*, 29(1), 46–52. Available from https://doi.org/10.1007/BF02427280.

Ng, A. C. T., Delgado, V., Borlaug, B. A., & Bax, J. J. (2021). Diabesity: The combined burden of obesity and diabetes on heart disease and the role of imaging. *Nature Reviews Cardiology*, 18(4), 291–304. Available from https://doi.org/10.1038/s41569-020-00465-5.

Oussaada, S. M., van Galen, K. A., Cooiman, M. I., Kleinendorst, L., Hazebroek, E. J., van Haelst, M. M., ter Horst, K. W., & Serlie, M. J. (2019). The pathogenesis of obesity. *Metabolism: Clinical and Experimental*, 92, 26–36. Available from https://doi.org/10.1016/j.metabol.2018.12.012.

Panwar, H., Rashmi, H. M., Batish, V. K., & Grover, S. (2013). Probiotics as potential biotherapeutics in the management of type 2 diabetes - prospects and perspectives. *Diabetes/Metabolism Research and Reviews*, 29(2), 103–112. Available from https://doi.org/10.1002/dmrr.2376.

Papatheodorou, K., Banach, M., Bekiari, E., Rizzo, M., & Edmonds, M. (2017). Complications of diabetes. *Journal of Diabetes Research*.

Paszti-Gere, E., Csibrik-Nemeth, E., Szeker, K., Csizinszky, R., Palocz, O., Farkas, O., & Galfi, P. (2013). Lactobacillus plantarum 2142 prevents intestinal oxidative stress in optimized in vitro systems. *Acta Physiologica Hungarica*, 100(1), 89–98. Available from https://doi.org/10.1556/APhysiol.100.2013.1.9.

Pedret, A., Valls, R. M., Calderón-Pérez, L., Llauradó, E., Companys, J., Pla-Pagà, L., & Solà, R. (2019). Effects of daily consumption of the probiotic Bifidobacterium animalis subsp. lactis CECT 8145 on anthropometric adiposity biomarkers in abdominally obese subjects: a randomized controlled trial. *International Journal of Obesity*, 43(9), 1863–1868.

Phillips, L. S., Ratner, R. E., Buse, J. B., & Kahn, S. E. (2014). We can change the natural history of type 2 diabetes. *Diabetes Care*, 37(10), 2668–2676. Available from https://doi.org/10.2337/dc14-0817.

Ruan, Y., Sun, J., He, J., Chen, F., Chen, R., & Chen, H. (2015). Effect of probiotics on glycemic control: A systematic review and meta-analysis of randomized, controlled trials. *PLoS One*, 10(7). Available from https://doi.org/10.1371/journal.pone.0132121.

Sanborn, V. E., Azcarate-Peril, M. A., & Gunstad, J. (2020). Lactobacillus rhamnosus GG and HbA1c in middle age and older adults without type 2 diabetes mellitus: A preliminary randomized study. *Diabetes and Metabolic Syndrome: Clinical Research and Reviews*, 14(5), 907–909. Available from https://doi.org/10.1016/j.dsx.2020.05.034.

Sanchez-Alcoholado, L., Castellano-Castillo, D., Jordán-Martínez, L., Moreno-Indias, I., Cardila-Cruz, P., Elena, D., & Jimenez-Navarro, M. (2017). Role of gut microbiota on cardio-metabolic parameters and immunity in coronary artery disease patients with and without type-2 diabetes mellitus. *Frontiers in Microbiology*, 8, 1936.

Schlauch, K. A., Read, R. W., Lombardi, V. C., Elhanan, G., Metcalf, W. J., Slonim, A. D., & Grzymski, J. J. (2020). A comprehensive genome-wide and phenome-wide examination of BMI and obesity in a Northern Nevadan Cohort. *G3: Genes|Genomes|Genetics*, 10(2), 645–664. Available from https://doi.org/10.1534/g3.119.400910.

Shah, N. J., & Swami, O. C. (2017). Role of probiotics in diabetes: A review of their rationale and efficacy. *Diabetes*, 5, 104–110.

Sheikh, A. B., Nasrullah, A., Haq, S., Akhtar, A., Ghazanfar, H., Nasir, A., et al. (2017). The Interplay of genetics and environmental factors in the development of obesity. *Cureus*, 9.

Shen, X., Miao, J., Wan, Q., Wang, S., Li, M., Pu, F., Wang, G., Qian, W., Yu, Q., Marotta, F., & He, F. (2018). Possible correlation between gut microbiota and immunity among healthy middle-aged and elderly people in southwest China. *Gut Pathogens*, 10(1). Available from https://doi.org/10.1186/s13099-018-0231-3.

Sikalidis, A. K., & Maykish, A. (2020). The gut microbiome and type 2 diabetes mellitus: Discussing a complex relationship. *Biomedicines*, 8(1). Available from https://doi.org/10.3390/biomedicines8010008.

Siljander, H., Honkanen, J., & Knip, M. (2019). Microbiome and type 1 diabetes. *EBioMedicine*, 46, 512–521. Available from https://doi.org/10.1016/j.ebiom.2019.06.031.

Silva, Y. P., Bernardi, A., & Frozza, R. L. (2020). The role of short-chain fatty acids from gut microbiota in gut-brain communication. *Frontiers in Endocrinology*, 11. Available from https://doi.org/10.3389/fendo.2020.00025.

Sotoudegan, F., Daniali, M., Hassani, S., Nikfar, S., & Abdollahi, M. (2019). Reappraisal of probiotics' safety in human. *Food and Chemical Toxicology*, 129, 22–29.

Stojanov, S., Berlec, A., & Štrukelj, B. (2020). The influence of probiotics on the Firmicutes/Bacteroidetes ratio in the treatment of obesity and inflammatory bowel disease. *Microorganisms*, 8(11), 1715.

Sunita, G., RashmiH., M., Namita, R., RajKumar, D., Harsh, P., & VirenderKumar, B. (2012). Management of metabolic syndrome through probiotic and prebiotic interventions. *Indian Journal of Endocrinology and Metabolism*, 20. Available from https://doi.org/10.4103/2230-8210.91178.

Tenorio-Jiménez, C., Martínez-Ramírez, M. J., Tercero-Lozano, M., Arraiza-Irigoyen, C., Del Castillo-Codes, I., Olza, J., & Gomez-Llorente, C. (2018). Evaluation of the effect of Lactobacillus reuteri V3401 on biomarkers of inflammation, cardiovascular risk and liver steatosis in obese adults with metabolic syndrome: A randomized clinical trial (PROSIR). *BMC complementary and alternative medicine*, 18(1), 1–8.

Thomas, R. M., & Jobin, C. (2020). Microbiota in pancreatic health and disease: The next frontier in microbiome research. *Nature Reviews Gastroenterology and Hepatology*, 17(1), 53–64. Available from https://doi.org/10.1038/s41575-019-0242-7.

Tolhurst, G., Heffron, H., Lam, Y. S., Parker, H. E., Habib, A. M., Diakogiannaki, E., Cameron, J., Grosse, J., Reimann, F., & Gribble, F. M. (2012). Short-chain fatty acids stimulate glucagon-like peptide-1 secretion via the G-protein-coupled receptor FFAR2. *Diabetes*, 61(2), 364–371. Available from https://doi.org/10.2337/db11-1019.

Tomé-Castro, X. M., Rodriguez-Arrastia, M., Cardona, D., Rueda-Ruzafa, L., Molina-Torres, G., & Roman, P. (2021). Probiotics as a therapeutic strategy in obesity and overweight: A systematic review. *Beneficial Microbes*, 12(1), 5–15. Available from https://doi.org/10.3920/BM2020.0111.

Tonucci, L. B., Dos Santos, K. M. O., de Oliveira, L. L., Ribeiro, S. M. R., & Martino, H. S. D. (2017). Clinical application of probiotics in type 2 diabetes mellitus: A randomized, double-blind, placebo-controlled study. *Clinical Nutrition*, 36(1), 85–92.

Traversi, D., Rabbone, I., Scaioli, G., Vallini, C., Carletto, G., Racca, I., Ala, U., Durazzo, M., Collo, A., Ferro, A., Carrera, D., Savastio, S., Cadario, F., Siliquini, R., & Cerutti, F. (2020). Risk factors for type 1 diabetes, including environmental, behavioural and gut microbial factors: A case-—control study. *Scientific Reports*, 10(1). Available from https://doi.org/10.1038/s41598-020-74678-6.

Tundis, R., Loizzo, M. R., & Menichini, F. (2010). Natural products as α-amylase and α-glucosidase inhibitors and their hypoglycaemic potential in the treatment of diabetes: An update. *Mini-Reviews in Medicinal Chemistry*, 10(4), 315–331. Available from https://doi.org/10.2174/138955710791331007.

Vaarala, O. (2012). Gut microbiota and type 1 diabetes. *Review of Diabetic Studies*, 9(4), 251–259. Available from https://doi.org/10.1900/RDS.2012.9.251.

Valladares, R., Sankar, D., Li, N., Williams, E., Lai, K. K., Abdelgeliel, A. S., Gonzalez, C. F., Wasserfall, C. H., Larkin, J., III, Schatz, D., & Atkinson, M. A. (2010). Lactobacillus johnsonii N6. 2 mitigates the development of type 1 diabetes in BB-DP rats. *Plos one*, 5(5), e10507.

Vangay, P., Ward, T., Gerber, J. S., & Knights, D. (2015). Antibiotics, pediatric dysbiosis, and disease. *Cell Host and Microbe*, 17(5), 553–564. Available from https://doi.org/10.1016/j.chom.2015.04.006.

Wang, Y., Dilidaxi, D., Wu, Y., Sailike, J., Sun, X., & Nabi, X. H. (2020). Composite probiotics alleviate type 2 diabetes by regulating intestinal microbiota and inducing GLP-1 secretion in db/db mice. *Biomedicine & Pharmacotherapy*, 125, 109914.

Wang, Y., Wu, Y., Wang, Y., Xu, H., Mei, X., Yu, D., Wang, Y., & Li, W. (2017). Antioxidant properties of probiotic bacteria. *Nutrients*, 9(5). Available from https://doi.org/10.3390/nu9050521.

Wei, S. H., Chen, Y. P., & Chen, M. J. (2015). Selecting probiotics with the abilities of enhancing GLP-1 to mitigate the progression of type 1 diabetes in vitro and in vivo. *Journal of Functional Foods*, 18, 473–486. Available from https://doi.org/10.1016/j.jff.2015.08.016.

Wei-Zheng, L., Kyle, S., Jun-Jie, Y., & Lei, Z. (2020). Gut microbiota and diabetes: From correlation to causality and mechanism. *World Journal of Diabetes*, 293–308. Available from https://doi.org/10.4239/wjd.v11.i7.293.

Wen, L., & Wong, F. S. (2017). Dietary short-chain fatty acids protect against type 1 diabetes. *Nature Immunology*, 18(5), 484–486. Available from https://doi.org/10.1038/ni.3730.

Woldeamlak, B., Yirdaw, K., & Biadgo, B. (2019). Role of gut microbiota in type 2 diabetes mellitus and its complications: Novel insights and potential intervention strategies. *The Korean Journal of Gastroenterology = Taehan Sohwagi Hakhoe Chi*, 74(6), 314–320. Available from https://doi.org/10.4166/kjg.2019.74.6.314.

Yadav, R., Dey, D. K., Vij, R., Meena, S., Kapila, R., & Kapila, S. (2018). Evaluation of anti-diabetic attributes of Lactobacillus rhamnosus MTCC:5957, Lactobacillus rhamnosus MTCC:5897 and Lactobacillus fermentum MTCC:5898 in streptozotocin induced diabetic rats. *Microbial Pathogenesis*, 125, 454–462. Available from https://doi.org/10.1016/j.micpath.2018.10.015.

Zaccardi, F., Webb, D. R., Yates, T., & Davies, M. J. (2016). Pathophysiology of type 1 and type 2 diabetes mellitus: A 90-year perspective. *Postgraduate Medical Journal*, *92*(1084), 63–69. Available from https://doi.org/10.1136/postgradmedj-2015-133281.

Zheng, P., Li, Z., & Zhou, Z. (2018). Gut microbiome in type 1 diabetes: A comprehensive review. *Diabetes/Metabolism Research and Reviews*, *34*(7). Available from https://doi.org/10.1002/dmrr.3043.

Zhou, H., Zhao, X., Sun, L., Liu, Y., Lv, Y., Gang, X., & Wang, G. (2020). Gut microbiota profile in patients with type 1 diabetes based on 16S rRNA gene sequencing: A systematic review. *Disease Markers*, *2020*. Available from https://doi.org/10.1155/2020/3936247.

Chapter 23

Probiotics in the prevention and management of cardiovascular diseases with focus on dyslipidemia

Cíntia Lacerda Ramos[1,2], Elizabethe Adriana Esteves[1,2], Rodrigo Pereira Prates[3], Lauane Gomes Moreno[3] and Carina Sousa Santos[1]

[1]*Graduate Program in Nutrition Sciences, Faculty of Biological and Health Sciences/Federal University of Jequitinhonha and Mucuri Valeys, Diamantina, Brazil,* [2]*Graduate Program in Health Sciences, Faculty of Biological and Health Sciences/Federal University of Jequitinhonha and Mucuri Valeys, Diamantina, Brazil,* [3]*Multicentre Graduate Program in Physiological Sciences, Faculty of Biological and Health Sciences/Federal University of Jequitinhonha and Mucuri Valeys, Diamantina, Brazil*

23.1 Introduction

Cardiovascular diseases (CVDs) remain the leading cause of death in the world. According to the World Health Organization, they were responsible for 31.4% of deaths in 2016, being ischemic heart disease (IHD) the leading cause of mortality (16.6%), followed by stroke (10.2%) (WHO, 2018a). More than three-quarters were in low-income and middle-income countries (Roth et al., 2018). CVDs produce immense health and economic burdens. In the United States, it was predicted that between 2010 and 2030, the total direct medical costs of CVD would triplicate, from U$273 billion to U$818 billion (Heidenreich et al., 2011).

Several diseases and clinical conditions have been included as CVD in the 11th version of the International Statistical Classification of Diseases and Related Health Problems (WHO, 2018b), but those with atherosclerosis as an underlying pathogenic mechanism are the most prevalent worldwide. They include IHD, cerebrovascular diseases, aorta, or arterioles diseases, such as hypertension, and peripheral vascular diseases (Mendis et al., 2011).

Although genetics, microbiome, lifestyle (especially diet and physical activity), and metabolic syndrome are risk factors associated with CVD development, dyslipidemia is one of the major risk factors related to their incidence (Sun & Buys, 2015). Dyslipidemia is a dysfunction of lipoprotein metabolism and includes overproduction or deficiency. High blood levels of total cholesterol, low-density lipoprotein cholesterol (LDL-C) and triacylglycerol (TAG); and low levels of high-density lipoprotein cholesterol (HDL-C) are manifestations of dyslipidemia (National Cholesterol Education Program (NCEP) Expert Panel on Detection, Evaluation, and Treatment of High Blood Cholesterol in Adults (Adult Treatment Panel III), 2002).

More specifically, it has been shown that the most important causal agents of atherosclerosis are high blood levels of apolipoprotein (apo) B-containing lipoproteins, of which LDL-C is the main driver for the initiation and progression of atherosclerosis (Moss & Ramji, 2016; Moss et al., 2018). Therefore elevated LDL-C is a significant risk factor for CVD and is the primary target of lipid-lowering therapy (Grundy, 2008). Indeed, recent meta-analyses of genetic, epidemiological, and clinical studies have demonstrated a direct causality between blood LDL-C levels and atherosclerosis-associated CVD (Ference et al., 2017). Additional risk factors for CVD include the other biomarkers of dyslipidemia, such as elevated levels of serum TAG and TAG-rich lipoproteins and low HDL-C, and nonlipid-related risk factors, such as markers for inflammation. These risk factors are essential but targeting them for therapy is secondary to targeting LDL-C (National Cholesterol Education Program (NCEP) Expert Panel on Detection, Evaluation, and Treatment of High Blood Cholesterol in Adults (Adult Treatment Panel III), 2002).

LDL-C initiates and promotes CVD progression, including the formation, growth, destabilization, and rupture of the called "atherosclerotic plaques" (Mendis et al., 2011). Briefly, the atherosclerotic process, sometimes called "hardening of the arteries," starts when fat (especially cholesterol from LDL-C) and calcium build up inside the lining of the medium and large blood vessels, generating an inflammatory process that contributes to the formation of a substance called plaque (Mendis et al., 2011). Over time, the fat and calcium accumulation narrow the artery and block blood flow through it, impairing oxygen distribution to some parts of the body. In certain circumstances, this plaque can also break up and form a blood clot, which falls into the bloodstream and lodges in a coronary artery, or in cerebral blood vessels, causing a heart attack or a stroke, respectively (WHO, 2018b).

Preventing and treating those conditions properly, especially hypercholesterolemia, became a key strategy to avoid CVD (Gragnano & Calabrò, 2018). It has been suggested that for each 1 mmol/L of LDL-C reduced in the blood, there is a 22% lower risk for cardiovascular events in 5 years (Baigent et al., 2005, 2010). Therefore most current therapies aim to reduce plasma LDL-C (Moss & Ramji, 2016; Moss et al., 2018). Both pharmacological methods (such as statins and fibrate) (Cicero et al., 2017) and lifestyle therapies (such as dietary interventions and exercise) have been used to control serum cholesterol levels of hypercholesterolemic patients (Cicero et al., 2017; Dunn-Emke et al., 2001).

However, due to the side effects of lipid-reducing drugs, contraindications for these medical treatments, and personal preferences, most patients have been interested in knowing the potential of functional foods in the prevention of atherosclerosis and their use as add-ons with current pharmaceutical agents (Gallagher et al., 2019; Moss & Ramji, 2016; Moss et al., 2018). Therefore many recent studies have highlighted the potential for cardiovascular health of probiotic microorganisms.

Probiotics are living microorganisms (yeast or bacteria) that provide beneficial effects to the host when administered in adequate amounts (Colin et al., 2014; World Health Organization Food and Agriculture Organization of the United Nations, 2006). A strain belonging to *Bifidobacterium* genera was the first mentioned probiotic strain in 1899 (Hewitt & Rigby, 1976). From this fact, many studies have been performed to evaluate health benefits associated with the probiotic intake (George Kerry et al., 2018; Kiousi et al., 2019; Rondanelli et al., 2017; Sharifi-Rad et al., 2020).

Many probiotic strains are currently available in the market as dietary supplements (Lau et al., 2017), in preparations capable of persisting in (or transiently colonizing) the human intestinal tract and conferring a beneficial influence host physiology. *Lactobacillus*, *Bifidobacterium*, *Saccharomyces*, *Bacillus*, *Streptococcus*, and *Enterococcus* are the most popular probiotic genus sources, and their application as probiotics are extensive in fermented and nonfermented food products, as well as functional and nutraceutical dietary supplements (Kleerebezem et al., 2019).

Probiotics exert their health benefits in several ways. For example, they produce antimicrobial substances, such as organic acids or bacteriocins; regulate the immune response through the secretion of immunoglobulin A against pathogens; reduce the risk of developing allergies; and improve the intestinal mucosal barrier function. In addition, they increase the stability or promote the recovery of the commensal microbiota when it is disturbed; modulate the expression of host genes; release functional proteins, such as lactase or natural enzymes; and decrease the adhesion of pathogens (revised by Sharifi-Rad et al., 2020). In addition, hypolipidemic effect, especially lowering serum LDL-C as one of the leading probiotic functions, has been proved by many experiments in vivo and clinical trials (revised by Jiang et al., 2020; O'Morain & Ramji, 2020). So, they are potential nutraceuticals in fighting CVD.

This chapter presents several probiotic strains with potential in protecting against CVD, including lactic and nonlactic bacteria and yeast strains. It will be presented their probiotics characteristics, especially scientific evidence regarding their protection against CVD in the context of dyslipidemia based on clinical trials and systematic reviews and meta-analyses. The main underlying mechanisms suggested for supporting their hypolipidemic effects, especially their cholesterol-lowering properties, are also discussed.

23.2 Probiotic bacteria

Probiotic bacteria are beneficial to the host because they produce vitamins, such as K and riboflavin and short-chain fatty acids (SCFAs), such as acetate, butyrate, or propionate, which are used as fuel by the intestinal microbiota and colonocytes (Lau et al., 2017). Notably, probiotic bacteria are known to improve gut barrier function by strengthening the epithelial tight junctions (Rao & Samak, 2013), reducing gut leakage, strengthening immunological and nonimmunological gut barrier function, and reducing the translocation of microbial immunogens (Mennigen & Bruewer, 2009).

Probiotic bacteria's ability to promote gut health has led to an explosion of research showing therapeutic benefits in a wide range of diseases. Indeed, probiotic bacteria are currently used to prevent and treat inflammatory bowel diseases, irritable bowel syndrome, gluten intolerance, gastroenteritis, and antibiotic-associated diarrhea (Rao & Samak, 2013). Species of lactic acid bacteria (LAB) (e.g., *Lactococcus*, *Lactobacillus*, *Streptococcus*, and *Enterococcus*), *Bifidobacterium*, and the yeasts (e.g., *Saccharomyces boulardii* and *Kluyveromyces fragilis*) are among the most studied probiotic microorganisms (Boddy et al., 1991; Bomhof et al., 2014; Czerucka et al., 2007; Ramos et al., 2013; Stenman et al., 2014). Also, non-LAB, such as sporing forming bacteria and *Propionibacterium*, have been reported as probiotic (Houem et al., 2017; Ma et al., 2020). In this context, probiotic LAB and no-LAB have been shown to beneficially modify several major atherosclerosis-associated cardiovascular risk factors, including chronic inflammation, hypertension, and hypercholesterolemia (O'Morain & Ramji, 2020).

23.2.1 Probiotic LAB

LAB are characterized by being Gram-positive, nonsporulating, and aerotolerant bacteria that produce lactic acid as the primary fermentation product. In addition, they are divided into three groups, based their carbohydrate metabolism: (1) obligatory homofermentative, when the bacteria can metabolize hexoses by glycolysis pathway, yielding only lactic acid; (2) obligatory heterofermentative, when the bacteria uses the phosphoketolase pathway, generating lactate and ethanol or acetate from hexoses and pentoses; and (3) facultative heterofermentative, when the bacteria degrade hexoses via glycolysis pathway or pentoses through the phosphoketolase pathway.

LAB belong to Firmicutes phylum, Bacilli class, and Lactobacillales order and are included in different families, such as Aerococcaceae, Carnobacteriaceae, Enterococcaceae, Lactobacillaceae, Leuconostocaceae, and Streptococcaceae (http://www.uniprot.org/taxonomy/186826). These bacteria have been isolated from a great diversity of environments and have a long history of fermentation and preservation applications in the food industry. This feature is because their metabolic products that can improve the nutritional and sensory aspects of foods and their antimicrobial compounds, including lactic acid production that contribute to extend the shelf life of food products.

Probiotics belonging to the LAB group have been primarily produced by various companies and are worldwide commercialized. Among these commercialized strains, it is highlighted the *Bifidobacterium lactis* BB-12 strain, which was developed by Chr. Hansen (Denmark) and *Lactobacillus casei* strain Shirota, produced by Yakult Company (Japan) (Terue et al., 2006; Wang et al., 2015). *Bifidobacterium lactis* BB-12 strain is one of the most thoroughly studied strains in the world (George Kerry et al., 2018; Työppönen et al., 2003), followed by *L. casei* strain Shirota (Terue et al., 2006; Wang et al., 2015).

In general, the LAB can withstand adverse conditions in the gastrointestinal tract, such as enzymatic action and acidity. They may colonize the host intestinal mucosa and contribute to health because they can regulate the microbiome and the immune system and possess antimicrobial activity, among other biological functions (Maria et al., 2013).

In this context, several in vitro and animal studies reported the cholesterol-lowering activity of probiotic LAB (Le & Yang, 2019; Nami et al., 2019; Ooi & Liong, 2010), which is of great interest to prevent CVD. In humans, the cholesterol-lowering effect of probiotic LAB was first reported in the 1970s due to the regular consumption of an *L. acidophilus*-fermented milk (Mann & Spoerry, 1974). In the following years, numerous LAB were related to reducing blood triglycerides, total cholesterol, and LDL-C (Houem et al., 2017; Ma et al., 2020).

In addition, numerous clinical trials have been accomplished to investigate the probiotic effects of LAB, especially their hypolipidemic effects. Because of that, several systematized reviews and meta-analyses on this subject were published in the last decade. In general, their conclusions point out many LAB strains as cholesterol-lowering probiotics. For example, in 2014, 26 clinical trials investigating the effects of several strains of probiotics on serum LDL-C were analyzed in a systematic review. The main conclusion was that *Lactobacillus reuteri* NCIMB 30242 and the combination of *Lactobacillus acidophilus* La5 and *Bifidobacterium lactis* Bb12 could significantly reduce serum LDL-C in hypercholesterolemic subjects. In addition, it concluded that *L. acidophilus* CHO-220 plus inulin and *L. acidophilus* plus fructooligosaccharides also significantly decreased LDL-C (Dirienzo, 2014). A meta-analysis of randomized controlled trials was recently accomplished to assess probiotic's efficacy in lowering serum lipid concentrations. The authors concluded that *L. acidophilus*, *L. plantarum*, and *L. reuteri* significantly decreased the total serum cholesterol. *L. plantarum* and a mixture of *L. helveticus* and *Enterococus faecium* significantly reduced serum LDL-C. There were no effects in TAG or HDL-C from any strain evaluated. Furthermore, the effects of probiotics on decreasing total cholesterol and LDL-C levels were more remarkable for longer intervention times (>6 weeks) and in younger mildly hypercholesterolemic subjects (Rui et al., 2019).

Therefore some probiotic LAB supplementation could be taken as a novel therapy for hypercholesterolemia. However, although enough evidence of their hypocholesterolemic effect is available from in vitro and in vivo studies and clinical trials, their exact cholesterol-lowering mechanisms are still obscure and need more profound studies. In general, the strain-specific effects, dosage, metabolic and enzymatic potential, carrier, viable number, the discreet and specific physiology and metabolism of individual hosts, and their responsiveness to probiotic could mediate the probiotic cholesterol-lowering ability of microorganisms (Bhat & Bajaj, 2019).

23.2.2 Probiotic non-LAB

Some non-LAB have also been described as probiotics, such as *Bacillus* and *Propionibacterium* species. *Bacillus* spp. are Gram-positive bacteria and form spores as a survival strategy in response to adverse environmental conditions. These bacteria belong to the Firmicutes phylum, and due to their resistance feature, they have shown increased interest for human and animal use as probiotics.

Lactobacillus and *Bifidobacterium* are the most studied and employed general as probiotics since they are part of natural gut microbiota (Hardy et al., 2013). However, these microorganisms may show low viability for a long storage period at environmental temperature (Corona-Hernandez et al., 2013; Succi et al., 2017). Conversely, due to spore formation, *Bacillus* spp. may survive for long periods of storage, representing an advantage for probiotic action.

Several spore-forming *Bacillus* species have been studied and applied as probiotics for both animals and humans, such as *B. coagulans*, *B. subtilis*, *B. licheniformis*, *B. pumilus*, *B. amyloliquefaciens*, *B. clausii*, and *B. polyfermentans* (Elshaghabee et al., 2017). They have been shown to prevent several gastrointestinal conditions and diseases, and the diversity of species and their applications are remarkable. The interest in these species for humans is due to their tolerance and ability to survive in gastric acid and the hostile intestinal environment (Hong et al., 2005).

Among the probiotic *Bacillus* species, *B. coagulans* and *B. subtillis* have been studied for a long time. Animal and preclinical studies of *Bacillus* strains have mainly focused on the prevention and treatment of gastrointestinal tract disorders, such as irritable bowel syndrome (IBS), antibiotic-associated diarrhea, inflammatory bowel disease, and colorectal cancer (Dolin, 2009; Marzorati et al., 2020; Sudha et al., 2018). They have also been used to treat and/or prevent nongastrointestinal conditions, including bacterial vaginosis, obesity, and major depression induced by IBS (Jäger et al., 2018; Ratna Sudha et al., 2012; Wu et al., 2018).

The cholesterol-lowering potential of *Bacillus* strains has been shown in vitro and animal models. The *B. coagulans* MTCC 5856 strain, in vitro, deconjugated bile salts and liberated deoxycholic acid, confirming its bile salt hydrolase activity. It also reduced cholesterol levels in culture media under growing, resting, and even heat-killed conditions. In addition, it reduced the cholesterol levels in cholesterol-rich foods, such as egg yolk, chicken liver, and butter, when incubated for 24 h in conditions mimicking the in vivo environment. Nevertheless, *B. coagulans* MTCC 5856 also produced significant amounts of propionic acid and butyric acid (SCFAs) while fermenting cholesterol-rich foods (Majeed et al., 2019). All those findings indicated the cholesterol-lowering potential of this strain. More recently, another strain, *B. coagulans* T242, showed good cholesterol assimilation potential (Sui et al., 2020). Moreover, in hypercholesterolemic rats, *B. coagulans* reduced the levels of triglycerides, cholesterol, LDL-C, VLDL-C, and the atherogenic index in the serum of these animals (Aminlari et al., 2019). The oral administration of both *B. coagulans* B37 and *B. pumilus* B9 resulted in decreased plasma cholesterol, LDL-C, and atherogenic index in hypercholesterolemic rats (Lopamudra & Gandhi, 2018).

In addition, some *Bacillus* strain metabolites could be considered for cholesterol-lowering management. For example, Zouari et al. (2015) explored the antidiabetic and antilipidemic properties of a biosurfactant produced by *B. subtilis* (SPB1) in alloxan-induced diabetic rats. Upon oral administration, the biosurfactant reduced the plasma alpha-amylase activity, protecting pancreatic β cells, and reduced serum total cholesterol, LDL-C, and TAG, while increased HDL-C. In another study, a purified exopolysaccharide from *B. subtilis* (BSEPS) reduced blood glucose, troponin, total serum cholesterol, LDL-C, and VLDL-C in streptozotocin-induced diabetic rats (Ghoneim et al., 2016).

Although there is evidence regarding the hypocholesterolemic potential of *Bacillus* strains from in vitro and in vivo studies, clinical trials investigating their cholesterol-lowering properties are scarce. In 1990 Mohan et al. conducted a nonrandomized study of 17 hyperlipidemic patients, in which two tablets, each containing 3.6×10^8 spores of *B. coagulans*, were given to patients three times per day for 12 weeks. In this study, which, unfortunately, did not carry dietary controls, reductions in serum total cholesterol were observed (Mohan et al., 1990). More recently, a randomized, double-blind, placebo-controlled 4-week intervention conducted in individuals 18–65 years of age showed that *B. subtillis* supplementation significantly reduced total cholesterol and non-HDL-C. Also, there were trending improvements in endothelial function and in LDL-C (Trotter et al., 2020). These data suggested that *B. subtilis* supplementation may be beneficial for improving risk factors associated with CVD. Therefore studies mentioned above support the cholesterol-lowering potential of spore-forming *Bacillus* strains, but further validation in human clinical trials is needed.

23.2.3 Hypolipidemic mechanisms of action of probiotic bacteria

Probiotic bacteria produce a lipid-lowering effect via various mechanisms (Fig. 23.1). The probiotic action mode is likely to be multifactorial and strain specific but usually includes microbial physiology, microbial ecology, and host

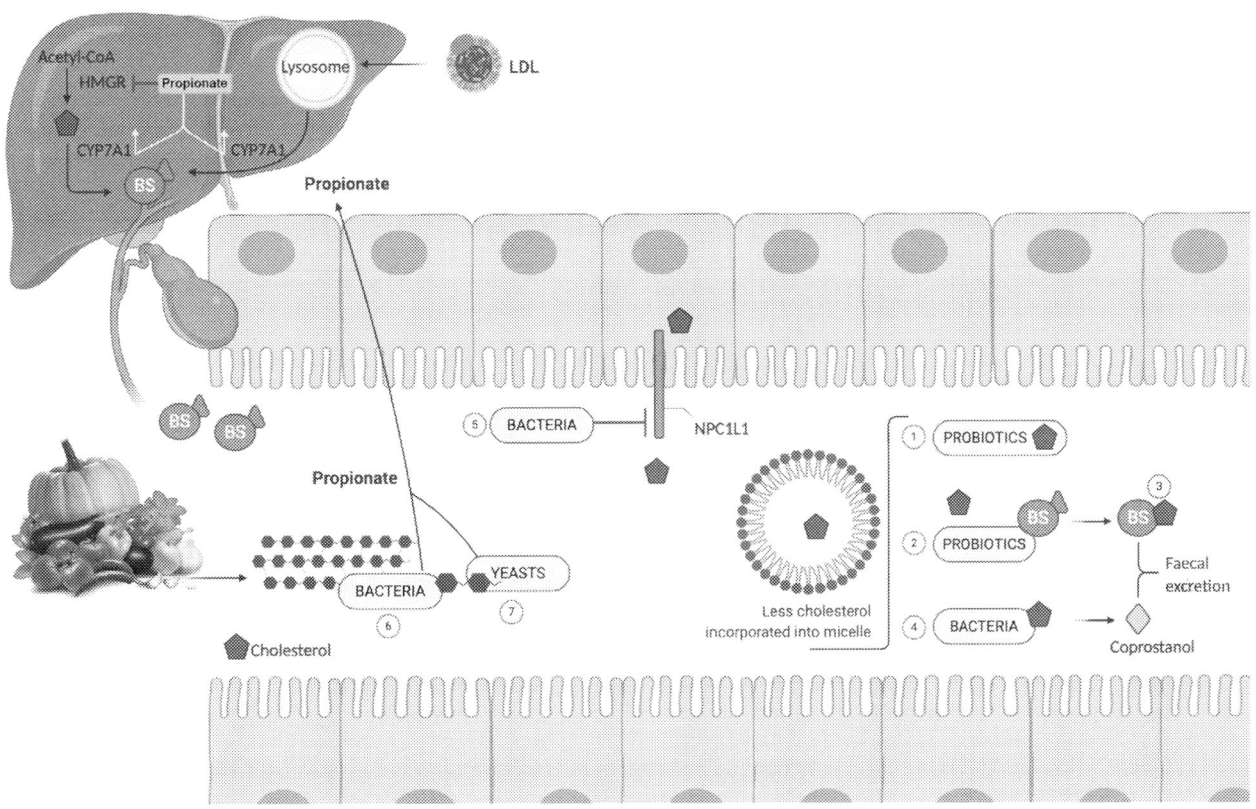

FIGURE 23.1 Proposed mechanisms of action for probiotic bacteria and yeasts: probiotic bacteria and yeasts can (1) assimilate and incorporate cholesterol into their cell membranes, (2) deconjugate bile salts (*BS*) by the action of the *BS* hydrolase enzyme, (3) coprecipitate cholesterol with deconjugated BS. Probiotic bacteria also can (4) convert cholesterol to coprostanol by the cholesterol reductase and (5) inhibit gene expression of the intestinal cholesterol transporter Niemann–Pick C1 Like 1. All those mechanisms reduce the absorption of intestinal cholesterol and lipids. Probiotic bacteria (6) fermentate indigestible carbohydrates leading to propionate production, which inhibits the hepatic activity of HMGR and stimulates CYP7A1, reducing cholesterol synthesis and increasing BS production. Also, the intake of polysaccharides extracted from yeast cell walls (7) can be used as substrate by the intestinal microbiota, which may increase the production of propionate, inhibiting the activity of the hepatic HMGR and reducing the cholesterol synthesis. Created in BioRender.com.

physiological response (Fava et al., 2006). Therefore based on in vitro and animal studies, several hypolipidemic mechanisms of action of probiotics have been suggested, such as (1) deconjugation of bile salts; (2) bacterial conversion of cholesterol into coprostanol; (3) incorporation and assimilation of cholesterol into the membrane; (4) coprecipitation of cholesterol; (5) inhibition of cholesterol transmembrane transporter [Niemann–Pick type-C1 Like-1 (NPC1L1)] expression in enterocytes; and (6) modulation of lipid metabolism by SCFAs: inhibition of hepatic synthesis of cholesterol (Hassan et al., 2019; Reis et al., 2017).

23.2.3.1 Deconjugation of bile salts

Hepatocytes produce bile salts from cholesterol, and they are used in the digestive process. After playing their role in the digestion, bile salts are reabsorbed by passive diffusion along the small intestine and by active transport in the terminal ileum, being recycled back to the liver (enterohepatic circulation). However, up to 5% of the total bile salt pool remains in the lumen and serves as a substrate for bacterial metabolism in the gastrointestinal tract (Gérard, 2013). Therefore bile salts are deconjugated by the action of the enzyme bile salt hydrolase (BSH).

In the enterohepatic circulation, BSH hydrolyzes the amide bond (C-24N-acyl amide) of the bile salts, which leads to hydroxylation of conjugated glycodeoxycholic and taurodeoxycholic, releasing glycine or taurine from the steroid nucleus. In this form, the steroid nucleus is called deconjugated or unconjugated bile salt. This mechanism results in glyco- and tauro-bile acids release (Marimuthu et al., 2020). The deconjugated bile salts have low solubility and are absorbed in lower amounts by the enterocytes than the conjugated form. In addition, they are eliminated with the feces (Kumar et al., 2012). As fecal excretion of bile salts increases, fewer of them are carried back to the liver by the enterohepatic circulation. Therefore the demand for cholesterol for de novo synthesis of bile salts in the liver also increases.

The liver increases the LDL receptor expression, increasing the hepatic uptake of LDL-C from the circulation. Thereby, total serum cholesterol and LDL-C concentrations are reduced (Lecerf & De Lorgeril, 2011).

This mechanism has been considered as the main responsible for the hypocholesterolemic effect of the regular consumption of probiotics, especially bacteria, since cholesterol and bile salt metabolism are closely related (Ishimwe et al., 2015). So far, many bacterial genera, such as *Clostridium*, *Bifidobacterium*, *Lactobacillus*, *Bacteroides*, *Enterococcus* (Ridlon et al., 2014; Tanaka et al., 1999), *Bacillus* (Majeed et al., 2019), and possibly many others, have BSH-positive activity.

23.2.3.2 Bacterial conversion of cholesterol into coprostanol

Dietary and endogenous cholesterol excreted by the transintestinal cholesterol efflux can be metabolized by the colonic microbiota in the intestinal lumen. By this mechanism, cholesterol is reduced mainly to coprostanol (5β-cholestan-3β-ol), and coprostanone. Both have low intestinal absorption and are eliminated with the feces. This process decreases in the cholesterol intestinal absorption or re-absorption (Gérard, 2013), which may contribute to reduce serum cholesterol. Indeed, the presence of coprostanol-forming bacteria in stool samples is associated with lower levels of fecal cholesterol (Kenny et al., 2020).

The efficiency of conversion of cholesterol to coprostanol is due to the abundance and activity of cholesterol-reducing bacteria in the intestinal microbiota. This ability was first reported in the 1930s (Schoenheimer, 1931). From that on, *Bifidobacterium*, *Lactobacillus*, and *Peptostreptococcus* strains were reported to reduce cholesterol to coprostanol (Crowther et al., 1973; Lye, Rusul, et al., 2010). *Lactobacillus* probiotic strains, such as *L. bulgaricus* FTCC 0411, *L. casei* 1311 FTDC ATCC 393, *B. bifidum* PRL2010, *L. acidophilus* ATCC 314, *L. acidophilus* FTCC 0291, and *Eubacterium coprostanoligenes* ATCC 51222, can convert cholesterol to coprostanol (Gérard, 2013; Lye, Rusul, et al., 2010; Zanotti et al., 2015). It seems that these strains have the cholesterol reductase, both in intracellular and extracellular compartments, which catalyzes the reduction of cholesterol in coprostanol (Lye, Rusul, et al., 2010). Interestingly, there is little information in the scientific literature about the strains positive for this enzyme; however, its activity is strain specific (Reis et al., 2017).

It is important to highlight that the cholesterol reductase enzyme expression and activity is affected by bile salts and by the type of bile salts present in the medium, as well as cholesterol. For example, the conversion is reduced in the medium supplemented with oxgall and taurocholic acid (Lye, Rusul, et al., 2010). Therefore the utilization of a strain positive for the cholesterol reductase enzyme may not be sufficient to significantly increase the conversion of cholesterol to coprostanol (Reis et al., 2017).

23.2.3.3 Incorporation and assimilation of cholesterol into the membrane

Cholesterol assimilation and incorporation into bacterial membranes was first noted in the early 1970s. By that time, mycoplasmas and several strains had shown to require exogenous cholesterol for growth and were able to incorporate large amounts into their cell membranes (Gilliland et al., 1985; Razin, 1975).

Many studies have investigated the mechanisms of cholesterol assimilation by probiotic bacteria. It has been proposed that cholesterol removal from culture media may be due to cholesterol precipitation and cholesterol binding to bacterial cell walls or its assimilation during growth (Noh et al., 1997; Tahri et al., 1996).

So far, the ability of bacterial uptake of cholesterol has been shown in vitro in several strains of *Lactobacillus*, including *L. acidophilus*, *L. delbrueckii* subsp. *bulgaricus*, *L. casei* and *L. gasseri* (Gilliland et al., 1985; Lye, Rahmat-Ali, et al., 2010; Walker & Gilliland, 1993) and distinct strains of *Bifidobacterium* (Liong & Shah, 2005; Tahri et al., 1996). *Bacillus coagulans* T242 also showed good cholesterol assimilation (Sui et al., 2020).

The amount of cholesterol uptake is strain specific and could be the consequence of the differences in the production capacity of exopolysaccharides. Therefore the amount of exopolysaccharide produced is strongly associated to the quantity of cholesterol assimilated by the strain. It seems the ability of each strain to assimilate cholesterol depends on the composition and structure of the peptidoglycan of the bacterial cell walls. Also, it is possible that differences in the expression of genes involved in intracellular cholesterol transport could contribute to the differences between strains (Tok & Aslim, 2010).

23.2.3.4 Coprecipitation of cholesterol

Intestinal absorption of cholesterol depends on the action of bile salts. Cholesterol is a hydrophobic molecule, so it needs to be emulsified by the bile salts to be absorbed. However, as previously discussed, some probiotic bacteria can deconjugate bile salts in the intestinal lumen. Furthermore, bile salts are less effective as emulsifiers in the deconjugated form than conjugated bile salts and do not form stable micelles. Therefore by producing deconjugated bile salts in the small intestine, probiotics prevent stable micelles' production, impairing the cholesterol uptake by enterocytes (Lye, Rahmat-Ali, et al., 2010).

Deconjugated bile salts are protonated and precipitated at acidic pH. Therefore intestinal cholesterol can be coprecipitated with deconjugated bile salts and will not be absorbed (Ahn et al., 2003; Fava et al., 2006). For the coprecipitation, it is necessary the presence of bile salts in the deconjugated form in the medium (Klaver & van der Meer, 1993).

Thereafter, pH of the medium is determinant of the coprecipitation of cholesterol with deconjugated bile salts. BSH needs a pH usually between 5 and 6, to have optimum performance (Guo et al., 2011) and deconjugated bile salts precipitate at a pH of lower than 6. Furthermore, the precipitation of cholesterol is codependent on the precipitation of bile salts (Klaver & van der Meer, 1993). Also, when the medium's pH reaches 7, cholesterol can re-dissolve (Tahri et al., 1996). Therefore due to the variability of pH along the intestine, it has been suggested that the coprecipitation of cholesterol with the unconjugated bile salts contributes little to the decrease of the absorption of cholesterol in vivo (Klaver & van der Meer, 1993).

Despite that, in vitro studies show the ability of several strains in coprecipitate cholesterol with the unconjugated bile salts, such as *L. acidophilus* SNUL020, SNUL01, and FM01 (Ahn et al., 2003), and *L. plantarum* Lp91, *L. plantarum* Lp21, and NCDO82 (Kumar et al., 2011).

23.2.3.5 Inhibition of cholesterol transmembrane transporter expression in enterocytes

The NPC1L1 sterol transporter is a polytopic transmembrane protein (Davies et al., 2000) from the apical membrane of the enterocytes and mediates the intestinal absorption of dietary and biliary cholesterol (Altmann et al., 2004). Therefore this protein has an essential role in maintaining cholesterol homeostasis (Betters & Yu, 2010). Several strains of probiotic bacteria have been shown to decrease these transporters' expression, in vitro and in vivo, such as *L. plantarum* Lp27 (Huang et al., 2013), *L. acidophilus* ATCC 4356 (Huang & Zheng, 2010), *L. acidophilus* La5, and *B. animalis* subsp. *lactis* Bb12 (Stancu et al., 2014).

The central hypothesis for probiotic bacteria to reduce NPC1L1 expression is that some molecules produced by them would connect and stimulate liver X receptors (LXR). LXR are regulators of cholesterol homeostasis and belong to the nuclear receptor superfamily (Nomiyama & Bruemmer, 2008). Their activation reduces whole-body cholesterol and decreases atherosclerosis (Bradley et al., 2007; Repa et al., 2000). Therefore it has been proposed that molecules produced by the probiotic bacteria could activate and stimulate LXR, downregulating NPC1L1 protein expression in the gut (Huang & Zheng, 2010).

For example, Caco-2 cells stimulated with *L. acidophilus* ATCC 4356, increased their expression of the LXR. When LXR were depleted by short interfering RNA (siRNA), NPC1L1 expression was no longer decreased by *L. acidophilus* ATCC 4356. Also, there was no reduction in micellar cholesterol uptake (Huang & Zheng, 2010).

23.2.3.6 Inhibition of hepatic cholesterol synthesis and stimulation of bile acid synthesis

Cholesterol is produced from acetyl-CoA. In mammalian cells, the biosynthetic pathway is complex and involves more than 40 cytosolic and membrane-bound enzymes. In this pathway, the 3-hydroxy-3-methylglutaryl-CoA (HMGCoA) reduction to mevalonate, is catalyzed by the HMGCoA reductase (HMGR), which is the rate-limiting enzyme of the cholesterol biosynthesis. Therefore it is a specific therapeutic target in hypercholesterolemia studies and treatment strategies (Ikonen, 2006).

Inhibition of the activity of the hepatic HMGR is another mechanism described in the literature as responsible for the hypocholesterolemic effect of the regular consumption of probiotic bacteria. The inhibition of the hepatic activity of HMGR may occur as a consequence of the action of SCFAs (Hassan et al., 2019). Several probiotic bacteria can fermentate nondigestible carbohydrates in the host producing, at last, SCFAs (Guilloteau et al., 2010). The major SCFAs produced are acetate, propionate, and butyrate. Other end products can be produced in minor amounts, such as lactate, succinate, formate, valerate, caproate, isobutyrate, 2-methyl-butyrate, and isovalerate (Vipperla & O'Keefe, 2012).

Among SCFAs, it seems propionate and is the main one involved in hypocholesterolemic effects. Propionate is an inhibitor of lipogenesis and cholesterogenesis. It inhibits the HMGR activity because it impairs the incorporation of acetate into the molecules of steroids, which, at last, reduces whole-body cholesterol (Wolever et al., 1995).

Furthermore, propionate can stimulate the hepatic synthesis of bile salts. Degradation of cholesterol into bile acid in the liver proceeds via a neutral (classical) or an acidic (alternative) pathway. Only the classical pathway of bile acid synthesis occurs in the hepatocytes, while the peripheral tissues mostly use the alternative pathway. In the case of the neutral pathway, carbon 7 of the cholesterol steroid ring is first hydroxylated. This reaction is facilitated by the rate-imitating cholesterol 7α-hydroxylase (CYP7A1) enzyme and is the most crucial step of bile acids' biosynthesis. Propionate also seems to be able to increase the activity of the CYP7A1, leading to an increase in the conversion of cholesterol in bile salts (Arora et al., 2011).

In this sense, in vivo studies have shown that several bacterial strains have their hypocholesterolemic effects mediated by propionate, such as *L. plantarum* MA2, *L. casei* F0822, and *L. plantarum* KCTC3928 (Jeun et al., 2010). Moreover, *L. acidophilus* ATCC 43121 showed to increase the expression of the hepatic CYP7A1 (Park et al., 2007). Similarly, *L. plantarum* KCTC3928 also increased bile acid levels in mice's feces and upregulated gene expression and CYP7A1 levels (Jeun et al., 2010).

It is essential to consider that the hypocholesterolemic effect of the bacterial SCFAs depends on the amount of propionate and acetate produced by the probiotic bacteria in the intestinal lumen since they have opposite effects on the hepatic cholesterol synthesis. As described, propionate can reduce the hepatic biosynthesis of cholesterol. However, in the liver, acetate, another SCFA produced by probiotic bacteria, is converted to acetyl-CoA, which can be used to synthesize cholesterol by the activity of the HMGR. Thus acetate could increase serum cholesterol concentration (Henningsson et al., 2001). Thus to have the hypocholesterolemic effect, it is necessary to consume probiotic bacteria that produce more propionate than acetate. In addition, the production of SCFAs can be increased when the host consumes a prebiotic (Reis et al., 2017).

23.3 Probiotic yeasts

Based on its diverse fermentative activities, yeasts have been used to produce many kinds of fermented foods. Three species of yeasts, *Saccharomyces cerevisiae*, *Candida utilis*, and *Kluyveromyces marxianus*, are widely used as dried yeasts for a different purpose (Yoshida et al., 2004). Among them, *Saccharomyces cerevisiae* var. *boulardii*, also known as *S. boulardii* or *S. cerevisiae* Hansen CBS 5926, is the most studied as probiotic yeast.

Historically, research on probiotic microorganisms has been performed using bacterial systems, although *S. boulardii* has been described as probiotic since 1923 (Mcfarland & Bernasconi, 1993). The presence of commensal fungal species in the human gut indicates that yeasts can benefit the host as well. Due to some characteristics, such as natural resistance to antibiotics, no association with genes' transfer related to antibiotic resistance and elimination after the interruption of probiotic consumption, yeast studies as probiotics have extensively increased lately (Czerucka et al., 2007).

Therefore *S. boulardii* has been commonly employed as a therapeutic and preventive agent in the world (Kelesidis & Pothoulakis, 2012). Many preparations of this yeast are typically recommended to treat acute gastrointestinal diseases, such as rotaviral and bacterial diarrhea, (Kelesidis & Pothoulakis, 2012) and chronic conditions, such as inflammatory bowel disease (Madsen, 2001). In addition, other yeast species have been reported to possess probiotic properties, including *Kluyveromyces marxianus*, *Kluyveromyces lactis*, *Debaryomyces hansenii*, *Torulaspora delbrueckii*, *Candida krusei*, *Candida utilis*, *Isaatchenkia orientalis*, *Yarrowia lipolytica*, *Pichia fermentase*, *Pichia kudriavzevii*, and others (Kumura et al., 2004; Psomas et al., 2003; Romanin et al., 2016; Saber et al., 2017).

Several yeasts isolated from raw milk and a wide range of fermented foods have demonstrated the ability to assimilate cholesterol in vitro, indicating a promising hypocholesterolemic potential for them (Şanlidere Aloğlu et al., 2016). In animal models, there are several studies with different lineages. For example, *S. cerevisiae* ARDMC1 isolated from traditional rice beer reduced serum LDL-C, VLDL-C, total cholesterol, and TAG of Wistar rats fed a high-cholesterol diet without affecting HDL-C (Saikia et al., 2018). In hamsters fed a 0.3% cholesterol-diet, the daily administration (3 g/kg) of *S. boulardii* CNCM I-745 for 21 or 39 days significantly reduced total plasma cholesterol and increased fecal total cholesterol compared to vehicle-treated animals (Briand et al., 2019).

In humans, scientific evidence on the hypocholesterolemic effects of yeasts is still lacking. A significant reduction in remnant lipoprotein particle (RLP-P) content was observed in the hypercholesterolemic patients who had probiotic supplementation with *S. cerevisiae* var. *boulardii* CNCM I-1079 for 8 weeks (four probiotic capsules at 1.4×10^9 CFU/capsule, twice per day). Although there was no modification for total cholesterol, LDL-C, VLDL-C, HDL-C, and TG levels, the results suggested that CNCM I-1079 supplementation could prevent and treat coronary artery disease (Ryan et al., 2015).

The hypocholesterolemic effect of probiotic yeasts is strain specific and depends on the differences in the composition of the cell wall. Cell walls of many yeasts are mainly composed of β-glucan and α-mannan, two types of dietary fibers, but their structures are strain specific (Yoshida et al., 2005). In this sense, rats fed a cholesterol-enriched diet, supplemented with β-glucan (30 g/kg of diet; for eight weeks) isolated from the baker's yeast *S. cerevisiae* exhibited a reduction in serum total cholesterol and LDL-C concentrations, while HDL-C and TAG concentrations were not affected by the treatment (El-Arab et al., 2009). Similar results were observed in the study performed by Wilson, Barbato, and Nicolosi (Klaver & van der Meer, 1993) in Syrian golden hamsters fed on a hypercholesterolemic diet supplemented with 10 g of yeast β-glucan/100 g of diet for 12 weeks.

In humans, the hypocholesterolemic effect of these polysaccharides has also been observed. Mildly hypercholesterolaemic subjects consumed a cell wall extract of *K. marxuanus* YIT 8292 (2 and 4 g/day, for 4 weeks) and they had serum total cholesterol and LDL-C concentrations, reduced. A similar effect was observed when a yogurt containing with 3 or 4 g/day of polysaccharides from the cell wall of *K. marxuanus* YIT 8292 was consumed for normal and hypercholesterolaemic subjects for 8 weeks (Yoshida et al., 2007).

23.3.1 Proposed hypocholesterolemic mechanisms of action for probiotic yeasts

Although many yeasts are used in the food industry, few studies have been evaluated the hypocholesterolemic effect of the regular consumption of probiotic yeasts. Thus little is known about the mechanisms for the hypocholesterolemic effect of regular probiotic yeast consumption (Fig. 23.1).

It has been shown that the intake of the polysaccharides extracted from the several yeast cell walls increases bile salts' fecal excretion. In addition, yeasts have fibers into their cell walls, like β-glucans, that bind to bile salts in the intestine, resulting in decreased bile acid pool and enhanced cholesterol breakdown (Yoshida et al., 2005). As previously discussed, the increase in bile salts' fecal excretion increases the demand for cholesterol for the hepatic synthesis of more bile salts. Moreover, yeasts polysaccharides can be used as a substrate by the intestinal microbiota, increasing the production of SCFAs, especially propionate, which, as previously described, can decrease the hepatic synthesis of cholesterol (Yoshida et al., 2005).

Like probiotic bacteria, some strains of yeasts can produce the BSH enzyme and, consequently, deconjugate bile salts (Liu et al., 2012), increasing the excretion of endogenous cholesterol and, in turn, stimulate the hepatic synthesis of bile salts and consequently reduce the amount of absorbed intestinal cholesterol; furthermore, the formation of micelles will be compromised (Kumar et al., 2011). BSH activity was observed for *K. marxianus* K1 and M3, as well as it was proportional to the amount of cholesterol removed from the culture medium. In addition, the lower concentration of cholesterol was due to its coprecipitation with the deconjugated bile salts (Liu et al., 2012).

Yeast cholesterol-lowering ability could also be due to cholesterol uptake; however, this mechanism is highly strain specific and growth-dependent. *S. cerevisiae* 832, *S. boulardii*, *Cryptococcus humicola* M5−2, *S. cerevisiae* KK1, and *I. orientalis* KK5.Y.1 were able to assimilate cholesterol from culture medium, compared to other strains. It seems that the cholesterol assimilation mechanism of probiotic yeasts is also similar to that of probiotic bacteria (Psomas et al., 2003).

Although in vitro and in vivo results on hypocholesterolemic effects of yeasts are promising, results from clinical trials are scarce. Therefore through more studies, it will be possible to identify hypocholesterolemic effects of yeasts in humans and to uncover more mechanisms through which yeast's regular consumption can cause those effects.

23.4 Conclusion

In the last decades probiotic bacteria and yeasts have awakened the scientific interest regarding their potential as protectors against CVD. The primary way in this protection is its hypocholesterolemic effects. Elevated LDL-C levels are the main risk of CVD since the aggregation of LDL-C in the blood and vessels may cause hypertension and hyperlipidemia and, consequently, lead to atherosclerotic lesions in the blood vessels. The hypocholesterolemic effect of probiotics is species and strain specific, with several hypothesized modes of action (Fig. 23.1).

Therefore specific probiotics might potentially decrease serum cholesterol and LDL-C levels in humans. However, additional studies are needed to investigate the fundamental mechanisms underlying the cholesterol-lowering effect of probiotics. It is also necessary to test the probiotic effect with different doses of various probiotics and long-term periods, to evaluate their long-term and strain-specific effects.

References

Ahn, Y. T., Kim, G. B., Lim, K. S., Baek, Y. J., & Kim, H. U. (2003). Deconjugation of bile salts by Lactobacillus acidophilus isolates. *International Dairy Journal*, *13*(4), 303−311. Available from https://doi.org/10.1016/S0958-6946(02)00174-7.

Altmann, S. W., Davis, H. R., Zhu, L. J., Yao, X., Hoos, L. M., Tetzloff, G., Iyer, S. P. N., Maguire, M., Golovko, A., Zeng, M., Wang, L., Murgolo, N., & Graziano, M. P. (2004). Niemann-Pick C1 Like 1 protein is critical for intestinal cholesterol absorption. *Science (New York, N.Y.), 303*(5661), 1201−1204. Available from https://doi.org/10.1126/science.1093131.

Aminlari, L., Shekarforoush, S. S., Hosseinzadeh, S., Nazifi, S., Sajedianfard, J., & Eskandari, M. H. (2019). Effect of probiotics Bacillus coagulans and Lactobacillus plantarum on lipid profile and feces bacteria of rats fed cholesterol-enriched diet. *Probiotics and Antimicrobial Proteins, 11*(4), 1163−1171. Available from https://doi.org/10.1007/s12602-018-9480-1.

Arora, T., Sharma, R., & Frost, G. (2011). Propionate. Anti-obesity and satiety enhancing factor? *Appetite, 56*(2), 511−515. Available from https://doi.org/10.1016/j.appet.2011.01.016.

Baigent, C., Blackwell, L., Emberson, J., Holland, L. E., Reith, C., Bhala, N., Peto, R., Barnes, E. H., Keech, A., Simes, J., Collins, R., De Lemos, J., Braunwald, E., Blazing, M., Murphy, S., Downs, J. R., Gotto, A., Clearfield, M., . . . Holdaas, H. (2010). Efficacy and safety of more intensive lowering of LDL cholesterol: A meta-analysis of data from 170 000 participants in 26 randomised trials. *The Lancet, 376*(9753), 1670−1681. Available from https://doi.org/10.1016/S0140-6736(10)61350-5.

Baigent, C., Keech, A., Kearney, P. M., Blackwell, L., Buck, G., Pollicino, C., Kirby, A., Sourjina, T., Peto, R., Collins, R., Simes, R., & Cholesterol Treatment Trialists' (CTT) Collaborators. (2005). Efficacy and safety of cholesterol-lowering treatment: Prospective meta-analysis of data from 90 056 participants in 14 randomised trials of statins. *The Lancet*, 1267−1278. Available from https://doi.org/10.1016/s0140-6736(05)67394-1.

Betters, J. L., & Yu, L. (2010). NPC1L1 and cholesterol transport. *FEBS Letters, 584*(13), 2740−2747. Available from https://doi.org/10.1016/j.febslet.2010.03.030.

Bhat, B., & Bajaj, B. (2019). Hypocholesterolemic potential of probiotics: Concept and mechanistic insights. *Indian Journal of Experimental Biology, 57*(2), 86−95.

Boddy, A. V., Elmer, G. W., McFarland, L. V., & Levy, R. H. (1991). Influence of antibiotics on the recovery and kinetics of Saccharomyces boulardii in rats. *Pharmaceutical Research: An Official Journal of the American Association of Pharmaceutical Scientists, 8*(6), 796−800. Available from https://doi.org/10.1023/A:1015822605815.

Bomhof, M. R., Saha, D. C., Reid, D. T., Paul, H. A., & Reimer, R. A. (2014). Combined effects of oligofructose and Bifidobacterium animalis on gut microbiota and glycemia in obese rats. *Obesity, 22*(3), 763−771. Available from https://doi.org/10.1002/oby.20632.

Bradley, M. N., Hong, C., Chen, M., Joseph, S. B., Wilpitz, D. C., Wang, X., Lusis, A. J., Collins, A., Hseuh, W. A., Collins, J. L., Tangirala, R. K., & Tontonoz, P. (2007). Ligand activation of LXRβ reverses atherosclerosis and cellular cholesterol overload in mice lacking LXRα and apoE. *Journal of Clinical Investigation, 117*(8), 2337−2346. Available from https://doi.org/10.1172/JCI31909.

Briand, F., Sulpice, T., Giammarinaro, P., & Roux, X. (2019). Saccharomyces boulardii CNCM I-745 changes lipidemic profile and gut microbiota in a hamster hypercholesterolemic model. *Beneficial Microbes, 10*(5), 555−567. Available from https://doi.org/10.3920/BM2018.0134.

Cicero, A. F. G., Colletti, A., Bajraktari, G., Descamps, O., Djuric, D. M., Ezhov, M., Fras, Z., Katsiki, N., Langlois, M., Latkovskis, G., Panagiotakos, D. B., Paragh, G., Mikhailidis, D. P., Mitchenko, O., Paulweber, B., Pella, D., Pitsavos, C., Reiner, Ž., Ray, K. K., & Banach, M. (2017). Lipid lowering nutraceuticals in clinical practice: Position paper from an International Lipid Expert Panel. *Archives of Medical Science, 13*(5), 965−1005. Available from https://doi.org/10.5114/aoms.2017.69326.

Colin, H., Francisco, G., Gregor, R., Gibson, G. R., Merenstein, D. J., Bruno, P., Lorenzo, M., Berni, C. R., Flint, H. J., Seppo, S., Calder, P. C., & Ellen, S. M. (2014). The International Scientific Association for Probiotics and Prebiotics consensus statement on the scope and appropriate use of the term probiotic. *Nature Reviews Gastroenterology & Hepatology*, 506−514. Available from https://doi.org/10.1038/nrgastro.2014.66.

Corona-Hernandez, R. I., Álvarez-Parrilla, E., Lizardi-Mendoza, J., Islas-Rubio, A. R., de la Rosa, L. A., & Wall-Medrano, A. (2013). Structural stability and viability of microencapsulated probiotic bacteria: A review. *Comprehensive Reviews in Food Science and Food Safety, 12*(6), 614−628. Available from https://doi.org/10.1111/1541-4337.12030.

Crowther, J. S., Drasar, B. S., Goddard, P., Hill, M. J., & Johnson, K. (1973). The effect of a chemically defined diet on the faecal flora and faecal steroid concentration. *Gut, 14*(10), 790−793. Available from https://doi.org/10.1136/gut.14.10.790.

Czerucka, D., Piche, T., & Rampal, P. (2007). Review article: Yeast as probiotics—Saccharomyces boulardii. *Alimentary Pharmacology and Therapeutics, 26*(6), 767−778. Available from https://doi.org/10.1111/j.1365-2036.2007.03442.x.

Davies, J. P., Levy, B., & Ioannou, Y. A. (2000). Evidence for a Niemann-pick C (NPC) gene family: Identification and characterization of NPC1L1. *Genomics, 65*(2), 137−145. Available from https://doi.org/10.1006/geno.2000.6151.

Dirienzo, D. B. (2014). Effect of probiotics on biomarkers of cardiovascular disease: Implications for heart-healthy diets. *Nutrition Reviews, 72*(1), 18−29. Available from https://doi.org/10.1111/nure.12084.

Dolin, B. J. (2009). Effects of a proprietary Bacillus coagulans preparation on symptoms of diarrhea-predominant irritable bowel syndrome. *Methods and Findings in Experimental and Clinical Pharmacology, 31*(10), 655−659. Available from https://doi.org/10.1358/mf.2009.31.10.1441078.

Dunn-Emke, S., Weidner, G., & Ornish, D. (2001). Benefits of a low-fat plant-based diet. *Obesity Research, 9*(11), 731. Available from https://doi.org/10.1038/oby.2001.100.

El-Arab, A. E., Foheid, S., & El-Said, M. (2009). Effect of yeast and botanical β-glucan on serum lipid profile and cecum probiotic bacteria using rats fed cholesterol diet. *Polish Journal of Food and Nutrition Sciences, 59*(2), 169−174.

Elshaghabee, F. M. F., Rokana, N., Gulhane, R. D., Sharma, C., & Panwar, H. (2017). Bacillus as potential probiotics: Status, concerns, and future perspectives. *Frontiers in Microbiology, 8*. Available from https://doi.org/10.3389/fmicb.2017.01490.

Fava, F., Lovegrove, J. A., Gitau, R., Jackson, K. G., & Tuohy, K. M. (2006). The gut microbiota and lipid metabolism: Implications for human health and coronary heart disease. *Current Medicinal Chemistry, 13*(25), 3005−3021. Available from https://doi.org/10.2174/092986706778521814.

Ference, B. A., Ginsberg, H. N., Graham, I., Ray, K. K., Packard, C. J., Bruckert, E., Hegele, R. A., Krauss, R. M., Raal, F. J., Schunkert, H., Watt, G. F., Borén, J., Fazio, S., Horton, J. D., Masana, L., Nicholls, S. J., Nordestgaard, B. G., Van De Sluis, B., Taskinen, M. R., ... Catapano, A. L. (2017). Low-density lipoproteins cause atherosclerotic cardiovascular disease. 1. Evidence from genetic, epidemiologic, and clinical studies. A consensus statement from the European Atherosclerosis Society Consensus Panel. *European Heart Journal*, *38*(32), 2459–2472. Available from https://doi.org/10.1093/eurheartj/ehx144.

Gallagher, H., Williams, J. O., Ferekidis, N., Ismail, A., Chan, Y. H., Michael, D. R., Guschina, I. A., Tyrrell, V. J., O'Donnell, V. B., Harwood, J. L., Khozin-Goldberg, I., Boussiba, S., & Ramji, D. P. (2019). Dihomo-γ-linolenic acid inhibits several key cellular processes associated with atherosclerosis. *Biochimica et Biophysica Acta - Molecular Basis of Disease*, *1865*(9), 2538–2550. Available from https://doi.org/10.1016/j.bbadis.2019.06.011.

George Kerry, R., Patra, J. K., Gouda, S., Park, Y., Shin, H. S., & Das, G. (2018). Benefaction of probiotics for human health: A review. *Journal of Food and Drug Analysis*, *26*(3), 927–939. Available from https://doi.org/10.1016/j.jfda.2018.01.002.

Gérard, P. (2013). Metabolism of cholesterol and bile acids by the gut microbiota. *Pathogens*, *3*(1), 14–24. Available from https://doi.org/10.3390/pathogens3010014.

Ghoneim, M. A. M., Hassan, A. I., Mahmoud, M. G., & Asker, M. S. (2016). Effect of polysaccharide from bacillus subtilis sp. on cardiovascular diseases and atherogenic indices in diabetic rats. *BMC Complementary and Alternative Medicine*, *16*(1). Available from https://doi.org/10.1186/s12906-016-1093-1.

Gilliland, S. E., Nelson, C. R., & Maxwell, C. (1985). Assimilation of cholesterol by Lactobacillus acidophilus. *Applied and Environmental Microbiology*, *49*(2), 377–381. Available from https://doi.org/10.1128/aem.49.2.377-381.1985.

Gragnano, F., & Calabrò, P. (2018). Role of dual lipid-lowering therapy in coronary atherosclerosis regression: Evidence from recent studies. *Atherosclerosis*, *269*, 219–228. Available from https://doi.org/10.1016/j.atherosclerosis.2018.01.012.

Grundy, S. M. (2008). Is lowering low-density lipoprotein an effective strategy to reduce cardiac risk?: Promise of low-density lipoprotein-lowering therapy for primary and secondary prevention. *Circulation*, *117*(4), 569–573. Available from https://doi.org/10.1161/CIRCULATIONAHA.107.720300.

Guilloteau, P., Martin, L., Eeckhaut, V., Ducatelle, R., Zabielski, R., & Van Immerseel, F. (2010). From the gut to the peripheral tissues: The multiple effects of butyrate. *Nutrition Research Reviews*, *23*(2), 366–384. Available from https://doi.org/10.1017/S0954422410000247.

Guo, Z., Liu, X. M., Zhang, Q. X., Shen, Z., Tian, F. W., Zhang, H., Sun, Z. H., Zhang, H. P., & Chen, W. (2011). Influence of consumption of probiotics on the plasma lipid profile: A meta-analysis of randomised controlled trials. *Nutrition, Metabolism and Cardiovascular Diseases*, *21*(11), 844–850. Available from https://doi.org/10.1016/j.numecd.2011.04.008.

Hardy, H., Harris, J., Lyon, E., Beal, J., & Foey, A. D. (2013). Probiotics, prebiotics and immunomodulation of gut mucosal defences: Homeostasis and immunopathology. *Nutrients*, *5*(6), 1869–1912. Available from https://doi.org/10.3390/nu5061869.

Hassan, A., Din, A. U., Zhu, Y., Zhang, K., Li, T., Wang, Y., Luo, Y., & Wang, G. (2019). Updates in understanding the hypocholesterolemia effect of probiotics on atherosclerosis. *Applied Microbiology and Biotechnology*, *103*(15), 5993–6006. Available from https://doi.org/10.1007/s00253-019-09927-4.

Heidenreich, P. A., Trogdon, J. G., Khavjou, O. A., Butler, J., Dracup, K., Ezekowitz, M. D., Finkelstein, E. A., Hong, Y., Johnston, S. C., Khera, A., Lloyd-Jones, D. M., Nelson, S. A., Nichol, G., Orenstein, D., Wilson, P. W. F., & Woo, Y. J. (2011). Forecasting the future of cardiovascular disease in the United States: A policy statement from the American Heart Association. *Circulation*, *123*(8), 933–944. Available from https://doi.org/10.1161/CIR.0b013e31820a55f5.

Henningsson, A., Björck, I., & Nyman, M. (2001). Short-chain fatty acid formation at fermentation of indigestible carbohydrates. *Scandinavian Journal of Nutrition/Naringsforskning*, *45*(4), 165–168.

Hewitt, J. H., & Rigby, J. (1976). Effect of various milk feeds on numbers of Escherichia coli and Bifidobacterium in the stools of new-born infants. *Journal of Hygiene*, *77*(1), 129–139. Available from https://doi.org/10.1017/S0022172400055601.

Hong, H. A., Le, H. D., & Cutting, S. M. (2005). The use of bacterial spore formers as probiotics. *FEMS Microbiology Reviews*, *29*(4), 813–835. Available from https://doi.org/10.1016/j.femsre.2004.12.001.

Houem, R., Fillipe, R., do, C., & Gwénaël, J. (2017). Dairy propionibacteria: Versatile probiotics. *Microorganisms*, *24*. Available from https://doi.org/10.3390/microorganisms5020024.

Huang, Y., & Zheng, Y. (2010). The probiotic Lactobacillus acidophilus reduces cholesterol absorption through the down-regulation of Niemann-Pick C1-like 1 in Caco-2 cells. *British Journal of Nutrition*, *103*(4), 473–478. Available from https://doi.org/10.1017/S0007114509991991.

Huang, Y., Wu, F., Wang, X., Sui, Y., Yang, L., & Wang, J. (2013). Characterization of Lactobacillus plantarum Lp27 isolated from Tibetan kefir grains: A potential probiotic bacterium with cholesterol-lowering effects. *Journal of Dairy Science*, *96*(5), 2816–2825. Available from https://doi.org/10.3168/jds.2012-6371.

Ikonen, E. (2006). Mechanisms for cellular cholesterol transport: Defects and human disease. *Physiological Reviews*, *86*(4), 1237–1261. Available from https://doi.org/10.1152/physrev.00022.2005.

Ishimwe, N., Daliri, E. B., Lee, B. H., Fang, F., & Du, G. (2015). The perspective on cholesterol-lowering mechanisms of probiotics. *Molecular Nutrition and Food Research*, *59*(1), 94–105. Available from https://doi.org/10.1002/mnfr.201400548.

Jäger, R., Purpura, M., Farmer, S., Cash, H. A., & Keller, D. (2018). Probiotic Bacillus coagulans GBI-30, 6086 improves protein absorption and utilization. *Probiotics and Antimicrobial Proteins*, *10*(4), 611–615. Available from https://doi.org/10.1007/s12602-017-9354-y.

Jeun, J., Kim, S., Cho, S. Y., Jun, H. J., Park, H. J., Seo, J. G., Chung, M. J., & Lee, S. J. (2010). Hypocholesterolemic effects of Lactobacillus plantarum KCTC3928 by increased bile acid excretion in C57BL/6 mice. *Nutrition (Burbank, Los Angeles County, Calif.)*, *26*(3), 321–330. Available from https://doi.org/10.1016/j.nut.2009.04.011.

Jiang, J., Wu, C., Zhang, C., Zhao, J., Yu, L., Zhang, H., Narbad, A., Chen, W., & Zhai, Q. (2020). Effects of probiotic supplementation on cardiovascular risk factors in hypercholesterolemia: A systematic review and meta-analysis of randomized clinical trial. *Journal of Functional Foods, 74*. Available from https://doi.org/10.1016/j.jff.2020.104177.

Kelesidis, T., & Pothoulakis, C. (2012). Efficacy and safety of the probiotic Saccharomyces boulardii for the prevention and therapy of gastrointestinal disorders. *Therapeutic Advances in Gastroenterology, 5*(2), 111–125. Available from https://doi.org/10.1177/1756283X11428502.

Kenny, D. J., Plichta, D. R., Shungin, D., Koppel, N., Hall, A. B., Fu, B., Vasan, R. S., Shaw, S. Y., Vlamakis, H., Balskus, E. P., & Xavier, R. J. (2020). Cholesterol metabolism by uncultured human gut bacteria influences host cholesterol level. *Cell Host and Microbe, 28*(2), 245–257.e6. Available from https://doi.org/10.1016/j.chom.2020.05.013.

Kiousi, D. E., Karapetsas, A., Karolidou, K., Panayiotidis, M. I., Pappa, A., & Galanis, A. (2019). Probiotics in extraintestinal diseases: Current trends and new directions. *Nutrients, 11*(4). Available from https://doi.org/10.3390/nu11040788.

Klaver, F. A., & van der Meer, R. (1993). The assumed assimilation of cholesterol by Lactobacilli and Bifidobacterium bifidum is due to their bile salt-deconjugating activity. *Applied and Environmental Microbiology*, 1120–1124. Available from https://doi.org/10.1128/aem.59.4.1120-1124.1993.

Kleerebezem, M., Binda, S., Bron, P. A., Gross, G., Hill, C., van Hylckama Vlieg, J. E., Lebeer, S., Satokari, R., & Ouwehand, A. C. (2019). Understanding mode of action can drive the translational pipeline towards more reliable health benefits for probiotics. *Current Opinion in Biotechnology, 56*, 55–60. Available from https://doi.org/10.1016/j.copbio.2018.09.007.

Kumar, M., Nagpal, R., Kumar, R., Hemalatha, R., Verma, V., Kumar, A., Chakraborty, C., Singh, B., Marotta, F., Jain, S., & Yadav, H. (2012). Cholesterol-lowering probiotics as potential biotherapeutics for metabolic diseases. *Experimental Diabetes Research, 2012*. Available from https://doi.org/10.1155/2012/902917.

Kumar, R., Grover, S., & Batish, V. K. (2011). Hypocholesterolaemic effect of dietary inclusion of two putative probiotic bile salt hydrolase-producing Lactobacillus plantarum strains in Sprague-Dawley rats. *British Journal of Nutrition, 105*(4), 561–573. Available from https://doi.org/10.1017/S0007114510003740.

Kumura, H., Tanoue, Y., Tsukahara, M., Tanaka, T., & Shimazaki, K. (2004). Screening of dairy yeast strains for probiotic applications. *Journal of Dairy Science, 87*(12), 4050–4056. Available from https://doi.org/10.3168/jds.S0022-0302(04)73546-8.

Lau, K., Srivatsav, V., Rizwan, A., Nashed, A., Liu, R., Shen, R., & Akhtar, M. (2017). Bridging the gap between gut microbial dysbiosis and cardiovascular diseases. *Nutrients, 9*(8). Available from https://doi.org/10.3390/nu9080859.

Le, B., & Yang, S. H. (2019). Identification of a novel potential probiotic Lactobacillus plantarum FB003 isolated from salted-fermented shrimp and its effect on cholesterol absorption by regulation of NPC1L1 and PPARα. *Probiotics and Antimicrobial Proteins, 11*(3), 785–793. Available from https://doi.org/10.1007/s12602-018-9469-9.

Lecerf, J. M., & De Lorgeril, M. (2011). Dietary cholesterol: From physiology to cardiovascular risk. *British Journal of Nutrition, 106*(1), 6–14. Available from https://doi.org/10.1017/S0007114511000237.

Liong, M. T., & Shah, N. P. (2005). Acid and bile tolerance and cholesterol removal ability of lactobacilli strains. *Journal of Dairy Science, 88*(1), 55–66. Available from https://doi.org/10.3168/jds.S0022-0302(05)72662-X.

Liu, H., Xie, Y., Xiong, L., Dong, R., Pan, C., Teng, G., & Zhang, H. (2012). Effect and mechanism of cholesterol-lowering by Kluyveromyces from Tibetan kefir. *Advanced Materials Research, 343–344*, 1290–1298. Available from https://doi.org/10.4028/http://www.scientific.net/AMR.343-344.1290.

Lopamudra, H., & Gandhi, D. N. (2018). Cholesterol-lowering effects of Bacillus coagulans B37 and Bacillus pumilus B9 strains in a rat animal model. *Indian Journal of Animal Research*. Available from https://doi.org/10.18805/ijar.b-3549.

Lye, H. S., Rahmat-Ali, G. R., & Liong, M. T. (2010). Mechanisms of cholesterol removal by lactobacilli under conditions that mimic the human gastrointestinal tract. *International Dairy Journal, 20*(3), 169–175. Available from https://doi.org/10.1016/j.idairyj.2009.10.003.

Lye, H.-S., Rusul, G., & Liong, M.-T. (2010). Removal of cholesterol by lactobacilli via incorporation and conversion to coprostanol. *Journal of Dairy Science*, 1383–1392. Available from https://doi.org/10.3168/jds.2009-2574.

Ma, S., Yeom, J., & Lim, Y. H. (2020). Dairy Propionibacterium freudenreichii ameliorates acute colitis by stimulating MUC2 expression in intestinal goblet cell in a DSS-induced colitis rat model. *Scientific Reports, 10*(1). Available from https://doi.org/10.1038/s41598-020-62497-8.

Madsen, K. L. (2001). The use of probiotics in gastrointestinal disease. *Canadian Journal of Gastroenterology, 15*(12), 817–822. Available from https://doi.org/10.1155/2001/690741.

Majeed, M., Majeed, S., Nagabhushanam, K., Arumugam, S., Beede, K., & Ali, F. (2019). Evaluation of the in vitro cholesterol-lowering activity of the probiotic strain Bacillus coagulansMTCC 5856. *International Journal of Food Science and Technology, 54*(1), 212–220. Available from https://doi.org/10.1111/ijfs.13926.

Mann, G. V., & Spoerry, A. (1974). Studies of a surfactant and cholesteremia in the Maasai. *American Journal of Clinical Nutrition, 27*(5), 464–469. Available from https://doi.org/10.1093/ajcn/27.5.464.

Maria, K., Dimitrios, B., Stavroula, K., Dimitra, D., Konstantina, G., Nikoletta, S., & Maria, F. E. (2013). Health benefits of probiotics: A review. *ISRN Nutrition*, 1–7. Available from https://doi.org/10.5402/2013/481651.

Marimuthu, A., Balayogan, S., & Parveen, R. R. (2020). Corrigendum to "Effects of probiotics, prebiotics, and synbiotics on hypercholesterolemia: A review.". *Chinese Journal of Biology*, 1–8. Available from https://doi.org/10.1155/2020/8236703.

Marzorati, M., Van den Abbeele, P., Bubeck, S. S., Bayne, T., Krishnan, K., Young, A., Mehta, D., & Desouza, A. (2020). Bacillus subtilis HU58 and bacillus coagulans SC208 probiotics reduced the effects of antibiotic-induced gut microbiome dysbiosis in an M-SHIME® model. *Microorganisms, 8*(7), 1–15. Available from https://doi.org/10.3390/microorganisms8071028.

Mcfarland, L. V., & Bernasconi, P. (1993). Saccharomyces boulardii'. A review of an innovative biotherapeutic agent. *Microbial Ecology in Health and Disease*, *6*(4), 157–171. Available from https://doi.org/10.3109/08910609309141323.

Mendis, S., Puska, P., & Norrving, B. (2011). Global atlas on cardiovascular disease prevention and control. In S. Mendis (Ed.), *World Health Organization*. Available from https://apps.who.int/iris/handle/10665/44701.

Mennigen, R., & Bruewer, M. (2009). Effect of probiotics on intestinal barrier function. *Annals of the New York Academy of Sciences*, *1165*, 183–189. Available from https://doi.org/10.1111/j.1749-6632.2009.04059.x.

Mohan, J. C., Arora, R., & Khalilullah, M. (1990). Preliminary observations on effect of Lactobacillus sporogenes on serum lipid levels in hypercholesterolemic patients. *Indian Journal of Medical Research - Section B Biomedical Research Other Than Infectious Diseases*, *92*, 431–432.

Moss, J. W. E., & Ramji, D. P. (2016). Nutraceutical therapies for atherosclerosis. *Nature Reviews Cardiology*, *13*(9), 513–532. Available from https://doi.org/10.1038/nrcardio.2016.103.

Moss, J. W. E., Williams, J. O., & Ramji, D. P. (2018). Nutraceuticals as therapeutic agents for atherosclerosis. *Biochimica et Biophysica Acta - Molecular Basis of Disease*, *1864*(5), 1562–1572. Available from https://doi.org/10.1016/j.bbadis.2018.02.006.

Nami, Y., Vaseghi Bakhshayesh, R., Manafi, M., & Hejazi, M. A. (2019). Hypocholesterolaemic activity of a novel autochthonous potential probiotic Lactobacillus plantarum YS5 isolated from yogurt. *LWT*, *111*, 876–882. Available from https://doi.org/10.1016/j.lwt.2019.05.057.

National Cholesterol Education Program (NCEP) Expert Panel on Detection, Evaluation, and Treatment of High Blood Cholesterol in Adults (Adult Treatment Panel III). (2002). Third Report of the National Cholesterol Education Program (NCEP) Expert Panel on Detection, Evaluation, and Treatment of High Blood Cholesterol in Adults (Adult Treatment Panel III) final report. *Circulation*, *106*(25), 3143–3421. Available from https://doi.org/10.1161/circ.106.25.3143.

Noh, D. O., Kim, S. H., & Gilliland, S. E. (1997). Incorporation of cholesterol into the cellular membrane of Lactobacillus acidophilus ATCC 43121. *Journal of Dairy Science*, *80*(12), 3107–3113. Available from https://doi.org/10.3168/jds.S0022-0302(97)76281-7.

Nomiyama, T., & Bruemmer, D. (2008). Liver X receptors as therapeutic targets in metabolism and atherosclerosis. *Current Atherosclerosis Reports*, *10*(1), 88–95. Available from https://doi.org/10.1007/s11883-008-0013-3.

O'Morain, V. L., & Ramji, D. P. (2020). The potential of probiotics in the prevention and treatment of atherosclerosis. *Molecular Nutrition and Food Research*, *64*(4). Available from https://doi.org/10.1002/mnfr.201900797.

Ooi, L. G., & Liong, M. T. (2010). Cholesterol-lowering effects of probiotics and prebiotics: A review of in vivo and in vitro findings. *International Journal of Molecular Sciences*, *11*(6), 2499–2522. Available from https://doi.org/10.3390/ijms11062499.

Park, Y. H., Kim, J. G., Shin, Y. W., Kim, S. H., & Whang, K. Y. (2007). Effect of dietary inclusion of Lactobacillus acidophilus ATCC 43121 on cholesterol metabolism in rats. *Journal of Microbiology and Biotechnology*, *17*(4), 655–662.

Psomas, E. I., Fletouris, D. J., Litopoulou-Tzanetaki, E., & Tzanetakis, N. (2003). Assimilation of cholesterol by yeast strains isolated from infant feces and feta cheese. *Journal of Dairy Science*, *86*(11), 3416–3422. Available from https://doi.org/10.3168/jds.S0022-0302(03)73945-9.

Ramos, C. L., Thorsen, L., Schwan, R. F., & Jespersen, L. (2013). Strain-specific probiotics properties of Lactobacillus fermentum, Lactobacillus plantarum and Lactobacillus brevis isolates from Brazilian food products. *Food Microbiology*, *36*(1), 22–29. Available from https://doi.org/10.1016/j.fm.2013.03.010.

Rao, R. K., & Samak, G. (2013). Protection and restitution of gut barrier by probiotics: Nutritional and clinical implications. *Current Nutrition and Food Science*, *9*(2), 99–107. Available from https://doi.org/10.2174/1573401311309020004.

Ratna Sudha, M., Yelikar, K. A., & Deshpande, S. (2012). Clinical study of Bacillus coagulans unique IS-2 (ATCC PTA-11748) in the treatment of patients with bacterial vaginosis. *Indian Journal of Microbiology*, *52*(3), 396–399. Available from https://doi.org/10.1007/s12088-011-0233-z.

Razin, S. (1975). Cholesterol incorporation into bacterial membranes. *Journal of Bacteriology*, 570–572. Available from https://doi.org/10.1128/jb.124.1.570-572.1975.

Reis, S. A., Conceição, L. L., Rosa, D. D., Siqueira, N. P., & Peluzio, M. C. G. (2017). Mechanisms responsible for the hypocholesterolaemic effect of regular consumption of probiotics. *Nutrition Research Reviews*, *30*(1), 36–49. Available from https://doi.org/10.1017/S0954422416000226.

Repa, J. J., Turley, S. D., Lobaccaro, J. M. A., Medina, J., Li, L., Lustig, K., Shan, B., Heyman, R. A., Dietschy, J. M., & Mangelsdorf, D. J. (2000). Regulation of absorption and ABC1-mediated efflux of cholesterol by RXR heterodimers. *Science (New York, N.Y.)*, *289*(5484), 1524–1529. Available from https://doi.org/10.1126/science.289.5484.1524.

Ridlon, J. M., Kang, D. J., Hylemon, P. B., & Bajaj, J. S. (2014). Bile acids and the gut microbiome. *Current Opinion in Gastroenterology*, *30*(3), 332–338. Available from https://doi.org/10.1097/MOG.0000000000000057.

Romanin, D. E., Llopis, S., Genovés, S., Martorell, P., Ramón, V. D., Garrote, G. L., & Rumbo, M. (2016). Probiotic yeast Kluyveromyces marxianus CIDCA 8154 shows anti-inflammatory and anti-oxidative stress properties in in vivo models. *Beneficial Microbes*, *7*(1), 83–93. Available from https://doi.org/10.3920/BM2015.0066.

Rondanelli, M., Faliva, M. A., Perna, S., Giacosa, A., Peroni, G., & Castellazzi, A. M. (2017). Using probiotics in clinical practice: Where are we now? A review of existing meta-analyses. *Gut Microbes*, *8*(6), 521–543. Available from https://doi.org/10.1080/19490976.2017.1345414.

Roth, G. A., Abate, D., Abate, K. H., Abay, S. M., Abbafati, C., Abbasi, N., ... Murray, C. J. L. (2018). Global, regional, and national age-sex-specific mortality for 282 causes of death in 195 countries and territories, 1980–2017: A systematic analysis for the Global Burden of Disease Study 2017. *The Lancet*, *392*(10159), 1736–1788. Available from https://doi.org/10.1016/S0140-6736(18)32203-7.

Rui, M., Xingwei, Z., & Yunsheng, Y. (2019). Effect of probiotics on lipid profiles in hypercholesterolaemic adults: A meta-analysis of randomized controlled trials. *Medicina Clínica*, 473–481. Available from https://doi.org/10.1016/j.medcli.2018.09.007.

Ryan, J. J., Hanes, D. A., Schafer, M. B., Mikolai, J., & Zwickey, H. (2015). Effect of the probiotic saccharomyces boulardii on cholesterol and lipoprotein particles in hypercholesterolemic adults: A single-arm, open-label pilot study. *Journal of Alternative and Complementary Medicine*, 21(5), 288–293. Available from https://doi.org/10.1089/acm.2014.0063.

Saber, A., Alipour, B., Faghfoori, Z., Mousavi Jam, A., & Yari Khosroushahi, A. (2017). Secretion metabolites of probiotic yeast, Pichia kudriavzevii AS-12, induces apoptosis pathways in human colorectal cancer cell lines. *Nutrition Research*, 41, 36–46. Available from https://doi.org/10.1016/j.nutres.2017.04.001.

Saikia, D., Manhar, A. K., Deka, B., Roy, R., Gupta, K., Namsa, N. D., Chattopadhyay, P., Doley, R., & Mandal, M. (2018). Hypocholesterolemic activity of indigenous probiotic isolate Saccharomyces cerevisiae ARDMC1 in a rat model. *Journal of Food and Drug Analysis*, 26(1), 154–162. Available from https://doi.org/10.1016/j.jfda.2016.12.017.

Şanlidere Aloğlu, H., Demir Özer, E., & Öner, Z. (2016). Assimilation of cholesterol and probiotic characterisation of yeast strains isolated from raw milk and fermented foods. *International Journal of Dairy Technology*, 69(1), 63–70. Available from https://doi.org/10.1111/1471-0307.12217.

Schoenheimer, R. (1931). New contributions in sterol metabolism. *Science (New York, N.Y.)*, 74(1928), 579–584. Available from https://doi.org/10.1126/science.74.1928.579.

Sharifi-Rad, J., Rodrigues, C. F., Stojanović-Radić, Z., Dimitrijević, M., Aleksić, A., Neffe-Skocińska, K., Zielińska, D., Kołożyn-Krajewska, D., Salehi, B., Prabu, S. M., Schutz, F., Docea, A. O., Martins, N., & Calina, D. (2020). Probiotics: Versatile bioactive components in promoting human health. *Medicina (Lithuania)*, 56(9), 1–30. Available from https://doi.org/10.3390/medicina56090433.

Stancu, C. S., Sanda, G. M., Deleanu, M., & Sima, A. V. (2014). Probiotics determine hypolipidemic and antioxidant effects in hyperlipidemic hamsters. *Molecular Nutrition and Food Research*, 58(3), 559–568. Available from https://doi.org/10.1002/mnfr.201300224.

Stenman, L. K., Waget, A., Garret, C., Klopp, P., Burcelin, R., & Lahtinen, S. (2014). Potential probiotic Bifidobacterium animalis ssp. lactis 420 prevents weight gain and glucose intolerance in diet-induced obese mice. *Beneficial Microbes*, 5(4), 437–445. Available from https://doi.org/10.3920/BM2014.0014.

Succi, M., Tremonte, P., Pannella, G., Tipaldi, L., Cozzolino, A., Coppola, R., & Sorrentino, E. (2017). Survival of commercial probiotic strains in dark chocolate with high cocoa and phenols content during the storage and in a static in vitro digestion model. *Journal of Functional Foods*, 35, 60–67. Available from https://doi.org/10.1016/j.jff.2017.05.019.

Sudha, M. R., Jayanthi, N., Aasin, M., Dhanashri, R. D., & Anirudh, T. (2018). Efficacy of Bacillus coagulans Unique IS2 in treatment of irritable bowel syndrome in children: A double blind, randomised placebo controlled study. *Beneficial Microbes*, 9(4), 563–572. Available from https://doi.org/10.3920/BM2017.0129.

Sui, L., Zhu, X., Wu, D., Ma, T., Tuo, Y., Jiang, S., Qian, F., & Mu, G. (2020). In vitro assessment of probiotic and functional properties of Bacillus coagulans T242. *Food Bioscience*, 36. Available from https://doi.org/10.1016/j.fbio.2020.100675.

Sun, J., & Buys, N. (2015). Effects of probiotics consumption on lowering lipids and CVD risk factors: A systematic review and meta-analysis of randomized controlled trials. *Annals of Medicine*, 47(6), 430–440. Available from https://doi.org/10.3109/07853890.2015.1071872.

Tahri, K., Grill, J. P., & Schneider, F. (1996). Bifidobacteria strain behavior toward cholesterol: Coprecipitation with bile salts and assimilation. *Current Microbiology*, 33(3), 187–193. Available from https://doi.org/10.1007/s002849900098.

Tanaka, H., Doesburg, K., Iwasaki, T., & Mierau, I. (1999). Screening of lactic acid bacteria for bile salt hydrolase activity. *Journal of Dairy Science*, 82(12), 2530–2535. Available from https://doi.org/10.3168/jds.S0022-0302(99)75506-2.

Terue, S., Keiko, Y., Sachie, N., Takashi, A., Norikatsu, Y., Koji, K., Yoshitaku, Y., Yuko, S., Koji, N., & Masumi, T. (2006). The effects of a synbiotic fermented milk beverage containing Lactobacillus casei Strain Shirota and transgalactosylated oligosaccharides on defecation frequency, intestinal microflora, organic acid concentrations, and putrefactive metabolites of sub-optimal health state volunteers: A randomized placebo-controlled cross-over study. *Bioscience and Microflora*, 137–146. Available from https://doi.org/10.12938/bifidus.25.137.

Tok, E., & Aslim, B. (2010). Cholesterol removal by some lactic acid bacteria that can be used as probiotic. *Microbiology and Immunology*, 54(5), 257–264. Available from https://doi.org/10.1111/j.1348-0421.2010.00219.x.

Trotter, R. E., Vazquez, A. R., Grubb, D. S., Freedman, K. E., Grabos, L. E., Jones, S., Gentile, C. L., Melby, C. L., Johnson, S. A., & Weir, T. L. (2020). Bacillus subtilis DE111 intake may improve blood lipids and endothelial function in healthy adults. *Beneficial Microbes*, 11(7), 621–630. Available from https://doi.org/10.3920/BM2020.0039.

Työppönen, S., Petäjä, E., & Mattila-Sandholm, T. (2003). Bioprotectives and probiotics for dry sausages. *International Journal of Food Microbiology*, 83(3), 233–244. Available from https://doi.org/10.1016/S0168-1605(02)00379-3.

Vipperla, K., & O'Keefe, S. J. (2012). The microbiota and its metabolites in colonic mucosal health and cancer risk. *Nutrition in Clinical Practice*, 27(5), 624–635. Available from https://doi.org/10.1177/0884533612452012.

Walker, D. K., & Gilliland, S. E. (1993). Relationships among bile tolerance, bile salt deconjugation, and assimilation of cholesterol by Lactobacillus acidophilus. *Journal of Dairy Science*, 76(4), 956–961. Available from https://doi.org/10.3168/jds.S0022-0302(93)77422-6.

Wang, R., Chen, S., Jin, J., Ren, F., Li, Y., Qiao, Z., Wang, Y., & Zhao, L. (2015). Survival of Lactobacillus casei strain Shirota in the intestines of healthy Chinese adults. *Microbiology and Immunology*, 59(5), 268–276. Available from https://doi.org/10.1111/1348-0421.12249.

WHO. (2018a). *World health statistics 2018: Monitoring health for the SDGs, sustainable development goals*. Geneva: World Health Organization; 2018. Licence: CC BY-NC-SA 3.0 IGO.

WHO. (2018b). ICD-11 for mortality and morbidity statistics. Diseases of the circulatory system. Available in https://icd.who.int/dev11/l-m/en#/http%3a%2f%2fid.who.int%2ficd%2fentity%2f426429380.

Wolever, T. M. S., Spadafora, P. J., Cunnane, S. C., & Pencharz, P. B. (1995).). Propionate inhibits incorporation of colonic [1,2–13C]acetate into plasma lipids in humans. *American Journal of Clinical Nutrition*, 61(6), 1241–1247. Available from https://doi.org/10.1093/ajcn/61.6.1241.

World Health Organization Food and Agriculture Organization of the United Nations. (2006). Probiotics in food: Health and nutritional properties and guidelines for evaluation. Rome: FAO, p. 56.

Wu, T., Zhang, Y., Lv, Y., Li, P., Yi, D., Wang, L., Zhao, D., Chen, H., Gong, J., & Hou, Y. (2018). Beneficial impact and molecular mechanism of Bacillus coagulans on piglets' intestine. *International Journal of Molecular Sciences, 19*(7). Available from https://doi.org/10.3390/ijms19072084.

Yoshida, Y., Naito, E., Ohishi, K., Okumura, T., Ito, M., Sato, T., & Sawada, H. (2007). Effect of Kluyveromyces marxianus YIT 8292 crude cell wall fraction on serum lipids in normocholesterolemic and mildly hypercholesterolemic subjects. *Bioscience, Biotechnology, and Biochemistry, 71*(4), 900–905. Available from https://doi.org/10.1271/bbb.60539.

Yoshida, Y., Yokoi, W., Ohishi, K., Ito, M., Naito, E., & Sawada, H. (2005). Effects of the cell wall of Kluyveromyces marxianus YIT 8292 on the plasma cholesterol and fecal sterol excretion in rats fed on a high-cholesterol diet. *Bioscience, Biotechnology, and Biochemistry, 69*(4), 714–723. Available from https://doi.org/10.1271/bbb.69.714.

Yoshida, Y., Yokoi, W., Wada, Y., Ohishi, K., Ito, M., & Sawada, H. (2004). Potent hypocholesterolemic activity of the yeast Kluyveromyces marxianus YIT 8292 in rats fed a high cholesterol diet. *Bioscience, Biotechnology, and Biochemistry, 68*(6), 1185–1192. Available from https://doi.org/10.1271/bbb.68.1185.

Zanotti, I., Turroni, F., Piemontese, A., Mancabelli, L., Milani, C., Viappiani, A., Prevedini, G., Sanchez, B., Margolles, A., Elviri, L., Franco, B., van Sinderen, D., & Ventura, M. (2015). Evidence for cholesterol-lowering activity by Bifidobacterium bifidum PRL2010 through gut microbiota modulation. *Applied Microbiology and Biotechnology, 99*(16), 6813–6829. Available from https://doi.org/10.1007/s00253-015-6564-7.

Zouari, R., Ben Abdallah-Kolsi, R., Hamden, K., Feki, A. E., Chaabouni, K., Makni-Ayadi, F., Sallemi, F., Ellouze-Chaabouni, S., & Ghribi-Aydi, D. (2015). Assessment of the antidiabetic and antilipidemic properties of bacillus subtilis spb1 biosurfactant in alloxan-induced diabetic rats. *Biopolymers, 104*(6), 764–774. Available from https://doi.org/10.1002/bip.22705.

Chapter 24

Gut—brain axis: role of probiotics in neurodevelopmental disorders including autism spectrum disorder

Ranjith Kumar Manokaran and Sheffali Gulati

Center of Excellence and Advanced Research for Childhood Neurodevelopmental Disorders, Child Neurology Division, Department of Pediatrics, AIIMS, New Delhi, India

24.1 Introduction

The microbiota, the biological community of commensal, symbiotic, and pathogenic microbes coinhabiting the human body, outnumbers the host cells to human cells by a vast majority. The majority of the microbiota resides in the gastro-intestinal (GI) tract and they range from 10 to 100 trillion microorganisms. A symbiosis of the gut microbiota (GM) can maintain normal physiology in the host, while disturbance of the GM can tilt the balance and may induce disorders. A healthy microbial composition is important to health, as dysbiosis is often observed in many gut-related diseases, but also unconventional diseases, such as allergy, cardiovascular disease, stress, depression, Alzheimer's disease, multiple sclerosis, Parkinson's, and autism spectrum disorder (ASD). Dysbiosis is an altered microbial composition favoring pathogenic microbes over beneficial ones in the gut.

The microbiota—gut—brain—axis describes the two-directional physiological exchange of signals between the microbiota, the gut, and the brain. Recent studies have explored the role of GM in the gut—brain axis, which can alter the mental state through the central nervous system (CNS). Hence, GM symbiosis is important for retaining healthy CNS functions. Sudo's study was the first to show evidence of a link between the GM and CNS, showing an enhanced hypothalamic—pituitary—adrenal (HPA) stress response and decreased brain-derived neurotrophic factor (BDNF) levels in the hippocampi of germ-free mice (Sudo et al., 2004). With the increasing prevalence of neurodevelopmental disorders, there has been a major push for basic sciences research in the field of neurodevelopmental disorders. This explosion of research has led to diverse opinions and the pooling of knowledge. This chapter discusses the role of GM and probiotics with regard to neurodevelopmental disorders with a special focus on ASDs.

24.2 Colonization of the intestinal ecosystem in early life and its evolution

The composition of the GM differs widely from fetal life to adult age. Until recently, it was thought that babies were born sterile and only colonized by microbes on exposure to their immediate extrauterine environments. Recent research suggests that the process of microbial colonization of the GI tract begins in utero as the acquisition of maternal microbiota might occur during intrauterine life through the placenta (Sudo et al., 2004). Neonates show dynamic intestinal microbiota with low microbial diversity. The first colonizers in healthy neonates are enterobacteria, *Staphylococcus*, and *Streptococcus*, followed by anaerobes, such as *Bacteroides*, *Bifidobacterium*, and *Clostridium*. This pattern of microbial diversity provides an efficient means for adaptation to the variable circumstances over a lifetime, such as changes in lifestyle, illness, puberty, and others. Over the first few years of life, GM matures and stabilizes to a more balanced "adult-like" composition at around the end of the third year.

Interestingly, the brain of neonates grows to approximately 90% of its future adult volume until the age of two, and the process of synaptogenesis in the brain overlaps with this phase of GM stabilization. Thus the critical window for the establishment of a healthy microbial composition falls into the same critical time window for cerebral development.

Therefore understanding the GM establishment and its critical developmental window in early childhood is important because any disturbance during this period causes long-lasting effects on the development of the CNS.

24.3 Gut microbiota

The entirety of microorganisms in a particular habitat is termed microbiota or microflora. The collective genomes of all the microorganisms in the microbiota are termed the microbiome. Microbial colonization may begin even in utero via the placenta, and the mother's microbiome can influence the infant's microbial colonization during pregnancy. It is unique to every individual. Some of the supporting functions of the human GM are the degradation of otherwise nondigestible food compounds; the conversion of toxic compounds; and the production of essential vitamins, important metabolic end-products, and defending bacteriocins. Microbial metabolic end-products, which account for one-third of the metabolites present in the human system, play an important role in gut homeostasis and have an impact on host metabolism and health. A symbiosis of the GM can maintain normal physiology in the host, while dysbiosis of the GM can shift the balance and may induce diseases.

24.4 What are probiotics?

Probiotics are defined as "live microorganisms which, when administered in adequate amounts, confer a health benefit on the host." Recently they have been reported to influence the CNS by altering the GM composition. Studies using probiotics to change CNS functions have skyrocketed tremendously over the last decade. Animals and human studies have found the potential mechanisms underlining these probiotic effects. First, probiotics may directly modify CNS biochemistry, such as by affecting levels of BDNF, γ-aminobutyric acid (GABA), serotonin [5 hydroxytryptamine (5HT)], and dopamine, thus influencing mind and behavior. Both the vagus and the enteric nerves are involved in this gut–brain interaction and can be affected by certain probiotics. The HPA stress response, which regulates mood and emotion, has frequently been shown to be mitigated by probiotics, reducing corticosteroid levels. The immune system can be influenced by probiotics, limiting proinflammatory cytokine production and inflammation, which, in turn, can affect the endocrine and nervous systems. Probiotics manipulate GM by increasing microbial diversity and altering the beneficial bacteria compositions. Favorable GM changes metabolites, such as short-chain fatty acids and tryptophan, which can indirectly improve CNS function. This complex interplay has been pictorially depicted in the cartoon as shown in Fig. 24.1.

24.5 Psychobiotics, prebiotics, and synbiotics

Psychobiotics are defined as live microorganisms that, when ingested in adequate amounts, produce beneficial health effects to patients with psychiatric illness. Prebiotic is a substrate that is selectively consumed by host microorganisms and confers a health benefit. The term synbiotic was proposed for a product that combines prebiotics and probiotics and in which the prebiotic compounds selectively favor the probiotic strains.

24.6 Autism and probiotics

ASD is a specific neurodevelopmental condition during the first 2 years of life that typically exhibits qualitative impairments in socialization and communication and restricted, repetitive, and stereotyped behaviors and activities. The etiopathogenesis of ASD is not yet clearly expounded. Many family studies point out the importance of both genetic and inherited predispositions, although epidemiological studies suggest a strong role of perinatal environmental factors. Genetic factors contribute to about 20%–30% of all cases, whereas the remaining 70%–80% of the cases are the results of a complex interplay between environmental risk factors and genetic susceptibility. Autism can be primarily divided into two subtypes, idiopathic autism or primary autism where the exact cause of the disorder is unknown (85%) and secondary autism (15%) where the specific etiology can be identified.

24.7 ASD and GI disorders

Whether patients with ASD have an increased prevalence of GI disorders has been discussed and debated in the literature. While there are many cases of ASD who may not have GI symptoms, recent studies confirm that children with ASD experience significantly more GI symptoms with a higher rate of diarrhea, constipation, chronic reflux, and

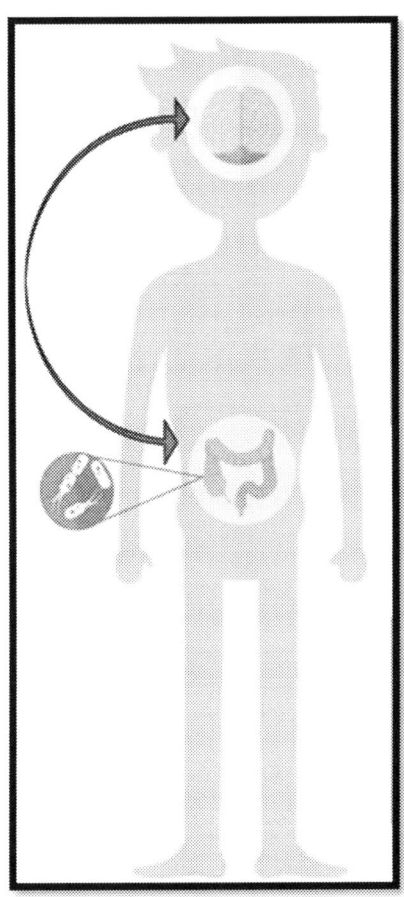

FIGURE 24.1 Complex interplay between the gut microbiota and the host brain.

abdominal pain. The prevalence of GI problems in patients with ASD based on published literature range from 9% to 91%. So, it can be concluded that GI disturbances are more commonly seen in ASD children, and the exact reason is poorly understood. Moreover, an increased risk of problem behaviors has been reported in individuals with ASD and gut symptoms and these problem behaviors may be the manifestations of the GI symptoms. The GI disturbances in ASD might be linked to gut dysbiosis representing the phenotype of a "gut–brain axis" disruption characterized by intestinal inflammation and disturbance in GI function. This is often referred to as "leaky gut syndrome."

24.8 The gut–brain axis

Gut–brain axis is a complex interface between the gut and the brain of an individual and has a central role in the positive effects of probiotics in ASD. The complex interplay between the central and enteric nervous systems forms the major part of the gut–brain axis. Gut–brain axis involves other pathways as well, among them are immune regulation, intestinal barrier maintenance, and gut–endocrine signaling. These communication channels are bidirectional and involve neuro-immuno-endocrine mediators. In recent times the role of gut flora, or microbiota, has been identified as a part of this axis. The GM can alter CNS functions, forming a critical link in the bidirectional interactions between the gut and the brain. The brain also influences the microbiota by multiple mechanisms. They include direct effects of GI motility and secretory functions. Signaling molecules released into the gut by the cells in the lamina propria (enterochromaffin cells, neurons, immune cells) play a role in regulating the gut microme. The reciprocal communication from the GM to the host can occur through epithelial cells and receptor molecule-mediated signaling. Intestinal permeability is a key factor in this reciprocal relationship between the host and the enteric microbiota.

Thus the modality of communication of microbiota–gut–brain is mainly through three pathways: (1) neural pathway—Vagus nerve stimulation by several neurotransmitters; (2) endocrinal pathway—through regulation of HPA axis; (3) metabolic pathway—commensal produced neuroactive substances, such as GABA, CA, 5HT, melatonin, histamine, and Ach; and (4) immunological pathway—through the role of microbiota in shaping the host immune system. The

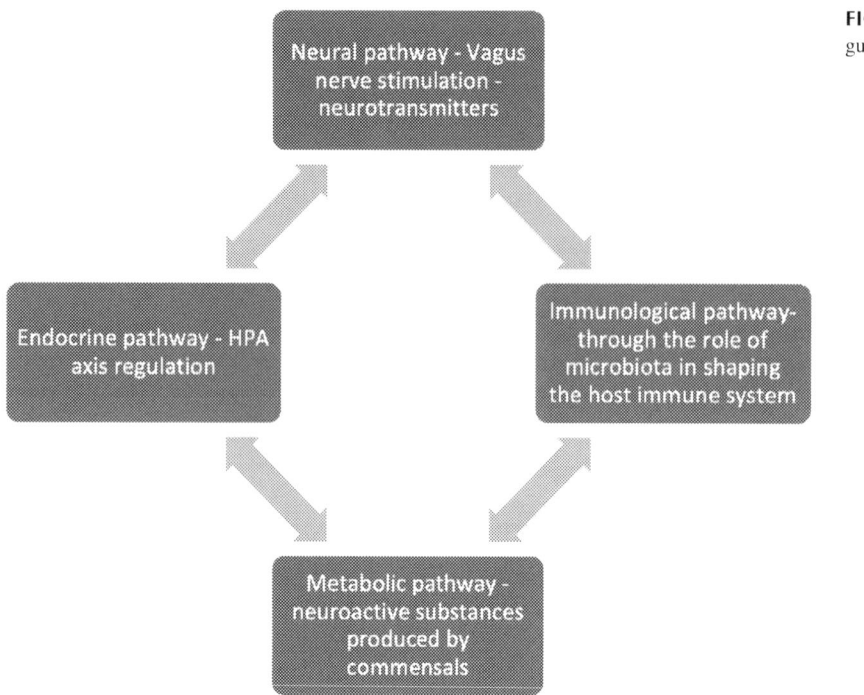

FIGURE 24.2 The complex mechanisms of gut—brain axis.

imbalance in the microbiota is termed as "dysbiosis." Alterations in the gut microbial composition have been associated with disturbed gut barrier functions, enhanced gut permeability, and increased plasma lipopolysaccharide concentrations, which results in inflammation that predisposes the host for obesity and metabolic syndrome. Many other GI disorders, such as inflammatory bowel disease, irritable bowel syndrome, GI cancers, and allergies, have been associated with gut dysbiosis. Over the years, the evidence of associations between the GM composition and neurobehavioral and neuropsychiatric disorders, such as depression, anxiety disorder, ASD, and schizophrenia, has grown stronger. The gut—brain axis is depicted in Fig. 24.2.

With the increasing evidence connecting certain disorders of the human body to the altered GM, there is a quest for chemicals that positively influence its composition and activity through dietary intake. These compounds are either probiotics or prebiotics. There are diverse mechanisms by which probiotics act. Probiotics influence the composition and dynamics of microbiota, the interaction with visceral hypersensitivity, mucosal inflammation and motility, intestinal permeability, and the gut—brain axis, thereby regulating several vital neurological functions. A recent metagenomic and metatranscriptomic study of feces of 12 healthy individuals has demonstrated that the oral administration of the probiotic strain *Lactobacillus rhamnosus* GG profoundly alters the activity of the GM, without changing its composition. Especially genes involved in adhesion, chemotaxis, and/or motility of *Bifidobacterium* spp., *Eubacterium* spp., and *Roseburia* spp. are overexpressed during probiotic consumption, suggesting that the oral consumption of the probiotic strains promote interactions between the GM and the host. The HPA stress response, which controls mood and emotions, has frequently been shown to be lessened by probiotics, decreasing corticosteroid levels. The immune system can be influenced by probiotics, limiting proinflammatory cytokine synthesis and inflammation, which, in turn, can affect the endocrine and nervous systems. This favorable role played by probiotics in modulating the gut—brain axis is recently being studied in various neurological disorders, including ASD, depression, anxiety, cognition, ASD, OCD, stress responses, and memory abilities. The mechanisms of effects of probiotics on the CNS have been depicted in Fig. 24.3.

24.9 Neurodevelopmental disorders

A child's brain is not a miniature model of an adult brain, but rather a brain in continual development, growing, at times immensely, subject to infinite modifications and connections due to the continual stimulation and fostering provided by the environment in which it grows. It is crucial to understand the development of the brain and its various stages to understand the deficits that can arise from abnormal brain development or be caused by insults at an early age.

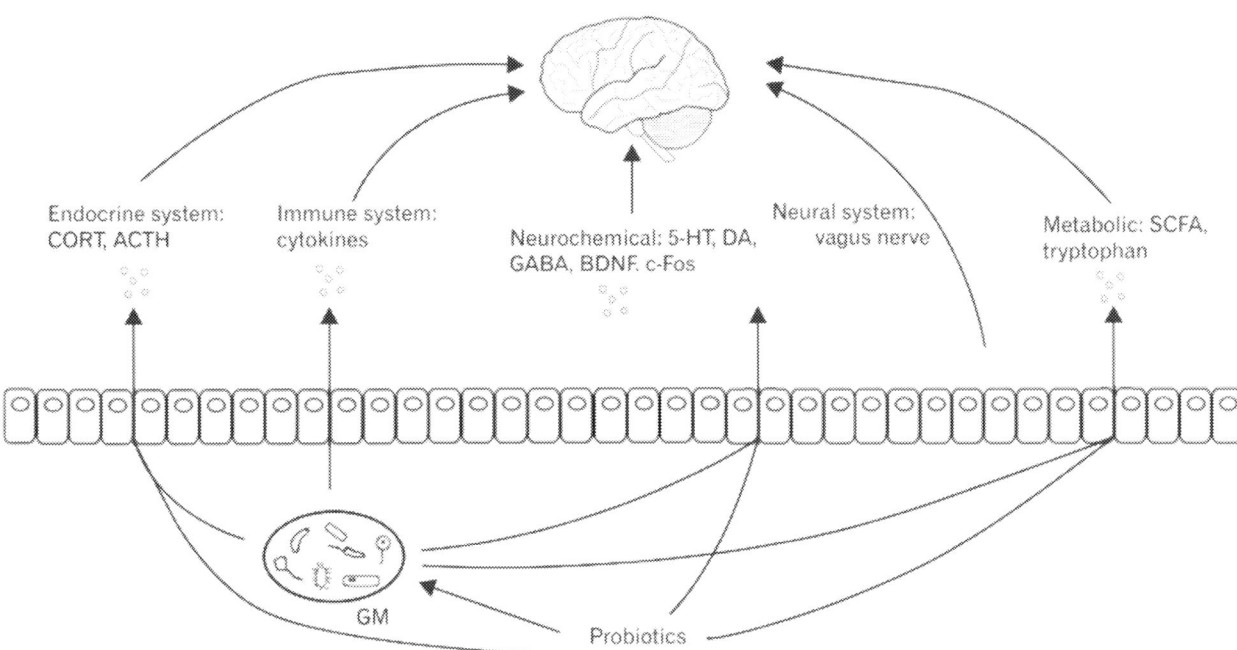

FIGURE 24.3 Mechanisms of action of probiotics. Source: *From Wang H, Lee, I. S., Braun, C., & Enck, P. (2016). Effect of probiotics on central nervous system functions in animals and humans: A systematic review.* Journal of Neurogastroenterology and Motility, 22(4), 589–605. https://doi.org/10.5056/jnm16018.

Depending upon the time when these abnormalities or damage happen (during the antenatal period, the perinatal period, or infancy/early childhood), the consequences will differ. Neurodevelopmental disorders include attention-deficit/hyperactivity disorder (ADHD), ASD, specific learning disability (SLD), and other related conditions. The role of GM will be further elucidated.

24.10 Is the gut microbiota of children with autism spectrum disorder different?

There has been growing evidence that the microbiota of children with autism is different when compared to normal children. A recent meta-analysis of the various studies regarding autism and microbiota suggests that there is a significant difference in GM of ASD children compared with typically developing children and that this difference may substantially contribute to the pathobiology of ASD (Xu et al., 2019). These ASD-related microbial species mainly belonged to phyla viz. *Bacteriodetes* (*Bacteroides*, *Prevotella*), *Firmicutes* (*Clostridium*, *Lactobacillus*, *Ruminococcus*), *Proteobacteria* (*Sutterella*, *Desulfovibrio*), and *Actinobacteria* (*Bifidobacterium*). The major bacterial genera that have been reported to increase in Autism include *Clostridium*, *Desulfovibrio*, *Sutterella*, *Bacteroides*, and *Prevotella*. Higher counts of *Clostridium* spp. in stool, gastric, and duodenal specimens have been reported in individuals with ASD. In larger studies by Parracho et al. (2010), *Clostridium histolyticum* species was higher among autistic children. Finegold et al. (2010) found a higher prevalence of Bacteroidetes (Finegold et al., 2010) and Adams et al. (2011) found a low level of Bifidobacterium species. However, Gondalia et al. (2010) did not find a difference in the microbiota composition of autistic and nonautistic children and also did not find any association between the GI symptoms and the microbiota composition. Gulati et al. (2020) studied the comparative abundance of major gut microflora between children with ASD and typically developing (TD) children.

There was decreased gut bacterial diversity in the gut microflora of children with ASD. The phylum *Firmicutes* was significantly less and the phylum *Bacteroidetes* was significantly more in children with ASD as compared to TD siblings. In addition, *Clostridium perfringens* was significantly higher in the GM of children with ASD.

Wang et al. (2016) reviewed the interventional studies undertaken in humans (adult) with probiotics. In their review among the fifteen studies, eight studies have used a single-strain probiotic (*Lactobacillus casei*, *L. casei*. subsp. *rhamnosus*, *L. casei*. Shirota, *Lactobacillus plantarum*, and *Bifidobacterium infantis*), of which two used novel intervention technique in the form of probiotic-containing milk, and the remaining seven studies used multiple strain probiotics. Eight of the 15 studies reported significant effects of probiotics. Doses of the effective interventions ranged from 10^7 to

3.63×10^{10}, and the duration of the interventions ranged from 20 days to 8 weeks. Doses that are most often administered were 10^9 (5/8) and 10^{10} (3/8). Durations were most commonly 4 (6/15) and 8 (4/15) weeks. Probiotics were found to alleviate psychiatric conditions with mood affection (depression/anxiety) and chronic fatigue syndrome. They affected memory and cognition but did not affect schizophrenia. A neuroimaging study using functional MRI sequence evaluating the modifications in brain activity to emotional stimuli and basal brain activation after ingestion of a fermented milk product with probiotic (FMPP) containing *Bifidobacterium lactis* with yogurt starters, *Streptococcus thermophilus*, *Lactobacillus bulgaricus*, and *Lactococcus lactis* subsp. *Lactis* showed that the FMPP reduced activity of a large distributed network, including affective, viscerosensory, and somatosensory cortical areas, to showing emotional faces and also modulated midbrain connectivity during the resting state.

Both GI disturbances and altered gut microbiome could predispose a child with a genetic susceptibility for ASD to express the autistic phenotype or increase the severity of the autism. This hypothesis confers biological plausibility to the strategies, which aim at normalizing the GM. These strategies, such as probiotics supplementation in diet, may provide a nonpharmacological option not only for GI disturbances but also for the core features of ASD.

24.11 Literature evidence in ASD

There are only a handful of studies conducted in ASD in children. In a recent RCT by Santocchi et al. (2016) in a group of 100 preschool children with ASD, the improvement of severity level by the administration of probiotics for 6 months was assessed. The probiotic preparation which was chosen for this study was a mixture (Vivomixx), each sachet of which contained 450 billions of lyophilized bacterial cells belonging to eight strains: one strain of *S. thermophilus* DSM 24731, three strains of *Bifidobacterium* (*B. breve* DSM 24732, *B. longum* DSM 24736, *B. infantis* DSM 24737), and four strains of *Lactobacillus* (*L. acidophilus* DSM 24735, *L. plantarum* DSM 24730, *L. paracasei* DSM 24733, *L. delbrueckii* subsp. *bulgaricus* DSM 24734). Vivomixx is a patented and marketed product and it has been approved for use in children. The primary outcome of this study was the improvement of the ASD symptom severity level. They discerned that the treatment with probiotics in children with ASD and GI symptoms produced more profound improvements in symptomatology, behavioral scores, adaptive functioning, and cognitive and linguistic function in comparison with children with ASD and GI symptoms who were treated with placebo.

Parracho et al. (2010) detected significant behavioral improvements in ASD patients treated with probiotics compared to ASD individuals treated with placebo. Kałuzna-Czaplińska and Błaszczyk (2012) observed significant metabolic modifications in ASD after probiotic administration. Adams et al. (2011) and Tomova et al. (2015) limited their findings to a strong positive correlation between autism severity and the severity of GI dysfunction without studying the effects of probiotics on ASD core features. Adams et al. (2011) compared GI flora and GI status from stool samples of 58 children with ASD and 39 typically developing children of similar ages and found lower levels of total SCFAs in the ASD group with a larger difference in children with autism taking probiotics. In that study, GI symptoms were positively correlated with the severity of autism. Nevertheless, information regarding the type of probiotic oral supplementation was only partially revealed. Kałuzna-Czaplińska and Błaszczyk (2012) administered oral supplementation of *Lactobacillus acidophilus* twice a day for 2 months to a group of ASD children and found significant metabolic modifications, and an improvement in the ability to perform tasks and concentration, but no other behavioral or emotional effects. Parracho et al. (2010) reported in a large sample of children with ASD a significant behavioral improvement in the ASD group treated with *L. plantarum* WCSF1 compared to the ASD group treated with placebo. Tomova et al. (2015) reported a strong positive correlation of autism symptom severity with the severity of GI dysfunction. In their study, probiotic diet supplementation (a combination of *Lactobacillus*, *Bifidobacter*, and *Streptococci*, three times a day for 4 months) restored the microflora of children with ASD. The effects of probiotic diet supplementation on behaviors were not studied by Tomova et al. (2015). The effect of probiotic supplementation on the health status of individuals with ASD is summarized in Table 24.1.

24.12 Newer techniques involving microbiota

Innovative treatment strategies, such as fecal microbiota transplantation (FMT) and microbiota transfer therapy (MTT), are also being researched. FMT is a novel intervention in which the fecal microbiota from a healthy person is transferred to a patient with altered GM and is now being explored in ASD. MTT is a newer way of administering FMT and encompasses 14 days of antibiotic treatment, which is subsequently followed by cleaning the gut and administering a high initial dose of standardized human GM for 7–8 weeks. Kang et al. (2019) have demonstrated that MTT has improved both GI symptoms and ASD symptoms and normalized the microbiota of ASD patients.

TABLE 24.1 Summary of studies showing the effects of probiotics supplementation on the health status of individuals with ASD.

Authors	Subjects	Probiotics	Dose and duration	Key findings
Adams et al. (2011)	ASD children (2.5–18 years old)	Any type of probiotic	Daily usage (33%)	A strong correlation of autism severity with gastrointestinal symptoms. Low level of short-chain fatty acids
Parracho et al. (2010)	ASD children (4–16 years old)	*Lactobacillus plantarum* WCSF1	4.5×10^{10} CFU per capsule per day for 3 weeks in the 12-week study duration	↑ *Enterococci* and *Lactobacilli* group. ↓ *Clostridium* cluster XIVa Improved the stool consistency compared to placebo, and behavioral scores compared to baseline
Tomova et al. (2015)	ASD children (2–9 years old): their siblings (5–7 years old); children in control group (2–11 years old)	3 *Lactobacillus* strains, 2 *Bifidobacterium* strains, and a *Streptococcus* strain (60:25:15 ratio)	3 capsules per day (1 capsule thrice a day) for 4 months	In ASD children, probiotic supplementation normalized *Bacteroidetes/Firmicutes* ratio ↓ *Desulfovibrio* spp. ↓ TNFα level in feces
Kałuzna-Czaplińska and Błaszczyk (2012)	ASD children (4–10 years old)	*L. acidophilus* Rosell-11	5×10^9 CFU per gram; twice a day for 2 months	↓ D-Arabinitol and D-arabinitol/L-arabinitol ratio in urine
Grossi et al. (2016)	ASD children (12 years old)	VSL # 3 (a mixture of live cells of *Lactobacillus delbrueckii* subsp. *Bulgaricus*, *L. acidophilus*, *B. breve*, *B. longum*, *B. infantis*, *L. paracasei*, *L. plantarum*, *S. thermophiles*)	5 months of treatment period (4 weeks of initial treatment + 4 months of follow up treatment); 10 months of follow up period	↓ Severity of abdominal symptoms Improvement in autistic core symptoms
Shaaban et al. (2018)	ASD children (5–9 years old)	*B. longum*, *L. rhamnosus*, *L. acidophilus*	1×10^8 CFU per gram; 5 g per day for 3 months	↑ Bifidobacteria and Lactobacilli level ↓ Severity of the ASD and GI symptoms
Santocchi et al. (2016)	ASD children (preschool)	Vivomixx, *Streptococcus thermophilus*, *B. longum*, *B. infantis*, *B. breve*, *Lactobacillus*	450 billions of lyophilized bacterial cells	Probiotics in individuals with ASD and GI symptoms produced more significant improvement in autistic symptoms, behavioral profiles, adaptive functioning, and cognitive and linguistic development in comparison with placebo

ASD, Autism spectrum disorder; *GI*, gastrointestinal.

Currently approved and recommended treatments for ASD are mainly based on rehabilitation, psycho-educational interventions, and psycho-pharmacological treatments. In children with ASD, GI dysfunction may be associated with a higher rate of irritability, anger, aggressive behaviors, and sleep disturbances. Hence, the treatment of these symptoms by probiotics administration could not only reduce overall costs for this disorder but also improve compliance and adherence of these patients and families to educational and rehabilitation treatments, thereby improving their quality of life.

24.13 ADHD

ADHD is emerging as the most prevalent neurodevelopmental disorder with an estimated worldwide prevalence of 5.29% among children up to and including 18 years of age. According to the Diagnostic and Statistical Manual of Mental Disorders-Fifth Edition, the diagnosis of ADHD is based on clinical symptoms. The recommended treatment for ADHD is behavioral therapy.

Pharmacological treatments are effective and are widely used, albeit with some limitations. For many reasons, but mostly because of adverse effects, parents choose to avoid pharmacotherapy, and nonadherence to therapy is quite high. Henceforth, more research is needed to explore the pathobiology of ADHD and the possible role of nonpharmacological therapies. A variety of nonpharmacological interventions are available, but their efficacy remains unproven. There has been a growing interest in dietary and probiotic interventions.

The quest for etiopathogenetic factors has been magnified in recent years to include the GM. There is evidence from preclinical studies that the GM might also be a therapeutic target in ADHD, mediated by the modulation of neurotransmitters.

Proposed mechanisms by which the GM may regulate brain development, function, and behavior are immune (cytokines), metabolic (short-chain fatty acids), hormonal (cortisol), and neuronal (the vagus nerve and the enteric nervous system) pathways. For example, human stress hormones, such as norepinephrine, might influence microbial gene expression or signaling between microbes and thus modify their composition and activity. GM can produce neuroactive compounds, such as neurotransmitters. *Lactobacillus* spp. and *Bifidobacterium* spp. can produce GABA and *Lactobacillus* spp. also produces acetylcholine, etc.

Multiple studies have hypothesized an immune pathway by which GM could modulate brain function in ADHD and these are backed by findings of increased levels of proinflammatory cytokines, such as IFN-γ and IL-16, in the serum of ADHD patients. Biochemical markers CRP, B-12, folate, iron, ferritin, transferrin, and the cytokines IL-6, IL-10, and IL-16 are found to be altered in children with ADHD (Al Aidy et al., 2014).

A study by Isolauri et al. (2008) on the modulation of the maturing gut barrier showed that *Lactobacillus Rhamnosus* (LGG) stabilizes the gut permeability barrier by its effects on intercellular tight junctions, mucin production, and antigen-specific immunoglobulin A production. Bravo et al. (2011) have demonstrated that LGG, via the vagus nerve, regulates emotional behavior and the central GABAergic system, which is also associated with neuropsychiatric disorders.

In a recent study by Pärtty et al. (2015) initial results showed that specific probiotics may reduce the risk of ADHD and other neurodevelopmental/neurobehavioral disorders. The study demonstrated that the administration of LGG during the first 6 months of life may reduce the risk of development of ADHD, Asperger syndrome (AS), and ASD later (Pärtty et al., 2015).

Kumperscak et al. (2020) in a recent randomized controlled study demonstrated that children with ADHD who received LGG supplementation reported better health-related quality of life compared to their peers who received the placebo, suggesting that LGG supplementation could be beneficial.

Pärtty et al. (2015) supplemented *L. rhamnosus* GG (10^{10} CFU per day) to pregnant women for 4 weeks in the antenatal period before delivery and continued the probiotic supplementation for 6 months to the mother (if breastfeeding) or to the infant. The clinical evaluation and behavioral assessments were done at 3 weeks and 3, 6, 12, 18, and 24 months of age, and final ADHD and AS records were made at the age of 13. The study demonstrated that probiotic supplementation reduced the risk of the development of a neurobehavioral disorder compared to that of the placebo group (Pärtty et al., 2015).

This is one of the few clinical studies on the possible effect of probiotics on ADHD. Even though the results are encouraging, they should be interpreted with a great deal of caution and need to be confirmed by further studies. Future double-blind randomized controlled trials in a large and diverse population of ADHD children are desirable.

24.14 Other neurodevelopmental disorders

In addition to ASD and ADHD, neurodevelopmental disorders, such as specific learning disabilities, intellectual disabilities, and communication disorders, also contribute to a huge burden of developmental disabilities in the community. There are no systematic intervention studies assessing the effect of probiotics in this set of neurodevelopmental disabilities. Future studies in these specific set of neurodevelopmental disabilities are desirable.

24.15 Future perspectives

In the last 10 years, many studies have investigated the effect of probiotics and prebiotics in human systems. It has been concluded that GM may modulate inflammation, adiposity, energy dynamics, and glycaemic control. Most efforts have focused on studying the mechanisms by which certain probiotics regulate the colonization of and protect against pathogens through the activation of the mucosal immune system and competition for limited nutrients. Novel therapeutic approaches, such as recombinant probiotics expressing therapeutic biomolecules, FMT, and phage therapy, need to be explored for the manipulation of the gut ecosystem. Customized phage cocktails may be a novel alternative for future therapies. These customized phages would precisely target preidentified bacterial pathogens, though the main disadvantage would be the high interindividual variation of the gut microbiome.

24.16 Conclusion

In conclusion, this chapter summarizes the gathering evidence on the modulation of gut microbial flora and metabolism as a potential strategy for early-onset neurodevelopmental disorders. Despite this enormous wealth of information, many lacunae gaps and inconsistencies exist when the studies are compared. Differences in the quantity of dose, type of strain, type of prebiotic, assessment of GM, duration of intervention, standardization of neurological measurements, variety and complexity of neurological symptoms, study design, and cohort size make it difficult to confirm evidence of efficacy. To this end, in vivo studies that exploit the power of the latest robust high-throughput multiomic technologies are required to precisely identify the molecular mechanisms of the gut's microbial modulation of neurodevelopmental disorders and ultimately to design effective probiotic and prebiotic therapies.

References

Adams, J. B., Johansen, L. J., Powell, L. D., Quig, D., & Rubin, R. A. (2011). Gastrointestinal flora and gastrointestinal status in children with autism—Comparisons to typical children and correlation with autism severity. *BMC Gastroenterology, 11*. Available from https://doi.org/10.1186/1471-230X-11-22.

Al Aidy, S. E., Dinan, T. G., & Cryan, J. F. (2014). Immune modulation of the brain-gut-microbe axis. *Frontiers in Microbiology, 5*. Available from https://doi.org/10.3389/fmicb.2014.00146.

Bravo, J. A., Forsythe, P., Chew, M. V., Escaravage, E., Savignac, H. M., Dinan, T. G., Bienenstock, J., & Cryan, J. F. (2011). Ingestion of Lactobacillus strain regulates emotional behavior and central GABA receptor expression in a mouse via the vagus nerve. *Proceedings of the National Academy of Sciences of the United States of America, 108*(38), 16050–16055. Available from https://doi.org/10.1073/pnas.1102999108.

Finegold, S., Dowd, S., Gontcharova, V., Liu, C., Henley, K., Wolcott., Youn, E., Summanen, P., Granpeesheh, D., Dixon, D., Molitoris, D., & Green, J., III. (2010). Pyrosequencing study of fecal microflora of autistic and control children. *Anaerobe, 16*(4), 444–453.

Gondalia, S., Palombo, E., Knowles, S., & Austin, D. (2010). Faecal microbiota of individuals with autism spectrum disorder. *European Journal of Applied Physiology, 6*, 24–29. Available from https://doi.org/10.7790/ejap.v6i2.213.

Gulati, S., Aparna, S. V., Rashmi, H. M., Batish, V. K., Sharma, S., Sondhi, V., & Grover. (2020). Comparative analysis of gut microbiota between children with autism spectrum disorder and typically developing children: A PCR and metagenomic approach: Poster 13. In: *Proceedings of the 16th international child neurology virtual congress: JICNA*, October.

Grossi E., Melli S., Dunca D., & Terruzzi V. (2016). Unexpected improvement in core autism spectrum disorder symptoms after long-term treatment with probiotics. *SAGE Open* Medical *Case Reports, 4*, 2050313X16666231. Published 2016 Aug 26. https://doi.org/10.1177/2050313X16666231.

Isolauri, E., Kalliomäki, M., Laitinen, K., & Salminen, S. (2008). Modulation of the maturing gut barrier and microbiota: A novel target in allergic disease. *Current Pharmaceutical Design, 14*(14), 1368–1375. Available from https://doi.org/10.2174/138161208784480207.

Kałużna-Czaplińska, J., & Błaszczyk, S. (2012). The level of arabinitol in autistic children after probiotic therapy. *Nutrition (Burbank, Los Angeles County, Calif.), 28*(2), 124–126. Available from https://doi.org/10.1016/j.nut.2011.08.002.

Kang, D. W., Adams, J. B., Coleman, D. M., Pollard, E. L., Maldonado, J., McDonough-Means, S., Caporaso, J. G., & Krajmalnik-Brown, R. (2019). Long-term benefit of microbiota transfer therapy on autism symptoms and gut microbiota. *Scientific Reports, 9*(1). Available from https://doi.org/10.1038/s41598-19-42183-0.

Kumperscak, H., Gricar, a, Ülen, I., & Micetic-Turk, D. (2020). A pilot randomized control trial with the probiotic strain Lactobacillus rhamnosus GG (LGG) in ADHD: Children and adolescents report better health-related quality of life. *Frontiers in Psychiatry, 11*.

Parracho, H. M. R. T., Gibson, G. R., Knott, F., Bosscher, D., Kleerebezem, M., & McCartney, A. L. (2010). A double-blind, placebo-controlled, crossover-designed probiotic feeding study in children diagnosed with autistic spectrum disorders. *International Journal of Probiotics and Prebiotics, 5*.

Pärtty, A., Kalliomäki, M., Wacklin, P., Salminen, S., & Isolauri, E. (2015). A possible link between early probiotic intervention and the risk of neuropsychiatric disorders later in childhood: A randomized trial. *Pediatric Research, 77*(6), 823–828. Available from https://doi.org/10.1038/pr.2015.51.

Shaaban, S. Y., El Gendy, Y. G., Mehanna, N. S., El-Senousy, W. M., El-Feki, H. S. A., Saad, K., & El-Asheer, O. M. (2018). The role of probiotics in children with autism spectrum disorder: A prospective, open-label study. *Nutritional Neuroscience, 21*(9), 676–681. Available from https://doi.org/10.1080/1028415X.2017.1347746, Epub 2017 Jul 7. PMID: 28686541.

Santocchi, E., Guiducci, L., Fulceri, F., Billeci, L., Buzzigoli, E., Apicella, F., Calderoni, S., Grossi, E., Morales, M. A., & Muratori, F. (2016). Gut to brain interaction in autism spectrum disorders: A randomized controlled trial on the role of probiotics on clinical, biochemical and neurophysiological parameters. *BMC Psychiatry, 16*(1). Available from https://doi.org/10.1186/s12888-016-0887-5.

Sudo, N., Chida, Y., Aiba, Y., Sonoda, J., Oyama, N., Yu, X. N., Kubo, C., & Koga, Y. (2004). Postnatal microbial colonization programs the hypothalamic-pituitary-adrenal system for stress response in mice. *Journal of Physiology, 558*(1), 263–275. Available from https://doi.org/10.1113/jphysiol.2004.063388.

Tomova, A., Husarova, V., Lakatosova, S., Bakos, J., Vlkova, B., Babinska, K., & Ostatnikova, D. (2015). Gastrointestinal microbiota in children with autism in Slovakia. *Physiology and Behavior, 138*, 179–187. Available from https://doi.org/10.1016/j.physbeh.2014.10.033.

Wang, H., Lee, I. S., Braun, C., & Enck, P. (2016). Effect of probiotics on central nervous system functions in animals and humans: A systematic review. *Journal of Neurogastroenterology and Motility, 22*(4), 589–605. Available from https://doi.org/10.5056/jnm16018.

Xu, M., Xu, X., Li, J., & Li, F. (2019). Association between gut microbiota and autism spectrum disorder: A systematic review and meta-analysis. *Frontiers in Psychiatry, 10*. Available from https://doi.org/10.3389/fpsyt.2019.00473.

Chapter 25

Probiotics in the prevention and control of foodborne diseases in humans

Atef A. Hassan[1], Rasha M. H. Sayed-ElAhl[1], Ahmed M. El Hamaky[1], Noha H. Oraby[1] and Mahmoud H. Barakat[2]

[1]*Mycology department, Animal Health Research Institute (AHRI), Agriculture Research Center (ARC), Giza, Egypt,* [2]*Faculty of Medicine, Cairo University (Al Kasr Al Ainy), Cairo, Egypt*

25.1 Introduction

Nowadays, foodborne diseases are worldwide problem and in spite of the progressive advancement in medical field, nutrition, and food preservation, they still potentiate diseases hazard and economic losses (Hossain et al., 2017). The diseases that resulted from infected food are very risky due to the high morbidity and mortality rates' occurrence (Budden et al., 2009). It is reported that the morbidity of diseases was 2 billion persons, 1 million were died, and 22 pathogens were recovered from infections (Kirk et al., 2015). The occurrence of antibiotic resistant in human pathogens initiated the search and spread use of synthetic antibiotics (Chammem et al., 2018). The gut is the target organs for infection and caused diarrhea, vomiting, fever, headache, and other adverse effects (Duarte et al., 2018). These pathogens cause various diseases resulted from a misbalanced gastrointestinal (GIT) microbiota and all methods of treatment directed to return of balance of microbiota (Danneskiold-Samsøe et al., 2019). In the past decades probiotics are widely used in food technology due to their benefits to human and animal health. The worldwide probiotics include *Lactobacillus* spp., *Streptococcus* spp., *Enterococcus* spp., and *Saccharomyces* spp. (Fredua-Agyeman et al., 2017). The availability of probiotic products occurred by combined effects of phytochemicals and probiotic strains (Boricha et al., 2019). The administration of probiotics in food products is the main important activity in the prevention and control of foodborne pathogens (Esaiassen et al., 2018; Hassan et al., 2016). The probiotics, especially probiotic strains of lactic acid bacteria (LAB), which have the ability to change the human GIT microbiota via inhibition the growth of bacteria (Lau & Chye, 2018; Lievin Moal, 2016). However, studies have reported that the probiotics strains (*L. rhamnosus*, *L. plantarum*, and *Bacillus* sp.) activate the GIT functions and release in food and help to improve the human health (Samedi & Charles, 2019; Singh et al., 2017; Soares et al., 2019). Moreover, probiotic activity of *L. casei* strain in yogurt food was also detected (Reissig Soares Vitola et al., 2018; Terpou et al., 2019). However, the fermented grains contain benefit yeast strains and have a probiotic activity (Abraham et al., 2019). Another study reported that the use of *Lactobacillus* strains that isolated from breast milk has antioxidant and antibiome activities against GI pathogens (Bhat & Bajaj, 2019; Gunyakti & Asan-Ozusaglam, 2019). Hence, the probiotic strains; particularly *Lactobacillus* species, have huge benefits for the prevention and therapy of pathogens in GIT (Peng & Biswas, 2017). They have various mechanisms of action against foodborne pathogens in GIT. The activities of probiotics are due to production or release various active biochemical materials, which suppress the activity of GIT pathogens (Gunyakti & Asan-Ozusaglam, 2019). Also, studies have reported that probiotic strains produce bacitracin-like inhibitory substances, which play a role in food protection by inhibiting and preventing the entrance of microbial strains (Martinez et al., 2015; Plaza-Diaz et al., 2019). Moreover, the probiotics prevent the gene expression of GIT pathogens (Peng & Biswas, 2017; Sun et al., 2012). The continuous awareness of foodborne diseases and benefits of probiotics gained huge interest for their supplementation in food and food products (Marcial-Coba et al., 2019; Roobab et al., 2020). Therefore this chapter highlights the foodborne diseases, sources of pollutions, and actions of probiotics against different infections of pathogens. Moreover, different mechanisms of action, methods of delivery, and factors required for ideal benefits of probiotics are fully discussed. In addition, the safety and risk hazard of their use in human health have also been illustrated.

25.2 Foodborne diseases

25.2.1 Foodborne pathogens and diseases

The worldwide problem of foodborne diseases occurred due to food contamination by pathogenic microorganisms during preparation, processing, and storage of food. They are occurred in aged human and children, and the mortality rate reach to 2.2 million every year between the user of contaminated food and water with pathogens (World Health Organization, 2015). These pathogens include wide range of bacterial, fungal, viral, and parasitic pathogens and their toxins (Smith & Fratamico, 2018; Sugrue et al., 2019). Foodborne pathogen to cause human diseases must have the potential to potentiate illness even at a relatively low infectious dose and persist or multiply in food (Table 25.1).

The *Salmonella* and *Escherichia coli* are the most pathogens recovered from cases of human food poisoning, which resulted from the consumption of contaminated foods (Carrasco et al., 2012). They are of zoonotic importance where the reservoirs are the infected animals and their products as poultry, meat, and milk that can be infected the GIT of consumers (Das et al., 2013). Hence, several methods are used to preserve and protect foods from infections with these pathogens (Vandeplas et al., 2010). The GIT is the targeted site of pathogens causing abdominal pain, vomiting, diarrhea, and dysentery due to microbial infections. The main source of infections with foodborne human pathogens is the consumption of contaminated poultry meat that grown and multiplied in GIT resulted in gastritis (Dasti et al., 2010; Young et al., 2007). Their action can be occurred as a result of penetration of pathogens to the GIT epithelial mucosa of infected human, hemolytic colitis, and renal failure (Boehm et al., 2011). This resulted from infection with Shiga toxins, *E. coli*, and *Shigella* spp. (Beutin & Martin, 2012; Muniesa et al., 2012). The infections could occur due to the ingestion of contaminated food. The pathogens produced Shiga toxin (STX) in the intestine and penetrated epithelial cells to the blood and caused kidney failure (Davis et al., 2013). Moreover, the infection of food and drinking water with hepatitis A and E resulted in human jaundice and hepatitis infections. There are some foodborne pathogens that can be affected pregnancy in women as *Listeria monocytogenes* and *Toxoplasma gondii* (Swaminathan & Gerner-Smidt, 2007) and they are of low incidence than other GIT pathogens as *Salmonella* and *E. coli* and sometimes cause death (Voetsch et al., 1996). Similarly, studies have reported that after *L. monocytogenes* entry into the intestinal tract, it crossed the blood barriers and resulted in abortion (Jiao et al., 2011; Kirk et al., 2015; Ribet & Cossart, 2015). Moreover, the consumption of contaminated food with *Campylobacter*, *Clostridium* sp., and their toxins caused nervous diseases and may cause paralysis (Amalaradjou & Bhunia, 2012). Whereas, the administration of mycotoxigenic fungi and mycotoxins in food resulted in the necrosis of liver and kidney and immunosuppression effects (Esaiassen et al., 2018; Hassan et al., 2016). Another cause included Norovirus (NoV), a world cause of water and food contamination, resulting in the gastroenteritis and even death (Rodríguez-Lázaro et al., 2012; Rubio-del-Campo et al., 2014).

25.2.2 Pathogenicity mechanisms of foodborne pathogens

There are several roles illustrating the mode of actions of foodborne pathogens in human. The popular mechanism is the penetration and adhesion to GIT mucosa and leads to the destruction of human tissues but immune system not affected (Dittoe et al., 2018). The pathogens should have the ability to act against normal gut microbiota (Verdu et al., 2015). The foodborne infectious diseases are occurred in all countries during food preparation and proceeding (Lake & Barker, 2018). Also, one study reported that after ingestion of contaminated food, the pathogen adhere GIT and penetrated tissues of intestine and distributed in all body tissues via blood supply (Martens et al., 2018). This mechanism was detected in many cases as *Cronobacter* spp. infection that causing meningitis (Chen et al., 2019).

The attachment of pathogen to human GIT followed by some changes in each of them. The outer bacterial cell wall proteins (OmpA) and human enable penetration and entrance of bacterial cells and transferred through blood to other body tissues. This is associated with gene expression of OmpA where the high-expressed OmpA pathogen have the ability for division in blood supply and vice-versa (Lehner et al., 2018). There are differences between GIT bacteria due to physiological defenses of GIT organs (stomach, colon, and intestine) (Wan et al., 2019). In addition, some GIT organs secreted enzyme and pH condition affecting the microbiota balance, which causes the degradation of food components (Sonnenburg & Bäckhed, 2016).

25.3 Probiotics

The probiotics have various benefits for human heath gut microbiota and hence general health can be improved (Hossain et al., 2017; Mackowiak, 2013; Wan et al., 2019). Probiotic organism mainly causes inhibition of the activity of food pathogen and hence GIT microbiota will be normally activated (Aureli et al., 2011) and help to compact enteric

TABLE 25.1 Common foodborne pathogens, possible food sources, incubation period, and symptoms.

Foodborne pathogens	Examples of food sources	Incubation period	Symptoms
Bacillus cereus	Meat, milk, rice, potatoes, pasta, vegetables, and cheese	30 min to 15 h	Diarrhea, abdominal cramps, vomiting
Campylobacter Jejuni	Raw milk, eggs, poultry, raw beef, water, and cake icing	1–7 days	Diarrhea, abdominal cramps, nausea
Clostridium botulinum	Low-acid, canned food, meat, sausage, and fish	12–36 h	Diarrhea, nausea, headache, vomiting, dry mouth, fatigue, double vision, slurred speech, repertory distress, flaccid paralysis
Clostridium	Undercooked, meats, roast beef, and gravies	8–24 h	Diarrhea, abdominal
Cryptosporidium parvum	Contaminated, water or milk, person-to-person transmission, or undercooked food	2–10 days	Watery diarrhea accompanied by mild hemorrhagic colitis
Escherichia coli O157:H7 and Shiga toxin-producing *E. coli*	Ground or undercooked beef, raw milk, apple, and green leafy vegetables	2–4 days	
Fungi (species of: *Asperagillus, Fusarium, Penicillium*, and others) and mycotoxins (aflatoxins, ochratoxins, and others)	Cereals, spices, meat and meat products, milk and milk products, vegetables, and fruits	3–5 days in case of fungi and 1–2 months in mycotoxins	Diarrhea, nausea, headache, vomiting, dry mouth, fatigue
Giardia lamblia	Contaminated, soil, water food, or surfaces	1–2 weeks	Diarrhea, loose or watery stool, stomach cramps, lactose intolerance
Hepatitis A	Water fruits, vegetables, ice drinks, shellfish, and salads	4–6 weeks	Fever, malaise, nausea, abdominal discomfort, hepatitis, jaundice
Listeria monocytogenes	Contaminated vegetables, milk, cheese, meats, sea food, smoked fish, and ready-to-eat foods	Days to weeks	Meningitis, septicemia, miscarriage, stillbirth, neonatal listeriosis
Norwalk virus, Norwalk-like virus or Norovirus	Raw oysters, shellfish, water and ice, salads, frosting, and person-to-person contact	12–60 h	Diarrhea, abdominal cramps, vomiting, nausea
Nontyphoidal *Salmonella* serovars	Meat, poultry, eggs, and milk products	12–24 h	Diarrhea, abdominal cramps, headache, fever, chills, prostration
Staphylococcus aureus	Custard or cream-filled baked goods, ham, poultry dressing, gravy, eggs, potato salad, cream sauces, and sandwich filling	1–6 h	Severe vomiting, abdominal cramps, diarrhea
Shigella spp.	Salad, raw vegetables, dairy products, and poultry	12–50 h	Fever, cramps, abdominal pain, vomiting
Toxoplasma gondii	Domestic cat, bird, rodent feces, and raw or undercooked foods	5–23 days	Swollen lymph glands, fever, headache, muscle ache, spontaneous abortion. Severe infection in the immunocompromised

Source: Adapted from Amalaradjou, M. A. R., & Bhunia, A. K. (2012). Modern approaches in probiotics research to control foodborne pathogens. In *Advances in food and nutrition research* (Vol. 67, pp. 185–239). Academic Press Inc. https://doi.org/10.1016/B978-0-12-394598-3.00005-8.

diseases (Saha, 2017). Various microbial strains have probiotic activity like LAB (Khaneghah & Fakhri, 2019). The major species of LAB used are belong to *Lactobacillus* spp., *Lactococcus* spp., and *Carnobacterium* spp. and the popular species as *Lactobacillus acidophilus, L. casei, L. lactis, L. plantarum*, and *L. reuteri* (Yadav & Srikanth, 2018). They are active and viable organisms and have used as an alternative to traditional antibiotic and improve food contents for good human health (Roobab et al., 2020). Furthermore, one study illustrated several ways of action of probiotics used in the prevention and therapy of GIT infections (Mousavi Khaneghah et al., 2020).

25.3.1 Factors affecting probiotic activity and benefits

25.3.1.1 Sources

Several sources can be used for obtaining probiotic activity (as *Lactobacillus* sp.) from fruits (Santos et al., 2017), *L. paraplantarum* (Son et al., 2018), and *S. cerevisiae* (Lee et al., 2019) isolated from traditional fermented foods. The release of *exo*-polysaccharides by the action of probiotics during fermentation produced antimicrobial effects (Chen et al., 2019). The probiotics yogurt supplemented with fruit extract, provide a new highly nutritional, bioactive value, antioxidant, and antibacterial activity (Abdel-Hamid et al., 2020). One study detected that during entrance of probiotics in GI, the substrates of probiotics affected its survival (*L. acidophilus* and *Bifidobacterium*), particularly in fermented milk contents (Rodrigues et al., 2019). A *B. tequilensis*-GM (an exopolysaccharide-producing strain) (Abid et al., 2019), *Lactobacterium* (Nami et al., 2019), *Lactobacillus* strains in fermented milk (Papadopoulou et al., 2019), and laboratory-dried sausages (Han et al., 2017). The probiotics strains in cheeses not cause any changes in their physicochemical properties as *Bacillus* strains (Soares et al., 2019) and *Lactobacillus* strains (Mushtaq et al., 2019; Reale et al., 2019). Fig. 25.1 shows sources of probiotic preparations.

25.3.1.2 Probiotics formulations and encapsulation

The addition of encapsulated probiotics in food causes the preservation during long time storage, such as refrigerated storage with beta-glucan (Ningtyas et al., 2019). The addition of beneficial organism as *Propionibacterium freudenreichii* for sweet whey, caused significant useful as a probiotic functional food (Huang et al., 2019). However, the capsulated cow milk probiotics provided higher viable effect than camel milk capsules (Ahmad et al., 2019). The capsulated probiotics kept their viability from adverse effect of gastric pH (Wu et al., 2018). One study detected the ability of gel-encapsulated probiotics with agar in the prevention of the growth of food pathogens (Alehosseini et al., 2018), and the microencapsulated spray drying juice with probiotics was formed and used for the preservation of food (Colín-Cruz et al., 2019). Researchers found that gum Arabic encapsulated probiotics used in the food processing and preserving activity of contents (Arepally & Goswami, 2019). Recently, researchers have developed probiotics (*L. paracasei*) with dried apple snack and used instead of dairy probiotic foods (Akman et al., 2019). Another group combined a sugar-free, chocolate-containing probiotics and gained the palatability consumers (Konar et al., 2018). Other researchers reported that the beta-glucan extracted from waste beer *S. cerevisiae* was used in preserving the probiotic *Lactobacilli* during freeze-drying storage (Guedes et al., 2019; Sampaolesi et al., 2019). Moreover, one study revealed that the preparation of probiotics of *Pediococcus pentosaceus* with Mg NPs resulted in effective encapsulation and release of active

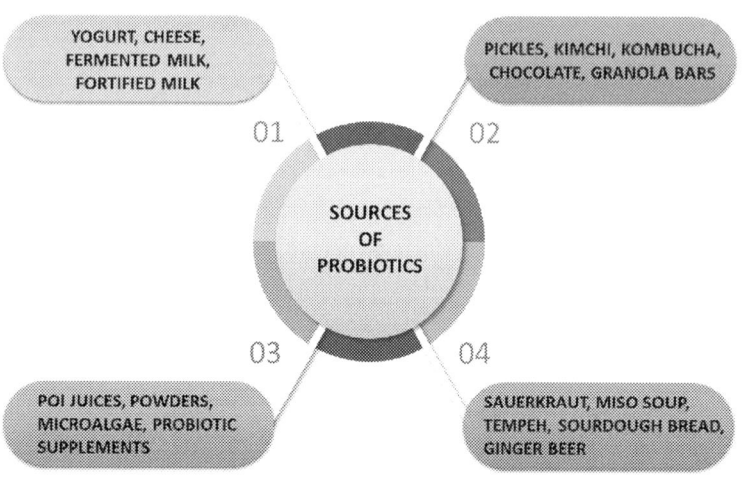

FIGURE 25.1 Sources of probiotics preparations.

probiotics in food (Yao et al., 2018). Also, researchers detected that the nanoencapsulated probiotics into polyvinyl alcohol sodium have used to keep its activity and used for preservation of fish fillets (Ceylan et al., 2018). The iron−pectin NPs have significant ability to preserve the activity of probiotic strains and prevent the loss of iron contents (Ghibaudo et al., 2019).

25.4 Antimicrobial potential of probiotics against foodborne pathogens

25.4.1 *Salmonella*

The significant economic importance of human *Salmonella* infections gained the attention of all authorities to measure the activities of probiotics against this infection. The supplementation of probiotics to chicken resulted in the inhibition and control of *Salmonella* infection hence preventing the health hazard of consumer of chicken products (Van Coillie et al., 2007). The probiotics of *L. rhamnosus* have the potential to remove the accumulation of attached *S. typhimurium* and penetration of epithelial cell (Burkholder & Bhunia, 2010). The probiotics of *L. plantarum* activated the health status of pigs that infected with *S. typhimurium* (Gebru et al., 2010). Also, they prevent the entrance of *S. typhimurium* to internal organs from GIT in chickens (Franchi et al., 2012). Whereas the conjugation of probiotics of different strains given in feed to chickens had not affected the infection with *S. Enteritidis* (Murate et al., 2015). Studies have reported that the probiotics of *L. casei* decreased the acidity of intestinal content and reduced the pH in intestine, which caused the growth suppression of *S. typhimurium* pathogen in mice (Asahara et al., 2011; Dobson et al., 2012). Moreover, probiotics of *L. casei* decreased the growth of *Salmonella* in GIT in mice by activating the stimulation of the activity of phagocyte and elevated humeral immunity (de Moreno de LeBlanc et al., 2010; Dobson et al., 2012). Hence, probiotic preparation prevents growth and suppresses *Salmonella* infection in GIT of human and animals with the improvement of their health status.

25.4.2 *Campylobacter*

In the past decade, it was reported that the probiotics of *Lactobacillus* spp. are able to prevent *C. jejuni* attachment and penetration to the intestinal cells (Neal-McKinney et al., 2012; Tareb et al., 2013). Similarly, the cell wall protein of *L. helveticus* and *L. gasseri* prevents *C. jejuni* attachment and entrance to GIT cells (Wine et al., 2009; Nishiyama et al., 2014). The oral administration *Lactobacilli* in mice given *Salmonella* or *C. jejuni*; the results revealed the significant suppression of both pathogens by probiotics (Wagner et al., 2009). Another study reported that the attachment of *Campylobacter* with intestinal tracts was successfully prevented by the probiotics of *Bacillus subtilis* in chickens (Aguiar et al., 2013).

25.4.3 Shiga toxin-producing *Escherichia coli*

During past years, the administration of probiotics preparations to the *E. coli*-infected human or animals resulted in their growth inhibition and the prevention of production of *Stx* toxin in GIT of pig (Hostetter et al., 2014). When the probiotics of *Lactobacillus*, given to mice prior to infection with *E. coli*, significant suppression of this infection will be occurred (Eaton et al., 2011; Tsai et al., 2010). Moreover, the probiotics of *L. lactis*-secreted alyteserin-1a inhibited the growth of *E. coli* O157:H7 (Volzing et al., 2013). Hence, the probiotic bacterium has significant effects in the prevention of the activity of Shiga toxin-producing *E. coli* (STEC) in both human and animals.

25.4.4 *Listeria monocytogenes*

The use of probiotics in the prevention and control of *listeria* was investigated. The supplementation of rats feed with *L. casei* had inhibited the growth of *L. monocytogenes* infection in GIT and elevated cell-mediated immunity and elevated interleukin levels (De Waard et al., 2002; Dos Santos et al., 2011). Hence, the main effects of probiotics against *Listeria* were changes in immune response. The level of cytokines was decreased after the addition of probiotics of *L. plantarum* and this decreased cytotoxic hazard of *Listeria* infection (Puertollano et al., 2008). The probiotic *Lactobacilli* produced bacitracin, which suppressed the activity of listeria infection (Corr et al., 2007). On the other hand, *Lactococcus lactis* secreted lacticin that gave significant inhibition of *Listeria* in vitro but no action against infection in vivo (Dobson et al., 2011; Rea et al., 2011). Also, one study detected that pediocin producer probiotic bacteria increase the activities of inactive microbiota in vivo but not affected the *L. monocytogenes* growth in vitro (Fernandez et al., 2016).

These variations in probiotics activities depend on the species and strains of bacteria used and no relation between in vivo and in vitro action.

25.4.5 Antiviral activity of probiotics

Some probiotics bacteria secreted antineuclic acid antibodies as *Lactobacillus paracasei* that are able to invade viral cells and damage the DNA in vitro (cell culture) and in vivo (mouse) (Hoang et al., 2015). They also added that the treated mice showed a significant decrease in mRNA expression in viral genes and no effect on cytokine concentration in mice. In a clinical human study, the patients of viral infection administrated milk contained (*L. casei* Shirota) and the results revealed that there is a reduction in period of fever and GIT disorders (Nagata et al., 2011).

25.4.6 Antifungal and antimycotoxin activities of probiotics

Several studies illustrated the efficacy of probiotics against fungal infection of different foods and degradation and eliminated their toxins. One study detected that the supplementation of ochratoxicated broiler chickens feed with probiotics resulted in the improvement of the health status of chickens and degradation of the toxic effects of O.A. (Awaad et al., 2011). They also eliminated the carcinogenic potential of aflatoxins on liver and kidney in rabbits (Esaiassen et al., 2018; Hassan et al., 2016). While other researchers found that *S. cerevisiae* yeast administration stimulated GIT and attach mycotoxins (Armando et al., 2012; Bejaoui et al., 2004). It was also observed that toxin binding was a function of cell wall thickness and binding occurs through the physical adsorption of toxins by probiotic, whereas it was reported that the probiotics of *Lactobacilli* have the ability to suppress the growth of mycotoxigenic fungi and hence prevent mycotoxins' production (Nabawy et al., 2014). In addition, the strains of *B. subtillis* prevent the viability of *A. flavus* and suppress their potential for aflatoxin production and damaged the biosynthetic gene *AflR* (Hossain et al., 2017). Moreover, the administration of probiotics of *Lactobacilli* to aflatoxicated rats and rabbits resulted in the elimination of the toxic effects induced by aflatoxins (Esaiassen et al., 2018; Hassan et al., 2016). They added that lower aflatoxin residues were detected in liver and kidney than the untreated control; this is indicated that the probiotic strains conjugated with mycotoxin in GIT and hence prevent its toxicity (Esaiassen et al., 2018; Hassan et al., 2016).

25.5 Probiotics mechanisms of action in the control and prevention of foodborne pathogens

Nowadays the strategies of treatments of foodborne diseases are needed to understand the mode of action probiotics bacteria for illustrating its therapeutic efficacy of GIT foodborne infections in human (Amalaradjou & Bhunia, 2012; Fijan, 2014; Hossain et al., 2017). The activity of probiotics may interact with pathogens in different ways; hence, several mechanisms of probiotic action have been proposed (Figs. 25.2 and 25.3).

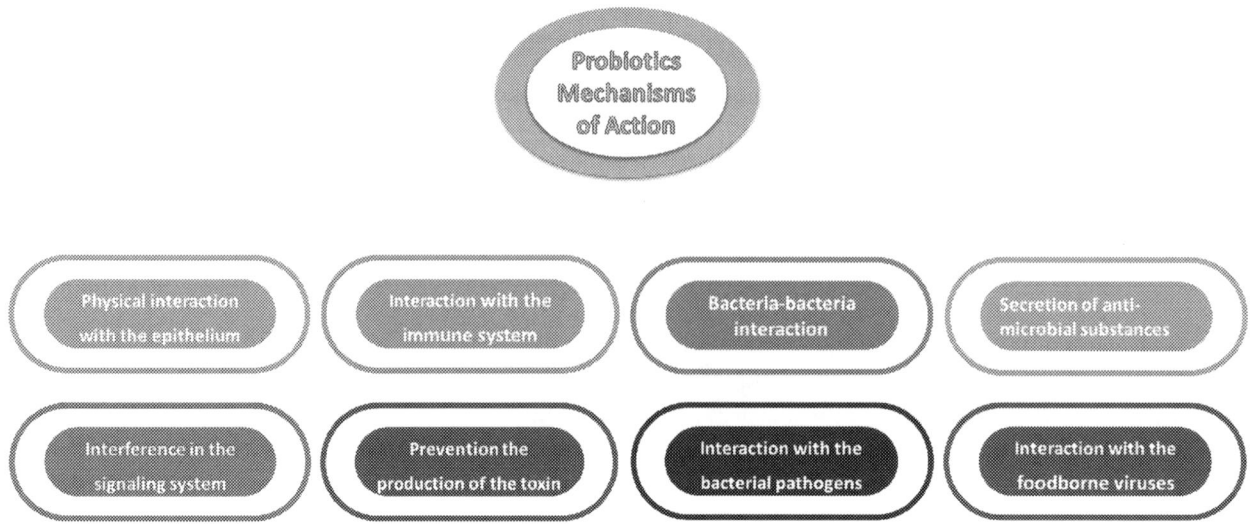

FIGURE 25.2 Mechanisms of action of probiotics.

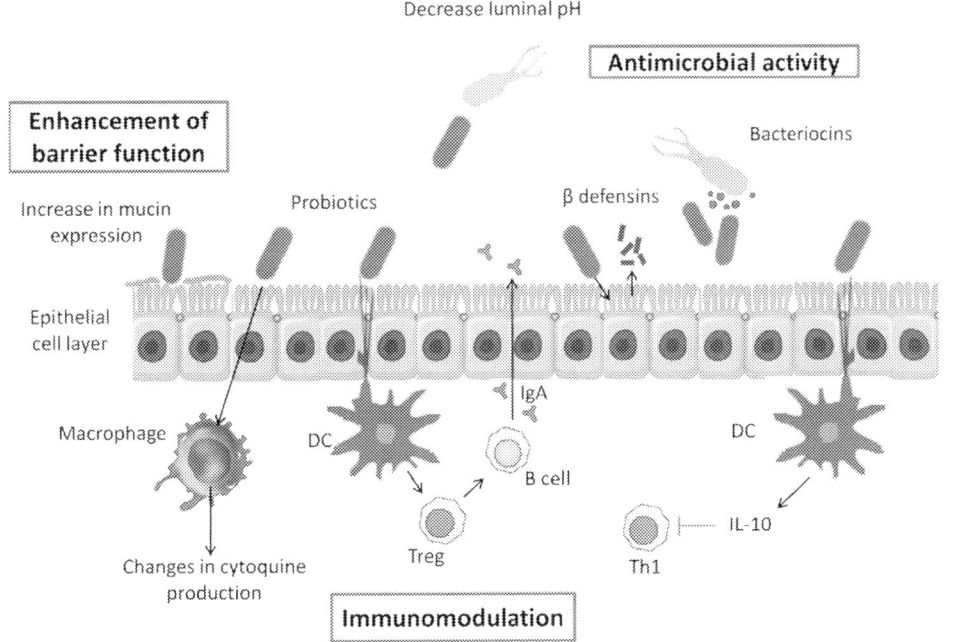

FIGURE 25.3 Mechanisms of probiotic action against foodborne pathogens in the gastrointestinal tract depicting immunological and cellular responses. A schematic diagram about potential mechanisms whereby probiotic bacteria might perform within the intestine. These mechanisms include antagonistic effects on various foodborne pathogens, competitive adherence to the mucosa and epithelium (antimicrobial activity), increased mucus production and enhanced barrier integrity (enhancement of barrier function), and modulation of the human immune system (immunomodulation). *Adapted from Cerdó, T., García-Santos, J., Bermúdez, M. G., & Campoy, C. (2019). The role of probiotics and prebiotics in the prevention and treatment of obesity. Nutrients, 11(3), 635. https://doi.org/10.3390/nu11030635.*

25.5.1 Physical interaction with the epithelium

As the first step in junction between probiotics strains and human intestinal tract, production of mucus and enhancement of the intestinal barrier (Misra et al., 2019).

25.5.1.1 Adherence capacity

The ability of adhesion by producing high amount of mucus is the essential function of probiotic strains and prevents the penetration of intestinal pathogens for GIT (Campaniello et al., 2018). The presence of several strains in probiotics causes more suppression of the activities of pathogens on GIT (Singh et al., 2017). The hydrophilic proteins on *Lactobacillus* cell walls significantly attracted with mucus of GIT epithelium and hence reduced adhesion of pathogens (Jia et al., 2017; Valeriano et al., 2014).

25.5.1.2 Production of mucus

The GIT epithelium produced mucins, a protein-like material, for producing mucus against colonization and penetration of infection agents. They added that any adverse condition in the production of mucins resulted in the occurrence of infections. As the ability of probiotics bacteria to prevent the adhesion of pathogens increased, the gene expression of mucins (Rokana et al., 2017) and activation of the intestine's enterocytes (Khoder et al., 2016) increased. The administration of probiotics consisted of different *Lactobacillus* strains secreted large amount of mucins (Maldonado Galdeano et al., 2019). Similarly, probiotics can raise the level of IgA, which assists in the GIT mucosa and prevents the entrance and growth of infection agents (Pahumunto et al., 2019).

25.5.1.3 Reinforcement of the intestinal barrier

The GIT epithelium barriers are the ability to detect the harmful foreign material as pathogens. It stimulates several barriers as rising in mucus amount, chloride, and water (Thomas & Versalovic, 2010; Raja, 2017). The dysfunction of these activities resulted in several diseases as bowel disease, diarrhea, and other GIT infections (Xavier & Podolsky, 2007). It is interesting to report here that probiotic bacteria have the ability to activate the barriers in GIT against any pathogenic materials (O'Hara & Shanahan, 2007).

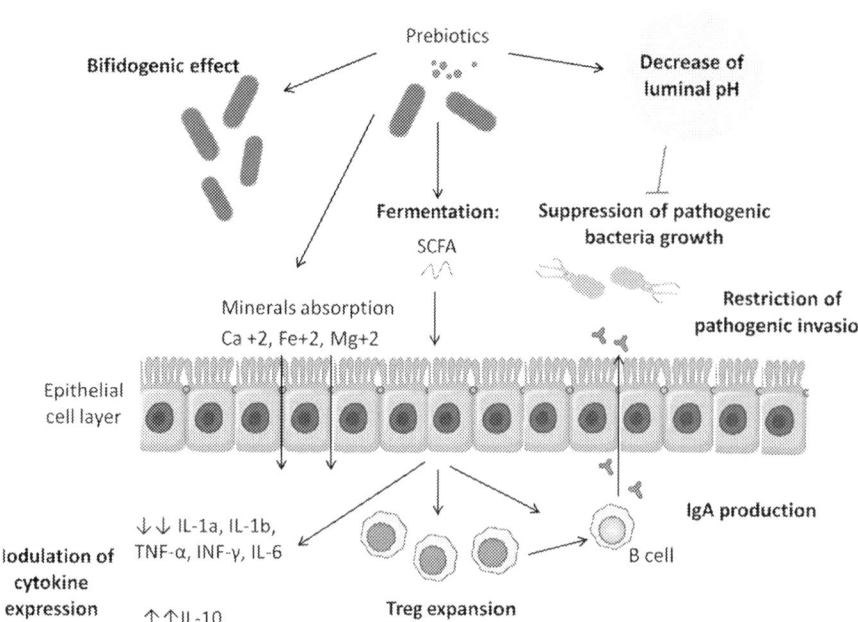

FIGURE 25.4 Mechanisms of prebiotic action. These mechanisms include the production of microbial metabolic products, noting short-chain fatty acids, the promotion of ion and trace element absorption (such as that of calcium, iron, and magnesium), a decrease in luminal pH, and the regulation of the immune system (increasing IgA production and modulating cytokine production). *Adapted from Cerdó, T., García-Santos, J., Bermúdez, M. G., & Campoy, C. (2019). The role of probiotics and prebiotics in the prevention and treatment of obesity. Nutrients, 11(3), 635. https://doi.org/10.3390/nu11030635.*

25.5.2 Interaction between probiotics and the immune system

Recently the normal GIT microbiota has been detected to significantly influence the immune response against infection (Shi et al., 2017). The probiotics bacteria conjugated and attached to GIT epithelial cells and hence stimulated immune systems as elevated release of mucin in human and rats (Caballero-Franco et al., 2007; Hemaiswarya et al., 2013). The probiotics influence the inflammatory signaling pathway after conjugation with gut epithelial cells and prevent phosphorylation and release of the nuclear factor kappa B (NF-κB) inhibitor (Mousavi Khaneghah et al., 2020). The use of antibiotic, NF-κB, is combined with an inhibitor molecule and becomes inactive, but under inflammation, the inhibitor molecule is phosphorylated and activated NF-κB and proinflammatory genes in the nucleus (Plaza-Díaz et al., 2017; Ryan & Bhunia, 2017). This activity also prevents release of IL-8 and stimulated the function of natural killer (NK) cells, which prevent apoptotic effect in epithelial cells and raise mucus amount (Esaiassen et al., 2018; Hassan et al., 2016). They also reinforced the production of cytokines, IgA, macrophages, T cells, interferon, and polysaccharides to increase immune responses (Kaji et al., 2018; Pahumunto et al., 2019) (Fig. 25.4).

25.5.3 Bacteria—bacteria interaction (competition by exclusion)

The competition between probiotic bacteria and pathogens is accompanied by competition on adhesion sites or nutrients in GIT (competition by exclusion). This is due to the probiotic bacteria closing the targeting sites of GIT pathogens as intestinal villi and cryptal. Hence, formation of barrier prevents pathogen penetration of epithelial cells due to (1) prevention of pathogens from obtaining requirement of nutrients and energy for the growth and penetration of epithelium; (2) release of acids that decrease GIT pH, which prevents the viability of pathogens; and (3) packing of intestinal epithelial surface by probiotics that prevent the attachment of pathogens; these mechanisms of action enable probiotics to prevent GIT infections, such as *Clostridium* spp., *Listeria monocytogenes*, *Salmonella*, and *E. coli* (Goldenberg et al., 2017; Liu et al., 2016).

25.5.4 Secretion of antimicrobial substances

The probiotics bacteria can produce bacteriocins (acidocin, enterocin, enterolysin, and lysostaphin) to prevent the growth of pathogens and their penetration to intestinal epithelium cells (Abengózar et al., 2017; Gaspar et al., 2018). Another material secreted by probiotics bacteria is pediocin (*Pediococcus pentosaceus*) that has antimicrobial potential against *Listeriasis* (Cavera et al., 2015). The pediocin penetrates the cells of pathogens and cytoplasm and damage its DNA. Furthermore, *L. acidophilus* secretes suppress the growth of *H. pylori* (Fang et al., 2019), and *L. rhamnosus* produces an antimicrobial agent and prevents the adhesion of pathogens of GIT cells (Dutra et al., 2016).

25.5.5 Interference in the signaling system to express virulence

The accumulation of probiotics bacteria and pathogen causes communication of each other and also with other materials in GIT that influenced the virulence expression of each and their multiplication (Kiymaci et al., 2018). However, probiotic bacteria secrete molecules depred virulence genes in *E. coli* O157:H7 (Gómez et al., 2016) and *Salmonella* (Bayoumi & Griffiths, 2012). One study detected that *Bacillus* species probiotics secreted lipopeptides, which suppress the growth of *S. aureus* (Piewngam & Otto, 2020).

25.5.6 Preventing the production of the toxin

The potentials of toxin production by pathogenic bacteria and fungi are of great health hazard due to the carcinogenic effects of these toxins as aflatoxins (*AflR*) and Shiga toxin (*Stx*) (Esaiassen et al., 2018; Hassan et al., 2016). Several studies used probiotics to ameliorate the toxic effects of these toxins. The drinking of probiotics strain in mice prevents their toxicity by Shiga toxin-producing *E. coli* O157:H7 (Asahara et al., 2004). Shiga toxins have inhibited the protein synthesis of host cells and DNA damage with apoptosis (Pacheco & Sperandio, 2012). On the other hand, the addition of probiotic bacteria to aflatoxicated feed of rabbits resulted in the prevention of the toxic carcinogenic effects on liver cells (Esaiassen et al., 2018; Hassan et al., 2016). They inhibit the growth of aflatoxigenic and ochratoxigenic fungi and prevent the production of respective mycotoxins (Mouhamed et al., 2015; Nabawy et al., 2014).

25.5.7 Interaction between probiotics and bacterial pathogens

Recently the use of beneficial bacteria as probiotics in the prevention and control of foodborne diseases is an alternative strategy for safe uses in human health than chemical methods. Few researchers detected that the addition of probiotic strain of *L. rhamnosus* to food matrix infected with *L. monocytogenes* pathogen causes the prevention of the penetration of pathogens into intestinal epithelium (Collazo et al., 2017; Iglesias et al., 2017). They added that the probiotic bacteria produce several agents that antagonize activities of pathogens. There are several benefits of biopreservation of food by probiotics that can be summarized in Fig. 25.5.

In addition, the agents that secreted by probiotics (surfactants, proteases, and antibiotics) prevent the contact adhesion of intestinal pathogens to the human intestinal epithelial cells and also influence the genes' expression of pathogens (Collazo et al., 2017).

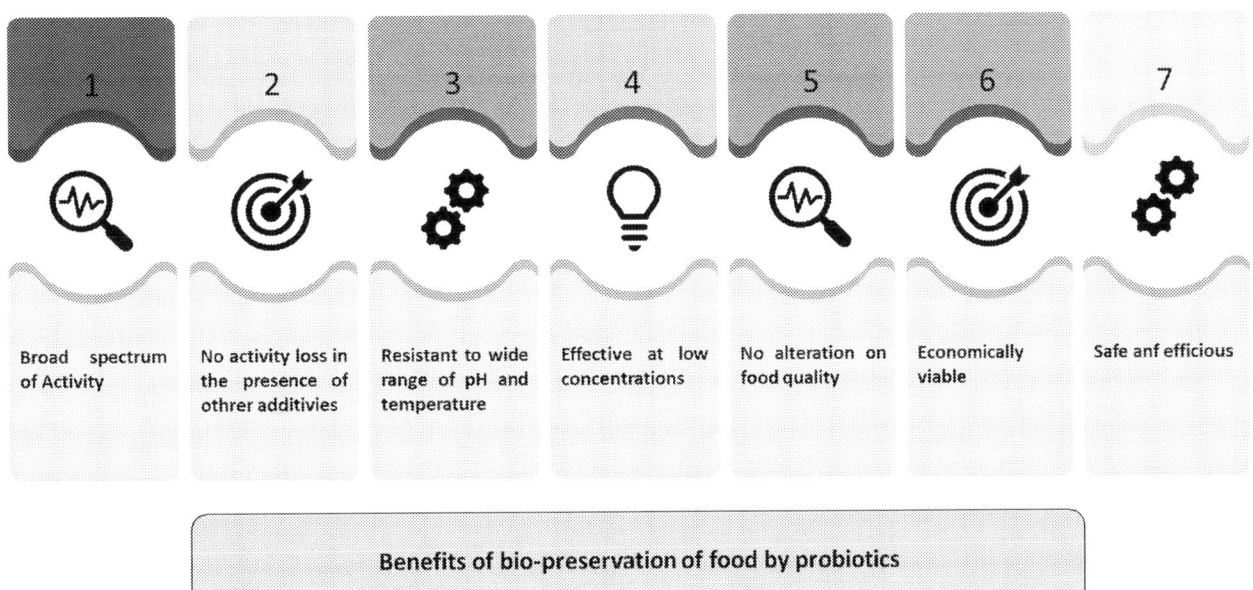

FIGURE 25.5 Biopreservation of food by probiotics.

25.5.8 Interaction between probiotics and foodborne viruses

The viral enteric infections caused by noro and rota viruses are worldwide problem particularly in children. They are resulted in diarrhea and dehydration and general loss in the health of child and even death. The administration of probiotics improved the risk of this illness and decreased the period of diarrhea (Mousavi Khaneghah et al., 2020). The mechanism of probiotic action against viral infection is related to the prevention of viral replication, adhesion, secreted material inhibited their growth, activated epithelial barrier action and potentiated immune-response (Rubio-del-Campo et al., 2014; Wan et al., 2019).

25.6 Supplementation of probiotics in food materials

Today food industries used probiotics in most of the products, especially dairy products as whey, cheeses, yogurt, and fermented milk (Martins et al., 2018; Ranadheera et al., 2017). This is due to their high water contents, low salts, no preservative, the probiotic bacteria persist as carrier's active and their benefits occur. In spite of this, the large levels of fats in cheeses as a carrier for probiotics are more efficient than recently prepared fermented milk, such as whey and yogurt (Martins et al., 2018). They found that the addition of probiotic bacteria in cheeses is ineffective because of their losses during storage and changes in flavor microbiota of milk. Moreover, milk and their products contain several kinds of *Lactobacilli*, which have produced significant proteolytic activities when amino acids' requirement is available (Brown et al., 2017). Hence, the accepted flavor, color, and texture are required to control the proteolytic and lipolytic activities of *Lactobacilli* in milk; these are achieved by the supplementation of dairy product with proper strains of probiotic bacteria (Mousavi Khaneghah et al., 2020). Moreover, the reaction of probiotic bacteria and food carriers produced organic acids, peptides, amino acids, bacteriocins, and free fatty acid, which affected the physicochemical properties of food (flavor and texture) as well as helped to conserve them (Mousavi Khaneghah et al., 2020).

25.7 Delivery system of probiotics

The probiotic supplementation and their activities in food preservation required suitable method of delivery (such as capsules, tablets, or powders) (Hajela et al., 2012). The encapsulation is the main method for the delivery of probiotics, such as gelatin, chitosan, whey proteins, gum, and starches, which stabilized bacterial cells and their activities during different steps of processing (Anal & Singh, 2007; Gbassi et al., 2009). Another method used freeze-drying producing dry powder, which has long storage time and preserves probiotics from intestinal juices (Rokka & Rantamäki, 2010). Extrusion method included addition of probiotics to hydrocolloid and yielded gelled droplets (beads) (Gouin, 2004), while emulsification consisted of probiotics and water leading to water-in-oil emulsion. The water/oil emulsion used for obtaining encapsulated probiotics (Gbassi & Vandamme, 2012). The microcapsules covered with chitosan elevated the viability of probiotic bacteria in the intestinal fluid and pH (Cook et al., 2011). The formation of tablet consisted of carboxylate methyl high amylose starch and chitosan used for probiotic colon delivery and this cause increased rates of released bacteria in GIT (Calinescu & Mateescu, 2008). Core mucoadhesive is another method used for probiotic delivery and coated with hypermellose which have mucoadhesive activity initiated intestinal activities and significant attachment of mucous higher than freeze dried bacteria (Calinescu & Mateescu, 2008). Furthermore, DNA-based gel method for oral delivery of probiotics and used to keep LAB against adverse factors in yogurts (Jonganurakkun et al., 2003, 2006). In this method, DNA conjugated with gelatin leading to the production of hydrogels and complex gels when the probiotic bacteria adhered to gal and yogurt and added to cooled DNA and gelling agent; this is called hydrogel. While the complex gel formed of yogurt and cacao oil mixed with gel solution that have DNA and gelling agents to form encapsulated probiotic. Moreover, the complexes gel has to preserve probiotics against disordered conditions in activated GIT. Hydrogels enable keeping probiotics against acidity in gastric tract and prolonged storage at low temperature (4°C) (Jonganurakkun et al., 2006). Therefore the later DNA-based gel methods are more desirable and accepted by human for probiotic delivery for the oral administration of probiotics.

25.8 The safety of probiotic therapy in host

Worldwide use of probiotics bacteria in the prevention and control foodborne diseases increased the need that the employed bacteria should not cause any infections in consumers. Most of the probiotics LAB (such as *Lactobacillus*) are nonpathogenic to host, while some strains are opportunistic pathogens in patient with low immunity (Boyle et al., 2006; Hempel et al., 2011).

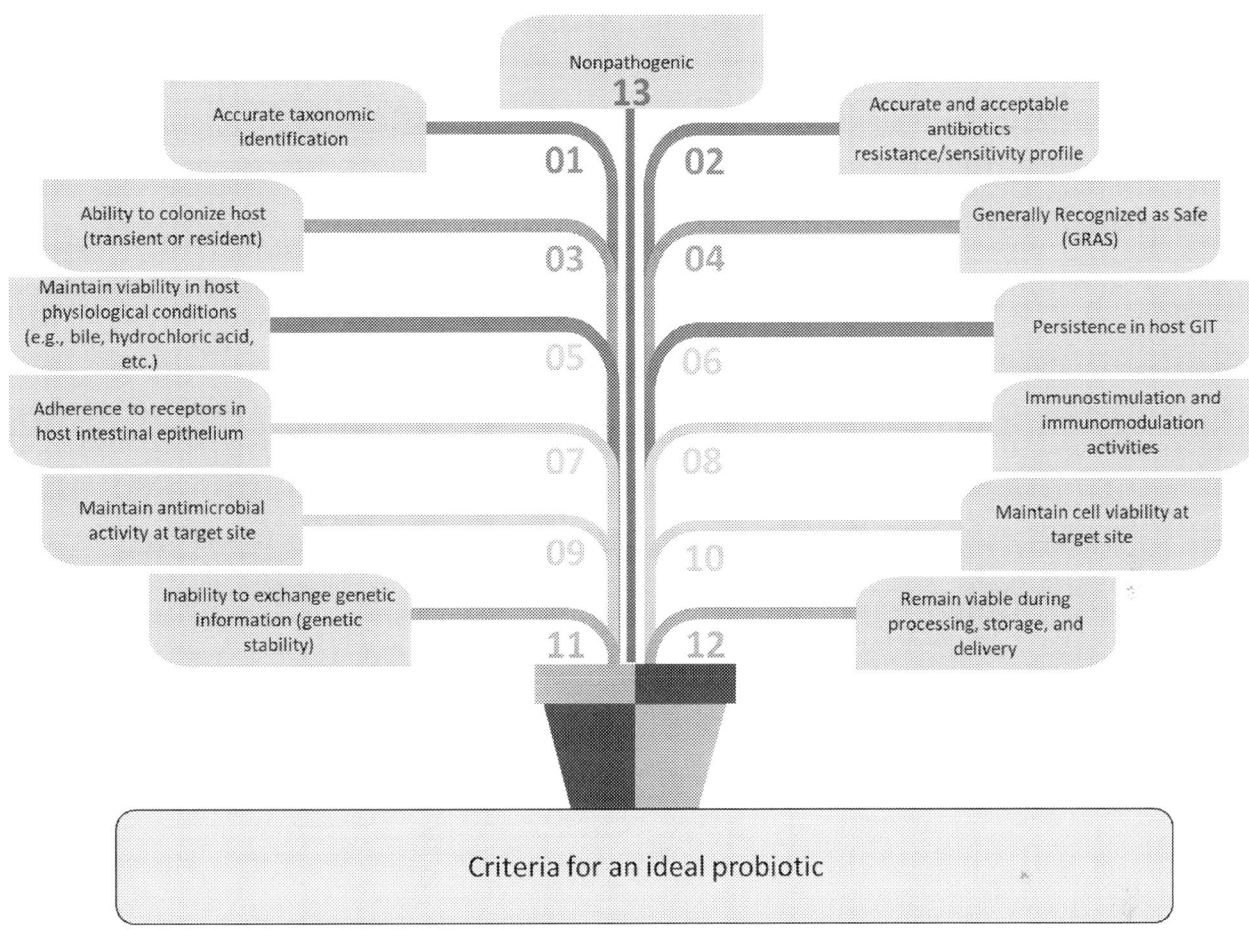

FIGURE 25.6 Criteria of an ideal probiotic.

It is interesting to report here that the genes transfer to GIT microbiota resulted in their conversion to pathogenic bacteria to the host. The most common example illustrating this problem is the transportation of multidrug-resistant (MDR) genes to commensal gut microbiota and lactic acidosis in host (Doron & Snydman, 2015). Therefore the evaluation of used probiotics bacteria for different virulence factors must be undertaken before their administration for the treatment of GIT pathogens. These virulence factors included sensitivity and resistance to antibiotics, genotyping absence of MDR genes, and ability to acquire pathogenic virulence genes from GIT pathogens (Amalaradjou & Bhunia, 2012; Didari et al., 2014). From the forgoing results, it becomes apparent that the use of probiotics bacteria may have been caused harmful health hazard more than benefits effects. Therefore the used probiotic bacteria should have the useful properties for human health without occurrence of any harmful (Fig. 25.6) (Hill et al., 2014; Mousavi Khaneghah et al., 2020).

25.9 Health significance of probiotics in the prevention of foodborne diseases

Probiotics preparations have the ability to suppress the viability of GIT pathogens and prevent microbial food contamination. Hence, they are used in the therapy of foodborne infections and improvement of health (Valdovinos-García et al., 2019). Probiotic strain (*S. cerevisiae*) has the activity against arterial sclerosis (Banik et al., 2019; Mohammadsadeghi et al., 2019) and competes *Salmonella* and *clostridium* infections (Misra et al., 2019; Moens et al., 2019). Moreover, probiotics have significant activity against inflammation in different diseases (Kazemi et al., 2020). Some examples of controlled diseases by probiotics are the antiinflammatory activity of *Bifidobacterium* (Devi et al., 2018) and bowel disease (Chopade et al., 2019); food allergies in pediatric (Ma et al., 2019) have also been recorded. Furthermore, the conjugation of polymer NPs and probiotics showed significant antimicrobial effects against bacterial resistant (Kim et al., 2017). One study revealed the ability of whey pearl probiotics in the suppression of the adverse effects of *Shigella* in mouse (Ganguly et al., 2019), while another study reported that the supplementation of probiotics in food improves brain depression in men rather than women (Chahwan et al., 2019). In addition, researchers prepared probiotics from *Lactobacilli* and can keep child from adverse conditions at early ages (Peng & Biswas, 2017). The probiotics decreased the absorption of toxic materials and prevent their reach to breast milk and hence improved health of children (Astolfi et al., 2019). There is little knowledge about activities' potential and therapeutic effects of probiotics in children (Browne et al., 2019). They are having significant effects as additive in the food processing to overcome the GIT infections and the immunosuppression (Shakibaie et al., 2016). The probiotic strains should resist the pH, enzyme secretion, and other conditions in GIT (Saha, 2017). These strains must have the ability to eliminate the DNA expression of the virulence gene, such as *Stx* and *AflR* production gens (Hassan et al., 2020).

25.10 Conclusion and future perspectives

The foodborne diseases in human are progressively increasing problems related to the huge consumption of ready-to-eat meals, which may be contaminated with pathogens to GIT. Sources of infections mainly related to polluted food and food products with pathogens and their toxins; hence, the intestinal barrier must have the ability to compete and prevent adverse effects of pathogens. Today, the use of biopreservation of food as probiotics bacteria in the prevention and control of GIT infection showed interesting advances. They have the ability to activate the immunity and the epithelial barrier of host to prevent adhesion of pathogens to GIT via secretion of specific antagonizing materials are observed here. The mechanisms of probiotics bacteria against pathogens as the numbers of strain increased, a desirable activity of probiotics is increased. This is related to the production of abundant substances by different bacterial strains of probiotics bacteria in food, which elevated the defense against intestinal pathogens. The DNA-based gels are the most suitable method for oral administration of probiotics. The safety addition in food required evaluation of all virulence factors for bacteria, which are used as probiotics. They must be not having any adverse harmful effects to the consumers and showed significant benefits. In future, a brief genotyping and phenotyping characterization of bacterial strains that used as probiotics must be undertaken to prevent their harmful effects on human health.

Acknowledgment

Grateful appreciation and heart thank to Pro. Dr. M.K. Refai, Professor of Microbiology, Cairo University, for his continuous assistance and advice in initiating the achievement of this work.

References

Abdel-Hamid, M., Romeih, E., Huang, Z., Enomoto, T., Huang, L., & Li, L. (2020). Bioactive properties of probiotic set-yogurt supplemented with Siraitia grosvenorii fruit extract. *Food Chemistry*, 303. Available from https://doi.org/10.1016/j.foodchem.2019.125400.

Abengózar, M. Á., Cebrián, R., Saugar, J. M., Gárate, T., Valdivia, E., Martínez-Bueno, M., Maqueda, M., & Rivas, L. (2017). Enterocin AS-48 as evidence for the use of bacteriocins as new leishmanicidal agents. *Antimicrobial Agents and Chemotherapy*, 61(4). Available from https://doi.org/10.1128/AAC.02288-16.

Abid, Y., Azabou, S., Casillo, A., Gharsallah, H., Jemil, N., Lanzetta, R., Attia, H., & Corsaro, M. M. (2019). Isolation and structural characterization of levan produced by probiotic Bacillus tequilensis-GM from Tunisian fermented goat milk. *International Journal of Biological Macromolecules*, 133, 786–794. Available from https://doi.org/10.1016/j.ijbiomac.2019.04.130.

Abraham, D., Feher, J., Scuderi, G. L., Szabo, D., Dobolyi, A., Cservenak, M., Juhasz, J., Ligeti, B., Pongor, S., Gomez-Cabrera, M. C., Vina, J., Higuchi, M., Suzuki, K., Boldogh, I., & Radak, Z. (2019). Exercise and probiotics attenuate the development of Alzheimer's disease in transgenic mice: Role of microbiome. *Experimental Gerontology*, 115, 122–131. Available from https://doi.org/10.1016/j.exger.2018.12.005.

Aguiar, V. F., Donoghue, A. M., Arsi, K., Reyes-Herrera, I., Metcalf, J. H., De Los Santos, F. S., Blore, P. J., & Donoghue, D. J. (2013). Targeting motility properties of bacteria in the development of probiotic cultures against campylobacter jejuni in Broiler Chickens. *Foodborne Pathogens and Disease*, 10(5), 435–441. Available from https://doi.org/10.1089/fpd.2012.1302.

Ahmad, M., Mudgil, P., & Maqsood, S. (2019). Camel whey protein microparticles for safe and efficient delivery of novel camel milk derived probiotics. *LWT*, 108, 81–88. Available from https://doi.org/10.1016/j.lwt.2019.03.008.

Akman, P. K., Uysal, E., Ozkaya, G. U., Tornuk, F., & Durak, M. Z. (2019). Development of probiotic carrier dried apples for consumption as snack food with the impregnation of Lactobacillus paracasei. *LWT*, 103, 60–68. Available from https://doi.org/10.1016/j.lwt.2018.12.070.

Alehosseini, A., Gomez del Pulgar, E. M., Gómez-Mascaraque, L. G., Martínez-Sanz, M., Fabra, M. J., Sanz, Y., Sarabi-Jamab, M., Ghorani, B., & Lopez-Rubio, A. (2018). Unpurified Gelidium-extracted carbohydrate-rich fractions improve probiotic protection during storage. *LWT*, 96, 694–703. Available from https://doi.org/10.1016/j.lwt.2018.06.043.

Amalaradjou, M. A. R., & Bhunia, A. K. (2012). *Modern approaches in probiotics research to control foodborne pathogens. Advances in food and nutrition research* (Vol. 67, pp. 185–239). Academic Press Inc. Available from https://doi.org/10.1016/B978-0-12-394598-3.00005-8.

Anal, A. K., & Singh, H. (2007). Recent advances in microencapsulation of probiotics for industrial applications and targeted delivery. *Trends in Food Science and Technology*, *18*(5), 240–251. Available from https://doi.org/10.1016/j.tifs.2007.01.004.

Arepally, D., & Goswami, T. K. (2019). Effect of inlet air temperature and gum Arabic concentration on encapsulation of probiotics by spray drying. *LWT*, *99*, 583–593. Available from https://doi.org/10.1016/j.lwt.2018.10.022.

Armando, M. R., Pizzolitto, R. P., Dogi, C. A., Cristofolini, A., Merkis, C., Poloni, V., Dalcero, A. M., & Cavaglieri, L. R. (2012). Adsorption of ochratoxin A and zearalenone by potential probiotic Saccharomyces cerevisiae strains and its relation with cell wall thickness. *Journal of Applied Microbiology*, *113*(2), 256–264. Available from https://doi.org/10.1111/j.1365-2672.2012.05331.x.

Asahara, T., Shimizu, K., Nomoto, K., Hamabata, T., Ozawa, A., & Takeda, Y. (2004). Probiotic Bifidobacteria Protect Mice from Lethal Infection with Shiga Toxin-Producing *Escherichia coli* O157:H7. *Infection and Immunity*, *72*(4), 2240–2247. Available from https://doi.org/10.1128/IAI.72.4.2240-2247.2004.

Asahara, T., Shimizu, K., Takada, T., Kado, S., Yuki, N., Morotomi, M., Tanaka, R., & Nomoto, K. (2011). Protective effect of Lactobacillus casei strain Shirota against lethal infection with multi-drug resistant Salmonella enterica serovar Typhimurium DT104 in mice. *Journal of Applied Microbiology*, *110*(1), 163–173. Available from https://doi.org/10.1111/j.1365-2672.2010.04884.x.

Astolfi, M. L., Protano, C., Schiavi, E., Marconi, E., Capobianco, D., Massimi, L., Ristorini, M., Baldassarre, M. E., Laforgia, N., & Vitali, M. (2019). A prophylactic multi-strain probiotic treatment to reduce the absorption of toxic elements: In-vitro study and biomonitoring of breast milk and infant stools. *Environment International*, *130*.

Aureli, P., Capurso, L., Castellazzi, A. M., Clerici, M., Giovannini, M., Morelli, L., Poli, A., Pregliasco, F., Salvini, F., & Zuccotti, G. V. (2011). Probiotics and health: An evidence-based review. *Pharmacological Research*, *63*(5), 366–376. Available from https://doi.org/10.1016/j.phrs.2011.02.006.

Awaad, M. H. H., Atta, A., Wafaa, A., Ghany., Elmenawy, M., Ahmed, K., Hassan, A. A., Nada, A. A., et al. (2011). Effect of a specific combination of mannan-oligosaccharides and β-glucans extracted from yeast cells wall on the health status and growth performance of ochratoxicated broiler chickens. *The Journal of American Science*, *7*(3), 82–96.

Banik, A., Mondal, J., Rakshit, S., Ghosh, K., Sha, S. P., Halder, S. K., Ghosh, C., & Mondal, K. C. (2019). Amelioration of cold-induced gastric injury by a yeast probiotic isolated from traditional fermented foods. *Journal of Functional Foods*, *59*, 164–173. Available from https://doi.org/10.1016/j.jff.2019.05.039.

Bayoumi, M. A., & Griffiths, M. W. (2012). In vitro inhibition of expression of virulence genes responsible for colonization and systemic spread of enteric pathogens using Bifidobacterium bifidum secreted molecules. *International Journal of Food Microbiology*, *156*(3), 255–263. Available from https://doi.org/10.1016/j.ijfoodmicro.2012.03.034.

Bejaoui, H., Mathieu, F., Taillandier, P., & Lebrihi, A. (2004). Ochratoxin A removal in synthetic and natural grape juices by selected oenological Saccharomyces strains. *Journal of Applied Microbiology*, 1038–1044. Available from https://doi.org/10.1111/j.1365-2672.2004.02385.x.

Beutin, L., & Martin, A. (2012). Outbreak of Shiga toxin-producing Escherichia coli (STEC) O104:H4 infection in Germany causes a paradigm shift with regard to human pathogenicity of STEC strains. *Journal of Food Protection*, *75*(2), 408–418. Available from https://doi.org/10.4315/0362-028X.JFP-11-452.

Bhat, B., & Bajaj, B. K. (2019). Hypocholesterolemic potential and bioactivity spectrum of an exopolysaccharide from a probiotic isolate Lactobacillus paracasei M7. *Bioactive Carbohydrates and Dietary Fibre*, *19*. Available from https://doi.org/10.1016/j.bcdf.2019.100191.

Boehm, M., Krause-Gruszczynska, M., Rohde, M., Tegtmeyer, N., Takahashi, S., Oyarzabal, O. A., & Backert, S. (2011). Major host factors involved in epithelial cell invasion of Campylobacter jejuni: Role of fibronectin, integrin beta1, FAK, Tiam-1, and DOCK180 in activating Rho GTPase Rac1. *Frontiers in Cellular and Infection Microbiology*, *1*, 17. Available from https://doi.org/10.3389/fcimb.2011.00017.

Boricha, A. A., Shekh, S. L., Pithva, S. P., Ambalam, P. S., & Manuel Vyas, B. R. (2019). In vitro evaluation of probiotic properties of Lactobacillus species of food and human origin. *LWT*, *106*, 201–208. Available from https://doi.org/10.1016/j.lwt.2019.02.021.

Boyle, R. J., Robins-Browne, R. M., & Tang, M. L. K. (2006). Probiotic use in clinical practice: What are the risks? *American Journal of Clinical Nutrition*, *83*(6), 1256–1264. Available from https://doi.org/10.1093/ajcn/83.6.1256.

Brown, L., Villegas, J. M., Elean, M., Fadda, S., Mozzi, F., Saavedra, L., & Hebert, E. M. (2017). YebC, a putative transcriptional factor involved in the regulation of the proteolytic system of Lactobacillus. *Scientific Reports*, *7*(1). Available from https://doi.org/10.1038/s41598-017-09124-1.

Browne, P. D., de Groen, A. C., Claassen, E., & Benninga, M. A. (2019). Probiotics for childhood functional gastrointestinal disorders: Do we know what we advise? *PharmaNutrition*, 100160. Available from https://doi.org/10.1016/j.phanu.2019.100160.

Budden, K. F., Gellatly, S. L., Wood, D. L. A., Cooper, M. A., Morrison, M., Hugenholtz, P., Burkholder, K., & Bhunia, A. (2009). Salmonella enterica serovar Typhimurium adhesion and cytotoxicity during epithelial cell stress is reduced by Lactobacillus rhamnosus GG. *Gut Pathogens*, *1*(1), 1–10.

Burkholder, K. M., & Bhunia, A. K. (2010). Listeria monocytogenes uses Listeria adhesion protein (LAP) to promote bacterial transepithelial translocation and induces expression of LAP receptor Hsp60. *Infection and Immunity*, *78*(12), 5062–5073. Available from https://doi.org/10.1128/IAI.00516-10.

Caballero-Franco, C., Keller, K., Simone., & Chadee, K. (2007). The VSL#3 probiotic formula induces mucin gene expression and secretion in colonic epithelial cells. *American Journal of of Physiology-Gastrointestinal and Liver Physiology*, *292*(1), 315–322.

Calinescu, C., & Mateescu, M. A. (2008). Carboxymethyl high amylose starch: Chitosan self-stabilized matrix for probiotic colon delivery. *European Journal of Pharmaceutics and Biopharmaceutics*, *70*(2), 582–589. Available from https://doi.org/10.1016/j.ejpb.2008.06.006.

Campaniello, D., Speranza, B., Petruzzi, L., Bevilacqua, A., & Corbo, M. R. (2018). How to routinely assess transition, adhesion and survival of probiotics into the gut: A case study on propionibacteria. *International Journal of Food Science and Technology*, *53*(2), 484–490. Available from https://doi.org/10.1111/ijfs.13607.

Carrasco, E., Morales-Rueda, A., & García-Gimeno, R. M. (2012). Cross-contamination and recontamination by Salmonella in foods: A review. *Food Research International*, *45*(2), 545–556. Available from https://doi.org/10.1016/j.foodres.2011.11.004.

Cavera, V. L., Arthur, T. D., Kashtanov, D., & Chikindas, M. L. (2015). Bacteriocins and their position in the next wave of conventional antibiotics. *International Journal of Antimicrobial Agents*, *46*(5), 494–501. Available from https://doi.org/10.1016/j.ijantimicag.2015.07.011.

Ceylan, Z., Meral, R., Karakaş, C. Y., Dertli, E., & Yilmaz, M. T. (2018). A novel strategy for probiotic bacteria: Ensuring microbial stability of fish fillets using characterized probiotic bacteria-loaded nanofibers. *Innovative Food Science and Emerging Technologies*, *48*, 212–218. Available from https://doi.org/10.1016/j.ifset.2018.07.002.

Chahwan, B., Kwan, S., Isik, A., van Hemert, S., Burke, C., & Roberts, L. (2019). Gut feelings: A randomised, triple-blind, placebo-controlled trial of probiotics for depressive symptoms. *Journal of Affective Disorders*, *253*, 317–326. Available from https://doi.org/10.1016/j.jad.2019.04.097.

Chammem, N., Issaoui, M., De Almeida, A. I. D., & Delgado, A. M. (2018). Food crises and food safety incidents in European Union, United States, and Maghreb Area: Current risk communication strategies and new approaches. *Journal of AOAC International*, *101*(4), 923–938. Available from https://doi.org/10.5740/jaoacint.17-0446.

Chen, Y., Wang, D., Wu, Y., Zhao, D., Zhang, J., Xie, H., & Zhang, J. (2019). The feasibility of metagenomic next-generation sequencing to identify pathogens causing tuberculous meningitis in cerebrospinal fluid. *Frontiers in Microbiology*, *10*(1993), 1–8.

Chopade, L. R., Paradeshi, J. S., Amrutkar, K. P., & Chaudhari, B. L. (2019). Finding out potent probiotic cultures from ayurvedic formulation Takrarishta through in-vitro probiotic characterization and principal component analysis. *LWT*, *100*, 205–212. Available from https://doi.org/10.1016/j.lwt.2018.10.061.

Colín-Cruz, M. A., Pimentel-González, D. J., Carrillo-Navas, H., Alvarez-Ramírez, J., & Guadarrama-Lezama, A. Y. (2019). Co-encapsulation of bioactive compounds from blackberry juice and probiotic bacteria in biopolymeric matrices. *LWT*, *110*, 94–101. Available from https://doi.org/10.1016/j.lwt.2019.04.064.

Collazo, C., Abadías, M., Colás-Medà, P., Iglesias, M. B., Granado-Serrano, A. B., Serrano, J., & Viñas, I. (2017). Effect of Pseudomonas graminis strain CPA-7 on the ability of Listeria monocytogenes and Salmonella enterica subsp. enterica to colonize Caco-2 cells after pre-incubation on fresh-cut pear. *International Journal of Food Microbiology*, *262*, 55–62. Available from https://doi.org/10.1016/j.ijfoodmicro.2017.09.003.

Cook, M. T., Tzortzis, G., Charalampopoulos, D., & Khutoryanskiy, V. V. (2011). Production and evaluation of dry alginate-chitosan microcapsules as an enteric delivery vehicle for probiotic bacteria. *Biomacromolecules*, *12*(7), 2834–2840. Available from https://doi.org/10.1021/bm200576h.

Corr, S. C., Li, Y., Riedel, C. U., O'Toole, P. W., Hill, C., & Gahan, C. G. M. (2007). Bacteriocin production as a mechanism for the antiinfective activity of Lactobacillus salivarius UCC118. *Proceedings of the National Academy of Sciences of the United States of America*, *104*(18), 7617–7621. Available from https://doi.org/10.1073/pnas.0700440104.

Danneskiold-Samsøe, N. B., Dias de Freitas Queiroz Barros, H., Santos, R., Bicas, J. L., Cazarin, C. B. B., Madsen, L., Kristiansen, K., Pastore, G. M., Brix, S., & Maróstica Júnior, M. R. (2019). Interplay between food and gut microbiota in health and disease. *Food Research International*, *115*, 23–31. Available from https://doi.org/10.1016/j.foodres.2018.07.043.

Das, J. K., Mishra, D., Ray, P., Tripathy, P., Beuria, T. K., Singh, N., & Suar, M. (2013). In vitro evaluation of anti-infective activity of a Lactobacillus plantarum strain against Salmonella enterica serovar Enteritidis. *Gut Pathogens*, *5*(1). Available from https://doi.org/10.1186/1757-4749-5-11.

Dasti, J. I., Tareen, A. M., Lugert, R., Zautner, A. E., & Groß, U. (2010). Campylobacter jejuni: A brief overview on pathogenicity-associated factors and disease-mediating mechanisms. *International Journal of Medical Microbiology*, *300*(4), 205–211. Available from https://doi.org/10.1016/j.ijmm.2009.07.002.

Davis, T. K., McKee, R., Schnadower, D., & Tarr, P. I. (2013). Treatment of shiga toxin-producing escherichia coli infections. *Infectious Disease Clinics of North America*, *27*(3), 577–597. Available from https://doi.org/10.1016/j.idc.2013.05.010.

de Moreno de LeBlanc, A., Castillo, N. A., & Perdigon Gabriela, G. (2010). Anti-infective mechanisms induced by a probiotic Lactobacillus strain against Salmonella enterica serovar Typhimurium infection. *International Journal of Food Microbiology*, *138*(3), 223–231. Available from https://doi.org/10.1016/j.ijfoodmicro.2010.01.020.

De Waard, R., Garssen, J., Bokken, G. C. A. M., & Vos, J. G. (2002). Antagonistic activity of Lactobacillus casei strain Shirota against gastrointestinal Listeria monocytogenes infection in rats. *International Journal of Food Microbiology*, *73*(1), 93–100. Available from https://doi.org/10.1016/S0168-1605(01)00699-7.

Devi, S. M., Kurrey, N. K., & Halami, P. M. (2018). In vitro anti-inflammatory activity among probiotic Lactobacillus species isolated from fermented foods. *Journal of Functional Foods*, *47*, 19–27. Available from https://doi.org/10.1016/j.jff.2018.05.036.

Didari, T., Solki, S., Mozaffari, S., Nikfar, S., & Abdollahi, M. (2014). A systematic review of the safety of probiotics. *Expert Opinion on Drug Safety*, *13*(2), 227–239. Available from https://doi.org/10.1517/14740338.2014.872627.

Dittoe, D. K., Ricke, S. C., & Kiess, A. S. (2018). Organic acids and potential for modifying the avian gastrointestinal tract and reducing pathogens and disease. *Frontiers in Veterinary Science*, 5. Available from https://doi.org/10.3389/fvets.2018.00216.

Dobson, A., Cotter, P. D., Paul Ross, R., & Hill, C. (2012). Bacteriocin production: A probiotic trait? *Applied and Environmental Microbiology*, *78*(1), 1–6. Available from https://doi.org/10.1128/AEM.05576-11.

Dobson, A., Crispie, F., Rea, M. C., O'Sullivan, O., Casey, P. G., Lawlor, P. G., Cotter, P. D., Ross, P., Gardiner, G. E., & Hill, C. (2011). Fate and efficacy of lacticin 3147-producing Lactococcus lactis in the mammalian gastrointestinal tract. *FEMS Microbiology Ecology*, *76*(3), 602–614. Available from https://doi.org/10.1111/j.1574-6941.2011.01069.x.

Doron, S., & Snydman, D. R. (2015). Risk and safety of probiotics. *Clinical Infectious Diseases*, *60*, S129–S134. Available from https://doi.org/10.1093/cid/civ085.

Dos Santos, L. M., Santos, M. M., De Souza Silva, H. P., Arantes, R. M. E., Nicoli, J. R., & Vieira, L. Q. (2011). Monoassociation with probiotic Lactobacillus delbrueckii UFV-H2b20 stimulates the immune system and protects germfree mice against Listeria monocytogenes infection. *Medical Microbiology and Immunology, 200*(1), 29–38. Available from https://doi.org/10.1007/s00430-010-0170-1.

Duarte, A. I., Sjögren, M., Santos, M. S., Oliveira, C. R., Moreira, P. I., & Björkqvist, M. (2018). Dual therapy with liraglutide and ghrelin promotes brain and peripheral energy metabolism in the R6/2 mouse model of Huntington's disease. *Scientific Reports, 8*(1). Available from https://doi.org/10.1038/s41598-018-27121-w.

Dutra, V., Silva, A. C., Cabrita, P., Peres, C., Malcata, X., & Brito, L. (2016). Lactobacillus plantarum LB95 impairs the virulence potential of Grampositive and Gram-negative food-borne pathogens in HT-29 and vero cell cultures. *Journal of Medical Microbiology, 65*(1), 28–35. Available from https://doi.org/10.1099/jmm.0.000196.

Eaton, K. A., Honkala, A., Auchtung, T. A., & Britton, R. A. (2011). Probiotic lactobacillus reuteri ameliorates disease due to enterohemorrhagic escherichia coli in germfree mice. *Infection and Immunity, 79*(1), 185–191. Available from https://doi.org/10.1128/IAI.00880-10.

Esaiassen, E., Hjerde, E., Cavanagh, J. P., Pedersen, T., Andresen, J. H., & Rettedal, S. I. (2018). The effect of probiotic supplementation on the gut microbiota and antibiotic resistome development in preterm infants. *Frontiers in Pediatrics, 6*.

Fang, H. R., Zhang, G. Q., Cheng, J. Y., & Li, Z. Y. (2019). Efficacy of Lactobacillus-supplemented triple therapy for Helicobacter pylori infection in children: A *meta*-analysis of randomized controlled trials. *European Journal of Pediatrics, 178*(1), 7–16. Available from https://doi.org/10.1007/s00431-018-3282-z.

Fernandez, B., Savard, P., & Fliss, I. (2016). Survival and metabolic activity of pediocin producer Pediococcus acidilactici UL5: Its impact on intestinal microbiota and Listeria monocytogenes in a model of the human terminal ileum. *Microbial Ecology, 72*(4), 931–942. Available from https://doi.org/10.1007/s00248-015-0645-0.

Fijan, S. (2014). Microorganisms with claimed probiotic properties: An overview of recent literature. *International Journal of Environmental Research and Public Health, 11*(5), 4745–4767. Available from https://doi.org/10.3390/ijerph110504745.

Franchi, L., Kamada, N., Nakamura, Y., Burberry, A., Kuffa, P., Suzuki, S., Shaw, M. H., Kim, Y. G., & Núñez, G. (2012). NLRC4-driven production of IL-1β discriminates between pathogenic and commensal bacteria and promotes host intestinal defense. *Nature Immunology, 13*(5), 449–456. Available from https://doi.org/10.1038/ni.2263.

Fredua-Agyeman, M., Stapleton, P., Basit, A. W., & Gaisford, S. (2017). Microcalorimetric evaluation of a multi-strain probiotic: Interspecies inhibition between probiotic strains. *Journal of Functional Foods, 36*, 357–361. Available from https://doi.org/10.1016/j.jff.2017.07.018.

Ganguly, S., Sabikhi, L., & Singh, A. K. (2019). Effect of whey-pearl millet-barley based probiotic beverage on Shigella-induced pathogenicity in murine model. *Journal of Functional Foods, 54*, 498–505. Available from https://doi.org/10.1016/j.jff.2019.01.049.

Gaspar, C., Donders, G. G., Palmeira-de-Oliveira, R., Queiroz, J. A., Tomaz, C., Martinez-de-Oliveira, J., & Palmeira-de-Oliveira, A. (2018). Bacteriocin production of the probiotic Lactobacillus acidophilus KS400. *AMB Express, 8*(1). Available from https://doi.org/10.1186/s13568-018-0679-z.

Gbassi, G. K., & Vandamme, T. (2012). Probiotic encapsulation technology: From microencapsulation to release into the gut. *Pharmaceutics, 4*(1), 149–163. Available from https://doi.org/10.3390/pharmaceutics4010149.

Gbassi, G. K., Vandamme, T., Ennahar, S., & Marchioni, E. (2009). Microencapsulation of Lactobacillus plantarum spp in an alginate matrix coated with whey proteins. *International Journal of Food Microbiology, 129*(1), 103–105. Available from https://doi.org/10.1016/j.ijfoodmicro.2008.11.012.

Gebru, E., Lee, J. S., Son, J. C., Yang, S. Y., Shin, S. A., Kim, B., Kim, M. K., & Park, S. C. (2010). Effect of probiotic-, bacteriophage-, or organic acid-supplemented feeds or fermented soybean meal on the growth performance, acute-phase response, and bacterial shedding of grower pigs challenged with Salmonella enterica serotype typhimurium. *Journal of Animal Science, 88*(12), 3880–3886. Available from https://doi.org/10.2527/jas.2010-2939.

Ghibaudo, F., Gerbino, E., Copello, G. J., Campo Dall' Orto, V., & Gómez-Zavaglia, A. (2019). Pectin-decorated magnetite nanoparticles as both iron delivery systems and protective matrices for probiotic bacteria. *Colloids and Surfaces B: Biointerfaces, 180*, 193–201. Available from https://doi.org/10.1016/j.colsurfb.2019.04.049.

Goldenberg, J. Z., Yap, C., Lytvyn, L., Lo, C. K. F., Beardsley, J., Mertz, D., & Johnston, B. C. (2017). Probiotics for the prevention of Clostridium difficile-associated diarrhea in adults and children. *Cochrane Database of Systematic Reviews, 2017*(12). Available from https://doi.org/10.1002/14651858.CD006095.pub4.

Gómez, N. C., Ramiro, J. M., Quecanm., Franco, X., & de Melo. (2016). Use of potential probiotic lactic acid bacteria (LAB) biofilms for the control of Listeria monocytogenes, Salmonella typhimurium, and Escherichia coli O157:H7 biofilms formation. *Frontiers in Microbiology, 7*(863).

Gouin, S. (2004). Microencapsulation: Industrial appraisal of existing technologies and trends. *Trends in food science and technology, 15*(7–8), 330–347. Available from https://doi.org/10.1016/j.tifs.2003.10.005.

Guedes, da S., Pimentel, T. C., Diniz-Silva., Almeida, T., da Cruz., Tavares, J. F., Souza., Garcia, E. F., & Magnani, M. (2019). Protective effects of b-glucan extracted from spent brewer yeast during freeze-drying, storage and exposure to simulated gastrointestinal conditions of probiotic lactobacilli. *LWT, 116*.

Gunyakti, A., & Asan-Ozusaglam, M. (2019). Lactobacillus gasseri from human milk with probiotic potential and some technological properties. *LWT, 109*, 261–269. Available from https://doi.org/10.1016/j.lwt.2019.04.043.

Hajela, N., Nair, G. B., Abraham, P., & Ganguly, N. K. (2012). Health impact of probiotics—Vision and opportunities. *Gut Pathogens, 4*(1). Available from https://doi.org/10.1186/1757-4749-4-1.

Han, Q., Kong, B., Chen, Q., Sun, F., & Zhang, H. (2017). In vitro comparison of probiotic properties of lactic acid bacteria isolated from Harbin dry sausages and selected probiotics. *Journal of Functional Foods, 32*, 391–400. Available from https://doi.org/10.1016/j.jff.2017.03.020.

Hassan, A. A., Abo-Zaid, K. F., & Oraby, N. H. (2020). Molecular and conventional detection of antimicrobial activity of zinc oxide nanoparticles and cinnamon oil against escherichia coli and aspergillus flavus. *Advances in Animal and Veterinary Sciences*, *8*(8), 839−847. Available from https://doi.org/10.17582/JOURNAL.AAVS/2020/8.8.839.847.

Hassan, A. A., Mogda, K., Mansour., Essam, M., Ibrahim., Naglaam, M., Al-Kalamawy, A., Flourage, M. A., Rady, M., & Darwish, A. S. (2016). Aflatoxicosis in rabbits with particular reference to their control by N. acetyl cysteine and probiotic. *International Journal of Current Research*, *8* (1), 25547−25560.

Hemaiswarya, S., Raja, R., Ravikumar, R., & Carvalho, I. S. (2013). Mechanism of action of probiotics. *Brazilian Archives of Biology and Technology*, *56*(1), 113−119. Available from https://doi.org/10.1590/S1516-89132013000100015.

Hempel, S., Newberry, S., Ruelaz, A., Wang, Z., Miles, J. N. V., Suttorp, M. J., Johnsen, B., Shanman, R., Slusser, W., Fu, N., Smith, A., Roth, B., Polak, J., Motala, A., Perry, T., & Shekelle, P. G. (2011). Safety of probiotics used to reduce risk and prevent or treat disease. *Evidence Report/Technology Assessment*, *200*, 1−645.

Hill, C., Guarner, F., Reid, G., Gibson, G. R., Merenstein, D. J., Pot, B., Morelli, L., Canani, R. B., Flint, H. J., Salminen, S., Calder, P. C., & Sanders, M. E. (2014). Expert consensus document: The international scientific association for probiotics and prebiotics consensus statement on the scope and appropriate use of the term probiotic. *Nature Reviews Gastroenterology and Hepatology*, *11*(8), 506−514. Available from https://doi.org/10.1038/nrgastro.2014.66.

Hoang, P. M., Cho, S., Kim, K. E., Byun, S. J., Lee, T. K., & Lee, S. (2015). Development of Lactobacillus paracasei harboring nucleic acid-hydrolyzing 3D8 scFv as a preventive probiotic against murine norovirus infection. *Applied Microbiology and Biotechnology*, *99*(6), 2793−2803. Available from https://doi.org/10.1007/s00253-014-6257-7.

Hossain, M. I., Sadekuzzaman, M., & Ha, S. D. (2017). Probiotics as potential alternative biocontrol agents in the agriculture and food industries: A review. *Food Research International*, *100*, 63−73. Available from https://doi.org/10.1016/j.foodres.2017.07.077.

Hostetter, S. J., Helgerson, A. F., Paton, J. C., Paton, A. W., & Cornick, N. A. (2014). Therapeutic use of a receptor mimic probiotic reduces intestinal Shiga toxin levels in a piglet model of hemolytic uremic syndrome. *BMC Research Notes*, *7*(1). Available from https://doi.org/10.1186/1756-0500-7-331.

Huang, S., Rabah, H., Ferret-Bernard, S., Le Normand, L., Gaucher, F., Guerin, S., Nogret, I., Le Loir, Y., Chen, X. D., Jan, G., Boudry, G., & Jeantet, R. (2019). Propionic fermentation by the probiotic Propionibacterium freudenreichii to functionalize whey. *Journal of Functional Foods*, *52*, 620−628. Available from https://doi.org/10.1016/j.jff.2018.11.043.

Iglesias, M. B., Viñas, I., Colás-Medà, P., Collazo, C., Serrano, J. C. E., & Abadias, M. (2017). Adhesion and invasion of Listeria monocytogenes and interaction with Lactobacillus rhamnosus GG after habituation on fresh-cut pear. *Journal of Functional Foods*, *34*, 453−460. Available from https://doi.org/10.1016/j.jff.2017.05.011.

Jia, F. F., Zhang, L. J., Pang, X. H., Gu, X. X., Abdelazez, A., Liang, Y., Sun, S. R., & Meng, X. C. (2017). Complete genome sequence of bacteriocin-producing Lactobacillus plantarum KLDS1.0391, a probiotic strain with gastrointestinal tract resistance and adhesion to the intestinal epithelial cells. *Genomics*, *109*(5−6), 432−437. Available from https://doi.org/10.1016/j.ygeno.2017.06.008.

Jiao, Y., Zhang, W., Ma, J., Wen, C., Wang, P., Wang, Y., Xing, J., Liu, W., Yang, L., & He, J. (2011). Early onset of neonatal listeriosis. *Pediatrics International*, *53*(6), 1034−1037. Available from https://doi.org/10.1111/j.1442-200X.2011.03442.x.

Jonganurakkun, B., Liu, X. D., Nodasaka, Y., Nomizu, M., & Nishi, N. (2003). Survival of lactic acid bacteria in simulated gastrointestinal juice protected by a DNA-based complex gel. *Journal of Biomaterials Science, Polymer Edition*, *14*(11), 1269−1281. Available from https://doi.org/10.1163/156856203322553482.

Jonganurakkun, B., Nodasaka, Y., Sakairi, N., & Nishi, N. (2006). DNA-based gels for oral delivery of probiotic bacteria. *Macromolecular Bioscience*, *6*(1), 99−103. Available from https://doi.org/10.1002/mabi.200500199.

Kaji, R., Kiyoshima-Shibata, J., Tsujibe, S., Nanno, M., & Shida, K. (2018). Short communication: Probiotic induction of interleukin-10 and interleukin-12 production by macrophages is modulated by co-stimulation with microbial components. *Journal of Dairy Science*, *101*(4), 2838−2841. Available from https://doi.org/10.3168/jds.2017-13868.

Kazemi, A., Soltani, S., Ghorabi, S., Keshtkar, A., Daneshzad, E., Nasri, F., & Mazloomi, S. M. (2020). Effect of probiotic and synbiotic supplementation on inflammatory markers in health and disease status: A systematic review and *meta*-analysis of clinical trials. *Clinical Nutrition*, *39*(3), 789−819. Available from https://doi.org/10.1016/j.clnu.2019.04.004.

Khaneghah, A. M., & Fakhri, Y. (2019). Probiotics and prebiotics as functional foods: State of the art. *Current Nutrition and Food Science*, *15*(1), 20−30. Available from https://doi.org/10.2174/1573401314666180416120241.

Khoder, G., Al-Menhali, A. A., Al-Yassir, F., & Karam, S. M. (2016). Potential role of probiotics in the management of gastric ulcer. *Experimental and Therapeutic Medicine*, *12*(1), 3−17. Available from https://doi.org/10.3892/etm.2016.3293.

Kim, S., Covington, A., & Pamer, E. G. (2017). The intestinal microbiota: Antibiotics, colonization resistance, and enteric pathogens. *Immunological Reviews*, *279*(1), 90−105. Available from https://doi.org/10.1111/imr.12563.

Kirk, M. D., Pires, S. M., Black, R. E., Caipo, M., Crump, J. A., Devleesschauwer, B., Döpfer, D., Fazil, A., Fischer-Walker, C. L., Hald, T., Hall, A. J., Keddy, K. H., Lake, R. J., Lanata, C. F., Torgerson, P. R., Havelaar, A. H., & Angulo, F. J. (2015). World Health Organization estimates of the global and regional disease burden of 22 foodborne bacterial, protozoal, and viral diseases, 2010: A data synthesis. *PLoS Medicine*, *12*(12). Available from https://doi.org/10.1371/journal.pmed.1001921.

Kiymaci, M. E., Altanlar, N., Gumustas, M., Ozkan, S. A., & Akin, A. (2018). Quorum sensing signals and related virulence inhibition of Pseudomonas aeruginosa by a potential probiotic strain's organic acid. *Microbial Pathogenesis*, *121*, 190−197. Available from https://doi.org/10.1016/j.micpath.2018.05.042.

Konar, N., Palabiyik, I., Toker, O. S., Polat, D. G., Kelleci, E., Pirouzian, H. R., Akcicek, A., & Sagdic, O. (2018). Conventional and sugar-free probiotic white chocolate: Effect of inulin DP on various quality properties and viability of probiotics. *Journal of Functional Foods*, *43*, 206–213. Available from https://doi.org/10.1016/j.jff.2018.02.016.

Lake, I. R., & Barker, G. C. (2018). Climate change, foodborne pathogens and illness in higher-income countries. *Current Environmental Health Reports*, *5*(1), 187–196. Available from https://doi.org/10.1007/s40572-018-0189-9.

Lau, L. Y. J., & Chye, F. Y. (2018). Antagonistic effects of Lactobacillus plantarum 0612 on the adhesion of selected foodborne enteropathogens in various colonic environments. *Food Control*, *91*, 237–247. Available from https://doi.org/10.1016/j.foodcont.2018.04.001.

Lee, N. K., Hong, J. Y., Yi, S. H., Hong, S. P., Lee, J. E., & Paik, H. D. (2019). Bioactive compounds of probiotic Saccharomyces cerevisiae strains isolated from cucumber jangajji. *Journal of Functional Foods*, *58*, 324–329. Available from https://doi.org/10.1016/j.jff.2019.04.059.

Lehner, A., Tall, B. D., Fanning, S., & Srikumar, S. (2018). Cronobacter spp.—Opportunistic foodborne pathogens: An update on evolution, osmotic adaptation and pathogenesis. *Current Clinical Microbiology Reports*, *5*(2), 97–105. Available from https://doi.org/10.1007/s40588-018-0089-7.

Lievin Moal, V. (2016). A gastrointestinal anti-infectious biotherapeutic agent: The heat-treated Lactobacillus LB. *Therapeutic Advances in Gastroenterology*, *9*(1), 57–75. Available from https://doi.org/10.1177/1756283X15602831.

Liu, Y., Gibson, G. R., & Walton, G. E. (2016). An in vitro approach to study effects of prebiotics and probiotics on the faecal microbiota and selected immune parameters relevant to the elderly. *PLoS One*, *11*(9). Available from https://doi.org/10.1371/journal.pone.0162604.

Ma, J., Zhang, J., Li, Q., Shi, Z., Wu, H., Zhang, H., Tang, L., Yi, R., Su, H., & Sun, X. (2019). Oral administration of a mixture of probiotics protects against food allergy via induction of CD103 + dendritic cells and modulates the intestinal microbiota. *Journal of Functional Foods*, *55*, 65–75. Available from https://doi.org/10.1016/j.jff.2019.02.010.

Mackowiak, P. A. (2013). Recycling Metchnikoff: Probiotics, the intestinal microbiome and the quest for long life. *Frontiers in Public Health*, 1. Available from https://doi.org/10.3389/fpubh.2013.00052.

Maldonado Galdeano, C., Cazorla, S., Lemme Dumit, J., Vélez, E., & Perdigón, G. (2019). Beneficial effects of probiotic consumption on the immune system. *Annals of Nutrition & Metabolism*, *74*(2), 115–124. Available from https://doi.org/10.1159/000496426.

Marcial-Coba, M. S., Pjaca, A. S., Andersen, C. J., Knøchel, S., & Nielsen, D. S. (2019). Dried date paste as carrier of the proposed probiotic Bacillus coagulans BC4 and viability assessment during storage and simulated gastric passage. *LWT*, *99*, 197–201. Available from https://doi.org/10.1016/j.lwt.2018.09.052.

Martens, E. C., Neumann, M., & Desai, M. S. (2018). Interactions of commensal and pathogenic microorganisms with the intestinal mucosal barrier. *Nature Reviews. Microbiology*, *16*(8), 457–470. Available from https://doi.org/10.1038/s41579-018-0036-x.

Martinez, F. A. C., Domínguez, J. M., Converti, A., & De Souza Oliveira, R. P. (2015). Production of bacteriocin-like inhibitory substance by Bifidobacterium lactis in skim milk supplemented with additives. *Journal of Dairy Research*, *82*(3), 350–355. Available from https://doi.org/10.1017/S0022029915000163.

Martins, I. B. A., Deliza, R., dos Santos, K. M. O., Walter, E. H. M., Martins, J. M., & Rosenthal, A. (2018). Viability of probiotics in goat cheese during storage and under simulated gastrointestinal conditions. *Food and Bioprocess Technology*, *11*(4), 853–863. Available from https://doi.org/10.1007/s11947-018-2060-2.

Misra, S., Mohanty, D., & Mohapatra, S. J. (2019). Applications of probiotics as a functional ingredient in food and gut health. *Journal of Food and Nutrition Research*, *7*, 213–223.

Moens, F., Van den Abbeele, P., Basit, A. W., Dodoo, C., Chatterjee, R., Smith, B., & Gaisford, S. (2019). A four-strain probiotic exerts positive immunomodulatory effects by enhancing colonic butyrate production in vitro. *International Journal of Pharmaceutics*, *555*, 1–10. Available from https://doi.org/10.1016/j.ijpharm.2018.11.020.

Mohammadsadeghi, F., Afsharmanesh, M., & Ebrahimnejad, H. (2019). The substitution of humic material complex with mineral premix in diet and interaction of that with probiotic on performance, intestinal morphology and microflora of chickens. *Livestock Science*, *228*, 1–4. Available from https://doi.org/10.1016/j.livsci.2019.07.010.

Mouhamed, A. E., Hassan, A. A., Hassan, M. A., El Hariri, M., & Refai, M. K. (2015). Effect of metal nanoparticles on the growth of ochratoxigenic moulds and ochratoxin a production isolated from food and feed. *International Journal of Reseaech Studies in Biosciences*, *3*(9), 1–14.

Mousavi Khaneghah, A., Abhari, K., Eş, I., Soares, M. B., Oliveira, R. B. A., Hosseini, H., Rezaei, M., Balthazar, C. F., Silva, R., Cruz, A. G., Ranadheera, C. S., & Sant'Ana, A. S. (2020). Interactions between probiotics and pathogenic microorganisms in hosts and foods: A review. *Trends in Food Science and Technology*, *95*, 205–218. Available from https://doi.org/10.1016/j.tifs.2019.11.022.

Muniesa, M., Hammerl, J. A., Hertwig, S., Appel, B., & Brüssow, H. (2012). Shiga toxin-producing Escherichia coli O104:H4: A new challenge for microbiology. *Applied and Environmental Microbiology*, *78*(12), 4065–4073. Available from https://doi.org/10.1128/AEM.00217-12.

Murate, L. S., Paião, F. G., de Almeida, A. M., Berchieri, A., & Shimokomaki, M. (2015). Efficacy of prebiotics, probiotics, and synbiotics on laying hens and broilers challenged with Salmonella enteritidis. *Journal of Poultry Science*, *52*(1), 53–56. Available from https://doi.org/10.2141/jpsa.0130211.

Mushtaq, M., Gani, A., & Masoodi, F. A. (2019). Himalayan cheese (Kalari/Kradi) fermented with different probiotic strains: In vitro investigation of nutraceutical properties. *LWT*, *104*, 53–60. Available from https://doi.org/10.1016/j.lwt.2019.01.024.

Nabawy, G. A., Hassan, A. A., Sayed-ElAhl, R. H., & Refai, M. K. (2014). Effect of metal nanoparticles in comparison with commericial antifungal feed additives on the growth of Aspergillus flavus and aflatoxin B1 production. *Journal of Global Biosciences*, *3*(6), 954–971.

Nagata, S., Asahara, T., Ohta, T., Yamada, T., Kondo, S., Bian, L., Wang, C., Yamashiro, Y., & Nomoto, K. (2011). Effect of the continuous intake of probiotic-fermented milk containing Lactobacillus casei strain Shirota on fever in a mass outbreak of norovirus gastroenteritis and the faecal microflora in a health service facility for the aged. *British Journal of Nutrition*, *106*(4), 549–556. Available from https://doi.org/10.1017/S000711451100064X.

Nami, Y., Bakhshayesh, R. V., Jalaly, H. M., Lotfi, H., Eslami, S., & Hejazi, M. A. (2019). Probiotic properties of Enterococcus isolated from artisanal dairy products. *Frontiers in Microbiology*, 10. Available from https://doi.org/10.3389/fmicb.2019.00300.

Neal-McKinney, J. M., Lu, X., Duong, T., Larson, C. L., Call, D. R., Shah, D. H., & Konkel, M. E. (2012). Production of organic acids by probiotic Lactobacilli can be used to reduce pathogen load in poultry. *PLoS One*, *7*(9). Available from https://doi.org/10.1371/journal.pone.0043928.

Ningtyas, D. W., Bhandari, B., Bansal, N., & Prakash, S. (2019). The viability of probiotic Lactobacillus rhamnosus (non-encapsulated and encapsulated) in functional reduced-fat cream cheese and its textural properties during storage. *Food Control*, *100*, 8–16. Available from https://doi.org/10.1016/j.foodcont.2018.12.048.

Nishiyama, K., Seto, Y., Yoshioka, K., Kakuda, T., Takai, S., Yamamoto, Y., & Mukai, T. (2014). Lactobacillus gasseri sbt2055 reduces infection by and colonization of campylobacter jejuni. *PLoS One*, *9*(9). Available from https://doi.org/10.1371/journal.pone.0108827.

O'Hara, A. M., & Shanahan, F. (2007). Gut microbiota: Mining for therapeutic potential. *Clinical Gastroenterology and Hepatology*, *5*(3), 274–284. Available from https://doi.org/10.1016/j.cgh.2006.12.009.

Pacheco, A. R., & Sperandio, V. (2012). Shiga toxin in enterohemorrhagic E. coli: Regulation and novel anti-virulence strategies. *Frontiers in Cellular and Infection Microbiology*, *2*, 81. Available from https://doi.org/10.3389/fcimb.2012.00081.

Pahumunto, N., Sophatha, B., Piwat, S., & Teanpaisan, R. (2019). Increasing salivary IgA and reducing Streptococcus mutans by probiotic Lactobacillus paracasei SD1: A double-blind, randomized, controlled study. *Journal of Dental Sciences*, *14*(2), 178–184. Available from https://doi.org/10.1016/j.jds.2019.01.008.

Papadopoulou, O. S., Argyri, A. A., Varzakis, E., Sidira, M., Kourkoutas, Y., Galanis, A., Tassou, C., & Chorianopoulos, N. G. (2019). Use of lactobacilli strains with probiotic potential in traditional fermented milk and their impact on quality and safety related to Listeria monocytogenes. *International Dairy Journal*, *98*, 44–53. Available from https://doi.org/10.1016/j.idairyj.2019.06.006.

Peng, M., & Biswas, D. (2017). Short chain and polyunsaturated fatty acids in host gut health and foodborne bacterial pathogen inhibition. *Critical Reviews in Food Science and Nutrition*, *57*(18), 3987–4002. Available from https://doi.org/10.1080/10408398.2016.1203286.

Piewngam, P., & Otto, M. (2020). Probiotics to prevent Staphylococcus aureus disease? *Gut Microbes*, *11*(1), 94–101. Available from https://doi.org/10.1080/19490976.2019.1591137.

Plaza-Diaz, J., Ruiz-Ojeda, F. J., Gil-Campos, M., & Gil, A. (2019). Mechanisms of action of probiotics. *Advances in Nutrition*, *10*, S49–S66. Available from https://doi.org/10.1093/advances/nmy063.

Plaza-Díaz, J., Ruiz-Ojeda, F. J., Vilchez-Padial, L. M., & Gil, A. (2017). Evidence of the anti-inflammatory effects of probiotics and symbiotic in intestinal chronic diseases. *Nutrients*, *9*(6).

Puertollano, E., Puertollano, M. A., Cruz-Chamorro, L., de Cienfuegos, G. A., Ruiz-Bravo, A., & de Pablo, M. A. (2008). Orally administered Lactobacillus plantarum reduces pro-inflammatory interleukin secretion in sera from Listeria monocytogenes infected mice. *British Journal of Nutrition*, *99*(4), 819–825. Available from https://doi.org/10.1017/S0007114507832533.

Raja, S. (2017). *Evaluation of potential antioxidant probiotics in vitro models of the gut epithelium* (Doctoral dissertation). Harvard Medical School, United States.

Ranadheera, C. S., Vidanarachchi, J. K., Rocha, R. S., Cruz, A. G., & Ajlouni, S. (2017). Probiotic delivery through fermentation: Dairy vs. non-dairy beverages. *Fermentation*, *3*(4). Available from https://doi.org/10.3390/fermentation3040067.

Rea, M. C., Dobson, A., O'Sullivan, O., Crispie, F., Fouhy, F., Cotter, P. D., Shanahan, F., Kiely, B., Hill, C., & Ross, R. P. (2011). Effect of broad- and narrow-spectrum antimicrobials on Clostridium difficile and microbial diversity in a model of the distal colon. *Proceedings of the National Academy of Sciences of the United States of America*, *108*, 4639–4644. Available from https://doi.org/10.1073/pnas.1001224107.

Reale, A., Di Renzo, T., & Coppola, R. (2019). Factors affecting viability of selected probiotics during cheese-making of pasta filata dairy products obtained by direct-to-vat inoculation system. *LWT*, 116. Available from https://doi.org/10.1016/j.lwt.2019.108476.

Reissig Soares Vitola, H., da Silva Dannenberg, G., de Lima Marques, J., Völz Lopes, G., Padilha da Silva, W., & Fiorentini, Â. M. (2018). Probiotic potential of Lactobacillus casei CSL3 isolated from bovine colostrum silage and its viability capacity immobilized in soybean. *Process Biochemistry*, *75*, 22–30. Available from https://doi.org/10.1016/j.procbio.2018.09.011.

Ribet, D., & Cossart, P. (2015). How bacterial pathogens colonize their hosts and invade deeper tissues. *Microbes and Infection*, *17*(3), 173–183. Available from https://doi.org/10.1016/j.micinf.2015.01.004.

Rodrigues, V. C. d C., Silva, L. G. S. d, Simabuco, F. M., Venema, K., & Antunes, A. E. C. (2019). Survival, metabolic status and cellular morphology of probiotics in dairy products and dietary supplement after simulated digestion. *Journal of Functional Foods*, *55*, 126–134. Available from https://doi.org/10.1016/j.jff.2019.01.046.

Rodríguez-Lázaro, D., Cook, N., Ruggeri, F. M., Sellwood, J., Nasser, A., Nascimento, M. S. J., D'Agostino, M., Santos, R., Saiz, J. C., Rzezutka, A., Bosch, A., Gironés, R., Carducci, A., Muscillo, M., Kovač, K., Diez-Valcarce, M., Vantarakis, A., von Bonsdorff, C. H., de Roda Husman, A. M., & van der Poel, W. H. M. (2012). Virus hazards from food, water and other contaminated environments. *FEMS Microbiology Reviews*, *36*(4), 786–814. Available from https://doi.org/10.1111/j.1574-6976.2011.00306.x.

Rokana, N., Mallappa, R. H., Batish, V. K., & Grover, S. (2017). Interaction between putative probiotic Lactobacillus strains of Indian gut origin and Salmonella: Impact on intestinal barrier function. *LWT—Food Science and Technology*, *84*, 851–860. Available from https://doi.org/10.1016/j.lwt.2016.08.021.

Rokka, S., & Rantamäki, P. (2010). Protecting probiotic bacteria by microencapsulation: Challenges for industrial applications. *European Food Research and Technology*, *231*(1), 1–12. Available from https://doi.org/10.1007/s00217-010-1246-2.

Roobab, U., Batool, Z., Manzoor, M. F., Shabbir, M. A., Khan, M. R., & Aadil, R. M. (2020). Sources, formulations, advanced delivery and health benefits of probiotics. *Current Opinion in Food Science*, *32*, 17–28. Available from https://doi.org/10.1016/j.cofs.2020.01.003.

Rubio-del-Campo, A., Coll-Marqués, J. M., Yebra, M. J., Buesa, J., Pérez-Martínez, G., Monedero, V., & Rodríguez-Díaz, J. (2014). Noroviral P-particles as an in vitro model to assess the interactions of noroviruses with probiotics. *PLoS One*, *9*(2). Available from https://doi.org/10.1371/journal.pone.0089586.

Ryan, V., & Bhunia, A. K. (2017). *Mitigation of foodborne illnesses by probiotics* (pp. 603–634). Springer Science and Business Media LLC. Available from https://doi.org/10.1007/978-3-319-56836-2_21.

Saha, R. (2017). *A study of the effects of diet on human gut microbial community structure and mercury metabolism* (Doctoral dissertation).

Samedi, L., & Charles, A. L. (2019). Isolation and characterization of potential probiotic Lactobacilli from leaves of food plants for possible additives in pellet feeding. *Annals of Agricultural Sciences*, *64*(1), 55–62. Available from https://doi.org/10.1016/j.aoas.2019.05.004.

Sampaolesi, S., Gamba, R. R., De Antoni, G. L., & Leon, A. (2019). Potentiality of yeasts obtained as beer fermentation residue to be used as probiotics. *LWT—Food Science and Technology*, *113*(2). Available from https://doi.org/10.1016/j.lwt.2019.108251.

Santos, E., Andrade, R., & Gouveia, E. (2017). Utilization of the pectin and pulp of the passion fruit from Caatinga as probiotic food carriers. *Food Bioscience*, *20*, 56–61. Available from https://doi.org/10.1016/j.fbio.2017.08.005.

Shakibaie, M., Mohammadi-Khorsand, T., Mahboubeh, a-s, & Jafari, M. (2016). Probiotic and antioxidant properties of selenium-enriched Lactobacillus brevis LSe isolated from an Iranian traditional dairy product. *Journal of Trace Elements in Medicine and Biology*, *40*. Available from https://doi.org/10.1016/j.jtemb.2016.11.013.

Shi, N., Li, N., Duan, X., & Niu, H. (2017). Interaction between the gut microbiome and mucosal immune system. *Military Medical Research*, *4*(1). Available from https://doi.org/10.1186/s40779-017-0122-9.

Singh, P., Medronho, B., Alves, L., da Silva, G. J., Miguel, M. G., & Lindman, B. (2017). Development of carboxymethyl cellulose-chitosan hybrid micro- and macroparticles for encapsulation of probiotic bacteria. *Carbohydrate Polymers*, *175*, 87–95. Available from https://doi.org/10.1016/j.carbpol.2017.06.119.

Smith, J. L., & Fratamico, P. M. (2018). Emerging and re-emerging foodborne pathogens. *Foodborne Pathogens and Disease*, *15*(12), 737–757. Available from https://doi.org/10.1089/fpd.2018.2493.

Soares, M. B., Martinez, R. C., Pereira, E. P., Balthazar, C. F., Cruz, A. G., Ranadheera, C. S., & Sant'Ana, A. S. (2019). The resistance of Bacillus, Bifidobacterium, and Lactobacillus strains with claimed probiotic properties in different food matrices exposed to simulated gastrointestinal tract conditions. *Food Research International*, *125*.

Son, S. H., Yang, S. J., Jeon, H. L., Yu, H. S., Lee, N. K., Park, Y. S., & Paik, H. D. (2018). Antioxidant and immunostimulatory effect of potential probiotic Lactobacillus paraplantarum SC61 isolated from Korean traditional fermented food, jangajji. *Microbial Pathogenesis*, *125*, 486–492. Available from https://doi.org/10.1016/j.micpath.2018.10.018.

Sonnenburg, J. L., & Bäckhed, F. (2016). Diet-microbiota interactions as moderators of human metabolism. *Nature*, *535*(7610), 56–64. Available from https://doi.org/10.1038/nature18846.

Sugrue, I., Tobin, C., Ross, R. P., Stanton, C., & Hill, C. (2019). *Foodborne pathogens and zoonotic diseases* (pp. 259–272). Elsevier BV. Available from https://doi.org/10.1016/b978-0-12-810530-6.00012-2.

Sun, Y., Wilkinson, B. J., Standiford, T. J., Akinbi, H. T., & O'Riordan, M. X. D. (2012). Fatty acids regulate stress resistance and virulence factor production for Listeria monocytogenes. *Journal of Bacteriology*, *194*(19), 5274–5284. Available from https://doi.org/10.1128/JB.00045-12.

Swaminathan, B., & Gerner-Smidt, P. (2007). The epidemiology of human listeriosis. *Microbes and Infection*, *9*(10), 1236–1243. Available from https://doi.org/10.1016/j.micinf.2007.05.011.

Tareb, R., Bernardeau, M., Gueguen, M., & Vernoux, J. P. (2013). In vitro characterization of aggregation and adhesion properties of viable and heat-killed forms of two probiotic Lactobacillus strains and interaction with foodborne zoonotic bacteria, especially Campylobacter jejuni. *Journal of Medical Microbiology*, *62*(4), 637–649. Available from https://doi.org/10.1099/jmm.0.049965-0.

Terpou, A., Papadaki, A., Bosnea, L., Kanellaki, M., & Kopsahelis, N. (2019). Novel frozen yogurt production fortified with sea buckthorn berries and probiotics. *LWT*, *105*, 242–249. Available from https://doi.org/10.1016/j.lwt.2019.02.024.

Thomas, C. M., & Versalovic, J. (2010). Probiotics-host communication: Modulation of signaling pathways in the intestine. *Gut Microbes*, *1*(3), 148–163.

Tsai, Y. T., Cheng, P. C., & Pan, T. M. (2010). Immunomodulating activity of lactobacillus paracasei subsp. paracasei NTU 101 in enterohemorrhagic escherichia coli O157H7-infected mice. *Journal of Agricultural and Food Chemistry*, *58*(21), 11265–11272. Available from https://doi.org/10.1021/jf103011z.

Valdovinos-García, L. R., Abreu, A. T., & Valdovinos-Díaz, M. A. (2019). Probiotic use in clinical practice: Results of a national survey of gastroenterologists and nutritionists. *Revista de Gastroenterología de México (English Edition)*, 303–309. Available from https://doi.org/10.1016/j.rgmxen.2018.10.001.

Valeriano, V. D., Parungao-Balolong, M. M., & Kang, D. K. (2014). In vitro evaluation of the mucin-adhesion ability and probiotic potential of Lactobacillus mucosae LM1. *Journal of Applied Microbiology*, *117*(2), 485–497. Available from https://doi.org/10.1111/jam.12539.

Van Coillie, E., Goris, J., Cleenwerck, I., Grijspeerdt, K., Botteldoorn, N., Van Immerseel, F., De Buck, J., Vancanneyt, M., Swings, J., Herman, L., & Heyndrickx, M. (2007). Identification of lactobacilli isolated from the cloaca and vagina of laying hens and characterization for potential use as probiotics to control Salmonella Enteritidis. *Journal of Applied Microbiology*, *102*(4), 1095–1106. Available from https://doi.org/10.1111/j.1365-2672.2006.03164.x.

Vandeplas, S., Dubois Dauphin, R., Beckers, Y., Thonart, P., & Théwis, A. (2010). Salmonella in chicken: Current and developing strategies to reduce contamination at farm level. *Journal of Food Protection, 73*(4), 774–785. Available from https://doi.org/10.4315/0362-028X-73.4.774.

Verdu, E. F., Galipeau, H. J., & Jabri, B. (2015). Novel players in coeliac disease pathogenesis: Role of the gut microbiota. *Nature Reviews Gastroenterology and Hepatology, 12*(9), 497–506. Available from https://doi.org/10.1038/nrgastro.2015.90.

Voetsch, A. C., Angulo, F. J., Jones, T. F., Moore, M. R., Nadon, C., McCarthy, P., Shiferaw, B., Megginson, M. B., Hurd, S., Anderson, B. J., & Cronquist, A. (1996). Centers for Disease Control and Prevention Emerging Infections Program Foodborne Diseases Active Surveillance Network Working Group. Reduction in the incidence of invasive listeriosis in foodborne diseases active surveillance network sites. *Clinical Infectious Diseases, 44*(4), 513–520.

Volzing, K., Borrero, J., Sadowsky, M. J., & Kaznessis, Y. N. (2013). Antimicrobial peptides targeting gram-negative pathogens, produced and delivered by lactic acid bacteria. *ACS Synthetic Biology, 2*(11), 643–650. Available from https://doi.org/10.1021/sb4000367.

Wagner, R. D., Johnson, S. J., & Rubin, D. K. (2009). Probiotic bacteria are antagonistic to Salmonella enterica and Campylobacter jejuni and influence host lymphocyte responses in human microbiota-associated immunodeficient and immunocompetent mice. *Molecular Nutrition and Food Research, 53*(3), 377–388. Available from https://doi.org/10.1002/mnfr.200800101.

Wan, M., Forsythe, S., & El-Nezami, H. (2019). Probiotics interaction with foodborne pathogens: A potential alternative to antibiotics and future challenges. *Critical Reviews in Food Science and Nutrition, 59*(20), 3320–3333. Available from https://doi.org/10.1080/10408398.2018.1490885.

Wine, E., Gareau, M. G., Johnson-Henry, K., & Sherman, P. M. (2009). Strain-specific probiotic (Lactobacillus helveticus) inhibition of Campylobacter jejuni invasion of human intestinal epithelial cells. *FEMS Microbiology Letters, 300*(1), 146–152. Available from https://doi.org/10.1111/j.1574-6968.2009.01781.x.

World Health Organization. (2015). *WHO estimates of the global burden of foodborne diseases: Foodborne disease burden epidemiology reference group 2007–2015*. World Health Organization. Available from https://apps.who.int/iris/handle/10665/199350.

Wu, L., Qin, W., He, Y., Zhu, W., Ren, X., York, P., Xiao, T., Yin, X., & Zhang, J. (2018). Material distributions and functional structures in probiotic microcapsules. *European Journal of Pharmaceutical Sciences, 122*, 1–8. Available from https://doi.org/10.1016/j.ejps.2018.06.013.

Xavier, R. J., & Podolsky, D. K. (2007). Unravelling the pathogenesis of inflammatory bowel disease. *Nature, 448*(7152), 427–434. Available from https://doi.org/10.1038/nature06005.

Yadav, D., & Srikanth, K. (2018). *Flavors in probiotics and prebiotics. Flavors for nutraceutical and functional foods* (pp. 51–74).

Yao, M., Li, B., Ye, H., Huang, W., Luo, Q., Xiao, H., McClements, D. J., & Li, L. (2018). Enhanced viability of probiotics (Pediococcus pentosaceus Li05) by encapsulation in microgels doped with inorganic nanoparticles. *Food Hydrocolloids, 83*, 246–252. Available from https://doi.org/10.1016/j.foodhyd.2018.05.024.

Young, K. T., Davis, L. M., & DiRita, V. J. (2007). Campylobacter jejuni: Molecular biology and pathogenesis. *Nature Reviews Microbiology, 5*(9), 665–679. Available from https://doi.org/10.1038/nrmicro1718.

Chapter 26

Role of probiotics in the management of respiratory infections

Cristina Méndez-Malagón[1], Alejandro Egea-Zorrilla[2], Pedro Perez-Ferrer[3] and Julio Plaza-Diaz[4]

[1]Center of Biomedical Research, University of Granada, Granada, Spain, [2]Laboratory of Cardiovascular Development and Disease, Andalusian Centre for Nanomedicine and Biotechnology (Bionand), Technological Park of Andalusia C/ Severo Ochoa, Málaga, Spain, [3]Department of Molecular and Cell Biology, School of Natural Sciences, University of California, Merced, Merced, CA, United States, [4]Children's Hospital of Eastern Ontario Research Institute, Ottawa, ON, Canada

26.1 Introduction

The lung is the internal organ most vulnerable to infection and injury from the external environment because of its constant exposure to particles, chemicals, and infectious organisms in ambient air. One of the most important systems of our body is the respiratory tract, a complex organ responsible for the exchange of oxygen and carbon dioxide. Globally, at least 2 billion people are exposed to the toxic smoke of biomass fuel, typically burned inefficiently in poorly ventilated indoor stoves or fireplaces. One billion people inhale polluted outdoor air, and 1 billion are exposed to tobacco smoke. Although respiratory impairment causes disability and death in all regions of the world and all social classes, poverty, crowding, environmental exposures, and generally poor living conditions increase vulnerability to this large group of disorders (Wang, Naghavi, et al., 2016).

Respiratory diseases are a group of pathologies that affects the respiratory tract. There is a wide range of respiratory diseases, from acute respiratory infections, such as pneumonia and bronchitis, to chronic diseases, such as asthma and chronic obstructive pulmonary disease. Among these diseases, respiratory tract infections (RTIs) are defined as any infectious disease that affects the upper or lower respiratory tract. RTIs represent one of the main health problems in children. Upper respiratory tract infections (URTIs) are the common cold, laryngitis, pharyngitis, acute rhinitis, acute rhinosinusitis, and otitis media. On the other hand, lower respiratory tract infections (LRTIs) are acute bronchitis, bronchiolitis, pneumonia, and tracheitis (Velilla et al., 2007). Symptoms of an RTI include, a cough—mucus (phlegm), sneezing, a stuffy or runny nose, a sore throat, headaches, muscle aches, breathlessness, tight chest or wheezing, a high temperature (fever), and feeling generally unwell (Velilla et al., 2007).

An estimated 65 million people have moderate-to-severe chronic obstructive pulmonary disease, from which about 3 million die each year, making it the third leading cause of death worldwide—and the numbers are increasing (Burney et al., 2015; Cruz, 2007). About 334 million people suffer from asthma (Asher et al., 2017), which is the most common chronic disease of childhood, affecting 14% of children globally. The prevalence of asthma in children is rising (Pearce et al., 2007). Acute lower RTIs have been among the top three causes of death and disability among both children and adults. Although the burden is difficult to quantify, it is estimated that LRTIs cause nearly 4 million deaths annually and is a leading cause of death among children under 5 years old (WHO & UNICEF, 2006). Moreover, acute LRTIs in children predisposed to chronic respiratory diseases later in life. RTIs caused by influenza kill between 250,000 and 500,000 people and cost between US$71 and 167 billion annually (Nguyen et al., 2016). A total of 10.4 million people developed tuberculosis and 1.4 million people died from it (World Health Organization, 2013).

The most common lethal neoplasm in the world is lung cancer, which kills 1.6 million people each year (Torre et al., 2015); and the numbers are growing. In addition to these five, there are several respiratory disorders whose burden is great but less well quantified. More than 100 million people suffer from sleep-disordered breathing (Cruz, 2007). Million of people live with pulmonary hypertension (Cruz, 2007). More than 50 million people struggle with occupational lung diseases. Respiratory diseases account for more than 10% of all disability-adjusted life-years, a metric that estimates the amount of active and productive life lost due to a condition. Respiratory diseases are second only to cardiovascular diseases (including stroke) (Fitzmaurice et al., 2017). The objective of the present chapter is to comprehend the RTIs, the different types of pathologies, treatments with special emphasis on the effects of probiotic administration, and finally, the current investigation in this field.

26.2 Respiratory tract infections

RTIs can be classified based on their location and etiology. In terms of location, we can differentiate two types of respiratory infections, those that affect the upper respiratory tract (nasopharynx, oropharynx, larynx, trachea, ear and paranasal sinuses), or those that affect the lower one (trachea, lung, bronchi, bronchioles). Furthermore, depending on the etiology of the infection, we can classify the RTIs into bacterial, viral, fungal, and parasitic, depending on which the infectious agent is responsible for the disease (Velilla et al., 2007). RTIs are among the leading causes of death worldwide, assuming a high health burden. Lower respiratory infections alone cause about 4 million deaths a year (Swedberg et al., 2020). RTIs have also a significant economic impact among countries (Ehlken et al., 2005; Lambert et al., 2008). The pediatric population is the most affected by these diseases, as they are the most common diseases in children around the world (Black et al., 2010), being the main cause of death in children under 5 years of age. Apart from this, they are the main reason for prescribing antibiotics in children (van der Gaag & Hummel, 2020). RTIs are also among the more usual causes for parental concern and medical visits in preschool and elementary school children, resulting in school absenteeism and hospitalizations (Massin et al., 2006; Nicholson et al., 2006).

Common colds are the most prevalent entity of all respiratory infections and are the leading cause of patient visits to the physician, as well as work and school absenteeism. Most colds are caused by viruses. Rhinoviruses with more than 100 serotypes are the most common pathogens, causing at least 25% of colds in adults. Coronaviruses may be responsible for more than 10% of the cases. Parainfluenza viruses, respiratory syncytial virus, adenoviruses, and influenza viruses have been linked to the common cold syndrome. All of these organisms show seasonal variations in incidence. The cause of 30%–40% of cold syndromes has not been yet determined (Dasaraju & Liu, 1996). After an incubation period of 48–72 h, classic symptoms of nasal discharge and obstruction, sneezing, sore throat, and cough occur in both adults and children. Myalgia and headache may also be present. Fever is rare. The duration of symptoms and viral shedding varies with the pathogen and the age of the patient. Complications are usually rare, but sinusitis and otitis media may follow (Dasaraju & Liu, 1996).

Infections of the lower respiratory tract include bronchitis, bronchiolitis, and pneumonia. These syndromes, especially pneumonia, can be severe or fatal. Although viruses, mycoplasma, rickettsiae, and fungi can all cause LRTIs, bacteria are the dominant pathogens; accounting for a much higher percentage of LRTIs than of URTIs. Bronchitis and bronchiolitis involve inflammation of the bronchial tree. Bronchitis is usually preceded by an URTIs or forms part of a clinical syndrome in diseases, such as influenza, rubeola, rubella, pertussis, scarlet fever, and typhoid fever. Chronic bronchitis with a persistent cough and sputum production appears to be caused by a combination of environmental factors, such as smoking, and bacterial infection with pathogens, such as *H. influenzae* and *S. pneumoniae*. Bronchiolitis is a viral respiratory disease of infants and is caused primarily by respiratory syncytial virus. Other viruses, including parainfluenza viruses, influenza viruses, and adenoviruses (as well as occasionally *M. pneumoniae*), are also known to cause bronchiolitis (Dasaraju & Liu, 1996).

26.2.1 Treatment

Most acute respiratory infections are self-limited. However, there is currently an excessive and inappropriate use of antimicrobials, which has led to an increase in bacterial resistance to these drugs. As a result, antibiotics are losing their effectiveness. It is important to note that antibiotics are not effective against viral infections. Furthermore, the use of antibiotics can disturb the fitness of human microbiota, making easier pathogen colonization and reducing the availability of vaccines for viruses (Andrews et al., 2012; Lange et al., 2016). Besides, we must remember that the great majority of respiratory infections are caused by viral agents, whose evolution is faster every day. This means that they are agents capable of crossing barriers between species, such as the influenza A virus and coronavirus. Such evolution has been so great that they have caused epidemics and pandemics throughout history, thus being associated with more severe clinical diseases and with a higher mortality rate (Mahooti et al., 2020). Other therapies could be hydration (oral or intravenous), oxygen therapy, and/or bronchodilator treatments, additional nursing supervision for symptom assessment and management (vital sign monitoring, lab/diagnostic test coordination, and reporting).

The coronavirus disease (Covid-19) caused by severe acute respiratory syndrome coronavirus 2 (SARS-CoV-2) is currently a World Public Health Emergency. This viral agent causes RTIs and is associated with pneumonia (Mahooti et al., 2020). For all the above, we must ensure the protection of the respiratory tract against infections and, for this, the development of new therapeutic strategies is necessary.

26.3 In search of new therapeutic strategies: microbiota and gut-lung axis

The microbiota is the "set of microorganisms that inhabit our body." This community is made up of bacteria, viruses, fungi, and protozoa. Many organs and tissues of our body coexist with these microbial ecosystems (e.g., gastrointestinal, genitourinary, and respiratory tracts, or the oral and nasopharyngeal cavity). There is continuously an interaction between the microbiota and the host, which must be kept in balance. However, this balance is susceptible to becoming unbalanced as it depends on many factors, both intrinsic and environmental. These factors are genetics, use of antibiotics, diet, presence of infectious agents, allergens, etc. All of them can alter the microbiota, allowing a state of imbalance or "dysbiosis" (Levy et al., 2017). Because of that dysbiosis, diseases can be aggravated or make the host more susceptible to other types of disorders.

Many organs and tissues of our body coexist with these microorganisms. However, the organ whose microbiota role is best studied is the intestine. The gut microbiota is the largest and most diverse of the human microbiome (Brestoff & Artis, 2013) and plays an important role in the maintenance of homeostasis, as well as in the modulation of the immune system among other things. Despite the gut is the best-studied organ in terms of microbiota, the lung has been an object of study in last years, and even more recently due to the Covid-19 pandemic. Years ago, it was thought that the lungs were sterile organs, in which commensal microorganisms did not coexist. However, metagenomic studies have revealed that commensal microorganisms do exist in the lungs, allowing us to study their abundance and composition (Dumas et al., 2018).

In this way, there are pathological conditions in which an alteration in the pulmonary microbiota exists, such as chronic obstructive pulmonary disease, cystic fibrosis, and asthma (Hilty et al., 2010; Pragman et al., 2012; Willner et al., 2012). The pulmonary microbial community, described only a few years ago, forms a discreet part of the human host microbiota. The airway microbiota is substantially altered in the context of numerous respiratory disorders; nonetheless, its role in health and disease is as yet only poorly understood (Dumas et al., 2018). This indicates that the lung microbiota influences the optimal and/or pathological lung status.

Also, it exists a possible relationship between the intestinal microbiota and lung immunity, which is called the "gut–lung axis." This axis allows crosstalk between both organs, the gut and lung, which are distally located. Thus endotoxins, microbial metabolites, cytokines, and hormones can be released from the intestinal niche, passing into the lymphatic and/or bloodstream, and finally reaching the lung, affecting the lung niche (Fig. 26.1). In the same way, this

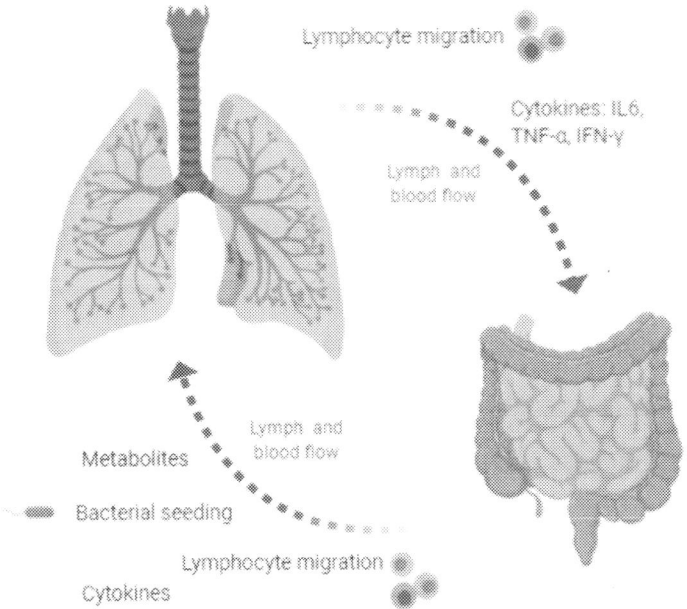

FIGURE 26.1 Intestinal-pulmonary crosstalk. A bidirectional crosstalk between these two microbiota compartments has been proposed. The intestinal microbiota influences pulmonary microbial composition and immune responses.

crosstalk can occur in the opposite direction, that is, from the lung to the gut. For example, when there is an inflammation in the lung, the lung–gut axis can induce changes in the gut microbiota (Zhang et al., 2020).

26.4 Pulmonary microbiota in diseases

Historically, the lower respiratory tract was considered to be sterile. However, recent studies identified a lung microbiome and there are reports that this is altered in patients with idiopathic pulmonary fibrosis (Bordon, 2019). The lungs are inhabited by microbial populations whose species are different from those that inhabit the intestine (Man et al., 2017). In addition, the lung microbiota is variable and different from the microbiota in other parts of the body, as confirmed by studies in mice. There are alterations in the lung and intestinal microbiota (dysbiosis) in many respiratory diseases. However, it is not yet known whether this dysbiosis is a cause or consequence of the disease.

On the other hand, we know that the gut microbiota can play an important role in the immunity of the lungs. However, to date, we do not know the contribution of the pulmonary microbiota to host immunity (Dumas et al., 2018).

26.4.1 Role of microbiota during respiratory disorders

The microbiota of the respiratory tract has been extensively studied in patients with chronic respiratory diseases of infectious origin, such as tuberculosis. However, the study of acute respiratory infections, such as pneumonia, has not been as extensive, probably due to their short duration (Dumas et al., 2018). Although studies in humans are limited, in germ-free mice (lacking microbiota) commensal microorganisms have been shown to play an important role in coping with acute respiratory infections. In this way, a dysbiosis can alter that response to infection, which can be harmful to the individual (Dumas et al., 2018).

Authors intranasally inoculated microbiota-depleted mice with different bacterial species before bleomycin challenge and identified three *Bacteroidetes* species—*B. ovatus*, *B. stercoris*, and *Prevotella melaninogenica*—that markedly increased lung fibrosis and mouse mortality. All of these species were expanded in the lungs of wild-type mice following bleomycin treatment; the authors linked this to an increase in host metabolites that support bacterial growth in the bleomycin-damaged lung. The three *Bacteroidetes* species did not induce the expression of interleukin (IL)-17 family cytokines in the lungs of resting mice but were found to induce IL-17B and IL-17A following bleomycin treatment (Bordon, 2019).

Dysbiosis is defined as the alteration in the composition and function of the microbiota of an organism. This can be caused by a wide variety of factors (environmental, genetic and/or pathological). Due to this dysbiosis, there is an alteration in the level and/or activation of the cells of the immune system, such as leukocytes. This alteration may lead to lung damage. We are only just beginning to understand the functional implications of lung microbiota in health and disease. It is clear that a much greater research effort needs to be dedicated to uncovering how the lung microbiota interacts and collaborates (or antagonizes) with the now increasingly well-studied gut microbiota (Dumas et al., 2018).

26.5 History of probiotics

Several medical and popular sources indicate that the first use of probiotics in human history dates back to 2000 BCE, when man first discovered how milk could be preserved for longer periods. Moreover, the first food-makers, although unaware of their existence, used bacteria and yeasts to transform milk into fermented dairy products (Hosono, 1992). However, it was in 2011 when Sicard and Legrad clarified that it was much earlier than 2000 BCE that our ancestors were already producing beverages using yeasts (Sicard & Legras, 2011). In fact, from an analysis performed by archeologists, we can say that microorganisms were already being used in the production of fermented beverages back in 7000 BCE (Zhang et al., 1999).

As said above, the use of probiotics is not recent, and the knowledge of an existing microbiota linked with health and disease was also known a long time ago. Many different nations were aware of the healthy outcomes elicited by the ingestion of milk and its derived products, like the Romans, being in 76 BCE, when the historian Plinio recommended the intake of milk products to treat various digestive problems (Ozen & Dinleyici, 2015). More recently, at the beginning of the 20th century, the pediatrician Henry Tissier observed a larger number of bacteria with Y-shaped morphology that was present in healthy children when compared with children with diarrhea (Tissier, 1906).

Some years later the microbiologist Ilja Metchnikoff suggested that the longevity of Bulgarians was due to the consumption of fermented milk products (Metchnikoff & Chalmers-Mitchell, 1908). Furthermore, during World War I, Professor Alfred Nissle isolated a special *Escherichia coli* strain from the stool of a war participant that remained completely healthy, as opposed to most of his comrades, who contracted different diseases like dysentery or typhoid fever (Sonnenborn & Schulze, 2009). However, it was not until 1965 when the term "probiotic" itself was introduced by Lilly and Stillwell, who described it as a microbial substance that is produced by one microorganism and has a growth-promoting effect on another microorganism, thus being the opposite of how antibiotics work (Lilly & Stillwell, 1965).

The first available probiotics were composed of just one species of microorganisms, being *Saccharomyces* or *Lactobacillus* the main genera used (Wieërs et al., 2020). However, subsequent forms of probiotics contained not only a larger number of microorganisms but also bacteria that belonged to other strains. These probiotics were developed mainly for their capacity to resist the low pH of the gastric, but this variety of microorganisms poses a great problem when it comes to assessing which strand is the one eliciting the possible beneficial changes in the patient (de Simone, 2019).

Nowadays, according to the World Health Organization and the Food and Agriculture Organization of the United Nations, probiotics are "live microorganisms which, when administered in adequate amounts, confer health and benefit on the host" (Food and Agriculture Organization of the United Nations, 2002). Synbiotics, which are primarily composed of prebiotics and probiotics, are defined as a kind of dietary intervention approach to targeting gut microbiota, which is now gaining growing attention (Chan et al., 2020).

26.6 Probiotic usage and safety

Probiotics, by definition, as mentioned above, are live microorganisms that, when administered in adequate amounts, confer a health benefit on the host (Hill et al., 2014). These live microorganisms are often present naturally on the human microbiota in healthy individuals; however, the composition of this can change both qualitatively and quantitatively depending on different factors, among which are the presence of a disease or disorder (Pascale et al., 2018). The main usage of probiotics is centered on acid bacteria, belonging to *Lactobacillus* spp. or *Bifidobacterium* spp. (Zheng et al., 2020).

These bacteria are known to be safe and suitable for human consumption since several studies have proven not only their efficacy but also their safety in both mice and humans and also in different ages, reporting just a few number of infections or adverse effects (Didari et al., 2014; Tapiovaara, Lehtoranta, et al., 2016).

Furthermore, some strains of other microbial genera, such as *Propionibacterium* spp. and *Bacillus* spp., are also used since their beneficial properties when administered as probiotics have been proven.

When it comes to probiotics safety in RTIs, the evidence obtained from meta-analyses and reviews gives the conclusion that the side effects upon probiotic consumption are minor (Hao et al., 2015; King et al., 2014).

In fact, probiotics are one of the most commonly consumed food supplements worldwide nowadays (Clarke et al., 2015) and are mostly consumed orally in the form of dietary supplements and food, so they are commercialized in different formats, among which are lyophilized pills and as supplements in various kinds of food such as yogurt, cheese, ice cream, nutrition bars, and infant formulas (Hoffmann et al., 2014), thus making the gastrointestinal tract their primary site of action (Pot et al., 2013). However, PCR-based methods in other parts of the body, such as the nasopharyngeal mucosa, adenoids and tonsils, have detected probiotics after oral consumption (Kumpu, Swanljung, et al., 2013; Lehtinen et al., 2018; Swanljung et al., 2015).

Probiotics play a role in balancing the host defensive immune response, thereby stimulating mucosal barrier function and modulating the immune system (El Hage et al., 2017). The small intestine is naturally exposed to microbes and nutrients because of the existence of a thin mucosal layer. This seems to play an important role in immune stimulation upon probiotics consumption since it has been shown that lymphocytes circulate between mucosal tissues, which gives us the idea that local mucosal stimulation on the lymphocytes may influence immune responses at other mucosal tissues and contribute to immunity in general (Brandtzaeg, 2009). Orally consumed probiotics are taken up by M cells or by CXCR3 + macrophages that are present in the gut epithelium; then, they are transferred to the dendritic cells (DCs) located in the subepithelial tissue, modulating DCs polarization and function (Christensen et al., 2002), which influence T- and B-cell responses in Peyer's patches and mesenteric lymph nodes (Fink et al., 2007); then, these activated lymphocytes can enter the circulation and migrate to other parts of the body, such as the respiratory tract (Baaten et al., 2013).

The fact that these ingested probiotics also stimulate the intestinal immune system makes it difficult to elucidate the contribution to URTIs' immune stimulation against RTIs (van Baarlen et al., 2013). However, probiotic components exert beneficial effects on immune responses, particularly on those that occur in both the upper and lower respiratory tract, that is, why its usage has increased in the past few years (Mahooti et al., 2020). In parallel, assessing the contributions of both small and large intestine and upper gastrointestinal tract on immune stimulation against RTIs is quite challenging with all the knowledge up to date.

Another important thing to take under consideration when assessing how probiotics exert their beneficial effects is that closely related bacteria have differences in their antigenic structures, which is important because this means that each strain may influence the immune system uniquely and thus elicit different responses depending on the strain (Hill et al., 2014). In other words, probiotics are thought to be able to alter the immune system in a strain-specific manner. However, they also share the mechanism of immune stimulation, for example, the secretion of metabolites like short-chain fatty acids (SCFAs), and in particular, butyrate, which have important immunomodulatory functions because it has been shown that they may signal through cell surface G-protein-coupled receptors (GPCRs), such as GPR41, GPR43, and GPR109A, to activate signaling cascades that control immune functions (Parada Venegas et al., 2019). The bacterial wall or the metabolites secreted can interact, through different receptors, like toll-like receptors, with the immune cells when these or the epithelial cells sample the digestive microenvironment, but it is important to know that in case of a condition that alters gut barrier permeability, instead of the immunoregulatory functions elicited normally, this could lead to endotoxemia (Wieërs et al., 2020).

Apart from the direct effects obtained by the interaction among the cells, probiotics may also influence immune function indirectly by changing the host-microbiota (Bermudez-Brito et al., 2012).

The role of the vitamin D (VITD) is of great interest in lung disease, this includes not only VITD itself but also VITD receptor and VITD-binding protein (Chishimba et al., 2010). In fact, VITD deficiency has been suggested to alter SARS-CoV-2 susceptibility and the course of the disease (Pizzini et al., 2020), and this must not be ignored since VITD insufficiency and deficiency are common in the general population (Al-Tarrah et al., 2018).

Interestingly, intestinal bacteria have been shown to exert beneficial effects through modulation of VITD axis (Del Pinto et al., 2017) since probiotic strains, such as *Lactobacillus rhamnosus* and *Lactobacillus plantarum*, have been shown to increase VDR expression in human intestinal epithelial cells (Wu et al., 2015), which is important for VITD intake and thus to prevent its deficiency, which could compromise the mucosal barrier, leading to increased intestinal permeability and potentially chronic low-grade inflammation (Rizzoli & Biver, 2020).

Through the VITD axis, probiotics can regulate both innate and adaptive immune systems and thus help to maintain mucosal barrier integrity and suppress gut mucosal inflammation (Li et al., 2015). All of this can be done by decreasing Th1 and Th17 T cells and proinflammatory cytokines, such as IL-1, IL-6, IL-8, IFN-γ, and TNFα (Del Pinto et al., 2017), favoring at the same time Th2 and Treg differentiation (Al-Tarrah et al., 2018), downregulating T-cell-driven IgG production, inhibiting DC differentiation, and helping maintain self-tolerance, while enhancing protective innate immune responses (Del Pinto et al., 2017).

All in all, the exact mechanisms by which probiotics may exert the beneficial effect in respiratory infections are still not completely understood. However, there is a high probability that they may be influenced by the probiotic strain used and, also really important, the microbiota composition and immunological status of the individual treated.

26.7 Probiotic administration in respiratory infections

26.7.1 Methodological and clinical aspects

The effects of probiotics on humans have been extensively studied both by scientists and the food and drug industry for decades. This has led to multiple suggested prophylactic and therapeutic health indications and claims, such as prevention or treatment of acute, antibiotic-associated and *Clostridium difficile*-associated diarrhea; amelioration of inflammatory bowel disease and irritable bowel syndrome; and reduction of risk for neonatal late-onset sepsis and necrotizing enterocolitis (Suez et al., 2019). There are many other applications, including relief of depression, reduction in morbidity and seriousness of respiratory infections, therapy and prevention of atopic dermatitis, and decrease of cardiovascular risk factors, which are associated with the cardiometabolic syndrome (Sniffen et al., 2018).

Despite all these studies and trials that have been developed with high methodological validity and quality, there are also studies with the same validity that show contrary or negative results, leading to an unavoidable discussion from both points of view (Canani et al., 2007; Gao et al., 2010; Panigrahi et al., 2017; Ruszczyński et al., 2008; Ukena et al., 2007).

Empirical clinical data are collected following a variety of methodologies, analytical rigor, and clinical endpoints, being the base of many readouts from probiotic trials. There are reports that use qualitative parameters, such as mood, cognition, or self-reported quality of life (Benton et al., 2007; Fujimori et al., 2009). Other trials are based on the measurement of markers that do not have clinical significance in these studies, for example, the rising of glucose-stimulated glucagon-like peptide 1 in glucose-tolerant individuals (Kekkonen et al., 2008) or the clinically irrelevant decrease in the inflammatory marker C-reactive protein in healthy individuals (Simon et al., 2015).

In addition, in these trials, there is an enormous diversity in the parameters and factors that are analyzed and which include in vitro studies, merely observational and subjective trials in both animal and human models, placebo-controlled trials. Sometimes, within a set of high-quality and fidelity trials, their results are contradictory and lead to conflicting conclusions about the benefits of probiotics (Dietrich et al., 2014; Pereg et al., 2005).

There is a wide variety of strains studied, which further contribute to the variability that exists in studies of probiotics. The microorganisms most used in the probiotic industry belong to two genera, *Lactobacillus* spp. and *Bifidobacterium* spp., in addition to strains, such as *Lactococcus* spp., *Streptococcus thermophilus*, *Escherichia coli* Nissle 1917, and the yeast *Saccharomyces boulardii* (Gareau et al., 2010).

There is homogeneity regarding the mechanisms of action of these microorganisms that have to do with human health, many of them being between multiple genera and species of probiotics (e.g., the production of bile salt hydrolases) (Begley et al., 2006).

Researchers and clinicians try to overcome these analytical and methodological limitations, also highlighting studies that may have gone unnoticed, integrating the results of a battery of studies in the form of systematic reviews and meta-analyses. This method is a good way to reveal general trends and observe the results from a more practical point of view; however, it is also susceptible to the introduction of biases in each analytical step (de Vrieze, 2018), such as the inclusion of atypical studies that are questioned, standing out in a homogeneous work and obscuring the actual effects, or lack thereof. Specifically, meta-analyses that have to do with probiotics tend, on occasions, to group studies where several supplemented microorganisms are tested that have little or nothing to do with each other under the same conditions, giving rise to possible erroneously interpreted results (Marteau, 2010; Shimizu et al., 2015).

This situation leads to meta-analyses that address the same topic in conflict with each other (Lu, Sang, et al., 2016; Lu, Yu, et al., 2016). Therefore large-scale, high-quality, randomized controlled clinical trials can be complementary to, but not replaced by, meta-analyses. As discussed below, it is important to bear in mind that the degree of colonization of probiotics varies from one host to another, so the effects on the gut microbiota or the hosts may change within the same experimental group. Finally, industry and commercial entities are, in many cases, those that finance, support, and promote studies on probiotics, and the professional groups that carry them out are paid by the industry itself (Kolber et al., 2014). This fact does not mean that the results obtained from these studies are not valid, or that they are misrepresented by various interests, but it would be interesting to have research that was not associated with the industry or medical-scientific societies.

Next, different meta-analyses that carry out the efficacy or not of the use of probiotics in the treatment of RTIs will be analyzed. In this case, we are going to use a comparison between meta-analyses, which is more visual and comprehensive. Starting with the meta-analysis by Wang, Li, et al. (2016) and Wang, Naghavi, et al. (2016), it was found that the use of probiotics significantly decreased the number of subjects who suffered at least one episode of RTI, with the duration of this episode being fewer days per person and fewer days absent from daycare or school, compared to placebo (Wang, Li, et al., 2016). However, this meta-analysis did not find a statistically significant difference in disease duration between the probiotic and placebo group. In the meta-analysis carried out by Laursen and Hojsak (2018), the age of the children was limited to 7 years, but the consumption of probiotics was not associated with a reduction in the duration of RTIs, nor with a reduction in the number of days missed to class due to RTIs. Was observed a reduction in the use of antibiotics and the risk of suffering at least one URTI. The effect of individually dispensed strains on RTIs results was also addressed in this meta-analysis. Specifically, *L. rhamnosus* GG had an impact on the duration of RTIs and *L. acidophilus* NCFM as a single supplement and in combination with *L. lactis* Bi-07 on the duration of RTIs and the use of antibiotics.

In addition, these strains have shown in vitro the ability to induce antiviral IFN-signaling pathways, which could explain their positive effect on the duration of RTIs (Miettinen et al., 2012). However, given the low number of studies of other strains compared to *L. rhamnosus* GG, these data should be treated with care.

There is consensus that the use of probiotics may have the potential to reduce the risk of RTI, but it should be noted that the clinical trials that are analyzed in the meta-analyses have been carried out in populations of different age ranges, with different genetic backgrounds and with various strains and combinations thereof. Furthermore, in these trials, procedures and data collection have not followed the same pattern, they are not harmonized and may vary substantially. Consequently, the combination of data obtained from clinical trials creates a bias since the effect of the probiotic is dependent on the strain, population and the dose.

26.7.2 Probiotic and respiratory infections

URTIs are common in children and adults. Antiviral treatments are only available for specific groups of patients. The incidence of respiratory infections or symptoms was shown to be reduced in some studies when probiotics, prebiotics, growing-up milk, fish oil, kiwi, garlic, and xylitol were taken. The duration was favorably influenced by the intake of elderberry, kiwi, probiotics, and fish oil. When the risk of bias and repetition is taken into account, probiotics and elderberry repeatedly show favorable effects. Prudent conclusions can be made in selective patient groups (van der Gaag & Hummel, 2020).

Probiotic consumption has demonstrated a positive impact on health outcomes in flu-like RTIs by reducing the number of RTI episodes, the number of days patients spent with RTI symptoms, and the need for antibiotics. Improved patient outcomes translated into considerable cost savings for both the payer and society. These results suggest that recommending daily probiotic consumption may be justified for particular at-risk populations, such as children or individuals with a shared indoor environment, for which this study shows a higher incremental benefit (Lenoir-Wijnkoop et al., 2019).

Recurrent respiratory tract infection (RRTI) is a disease that occurs frequently in preschool children. A total of 120 RRTI children were randomly divided into active group, remission group, intervention group, and control group, meanwhile, 30 healthy children were selected as the healthy group. Children in the intervention group were given oral *Bifidobacterium tetravaccine* tablets for 2 months, while the control group received routine treatment. During the follow-up period, the average annual frequency of different acute RTI and the use of antibiotics were significantly reduced, and the average duration of cough, fever, and use of antibiotics at each episode were also significantly shortened in the intervention group compared to the control group (Li et al., 2019).

Several trials have reported that synbiotic therapy could help prevent RTIs or relieve symptoms of some diseases. Overall, synbiotic interventions reduced the incidence rate of RTIs by 16% and the proportion of participants experiencing RTIs by 16%. There was no significant evidence of publication bias. A subgroup analysis suggested more prominent effects of synbiotics among adults than infants and children for RTI prevention. The sensitivity analysis excluding trials with prebiotics or probiotics as controls was consistent with our primary analysis. This meta-analysis of clinical trials involving >10,000 individuals showed that synbiotic interventions could be an alternative nutrition strategy for conferring human health and preventing RTIs (Chan et al., 2020).

26.7.3 Probiotic and respiratory viral infections

Regarding the effects of probiotics on the incidence and behavior of specific respiratory virus infections in clinical settings, several trials have been performed on infants (Luoto et al., 2014), children (Kumpu, Lehtoranta, et al., 2013; Lehtoranta et al., 2012; Waki et al., 2014), adults (Lehtoranta et al., 2014), and the elderly (Wang et al., 2018). On the other hand, two clinical trials have tested the efficacy of two probiotic strains in an experimental model of exposure to rhinovirus (Table 26.1) (Kumpu et al., 2015; Lehtoranta et al., 2020; Tapiovaara, Kumpu, et al., 2016; Turner et al., 2017).

No consistent data have been obtained from clinical trials carried out on free-living subjects, showing that the use of specific probiotics reduces the incidence of infections caused by respiratory viruses that have been confirmed in the laboratory. In the case of premature infants, the application of *L. rhamnosus* GG for 60 days was associated with a lower incidence of episodes caused by rhinovirus, which is responsible for 80% of all RTI episodes, compared to placebo. However, no effect by *L. rhamnosus* GG on rhinovirus RNA load, duration or severity of infection, or RNA emergence in asymptomatic infants is reported (Luoto et al., 2014).

Nor does it apply to children attending daycare who were supplemented with *L. rhamnosus* GG for 28 weeks. It did not reduce the appearance of any common respiratory virus (Kumpu, Lehtoranta, et al., 2013). In a otitis-prone children, dispensing a combination of *L. rhamnosus* GG, *L. rhamnosus* Lc705, *B. brevis* 99, and *Propionibacterium jensenii* JS, for 6 months, reduced the titer of human bocavirus in positive nasopharyngeal samples, compared to placebo, but not the titer of rhinovirus/enterovirus samples positive (Lehtoranta et al., 2012). In addition, in schoolchildren, taking the probiotic *Lactobacillus brevis* KB290 during the flu season was associated with a lower incidence of diagnosed influenza virus cases (Waki et al., 2014). In the case of adult individuals attending military service, the application of a combination of *L. rhamnosus* GG and *B. lactis* BB-12 for 90–150 days was not associated with a reduction in the incidence of common respiratory viruses after presenting symptoms compatible with colds (Lehtoranta et al., 2014). However, in one subgroup, a lower incidence of rhinovirus/enterovirus was noted after 3 months in the probiotic group versus the placebo group. In nursing home residents, Wang et al. (2018) reported that the use of *L. rhamnosus* GG for 6 months did not appear to affect the appearance of diagnosed respiratory viral infections (Wang et al., 2018). The fact that these studies have been carried out in such different age groups (babies, children, healthy adults and the elderly) with the immune system in different states, seasons of the year, probiotic strains and combinations of them, different doses, and duration of application also makes them appreciate those highly variable results.

The effects of probiotics against specific viruses are difficult to identify in clinical trials directed at free individuals in the community. Trying to overcome all these problems, an experiment was designed in which the efficacy of two

TABLE 26.1 Clinical trials for testing the efficacy of probiotics against viral respiratory infections.

Study type and reference	Randomized subjects	Probiotic intervention	Analyzed viruses	Study outcomes: probiotics versus placebo
Community				
R BD PC (Luoto et al., 2014)	94 preterm infants (2 days to 2 months)	*L. rhamnosus* GG 1×10^9 CFU/day (1–30 days) and 2×10^9 CFU/day for 31–60 days or galacto-oligosaccharide or placebo for 60 days	From nasal swab: human bocavirus, rhinovirus/enterovirus, RSV A and B, adenovirus, coronaviruses types 229E/NL63 and OC43/HKU1, influenza A and B virus, human metapneumovirus, PIV 1–3	A lower incidence of rhinovirus-induced RTI episodes ($P = .04$). Lower number of rhinovirus findings in acute RTI over 12 months ($P = .015$). No significant difference in the mean duration of symptoms in rhinovirus episodes, severity scores of clinical symptoms in rhinovirus episodes, rhinovirus RNA load during infections, duration of rhinovirus RNA shedding, duration or severity of rhinovirus.
R BD PC (Lehtoranta et al., 2012)	269 otitis-prone children (9 months to 5.6 years)	*L. rhamnosus* GG, *L. rhamnosus* Lc705, *B. breve* 99, and *P. jensenii* JS $8–9 \times 10^9$ CFU/day of each strain, or placebo in a capsule for 6 months	From nasal swab: human bocavirus 1–4, rhinovirus/enterovirus	Lower number of human bocavirus 1 positive sample during the study (6.4% vs 19.0%, $P = .039$). No effect on rhinovirus/enterovirus occurrence.
R BD PC (Kumpu, Lehtoranta, et al., 2013)	97 daycare children (2–6 years) visiting healthcare practitioner due to RTI	*L. rhamnosus* GG approximately 10^8 CFU/day in milk for 28 weeks	From nasal swab: human bocavirus 1–4, rhinovirus/enterovirus, RSV, adenovirus, influenza A virus, PIV 1–2	Children had fewer days with respiratory symptoms per month (6.5 vs 7.2, $P < .001$). No effect on the occurrence of respiratory viruses during the study or respiratory symptoms associated with viral findings.
R BD PC (Lehtoranta et al., 2014)	192 military conscripts (18–30 years) visiting healthcare practitioner due to RTI	*L. rhamnosus* GG 5×10^9 CFU/day + *B. lactis* BB-12 2×10^9 CFU/day in a chewing tablet for either 3 or 6 months	From nasal swab: human bocavirus, rhinovirus/enterovirus, RSV A and B, adenovirus, coronavirus types 229E/NL63 and OC43/HKU1, influenza A and B virus, human metapneumovirus, PIV 1–4	Overall, no significant effect on the occurrence of common respiratory viruses. In a subgroup, there was a lower occurrence of rhino/enteroviruses after 3 months (5 vs 15, $P < .01$)
Open-label, parallel group (Waki et al., 2014)	2926 schoolchildren (6–12 years)	*L. brevis* KB290 in a nutrient drink 6×10^9 CFU/bottle 5 day/week for 8 weeks + no consumption for 8 weeks or vice versa (2 alternate study groups)	The physician diagnosed influenza virus infection	During the influenza epidemic, fewer influenza infections in the group consuming probiotic drink compared with the group not consuming the probiotic drink (15.7% vs 23.9%, $P < .001$)

(*Continued*)

TABLE 26.1 (Continued)

Study type and reference	Randomized subjects	Probiotic intervention	Analyzed viruses	Study outcomes: probiotics versus placebo
R DB PC (Wang et al., 2018)	209 nursing home residents aged ≥65 years	L. rhamnosus GG 2×10^{10} CFU/day in capsule or placebo for 6 months	From nasal swab: rhinovirus/enterovirus, RSV, influenza A and B virus, human metapneumovirus, PIV 1–3	No statistically significant difference in laboratory-confirmed viral respiratory infections.
Experimental virus challenge				
R DB PC (Kumpu et al., 2015; Tapiovaara, Kumpu, et al., 2016)	59 healthy adults (mean 22–24 years)	L. rhamnosus GG 10^9 CFU of live or heat inactivated (by spray drying) in 100 mL of fruit juice or control juice daily for 6 weeks	From nasal lavage: rhinovirus A39	No significant effect on rhinovirus infection rate. No significant effect on the occurrence and severity of cold symptoms during rhinovirus infection. No significant effect on viral loads.
R DB PC (Turner et al., 2017)	115 healthy adults with confirmed experimental infection (mean 22–23 years)	B. lactis Bl-04 2×10^9 CFU powder or placebo daily for 32 days	From nasal lavage: rhinovirus A39	Reduction in nasal rhinovirus titer and the proportion of subjects shedding the virus in nasal secretions (76% vs 91%, $P = .04$) during the infection. Significantly higher IL-8 levels in nasal lavage before infection (90 vs 58 pg/mL, $P = .04$). Significantly reduced IL-8 response to rhinovirus infection in nasal lavage ($P = .03$). No significant effect on symptom severity/scores or infection rate.

CFU, Colony-forming unit; *PIV*, parainfluenza virus; *R DB PC*, randomized double-blind placebo-controlled; *RSV*, respiratory syncytial virus; *RTI*, respiratory tract infection.

probiotic strains is tested against a rhinovirus, a specific viral pathogen. *B. lactis* Bl-04 was administered for 28 days to health volunteers after they were inoculated with a rhinovirus strain (type 39) and the probiotic strain continued to be administered for 5 more days (Turner et al., 2017). In the group supplemented with *B. lactis* Bl-04, there is a significant decrease in the viral titer from nasal washes, in addition to a lower number of participants who excrete the virus, compared to the placebo group. Also, in the group supplemented with *B. lactis* Bl-04, a significantly higher concentration of IL-8 is considered in the nasal washes after the 28 days of supplementation before infection. Given the low viral titer in this group, the elevation of the IL-8 concentration could be interpreted as a preparation of the immune tissue present in the nasopharyngeal mucosa before infection. The hypothesis used here is in agreement with a clinical study carried out in healthy adult individuals, where an application of *B. lactis* Bl-04 reduced the incidence of URTIs compared to placebo (West et al., 2014).

In another experiment carried out similarly with a type 39 rhinovirus, no significant antiviral effect was observed in the groups that were supplemented with *L. rhamnosus* GG compared to placebo (Kumpu et al., 2015; Tapiovaara, Kumpu, et al., 2016), strengthening the idea of specificity of the probiotic strain in the potential benefit against respiratory infections caused by viruses. In any case, the design of powerful and harmonized studies is very necessary to draw a clear conclusion about the efficacy of probiotics against respiratory infections caused by viruses.

26.8 Conclusion

Probiotics are safe microorganisms that when administered to human subjects in adequate doses and at appropriate periods confer some beneficial effects on the host. The effects of probiotics on gut microbiota composition are still in discussion. Since there are some gaps in the evidence related to the health effects of probiotics in nonhealthy populations, further studies are needed to elucidate the changes observed in the pulmonary microbiota in humans and to assess the effects of probiotics for which evidence is not available so far. In this regard, there is an actual need to perform well-designed, long-term, double-blind, placebo-controlled, randomized clinical trials with appropriate doses and adequate subject sizes to evaluate the potential impact of probiotics on intestinal microbiota and how they could affect major outcomes and risk biomarkers related to RTI diseases.

References

Al-Tarrah, K., Hewison, M., Moiemen, N., & Lord, J. M. (2018). Vitamin D status and its influence on outcomes following major burn injury and critical illness. *Burns & Trauma, 6*, 11.

Andrews, T., Thompson, M., Buckley, D. I., Heneghan, C., Deyo, R., Redmond, N., Lucas, P. J., Blair, P. S., & Hay, A. D. (2012). Interventions to influence consulting and antibiotic use for acute respiratory tract infections in children: A systematic review and meta-analysis. *PLoS One, 7*, e30334.

Asher, I., Haahtela, T., Selroos, O., Ellwood, P., Ellwood, E., & Group, G. A. N. S. (2017). Global Asthma Network survey suggests more national asthma strategies could reduce burden of asthma. *Allergologia et Immunopathologia, 45*, 105–114.

Baaten, B. J., Cooper, A. M., Swain, S. L., & Bradley, L. M. (2013). Location, location, location: The impact of migratory heterogeneity on T cell function. *Frontiers in Immunology, 4*, 311.

Begley, M., Hill, C., & Gahan, C. G. (2006). Bile salt hydrolase activity in probiotics. *Applied and Environmental Microbiology, 72*, 1729–1738.

Benton, D., Williams, C., & Brown, A. (2007). Impact of consuming a milk drink containing a probiotic on mood and cognition. *European Journal of Clinical Nutrition, 61*, 355–361.

Bermudez-Brito, M., Plaza-Díaz, J., Muñoz-Quezada, S., Gómez-Llorente, C., & Gil, A. (2012). Probiotic mechanisms of action. *Annals of Nutrition and Metabolism, 61*, 160–174.

Black, R. E., Cousens, S., Johnson, H. L., Lawn, J. E., Rudan, I., Bassani, D. G., Jha, P., Campbell, H., Walker, C. F., & Cibulskis, R. (2010). Global, regional, and national causes of child mortality in 2008: A systematic analysis. *The Lancet, 375*, 1969–1987.

Bordon, Y. (2019). Microbiota supports air attack. *Nature Reviews. Immunology, 19*, 203.

Brandtzaeg, P. (2009). Mucosal immunity: Induction, dissemination, and effector functions. *Scandinavian Journal of Immunology, 70*, 505–515.

Brestoff, J. R., & Artis, D. (2013). Commensal bacteria at the interface of host metabolism and the immune system. *Nature Immunology, 14*, 676–684.

Burney, P. G., Patel, J., Newson, R., Minelli, C., & Naghavi, M. (2015). Global and regional trends in COPD mortality, 1990–2010. *European Respiratory Journal, 45*, 1239–1247.

Canani, R. B., Cirillo, P., Terrin, G., Cesarano, L., Spagnuolo, M. I., de Vincenzo, A., Albano, F., Passariello, A., de Marco, G., Manguso, F., & Guarino, A. (2007). Probiotics for treatment of acute diarrhoea in children: Randomised clinical trial of five different preparations. *BMJ, 335*, 340.

Chan, C. K. Y., Tao, J., Chan, O. S., Li, H. B., & Pang, H. (2020). Preventing respiratory tract infections by synbiotic interventions: A systematic review and meta-analysis of randomized controlled trials. *Advances in Nutrition, 11*, 979–988.

Chishimba, L., Thickett, D. R., Stockley, R. A., & Wood, A. M. (2010). The vitamin D axis in the lung: A key role for vitamin D-binding protein. *Thorax, 65*, 456–462.

Christensen, H. R., Frokiaer, H., & Pestka, J. J. (2002). Lactobacilli differentially modulate expression of cytokines and maturation surface markers in murine dendritic cells. *Journal of Immunology, 168*, 171–178.

Clarke, T. C., Black, L. I., Stussman, B. J., Barnes, P. M., & Nahin, R. L. (2015). Trends in the use of complementary health approaches among adults: United States, 2002–2012. *National Health Statistics Report*, 1–16.

Cruz, A. A. (2007). *Global surveillance, prevention and control of chronic respiratory diseases: A comprehensive approach*. World Health Organization.

Dasaraju, P. V., & Liu, C. (1996). *Infections of the respiratory system. Medical microbiology* (4th ed.). Galveston: University of Texas Medical Branch at Galveston, Chapter 93.

de Simone, C. (2019). The unregulated probiotic market. *Clinical Gastroenterology and Hepatology, 17*, 809–817.

de Vrieze, J. (2018). The metawars. *Science (New York, N.Y.), 361*, 1184–1188.

Del Pinto, R., Ferri, C., & Cominelli, F. (2017). Vitamin D axis in inflammatory bowel diseases: Role, current uses and future perspectives. *International Journal of Molecular Sciences, 18*.

Didari, T., Solki, S., Mozaffari, S., Nikfar, S., & Abdollahi, M. (2014). A systematic review of the safety of probiotics. *Expert Opinion on Drug Safety, 13*, 227–239.

Dietrich, C. G., Kottmann, T., & Alavi, M. (2014). Commercially available probiotic drinks containing Lactobacillus casei DN-114001 reduce antibiotic-associated diarrhea. *World Journal of Gastroenterology: WJG, 20*, 15837–15844.

Dumas, A., Bernard, L., Poquet, Y., LUGO-Villarino, G., & Neyrolles, O. (2018). The role of the lung microbiota and the gut—lung axis in respiratory infectious diseases. *Cellular Microbiology, 20*, e12966.

Ehlken, B., Ihorst, G., Lippert, B., Rohwedder, A., Petersen, G., Schumacher, M., Forster, J., & Group, P. S. (2005). Economic impact of community-acquired and nosocomial lower respiratory tract infections in young children in Germany. *European Journal of Pediatrics, 164*, 607—615.

El Hage, R., Hernandez-Sanabria, E., & Van De wiele, T. (2017). Emerging trends in "smart probiotics": Functional consideration for the development of novel health and industrial applications. *Frontiers in Microbiology, 8*, 1889.

Fink, L. N., Zeuthen, L. H., Ferlazzo, G., & Frokiaer, H. (2007). Human antigen-presenting cells respond differently to gut-derived probiotic bacteria but mediate similar strain-dependent NK and T cell activation. *FEMS Immunology and Medical Microbiology, 51*, 535—546.

Fitzmaurice, C., Allen, C., Barber, R. M., Barregard, L., Bhutta, Z. A., Brenner, H., Dicker, D. J., Chimed-Orchir, O., Dandona, R., & Dandona, L. (2017). Global, regional, and national cancer incidence, mortality, years of life lost, years lived with disability, and disability-adjusted life-years for 32 cancer groups, 1990 to 2015: A systematic analysis for the global burden of disease study. *JAMA Oncology, 3*, 524—548.

Food and Agriculture Organization of the United Nations. (2002). Guidelines for the evaluation of probiotics in food. Joint FAO/WHO working group report on drafting guidelines for the evaluation of probiotics in food.

Fujimori, S., Gudis, K., Mitsui, K., Seo, T., Yonezawa, M., Tanaka, S., Tatsuguchi, A., & Sakamoto, C. (2009). A randomized controlled trial on the efficacy of synbiotic vs probiotic or prebiotic treatment to improve the quality of life in patients with ulcerative colitis. *Nutrition (Burbank, Los Angeles County, Calif.), 25*, 520—525.

Gao, X. W., Mubasher, M., Fang, C. Y., Reifer, C., & Miller, L. E. (2010). Dose—Response Efficacy of a Proprietary Probiotic Formula ofLactobacillus acidophilusCL1285 andLactobacillus caseiLBC80R for Antibiotic-Associated Diarrhea andClostridium difficile-Associated Diarrhea Prophylaxis in Adult Patients. *American Journal of Gastroenterology, 105*, 1636—1641.

Gareau, M. G., Sherman, P. M., & Walker, W. A. (2010). Probiotics and the gut microbiota in intestinal health and disease. *Nature Reviews Gastroenterology & Hepatology, 7*, 503.

Hao, Q., Dong, B. R., & Wu, T. (2015). Probiotics for preventing acute upper respiratory tract infections. *Cochrane Database of Systematic Reviews*.

Hill, C., Guarner, F., Reid, G., Gibson, G., & Merenstein, D. (2014). Expert consensus document. The International Scientific Association for Probiotics and Prebiotics consensus statement on the scope and appropriate use of the term probiotic. *Nature Reviews Gastroenterology & Hepatology, 11*, 506—514.

Hilty, M., Burke, C., Pedro, H., Cardenas, P., Bush, A., Bossley, C., Davies, J., Ervine, A., Poulter, L., & Pachter, L. (2010). Disordered microbial communities in asthmatic airways. *PLoS One, 5*, e8578.

Hoffmann, D. E., Fraser, C. M., Palumbo, F., Ravel, J., Rowthorn, V., & Schwartz, J. (2014). Probiotics: Achieving a better regulatory fit. *Food and Drug Law Journal, 69*, 237—272, ii.

Hosono, A. (1992). Fermented milk in the orient. In Y. Nakazawa, & A. Hosono (Eds.), *Functions of fermented milk, challenges for health science*. London: Elsevier Applied Science Publishers Ltd.

Kekkonen, R. A., Lummela, N., Karjalainen, H., Latvala, S., Tynkkynen, S., Jarvenpaa, S., Kautiainen, H., Julkunen, I., Vapaatalo, H., & Korpela, R. (2008). Probiotic intervention has strain-specific anti-inflammatory effects in healthy adults. *World Journal of Gastroenterology: WJG, 14*, 2029—2036.

King, S., Glanville, J., Sanders, M. E., Fitzgerald, A., & Varley, D. (2014). Effectiveness of probiotics on the duration of illness in healthy children and adults who develop common acute respiratory infectious conditions: A systematic review and meta-analysis. *British Journal of Nutrition, 112*, 41—54.

Kolber, M. R., Vandermeer, B., & Allan, G. M. (2014). Funding may influence trial results examining probiotics and Clostridium difficile diarrhea rates. *The American Journal of Gastroenterology, 109*, 1081—1082.

Kumpu, M., Kekkonen, R. A., Korpela, R., Tynkkynen, S., Jarvenpaa, S., Kautiainen, H., Allen, E. K., Hendley, J. O., Pitkaranta, A., & Winther, B. (2015). Effect of live and inactivated Lactobacillus rhamnosus GG on experimentally induced rhinovirus colds: Randomised, double blind, placebo-controlled pilot trial. *Benef Microbes, 6*, 631—639.

Kumpu, M., Lehtoranta, L., Roivainen, M., Ronkko, E., Ziegler, T., Soderlund-Venermo, M., Kautiainen, H., Jarvenpaa, S., Kekkonen, R., Hatakka, K., Korpela, R., & Pitkaranta, A. (2013). The use of the probiotic Lactobacillus rhamnosus GG and viral findings in the nasopharynx of children attending day care. *Journal of Medical Virology, 85*, 1632—1638.

Kumpu, M., Swanljung, E., Tynkkynen, S., Hatakka, K., Kekkonen, R. A., Järvenpää, S., Korpela, R., & Pitkäranta, A. (2013). Recovery of probiotic Lactobacillus rhamnosus GG in tonsil tissue after oral administration: Randomised, placebo-controlled, double-blind clinical trial. *British Journal of Nutrition, 109*, 2240—2246.

Lambert, S. B., Allen, K. M., Carter, R. C., & Nolan, T. M. (2008). The cost of community-managed viral respiratory illnesses in a cohort of healthy preschool-aged children. *Respiratory Research, 9*, 11.

Lange, K., Buerger, M., Stallmach, A., & Bruns, T. (2016). Effects of antibiotics on gut microbiota. *Digestive Diseases, 34*, 260—268.

Laursen, R. P., & Hojsak, I. (2018). Probiotics for respiratory tract infections in children attending day care centers-a systematic review. *European Journal of Pediatrics, 177*, 979—994.

Lehtinen, M. J., Hibberd, A. A., Männikkö, S., Yeung, N., Kauko, T., Forssten, S., Lehtoranta, L., Lahtinen, S. J., Stahl, B., & Lyra, A. (2018). Nasal microbiota clusters associate with inflammatory response, viral load, and symptom severity in experimental rhinovirus challenge. *Scientific Reports, 8*, 1—12.

Lehtoranta, L., Kalima, K., He, L., Lappalainen, M., Roivainen, M., Narkio, M., Makela, M., Siitonen, S., Korpela, R., & Pitkaranta, A. (2014). Specific probiotics and virological findings in symptomatic conscripts attending military service in Finland. *Journal of Clinical Virology: The Official Publication of the Pan American Society for Clinical Virology, 60*, 276—281.

Lehtoranta, L., Latvala, S., & Lehtinen, M. J. (2020). Role of probiotics in stimulating the immune system in viral respiratory tract infections: A narrative review. *Nutrients*, *12*.

Lehtoranta, L., Soderlund-Venermo, M., Nokso-Koivisto, J., Toivola, H., Blomgren, K., Hatakka, K., Poussa, T., Korpela, R., & Pitkaranta, A. (2012). Human bocavirus in the nasopharynx of otitis-prone children. *International Journal of Pediatric Otorhinolaryngology*, *76*, 206–211.

Lenoir-Wijnkoop, I., Merenstein, D., Korchagina, D., Broholm, C., Sanders, M. E., & Tancredi, D. (2019). Probiotics reduce health care cost and societal impact of flu-like respiratory tract infections in the USA: An economic modeling study. *Frontiers in Pharmacology*, *10*, 980.

Levy, M., Kolodziejczyk, A. A., Thaiss, C. A., & Elinav, E. (2017). Dysbiosis and the immune system. *Nature Reviews Immunology*, *17*, 219–232.

Li, K. L., Wang, B. Z., Li, Z. P., Li, Y. L., & Liang, J. J. (2019). Alterations of intestinal flora and the effects of probiotics in children with recurrent respiratory tract infection. *World Journal of Pediatrics: WJP*, *15*, 255–261.

Li, Y. C., Chen, Y., & Du, J. (2015). Critical roles of intestinal epithelial vitamin D receptor signaling in controlling gut mucosal inflammation. *The Journal of Steroid Biochemistry and Molecular Biology*, *148*, 179–183.

Lilly, D. M., & Stillwell, R. H. (1965). Probiotics: Growth-promoting factors produced by microorganisms. *Science (New York, N.Y.)*, *147*, 747–748.

Lu, C., Sang, J., He, H., Wan, X., Lin, Y., Li, L., Li, Y., & Yu, C. (2016). Probiotic supplementation does not improve eradication rate of Helicobacter pylori infection compared to placebo based on standard therapy: A meta-analysis. *Scientific Reports*, *6*, 23522.

Lu, M., Yu, S., Deng, J., Yan, Q., Yang, C., Xia, G., & Zhou, X. (2016). Efficacy of probiotic supplementation therapy for Helicobacter pylori eradication: A meta-analysis of randomized controlled trials. *PLoS One*, *11*, e0163743.

Luoto, R., Ruuskanen, O., Waris, M., Kalliomaki, M., Salminen, S., & Isolauri, E. (2014). Prebiotic and probiotic supplementation prevents rhinovirus infections in preterm infants: A randomized, placebo-controlled trial. *The Journal of Allergy and Clinical Immunology*, *133*, 405–413.

Mahooti, M., Miri, S. M., Abdolalipour, E., & Ghaemi, A. (2020). The immunomodulatory effects of probiotics on respiratory viral infections: A hint for COVID-19 treatment? *Microbial Pathogenesis*, 104452.

Man, W. H., De Steenhuijsen piters, W. A., & Bogaert, D. (2017). The microbiota of the respiratory tract: Gatekeeper to respiratory health. *Nature Reviews Microbiology*, *15*, 259–270.

Marteau, P. (2010). Probiotics in functional intestinal disorders and IBS: Proof of action and dissecting the multiple mechanisms. *Gut*, *59*, 285–286.

Massin, M., Montesanti, J., Gerard, P., & Lepage, P. (2006). Spectrum and frequency of illness presenting to a pediatric emergency department. *Acta Clinica Belgica*, *61*, 161–165.

Metchnikoff, E., & Chalmers-Mitchell, P. (1908). In P. Chalmers Mitchell (Ed.), *The prolongation of life optimistic studies*. New York: GP Putnam's Sons. The Knickerbocker Press.

Miettinen, M., Pietila, T. E., Kekkonen, R. A., Kankainen, M., Latvala, S., Pirhonen, J., Osterlund, P., Korpela, R., & Julkunen, I. (2012). Nonpathogenic Lactobacillus rhamnosus activates the inflammasome and antiviral responses in human macrophages. *Gut Microbes*, *3*, 510–522.

Nguyen, J. L., Yang, W., Ito, K., Matte, T. D., Shaman, J., & Kinney, P. L. (2016). Seasonal influenza infections and cardiovascular disease mortality. *JAMA Cardiology*, *1*, 274–281.

Nicholson, K. G., Mcnally, T., Silverman, M., Simons, P., Stockton, J. D., & Zambon, M. C. (2006). Rates of hospitalisation for influenza, respiratory syncytial virus and human metapneumovirus among infants and young children. *Vaccine*, *24*, 102–108.

Ozen, M., & Dinleyici, E. (2015). The history of probiotics: The untold story. *Beneficial Microbes*, *6*, 159–165.

Panigrahi, P., Parida, S., Nanda, N. C., Satpathy, R., Pradhan, L., Chandel, D. S., Baccaglini, L., Mohapatra, A., Mohapatra, S. S., & Misra, P. R. (2017). A randomized synbiotic trial to prevent sepsis among infants in rural India. *Nature*, *548*, 407–412.

Parada Venegas, D., De La fuente, M. K., Landskron, G., González, M. J., Quera, R., Dijkstra, G., Harmsen, H. J., Faber, K. N., & Hermoso, M. A. (2019). Short chain fatty acids (SCFAs)-mediated gut epithelial and immune regulation and its relevance for inflammatory bowel diseases. *Frontiers in Immunology*, *10*, 277.

Pascale, A., Marchesi, N., Marelli, C., Coppola, A., Luzi, L., Govoni, S., Giustina, A., & Gazzaruso, C. (2018). Microbiota and metabolic diseases. *Endocrine*, *61*, 357–371.

Pearce, N., Aït-Khaled, N., Beasley, R., Mallol, J., Keil, U., Mitchell, E., & Robertson, C. (2007). Worldwide trends in the prevalence of asthma symptoms: Phase III of the International Study of Asthma and Allergies in Childhood (ISAAC). *Thorax*, *62*, 758–766.

Pereg, D., Kimhi, O., Tirosh, A., Orr, N., Kayouf, R., & Lishner, M. (2005). The effect of fermented yogurt on the prevention of diarrhea in a healthy adult population. *American Journal of Infection Control*, *33*, 122–125.

Pizzini, A., Aichner, M., Sahanic, S., Bohm, A., Egger, A., Hoermann, G., Kurz, K., Widmann, G., Bellmann-Weiler, R., Weiss, G., Tancevski, I., Sonnweber, T., & Loffler-Ragg, J. (2020). Impact of vitamin D deficiency on COVID-19—A prospective analysis from the CovILD Registry. *Nutrients*, *12*.

Pot, B., Foligné, B., Daniel, C., & Grangette, C. (2013). *Understanding immunomodulatory effects of probiotics. The importance of immunonutrition*. Karger Publishers.

Pragman, A. A., Kim, H. B., Reilly, C. S., Wendt, C., & Isaacson, R. E. (2012). The lung microbiome in moderate and severe chronic obstructive pulmonary disease. *PLoS One*, *7*, e47305.

Rizzoli, R., & Biver, E. (2020). Are probiotics the new calcium and vitamin D for bone health? *Current Osteoporosis Reports*, *18*, 273–284.

Ruszczyński, M., Radzikowski, A., & Szajewska, H. (2008). Clinical trial: Effectiveness of Lactobacillus rhamnosus (strains E/N, Oxy and Pen) in the prevention of antibiotic-associated diarrhoea in children. *Alimentary Pharmacology & Therapeutics*, *28*, 154–161.

Shimizu, M., Hashiguchi, M., Shiga, T., Tamura, H. O., & Mochizuki, M. (2015). Meta-analysis: Effects of probiotic supplementation on lipid profiles in normal to mildly hypercholesterolemic individuals. *PLoS One*, *10*, e0139795.

Sicard, D., & Legras, J.-L. (2011). Bread, beer and wine: Yeast domestication in the Saccharomyces sensu stricto complex. *Comptes Rendus Biologies*, *334*, 229–236.

Simon, M. C., Strassburger, K., Nowotny, B., Kolb, H., Nowotny, P., Burkart, V., Zivehe, F., Hwang, J. H., Stehle, P., Pacini, G., Hartmann, B., Holst, J. J., Mackenzie, C., Bindels, L. B., Martinez, I., Walter, J., Henrich, B., Schloot, N. C., & Roden, M. (2015). Intake of Lactobacillus reuteri improves incretin and insulin secretion in glucose-tolerant humans: A proof of concept. *Diabetes Care, 38*, 1827−1834.

Sniffen, J. C., Mcfarland, L. V., Evans, C. T., & Goldstein, E. J. (2018). Choosing an appropriate probiotic product for your patient: An evidence-based practical guide. *PLoS One, 13*, e0209205.

Sonnenborn, U., & Schulze, J. (2009). The non-pathogenic Escherichia coli strain Nissle 1917—features of a versatile probiotic. *Microbial Ecology in Health and Disease, 21*, 122−158.

Suez, J., Zmora, N., Segal, E., & Elinav, E. (2019). The pros, cons, and many unknowns of probiotics. *Nature Medicine, 25*, 716−729.

Swanljung, E., Tapiovaara, L., Lehtoranta, L., Mäkivuokko, H., Roivainen, M., Korpela, R., & Pitkäranta, A. (2015). Lactobacillus rhamnosus GG in adenoid tissue: Double-blind, placebo-controlled, randomized clinical trial. *Acta Oto-Laryngologica, 135*, 824−830.

Swedberg, E., Shah, R., Sadruddin, S., & Soeripto, J. (2020). *Saving young children from forgotten killer: Pneumonia*. Bethesda, MD: American Physiological Society.

Tapiovaara, L., Kumpu, M., Makivuokko, H., Waris, M., Korpela, R., Pitkaranta, A., & Winther, B. (2016). Human rhinovirus in experimental infection after peroral Lactobacillus rhamnosus GG consumption, a pilot study. *International Forum of Allergy & Rhinology, 6*, 848−853.

Tapiovaara, L., Lehtoranta, L., Poussa, T., Mäkivuokko, H., Korpela, R., & Pitkäranta, A. (2016). Absence of adverse events in healthy individuals using probiotics—analysis of six randomised studies by one study group. *Beneficial Microbes, 7*, 161−169.

Tissier, H. (1906). Treatment of intestinal infections using bacterial flora of the intestine. *Critical Reviews in Society Biology, 60*, 359−361.

Torre, L. A., Bray, F., Siegel, R. L., Ferlay, J., Lortet-Tieulent, J., & Jemal, A. (2015). Global cancer statistics, 2012. *CA: A Cancer Journal for Clinicians, 65*, 87−108.

Turner, R. B., Woodfolk, J. A., Borish, L., Steinke, J. W., Patrie, J. T., Muehling, L. M., Lahtinen, S., & Lehtinen, M. J. (2017). Effect of probiotic on innate inflammatory response and viral shedding in experimental rhinovirus infection—A randomised controlled trial. *Beneficial Microbes, 8*, 207−215.

Ukena, S. N., Singh, A., Dringenberg, U., Engelhardt, R., Seidler, U., Hansen, W., Bleich, A., Bruder, D., Franzke, A., Rogler, G., Suerbaum, S., Buer, J., Gunzer, F., & Westendorf, A. M. (2007). Probiotic *Escherichia coli* Nissle 1917 inhibits leaky gut by enhancing mucosal integrity. *PLoS One, 2*, e1308.

van Baarlen, P., Wells, J. M., & Kleerebezem, M. (2013). Regulation of intestinal homeostasis and immunity with probiotic lactobacilli. *Trends in Immunology, 34*, 208−215.

Van Der Gaag, E., & Hummel, T. Z. (2020). Food or medication? The therapeutic effects of food on the duration and incidence of upper respiratory tract infections: A review of the literature. *Critical Reviews in Food Science and Nutrition*, 1−14.

Velilla, N. M., Apezteguía, I. I., Renedo, J. A., & Infante, B. F. (2007). Infecciones respiratorias. *Revista Española de Geriatría y Gerontología, 42*, 51−59.

Waki, N., Matsumoto, M., Fukui, Y., & Suganuma, H. (2014). Effects of probiotic Lactobacillus brevis KB290 on incidence of influenza infection among schoolchildren: An open-label pilot study. *Letters in Applied Microbiology, 59*, 565−571.

Wang, B., Hylwka, T., Smieja, M., Surrette, M., Bowdish, D. M. E., & Loeb, M. (2018). Probiotics to prevent respiratory infections in nursing homes: A pilot randomized controlled trial. *Journal of the American Geriatrics Society, 66*, 1346−1352.

Wang, H., Naghavi, M., Allen, C., Barber, R. M., Bhutta, Z. A., Carter, A., Casey, D. C., Charlson, F. J., Chen, A. Z., & Coates, M. M. (2016). Global, regional, and national life expectancy, all-cause mortality, and cause-specific mortality for 249 causes of death, 1980−2015: A systematic analysis for the Global Burden of Disease Study 2015. *The Lancet, 388*, 1459−1544.

Wang, Y., Li, X., Ge, T., Xiao, Y., Liao, Y., Cui, Y., Zhang, Y., Ho, W., Yu, G., & Zhang, T. (2016). Probiotics for prevention and treatment of respiratory tract infections in children: A systematic review and meta-analysis of randomized controlled trials. *Medicine (Baltimore), 95*, e4509.

West, N. P., Horn, P. L., Pyne, D. B., Gebski, V. J., Lahtinen, S. J., Fricker, P. A., & Cripps, A. W. (2014). Probiotic supplementation for respiratory and gastrointestinal illness symptoms in healthy physically active individuals. *Clinical Nutrition (Edinburgh, Scotland), 33*, 581−587.

WHO & UNICEF. (2006). *Pneummonia: The forgotten killer of children*. Geneva: World Health Organization.

Wieërs, G., Belkhir, L., Enaud, R., Leclercq, S., Philippart De foy, J.-M., Dequenne, I., De timary, P., & Cani, P. D. (2020). How probiotics affect the microbiota. *Frontiers in Cellular and Infection Microbiology, 9*, 454.

Willner, D., Haynes, M. R., Furlan, M., Schmieder, R., Lim, Y. W., Rainey, P. B., Rohwer, F., & Conrad, D. (2012). Spatial distribution of microbial communities in the cystic fibrosis lung. *The ISME Journal, 6*, 471−474.

World Health Organization. (2013). *Global tuberculosis report 2013*. World Health Organization.

Wu, S., Yoon, S., Zhang, Y. G., Lu, R., Xia, Y., Wan, J., Petrof, E. O., Claud, E. C., Chen, D., & Sun, J. (2015). Vitamin D receptor pathway is required for probiotic protection in colitis. *American Journal of Physiology. Gastrointestinal and Liver Physiology, 309*, G341−G349.

Zhang, D., Li, S., Wang, N., Tan, H.-Y., Zhang, Z., & Feng, Y. (2020). The cross-talk between gut microbiota and lungs in common lung diseases. *Frontiers in Microbiology, 11*.

Zhang, J., Harbottle, G., Wang, C., & Kong, Z. (1999). Oldest playable musical instruments found at Jiahu early Neolithic site in China. *Nature, 401*, 366−368.

Zheng, J., Wittouck, S., Salvetti, E., Franz, C. M., Harris, H. M., Mattarelli, P., O'toole, P. W., Pot, B., Vandamme, P., & Walter, J. (2020). A taxonomic note on the genus *Lactobacillus*: Description of 23 novel genera, emended description of the genus *Lactobacillus Beijerinck* 1901, and union of Lactobacillaceae and Leuconostocaceae. *International Journal of Systematic and Evolutionary Microbiology, 70*, 2782−2858.

Chapter 27

The role of probiotics in nutritional health: probiotics as nutribiotics

María Chávarri[1], Lucía Diez-Gutiérrez[1], Izaskun Marañón[1], María del Carmen Villarán[1] and Luis Javier R. Barrón[2]

[1]*Health and Food Area, Health Division, TECNALIA, Basque Research and Technology Alliance (BRTA), Parque Tecnológico de Álava, Miñano, Spain,*
[2]*Lactiker Research Group, Department of Pharmacy and Food Sciences, University of the Basque Country (UPV/EHU), Vitoria-Gasteiz, Spain*

27.1 Nutribiotics: ways to improve the nutritional status

In recent years the intestinal microbiota has been of great interest since it is involved in many functions in humans and animals (Kraimi et al., 2019). This intestinal microbiota is composed of a wide variety of microorganisms, such as bacteria, Archaea, viruses, and eukaryotes (including protozoa and fungi). For years, scientific studies carried out in this field have shown that the intestinal microbiota influences the immune function, having a strong impact on health (Alverdy & Luo, 2017; O'Mahony et al., 2014; Sampson et al., 2016; Williams et al., 2011). Likewise, gut microbiota performs a fundamental role in the control of homeostatic processes, such as nutrient metabolism or micronutrient synthesis. For this reason, the deterioration of the intestinal microbiota can cause an imbalance known as dysbiosis, and thus many intestinal diseases could be triggered due to inadequate homeostatic regulation (Cammarota et al., 2014). Consequently, the imbalance in the intestinal microbiota facilitates the generation of many pathological states that involve infections with pathogens or metabolic disorders (Alverdy & Luo, 2017; O'Mahony et al., 2014; Sampson et al., 2016; Williams et al., 2011). Furthermore, the intestinal microbiota also plays a very important role in many extraintestinal tissues and in various development and metabolism processes in organs, such as the liver, adipose tissue, and bone (Sommer & Bäckhed, 2013).

Moreover, evidence has shown that the balance of the intestinal microbiota could be restored using live microorganisms, known as probiotics, which when administered in adequate amounts confer a benefit for the host's health (FAO/WHO, 2006). For instance, Korpela et al. (2018) showed the beneficial effect of commercial probiotics, such as *Bifidobacterium breve* or *Lactobacillus rhamnosus*, conducting a study with infants who were likely to develop allergic diseases due to their microbiota disruption after using antibiotics.

Probiotics can also aid in the homeostasis preservation through the modulation of the immune system with the regulation of immunoglobulins and cytokines, the stimulation of macrophages, and the response against food antigens. As well as, probiotics can reinforce the intestinal epithelial barrier, promote nutrients absorption or enhance the proliferation of other beneficial microorganisms, and inhibit other pathogens (Sehrawat et al., 2020). Therefore these beneficial effects of probiotics may help in the prevention or treatment of diseases related to the gastrointestinal (GI) tract, alterations in the immune system, hepatic diseases, neoplastic proliferation, the cardiovascular system, or intolerances, among others (Brown & Valiere, 2004).

Due to the wide variety of potential health benefits of probiotics, Arora and Baldi (2015) proposed to split the classification of probiotics into pharmabiotics and nutribiotics. Considering pharmabiotics those microorganisms used to treat or prevent medical illnesses by giving physiological and pharmacological benefits. However, the concept of nutribiotics would be focused more on treating nutritional problems, enhancing the benefits of food or dietary supplements, and preserving human health. Hence, these authors indicated that the term nutribiotics would embrace the probiotic microorganisms, and the products obtained from these microorganisms with specific nutritional claims, currently known as postbiotics Fig. 27.1.

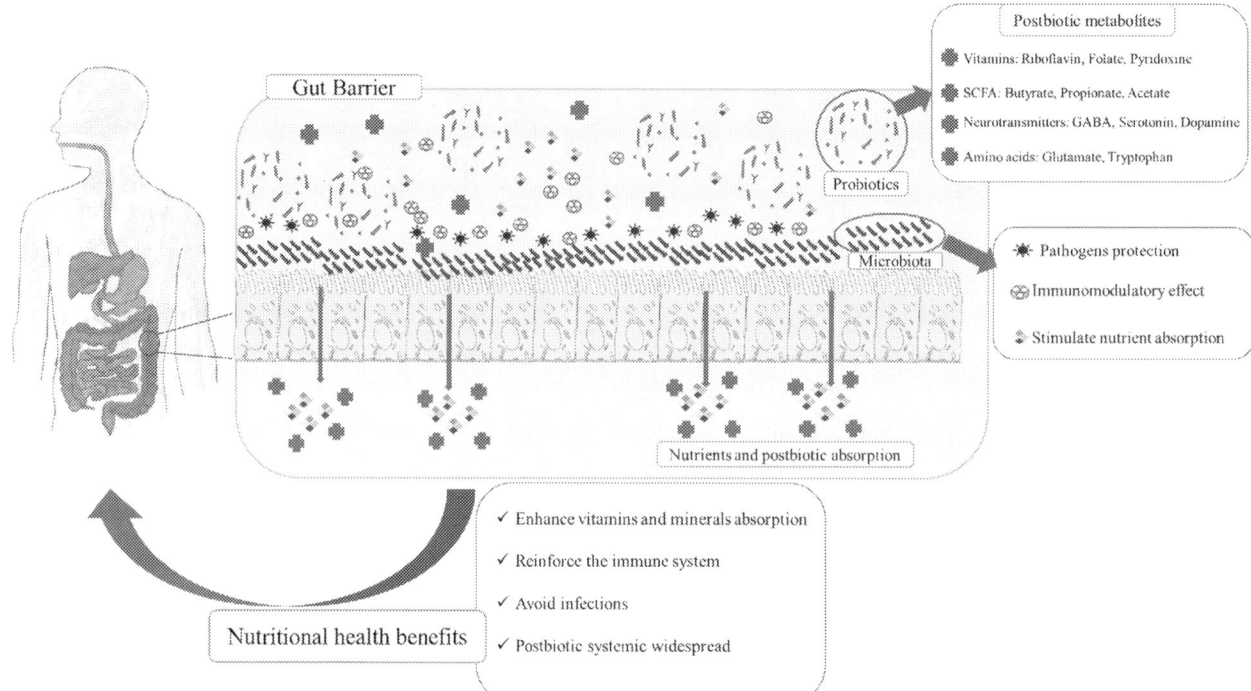

FIGURE 27.1 Overview of gut microbiota and probiotics health benefits. The figure shows how the probiotics in the intestinal microbiota produce postbiotics that are metabolites, such as vitamins, short-chain fatty acids, neurotransmitters, and amino acids. Probiotics and postbiotics allow maintaining a healthy intestinal barrier by generating protection against pathogens, as well as having an immunomodulatory effect and stimulating the absorption of nutrients. This combination allows healthy effects through nutrition through the intake of these compounds (probiotics and postbiotics). *From Diez-Gutiérrez L., San Vicente L., R. Barrón L.J., Villarán, M. del C. and Chávarri M., Gamma-aminobutyric acid and probiotics: Multiple health benefits and their future in the global functional food and nutraceuticals market, Journal of Functional Foods 64, 2020, 1–14. https://doi.org/10.1016/j.jff.2019.103669. Image edited by the author Lucía Diez-Gutiérrez.*

27.1.1 Probiotics: source, variety, and potential

Conventionally, probiotic microorganism has been isolated from dairy products, such as different types of cheeses, kefir, buttermilk and yogurt, and human GI tract or breast milk. According to the current demand of probiotics, the screening of these microorganisms has moved to unconventional raw materials focusing on traditional fermented foods, fruits, vegetables, or other natural sources (Sornplang & Piyadeatsoontorn, 2016). For instance, Yu et al. (2013) used traditional Chinese sauerkraut to isolate probiotics and identified their potential beneficial properties. Erginkaya et al. (2018) performed a similar isolation process of probiotic strains from traditional Turkish dairy products, for instance, Tulum cheese, yogurt, cokelek, camis cream, and kefir.

Currently, the variety of probiotics is mainly composed of lactic acid bacteria (LAB) that are classified as Gram-positive cocci or bacilli cytochrome and catalase-negative characterized by producing a large amount of lactic acid during the fermentation of sugars. This kind of microorganisms are also classified as nonspore-forming and aerotolerant, which could admit a low concentration of oxygen, or microaerophilic, or need a lack of oxygen, anaerobic. The LAB group is mostly composed by bacteria from genera *Lactobacillus, Streptococcus, Lactococcus, Leuconostoc, Weisella, Pediococcus*, and *Oenococcus* (Papadimitriou et al., 2016; Yépez & Tenea, 2015). Other probiotics closely linked to LAB are the *Bifidobacterium* genera. These bacteria are anaerobic gram-positive curved and bifurcated rod-shaped, which are generally classified as catalase negative and nonspore-forming (Shah, 2011). According to the sugar fermentation, *Bifidobacterium* strains also produce lactic acid but mainly produce acetic acid. Moreover, *Bifidobacterium* genome encodes the fructose-6-phosphate phosphoketolase that catalyzes the breakdown of hexose phosphate molecules into erythrose-4-phosphate plus acetyl phosphate. However, this pathway is not present in LAB being therefore a suitable test to distinguish both groups (Hoover, 2014).

Lee et al. (2018) made an overview of the *Lactobacillus* strains (*L. acidophilus, L. fermentum, L. reuteri*, or *L. plantarum*), *Bifidobacterium* strains (*Bifidobacterium bifidum, Bifidobacterium breve*, or *Bifidobacterium animalis*), or *Streptococcus thermophilus* that have been currently classified as nutribiotics.

Furthermore, several studies have reported that some yeasts, such as *Saccharomyces cerevisiae, D. hansenii, Kluyveromyces lactis, Yarrowia lipolitica,* or *Torulaspora delbrueckii,* could have the potential to be classified as probiotics. Nevertheless, none of these yeasts have been properly classified as probiotics (Hatoum et al., 2012). Palma et al. (2015) explained that *Saccharomyces boulardi*, belonging to the same species as *S. cerevisiae*, is the only yeast currently declared as a human probiotic, proved by different clinical trials. For a long time, probiotic activity research has mainly focused on bacteria but ongoing studies are trying to prove the probiotic effect of different types of yeasts and fungi (Chuang et al., 2020). For instance, Wang et al. (2019) studied the potential probiotic effect of the nonpathogenic yeast *Diutina rugosa*, which has resistance against GI environment and the ability to colonize and adhere to intestinal cells, considered proper probiotic characteristics. Karim et al. (2020) has reported that *Kluyveromyces marxianus* is a promising nonconventional probiotic yeast due to its potential health benefits, such as immune system and cholesterol modulation, antioxidative properties and resistance against adverse GI conditions. Moreover, the fungus *Aspergillus oryzae* also present potential probiotic effects, such as prevention of bacterial infection, potential to reconstruct the microbiota, or maintenance of the immune system, due to the studies performed with pigs, poultries, and fishes (Dawood et al., 2020). The same happens with *Eurotium cristatus (Aspergillus cristatus)*, which can modulate the gut microbiota of mice (Kang et al., 2019).

Despite the wide variety of potential probiotic microorganisms, specific characteristics are required to be considered as probiotics. Fontana et al. (2013) portrayed that probiotics should be Generally Regarded as Safe microorganisms for instance, they cannot present any pathogenic, toxic, or another potential side negative effect. In addition, they indicated that probiotics need to survive adverse environment conditions related to the GI tract, such as the high concentration of bile salts and the pH stress. FAO/WHO (2006) reported specific safety and functionality properties that need to be assayed in vitro, such as hemolytic activity, resistance against pH and salinity, microorganism aggregation, antibiotic resistance, antimicrobial activity, adhesion ability to gut cells, cholesterol modulation, or immunomodulatory effect. Angmo et al. (2016) reported that the resistance against acidic pH, lysozyme, and bile salts were relevant characteristics to survive the stressful environment of the GI tract. Moreover, they reported that aggregation and hydrophobicity are properties related to the ability of microorganisms to adhere to intestinal epithelial cells. In addition, these authors highlighted the importance of the characterization of probiotics without potential harmful properties related to hemolytic activity, pathogen inhibitory effect, or antibiotic resistance capacity.

27.1.2 Postbiotics: bioactive probiotic products

Nowadays, probiotic research is moving toward the importance of probiotic products due to their potential beneficial effect on health. These probiotic products have been defined as postbiotics, including metabolic compounds and the nonviable bacterial products that present a relevant biological activity (George et al., 2018). Cuevas-González et al. (2020) have even specified postbiotics are considered only soluble factors produced by bacteria metabolism or released after the probiotic breakdown. In this regard, they considered that dead probiotics are best classified as paraprobiotics.

Furthermore, among the metabolic compounds considered as postbiotics are organic acids, lipids, proteins, and other complex molecules, which can modulate the immune system, inflammatory response, cholesterol accumulation, or antioxidant effect (Aguilar-Toalá et al., 2018). Diez-Gutiérrez et al. (2020) summarized different compounds considered postbiotics due to their potential health benefit, such as short-chain fatty acids (SCFA) (acetate, butyrate, or propionate), vitamins (folate, biotin, or riboflavin), bacteriocins (nisin or glycocin), neurotransmitters [gamma-aminobutyric acid (GABA), serotonin, dopamine, or acetylcholine], or mediators of inflammation (lactocepin).

A good way to determine the ability of probiotics to produce postbiotic metabolites is using cell-free supernatants (CFS) obtained after probiotic in vitro fermentation under specific conditions. Thus supernatants obtained from probiotics, such as *L. acidophilus* and *L. casei*, could modulate the inflammatory response decreasing the TNF-α secretion and increasing the synthesis of IL-10 in the intestinal epithelia (Żółkiewicz et al., 2020). Moreover, Moradi et al. (2019) studied the potential benefits of CFS produced by *Lactobacillus* strains, such as *L. acidophilus*, *L. casei*, and *L. salivarius*. The characterization was based on the analysis of the antimicrobial effect of the lyophilized CFS against the pathogen *L. monocytogenes*, the influence of CFS in the formation of biofilms, and the potential cytotoxic effect. Promising results were shown for CFS produced by *L. salivarius* reporting high effectiveness against *L. monocytogenes*, resistance under stressful environments, and safe for consumption.

Likewise, researchers have analyzed the potential applications of postbiotics improving probiotics efficiency or, even, use postbiotics as active ingredients due to their potency against several types of diseases (Hernández-Granados & Franco-Robles, 2020). Singh et al. (2018) gather information about the beneficial implications of postbiotics. Their highlighted postbiotics effects, such as the modulation of neural diseases, alterations in the immune system, metabolic disorders, cardiovascular diseases, or pathogen infections.

27.2 Nutritional health benefits of probiotics and postbiotics

The wide variety of beneficial effects from probiotic supplementation could be reinforced with postbiotics, as they could enhance the crosstalk between the host and the gut microbiota. According to the huge amount of probiotic microorganisms and the substances included in the postbiotic term, diverse mechanisms of action are expected to undertake their beneficial effect on the gut microbiota (Żółkiewicz et al., 2020). Million et al. (2017) supported the relationship between the alteration of the gut microbiota and malnutrition situations. Malnutrition is considered a worldwide concern that affects millions of people every year mainly produced by low dietary intake, malabsorption of micro- or macronutrients or higher energy requirements. The malnutrition term includes the range of under- and overnutrition situations. Likewise, malnutrition situations could be related to other types of health problems worsening the symptomatology and decreasing the quality of life. For instance, malnutrition could be associated to gastroenterology illnesses (Norman et al., 2006), cancer (de Pinho et al., 2019), or infectious diseases (Rai et al., 2002). The potential beneficial effects that probiotics could have under several nutritional health disorders are shown in Table 27.1.

27.2.1 Undernutrition situations

Undernutrition embraces the deficit of several macronutrients, such as proteins, and micronutrients like vitamins and minerals. Generally, this kind of deficiencies produce the disruption of the body homeostasis and triggers health problems associated with skin alterations, liver disturbances, or diarrhea associated to the imbalanced microbiota (Million et al., 2017). Therefore several research have wonder how probiotics could improve the nutritional status of malnourished people. Sheridan et al. (2014) conducted an in-depth review of the most common malnutrition situations and the potential of probiotics to address these concerns in susceptible population, such as children, pregnant women, or elderly people.

27.2.1.1 Children nutritional deficiencies

Kambale et al. (2021) reported that around 200 million children are currently suffering undernutrition and this situation supposes the 45% of children death every year. They consider that diarrhea is one of the biggest problems as it leads to infections, increase the situation of severe malnutrition and raise the death rate. Therefore several studies have focused on severe acute malnutrition (SAM) due to its high incidence and the severe side effects produced, such as weak immune system, cognitive deficiencies or appearance of the nutritional edema called kwashiorkor. Also, this nutritional problem could enhance the development of other types of diseases such diabetes, coronary problems, pneumonia and infections produced by *S. aureus*, *Salmonella*, *Klebsiella*, or *E. coli* (Million et al., 2017; Sheridan et al., 2014). Kerac et al. (2009) performed the PRONUT study based on a randomized double-blind placebo-controlled trial with 795 children who suffered SAM and used a combination of four different well-known probiotics, *Pediococcus pentosaceus*, *Leuconostoc mesenteroides*, *Lactobacillus paracasei*, and *Lactobacillus plantarum*, combined with several prebiotics. The results of this study suggested that probiotics have the potential to improve the health of SAM children and decrease the mortality rate. Following this study, Grenov et al. (2017) developed another double-blind, randomized, placebo-controlled study with 400 SAM children and they evaluated how the probiotics *B. animalis* and *L. rhamnosus* influenced diarrhea and pneumonia caused by SAM. Likewise, the results showed that probiotics could reduce the time of suffering severe diarrhea and decrease the mortality rate. Castro-Mejía et al. (2020) also evaluated the probiotic effect of *L. rhamnosus* and *B. animalis* in SAM children. In this case, they analyzed the evolution of the gut microbiota when these probiotics were administered. The consumption of probiotics decreases the days with diarrhea associated to SAM; however, heterogenic results were shown if they presented kwashiorkor or not.

Following this trend, Alou et al. (2017) went one step further using metagenomic and culturomic techniques to accurately identify the microorganisms involved in SAM. For that purpose, the microbiota of SAM and healthy children were investigated to determine the deficient microorganisms, which could be characterized and potentially supplied as probiotics. The results showed a wide variety of potential probiotics, such as *Bacillus subtilis*, *B. adolescentis*, *Weisella confusa*, or *L. parabuchneri*, which presented different functions in the microbiota, such as antioxidant activity, antibacterial function, mutualism with other microorganisms, or production of postbiotics.

More recently, Kambale et al. (2021) carried out a systematic review of the trials performed since 1990 to 2020 in people affected by SAM. They indicated that gut microbiota alteration, mainly *B. longum* absence, affects the synthesis of vitamins, energy harvest, or immune system development, which is linked to malabsorption, pathogens' infection, and diarrhea. As well, the diarrhea decreases the absorption of proteins, potassium, zinc, or other micronutrients essentials for the correct body function. The probiotic supplementation increases the absorption of calcium, zinc, or different

TABLE 27.1 Representation of the probiotics that present a nutritional health benefit.

Nutritional health		Probiotic	Probiotic health	References
Undernutrition	Severe acute malnutrition in children	L. paracasei, L. plantarum, L. rhamnosus, B. animalis, B. adolescentis, W. confusa, P. pentosaceus, B. subtilis	• Alleviate diarrhea • Increase vitamins and minerals absorption • Synthetize of B group vitamins	Grenov et al. (2017), Kerac et al. (2009), and Leblanc et al. (2011)
	Pregnancy malnourishment	L. rhamnosus, B. lactis, L. acidophilus, L. plantarum, B. animalis, L. fermentum, L. reuteri, S. thermophilus	• Enhance iron assimilation • Stimulate folate production and metabolisms	Ballini et al. (2020) and Rusu et al. (2020)
	Frailty syndrome in the elderly	L. reuteri, B. longum, L. helveticus, L. paracasei, L. plantarum, L. brevis, L. zymae, B. bifidum, L. bulgaricus	• Increase vitamin D synthesis • Modulate inflammatory response • Synthetize neurotransmitters as GABA serotonin or dopamine	Diez-Gutiérrez et al. (2020), Lei et al. (2016), and Rizzoli and Biver (2020)
Overnutrition	Cardiovascular diseases	Enterococcus sp., L. plantarum	• Cholesterol modulation • Increase bile salts elimination	Liu et al. (2017) and Nuhwa et al. (2019)
	Metabolic disorders	L. rhamnosus, L. plantarum, L. gasseri, L. acidophilus, L. curvatus, B. breve	• Modulate glucose levels • Interfere in adipocytes functionality	Cani and Van Hul (2015) and Mallappa et al. (2012)
Malnutrition associated to other disorders	Irritable bowel diseases	L. rhamnosus, L. plantarum, L. bulgaricus, B. animalis, B. longum, S. boulardi, L. reuteri, L. fermentum	• Increase micronutrients absorption • Modulate the inflammatory response • Enhance the synthesis of amino acids and SCFA	Lee et al. (2018), Lichtenstein et al. (2016), Martínez-Abad et al. (2016), and Turroni et al. (2012)
	Pathogens infection	L. reuteri, L. acidophilus, L. bulgaricus, S. thermophilus, L. plantarum, S. faecium	• Enhance the immune system • Reinforce mucosal barrier • Increase the nutritional status avoiding longer illnesses	Goderska et al. (2018) and Ruggiero (2014)
	Food intolerances	B. lactis, L. casei, B. longum, L. acidophilus, S. thermophilus, B. infantis	• Protect against intestinal cell damage • Increase nutrients absorption	Gingold-Belfer et al. (2020) and Sousa Moraes et al. (2014)

vitamins and avoids pathogens' colonization. Hence, probiotics' potential leads to alleviate diarrhea, decrease the risk to develop anemia, and reduce hospitalization time. Moreover, probiotics could also alleviate SAM through the synthesis of useful postbiotic compounds, such as vitamins or bacteriocins. Leblanc et al. (2011) indicated the potential of several LAB to produce B group vitamins, such as riboflavin, folate, or vitamin B12.

27.2.1.2 Pregnant women nutritional deficiencies

Maternal and fetal health could be compromised due to the deficiency of micronutrients, such as vitamins and minerals, which are necessary to preserve the body homeostasis, cell functionality, and metabolic activity. Therefore these micronutrients have an essential influence on pregnancy through the materno-placental fetal axis. For instance, vitamins' deficiency in pregnant women could affect the organogenesis process or could trigger epigenetic disturbances due to the alteration in the DNA methylation leading to an increased likelihood that the fetus will develop insulin resistance, obesity, or hypertension (Gernand et al., 2016). Mantaring et al. (2018) reported that pregnant and breastfeeding women need to consume supplements, such as iron, folate, or vitamin B6, to enhance the proper development of the baby. Hence, this study was focused on assessing the beneficial effect of using probiotics combined with maternal nutritional supplements. Promising results were obtained after the oral consumption of *L. rhamnosus* and *B. lactis* combined with different kind of vitamins, minerals, proteins, and lipids due to the increase of the nutrient absorption and the energy density. Furthermore, Bisanz et al. (2015) used a yogurt fortified with the probiotic *L. rhamnosus* combined with Moringa plant characterized due to its high amount of vitamin A, iron, zinc, or calcium, among others. This combination could be a cheap way to preserve a healthy microbiota and avoid the micronutrients deficiency. Khalili et al. (2020) studied how to increase the folate content into yogurt by adding different types of probiotics, such as *S. thermophilus*, *B. lactis*, *L. acidophilus*, or *L. plantarum*, that could produce folate as a postbiotic. The results obtained showed a higher amount of folate with the fortification with *L. plantarum* strains, suggesting that some probiotics could be an alternative way to the synthetic folic acid. Following this trend, Bardosono et al. (2019) performed a clinical trial with pregnant women to evaluate how the probiotic *B. animalis* could modulate the plasma levels of vitamins B12, B6, and folate. This research showed that the supplementation of this probiotic increased the blood levels of these vitamins providing potential health benefits. For example, vitamin B12 enhances the metabolism of folate and decreases the risk of cardiovascular diseases (CAD) avoiding the synthesis of homocysteine and the combination of this vitamin with B6 and folate maintains the correct methylation process involved in the synthesis of DNA and thus in the development of the fetus. Ballini et al. (2020) carried out a pilot study with 20 pregnant women to determine the effect of a probiotic mix and the kiwi fruit powder in the availability of folate. The probiotics used in this experiment, *B. infantis*, *L. plantarum*, *L. rhamnosus*, *L. fermentum*, *L. reuteri*, and *L. acidophilus*, were selected according to their ability to increase the absorption of nutrients, the natural synthesis of folate, and the modulation of the immune system. Likewise, the consumption of these probiotics supposed an increase in the folate concentration coupled with the modulation of the levels of sugar in blood and the women weight during the gestational time.

Anemia is another health problem commonly associated to pregnant women who suffered micronutrients deficiency, and it is experienced by about half of pregnant women worldwide. Generally, this health problem is produced by the deficiency of vitamin A, considered essential for the embryogenesis process, cell maintenance, tissue synthesis or hematopoiesis, or iron needed for the immune system and neurological maintenance (Van Den Broek, 2003). Vonderheid et al. (2019) performed a wide analysis to determine how probiotics could increase the absorption of iron. A significant increase in the iron absorption was reported with the supplementation of *L. plantarum* strains. Rusu et al. (2020) also carried out a wide research of the most significant probiotics that could alleviate anemia through the increase in iron absorption and bioavailability. In this review, they highlighted the potential effect of *L. fermentum*, which could interact with enterocytes to improve the iron levels and enhance its absorption, *L. acidophilus*, involved in the ferritin formation and iron assimilation, or *S. thermophilus*, that influence the iron binding, hemoglobin and ferritin.

27.2.1.3 Elderly nutritional deficiencies

During the last decades, the ageing process has been directly linked to the modification of the gut microbiota through the decrease of beneficial microorganisms coupled with an increase of potentially pathogenic bacteria. Consequently, elderly people could suffer the deterioration of some essential biological functions required for a healthy microbiota, such as low levels of SCFA or reduction of macro and micronutrients absorption, which leads to malnutrition situations (Salazar et al., 2017). Poor nutritional status in elderly people could produce the frailty syndrome (FS) supposing the loss of organs functionality, increase the DNA damage, or enhance metabolic disorders (Salvatella-Flores & Bermúdez-Humarán, 2020). Lorenzo-López et al. (2017) evaluated the relation between FS and the nutritional status. They highlighted that the development of this syndrome is related to the low consumption and assimilation of essential micronutrients, such as vitamin B6, D, E, or C, folate, or macronutrients including proteins and thus amino acids. Salazar et al. (2017) agreed on the relationship between the deficiency of some vitamins, proteins, and iron and added that this kind of alterations could trigger neurological disorders, anorexia, loss of bone mass, depletion of the immune system, or gut alterations. Recently, Davinelli et al. (2021) supported that the improvement of the nutritional status using functional nutrients could decrease the likelihood to suffer FS. Based on their review, they considered functional nutrients those involved in specific physiological benefits including mineral and vitamins supplements, carotenoids, prebiotics, and probiotics. Patel et al. (2014) explained that probiotics could enhance the solubility of minerals like calcium and magnesium through the synthesis of SCFA, such as butyrate and lactate, which increase the absorption of these compounds and thus promote bone health. Rizzoli and Biver (2020) also supported the potential of probiotics to maintain the health of bone. For instance, probiotics, such as *L. reuteri*, *L. paracasei*, *B. longum* and *L. helveticus*, could reduce the osteoclastic bone resorption decreasing the response of proinflammatory cytokines. Likewise, those probiotics could also increase the levels of vitamin D by producing lactic acid, which indirectly stimulates the expression of vitamin D receptors. Lei et al. (2016) carried out a clinical trial with 417 elderly people who had suffered a distal radius fracture. In this case, *L. casei* was used to determine the effect of this microorganisms on the patient's recovery. The results indicated that the consumption of probiotics could decrease the recovery time.

Moreover, the FS has also been linked to cognitive deterioration associated to different types of dementia, Alzheimer's disease, and Parkinson's disease. The improvement of the nutritional status with the supplementation of antioxidants, flavonoids, and vitamins C, B, E, or D may prevent or delay the worsening of these diseases (Gómez-Gómez & Zapico, 2019). Also, scientific evidence currently remarks the important connection between the gut and brain, how the gut microbiota influences the development of neurological diseases and the phsychomodulatory effect of probiotic microorganisms. Therefore probiotic strains that can produce positive psychiatric effects on patients with psychopathologies are defined as psychobiotics (Tyagi et al., 2020). This type of probiotics influences the relation between the host and the brain exerting antidepressant effects that can alter emotional, cognitive, and neuronal indices (Dinan et al., 2013). As mentioned before, psychobiotics act by reducing host neurodegeneration by decreasing oxidative stress, modulating cytokine milieu and thus reducing circulating proinflammatory cytokines and/or altering brain hormones or neurotrophic factors. In addition, psychobiotic action is strain and species specific, as well as the mechanism of action with respect to reduction of mental stress (Talbott et al., 2019). For example, Lister (2020) analyzed the effect of nutrition and lifestyle on the development of Parkinson disease. This study suggested that nutritional supplements, such as vitamins B and D, probiotics, antioxidants, or flavonoids, could decrease the inflammation process. Szczechowiak et al. (2019) summarized the impact diet and nutritional status in the progression of Alzheimer disease, indicating the antiinflammatory effect of vitamins complexes, probiotics, flavonoids like resveratrol, polyphenols like curcumins, or alkaloids as caffeine. Diez-Gutiérrez et al. (2020) reported that postbiotics, such as GABA, serotonin, dopamine, or acetylcholine, could have a beneficial effect of neurological disorders.

27.2.2 Overnutrition situations

Overnutrition is considered another type of malnutrition associated to the excessive consumption of nutrients. This exaggerated nutrient intake produces the mitochondria and endoplasmic reticulum stress due to the high concentration of metabolites that need to be processed and assimilated. Therefore the imbalance between nutrient intake and the energy consumed have a side effect on the proper function of the enzymes involved in catabolism and triggers the stimulation of other enzymes which generates a metabolic imbalance. Also, this nutrient overload leads to the increased accumulation of fat or lipogenesis. Currently, overnutritions situations enhance the provability to develop cardiometabolic disorders, such as hypertension, diabetes, metabolic disorders, or obesity (Aggarwal et al., 2012; Qiu & Schlegel, 2018).

27.2.2.1 Cardiovascular diseases

CVD are an increasing cause of death generally caused by smoking, obesity, a sedentary routine, diabetes, stress, or lipid abnormalities. According to this information, alteration in the levels of body lipids, such as low- and high-density lipoprotein-cholesterol, LDL-C and HDLC-C, or triglycerides, could increase the likelihood to develop CVD (Thushara et al., 2016). DiRienzo (2014) explained that high levels of LDL-C could trigger coronary heart disease (CHD) through the formation of atherosclerotic plaques. Therefore therapies have been developed to decrease the risk to develop CHD focusing on lowering the LDL-C. In addition, low levels of HDL-C or high levels of triacylglycerol and triglyceride-rich proteins could increase the risk to develop CHD. Likewise, Nuhwa et al. (2019) reported how LABs isolated from flowers can modulate the cholesterol levels by testing the capacity of these LABs to assimilate cholesterol. The results showed that seven *Enterococcus* sp. and four *L. plantarum* presented bile salt hydrolase (BSH) activity coupled with high cholesterol assimilation. In addition, the assimilation of cholesterol and the BSH activity suggests that these probiotics are promising ways to prevent hypercholesterolemia diseases. Liu et al. (2017) performed an in vivo study to determine the ability of *L. plantarum* strainsto modulate the levels of cholesterol. Positive results were obtained because this probiotic reduced the liver and serum cholesterol, regulated the levels of triglycerides, and increased the bile acids elimination. Hence, *L. plantarum* could be considered as a tool to prevent CVD.

27.2.2.2 Metabolic disorders

The metabolic syndrome (Ms) is a worldwide concern mainly produced in obese people. This pathology could increase the risk to develop CVD, raise the blood pressure, or trigger insulin resistance (Grundy, 2016). Mallappa et al. (2012) presented the potential benefits of using probiotics in patients who suffered metabolic disorders, such as obesity, diabetes, and Ms. Probiotics, such as *L. rhamnosus*, *L. plantarum*, *Lactobacillus gasseri*, or *L. acidophilus*, were highlighted due to their ability to reduce the cholesterol, modulate adipocytes functionality, and thus maintain the body weight avoiding the fat accumulation. Cani and Van Hul (2015) added that *B. animalis*, *B. breve*, *L. curvatus*, or *L. reuteri* could have important metabolic effects through the modulation of glucose levels, cholesterol, and triglycerides concentration. Also, these probiotic could modulate the inflammatory response, decrease the accumulation of fats in the liver and preserve the body weight, essential characteristics to prevent Ms, diabetes, and obesity. The systematic review of Tenorio-Jiménez et al. (2020) analyzed the effect of probiotics in clinical trials performed in Ms patients. Beneficial effects were shown with the supplementation of probiotics and indicated that these microorganisms could be used as a good adjuvant to current therapies.

27.2.2.3 Malnutrition and other health disorders

27.2.2.3.1 Gastrointestinal disorders

For a long time, probiotics have been used as a complement to treat GI tract disorders. Disorders mainly produced by dysbiosis or other alterations in the microbiota that can affect the correct functioning of the GI tract. Generally, the available probiotics present interesting mechanisms which involve the regulation of inflammatory cascades, absorption of nutrients, modulation of hypersensitivity reactions, improvement of the GI barrier, and suppression of pathogens. Therefore Lee et al. (2018) explained that some probiotics, such as *L. rhamnosus*, *L. plantarum*, *L. bulgaricus*, or *B. animalis*, have been used to treat different nutritional problems that involved disorders, such as antibiotic-associated diarrhea, acute diarrhea, or food intolerances, among others. Hence, there is a wide variety of investigations that were conducted to test the effect of these probiotics in several GI disorders (Verna & Lucak, 2010).

Brown and Mullin (2011) supported that patients with irritable bowel disease (IBD), such as Crohn's disease (CD), or ulcerative colitis (UC), required specific dietary guidelines to maintain their life quality. Among these guidelines, they remarked the importance of consuming supplements, such as multivitamins, minerals, probiotics, or prebiotics, trying to avoid any nutritional deficiency. Judkins et al. (2020) remarked the importance of using probiotics IBD patients to enhance the permeability and nutrient absorption decreasing the malnutrition risk and improving the immune system.

For example, *B. longum* is considered the most common *Bifidobacterium* species found in the GI tract of adults and infants (Turroni et al., 2012). Palma et al. (2015) reported a lower level of *B. longum* in the stool of CD patients than in healthy individuals. In this sense, the oral administration of *B. longum* could provide beneficial effects on human health (Zhang et al., 2019). In the same way, Tamaki et al. (2016) evaluated the efficiency of *B. longum* in UC patients. The trial showed that the supplementation of this probiotic could modulate the production of cytokines and enhance the mucosal barrier, suggesting that this microorganism could be a promising complement for UC patients.

Furthermore, Lichtenstein et al. (2016) summarized how probiotic therapies could alleviate Crohn's patients and they highlighted that *S. boulardi* could be a promising probiotic for this disease compared to other probiotic microorganisms. Fedorak et al. (2015) also evaluated the benefits of probiotics in Crohn's patients. In this case, they found out that the supplementation of single strain probiotic was not significantly beneficial for patients. However, the consumption of the mixture called VSL#3, composed of four strains of *Lactobacillus*, three strains of *Bifidobacterium*, and a strain of *Streptococcus salivarius*, could be useful to decrease the inflammatory response.

Similarly, Martínez-Abad et al. (2016) focused on the immunomodulatory effect of the probiotics *L. rhamnosus*, *L. fermentum*, and *B. lactis*. Their mechanisms of action could be helpful to modulate the immune response of IBD patients. Similar modulation of the immune response in patients affected by IBD was shown by *L. plantarum* strains.

Also, the consumption of this probiotic could alleviate the symptomatology IBD, such as abdominal bloating and pain (Vries et al., 2006).

Studies have also focus on the potential effect of probiotic and postbiotics combination against GI disorders. Haileselassie et al. (2016) evaluated how immune cells responded after the supplementation of CFS rich in postbiotics produced by *L. reuteri*. These postbiotics had a strong effect on the regulation of dendritic cells followed by the influence on regulatory T cells. Moreover, an increase in the synthesis of IL-10 was shown along with a reduction in the expression of genes related to proinflammatory response. These results indicated that the identification of the postbiotics presented in the CFS was needed to use them in clinical assays based on necrotizing enterocolitis (NEC) or IBS. In this regard, Patel et al. (2014) concluded that probiotics are a good way to prevent NEC development as these microorganisms can fight against pathogen colonization, strengthen the intestinal epithelial barrier, and block inflammatory pathways. Therefore probiotics can be considered essential for the prevention of NEC and postbiotics could be used to enhance their effectiveness. Butyric acid is a promising postbiotic useful for NEC because this SCFA can suppress the inflammatory response, modulate apoptosis, and maintain the colon cell structure. Russo et al. (2019) also indicated that SCFAs and tryptophan are postbiotics with a potentially positive effect on CD and UC through the interconnection of the gut microbiota with the innate and adaptative immune cells.

27.2.2.3.2 Pathogens infection

Probiotic supplementation has also moved around the infection of the GI tract by *Helicobacter pylori*, characterized due to its high infection rate, which can trigger chronic gastritis, gastric adenocarcinoma, or peptic ulcer. Gonzalez and López-Carrillo (2010) indicated the importance of the nutritional status to decrease the likelihood to develop cancer. Likewise, several studies have been focused on using probiotics as a complementary treatment to this pathogen Goderska et al. (2018). Zhang et al. (2019) explained how *Lactobacillus*, *Streptococcus*, and *Bifidobacterium* strains could be useful to eradicate *H. pylori* as they could inhibit the urease activity, avoid cell adhesion, stimulate the immune system, and reinforce the mucosal barrier.

27.2.2.3.3 Food intolerances

As well as, studies were carried out trying to determine the benefits of probiotics in different types of food intolerances. Sousa Moraes et al. (2014) summarized how probiotic microorganisms could counteract the side effects produced by gluten proteins, such as gliadins and glutenins, which trigger the development of the celiac disease. They indicated that microorganisms, such as *B. lactis*, *L. casei*, and *B. longum*, could protect the epithelial cells against the damage caused by gliadins. Moreover, in this study, they highlighted the effectiveness of using a combination of probiotic strains, such as VSL#3, which hydrolyzes gliadins more efficiently than single-strain probiotics. Gingold-Belfer et al. (2020) performed a clinical trial with lactose-intolerant patients who were treated with a probiotic cocktail called Bio-25 composed by 11 different strains, including *L. acidophilus*, *L. rhamnosus*, *L. casei*, *B. breve*, *S. thermophilus*, *B. longum*, and *B. infantis*. Significant reduction of the symptoms and enhancement of the lactose absorption was shown due to the β-galactosidase activity of the probiotics supplied.

27.3 Encapsulation technology for the development of functional ingredients

As previously stated, intestinal microbiota influences immune functions and the development and metabolism processes in the different organs of body, including the brain. If the alteration of the microbiota leads to a disease development, triggered by an inadequate homeostatic regulation, the challenge is to manage the composition of the microbiota and compensate for any alterations that may occur to minimize the negative impact on the immune functions or metabolism processes in the host.

The restoration of the intestinal microbiota using live microorganisms requires the definition of dietary supplementation strategies that allow these microorganisms to reach the intestine alive (Ma et al., 2019; Roselino et al., 2020). Likewise, if the compounds of interest are postbiotics or parabiotics, the stability of these molecules must be guaranteed in the environment of the intestinal microbiota (Perez-Burgos et al., 2013; Wu et al., 2020). In both postbiotic and parabiotic cases, the formulation and processing of a food or nutritional or nutraceutical supplement can result in a loss of the desired functionality when the probiotic dies or the postbiotic or parabiotic is not functional.

Food matrix composition (pH, nutritional composition, water activity, natural antibiotic presence, etc.) may alter the probiotic cell viability during the processing and storage time, as well as during the GI transit after intake. Dairy products are considered as effective vector for the probiotic bacteria delivery into the GI tract, due to the high buffering capacity of milk proteins, which can protect the bacterial cells during gastric transit. Aljutaily et al. (2020) evaluated the influence of the food matrix on the mouse gut microbiota enriched with *Clostridium butyricum* used as probiotic. The presence of prebiotics, milk protein with high buffering capacity, or dense structure of dairy products were relevant factors for the bacteria viability. Chocolate is another interesting food matrix to improve the probiotic cell viability. The low water activity of this food matrix linked to the presence of protective substances, such as milk proteins and sugars, contributes to a high stability of probiotic bacteria, such as *Bacillus coagulans*, *Lactobacillus*, or *Bifidobacterium*, during storage (Cielecka-Piontek et al., 2020; Kobus-Cisowska et al., 2019). However, the convenience of other food matrices, such as fruits or vegetable matrices, depends on pH value, concentration of lactic and acetic acids and presence of antioxidant and antimicrobial substances. For example, the fermentation of a tomato juice with different *Lactobacillus* spp. leads to changes in pH, acidity, and sugar content that can affect probiotic viability, and in consequence, limiting the storage time and conditions (Yoon et al., 2004). Therefore the application of probiotic cultures in different food matrices is nowadays a great challenge for the food industry.

In this regard, the encapsulation of probiotics, prebiotics, postbiotics, and parabiotics is probably one of the most promising and successful strategies to achieve the protection of these components until their release in the large intestine. Microencapsulation may be defined as the process of enveloping or surrounding any substance (encapsulated material, in this case, bacteria, yeasts, postbiotics, etc.) within another substance (encapsulating material preferably biopolymers) on a very small scale, yielding microcapsules ranging from less than one micron to several hundred microns in size. The main purpose of microencapsulation is to produce particles that control mass transport behavior in some way. The microcapsule matrix or shell is designed to prevent diffusion of material from or into the microcapsule to achieve the protection of sensitive components in an oxidative o degradative environment. However, at the same time, the encapsulated material must be released in the large intestine and the mechanism should be controlled by pH change, transit time, or colonic microbiota enzymes.

Depending on the nature of encapsulated substances, the purpose of the encapsulation, and the release mechanism selected, different encapsulation technologies should be applied (Chávarri et al., 2012). The first aspect to be taken into account for selecting the encapsulation technology is the structure of the microcapsules that, in turn, will influence their functionality. Encapsulation technologies, such as spray-, freeze-, and vacuum drying and some extraction and coacervation processes generate regular or irregular geometry microcapsules containing small portions of encapsulated material (Fig. 27.2A). This multinuclear structure of the microcapsule allows a slow release of the encapsulated substances as the degradation of the matrix occurs, in comparison to the rapid release that would occur in the rupture of the mononuclear microcapsule obtained by some coacervation or emulsion processes (Fig. 27.2B). However, a well-established core−shell structure could offer a higher stability of the encapsulated active substances because they are not trapped onto the particle surface. Multinuclear microcapsules are usually more easily produced but the wall layer is not equally distributed over the multinuclear structures and it is difficult to achieve a standardization of the release kinetics in a set of these microcapsules as shown in Fig. 27.2 (Chávarri et al., 2012).

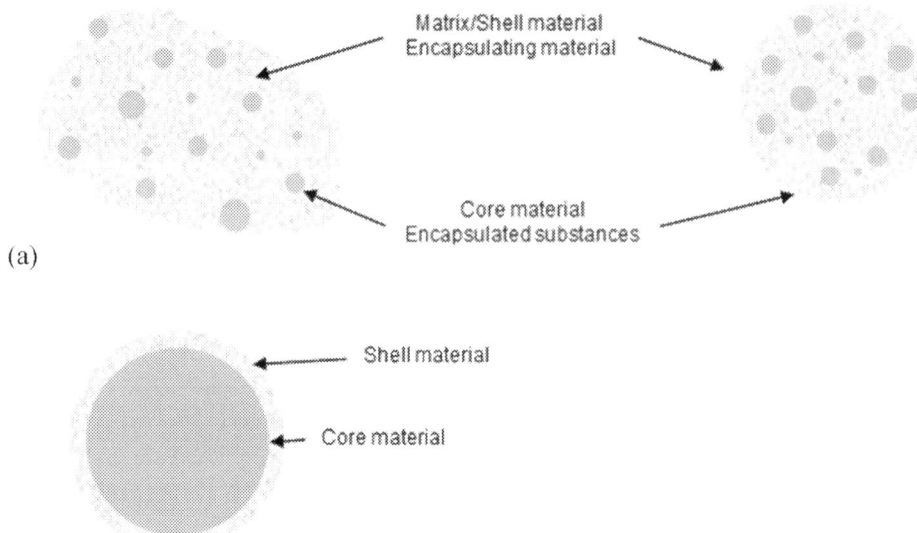

FIGURE 27.2 Multinuclear (A) and mononuclear (B) microcapsule structures. In the figure A, two different structures of microcapsules are observed, the corresponds to the multinuclear structure of a microcapsule where both the encapsulating material and the encapsulated compound are mixed. (B) A mononuclear structure where the center and the shell of the microcapsule are perfectly separated. *From Marañon, I., San Vicente, L., Hidalgo, N., & Chávarri, M., Multilayer probiotic microcapsules. Multilayer Probiotic Microcapsules." (EUROPE No. EP3205216A1). European Patent Application, 2016. Image edited by the author Izaskun Marañón.*

For example, a more cost-effective solution to improve the viability of some probiotic bacteria during food processing and along the product shelf life could be the use of spray-drying or chilling encapsulation technologies. The purpose of these techniques is to extend the survival of the bacteria, using the encapsulating material to isolate bacteria from the food matrix creating a barrier between them. *Lactobacillus acidophilus* and *B. animalis* subsp. *lactis* added to savory cereal bars improved their stability by microencapsulation compared to the incorporation of active or lyophilized bacteria. Encapsulated *Lactobacillus acidiphilus* ($>10^8$ CFU/g) remained stable for 30 days longer than lyophilized form did, until 90 days, and *B. animalis* remained stable for 105 days, 75 days longer than the lyophilized form, because the microorganisms inside the matrix were protected from the environment and remained in a latent state for longer (Bampi et al., 2016). Proper selection of the material of microcapsule shell not only can prolong the shelf life of the probiotic ingredient but also maximize the survival of probiotic cells as they pass through the gastric system. Bustamante et al. (2017) showed that the encapsulating material influenced the bacteria viability but also that this material did not protect in the same way the life of different types of bacteria encapsulated in a multinuclear structure not provided with a continuous shell. In this regard, the use of a combination of maltodextrin with vegetal soluble proteins as encapsulating material in a spray-drying process can improve the *Bifidobacterium infantis* and *Lactobacillus plantarum* viability during storage. Both probiotics showed an increase in resistance to simulated gastric conditions but *L. plantarum* cells were more sensitive to gastric juice than *B. infantis* cells probably due to the cell distribution into the microcapsule structure and the presence of cells on the particle surface.

The use of a three-fluid nozzle for spray-drying has improved the loading capacity and encapsulation efficiency of bioactive compounds due the core–shell droplet formation (Gorgannezhad et al., 2020). Tasch Holkem and Favaro-Trindade (2020) has also used a shell constituted by a mixture of protein complex and polysaccharide to increase the protection of *L. paracasei* and *B. animalis* encapsulated in solid lipid microparticles.

Up to now, the best encapsulation solutions usually require a combination of both types of structures to optimize the efficiency of microencapsulated products by maximizing the amount of active components that reach the large intestine intact. Thus a matrix structure that contains probiotics, postbiotics, parabiotics, or prebiotics covered by a continuous layer of a polymeric material that reduces matrix permeability from the inside to the outside of the microcapsules, or vice versa, can be an interesting solution to achieve functional ingredients more effective. Complex coacervation using chitosan coating on alginate or pectinate beads in which the active component is dispersed is an example of this matrix structure (Chávarri et al., 2012).

In this regard, a double-stage procedure (collection alginate beads from a calcium chloride bath and introducing them into a chitosan bath) to create an alginate-chitosan microcapsule shows a more structured chitosan coating layer (Zaeim, 2020). However, these scientific results require defining profitable and easily scalable processes to be commercially developed. Processes that involve a high number of stages do not usually fit with industrial requirements, so current research is focused on obtaining multilayer structures by applying concentric nozzles. This is the case of the stabilization of probiotics through extrusion in concentric nozzles (Oxley, 2012) or by one-step coaxial electrospinning procedure (Feng et al., 2020). Multilayer structures not only improve the stability of the active substances contained in the microcapsule core but also offer opportunities for more accurate controlled release systems. Furthermore, multilayer structure can achieve serial releases of the different components contained in each of the layers of the microcapsule increasing the dosage effectiveness of the active ingredient (Marañon et al., 2016). Fig. 27.3 depicts a scheme of a three-layer structure where the outer layer is a barrier that protects the inner layers during the gastric transit, the intermediate layer breaks down in the intestine first releasing the prebiotic component, and finally the microcapsule nucleus disintegrates to release a probiotic in the gut. This type of structure can serve for sequential release of different probiotics or for two different release times of the same encapsulated active component as shown in Fig. 27.3 (Oxley, 2012; Zaeim, 2020).

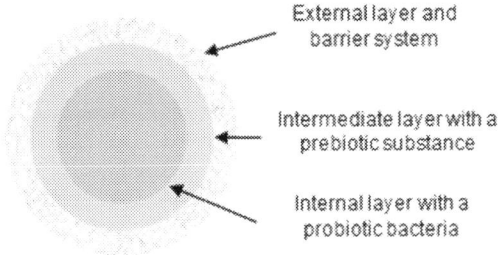

FIGURE 27.3 Multilayer microcapsule scheme. Scheme of a multilayer microcapsule where a probiotic bacterium can be included in the nucleus, in the intermediate layer a prebiotic compound, and in the outermost layer that acts as a barrier. *From Marañon, I., San Vicente, L., Hidalgo, N., & Chávarri, M., Multilayer probiotic microcapsules. Multilayer Probiotic Microcapsules." (EUROPE No. EP3205216A1). European Patent Application, 2016. Image edited by the author Izaskun Marañón.*

On the other hand, multilayer structures offer the possibility of combining separately active ingredients in a single microcapsule that, if found together, their stability would be negatively affected. (Bepeyeva et al., 2017; Chávarri et al., 2010) verified that the encapsulation of *L. gasseri* or *B. bifidum* together with quercetin causes the loss of viability of bacteria during encapsulation process and storage. To improve the bacteria survival, each component of the symbiotic formulation must be individually encapsulated. This procedure involves three individual encapsulation processes and a finished microcapsule mixing process. However, the development of a multilayer structure simplifies the procedure for obtaining the symbiotic. The isolation of quercetin and bacteria in different layers of the same microcapsule allows the symbiotic to develop in an one-stage process. Furthermore, multilayer structures can confine chemically incompatible substances in differentiated layers. In this way, the new microcapsule structure facilitates the dosage for a combination of probiotics, prebiotics, and/or postbiotics (Marañon et al., 2016).

Despite the efforts made to optimize the processes in terms of profitability, the inclusion of new stages in the manufacturing process to stabilize the active components entails a large increase in the total cost for developing of functional ingredients, foods or supplements. The success of encapsulation technologies lies in a greater product efficiency to reduce the dosage of the active components. Consequently, this can lead to a reduction in cost for the manufacturer and at the same time an increase in sales of the product due to greater consumer acceptance.

27.4 Current market of probiotics and future perspectives

The market of probiotic bacteria has experienced significant growth in recent years. Apart from the positive consumer perception due to their healthy properties, prescription of probiotics by healthcare professionals after a surgery or after taking antibiotics is contributing to the increasing consumption of functional foods and supplements containing probiotics.

As a result, and according to the study carried out by Fortune Business Insights (Fortune Business Insights, 2020), the global probiotic market achieved US$ 48.88 billion in 2019 and is expected to reach US$ 94.48 billion in 2027 with a Compound Annual Growth Rate (CAGR) of 7.9% during the forecast period (BCC Research, 2018). These products are becoming more popular for their health benefits and specially for the positive effect on improving the immune response. Last months, as a consequence of coronavirus pandemic, consumers are more conscious of their health and the demand of these products has experimented a notable increase.

According to the study carried out by Market Research Future (BCC Research, 2018), in 2025 the segment with the highest consumption of probiotics will be functional foods and beverages, followed by dietary supplements, animal nutrition and others as shown in Fig. 27.4.

In the food and beverage industry, as well as in dietary supplements and animal feed, the most widely used strains for probiotic ingredients in 2022 will be *Lactobacillus* followed by *Bifidobacterium* and *Streptococcus*. *Lactobacillus* will reach a share of 63%, followed by *Bifidobacterium* reach a share of 27%, *Streptococcus*, and *Bacillus* with shares of 4%, with a CAGR of 8%, 7.8%, and 7.7%, respectively. It is expected that this distribution of markets by bacteria genus will continue in the following years as shown in Fig. 27.5.

Growing consumer concern for health has led to increase demand for healthy food products. Probiotics have proven to have a positive effect on health, especially on digestive health and this makes them products highly demanded by the

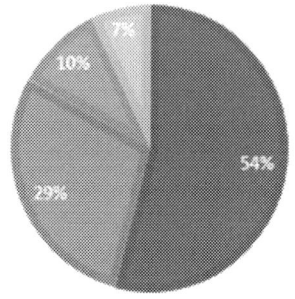

FIGURE 27.4 Distribution of probiotics consumption (%) by segments in 2025. The following figure shows the distribution of probiotic consumption by segments. Specifically, functional foods and beverages have 54%, dietary supplements 29%, animal nutrition 10%, and others 7%. *From Diez-Gutiérrez L., San Vicente L., R. Barrón L.J., Villarán, M. del C. and Chávarri M., Gamma-aminobutyric acid and probiotics: Multiple health benefits and their future in the global functional food and nutraceuticals market, Journal of Functional Foods 64, 2020, 1–14. https://doi.org/10.1016/j.jff.2019.103669. Image edited by the author María del Carmen Villarán.*

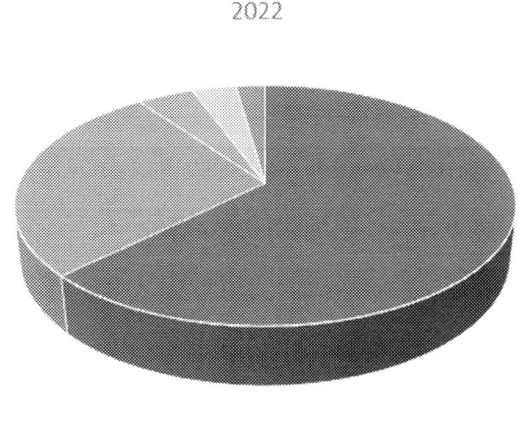

FIGURE 27.5 Global market shares (%) for probiotics forseen for 2022 (BCC Research, 2018). The following figure represents the world market share in % of probiotics forecast for 2022. Specifically, *Lactobacillus* will reach a share of 63%, followed by *Bifidobacterium* reach a share of 27% and *Streptococcus* and *Bacillus* with shares of 4%. From Diez-Gutiérrez L., San Vicente L., R. Barrón L.J., Villarán, M. del C. and Chávarri M., Gamma-aminobutyric acid and probiotics: Multiple health benefits and their future in the global functional food and nutraceuticals market, Journal of Functional Foods 64, 2020, 1–14. https://doi.org/10.1016/j.jff.2019.103669. Image edited by the author María del Carmen Villarán.

population. Consumers look for products that have a proven effect on health and they prefer natural products over drugs. The role of probiotics in the recovery of certain illness is causing the consumer to have high expectations in probiotics as possible products for the prevention of certain diseases.

In addition, probiotics can be incorporated without excessive additional costs into daily products, such as yogurts. Thus they present a low-cost, safe, and natural alternative to drugs for the prevention of certain diseases.

However, the development of the probiotics market and the obtention of new probiotic strains with specific health benefits require significant investment in R&D to respond to several challenges (Binda et al., 2020).

The correct characterization of probiotic strains. It would allow manufacturers to ensure and maintain the purity of their strains and avoid confusions. This complete strain characterization should support their probiotic activity.

Probiotic strains must comply with the safety requirements established by national regulatory entities.

The ability of a probiotics to provide a certain health benefit must be corroborated by at least one human clinical trial performed following recognized guidelines.

The final product, throughout its useful life, must contain the established probiotic dose to provide the declared health effect.

The perception of consumers toward food has changed from products that only provides nutritional value to other products that offer proven health benefits. Among other, consumers recognize the positive effect of probiotic enriched foods on health and on the immune system.

Increased investment by major players in the development of new food products will positively contribute to solve the challenges for new probiotics development with proved claims and to contribute to the increasing the probiotics market.

27.5 Conclusions

Nutribiotics are gaining importance due to their potential beneficial effects to improve the nutritional status of people suffering different disorders associates to malnutrition situations. Several probiotic microorganisms and postbiotics metabolites have been included in this new classification; nevertheless, new investigations could lead to find out new probiotics and postbiotics that could be included in this group. Furthermore, this could suppose an increase in nutribiotics demand to address nutritional problems that could result as even worse health problems.

References

Aggarwal, A., Mehta, S., Gupta, D., Sheikh, S., Pallagatti, S., Singh, R., & Singla, I. (2012). Clinical & immunological erythematosus patients characteristics in systemic lupus Maryam. *Journal of Dental Education, 76*(11), 1532–1539. Available from https://doi.org/10.4103/ijmr.IJMR.

Aguilar-Toalá, J. E., Garcia-Varela, R., Garcia, H. S., Mata-Haro, V., González-Córdova, A. F., Vallejo-Cordoba, B., & Hernández-Mendoza, A. (2018). Postbiotics: An evolving term within the functional foods field. *Trends in Food Science & Technology, 75*, 105–114. Available from https://doi.org/10.1016/J.TIFS.2018.03.009.

Aljutaily, T., Huarte, E., Martinez-Monteagudo, S., Gonzalez-Hernandez, J., Rovai, M., & Sergeev, I. (2020). Probiotic-enriched milk and dairy products increase the gut microbiota diversity: A comparative study. *Nutrition Research*. Available from https://doi.org/10.1016/j.nutres.2020.06.017.

Alou, M. T., Million, M., Traore, S. I., Mouelhi, D., Khelaifia, S., Bachar, D., Caputo, A., Delerce, J., Brah, S., Alhousseini, D., Sokhna, C., Robert, C., Diallo, B. A., Diallo, A., Parola, P., Golden, M., Lagier, J. C., & Raoult, D. (2017). Gut bacteria missing in severe acute malnutrition, can we identify potential probiotics by culturomics? *Frontiers in Microbiology*, 8, 1−17. Available from https://doi.org/10.3389/fmicb.2017.00899.

Alverdy, J. C., & Luo, J. N. (2017). The influence of host stress on the mechanism of infection: Lost microbiomes, emergent pathobiomes, and the role of interkingdom signaling. *Frontiers in Microbiology*, 08, 322. Available from https://doi.org/10.3389/fmicb.2017.00322.

Angmo, K., Kumari, A., Savitri., & Bhalla, T. C. (2016). Probiotic characterization of lactic acid bacteria isolated from fermented foods and beverage of Ladakh. *LWT—Food Science and Technology*, 66, 428−435. Available from https://doi.org/10.1016/j.lwt.2015.10.057.

Arora, M., & Baldi, A. (2015). Regulatory categories of probiotics across the globe: A review representing existing and recommended categorization. *Indian Journal of Medical Microbiology*, 33, S2−S10. Available from https://doi.org/10.4103/0255-0857.150868.

Ballini, A., Signorini, L., Inchingolo, A. D., Saini, R., Gnoni, A., Scacco, S., Cantore, S., Dipalma, G., Inchingolo, F., & Santacroce, L. (2020). Probiotics may improve serum folate availability in pregnant women: A pilot study. *Open Access Macedonian Journal of Medical Sciences*, 8, 1124−1130. Available from https://doi.org/10.3889/oamjms.2020.5494.

Bampi, G. B., Backes, G. T., Cansian, R. L., de Matos, F. E., Ansolin, I. M. A., Poleto, B. C., Corezzolla, L. R., & Favaro-Trindade, C. S. (2016). Spray chilling microencapsulation of Lactobacillus acidophilus and Bifidobacterium animalis subsp. lactis and its use in the preparation of savory probiotic cereal bars. *Food and Bioprocess Technology*, 9(8), 1422−1428. Available from https://doi.org/10.1007/s11947-016-1724-z.

Bardosono, S., Wibowo, N., Sutanto, L. B., Irwinda, R., Cannan, R., Rowan, A., & Dekker, J. (2019). Plasma folate, vitamin B6 and B12 in their relationship to the presence of probiotic strain Bifidobacterium animalis subsp. lactis HNO19 (DR10TM) among indonesian pregnant women in their third semester. *World Nutrition Journal*, 2(2), 56. Available from https://doi.org/10.25220/wnj.v02.i2.0009.

BCC Research. (2018). Global Market for Probiotics to Reach $36.7 Billion in 2018; Supplements Moving At 11.5% CAGR. *BCC Research*. https://www.bccresearch.com/pressroom/fod/global-market-for-probiotics-reach-$36.7-billion-2018.

Bepeyeva, A., de Barros, J., Albadran, H., Kakimov, A., Kakimova, Z., Charalampopoulos, D., & Khutoryanskiy, V. (2017). Encapsulation of Lactobacillus casei into calcium pectinate-chitosan beads for enteric delivery. *Journal of Food Science*, 82(12), 2954−2959. Available from https://doi.org/10.1111/1750-3841.13974.

Binda, S., Hill, C., Johansen, E., Obis, D., Pot, B., Sanders, M. E., Tremblay, A., & Ouwehand, A. C. (2020). Criteria to qualify microorganisms as "probiotic" in foods and dietary supplements. *Frontiers in Microbiology*, 11, 1662. Available from https://doi.org/10.3389/fmicb.2020.01662.

Bisanz, J. E., Enos, M. K., PrayGod, G., Seney, S., Macklaim, J. M., Chilton, S., Willner, D., Knight, R., Fusch, C., Fusch, G., Gloor, G. B., Burton, J. P., & Reid, G. (2015). Microbiota at multiple body sites during pregnancy in a rural tanzanian population and effects of Moringa-supplemented probiotic yogurt. *Applied and Environmental Microbiology*, 81(15), 4965−4975. Available from https://doi.org/10.1128/AEM.00780-15.

Brown, A. C., Rampertab, S. D., & Mullin, G. E. (2011). Existing dietary guidelines for Crohn's disease and ulcerative colitis. *Expert Rev. Gastroenterol. Hepatol.*, 5(3), 411−425.

Brown, A. C., & Valiere, A. (2004). Probiotics and medical nutrition therapy. *Nutrition in Clinical Care: An Official Publication of Tufts University*, 7(2), 56−68.

Bustamante, M., Oomah, B. D., Rubilar, M., & Shene, C. (2017). Effective Lactobacillus plantarum and Bifidobacterium infantis encapsulation with chia seed (Salvia hispanica L.) and flaxseed (Linum usitatissimum L.) mucilage and soluble protein by spray drying. *Food Chemistry*, 216, 97−105. Available from https://doi.org/10.1016/j.foodchem.2016.08.019.

Cammarota, G., Ianiro, G., Bibbò, S., & Gasbarrini, A. (2014). Gut microbiota modulation: Probiotics, antibiotics or fecal microbiota transplantation? *Internal and Emergency Medicine*, 9(4), 365−373. Available from https://doi.org/10.1007/s11739-014-1069-4.

Cani, P. D., & Van Hul, M. (2015). Novel opportunities for next-generation probiotics targeting metabolic syndrome. *Current Opinion in Biotechnology*, 32, 21−27. Available from https://doi.org/10.1016/j.copbio.2014.10.006.

Castro-Mejía, J. L., O'Ferrall, S., Krych, Ł., O'Mahony, E., Namusoke, H., Lanyero, B., Kot, W., Nabukeera-Barungi, N., Michaelsen, K. F., Mølgaard, C., Friis, H., Grenov, B., & Nielsen, D. S. (2020). Restitution of gut microbiota in Ugandan children administered with probiotics (Lactobacillus rhamnosus GG and Bifidobacterium animalis subsp. lactis BB-12) during treatment for severe acute malnutrition. *Gut Microbes*, 11(4), 855−867. Available from https://doi.org/10.1080/19490976.2020.1712982.

Chávarri, M., Marañón, I., & Villarán, M. C. (2012). *Encapsulation technology to protect probiotic bacteria. Probiotics*. InTech. Available from https://doi.org/10.5772/50046.

Chávarri, M., Marañón, I., Ares, R., Ibáñez, F. C., Marzo, F., Villarán, M., & del, C. (2010). Microencapsulation of a probiotic and prebiotic in alginate-chitosan capsules improves survival in simulated gastro-intestinal conditions. *International Journal of Food Microbiology*, 142(1−2), 185−189. Available from https://doi.org/10.1016/j.ijfoodmicro.2010.06.022.

Chuang, W. Y., Hsieh, Y. C., & Lee, T. T. (2020). The effects of fungal feed additives in animals: A review. *Animals*, 10(5), 1−15. Available from https://doi.org/10.3390/ani10050805.

Cielecka-Piontek, J., Dziedziński, M., Szczepaniak, O., Kobus-Cisowska, J., Telichowska, A., & Szymanowska, D. (2020). Survival of commercial probiotic strains and their effect on dark chocolate synbiotic snack with raspberry content during the storage and after simulated digestion. *Electronic Journal of Biotechnology*. Available from https://doi.org/10.1016/j.ejbt.2020.09.005.

Cuevas-González, P. F., Liceaga, A. M., & Aguilar-Toalá, J. E. (2020). Postbiotics and paraprobiotics: From concepts to applications. *Food Research International, 136*. Available from https://doi.org/10.1016/j.foodres.2020.109502.

Davinelli, S., Corbi, G., & Scapagnini, G. (2021). Frailty syndrome: A target for functional nutrients? *Mechanisms of Ageing and Development, 195*, 111441. Available from https://doi.org/10.1016/j.mad.2021.111441.

Dawood, M. A. O., Eweedah, N. M., Moustafa, E. M., & Farahat, E. M. (2020). Probiotic effects of Aspergillus oryzae on the oxidative status, heat shock protein, and immune related gene expression of Nile tilapia (Oreochromis niloticus) under hypoxia challenge. *Aquaculture (Amsterdam, Netherlands), 520*, 734669. Available from https://doi.org/10.1016/j.aquaculture.2019.734669.

de Pinho, N. B., Martucci, R. B., Rodrigues, V. D., D'Almeida, C. A., Thuler, L. C. S., Saunders, C., Jager-Wittenaar, H., & Peres, W. A. F. (2019). Malnutrition associated with nutrition impact symptoms and localization of the disease: Results of a multicentric research on oncological nutrition. *Clinical Nutrition, 38*(3), 1274–1279. Available from https://doi.org/10.1016/j.clnu.2018.05.010.

Diez-Gutiérrez, L., San Vicente, L., R. Barrón, L. J., Villarán., M. del, C., & Chávarri, M. (2020). Gamma-aminobutyric acid and probiotics: Multiple health benefits and their future in the global functional food and nutraceuticals market. *Journal of Functional Foods, 64*, 1–14. Available from https://doi.org/10.1016/j.jff.2019.103669.

Dinan, T. G., Stanton, C., & Cryan, J. F. (2013). Psychobiotics: A novel class of psychotropic. *Biological Psychiatry, 74*(10), 720–726. Available from https://doi.org/10.1016/j.biopsych.2013.05.001.

DiRienzo, D. (2014). Effect of probiotics on biomarkers of cardiovascular disease: Implications for heart-healthy diets. *Nutrition Reviews, 72*(1), 18–29.

Erginkaya, Z., Turhan, E. U., & Tatlı, D. (2018). Determination of antibiotic resistance of lactic acid bacteria isolated from traditional Turkish fermented dairy products. *Iranian Journal of Veterinary Research, Shiraz University, 19*(1), 53–56.

FAO/WHO. (2006). *Probiotics in food: Health and nutritional properties and guidelines for evaluation* (pp. 1–50). Food and Agriculture Organization of the United Nations, World Health Organization.

Fedorak, R. N., Feagan, B. G., Hotte, N., Leddin, D., Dieleman, L. A., Petrunia, D. M., Enns, R., Bitton, A., Chiba, N., Paré, P., Rostom, A., Marshall, J., Depew, W., Bernstein, C. N., Panaccione, R., Aumais, G., Steinhart, A. H., Cockeram, A., Bailey, R. J., & Madsen, K. (2015). The probiotic vsl#3 has anti-inflammatory effects and could reduce endoscopic recurrence after surgery for crohn's disease. *Clinical Gastroenterology and Hepatology, 13*(5), 928–935.e2. Available from https://doi.org/10.1016/j.cgh.2014.10.031.

Feng, K., Huang, R., Wu, R., Wei, Y., Zong, M., Linhardt, R., & Wu, H. (2020). A novel route for double-layered encapsulation of probiotics with improved viability under adverse conditions. *Food Chemistry, 310*, 125977. Available from https://doi.org/10.1016/j.foodchem.2019.125977.

Fontana, L., Bermudez-Brito, M., Plaza-Diaz, J., Muñoz-Quezada, S., & Gil, A. (2013). Sources, isolation, characterisation and evaluation of probiotics. *British Journal of Nutrition, 109*(Suppl. 2). Available from https://doi.org/10.1017/S0007114512004011.

Fortune Business Insights. 2020. "Probiotics Market Size, Share & Covid-19 Impact Analysis, by Microbial Genus (*Lactobacillus, Bifidobacterium* and Yeast) Application (Functional Foods & Beverages, Dietary Supplements and Animal Feed), Distribution Channel (Supermarkets/ Hypermarkets, Pharm." *Market Research report.* https://www.fortunebusinessinsights.com/industry-reports/infographics/probiotics-market-100083 (November 27, 2020).

George, R., Kumar, J., Gouda, S., Park, Y., Shin, H., & Das, G. (2018). Benefaction of probiotics for human health: A review. *Journal of Food and Drug Analysis, 26*(3), 927–939. Available from https://doi.org/10.1016/j.jfda.2018.01.002.

Gernand, A. D., Schulze, K. J., Stewart, C. P., West, K. P., & Christian, P. (2016). Micronutrient deficiencies in pregnancy worldwide: Health effects and prevention. *Nature Reviews Endocrinology, 12*(5), 274–289. Available from https://doi.org/10.1038/nrendo.2016.37.

Gingold-Belfer, R., Levy, S., Layfer, O., Pakanaev, L., Niv, Y., Dickman, R., & Perets, T. T. (2020). Use of a novel probiotic formulation to alleviate lactose intolerance symptoms—A pilot study. *Probiotics and Antimicrobial Proteins, 12*(1), 112–118. Available from https://doi.org/10.1007/s12602-018-9507-7.

Goderska, K., Agudo Pena, S., & Alarcon, T. (2018). Helicobacter pylori treatment: Antibiotics or probiotics. *Applied Microbiology and Biotechnology, 102*(1), 1–7. Available from https://doi.org/10.1007/s00253-017-8535-7.

Gómez-Gómez, M. E., & Zapico, S. C. (2019). Frailty, cognitive decline, neurodegenerative diseases and nutrition interventions. *International Journal of Molecular Sciences, 20*(11). Available from https://doi.org/10.3390/ijms20112842.

Gonzalez, C. A., & López-Carrillo, L. (2010). Helicobacter pylori, nutrition and smoking interactions: Their impact in gastric carcinogenesis. *Scandinavian Journal of Gastroenterology, 45*(1), 6–14. Available from https://doi.org/10.3109/00365520903401959.

Gorgannezhad, L., Sreejith, K., Christi, M., Jin, J., Ooi, C., Katouli, M., Stratton, H., & Nguyen, N. (2020). Core-shell beads as microreactors for phylogrouping of E. coli strains. *Micromachines (Basel), 11*(8), 761. Available from https://doi.org/10.3390/mi11080761.

Grenov, B., Namusoke, H., Lanyero, B., Nabukeera-Barungi, N., Ritz, C., Mølgaard, C., Friis, H., & Michaelsen, K. F. (2017). Effect of probiotics on diarrhea in children with severe acute malnutrition: A randomized controlled study in Uganda. *Journal of Pediatric Gastroenterology and Nutrition, 64*(3), 396–403. Available from https://doi.org/10.1097/MPG.0000000000001515.

Grundy, S. M. (2016). Overnutrition, ectopic lipid and the metabolic syndrome. *Journal of Investigative Medicine, 64*(6), 1082–1086. Available from https://doi.org/10.1136/jim-2016-000155.

Haileselassie, Y., Navis, M., Vu, N., Qazi, K. R., Rethi, B., & Sverremark-Ekström, E. (2016). Postbiotic modulation of retinoic acid imprinted mucosal-like dendritic cells by probiotic Lactobacillus reuteri 17938 in vitro. *Frontiers in Immunology, 7*. Available from https://doi.org/10.3389/fimmu.2016.00096.

Hatoum, R., Labrie, S., & Fliss, I. (2012). Antimicrobial and probiotic properties of yeasts: From fundamental to novel applications. *Frontiers in Microbiology, 3*, 1−12. Available from https://doi.org/10.3389/fmicb.2012.00421.

Hernández-Granados, M. J., & Franco-Robles, E. (2020). Postbiotics in human health: Possible new functional ingredients? *Food Research International, 137*. Available from https://doi.org/10.1016/j.foodres.2020.109660.

Hoover, D. G. (2014). Bifidobacterium. In *Encyclopedia of food microbiology* (2nd ed., Vol. 1, pp. 216−222). https://doi.org/10.1016/B978-0-12-384730-0.00033-1

Judkins, T. C., Archer, D. L., Kramer, D. C., & Solch, R. J. (2020). Probiotics, Nutrition and the Small Intestine. *Curr. Gastroenterol. Rep., 22*(2), 1−8.

Kambale, R. M., Nancy, F. I., Ngaboyeka, G. A., Kasengi, J. B., Bindels, L. B., & Van der Linden, D. (2021). Effects of probiotics and synbiotics on diarrhea in undernourished children: Systematic review with *meta*-analysis. *Clinical Nutrition*. Available from https://doi.org/10.1016/j.clnu.2020.12.026.

Kang, D., Su, M., Duan, Y., & Huang, Y. (2019). Eurotium cristatum, a potential probiotic fungus from Fuzhuan brick tea, alleviated obesity in mice by modulating gut microbiota. *Food and Function, 10*(8), 5032−5045. Available from https://doi.org/10.1039/c9fo00604d.

Karim, A., Gerliani, N., & Aïder, M. (2020). Kluyveromyces marxianus: An emerging yeast cell factory for applications in food and biotechnology. *International Journal of Food Microbiology, 333*, 108818. Available from https://doi.org/10.1016/j.ijfoodmicro.2020.108818.

Kerac, M., Bunn, J., Seal, A., Thindwa, M., Tomkins, A., Sadler, K., Bahwere, P., & Collins, S. (2009). Probiotics and prebiotics for severe acute malnutrition (PRONUT study): A double-blind efficacy randomised controlled trial in Malawi. *The Lancet, 374*(9684), 136−144. Available from https://doi.org/10.1016/S0140-6736(09)60884-9.

Khalili, M., Rad, A. H., Khosroushahi, A. Y., Khosravi, H., & Jafarzadeh, S. (2020). Application of probiotics in folate bio-fortification of yoghurt. *Probiotics and Antimicrobial Proteins, 12*(2), 756−763. Available from https://doi.org/10.1007/s12602-019-09560-7.

Kobus-Cisowska, J., Szymanowska, D., Maciejewska, P., Szczepaniak, O., Kmiecik, D., Gramza-Michałowska, A., Kulczyński, B., & Cielecka-Piontek, J. (2019). Enriching novel dark chocolate with Bacillus coagulans as a way to provide beneficial nutrients. *Food and Function, 10*(2), 997−1006. Available from https://doi.org/10.1039/c8fo02099j.

Korpela, K., Salonen, A., Vepsäläinen, O., Suomalainen, M., Kolmeder, C., Varjosalo, M., Miettinen, S., Kukkonen, K., Savilahti, E., Kuitunen, M., & De Vos, W. M. (2018). Probiotic supplementation restores normal microbiota composition and function in antibiotic-treated and in caesarean-born infants. *Microbiome, 6*(1), 1−11. Available from https://doi.org/10.1186/s40168-018-0567-4.

Kraimi, N., Dawkins, M., Gebhardt-Henrich, S. G., Velge, P., Rychlik, I., Volf, J., Creach, P., Smith, A., Colles, F., & Leterrier, C. (2019). Influence of the microbiota-gut-brain axis on behavior and welfare in farm animals: A review. *Physiology and Behavior, 210*. Available from https://doi.org/10.1016/j.physbeh.2019.112658.

Leblanc, J. G., Laiño, J. E., del Valle, M. J., Vannini, V., van Sinderen, D., Taranto, M. P., de Valdez, G. F., de Giori, G. S., & Sesma, F. (2011). B-Group vitamin production by lactic acid bacteria—Current knowledge and potential applications. *Journal of Applied Microbiology, 111*(6), 1297−1309. Available from https://doi.org/10.1111/j.1365-2672.2011.05157.x.

Lee, E. S., Song, E. J., Nam, Y. D., & Lee, S. Y. (2018). Probiotics in human health and disease: From nutribiotics to pharmabiotics. *Journal of Microbiology, 56*(11), 773−782. Available from https://doi.org/10.1007/s12275-018-8293-y.

Lei, M., Hua, L. M., & Wang, D. W. (2016). The effect of probiotic treatment on elderly patients with distal radius fracture: A prospective double-blind, placebo-controlled randomised clinical trial. *Benficial Microbes, 7*(5), 631−637.

Lichtenstein, L., Avni-Biron, I., & Ben-Bassat, O. (2016). Probiotics and prebiotics in Crohn's disease therapies. *Best Practice and Research: Clinical Gastroenterology, 30*(1), 81−88. Available from https://doi.org/10.1016/j.bpg.2016.02.002.

Lister, T. (2020). Nutrition and lifestyle interventions for managing parkinson's disease: A narrative review. *Journal of Movement Disorders, 13*(2), 97−104. Available from https://doi.org/10.14802/jmd.20006.

Liu, D. M., Guo, J., Zeng, X. A., Sun, D. W., Brennan, C. S., Zhou, Q. X., & Zhou, J. S. (2017). The probiotic role of Lactobacillus plantarum in reducing risks associated with cardiovascular disease. *International Journal of Food Science and Technology, 52*(1), 127−136. Available from https://doi.org/10.1111/ijfs.13234.

Lorenzo-López, L., Maseda, A., De Labra, C., Regueiro-Folgueira, L., Rodríguez-Villamil, J. L., & Millán-Calenti, J. C. (2017). Nutritional determinants of frailty in older adults: A systematic review. *BMC Geriatrics, 17*(1), 1−13. Available from https://doi.org/10.1186/s12877-017-0496-2.

Ma, J., Zhang, J., Li, Q., Shi, Z., Wu, H., Zhang, H., Tang, L., Yi, R., Su, H., & Sun, X. (2019). Oral administration of a mixture of probiotics protects against food allergy via induction of CD103 + dendritic cells and modulates the intestinal microbiota. *Journal of Functional Foods, 55*, 65−75. Available from https://doi.org/10.1016/j.jff.2019.02.010.

Mallappa, R. H., Rokana, N., Duary, R. K., Panwar, H., Batish, V. K., & Grover, S. (2012). Management of metabolic syndrome through probiotic and prebiotic interventions. *Indian Journal of Endocrinology and Metabolism, 16*(1), 20. Available from https://doi.org/10.4103/2230-8210.91178.

Mantaring, J., Benyacoub, J., Destura, R., Pecquet, S., Vidal, K., Volger, S., & Guinto, V. (2018). Effect of maternal supplement beverage with and without probiotics during pregnancy and lactation on maternal and infant health: A randomized controlled trial in the Philippines. *BMC Pregnancy and Childbirth, 18*(1), 1−12. Available from https://doi.org/10.1186/s12884-018-1828-8.

Marañon, I., San Vicente, L., Hidalgo, N., & Chavarri, M. (2016). Multilayer probiotic microcapsules. Multilayer Probiotic Microcapsules." (EUROPE No. EP3205216A1). European Patent Application.

Martínez-Abad, B., Garrote, J. A., Bernardo, D., Montalvillo, E., Escudero-Hernández, C., Vázquez, E., Rueda, R., & Arranz, E. (2016). Differential immunomodulatory effects of Lactobacillus rhamnosus DR20, Lactobacillus fermentum CECT 5716 and Bifidobacterium animalis subsp. lactis on monocyte-derived dendritic cells. *Journal of Functional Foods, 22*, 300–312. Available from https://doi.org/10.1016/j.jff.2016.01.033.

Million, M., Diallo, A., & Raoult, D. (2017). Gut microbiota and malnutrition. *Microbial Pathogenesis, 106*, 127–138. Available from https://doi.org/10.1016/j.micpath.2016.02.003.

Moradi, M., Mardani, K., & Tajik, H. (2019). Characterization and application of postbiotics of Lactobacillus spp. on Listeria monocytogenes in vitro and in food models. *LWT, 111*, 457–464. Available from https://doi.org/10.1016/j.lwt.2019.05.072.

Norman, K., Kirchner, H., Lochs, H., & Pirlich, M. (2006). Malnutrition affects quality of life in gastroenterology patients. *World Journal of Gastroenterology, 12*(21), 3380–3385. Available from https://doi.org/10.3748/wjg.v12.i21.3380.

Nuhwa, R., Tanasupawat, S., Taweechotipatr, M., Sitdhipol, J., & Savarajara, A. (2019). Bile salt hydrolase activity and cholesterol assimilation of lactic acid bacteria isolated from flowers. *Journal of Applied Pharmaceutical Science, 9*(6), 106–110. Available from https://doi.org/10.7324/JAPS.2019.90615.

O'Mahony, S. M., Felice, V. D., Nally, K., Savignac, H. M., Claesson, M. J., Scully, P., Woznicki, J., Hyland, N. P., Shanahan, F., Quigley, E. M., Marchesi, J. R., O'Toole, P. W., Dinan, T. G., & Cryan, J. F. (2014). Disturbance of the gut microbiota in early-life selectively affects visceral pain in adulthood without impacting cognitive or anxiety-related behaviors in male rats. *Neuroscience, 277*, 885–901. Available from https://doi.org/10.1016/j.neuroscience.2014.07.054.

Oxley, J. (2012). Spray cooling and spray chilling for food ingredient and nutraceutical encapsulation. *Encapsulation Technologies and Delivery Systems for Food Ingredients and Nutraceuticals*, 110–130. Available from https://doi.org/10.1016/B978-0-85709-124-6.50005-6.

Palma, M. L., Zamith-Miranda, D., Martins, F. S., Bozza, F. A., Nimrichter, L., Montero-Lomeli, M., Marques, E. T. A., & Douradinha, B. (2015). Probiotic Saccharomyces cerevisiae strains as biotherapeutic tools: Is there room for improvement? *Applied Microbiology and Biotechnology, 99*(16), 6563–6570. Available from https://doi.org/10.1007/s00253-015-6776-x.

Papadimitriou, K., Alegría, Á., Bron, P. A., de Angelis, M., Gobbetti, M., Kleerebezem, M., Lemos, J. A., Linares, D. M., Ross, P., Stanton, C., Turroni, F., van Sinderen, D., Varmanen, P., Ventura, M., Zúñiga, M., Tsakalidou, E., & Kok, J. (2016). Stress physiology of lactic acid bacteria. *Microbiology and Molecular Biology Reviews, 80*(3), 837–890. Available from https://doi.org/10.1128/mmbr.00076-15.

Patel, P. J., Singh, S. K., Panaich, S., & Cardozo, L. (2014). The aging gut and the role of prebiotics, probiotics, and synbiotics: A review. *Journal of Clinical Gerontology and Geriatrics, 5*(1), 3–6. Available from https://doi.org/10.1016/j.jcgg.2013.08.003.

Perez-Burgos, A., Wang, B., Mao, Y.-K., Mistry, B., Neufeld, K.-A. M., Bienenstock, J., & Kunze, W. (2013). Psychoactive bacteria Lactobacillus rhamnosus (JB-1) elicits rapid frequency facilitation in vagal afferents. *American Journal of Physiology-Gastrointestinal and Liver Physiology, 304*(2), G211–G220. Available from https://doi.org/10.1152/ajpgi.00128.2012.

Qiu, H., & Schlegel, V. (2018). Chronic nutrition overtake can lead to the onset of multiple diseases. *Nutrition Reviews*. https://academic.oup.com/nutritionreviews/pages/chronic_nutrition_overtake_can_lead_to_the_onset_of_multiple_diseases.

Rai, S. K., Kazuko, H., Ayako, A., & Yoshimi, O. (2002). Infectious diseases and malnutrition status in Nepal: An overview. *Malaysian Journal of Nutrition, 8*(2), 191–200.

Rizzoli, R., & Biver, E. (2020). Are probiotics the new calcium and vitamin D for bone health? *Current Osteoporosis Reports, 18*(3), 273–284. Available from https://doi.org/10.1007/s11914-020-00591-6.

Roselino, M. N., Sakamoto, I. K., Tallarico Adorno, M. A., Márcia Canaan, J. M., de Valdez, G. F., Rossi, E. A., Sivieri, K., & Umbelino Cavallini, D. C. (2020). Effect of fermented sausages with probiotic Enterococcus faecium CRL 183 on gut microbiota using dynamic colonic model. *LWT, 132*. Available from https://doi.org/10.1016/j.lwt.2020.109876.

Ruggiero, P. (2014). Use of probiotics in the fight against Helicobacter pylori. *World Journal of Gastrointestinal Pathophysiology, 5*(4), 384. Available from https://doi.org/10.4291/wjgp.v5.i4.384.

Russo, E., Giudici, F., Fiorindi, C., Ficari, F., Scaringi, S., & Amedei, A. (2019). Immunomodulating activity and therapeutic effects of short chain fatty acids and tryptophan post-biotics in inflammatory bowel disease. *Frontiers in Immunology, 10*, 1–10. Available from https://doi.org/10.3389/fimmu.2019.02754.

Rusu, I. G., Suharoschi, R., Vodnar, D. C., Pop, C. R., Socaci, S. A., Vulturar, R., & Pop, O. L. i (2020). Iron supplementation influence on the gut microbiota and probiotic intake effect in iron deficiency—A literature-based review. *Nutrien, 12*(7), 1993.

Salazar, N., Valdés-Varela, L., González, S., Gueimonde, M., & de los Reyes-Gavilán, C. G. (2017). Nutrition and the gut microbiome in the elderly. *Gut Microbes, 8*(2), 82–97. Available from https://doi.org/10.1080/19490976.2016.1256525.

Salvatella-Flores, M. J., & Bermúdez-Humarán, L. G. (2020). Malnutrition and fragility: From children to elderly with probiotics. *Archives of Clinical and Biomedical Research, 4*(6), 709–720. Available from https://doi.org/10.26502/acbr.50170136.

Sampson, T. R., Debelius, J. W., Thron, T., Janssen, S., Shastri, G. G., Ilhan, Z. E., Challis, C., Schretter, C. E., Rocha, S., Gradinaru, V., Chesselet, M. F., Keshavarzian, A., Shannon, K. M., Krajmalnik-Brown, R., Wittung-Stafshede, P., Knight, R., & Mazmanian, S. K. (2016). Gut microbiota regulate motor deficits and neuroinflammation in a model of parkinson's disease. *Cell, 167*(6), 1469–1480.e12. Available from https://doi.org/10.1016/j.cell.2016.11.018.

Sehrawat, N., Yadav, M., Singh, M., Kumar, V., Sharma, V. R., & Sharma, A. K. (2020). Probiotics in microbiome ecological balance providing a therapeutic window against cancer. *Seminars in Cancer Biology*. Available from https://doi.org/10.1016/j.semcancer.2020.06.009.

Shah, N.P. (2011). Bifidobacterium spp.: Morphology and physiology. In Encyclopedia of dairy sciences (2nd ed., pp. 381–387).

Sheridan, P. O., Bindels, L. B., Saulnier, D. M., Reid, G., Nova, E., Holmgren, K., Toole, P. W. O., Bunn, J., Delzenne, N., & Scott, K. P. (2014). Can prebiotics and probiotics improve therapeutic outcomes for undernourished individuals? 5(1), 74−82.

Singh, A., Vishwakarma, V., & Singhal, B. (2018). Metabiotics: The functional metabolic signatures of probiotics: Current state-of-art and future research priorities—Metabiotics: Probiotics effector molecules. *Advances in Bioscience and Biotechnology*, 9(4), 147−189. Available from https://doi.org/10.4236/abb.2018.94012.

Sommer, F., & Bäckhed, F. (2013). The gut microbiota-masters of host development and physiology. *Nature Reviews Microbiology*, 11(4), 227−238. Available from https://doi.org/10.1038/nrmicro2974.

Sornplang, P., & Piyadeatsoontorn, S. (2016). Probiotic isolates from unconventional sources: A review. *Journal of Animal Science and Technology*, 58(1), 1−11. Available from https://doi.org/10.1186/s40781-016-0108-2.

Sousa Moraes, L. F., de, Grzeskowiak, L. M., de Sales Teixeira, T. F., & do Carmo Gouveia Peluzio, M. (2014). Intestinal microbiota and probiotics in celiac disease. *Clinical Microbiology Reviews*, 27(3), 482−489. Available from https://doi.org/10.1128/CMR.00106-13.

Szczechowiak, K., Diniz, B. S., & Leszek, J. (2019). Diet and Alzheimer's dementia—Nutritional approach to modulate inflammation. *Pharmacology, Biochemistry, and Behavior*, 184, 172743. Available from https://doi.org/10.1016/j.pbb.2019.172743.

Talbott, S. M., Talbott, J. A., Stephens, B. J., & Oddou, M. P. (2019). Effect of coordinated probiotic/prebiotic/phytobiotic supplementation on microbiome balance and psychological mood state in healthy stressed adults. *Functional Foods in Health and Disease*, 9(4), 265−275. Available from https://doi.org/10.31989/ffhd.v9i4.599.

Tamaki, H., Nakase, H., Inoue, S., Kawanami, C., Itani, T., Ohana, M., Kusaka, T., Uose, S., Hisatsune, H., Tojo, M., Noda, T., Arasawa, S., Izuta, M., Kubo, A., Ogawa, C., Matsunaka, T., & Shibatouge, M. (2016). Efficacy of probiotic treatment with Bifidobacterium longum 536 for induction of remission in active ulcerative colitis: A randomized, double-blinded, placebo-controlled multicenter trial. *Digestive Endoscopy*, 28(1), 67−74. Available from https://doi.org/10.1111/den.12553.

Tasch Holkem, A., & Favaro-Trindade, C. (2020). Potential of solid lipid microparticles covered by the protein-polysaccharide complex for protection of probiotics and proanthocyanidin-rich cinnamon extract. *Food Res International*, 136, 109520. Available from https://doi.org/10.1016/j.foodres.2020.109520.

Tenorio-Jiménez, C., Martínez-Ramírez, M. J., Gil, Á., & Gómez-Llorente, C. (2020). Effects of probiotics on metabolic syndrome: A systematic review of randomized clinical trials. *Nutrients*, 12(1). Available from https://doi.org/10.3390/nu12010124.

Thushara, R. M., Gangadaran, S., Solati, Z., & Moghadasian, M. H. (2016). Cardiovascular benefits of probiotics: A review of experimental and clinical studies. *Food and Function*, 7(2), 632−642. Available from https://doi.org/10.1039/c5fo01190f.

Turroni, F., Peano, C., Pass, D. A., Foroni, E., Severgnini, M., Claesson, M. J., Kerr, C., Hourihane, J., Murray, D., Fuligni, F., Gueimonde, M., Margolles, A., de Bellis, G., O'Toole, P. W., van Sinderen, D., Marchesi, J. R., & Ventura, M. (2012). Diversity of bifidobacteria within the infant gut microbiota. *PLoS One*, 7(5), 20−24. Available from https://doi.org/10.1371/journal.pone.0036957.

Tyagi, P., Tasleem, M., Prakash, S., & Chouhan, G. (2020). Intermingling of gut microbiota with brain: Exploring the role of probiotics in battle against depressive disorders. *Food Research International*, 137. Available from https://doi.org/10.1016/j.foodres.2020.109489.

Van Den Broek, N. (2003). Anaemia and micronutrient deficiencies. *British Medical Bulletin*, 67, 149−160. Available from https://doi.org/10.1093/bmb/ldg004.

Verna, E. C., & Lucak, S. (2010). Use of probiotics in gastrointestinal disorders: What to recommend? *Therapeutic Advances in Gastroenterology*, 3(5), 307−319. Available from https://doi.org/10.1177/1756283X10373814.

Vonderheid, S. C., Tussing-Humphreys, L., Park, C., Pauls, H., Hemphill, N. O., Labomascus, B., McLeod, A., & Koenig, M. D. (2019). A systematic review and *meta*-analysis on the effects of probiotic species on iron absorption and iron status. *Nutrients*, 11(12). Available from https://doi.org/10.3390/nu11122938.

Vries, M. C., de, Vaughan, E. E., Kleerebezem, M., & de Vos, W. M. (2006). Lactobacillus plantarum-survival, functional and potential probiotic properties in the human intestinal tract. *International Dairy Journal*, 16(9), 1018−1028. Available from https://doi.org/10.1016/j.idairyj.2005.09.003.

Wang, J., Zhang, H., Du, H., Wang, F., Li, H., & Zhao, X. (2019). Identification and characterization of Diutina rugosa SD-17 for potential use as a probiotic. *LWT*, 109, 283−288. Available from https://doi.org/10.1016/j.lwt.2019.04.042, July 2018.

Williams, B. L., Hornig, M., Buie, T., Bauman, M. L., Cho Paik, M., Wick, I., Bennett, A., Jabado, O., Hirschberg, D. L., & Lipkin, W. I. (2011). Impaired carbohydrate digestion and transport and mucosal dysbiosis in the intestines of children with autism and gastrointestinal disturbances. *PLoS One*, 6(9), e24585. Available from https://doi.org/10.1371/journal.pone.0024585.

Wu, X., Teame, T., Hao, Q., Ding, Q., Liu, H., Ran, C., Yang, Y., Zhang, Y., Zhou, Z., Duan, M., & Zhang, Z. (2020). Use of a paraprobiotic and postbiotic feed supplement (HWFTM) improves the growth performance, composition and function of gut microbiota in hybrid sturgeon (Acipenser baerii × Acipenser schrenckii). *Fish and Shellfish Immunology*, 104, 36−45. Available from https://doi.org/10.1016/j.fsi.2020.05.054.

Yépez, L., & Tenea, G. N. (2015). Genetic diversity of lactic acid bacteria strains towards their potential probiotic application. *Romanian Biotechnological Letters*, 20(2), 10191−10199.

Yoon, K. Y., Woodams, E. E., & Hang, Y. D. (2004). Probiotication of tomato juice by lactic acid bacteria. *The Journal of Microbiology*, 42(4), 315−318.

Yu, Z., Zhang, X., Li, S., Li, C., Li, D., & Yang, Z. (2013). Evaluation of probiotic properties of Lactobacillus plantarum strains isolated from Chinese sauerkraut. *World Journal of Microbiology and Biotechnology*, *29*(3), 489–498. Available from https://doi.org/10.1007/s11274-012-1202-3.

Zaeim, D. (2020). Electro-hydrodynamic processing of probiotics: An innovative approach. https://doi.org/10.13140/RG.2.2.35372.90241.

Zhang, C., Yu, Z., Zhao, J., Zhang, H., Zhai, Q., & Chen, W. (2019). Colonization and probiotic function of Bifidobacterium longum. *Journal of Functional Foods*, *53*, 157–165. Available from https://doi.org/10.1016/j.jff.2018.12.022, December 2018.

Żółkiewicz, J., Marzec, A., Ruszczyński, M., & Feleszko, W. (2020). Postbiotics—A step beyond pre- and probiotics. *Nutrients*, *12*(8), 1–17. Available from https://doi.org/10.3390/nu12082189.

Chapter 28

Role of immunobiotic lactic acid bacteria as vaccine adjuvants

Maryam Dadar, Youcef Shahali and Naheed Mojgani

Razi Vaccine and Serum Research Institute, Agricultural Research, Education and Extension Organization (AREEO), Karaj, Iran

28.1 Introduction

Vaccination is one of the essential prevention tools that provide protection in humans and animals against harmful infectious diseases. However, suboptimal immunity could be achieved from different licensed vaccines such as diphtheria, anthrax, tetanus, and pertussis, that highlight the important role of multiple boosters to provide a potent immunoprotective response (Skowera et al., 2005; Trollfors et al., 2006). This issue suggests an urgent demand for more effective adjuvants to represent efficient responses for the production of vaccine-specific memory T and B cells (Barnes et al., 2007). The annual implementation of six standard vaccines including *Haemophil influenza* type b, hepatitis B, diphtheria, polio, yellow fever, and tetanus could save more than 5 million lives. However, there are different challenges in developing countries with difficulties in vaccine coverage that cause significant morbidity and mortality (Mojgani et al., 2020). Furthermore, the cost of these vaccines is also one of the main causes of inadequate and inappropriate vaccinations in these countries (Ward et al., 2020). Therefore the improvement of cost-effective vaccines that reduced vaccination schedules through the stimulation of a stronger immune response is of critical importance. According to numerous reports, relative immune response and improvement in cellular, humoral and innate immunity required for combatting pathogens like *Mycobacterium tuberculosis*, *Plasmodium falciparum*, and HIV depends on various host genetic factors and major histocompatibility complex (MHC) haplotype (Hill, 2006; Kaufmann, 2006). Therefore preventive vaccines against these pathogens must be efficient so as to induce CD8 + T cells supported by neutralizing antibodies and CD4 + T cells to load the various effector pathways. Adjuvants are essential immune-boosting substances required to boost the immune response of certain vaccines. Although, these immunogenic adjuvants used in vaccines have well-established safety records, they might also show several side effects like local and systemic symptoms. For such reasons, both new and existing vaccines may need the presence of improved adjuvant formulations that can both increase and instruct different polyvalent adaptive immune pathways and have lesser side effects compared to conventionally used adjuvants (Barnes et al., 2007; McMichael, 2006). Recently, different vaccine strategies have been evaluated, among which LAB have been extensively investigated as effective and safe vaccine approaches. These microorganisms are generally recognized as safe bacteria that have also attracted attention because of their efficient role as new vaccine adjuvants and/or delivery systems for mucosal vaccine development (Jung et al., 2020; Tonetti et al., 2020). In this regard, bacterium-like particles (BLPs) derived from the heat and acid treatments of *Lactococcus lactis* known as Gram-positive bacteria do not contain cytoplasmic proteins or DNA, but conserve the adjuvant activities of the *L. lactis*-derived BLPs (Audouy et al., 2006; Bosma et al., 2006). A significant capacity of these bacteria is the intrinsically possessive mucosal adjuvant activities (Mojgani et al., 2020). Additionally, as acid/heat treated bacterial are administered orally or nasally, they have a higher acceptance and increased safety related to the higher dose used a promising adjuvant for mucosal immunization. In this review, we highlight the effective role of immunobiotic LAB as novel vaccine adjuvants.

28.2 Vaccine adjuvants

Vaccination is an effective strategy for preventing a number of diseases caused by pathogenic microorganisms. To date, the majority of vaccines in use, such as live-attenuated and whole pathogen vaccines, are capable of inducing long-lived immunity in the host. Hence, for a vaccine to be effective it is essential that they are capable of generating and/or stimulating a strong immune response in the body, which consequently results in long-term protection against the infection (Coffman et al., 2010). However, unlike these live and attenuated vaccines—the nonliving vaccines antigens most importantly—purified or recombinant subunit vaccines are poor immunogens that cannot elicit a strong immune response and fail to provide long-term immunity (Geeraedts et al., 2008). In such circumstances, certain immunological active substances are added to these vaccines to accelerate and enhance the antigen-specific immune response that could provide long-term protection against the administered antigen (Endo & Manya, 2006). These immune provoking substances are referred to as adjuvants and have a long history of use in vaccinations. Among number of adjuvants being used, some are inorganic, such as alum (aluminum phosphate, aluminum hydroxide, aluminum potassium sulfate) organic adjuvants such as Freund's complete adjuvant, Squalene (Abreu, 2010; Clements & Griffiths, 2002), virosome, heat-labile enterotoxin and liposomes, etc. Although these adjuvants have a number of distinct immunological features and have demonstrated potential immunomodulatory roles (Barnes et al., 2007; Beran, 2008; Schwarz et al., 2009), yet compared to nonadjuvanted vaccines, these adjuvanted vaccines might cause local and systemic reactions. Some of these reactions include redness, swelling, and pain at the injection site (local reactions), fever, chills, and body aches (systemic reactions). It has been reported that aluminum adjuvant containing vaccines can cause postimmunization headache, arthralgia, and myalgia, which could reflect alum's propensity to induce IL-1, with IL-1 administration to human subjects reproducing these symptoms (Dinarello & van der Meer, 2013). Furthermore, high aluminum levels in the body have been shown to affect the brain and bone tissues, causing a fatal neurological syndrome and dialysis-associated dementia (Reusche & Seydel, 1993). Additionally, cerebral aluminum accumulation has also been observed in Alzheimer's disease (Miu & Benga, 2006). The adverse effects of some of these adjuvants have also been reported in animals like in cats, dogs, and ferrets. According to available reports, aluminum adjuvants cause local chronic granulomatous lesions, which can progress to malignant fibrosarcoma in the vaccinated animals (Vascellari et al., 2003).

Similar to aluminum adjuvants, oil emulsion adjuvants might also cause generalized systemic symptoms, including fever, headache, malaise, nausea, diarrhea, arthralgia, myalgia, and lethargy, reflecting the induction of inflammation (Petrovsky, 2008). A major recurring concern is a potential association between oil emulsion adjuvants and autoimmune disease induction, as seen in animal and fish models (Koppang et al., 2008; Vera-Lastra et al., 2012; Whitehouse, 2012). Although all these vaccine adjuvants have safety records and have been used for a long period of time in numerous vaccines in humans and animals, there is an ongoing urge for the search of novel adjuvants that are safer with lesser side effects, are natural, and with strong immune boosters.

28.3 Probiotic lactic acid bacteria

Nonpathogenic Gram-positive, LAB are evaluated to be effective candidates for the improvement of safe, novel delivery systems, and production of heterologous immunoproteins. At the end of the 19th century, natural gastrointestinal microbiota has been reorganized and microbiologists showed that LAB are amply found in the digestive tracts of healthy persons. These LAB have been called "probiotics" and defined by FAO and WHO experts as: "Live microorganisms which when administered in adequate amounts confer a health benefit on the host" (Morelli & Capurso, 2012; Tonetti et al., 2020). There is growing interest regarding probiotics from researchers, governmental organizations (like the FAO/WHO), the public, and food and medicinal companies. Furthermore, several randomized, placebo-controlled clinical trials (RCTs) have identified the effectiveness and promising effects of probiotics as a vehicle delivery in stimulating both mucosally and parenterally used vaccine-specific immune responses (Amdekar et al., 2010). In other words, probiotics induce immunomodulatory properties to preserve intestinal homeostasis, thereby developing gut immunity (Adel et al., 2017; Azcárate-Peril et al., 2011; Galdeano et al., 2019; Kałużna-Czaplińska et al., 2017; Mojgani et al., 2020). Adjuvant activities of probiotics could improve the immune responses for a vaccine antigen and stimulate the maximum protection in the low coverage of vaccine responses against infectious diseases (Licciardi & Tang, 2011; Soltani et al., 2019). On the other hand, the targeting and induction of particular immune pathways in the mucosa-associated lymphoid tissue, is most efficiently achieved by direct administration of a vaccine to mucosal surfaces, explaining the best initiation of a humoral and/or a cell-mediated mechanism (Dugas et al., 1999; Fujimura et al., 2012). For the first time, Lilly and Stillwell applied the term probiotic to describe substances released by protozoa, which improved the development and growth of other organisms (Lilly & Stillwell, 1965). Furthermore, Fuller, the father of modern immunology, wrote about the effective role of live bacteria in yogurt, including *Streptococcus thermophilus* and *Lactobacillus bulgaricus*, for general and gastrointestinal tract health conditions that could result in a long life (Fuller, 1992). Several studies have found evidence that also proved the important role of probiotic strains as hopeful supplements for antibiotic therapy by improving mucosal immunity, increasing antibiotic function, and limiting adverse effects (Amdekar et al., 2010; Anukam et al., 2008; Bahey-El-Din et al., 2010; Rolfe, 2000). It is now approved that probiotics help to improve health improvement, disease management, and remarkably restricts the adverse effects of antibiotics through their effective role on the digestive and immune systems (Cremon et al., 2018; Sartor, 2004). Therefore products of different probiotics are considered a helpful resource to the body because they can improve the function of different parts of the body, where other supplements particularly focus on a limited number organs (Bisanz et al., 2015; Varankovich et al., 2015). It also has been well-documented that probiotics show favorable effects on improving the bioavailability of essential nutrients (Pandey et al., 2015), increasing health conditions of the gastrointestinal system (Varankovich et al., 2015), preventing atopic sensitization among susceptible individuals (Allen et al., 2014), declining frequent symptoms of food intolerance (Oak & Jha, 2019), ameliorating the adaptive and innate immune mechanisms (Galdeano et al., 2019), and controlling the onset of specific cancers (Sharma, 2019). Therefore probiotics and their derivatives are evaluated as one of the most promising novel supplements in the treatment of several chronic disorders and improve immune responses (Amara & Shibl, 2015; Anand et al., 2019; Cervin, 2018; Neto et al., 2018).

28.3.1 Immunobiotics

Microorganisms that show immunomodulatory responses are referred to as immunobiotics. A number of bacterial immunobiotics have been shown to interact with different pattern recognition receptors expressed in nonimmune and immune cells and exert beneficial effects on the host health (Garcia-Castillo et al., 2019). In past few years, the focus of attention has been on the immunomodulatory capacity of certain probiotic LAB that activate the common mucosal system through the stimulation of gut antigen-presenting cells (APCs) and, hence, provide protection (Clancy, 2003). The beneficial properties of immunobiotics are strain dependent, and *Lactobacillus* strains that promote mucosal T-cell function are termed as immunobiotic lactobacillus strains (Marranzino et al., 2012).

28.3.2 Probiotic LAB as immunobiotics

A decline in the cellular immunity and malfunctioning of the immune system led to different diseases and infections in the body (Nikolich-Žugich, 2018). It has been broadly reported that the immune response directly or indirectly affected by gut microbiota have a beneficial effect in stimulation of the pathways contributed in the immune responses (Amara & Shibl, 2015; Frei et al., 2015; Hoseinifar et al., 2017). These pathways could regular both the adaptive and innate immune mechanisms in the gut systems. Thus it is anticipated that by development of the gut microbiota, a resistance to disease has occurred (Rosshart et al., 2017; Sánchez et al., 2017; Vlasova et al., 2019). According to different studies that clearly revealed a healthy gut microbiota improves the immune system. It has been reported that different HIV/AIDS patients suffered from gastrointestinal disorders and that probiotic consumption could improve the beneficial effects in the immune system (Anukam et al., 2008; Irvine et al., 2010). Following the consumption of yogurt supplemented with *Lactobacillus*, HIV/AIDS patients showed an elevation in CD4 cell counts (Anukam et al., 2008). Furthermore, a significant increase in the leukocyte counts has been reported in elderly individuals consuming milk with active *Bifidus* (*Bifidobacterium animalis* DN-173 010), resulting in improvement of immunity responses and counteractions with infection (Bouvier et al., 2001). Furthermore, a diet enriched with live *Bifidobacterium lactis* (HN019) could greatly improve the host immune responses (Arunachalam et al., 2000). Moreover, the benefits effects of probiotic bacteria on control of rotavirus has been reported (Korik et al., 1968). For example, it has been shown that *Bifidobacterium longum*, and *Lactobacillus acidophilus* decrease the diarrhea duration in pediatric patients and control the infection by rotavirus in vitro (Lee et al., 2015). Also, increased specific IgA response to rotavirus, was seen after treatment with *Lactobacillus reuteri* in young children (Shornikova et al., 1997). Similarly, strain GG of *Lactobacillus casei* show significant effects in increasing immune functions against acute diarrhea-associated rotavirus in children (Gombosova et al., 1986). The therapeutic activity exerted by LAB is directly associated with their immune-modulating (IL-10 and IL-6 production), and suppressor promotes IFN-γ producing, Treg cell or T-cell immune responses (Amdekar et al., 2010; Reid et al., 2003; Van Hoang et al., 2018). However, the various effects of LAB on the host immune responses are strain and species-specific that could stimulate specific mucosal cytokine profiles. Through the oral route, the probiotic LAB could enter the gut and induce systemic immune activities by the release of cytokines via lymphoid cells related to the mucosa. Numerous cells such as stromal cells, immune cells, fibroblasts, and endothelial cells produce cytokines that are associated with down or up modulation of the immune pathways.

The stimulation of gut mucosal immune pathways through the probiotic bacteria is related to the interaction between the gut epithelial cells and these bacteria. This interaction leads to the stimulation of inducing signals for immune responses (Amdekar et al., 2010; Galdeano & Perdigon, 2006). Probiotics can regulate the populations of DCs, B and T cells, and also cytokine and antibody responses (Konieczna et al., 2012; Kukkonen et al., 2010). It is worth mentioning that immunostimulating functions of probiotics might lead to an increase in the immune responses to vaccine antigens that would result in enhanced protection against infectious diseases. The nonspecific immune activities could be developed by the inflammatory functions with the effective participation of macrophages and the phagocytic cells [polymorphonuclear (PMN)] (Dvorožňáková et al., 2016; Isolauri et al., 2001; Rocha-Ramírez et al., 2017).

In these interactions, probiotics are immediately absorbed by the M cells overlying the normal epithelium, overlying the lamina propria or Peyer's patches of the small intestine. After that, the intact probiotic cells are transferred to the phagocytes by the macrophages—dendritic cells T and B lymphocytes, and the APC—to be phagocytized (Perdigón & Alvarez, 1992). Therefore probiotic strains show initial immunostimulatory responses that could be directly related to the early inflammation response in the human macrophages (Rocha-Ramírez et al., 2017). Miettinen and his colleague reported that both dead and viable *Lactobacillus rhamnosus* GG improved the functions of macrophages through the stimulation of STAT1, STAT3 DNA-binding, and NF-κB activity (Miettinen et al., 2000). However, the molecular pathways underlying these functions have not been reported. The mucosal immune epithelial cells correlate with the defense pathways by the release of IL-2, IL-6, and IL-10 that modulate both nonspecific and specific immune functions by their effects on the immune cells. One of the most important B-cell differentiation factor is IL-6 that probiotic bacteria could affect these B cells in axillary lymph nodes (Akira et al., 2001). Probiotics are capable of stimulating the release of cytokines by macrophages and T cells, resulting in the modulation of mucosal immune pathways (Galdeano et al., 2019; Li et al., 2019).

28.3.3 Probiotic LAB as novel vaccine adjuvants

Among all immune-stimulating factors that contributed to the improvement of efficient vaccine immune functions, adjuvants are of high importance. There is a critical requirement for effective, safe, and cheap vaccine adjuvants to mix with subunit antigens for improvement of their immunogenicity. To date, numerous compounds such as liposomes, mineral salts, particulate compounds, and saponins have been applied as possible vaccine adjuvants in the vaccine formulation (Pasquale et al., 2015). The most extensively applied vaccine adjuvant in humans is alum (aluminum-based compounds) (Bilyy et al., 2019; Freiberger et al., 2018). However, the restricted effectivity of alum in stimulating mucosal responses highlights the demand for a new vaccine adjuvant that could enhance and provoke local mucosal immune activates (Mohan et al., 2013; Reed et al., 2009). The capability of probiotics and their components to stimulate strong mucosal immune response has attracted the attention of most researchers for evaluation of bacterial-based adjuvants as promising means of mucosal immune stimulators (Licciardi & Tang, 2011). The use of immunostimulatory effects of probiotic strains for the treatment or prevention of different diseases, such as allergic diseases led to highlight that probiotic strain, could increase the antigen-specific immune responses as novel vaccine adjuvants (Barnes et al., 2007; Jung et al., 2020; Licciardi & Tang, 2011; Reed et al., 2009; Van Overtvelt et al., 2010). Several properties of probiotics such as improvement of mucosal sIgA responses, the ability to target specific immune cell types, and an approved safety profile make them promising candidates as vaccine adjuvants. Several clinical studies in humans and animals have reported the immune-adjuvant activities of various probiotic bacterial in response to parentally and mucosal used vaccines (Kukkonen et al., 2010; West et al., 2008). Most of these investigations showed the ability of probiotic bacteria to influence both mucosal and systemic immune functions (Ferreira et al., 2010; Jung et al., 2020; Licciardi & Tang, 2011). Probiotics could influence the innate immune cells, including intestinal DCs, or macrophages, and improve the antigen presentation and specific antibody production after vaccination (Licciardi & Tang, 2011). Probiotic bacteria also stimulate the signaling pathways and gene expression in the host cells and reveal important immunomodulatory effects (Yan & Polk, 2011). However, administration of the parenteral route of *Lactobacilli* could stimulate the production of an IgG class of antibodies in the experimental animals. In contrast, only low titers of antibodies could stimulate oral immunization with *Lactobacilli* (Pouwels et al., 1998). A different study demonstrated that *Lactobacilli* in combination with the antigen can nonspecifically induce antigen-specific immune activity after intraperitoneal injection (Perdigon et al., 1993). Furthermore, probiotics may be used as promising adjuvant systems for allergy treatment and prevention. Recently, a well-documented clinical and experimental investigation has confirmed the best candidates are probiotic strains for therapeutic and preventive immunomodulation (Schabussova & Wiedermann, 2008). A study with different strains of LAB for improvement of sublingual immunotherapy efficacy in a murine asthma model has been performed, and two types of bacterial strains including *Lactobacillus helveticus* and *L. casei* were revealed as powerful stimulators of IL-10 and IL-12p70 in dendritic cells, supporting the production of IL-10 and IFN-γ in CD4 + T cells as well as pure Th1 stimulators, respectively. Sublingual administration of *L. helveticus*, but not *L. casei*, in ovalbumin-sensitized mice decreased the proliferation of specific T cells in cervical lymph nodes, airways hyperresponsiveness, and bronchial inflammation, suggesting LAB as potent adjuvants for sublingual allergy vaccines (Van Overtvelt et al., 2010). Moreover, to determine the adjuvant properties of LAB, the nonspecific immune improvement responses were analyzed through the intraperitoneal injection administration of selected *Lactobacillus* strains together with a model antigen. The responses were evaluated as delayed-type hypersensitivity (DTH T-cell responses). DTH T-cell activities are clearly specific for various *Lactobacilli* (Boersma et al., 1992, 2000). It has been reported that strong adjuvant effects for *L. plantarum* ATCC 8014 and *L. casei* var. Shirota were equivalent to the common water-in-oil emulsion adjuvant of Specol (Boersma et al., 1992). However, *Lactobacillus fermentum* showed slight adjuvant properties. Barnes and his colleague also reported that *Bacillus subtilis* spores could instruct a balanced Th1 and Th2 immune response for a specific antigen as a novel microparticle adjuvant. They showed that *B. subtilis* spores not only improved T-cell and antibody responses in a combination used with soluble antigen but also increase noncomplement fixing antibody isotypes, complement and antigen-specific CD4 + and CD8 + T-cell responses (Barnes et al., 2007).

28.3.4 Experimental studies on adjuvant properties of probiotic LAB

Currently, new and existing vaccines may need to combine with potent new adjuvants to increase polyvalent responses of the adaptive immune system. Recently, it has been proposed that induction of the innate immune system is an important factor for the quality and strength of the adaptive immune responses (Luft et al., 2006; Medzhitov & Janeway Jr, 2000) and for recognition of pathogen-associated molecules, specifically by nuclear oligomerization receptors (NOD), scavenger receptors, and Toll-like receptor (TLR) (Iwasaki & Medzhitov, 2004). Numerous data propose that signaling via TLR leads to a Th1-polarized immune pathway. This finding of innate signaling revealed the improvement of synthetic molecular adjuvants according to the TLR agonists (Gorden et al., 2005; Weiner et al., 1997). The adjuvant functions of several probiotic bacterial against various viral and bacterial, parenteral, and mucosal used vaccines are described in Table 28.1. In a study, evaluation of lipopeptide biosurfactants generated from native strains of *Bacillus cereus* showed that this component could act as an adjuvant in inactivated avian influenza H9N2 vaccine (Basit et al., 2018). According to these researchers, 100% protection observed in vaccinated groups indicates that this immunogenic component was safe and had efficacy similar to adjuvant an the inactivated vaccine. They concluded that the obtained biosurfactant could be proposed as an adjuvant in the future. Probiotic lipopeptides constitute promising nonpyrogenic, nontoxic immunological adjuvants when combined with antigen vaccines. A greater humoral immune response was demonstrated in humans when low molecular mass antigens were used (Gharaei-Fathabad, 2011). Particular cellular components in probiotic bacteria could stimulate potent adjuvant functions such as stimulation of reticuloendothelial system, regulation of cell-mediated immune responses, enhancement of cytokine mechanisms and modulation of interleukins, and tumor necrosis factors (Naidu et al., 1999). In a study, it was shown that cellular components from the potential probiotic bacteria *B. subtilis* VSG1, *Pseudomonas aeruginosa* VSG2, and VSG3 in *Labeo rohita* fingerlings could remarkably increase the phagocytosis activity of serum lysozyme, respiratory bursts, and the alternative complement pathway. The results of these studies indicated that immune-associated genes such as COX-2, IL-10, IL-1β, and iNOS were significantly upregulated in fish immunized with cellular components (Giri et al., 2015). Based on these results, it was concluded that probiotic cellular components could be promising adjuvants for vaccines in aquaculture. Another animal study also reported that the subcellular components of probiotic *Bacillus* spp. could increase the immune responses against *Aeromonas hydrophila* (Ramesh et al., 2015). Therefore it could be proposed that probiotics and their components introduce as a microbial dietary adjuvant that helpfully affects the physiology of the host by improving microbial and nutritional balance in the gastrointestinal system, regulating systemic and mucosal immunity (Naidu et al., 1999).

28.3.5 Bacterium-like particles from LAB as mucosal adjuvants

BLPs are described as the nonviable of LAB with the potential to be improved as promising adjuvants for a mucosal candidate vaccine (Tonetti et al., 2020). BLPs derived from *L. lactis* could significantly stimulate the specific immune activities. It is well-known that the immunomodulatory functions of LAB are specific for each strain and thus, different adjuvant capacities could be derived from the BLPs of each individual strain (Li et al., 2019; Tonetti et al., 2020). Different genetically modified LAB were developed, as BLPs derived from the acid and heat treatments of *L. lactis* (Apostólico et al., 2016; Banzhoff et al., 2009; Barnes et al., 2007) could conserve the adjuvant activities of LAB

TABLE 28.1 The adjuvant functions of several probiotic bacterial against various viral and bacterial, parenteral, and mucosal used vaccines.

Probiotic bacteria	Vaccine antigen	Biological effect	Reference(s)
Bifidobacterium longum BL999, Lactobacillus rhamnosus LPR	Hepatitis B	Increased HBs Ag IgG concentrations	Maidens et al. (2013); Soh et al. (2010)
Bifidobacterium animalis ssp. lactis BB-12 and L. paracasei ssp. paracasei 431	Influenza	Increased influenza-specific IgG, IgG1, IgG3 No difference in influenza-specific IgG or IgA	Trachootham et al. (2017)
Lactobacillus fermentum CECT5716	Inactivated trivalent influenza	Elevated total IgG, IgM Elevated influenza-specific IgA responses	Bosch et al. (2012); Olivares et al. (2007)
L. rhamnosus GG (LGG)	Oral live-attenuated poliovirus	Higher neutralizing antibodies to serotype 1 and 2 Elevated polio-specific IgA levels	Licciardi and Tang (2011)
Streptococcus thermophilus and Bifidobacterium breve	Pentacoq	Increased poliovirus-specific IgA levels	Mullié et al. (2004)
L. rhamnosus GG, L. rhamnosus LC705, B. breve Bbi99, Propionibacterium freudenreichi ssp. shermanii	Hib, DTwP	Higher Hib specific IgG levels No effect on diphtheria or tetanus specific IgG	Kukkonen et al. (2006)
Lactobacillus paracasei F19	DTaP, Hib	No effect of diphtheria, tetanus or Hib IgG	West et al. (2008)
S. thermophilus, Lactobacillus casei CRL431, Lactobacillus acidophilus CRL730	Tetanus or pneumococcal vaccine	No effect on tetanus or pneumococcal IgG	Licciardi and Tang (2011)
L. casei strain GG (L. rhamnosus GG or LGG)	Rotavirus vaccine	Increase in IgM antibody-secreting cells in LGG group and higher IgA production in LGG group	Isolauri et al. (1995)
L. acidophilus strain ATCC4356, Bifidobacterium bifidum DSMZ20082, B. longum ATCC157078, Bifidobacterium infantis ATCC15697	Parenteral mumps, measles, rubella and varicella (MMRV) vaccine	Higher proportion of vaccinated infants reached protective IgG antibody titers 3 months after vaccination in probiotic vs. placebo group ($P = .052$)	Youngster et al. (2011)
L. rhamnosus GG (LGG)	Live-attenuated nasal influenza	Increased numbers with protective HAI titers	Davidson et al. (2011)
L. paracasei CRL431	Oral live-attenuated poliovirus	Higher neutralizing antibodies to serotype 3 Elevated polio-specific IgA levels	de Vrese et al. (2005); Valdez et al. (2014)
B. lactis (Bi-07 or Bl-04), L. plantarum Lp-115, L. paracasei Lpc-37, L. salivarius Ls-33 L. acidophilus La-14 and NCFM	Oral cholera vaccine	Increased vaccine-specific serum IgG antibody levels in B. lactis Bl-04 and L. acidophilus La-14 groups. No significant changes for other groups	Maidens et al. (2013); Paineau et al. (2008)
L. acidophilus La1 and B. lactis BB-12	Oral Ty21a typhoid	Increased proportion of subjects with S. typhi-specifc IgA ASCs	Ferreccio et al. (1990)
L. acidophilus LAVRI-A1 1	Parenteral tetanus vaccine	Lower IL-10 responses to tetanus antigen in newborn infants given probiotics	Taylor et al. (2006)
L. rhamnosus GG or L. lactis	Attenuated Salmonella typhi Ty21a oral vaccine	Increased specific IgA in LGG group and increased CR3 receptor expression in L. lactis group	Fang et al. (2000)

bacteria, although they do not contain any cytoplasmic or DNA proteins. The heat/acid treatment produces the dead bacteria that improve the immune-protective responses produced at the mucosal level by recombinant proteins from various pathogens fused to lysine motifs (LysM) (Apostólico et al., 2016). The pathogens are comprised of the influenza virus (de Haan et al., 2012), *Streptococcus pneumoniae* (Li et al., 2018), and *Plasmodium berghei* (Nganou-Makamdop et al., 2012; Velraeds et al., 1998). Those investigations clearly confirmed that *L. lactis*-derived BLPs are a potent adjuvant for mucosal immunization. Furthermore, immunomodulatory activities of BLP obtained from *Lactobacilli* were capable to develop the numbers of CD24 + B220 + B and CD4 + T cells in spleen and Peyer's patches, the production of IFN-γ by immune cells, and the levels of serum IgG and intestinal IgA, suggesting their potential role as mucosal adjuvants (Tonetti et al., 2020). It has been revealed that immunobiotics-derived BLPs of *L. rhamnosus* IBL027, *L. plantarum* CRL1506, and *L. rhamnosus* CRL1505 could show more effective responses in the systemic and intestinal humoral immune pathways regarding derived BLPs of other probiotic bacteria. This result highlights species-specific responses of BLPs for efficient adjuvant activities. However, it has been revealed that the BLP particles derived from the different *Lactobacillus* strains showed various adjuvant activities regarding their capability to increase the humoral and cellular immune functions triggered by rotavirus vaccination (Tonetti et al., 2020). The improvement of different expression of IFN-γ, IL-6, IL-1β as well as porcine CD172a-CD11R1^{low} and CD172a + CD11R1^{high} dendritic cells is more efficient for *L. rhamnosus* CRL1505 in compare with *L. plantarum* CRL1506 (Villena et al., 2014). Moreover, another study confirmed that oral vaccination with immunobiotic BLP derived from *L. rhamnosus* strains along with capsid protein of hepatitis E virus could stimulate the systemic and intestinal immunity in mice. BLP from *L. rhamnosus* strains was more efficient in stimulating specific secretory IgA in the gut. IL-4, TNF-α, and IFN-γ were generated by Peyer's plaque lymphocytes induced with ORF2 ex vivo revealing a mixed adaptive immune response of Th1/Th2-type in immunized BALB/c mice (Arce et al., 2019). Furthermore, nasal immunization with pneumococcal surface protein A (PspA) adjuvanted with BLPs from *Lactobacillus* could stimulate a high level of SIgA antibodies and a high level of serum IgG antibodies in the respiratory tract against heterogenous and homologous *S. pneumoniae* infection in mice (Li et al., 2018). Therefore characterization of mucosal adjuvants to increase the immune responses against pathogens is of fundamental importance to improve vaccine efficacy. For these reasons, the appropriate selection of BLPs obtained from immunomodulatory LAB is a promising adjuvant alternative.

28.3.6 Adjuvant potential of biosurfactants produced by LAB

Biosurfactants are amphiphilic naturally produced surfactants that diminish the surface tension between a liquid and a solid or two liquids (Aparna et al., 2012). A number of *Lactobacillus* species have been known as potential biosurfactant producers comprising various proportions of proteins and polysaccharides (Aparna et al., 2012; Velraeds et al., 1996a,b, 1998). An interesting characteristic of biosurfactants produced by a number of LAB bacteria is their strong immune-modulatory actions that have led to possible pharmaceutical applications. These bacterial lipopeptides are nonpyrogenic, nontoxic, and do not induce tissue damage when mixed with conventional antigens. They are potent immune-adjuvant compared to Freund's adjuvant. They enhance the humoral immune response without a decrease in specific IgG. Therefore they have a potential application as an immune-adjuvant in vaccine production (Kaloorazi & Choobari, 2013). They could change the surface energy and wettability properties of the original surface (Neu, 1996). Biosurfactants may affect the detachment and adhesion of bacteria through the interaction with the bacteria. Furthermore, the properties of the substratum surface could identify the orientation and composition of the surface of the molecule at the first time of exposure. The biosurfactant compounds of *Bacillus licheniformis* were recognized as lichenysin that showed nonpyrogenic and nontoxic immunological adjuvants (Grangemard et al., 2001; Jenny et al., 1991; Rodrigues et al., 2006). Promising applications of biosurfactants as emulsifying factors for adjuvant of vaccines were shown bacterial lipopeptides establish the powerful nontoxic and nonpyrogenic immunological adjuvants when mixed with different conventional antigens. A significant increase of the humoral immune functions was reported with the low molecular mass antigens microcystin (MLR) coupled to poly-L-lysine (MLR-PLL), herbicolin A, and iturin AL in chickens and rabbits. Conjugates of lipopeptide−Th-cell epitopes also created potent adjuvants for the in vitro immunization of mouse B cells as well as human mononuclear cells with MLR-PLL which induced a remarkably expanded yield of antibody-secreting hybridoma (Mittenbühler et al., 1997). Biosurfactants are the diverse polymeric molecules synthesized during the early stationary phase or late log of the growth cycle of an organism, secreted either cell wall-bound or extracellularly. These compounds are commonly made of amphiphilic molecules, comprising both hydrophilic and hydrophobic moieties (Banat et al., 2010). The major group of biosurfactants comprised of polymeric surfactants, phospholipids, glycolipids, fatty acids, particulate surfactants, lipoproteins, and lipopeptides as shown in Table 28.2. These bioactive compounds have recently emerged as promising molecules for their structural versatility, novelty, and

TABLE 28.2 Structural composition of biosurfactants derived from various LAB strains.

LAB strain	Biosurfactant composition	Reference
Lactobacillus acidophilus RC14	High amount of phosphate and polysaccharides content, rich in protein	Velraeds et al. (1996b)
Streptococcus thermophilus	Glycolipid	Busscher and Van der Mei (1997)
Lactobacillus acidophilus	Surlactin	Velraeds et al. (1996b)
Streptococcus mutans NS	Rhamnolipid like	van Hoogmoed et al. (2004)
Streptococcus thermophiles A	Glycolipid	Rodrigues et al. (2006)
Lactobacillus plantarum	Glycolipids	Sauvageau et al. (2012)
Lactobacillus pentosus	Glycolipids	Vecino et al. (2014)
Lactobacillus casei MRTL3	Glycolipids	Sharma et al. (2014)
Lactobacillus casei	Glycoprotein	Gol·ek et al. (2009)
Lactococcus lactis	Xylolipids	Saravanakumari and Mani (2010)
Lactobacillus acidophilus	Glycoprotein	Tahmourespour et al. (2011)
Lactobacillus plantarum	Glycoprotein	Madhu and Prapulla (2014)
Enterococcus faecium MRTL9	Xylolipids	Sharma et al. (2015)
Lactobacillus helveticus MRTL91	Glycolipids	Sharma et al. (2015)
Lactobacillus pentosus	Glycolipopeptide	Vecino et al. (2015)
Lactobacillus gasseri P_{65} and Lactobacillus jensenii P_{6A}	Glycolipioproteins	Morais et al. (2017)
Lactococcus lactis 53	Glycoprotein	Rodrigues et al. (2006)
Lactobacillus paracasei	Glycoprotein	Gudina et al. (2010)
Lactobacillus pentosus	Glycoprotein	Moldes et al. (2013)
Bacillus subtilis ATCC 6633	Lipopeptide	Dehghan-Noudeh et al. (2005)

diverse properties that are potentially useful for many therapeutic applications. One of the most important therapeutic effects of biosurfactants is their anticancer actions and their ability to regulate cancer progression processes (Gudiña et al., 2013).

28.3.7 Adjuvant potential of LAB ghost cells

Bacterial ghosts (BGs) are empty bacterial cell envelopes created by releasing the cytoplasmic contents through pores in the cell walls. As BGs retain their original cell shape and surface structures, much of their immunogenicity is also retained and hence are considered potential immunogens (Batah & Ahmad, 2020; Riedmann et al., 2007). Development of DNA vaccines is a major breakthrough in the vaccinology field. Although these vaccines may have many advantages compared to the traditional vaccines, their poor immunogenicity hampers their application (Ebensen et al., 2004). Thus many efforts have been put into boosting the DNA vaccine immune response to make its practical applications possible. It has been known that BGs have a strong capacity for carrying DNA and have the potential to target the DNA vaccine to APCs; BGs also act as adjuvants to promote activation and maturation of dendritic cells (Cai et al., 2010; Hou et al., 2018). Hou and colleagues (2018), for the very first time showed that *L. casei* BGs were constructed by expressing the lysis protein of *L. casei* phage, stimulated more efficient immune responses compared to naked DNA. These researchers concluded that as *L. casei* BG is bigger in size, they have the ability to carry more DNA and thus may overcome the problems associated with DNA vaccines, such as poor immunogenicity and high degradability, and improve the level of immune response elicited by them (Hou et al., 2018). Ghost-vaccine techniques enable the production of safer alternative-killed vaccines; there are platforms that express a wide number of antigens and DNA encoding epitopes, carrier envelopes for DNA vaccines and antigens, adjuvants, and dendritic cell enhancers.

28.4 Conclusions

To date a number of studies have proven the promising role of probiotic LAB as an effective adjuvant system for mucosal vaccine development. The role of probiotics as adjuvants, that could improve vaccine potency without compromising tolerability or safety, are proposed as safer alternatives to the conventional used adjuvants. Furthermore, the components of LAB have adjuvant properties, which can enhance the immune responses induced by the carried antigen. However, a hypothesis warranting further exploration as to whether it is possible to design a noninflammatory probiotic adjuvant that could enhance vaccine immunogenicity without causing reactogenicity or compromising vaccine safety.

References

Abreu, M. T. (2010). Toll-like receptor signalling in the intestinal epithelium: How bacterial recognition shapes intestinal function. *Nature Reviews Immunology, 10*, 131–144.

Adel, M., El-Sayed, A.-F. M., Yeganeh, S., Dadar, M., & Giri, S. S. (2017). Effect of potential probiotic *Lactococcus lactis* subsp. lactis on growth performance, intestinal microbiota, digestive enzyme activities, and disease resistance of *Litopenaeus vannamei*. *Probiotics and antimicrobial proteins, 9*, 150–156.

Akira, S., Takeda, K., & Kaisho, T. (2001). Toll-like receptors: Critical proteins linking innate and acquired immunity. *Nature Immunology, 2*, 675.

Allen, S. J., Jordan, S., Storey, M., Thornton, C. A., Gravenor, M. B., Garaiova, I., Plummer, S. F., Wang, D., & Morgan, G. (2014). Probiotics in the prevention of eczema: A randomised controlled trial. *Archives of Disease in Childhood, 99*, 1014–1019.

Amara, A., & Shibl, A. (2015). Role of Probiotics in health improvement, infection control and disease treatment and management. *Saudi Pharmaceutical Journal, 23*, 107–114.

Amdekar, S., Dwivedi, D., Roy, P., Kushwah, S., & Singh, V. (2010). Probiotics: Multifarious oral vaccine against infectious traumas. *FEMS Immunology and Medical Microbiology, 58*, 299–306.

Anand, A., Sato, M., & Aoyagi, H. (2019). Screening of phosphate-accumulating probiotics for potential use in chronic kidney disorder. *Food Science and Technology Research, 25*, 89–96.

Anukam, K. C., Osazuwa, E. O., Osadolor, H. B., Bruce, A. W., & Reid, G. (2008). Yogurt containing probiotic *Lactobacillus rhamnosus* GR-1 and L. reuteri RC-14 helps resolve moderate diarrhea and increases CD4 count in HIV/AIDS patients. *Journal of Clinical Gastroenterology, 42*, 239–243.

Aparna, A., Srinikethan, G., & Smitha, H. (2012). Production and characterization of biosurfactant produced by a novel *Pseudomonas* sp. 2B. *Colloids and Surfaces B: Biointerfaces, 95*, 23–29.

Apostólico, Jd. S., Lunardelli, V. A. S., Coirada, F. C., Boscardin, S. B., & Rosa, D. S. (2016). Adjuvants: Classification, modus operandi, and licensing. *Journal of immunology research, 2016*.

Arce, L., Tonetti, M. R., Raimondo, M., Müller, M., Salva, S., Álvarez, S., Baiker, A., Villena, J., & Pinto, M. V. (2019). Oral vaccination with Hepatitis E virus capsid protein and immunobiotic bacterium-like particles induce intestinal and systemic immunity in mice. *Probiotics and Antimicrobial Proteins*, 1–12.

Arunachalam, K., Gill, H., & Chandra, R. (2000). Enhancement of natural immune function by dietary consumption of *Bifidobacterium lactis* (HN019). *European Journal of Clinical Nutrition, 54*, 263.

Audouy, S. A., Van Roosmalen, M. L., Neef, J., Kanninga, R., Post, E., Van Deemter, M., Metselaar, H., Van Selm, S., Robillard, G. T., & Leenhouts, K. J. (2006). *Lactococcus lactis* GEM particles displaying pneumococcal antigens induce local and systemic immune responses following intranasal immunization. *Vaccine, 24*, 5434–5441.

Azcárate-Peril, M. A., Sikes, M., & Bruno-Bárcena, J. M. (2011). The intestinal microbiota, gastrointestinal environment and colorectal cancer: A putative role for probiotics in prevention of colorectal cancer? *American Journal of Physiology-Gastrointestinal and Liver Physiology, 301*, G401–G424.

Bahey-El-Din, M., Gahan, C. G., & Griffin, B. T. (2010). Lactococcus lactis as a cell factory for delivery of therapeutic proteins. *Current Gene Therapy, 10*, 34–45.

Banat, I. M., Franzetti, A., Gandolfi, I., Bestetti, G., Martinotti, M. G., Fracchia, L., Smyth, T. J., & Marchant, R. (2010). Microbial biosurfactants production, applications and future potential. *Applied Microbiology and Biotechnology, 87*, 427–444.

Banzhoff, A., Gasparini, R., Laghi-Pasini, F., Staniscia, T., Durando, P., Montomoli, E., Capecchi, P., Di Giovanni, P., Sticchi, L., & Gentile, C. (2009). MF59®-adjuvanted H5N1 vaccine induces immunologic memory and heterotypic antibody responses in non-elderly and elderly adults. *PLoS One, 4*, e4384.

Barnes, A. G., Cerovic, V., Hobson, P. S., & Klavinskis, L. S. (2007). *Bacillus subtilis* spores: A novel microparticle adjuvant which can instruct a balanced Th1 and Th2 immune response to specific antigen. *European Journal of Immunology, 37*, 1538–1547.

Basit, M., Rasool, M. H., Hassan, M. F., Khurshid, M., Aslam, N., Tahir, M. F., Waseem, M., & Aslam, B. (2018). Evaluation of lipopeptide biosurfactants produced from native strains of *Bacillus cereus* as adjuvant in inactivated low pathogenicity avian influenza H9N2 vaccine. *International Journal of Agriculture and Biology, 20*, 1419–1423.

Batah, A. M., & Ahmad, T. A. (2020). The development of ghosts vaccine trials. *Expert Review of Vaccines*.

Beran, J. (2008). Safety and immunogenicity of a new hepatitis B vaccine for the protection of patients with renal insufficiency including prehaemodialysis and haemodialysis patients. *Expert Opinion on Biological Therapy, 8*, 235–247.

Bilyy, R., Paryzhak, S., Turcheniuk, K., Dumych, T., Barras, A., Boukherroub, R., Wang, F., Yushin, G., & Szunerits, S. (2019). Aluminum oxide nanowires as safe and effective adjuvants for next-generation vaccines. *Materials Today*, 22, 58−66.

Bisanz, J. E., Enos, M. K., PrayGod, G., Seney, S., Macklaim, J. M., Chilton, S., Willner, D., Knight, R., Fusch, C., & Fusch, G. (2015). Microbiota at multiple body sites during pregnancy in a rural Tanzanian population and effects of Moringa-supplemented probiotic yogurt. *Applied and Environmental Microbiology*, 81, 4965−4975.

Boersma, W. J. A., Shaw, M., & Claassen, E. (2000). Probiotic bacteria as live oral vaccines Lactobacillus as the versatile delivery vehicle. In R. Fuller, & G. Perdigon (Eds.), *Probiotics 3: Immunomodulation by the gut microflora and probiotics* (pp. 234−270). Kluwer Academic Publ.

Boersma, W. A., Bogaerts, W. C., Bianchi, A. J., & Claassen, E. (1992). Adjuvant properties of stable water-in-oil emulsions: Evaluation of the experience with Specol. *Research in Immunology (Paris)*, 143, 503−512.

Bosch, M., Mendez, M., Perez, M., Farran, A., Fuentes, M., & Cune, J. (2012). *Lactobacillus plantarum* CECT7315 and CECT7316 stimulate immunoglobulin production after influenza vaccination in elderly. *Nutricion Hospitalaria: Organo Oficial de la Sociedad Espanola de Nutricion Parenteral y Enteral*, 27, 504−509.

Bosma, T., Kanninga, R., Neef, J., Audouy, S. A., van Roosmalen, M. L., Steen, A., Buist, G., Kok, J., Kuipers, O. P., & Robillard, G. (2006). Novel surface display system for proteins on non-genetically modified gram-positive bacteria. *Applied and Environmental Microbiology*, 72, 880−889.

Bouvier, M., Meance, S., Bouley, C., Berta, J.-L., & Grimaud, J.-C. (2001). Effects of consumptionof a milk fermented by the probiotic strain *Bifidobacterium animalis* DN-173 010 on colonic transit times in healthy humans. *Bioscience and Microflora*, 20, 43−48.

Busscher, H., & Van der Mei, H. (1997). Physico-chemical interactions in initial microbial adhesion and relevance for biofilm formation. *Advances in Dental Research*, 11, 24−32.

Cai, K., Gao, X., Li, T., Hou, X., Wang, Q., Liu, H., Xiao, L., Tu, W., Liu, Y., & Shi, J. (2010). Intragastric immunization of mice with enterohemorrhagic *Escherichia coli* O157: H7 bacterial ghosts reduces mortality and shedding and induces a Th2-type dominated mixed immune response. *Canadian Journal of Microbiology*, 56, 389−398.

Cervin, A. U. (2018). The potential for topical probiotic treatment of chronic rhinosinusitis, a personal perspective. *Frontiers in Cellular and Infection Microbiology*, 7, 530.

Clancy, R. (2003). Immunobiotics and the probiotic evolution. *FEMS Immunology and Medical Microbiology*, 38, 9−12.

Clements, C., & Griffiths, E. (2002). The global impact of vaccines containing aluminium adjuvants. *Vaccine*, 20, S24−S33.

Coffman, R. L., Sher, A., & Seder, R. A. (2010). Vaccine adjuvants: Putting innate immunity to work. *Immunity*, 33, 492−503.

Cremon, C., Barbaro, M. R., Ventura, M., & Barbara, G. (2018). Pre-and probiotic overview. *Current Opinion in Pharmacology*, 43, 87−92.

Davidson, L. E., Fiorino, A.-M., Snydman, D. R., & Hibberd, P. L. (2011). Lactobacillus GG as an immune adjuvant for live-attenuated influenza vaccine in healthy adults: A randomized double-blind placebo-controlled trial. Eur. *The Journal of Clinical Nutrition*, 65, 501.

de Haan, A., Haijema, B. J., Voorn, P., Meijerhof, T., van Roosmalen, M. L., & Leenhouts, K. (2012). Bacterium-like particles supplemented with inactivated influenza antigen induce cross-protective influenza-specific antibody responses through intranasal administration. *Vaccine*, 30, 4884−4891.

de Vrese, M., Rautenberg, P., Laue, C., Koopmans, M., Herremans, T., & Schrezenmeir, J. (2005). Probiotic bacteria stimulate virus−specific neutralizing antibodies following a booster polio vaccination. *European Journal of Nutrition*, 44, 406−413.

Dehghan-Noudeh, G., Housaindokht, M., & Bazzaz, B. S. F. (2005). Isolation, characterization, and investigation of surface and hemolytic activities of a lipopeptide biosurfactant produced by Bacillus subtilis ATCC 6633. The. *Journal of Microbiology*, 43, 272−276.

Dinarello, C. A., & van der Meer, J. W. (2013). Treating inflammation by blocking interleukin-1 in humans. *Seminars in Immunology*, 25(6), 469−484, Elsevier. Available from https://doi.org/10.1016/j.smim.2013.10.008.

Dugas, B., Mercenier, A., Lenoir-Wijnkoop, I., Arnaud, C., Dugas, N., & Postaire, E. (1999). Immunity and probiotics. *Immunology Today*, 20, 387−390.

Dvorožňáková, E., Bucková, B., Hurníková, Z., Revajová, V., & Lauková, A. (2016). Effect of probiotic bacteria on phagocytosis and respiratory burst activity of blood polymorphonuclear leukocytes (PMNL) in mice infected with *Trichinella spiralis*. *Veterinary Parasitology*, 231, 69−76.

Ebensen, T., Paukner, S., Link, C., Kudela, P., de Domenico, C., Lubitz, W., & Guzmán, C. A. (2004). Bacterial ghosts are an efficient delivery system for DNA vaccines. *The Journal of Immunology*, 172, 6858−6865.

Endo, T., & Manya, H. (2006). *O-mannosylation in mammalian cells. Glycobiology protocols* (pp. 43−56). Springer.

Fang, H., Elina, T., Heikki, A., & Seppo, S. (2000). Modulation of humoral immune response through probiotic intake. *FEMS Immunology and Medical Microbiology*, 29, 47−52.

Ferreccio, C., Ortiz, E., Cryz, S., & Levine, M. (1990). Comparison of enteric-coated capsules and liquid formulation of Ty21a typhoid vaccine in randomised controlled field trial. *The Lancet*, 336, 891−894.

Ferreira, R. B., Antunes, L. C. M., & Finlay, B. B. (2010). Should the human microbiome be considered when developing vaccines? *PLoS Pathogens*, 6, e1001190.

Frei, R., Akdis, M., & O'Mahony, L. (2015). Prebiotics, probiotics, synbiotics, and the immune system: Experimental data and clinical evidence. *Current Opinion in Gastroenterology*, 31, 153−158.

Freiberger, S. N., Leuthard, D. S., Duda, A., Contassot, E., Thallmair, M., Kündig, T. M., & Johansen, P. (2018). Intraperitoneal administration of aluminium-based adjuvants produces severe transient systemic adverse events in mice. *European Journal of Pharmaceutical Sciences: Official Journal of the European Federation for Pharmaceutical Sciences*, 115, 362−368.

Fujimura, S., Watanabe, A., Kimura, K., & Kaji, M. (2012). Probiotic mechanism of *Lactobacillus gasseri* OLL2716 strain against *Helicobacter pylori*. *Journal of Clinical Microbiology*, 50, 1134−1136.

Fuller, R. (1992). *History and development of probiotics*. Probiotics (pp. 1−8). Springer.
Galdeano, C. M., Cazorla, S. I., Dumit, J. M. L., Vélez, E., & Perdigón, G. (2019). Beneficial effects of probiotic consumption on the immune system. *Annals of Nutrition & Metabolism, 74*, 115−124.
Galdeano, C. M., & Perdigon, G. (2006). The probiotic bacterium *Lactobacillus casei* induces activation of the gut mucosal immune system through innate immunity. *Clinical and Vaccine Immunology: CVI, 13*, 219−226.
Garcia-Castillo, V., Albarracin, L., Kitazawa, H., & Villena, J. (2019). *Screening and characterization of immunobiotic lactic acid bacteria with porcine immunoassay systems*. Lactic acid bacteria (pp. 131−144). Springer.
Geeraedts, F., Goutagny, N., Hornung, V., Severa, M., de Haan, A., Pool, J., Wilschut, J., Fitzgerald, K. A., & Huckriede, A. (2008). Superior immunogenicity of inactivated whole virus H5N1 influenza vaccine is primarily controlled by Toll-like receptor signalling. *PLoS Pathogens, 4*, e1000138.
Gharaei-Fathabad, E. (2011). Biosurfactants in pharmaceutical industry: A mini-review. *American Journal of Drug Discovery and Development, 1*, 58−69.
Giri, S. S., Sen, S. S., Chi, C., Kim, H. J., Yun, S., Park, S. C., & Sukumaran, V. (2015). Effect of cellular products of potential probiotic bacteria on the immune response of *Labeo rohita* and susceptibility to Aeromonas hydrophila infection. *Fish & Shellfish Immunology, 46*, 716−722.
Gol·ek, P., Bednarski, W., Brzozowski, B., & Dziuba, B. (2009). The obtaining and properties of biosurfactants synthesized by bacteria of the genus Lactobacillus. *Annals of Microbiology, 59*, 119−126.
Gombosova, A., Demes, P., & Valent, M. (1986). Immunotherapeutic effect of the lactobacillus vaccine, Solco Trichovac, in trichomoniasis is not mediated by antibodies cross reacting with Trichomonas vaginalis. *Sexually Transmitted Infections, 62*, 107−110.
Gorden, K. B., Gorski, K. S., Gibson, S. J., Kedl, R. M., Kieper, W. C., Qiu, X., Tomai, M. A., Alkan, S. S., & Vasilakos, J. P. (2005). Synthetic TLR agonists reveal functional differences between human TLR7 and TLR8. *The Journal of Immunology, 174*, 1259−1268.
Grangemard, I., Wallach, J., Maget-Dana, R., & Peypoux, F. (2001). Lichenysin. *Applied Biochemistry and Biotechnology, 90*, 199−210.
Gudiña, E. J., Rangarajan, V., Sen, R., & Rodrigues, L. R. (2013). Potential therapeutic applications of biosurfactants. *Trends in Pharmacological Sciences, 34*, 667−675.
Gudina, E. J., Teixeira, J. A., & Rodrigues, L. R. (2010). Isolation and functional characterization of a biosurfactant produced by *Lactobacillus paracasei*. *Colloids and Surfaces B: Biointerfaces, 76*, 298−304.
Hill, A. V. (2006). Pre-erythrocytic malaria vaccines: Towards greater efficacy. *Nature Reviews Immunology, 6*, 21−32.
Hoseinifar, S. H., Dadar, M., & Ringø, E. (2017). Modulation of nutrient digestibility and digestive enzyme activities in aquatic animals: The functional feed additives scenario. *Aquaculture Research, 48*, 3987−4000.
Hou, R., Li, M., Tang, T., Wang, R., Li, Y., Xu, Y., Tang, L., Wang, L., Liu, M., & Jiang, Y. (2018). Construction of *Lactobacillus casei* ghosts by Holin-mediated inactivation and the potential as a safe and effective vehicle for the delivery of DNA vaccines. *BMC Microbiology, 18*, 80.
Irvine, S. L., Hummelen, R., Hekmat, S., Looman, C. W., Habbema, J. D. F., & Reid, G. (2010). Probiotic yogurt consumption is associated with an increase of CD4 count among people living with HIV/AIDS. *Journal of Clinical Gastroenterology, 44*, e201−e205.
Isolauri, E., Joensuu, J., Suomalainen, H., Luomala, M., & Vesikari, T. (1995). Improved immunogenicity of oral D x RRV reassortant rotavirus vaccine by *Lactobacillus casei* GG. *Vaccine, 13*, 310−312.
Isolauri, E., Sütas, Y., Kankaanpää, P., Arvilommi, H., & Salminen, S. (2001). Probiotics: Effects on immunity. *The American Journal of Clinical Nutrition, 73*, 444s−450s.
Iwasaki, A., & Medzhitov, R. (2004). Toll-like receptor control of the adaptive immune responses. *Nature Immunology, 5*, 987−995.
Jenny, K., Käppeli, O., & Fiechter, A. (1991). Biosurfactants from *Bacillus licheniformis*: Structural analysis and characterization. *Applied Microbiology and Biotechnology, 36*, 5−13.
Jung, Y.-J., Kim, K.-H., Ko, E.-J., Lee, Y., Kim, M.-C., Lee, Y.-T., Kim, C.-H., Jeeva, S., Park, B. R., & Kang, S.-M. (2020). Adjuvant effects of killed *Lactobacillus casei* DK128 on enhancing T helper type 1 immune responses and the efficacy of influenza vaccination in normal and CD4-deficient mice. *Vaccine, 38*, 5783−5792.
Kaloorazi, N. A., & Choobari, M. F. S. (2013). Biosurfactants: Properties and applications. *Journal of Biology and Today's World, 2*, 235−241.
Kałużna-Czaplińska, J., Gątarek, P., Chartrand, M. S., Dadar, M., & Bjørklund, G. (2017). Is there a relationship between intestinal microbiota, dietary compounds, and obesity? *Trends in Food Science & Technology, 70*, 105−113.
Kaufmann, S. H. (2006). Tuberculosis: Back on the immunologists' agenda. *Immunity, 24*, 351−357.
Konieczna, P., Groeger, D., Ziegler, M., Frei, R., Ferstl, R., Shanahan, F., Quigley, E. M., Kiely, B., Akdis, C. A., & O'Mahony, L. (2012). *Bifidobacterium infantis* 35624 administration induces Foxp3 T regulatory cells in human peripheral blood: Potential role for myeloid and plasmacytoid dendritic cells. *Gut, 61*, 354−366.
Koppang, E. O., Bjerkås, I., Haugarvoll, E., Chan, E. K., Szabo, N. J., Ono, N., Akikusa, B., Jirillo, E., Poppe, T. T., & Sveier, H. (2008). Vaccination-induced systemic autoimmunity in farmed Atlantic salmon. *The Journal of Immunology, 181*, 4807−4814.
Korik, L., Liubimova, L., & Tovstoles, K. (1968). Immediate and remote results of the treatment of male trichomonas infections with trichomonas vaccine. *Vestnik Dermatologii i Venerologii, 42*, 80−84.
Kukkonen, K., Kuitunen, M., Haahtela, T., Korpela, R., Poussa, T., & Savilahti, E. (2010). High intestinal IgA associates with reduced risk of IgE-associated allergic diseases. *Pediatric Allergy and Immunology: Official Publication of the European Society of Pediatric Allergy and Immunology, 21*, 67−73.
Kukkonen, K., Nieminen, T., Poussa, T., Savilahti, E., & Kuitunen, M. (2006). Effect of probiotics on vaccine antibody responses in infancy—a randomized placebo-controlled double-blind trial. *Pediatric Allergy and Immunology: Official Publication of the European Society of Pediatric Allergy and Immunology, 17*, 416−421.

Lee, D. K., Park, J. E., Kim, M. J., Seo, J. G., Lee, J. H., & Ha, N. J. (2015). Probiotic bacteria, B. longum and L. acidophilus inhibit infection by rotavirus in vitro and decrease the duration of diarrhea in pediatric patients. *Clinics and Research in Hepatology and Gastroenterology, 39*, 237−244.

Li, B., Chen, X., Yu, J., Zhang, Y., Mo, Z., Gu, T., Kong, W., & Wu, Y. (2018). Protection elicited by nasal immunization with pneumococcal surface protein A (PspA) adjuvanted with bacterium-like particles against *Streptococcus pneumoniae* infection in mice. *Microbial Pathogenesis, 123*, 115−119.

Li, E., Chi, H., Huang, P., Yan, F., Zhang, Y., Liu, C., Wang, Z., Li, G., Zhang, S., & Mo, R. (2019). A novel bacterium-like particle vaccine displaying the MERS-CoV receptor-binding domain induces specific mucosal and systemic immune responses in mice. *Viruses, 11*, 799. Available from https://doi.org/10.3390/v11090799.

Licciardi, P. V., & Tang, M. L. (2011). Vaccine adjuvant properties of probiotic bacteria. *Discovery Medicine, 12*, 525−533.

Lilly, D. M., & Stillwell, R. H. (1965). Probiotics: Growth-promoting factors produced by microorganisms. *Science (New York, N.Y.), 147*, 747−748.

Luft, T., Rodionova, E., Maraskovsky, E., Kirsch, M., Hess, M., Buchholtz, C., Goerner, M., Schnurr, M., Skoda, R., & Ho, A. D. (2006). Adaptive functional differentiation of dendritic cells: Integrating the network of extra-and intracellular signals. *Blood, 107*, 4763−4769.

Madhu, A. N., & Prapulla, S. G. (2014). Evaluation and functional characterization of a biosurfactant produced by *Lactobacillus plantarum* CFR 2194. *Applied Biochemistry and Biotechnology, 172*, 1777−1789.

Maidens, C., Childs, C., Przemska, A., Dayel, I. B., & Yaqoob, P. (2013). Modulation of vaccine response by concomitant probiotic administration. *British Journal of Clinical Pharmacology, 75*, 663−670.

Marranzino, G., Villena, J., Salva, S., & Alvarez, S. (2012). Stimulation of macrophages by immunobiotic Lactobacillus strains: Influence beyond the intestinal tract. *Microbiology and Immunology, 56*, 771−781.

McMichael, A. J. (2006). HIV vaccines. *Annual Review of Immunology, 24*, 227−255.

Medzhitov, R., & Janeway, C., Jr (2000). Innate immune recognition: Mechanisms and pathways. *Immunological Reviews, 173*, 89.

Miettinen, M., Lehtonen, A., Julkunen, I., & Matikainen, S. (2000). Lactobacilli and streptococci activate NF-κB and STAT signaling pathways in human macrophages. *The Journal of Immunology, 164*, 3733−3740.

Mittenbühler, K., Loleit, M., Baier, W., Fischer, B., Sedelmeier, E., Jung, G., Winkelmann, G., Jacobi, C., Weckesser, J., & Erhard, M. H. (1997). Drug specific antibodies: T-cell epitope-lipopeptide conjugates are potent adjuvants for small antigens in vivo and in vitro. *International Journal of Immunopharmacology, 19*, 277−287.

Miu, A. C., & Benga, O. (2006). Aluminum and Alzheimer's disease: A new look. *Journal of Alzheimer's Disease: JAD, 10*, 179−201.

Mohan, T., Verma, P., & Rao, D. N. (2013). Novel adjuvants & delivery vehicles for vaccines development: A road ahead. *The Indian Journal of Medical Research, 138*, 779.

Mojgani, N., Shahali, Y., & Dadar, M. (2020). Immune modulatory capacity of probiotic lactic acid bacteria and applications in vaccine development. *Beneficial Microbes, 11*, 213−226.

Moldes, A., Paradelo, R., Vecino, X., Cruz, J., Gudiña, E., Rodrigues, L., Teixeira, J., Domínguez, J. M., & Barral, M. (2013). Partial characterization of biosurfactant from Lactobacillus pentosus and comparison with sodium dodecyl sulphate for the bioremediation of hydrocarbon contaminated soil. *BioMed Research International, 2013*.

Morais, I., Cordeiro, A., Teixeira, G., Domingues, V., Nardi, R., Monteiro, A., Alves, R., Siqueira, E., & Santos, V. (2017). Biological and physicochemical properties of biosurfactants produced by *Lactobacillus jensenii* P 6A and Lactobacillus gasseri P 65. *Microbial Cell Factories, 16*, 155.

Morelli, L., & Capurso, L. (2012). FAO/WHO guidelines on probiotics: 10 years later. *Journal of Clinical Gastroenterology, 46*, S1−S2.

Mullié, C., Yazourh, A., Thibault, H., Odou, M.-F., Singer, E., Kalach, N., Kremp, O., & Romond, M.-B. (2004). Increased poliovirus-specific intestinal antibody response coincides with promotion of *Bifidobacterium longum*-infantis and *Bifidobacterium breve* in infants: A randomized, double-blind, placebo-controlled trial. *Pediatric Research, 56*, 791.

Naidu, A., Bidlack, W., & Clemens, R. (1999). Probiotic spectra of lactic acid bacteria (LAB). *Critical Reviews in Food Science and Nutrition, 39*, 13−126.

Neto, M. P. C., de Souza Aquino, J., da Silva, L. D. F. R., de Oliveira Silva, R., de Lima Guimaraes, K. S., de Oliveira, Y., de Souza, E. L., Magnani, M., Vidal, H., & de Brito Alves, J. L. (2018). Gut microbiota and probiotics intervention: A potential therapeutic target for management of cardiometabolic disorders and chronic kidney disease? *Pharmacological Research: The Official Journal of the Italian Pharmacological Society, 130*, 152−163.

Neu, T. R. (1996). Significance of bacterial surface-active compounds in interaction of bacteria with interfaces. *Microbiological Reviews, 60*, 151.

Nganou-Makamdop, K., van Roosmalen, M. L., Audouy, S. A., van Gemert, G.-J., Leenhouts, K., Hermsen, C. C., & Sauerwein, R. W. (2012). Bacterium-like particles as multi-epitope delivery platform for *Plasmodium berghei* circumsporozoite protein induce complete protection against malaria in mice. *Malaria Journal, 11*, 50.

Nikolich-Žugich, J. (2018). The twilight of immunity: Emerging concepts in aging of the immune system. *Nature Immunology, 19*, 10−19.

Oak, S. J., & Jha, R. (2019). The effects of probiotics in lactose intolerance: A systematic review. *Critical Reviews in Food Science and Nutrition, 59*, 1675−1683.

Olivares, M., Díaz-Ropero, M. P., Sierra, S., Lara-Villoslada, F., Fonollá, J., Navas, M., Rodríguez, J. M., & Xaus, J. (2007). Oral intake of *Lactobacillus fermentum* CECT5716 enhances the effects of influenza vaccination. *Nutrition (Burbank, Los Angeles County, Calif.), 23*, 254−260.

Paineau, D., Carcano, D., Leyer, G., Darquy, S., Alyanakian, M.-A., Simoneau, G., Bergmann, J.-F., Brassart, D., Bornet, F., & Ouwehand, A. C. (2008). Effects of seven potential probiotic strains on specific immune responses in healthy adults: A double-blind, randomized, controlled trial. *FEMS Immunology and Medical Microbiology, 53*, 107−113.

Pandey, K. R., Naik, S. R., & Vakil, B. V. (2015). Probiotics, prebiotics and synbiotics-a review. *Journal of Food Science and Technology, 52*, 7577–7587.

Pasquale, A. D., Preiss, S., Silva, F. T. D., & Garçon, N. (2015). Vaccine adjuvants: From 1920 to 2015 and beyond. *Vaccines, 3*, 320–343.

Perdigón, G., & Alvarez, S. (1992). *Probiotics and the immune state. Probiotics* (pp. 145–180). Springer.

Perdigon, G., Medici, M., Bibas Bonet de Jorrat, M., Valverde de Budeguer, M., & Pesce de Ruiz Holgado, A. (1993). Immunomodulating effects of lactic acid bacteria on mucosal and tumoral immunity. *International Journal of Immunotherapy, 9*, 29–52.

Petrovsky, N. (2008). Freeing vaccine adjuvants from dangerous immunological dogma. *Expert Review of Vaccines, 7*, 7–10.

Pouwels, P. H., Leer, R. J., Shaw, M., den Bak-Glashouwer, M.-J. H., Tielen, F. D., Smit, E., Martinez, B., Jore, J., & Conway, P. L. (1998). Lactic acid bacteria as antigen delivery vehicles for oral immunization purposes. *International Journal of Food Microbiology, 41*, 155–167.

Ramesh, D., Vinothkanna, A., Rai, A. K., & Vignesh, V. S. (2015). Isolation of potential probiotic *Bacillus* spp. and assessment of their subcellular components to induce immune responses in *Labeo rohita* against *Aeromonas hydrophila*. *Fish & Shellfish Immunology, 45*, 268–276.

Reed, S. G., Bertholet, S., Coler, R. N., & Friede, M. (2009). New horizons in adjuvants for vaccine development. *Trends in Immunology, 30*, 23–32.

Reid, G., Jass, J., Sebulsky, M. T., & McCormick, J. K. (2003). Potential uses of probiotics in clinical practice. *Clinical Microbiology Reviews, 16*, 658–672.

Reusche, E., & Seydel, U. (1993). Dialysis-associated encephalopathy: Light and electron microscopic morphology and topography with evidence of aluminum by laser microprobe mass analysis. *Acta Neuropathologica, 86*, 249–258.

Riedmann, E. M., Kyd, J. M., Cripps, A. W., & Lubitz, W. (2007). Bacterial ghosts as adjuvant particles. *Expert Review of Vaccines, 6*, 241–253.

Rocha-Ramírez, L., Pérez-Solano, R., Castañón-Alonso, S., Moreno Guerrero, S., Ramírez Pacheco, A., García Garibay, M., & Eslava, C. (2017). Probiotic Lactobacillus strains stimulate the inflammatory response and activate human macrophages. *Journal of Immunology Research, 2017*, 4607491.

Rodrigues, L., Banat, I. M., Teixeira, J., & Oliveira, R. (2006). Biosurfactants: Potential applications in medicine. *The Journal of Antimicrobial Chemotherapy, 57*, 609–618.

Rolfe, R. D. (2000). The role of probiotic cultures in the control of gastrointestinal health. *The Journal of Nutrition, 130*, 396S–402S.

Rosshart, S. P., Vassallo, B. G., Angeletti, D., Hutchinson, D. S., Morgan, A. P., Takeda, K., Hickman, H. D., McCulloch, J. A., Badger, J. H., & Ajami, N. J. (2017). Wild mouse gut microbiota promotes host fitness and improves disease resistance. *Cell, 171*, 1015–1028. e1013.

Sánchez, B., Delgado, S., Blanco-Míguez, A., Lourenço, A., Gueimonde, M., & Margolles, A. (2017). Probiotics, gut microbiota, and their influence on host health and disease. *Molecular Nutrition & Food Research, 61*, 1600240.

Saravanakumari, P., & Mani, K. (2010). Structural characterization of a novel xylolipid biosurfactant from *Lactococcus lactis* and analysis of antibacterial activity against multi-drug resistant pathogens. *Bioresource Technology, 101*, 8851–8854.

Sartor, R. B. (2004). Therapeutic manipulation of the enteric microflora in inflammatory bowel diseases: Antibiotics, probiotics, and prebiotics. *Gastroenterology, 126*, 1620–1633.

Sauvageau, J., Ryan, J., Lagutin, K., Sims, I. M., Stocker, B. L., & Timmer, M. S. (2012). Isolation and structural characterisation of the major glycolipids from *Lactobacillus plantarum*. *Carbohydrate Research, 357*, 151–156.

Schabussova, I., & Wiedermann, U. (2008). Lactic acid bacteria as novel adjuvant systems for prevention and treatment of atopic diseases. *Current Opinion in Allergy and Clinical Immunology, 8*, 557–564.

Schwarz, T. F., Horacek, T., Knuf, M., Damman, H.-G., Roman, F., Dramé, M., Gillard, P., & Jilg, W. (2009). Single dose vaccination with AS03-adjuvanted H5N1 vaccines in a randomized trial induces strong and broad immune responsiveness to booster vaccination in adults. *Vaccine, 27*, 6284–6290.

Sharma, A. (2019). *Importance of probiotics in cancer prevention and treatment. Recent developments in applied microbiology and biochemistry* (pp. 33–45). Elsevier.

Sharma, D., Saharan, B. S., Chauhan, N., Bansal, A., & Procha, S. (2014). Production and structural characterization of *Lactobacillus helveticus* derived biosurfactant. *The Scientific World Journal, 2014*.

Sharma, D., Saharan, B. S., Chauhan, N., Procha, S., & Lal, S. (2015). Isolation and functional characterization of novel biosurfactant produced by *Enterococcus faecium*. *SpringerPlus, 4*, 1–14.

Shornikova, A.-V., Casas, I. A., Isolauri, E., Mykkänen, H., & Vesikari, T. (1997). Lactobacillus reuteri as a therapeutic agent in acute diarrhea in young children. *Journal of Pediatric Gastroenterology and Nutrition, 24*, 399–404.

Skowera, A., de Jong, E. C., Schuitemaker, J. H., Allen, J. S., Wessely, S. C., Griffiths, G., Kapsenberg, M., & Peakman, M. (2005). Analysis of anthrax and plague biowarfare vaccine interactions with human monocyte-derived dendritic cells. *The Journal of Immunology, 175*, 7235–7243.

Soh, S. E., Ong, D. Q. R., Gerez, I., Zhang, X., Chollate, P., Shek, L. P.-C., Lee, B. W., & Aw, M. (2010). Effect of probiotic supplementation in the first 6 months of life on specific antibody responses to infant Hepatitis B vaccination. *Vaccine, 28*, 2577–2579.

Soltani, M., Lymbery, A., Song, S. K., & Hosseini Shekarabi, P. (2019). Adjuvant effects of medicinal herbs and probiotics for fish vaccines. *Reviews in Aquaculture, 11*, 1325–1341.

Tahmourespour, A., Salehi, R., & Kermanshahi, R. K. (2011). *Lactobacillus acidophilus*-derived biosurfactant effect on gtfB and gtfC expression level in *Streptococcus mutans* biofilm cells. *Brazilian Journal of Microbiology, 42*, 330–339.

Taylor, A., Hale, J., Wiltschut, J., Lehmann, H., Dunstan, J., & Prescott, S. (2006). Effects of probiotic supplementation for the first 6 months of life on allergen-and vaccine-specific immune responses. *Clinical and Experimental Allergy: Journal of the British Society for Allergy and Clinical Immunology, 36*, 1227–1235.

Tonetti, F. R., Arce, L., Salva, S., Alvarez, S., Takahashi, H., Kitazawa, H., Vizoso-Pinto, M. G., & Villena, J. (2020). Immunomodulatory properties of bacterium-like particles obtained from immunobiotic lactobacilli: Prospects for their use as mucosal adjuvants. *Frontiers in Immunology, 11*.

Trachootham, D., Chupeerach, C., Tuntipopipat, S., Pathomyok, L., Boonnak, K., Praengam, K., Promkam, C., & Santivarangkna, C. (2017). Drinking fermented milk containing *Lactobacillus paracasei* 431 (IMULUS™) improves immune response against H1N1 and cross-reactive H3N2 viruses after influenza vaccination: A pilot randomized triple-blinded placebo controlled trial. *Journal of Functional Foods, 33*, 1–10.

Trollfors, B., Knutsson, N., Taranger, J., Mark, A., Bergfors, E., Sundh, V., & Lagergård, T. (2006). Diphtheria, tetanus and pertussis antibodies in 10-year-old children before and after a booster dose of three toxoids: Implications for the timing of a booster dose. *European Journal of Pediatrics, 165*, 14–18.

Valdez, Y., Brown, E. M., & Finlay, B. B. (2014). Influence of the microbiota on vaccine effectiveness. *Trends in Immunology, 35*, 526–537.

Van Hoang, V., Ochi, T., Kurata, K., Arita, Y., Ogasahara, Y., & Enomoto, K. (2018). Nisin-induced expression of recombinant T cell epitopes of major Japanese cedar pollen allergens in *Lactococcus lactis*. *Applied Microbiology and Biotechnology, 102*, 261–268.

van Hoogmoed, C. G., van der Mei, H. C., & Busscher, H. J. (2004). The influence of biosurfactants released by S. mitis BMS on the adhesion of pioneer strains and cariogenic bacteria. *Biofouling, 20*, 261–267.

Van Overtvelt, L., Moussu, H., Horiot, S., Samson, S., Lombardi, V., Mascarell, L., Van de Moer, A., Bourdet-Sicard, R., & Moingeon, P. (2010). Lactic acid bacteria as adjuvants for sublingual allergy vaccines. *Vaccine, 28*, 2986–2992.

Varankovich, N. V., Nickerson, M. T., & Korber, D. R. (2015). Probiotic-based strategies for therapeutic and prophylactic use against multiple gastrointestinal diseases. *Frontiers in Microbiology, 6*, 685.

Vascellari, M., Melchiotti, E., Bozza, M., & Mutinelli, F. (2003). Fibrosarcomas at presumed sites of injection in dogs: Characteristics and comparison with non-vaccination site fibrosarcomas and feline post-vaccinal fibrosarcomas. *Journal of Veterinary Medicine Series A, 50*, 286–291.

Vecino, X., Barbosa-Pereira, L., Devesa-Rey, R., Cruz, J. M., & Moldes, A. B. (2015). Optimization of extraction conditions and fatty acid characterization of *Lactobacillus pentosus* cell-bound biosurfactant/bioemulsifier. *Journal of the Science of Food and Agriculture, 95*, 313–320.

Vecino, X., Devesa-Rey, R., Moldes, A., & Cruz, J. (2014). Formulation of an alginate-vineyard pruning waste composite as a new eco-friendly adsorbent to remove micronutrients from agroindustrial effluents. *Chemosphere, 111*, 24–31.

Velraeds, M., Van der Mei, H., Reid, G., & Busscher, H. J. (1996a). Inhibition of initial adhesion of uropathogenic *Enterococcus faecalis* by biosurfactants from Lactobacillus isolates. *Applied and Environmental Microbiology, 62*, 1958–1963.

Velraeds, M. M., Van de Belt-Gritter, B., Van der Mei, H., Reid, G., & Busscher, H. (1998). Interference in initial adhesion of uropathogenic bacteria and yeasts to silicone rubber by a *Lactobacillus acidophilus* biosurfactant. *Journal of Medical Microbiology, 47*, 1081–1085.

Velraeds, M. M., van der Mei, H. C., Reid, G., & Busscher, H. J. (1996b). Physicochemical and biochemical characterization of biosurfactants released by Lactobacillus strains. *Colloids and Surfaces B: Biointerfaces, 8*, 51–61.

Vera-Lastra, O., Medina, G., Cruz-Dominguez, M. D. P., Ramirez, P., Gayosso-Rivera, J., Anduaga-Dominguez, H., Lievana-Torres, C., & Jara, L. (2012). Human adjuvant disease induced by foreign substances: A new model of ASIA (Shoenfeld's syndrome). *Lupus, 21*, 128–135.

Villena, J., Chiba, E., Vizoso-Pinto, M. G., Tomosada, Y., Takahashi, T., Ishizuka, T., Aso, H., Salva, S., Alvarez, S., & Kitazawa, H. (2014). Immunobiotic *Lactobacillus rhamnosus* strains differentially modulate antiviral immune response in porcine intestinal epithelial and antigen presenting cells. *BMC Microbiology, 14*, 1–14.

Vlasova, A. N., Takanashi, S., Miyazaki, A., Rajashekara, G., & Saif, L. J. (2019). How the gut microbiome regulates host immune responses to viral vaccines. *Current Opinion in Virology, 37*, 16–25.

Ward, K., Mugenyi, K., MacNeil, A., Luzze, H., Kyozira, C., Kisakye, A., Matseketse, D., Newall, A. T., Heywood, A. E., & Bloland, P. (2020). Financial cost analysis of a strategy to improve the quality of administrative vaccination data in Uganda. *Vaccine, 38*, 1105–1113.

Weiner, G. J., Liu, H.-M., Wooldridge, J. E., Dahle, C. E., & Krieg, A. M. (1997). Immunostimulatory oligodeoxynucleotides containing the CpG motif are effective as immune adjuvants in tumor antigen immunization. *Proceedings of the National Academy of Sciences, 94*, 10833–10837.

West, C. E., Gothefors, L., Granström, M., Käyhty, H., Hammarström, M. L. K., & Hernell, O. (2008). Effects of feeding probiotics during weaning on infections and antibody responses to diphtheria, tetanus and Hib vaccines. *Pediatric Allergy and Immunology: Official Publication of the European Society of Pediatric Allergy and Immunology, 19*, 53–60.

Whitehouse, M. (2012). Oily adjuvants and autoimmunity: Now time for reconsideration? *Lupus, 21*, 217–222.

Yan, F., & Polk, D. (2011). Probiotics and immune health. *Current Opinion in Gastroenterology, 27*, 496.

Youngster, I., Kozer, E., Lazarovitch, Z., Broide, E., & Goldman, M. (2011). Probiotics and the immunological response to infant vaccinations: A prospective, placebo controlled pilot study. *Archives of Disease in Childhood, 96*, 345–349.

Chapter 29

Probiotics: past, present, and future challenges

Marieta Georgieva, Kaloyan Georgiev and Nadezhda Hvarchanova
Department of Pharmacology, Toxicology and Pharmacotherapy, Faculty of Pharmacy, Medical University of Varna, Varna, Bulgaria

29.1 Probiotics—the concept

Diseases existed long before evolution reached *Homo sapiens*. Over thousands of years, man has been immersed in an ocean of microorganisms invisible to him, which not only made him ill, but also helped him heal and survive. Only in the 19th century, called the "golden age of microbiology," did the great researchers R. Koch, L. Pasteur, I. Metchnikoff and others point out that there are pathogenic microorganisms visible under a microscope which are "enemies" of human health. Yet many centuries before these epoch-making discoveries, people knew about the beneficial effects of fermented foods; contemporaneous probiotics are derivatives of these ancient food stuffs. The use of fermented milk is a part of the history of human civilization. The term "fermentation" has a Latin root (fermentum—boiling), as the grapes crushed for wine have formed bubbles, characteristic of boiling liquid. The use of fermented milk has been known since ancient times (Sumer, Egypt, Greece, and Rome). Geographical differences and cultural traditions have coined its name: koumiss, kefir, yogurt, etc. The secret of fermentation was revealed by Louis Pasteur (20th century), who states that the process is due to the presence of yeasts, but does not make an association between these microorganisms and their possible health effects.

Professor I. Metchnikoff took the next big step in 1907 (Metchnikoff, 1907). He formulated the hypothesis of putrefactive microorganisms inhabiting the human colon, which leads to a kind of autointoxication with waste metabolites and thus shortens human life. Shortly before that (1905) the young Bulgarian doctor Stamen Grigorov discovered in Geneva the lactic acid bacillus, which leads to fermentation of milk and turns it into yogurt; he worked with an lactic acid starter sent to him directly from Bulgaria. Metchnikoff believed that *Lactobacillus bulgaricus* suppressed putrefactive pathogens in the colon and thus helped to prolong human life (the scientist himself consumed yogurt daily for the rest of his life). That marks the beginning to many studies on the healing and prophylactic properties of yogurt and *Lactobacilli*.

Two world wars and the discovery of antibiotics overshadowed Metchnikoff's ideas for decades. Yet in 1965, the name "probiotic" entered the medical literature and has no longer been off the stage. Of 176 publications in literature, there were 1476 (2014) articles and 477 randomized (medical) trials (according to PubMed). In February 2019, the number of publications related to probiotics was 20,315, which illustrates the great interest and human hope for modern application of lactic acid fermentation products.

Probiotics are a concept from the beginning of the 20th century, which modern humans need more and more frequently. Furthermore, today they are accepted and scientifically proven to be a useful component in nutrition, with an important role for good physiological status, healthy balance and disease prevention in humans and animals. The word "probiotic" comes from Latin ("pro" meaning for), and ancient Greek ("bios" meaning life), that is, "for life." It was first used in 1954 to compare the harmful effects of antibiotics with those beneficial to the bacteria probiotica. Today, the International Scientific Association for Probiotics and Prebiotics defines "probiotics" as "live microorganisms that, when administered in adequate amounts, confer a health benefit on the host" (Hill et al., 2014). Probiotics as "living microorganisms" have prophylactic and therapeutic effects that improve the internal microbial balance.

Today, the world is returning to natural remedies for health prevention. Probiotics take the leading place among them. It creates a new challenge for scientists, technologists, and physicians. A response to new requirements in the

21st century is the elaborateness of new technologies for the production of probiotics, and functional foods for the prevention and treatment of many diseases that lead to the genesis of the disturbed balance of gut microbiota (Anukam & Reid, 2007; McFarland, 2015).

The concept of functional foods was first created in Japan in 1980 (The American Dietetic Association). Functional or "biotherapeutic" foods include specific additives and substances that have a positive effect on human health, determine good health and, along with their nutritional qualities, contribute to the prevention of certain diseases (Salminen, 1996). Certain natural products can be classified as functional if they contain a nutritional component that positively affects any of the physiological functions in humans and/or has a protective, healing effect. Functional foods are various products containing probiotics, prebiotics, vitamins and, to some extent, specific supplements. The most significant and well-known group among them are probiotic foods containing live bacteria that have a positive effect on the human body. They have been shown to have a better health effect than traditional foods and most often this is directly related to the available living microorganisms with unique biological properties (Salminen & Marteau, 1997). Consequently, probiotics and products with their participation are gradually becoming an important element of the food chain and as such need to be monitored and evaluated very seriously.

New challenges in probiotic research include the creation of modern forms of food, supplements, and therapeutics, meeting the requirements of reliability—safety, convenience and usefulness, according to European regulatory frameworks—as well as providing knowledge about the genetic basis and molecular mechanisms of action to ensure optimal health for each individual. This will allow the creation of the so-called. targeted probiotic preparations that will best meet the needs of the target groups of consumers without risk in their application.

29.2 Probiotics—modern trends

29.2.1 Definition and classification of probiotics

Recent decades marked an evolution with the discovery that the human gastrointestinal tract is a host for a huge number of beneficial bacteria known as the intestinal microbiota. It includes at least 500–1000 species in each person, with about 100 trillion cells, which exceeds 3–10 times the number of human cells (Guarner & Malagelada, 2003; Human Microbiome Project Consortium, 2012). Bacteria make up 90% of human microbiome (HM) and are the best studied microorganisms in the intestinal ecosystem. With the development of high-performance gene sequencing technology, the study of HM currently includes two main steps: (1) 16S rRNA-based bacterial gene sequencing and (2) bioinformation analysis. Metabolomics is another rapidly evolving field of HM research that evaluates small molecules associated with the interaction between human metabolism and bacteria, which has an impact on health and disease. Data from the study of HM and metaboloma currently provide the strongest evidence for their association with health and various diseases (Cani & Delzenne, 2011; Dave et al., 2012; Lloyd-Price et al., 2016). In addition, the genes encoded by the bacterial genome are about 150 times the genes encoded by the human genome. These additional genes have added various types of enzymatic proteins that play an important role in facilitating the body's metabolism and thus contribute to the regulation of human physiology (Hooper & Gordon, 2001; Ursell et al., 2014).

For years, medicine has been fighting infections with the help of antibiotics and the lives of millions of people have been saved thanks to them. Today we know, however, that their use leads to an imbalance in the intestinal microbiota of the body, which has adverse consequences. Awareness of the importance of the microbiota for health has led to its largest study to date, the American Human Microbiome Project. That project, which lasted 5 years (2007–12) (Human Microbiome Project Consortium, 2012), aimed to study in detail the whole set of microorganisms inhabiting the human body—the so-called human microbiota—and collect complete information about their genetic material: the HM. As a result, a map of the human microbiota inhabiting the mouth, upper respiratory tract, gastrointestinal tract, urogenital tract, and skin was created. It turns out that we coexist with single-celled organisms that exceed the number of our own cells in a ratio of 10:1, that is, man is a macro-organism with 10 times more belonging to microorganisms.

The list of global microbiome studies is becoming increasingly impressive. In 2012, the Canadian Microbiome Initiative was launched, the European Metacardis project, mainly related to cardiovascular diseases, as well as the MegaHit project that implemented in collaboration with China. China is independently running an autonomous project called MegaGut, while Japan is focused on the Human Metagenome Consortium. This steady increase in global microbiome research projects is actually a logical echo of the human genome sequence we witnessed in the 1990s (Araya et al., 2002).

Each person has a unique microbiota, which they acquire at birth. It changes with age, health, and lifestyle. Its composition includes bacteria, fungi, and viruses that play different roles in our body. They help digest and assimilate food, communicate with the host's immune system, and serve as a shield against unwanted environmental pathogens. In turn, the human body offers them habitat and a nutritious environment.

These mutually beneficial relationships are fragile and the balance can easily be upset. Changes in the environment associated with malnutrition, decreased immunity, stress, and various diseases, lead to quantitative and qualitative changes in the microbiome. The huge differences in the modern way of life compared to the way of life of our ancestors barely a century ago have brought about drastic changes in the microbiome that has evolved with us for millions of years. Scientists link these changes to some of the most common chronic and autoimmune diseases today. More than ever, the role of microorganisms in human life needs to be rethought (Araya et al., 2002).

With the development of research on probiotics, the need for them to be correctly defined and validated increases. At the request of the Argentine government, in 2001 the FAO and WHO sponsored an expert advisory group. During the consultation, which was chaired by Dr. Gregor Reid, Director of the Canadian Center for Probiotics Research and Development, the group adopted by consensus the definition of "probiotics" as "live microorganisms that, when administered in adequate amounts, confer a health benefit on the host." Thus in 2002, the WHO officially defined probiotics. (Araya et al., 2002; Hansen, 2002). This is currently the most widely used and accepted definition, as it covers all applications of probiotics as live microbes, not just the benefits of intestinal homeostasis. Two main features are considered to be the most important:

1. Probiotic preparations must contain live microorganisms.
2. The desired effects should be related to the amount taken.

The main probiotics used in the present commercial preparations contain lactic acid bacteria (LAB), including *Lactobacilli*, and *Bifidobacteria* (Hansen, 2002).

The European institutions have the following requirements for functional foods:

- to be taken daily;
- be part of normal food;
- be obtained from natural products;
- have a positive healthy effect on the body; and
- reduce the risk of disease and improve the quality of life.

The effectiveness of probiotics depends on many factors: their composition, the state of the microbiome in the body, as well as the age, gender, and living conditions of the individual.

In general, probiotic strains can be divided into two groups:

1. resident
2. transiting

The strains of the first group are permanent and often found in the GIT. Preparations based on such microorganisms favor their recovery in the intestinal tract. Resident strains are more compatible and less antagonistic to other beneficial microorganisms permanently present in the human body; it is a kind of evolutionarily fixed microbial association with a positive effect on the host organism. The following species have been described as resident in humans: *Lactobacillus acidophilus*, *Lactobacillus salivarius*, *Lactobacillus fermentum*, *Lactobacillus gasseri*, *Lactobacillus crispatus*, *Bifidobacterium* spp. Transiting strains belonging to the species *Lactobacillus casei*, *Lactobacillus delbrueckii*, *Lactobacillus yogurti*, *Lactobacillus brevis*, *Lactobacillus kefir*, *Lactobacillus plantarum*, only temporarily reside in the intestinal tract, but during the transition can also have a positive effect. Therefore the use of multistrain preparations containing bacteria from both groups is recommended. Only individual strains meeting certain selection criteria are used in practice, however.

The International Research Group on New Antimicrobial Strategies (ISGNAS) is developing a concept for a detailed definition of probiotics in the following three categories (Rusch, 2002):

1. Medical probiotic—microbial preparation containing live and/or killed microorganisms, including their components or metabolites, formulated for therapeutic use, as a medicament for treatment and prophylaxis.
2. Pharmaceutical probiotic—a microbial preparation designed as a food supplement.
3. Food probiotic—a microbial preparation designed for use in food fermentation and food production. The mechanism of action of which includes immunomodulation, effective influence of the protective microflora and modulation of metabolic activity (Rusch, 2002).

This division, although still debatable, gives a more accurate picture of the scope of probiotics and can be adopted with a view to drafting legislation and regulations on probiotics.

Probiotics can be considered in groups according to the field of application and the host:

- Probiotics for stock-breeding.
- Food probiotics and food supplements for humans.
- Probiotics with a medical focus for prevention and treatment, which may include not only live microorganisms but also their active metabolites or components.

Regardless of their subdivision, both scientists and food experts on food safety and risk assessment are consolidating around the attitude that should be proven for each proposed probiotic:

- origin and identity;
- safety; and
- efficiency and effectiveness—that is, to demonstrate the physiological benefits of using a number of viable probiotic bacteria in the appropriate forms of administration (food, capsules, etc.) in a number of placebo-controlled patients and/or a standard treatment option if the final result is treatment of the disease.

These are the main indicators by which the practical acceptability of each probiotic is assessed today and they are complementary, but no less important, criteria. The next step in the development is to include these biologically active microorganisms and/or the active metabolites produced by them in the production of naturally protected and functional foods, probiotic food, and feed additives or in formulations with therapeutic applications.

Prospects for the development of probiotic products are closely dependent on scientific evidence of their safety, organoleptic properties, health, and therapeutic effects (Ward & German, 2004).

More detailed studies of the main groups of probiotic microorganisms (lactic and bifidobacteria, as well as some yeasts) and new biomarkers are needed to adequately reveal the physiological potential of functional foods and the lactic acid microflora involved in their production (Mattila-Sandholm et al., 2002).

29.2.1.1 Criteria, selection, and application of probiotic strains

The selection of probiotics includes two types of analysis:

1. in vitro analysis, which are important for the overall selection process and for the preselection from a large number of strains of potentially probiotic ones. This type of analysis is based on the use of different model systems.
2. controlled in vivo studies in healthy volunteers given a specific dose of a strain or strains selected by in vitro analysis (Morelli et al., 1986).

The direct addition of probiotic microorganisms to functional foods, nonpharmacological or medicinal products require a careful selection of strains suitable for industrial use. Their qualities and functional properties must be established. Three main aspects can be formulated that should be taken into account when selecting probiotic strains: (1) safety, (2) functionality, and (3) technological ability.

29.2.1.2 Characteristics of probiotic strains

Probiotics are determined by their specific strain, which includes the genus, species, subspecies (if applicable) and the alphanumeric designation of the strain (Guarner et al., 2017). The seven main genera of microbial organisms most commonly used in probiotic products are *Lactobacillus*, *Bifidobacterium*, *Saccharomyces*, *Streptococcus*, *Enterococcus*, *Escherichia* and *Bacillus*. Table 29.1 shows examples of the nomenclature used for several commercial strains of probiotic organisms.

TABLE 29.1 Nomenclature for sample commercial strains of probiotics.

Genus	Species	Subspecies	Strain designation	Strain nickname
Lactobacillus	rhamnosus	None	GG	LGG
Bifidobacterium	animalis	lactis	DN-173 010	Bifidus regularis
Bifidobacterium	longum	longum	35624	Bifantis

Lactobacillus and *Bifidobacterium* are the two main genera of Gram-positive bacteria widely used as probiotics. They are the two well-studied probiotic strains recommended for improvement of gut health and gut immunity (Sanders, 2008; Vajro et al., 2014). LAB are the most commonly used microorganisms as probiotics that can be isolated from humans, animals, plants, and the environment. The most common microorganisms used in the preparation of probiotics are those associated with the human gut flora. These include mainly LAB, *Bifidobacteria* spp. and *Propionibacteria* spp. They are often found in fermented foods, especially dairy products. They are quantitatively the most important ingested bacteria. Therefore most studies focus on the effects of these bacterial groups in probiotics on the gut microbiota and the health of the host (de Vrese & Schrezenmeir, 2008; Singh et al., 2013).

29.2.1.3 Lactobacillus bulgaricus—a unique probiotic

Lactobacillus bulgaricus is the only probiotic named after a specific people and geographical area. It is the first microorganism selected by man thousands of years ago and changed its evolution. *Lactobacillus bulgaricus* is of plant and aquatic origin and is isolated from green plants only on the territory of Bulgaria. Once in other parts of the world, it mutates and stops reproducing (Fig. 29.1A and B).

The territory of Bulgaria is host to the plants draca (*Paliuris aculateus*), sour (prickly) thorn (*Berberis vulgaris lam*), from the flowers of dogwood (*Cornus mas* L), the flowers of the Bulgarian rose (*Rosa damascena* var *trigintipetala*), in the roots and bark of oak trees (*Quercus robur* L).

Rods were isolated from *Calendula officinalis*, *Cornus mas*, *Galanthus nivalis*, *Prunus spinosa* and other unidentified plant species. Cocci were isolated from *Calendula officinalis*, *Capsella bursa-pastoris*, *Chrysanthemum*, *Cichorium intybus*, *Colchicum*, *C. mas*, *Dianthus*, *G. nivalis*, *Hedera*, *Nerium oleander*, *Plantago lanceolata*, *P. spinosa*, *Rosa*, *Tropaeolum*, and others. Both rods and cocci were simultaneously isolated from *C. officinalis*, *C. mas*, *G. nivalis*, and *P. spinosa* (Michaylova et al., 2007).

During the spring days, in the beginning of may, *L. bulgaricus* can be isolated from spring water in oak forests. With this spring water it is possible to ferment milk. These springs have been defined by the Bulgarian population as sacred for hundreds of years. For the first time in the world, in 2011, Bulgarian scientists (N. Alexandrov and D. Petrova) managed to isolate eight completely natural, original strains of *L. bulgaricus*, *Lactobacillus helveticus*, *Lactobacillus lactis*, and *Streptococcus thermophilus* from spring water in the Balkan Mountains, near a Thracian settlement (Fig. 29.1A and B). Using the method of modern biotechnology, these scientists managed to create a new probiotic formula, as an established probiotic cocktail (LDB-ST). All probiotics containing strains of aquatic origin are patented in the United States with an official patent number in 2015 (US Patent, 9,131,708B2/2015, September 15). Due to their all-natural origin, all these new strains have maximum resistance and survival when passing through the gastrointestinal tract and retain their number and viability under normal storage conditions for up to 2 years. (Georgiev et al., 2015).

It is well known that ST, an established yogurt-producing bacterium, is useful for improving and maintaining health, along with the protooperative LDB bacteria (Herve-Jimenez et al., 2009). LDB and ST work closely together, with the presence of ST stimulating the growth of LDB through the production of formic acid and carbon dioxide, while LDB promotes the growth of ST by providing the necessary amino acids by breaking down proteins (Driessen et al., 1982; Veringa et al., 1968). It has been reported that this cooperation between LDB and ST is one of the reasons for the production of products with specific qualities that cause effects in vivo and are clinically active against pathogens (Carper, 1994).

Probiotics belong to the GRAS (Generally Recognized As Safe bacteria) group, according to the US Food and Drug Administration (FDA). The experience gained by man over the millennia, as well as modern scientific research, show that the LAB used are harmless to the human and animal body.

29.3 Viability of probiotic bacteria in the gastrointestinal tract and their secondary reproduction: probiotic concentration

Oral probiotic bacteria are exposed to various factors—saliva, gastric juice, bile acids, etc.—which initially aim to stop the entry of various bacteria into the body. In addition, they are affected by food, water, beverages, and other microorganisms. The ability of probiotic bacteria to stay alive in sufficient quantities as they pass through the upper sections of the digestive system is one of their most important requirements. Not all types of probiotic bacteria have qualities that allow them to overcome these barriers. Probiotic bacteria are known to have a higher survival rate when taken as part

436 Probiotics in The Prevention and Management of Human Diseases

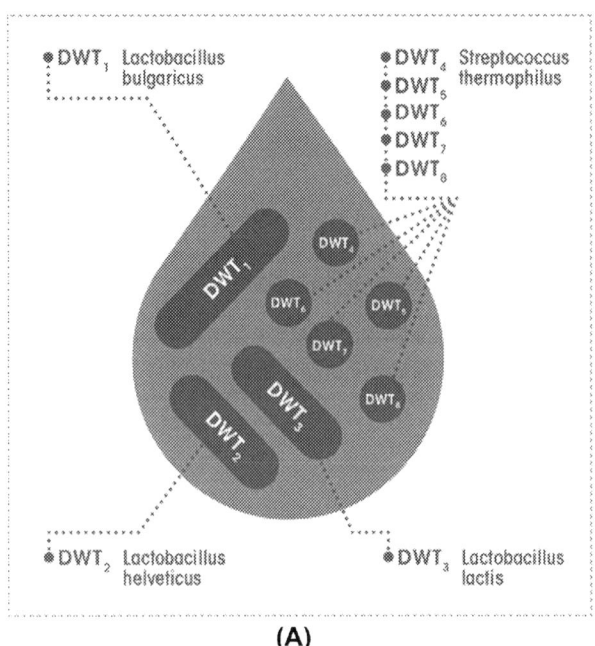

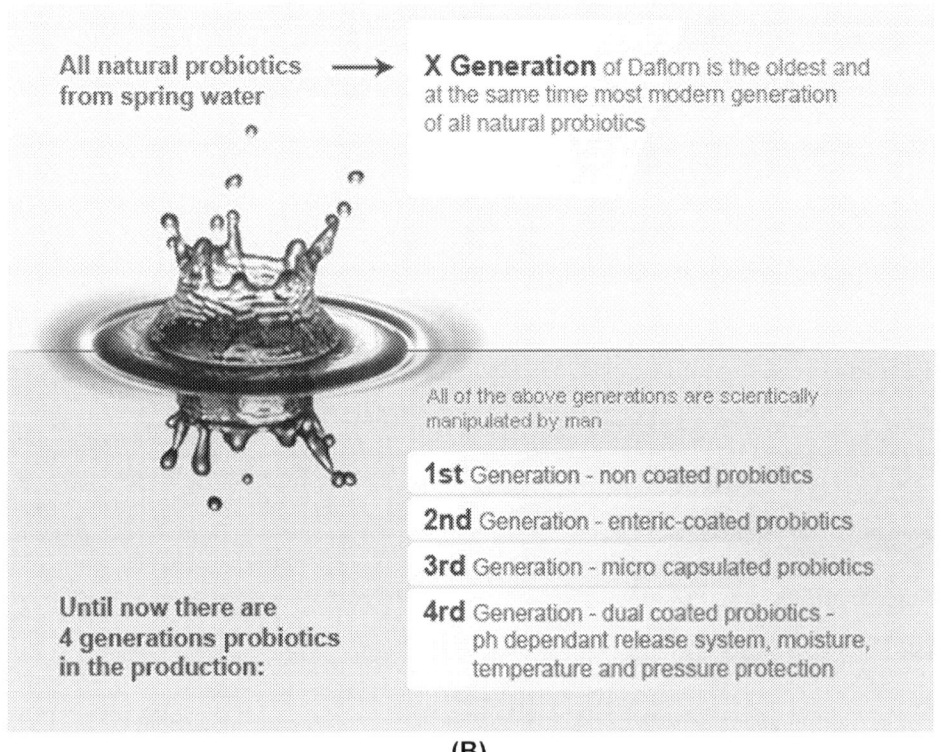

FIGURE 29.1 Probiotics from spring water: (A) all isolated probiotics from spring water; (B) generations.

of a lactic acid product than as a pure culture (Georgiev et al., 2015). The use of modern biotechnological processes for the production of new probiotic lactic acid products achieves a significantly higher survival rate of beneficial bacteria.

Different methods for quantifying probiotic bacteria have been established in different parts of the world.

In the countries of the European Union, a method for counting the number of live probiotic microorganisms in solid nutrient media at the time of sowing has become widespread. To define a product as probiotic, it must contain more than 10,000,000 (107) live probiotic microorganisms in 1 g of probiotic product. In the United States, Canada, Japan, Korea, and other countries, a method is used to enumerate colony-forming units (CFUs) in a liquid medium at 72 hours after inoculation. In Russia, a method is used to quantify probiotic bacteria as a weight fraction of 1 g milligrams of probiotic bacteria in 1 g of probiotic product. This leads to different results.

Mass manufacturers of probiotic products write on the labels the number of living cells or CFU at the date of manufacture. Their products should be stored in the refrigerator, because if they are not wrapped naturally or synthetically. The number of living cells in the products for several months decreases rapidly and then their health effects are minimal. Leading French companies in the field of probiotics are developing methods for wrapping probiotic bacteria with synthetic proteins.

29.4 Dose of probiotics

The beneficial effect of probiotic bacteria on the human body is associated with their intake in sufficient quantities. There is currently no consensus on the required single or daily dose. It is assumed that the amount of living cells of a certain type and strain should be consumed in order to obtain a clear health effect. Most authors assume that this amount should be between 3 and 5 billion living cells per day (Lee & Salminen, 2009).

Gibson et al. differentiates that if probiotic bacteria are taken in lactic acid products, their amount should be 2−3 billion per day, and if taken as pure cultures (only live cells), from 10 to 15 times more (15−30 billion) (Gibson et al., 2010). In some European countries, probiotic bacteria are thought to have minimal health effects at doses above 1 million. Studies show that this amount is too small to have a distinct health effect, and the daily dose should be significantly higher, on the order of several billion living cells. As mentioned, the health effects of probiotic bacteria depend on a number of factors, such as resistance to passing through the upper sections of the digestive system, the type of strain, and so on (Gibson et al., 2010).

29.5 Safety of probiotic bacteria

One of the main requirements for probiotic bacteria is that they are safe for the consumer. Intake of probiotic LAB by children, pregnant women, or the elderly is not considered a risk factor. Moreover, a number of observations and clinical studies have shown that taking probiotics strengthens their immune system and improves their health.

It is essential that the safety assessment of bacterial strains used as probiotics is thoroughly studied. Probiotics belong to the GRAS group, according to the FDA. The experience gained by man over the millennia, as well as modern scientific research, show that the LAB used are harmless to the human and animal body. They belong to the group of GRAS microorganisms, that is, generally accepted for safe bacteria. There is also no evidence that taking them in larger doses than usual will lead to side effects (Salminen & Marteau, 1997). However, both WHO and FAO stated that probiotics may results in several types of adverse events, at least theoretically. Microorganisms used as probiotics can cause systemic infections, stimulate the immune system, disrupt metabolism, and participate in horizontal gene transfer. Brown & Valiere (2004) and Salminen (1996) reported some methods for assessment the safety of LAB, using in vitro studies, experimental animal tests, and clinical trials. Their combination has proven that most of the current probiotic strains meet the required safety standards. According to Salminen and Marteau (1997) further studies are needed on the characteristic properties of probiotics, their pharmacokinetics, and the interactions between them and the host in order to assess their safety.

29.6 Health effects of probiotics

29.6.1 Prevention and treatment with probiotics

Probiotics play a responsible role, especially in the prevention of a large number of serious diseases, originating from a disturbed balance of the GIT microbiota such as gastrointestinal infections, dysbacteriosis, enteritis, gastritis, ulcers, high cholesterol, weakened immune system, tumors, and others. Through appropriate prevention, these diseases can be brought under control and society can save a huge resource (labor, material, financial, mental). Active scientific disclosure of the positive results of the evaluation of a large number of probiotic crops and the opportunities they provide to the health concerns of the consumer lead to increasing trust and increased demand. Not coincidentally, probiotics and probiotic foods are among the most sought after on the market in Europe.

The economic importance of probiotics is great: the global market for probiotics amounted to US$40 trillion in 2017 and is expected to grow to US$64 trillion by 2023 (Reid et al., 2019). Europe is a traditional market leader in

LAB with probiotic properties and mainly *Lactobacilli*. *Lactobacillus* and *Bifidobacterium* are the two main types of Gram-positive bacteria widely used as probiotics (Araya et al., 2002).

In today's global society, where people are exposed to daily stress, the widespread use of antibiotics, poor nutrition, and a number of harmful external factors, the balance of the gastrointestinal flora is constantly disturbed. The ability to control and predict the effects of probiotics based on rigorous research would allow both consumers and manufacturers to choose and offer products with proven curative properties and thus fully extend human life.

Understanding the mechanisms of probiotic bacteria action is perhaps the biggest challenge before us. There is currently very little information about the mechanisms by which probiotics provide their health effects. Probiotic strains are living microorganisms that most likely work through multiple mechanisms and molecules, yet there is a real need for more in-depth research. Researchers are trying to scientifically explain how probiotics work should be applauded, which will allow for more rational approaches to the selection and use of probiotics.

As you can see in Table 29.2, a significant number of health effects have been found as a result of taking probiotics: relieving lactose intolerance, stimulation of intestinal immunity; prevention of pathogen colonization; lowering serum cholesterol and blood pressure, reduction of inflammatory reactions, cancer prevention, reduction of food allergies, modification of the intestinal flora, and improving well-being. (Simmering & Blaut, 2001). Much of the research proves the essential role of probiotics in proper digestive function and healthy balance in the GIT and urogenital tract. At the same time, scientists focus on the functional effects of foods and their health properties associated with bioactive and probiotic crops (appetizer and/or supplements). Functional foods provide the body not only with essential nutrients (Table 29.3), but also with healthy bioactive components.

Recent research shows that people with psychoneurological diseases (depression, chronic fatigue, and other mental illnesses) suffer from severe dysbacteriosis. Correction of dysbiosis with probiotics has a beneficial effect on the underlying disease (Bercik et al., 2012; Boukthir et al., 2010; Kennedy et al., 2012). In the last year, a new challenge has emerged: The use of probiotics to prevent Covid -19? It is worth to be noted that probiotics, although harmless, are not a magic panacea. Continuous and adequate supervision of their use is necessary to prevent even the slightest risk to human health.

In recent years, probiotics have been studied as natural living carriers of vaccines, enzymes, antimicrobials, as they are biologically active molecules with a number of health and nutritional effects.

Further application of advanced "-omics" technologies will provide a better understanding of complex host-bacterial interactions, but research strategies need to be well planned to provide informative data that can be interpreted biologically. Once these biological mechanisms and physiological interactions are clarified and more confidently defined, the

TABLE 29.2 Health effects of probiotics.

Effects	Probable mechanism
1. Help digest lactose	Bacterial lactase breaks down lactose in the small intestine.
2. Resistance to internal pathogens	Auxiliary effect, increasing the production of antibodies. Systemic immune effect. Resistance to colonization. Creates unsuitable conditions for pathogens.
3. Antitumor effect of the colon	Antimutagenic activity. Alters the procarcinogenic activity of colonizing microbes. Stimulates immune function; Reduces the concentration of bile salts.
4. Reduce the overgrowth of pathogens in the small intestine	Lactobacilli affect the activity of overgrowth. Reduce toxic metabolites.
5. Modulation of the immune system	Auxiliary effect in antigen-specific immune response. Cytokinin production.
6. Antiallergic effect	Prevents translocation of antigens in the bloodstream.
7. Antisclerotic action	Assimilation of cholesterol by bacterial cells. Antioxidant effect. They change the hydrolase enzyme activity.
8. Antihypertensive effect	Cell wall components act as ACE inhibitors.
9. Infections caused by *Helicobacter pylori*	Competitive colonization.
10. Hepatic encephalopathy	Inhibit urease-producing flora.
11. Urogenital infections	Reduce bacterial adhesion to the urinary and vaginal tract.

ACE, angiotensin-converting enzyme.

TABLE 29.3 Nutritional effects of probiotics.

Increase the absorption of proteins, fats and carbohydrates.

Increase the absorption of minerals and trace elements—calcium, potassium, phosphorus, iron, magnesium, selenium, zinc.

Increase the synthesis and stabilize vitamins—A, B1, B2, B6, B12, C, D, E.

Increase and stabilize the enzymes protease, lipase, amylase, cellulase.

Increase synthesis and stabilize hormones.

Stimulate the secretion of digestive juices.

Stimulate growth.

extrapolation from laboratory science to clinical treatment with probiotic supplements will be significantly accelerated. The future of probiotic research offers exciting potential to influence human health and disease.

29.6.1.1 Probiotics and diseases of the gastrointestinal tract

The 2005 Nobel Prize in Physiology or Medicine by Robin Warren and Barry Marshall reminds us that the solution to some diseases lies not only within the human body, but rather can be found on the border with the microbial environment. Manipulation of CM (intestinal microbiota) is becoming a realistic therapeutic and prophylactic strategy for many infectious, inflammatory and even neoplastic diseases in the intestine, as well as for diseases outside the GIT. However, the promise of pharmabiotics is unlikely to be fulfilled without paying more attention to the secrets hidden in the neglected internal organ (the GIT). It is a rich repository of metabolites that can be used for therapeutic purposes. Therefore the deep penetration into the molecular details of the interactions between the organism and the intestinal microbiome is a prerequisite for the discovery of new therapeutic possibilities for many diseases. A number of stomach ailments, such as gastrointestinal infections, Crohn's disease, ulcerative colitis, food allergies, antibiotic and infectious diarrhea, all benefit from probiotics (Derwa et al., 2017; Kalliomäki et al., 2001).

One of the most thoroughly researched areas for probiotic use is the prevention of antibiotic-associated diarrhea (AAD). It is important to note that not all probiotic strains will be as effective for this purpose. For example, a recent systematic review comparing the efficacy and tolerability of different probiotics for AAD, where the authors examined 51 RCTs ($n = 9569$) and found that treatment with *Lactobacillus rhamnosus* GG (LGG) was significantly better than that of any other strain of AAD when used to prevent this condition. While *Lactobacillus casei* has a higher efficacy (Cai et al., 2018) in reducing the rate of *Clostridium difficile* infection, it should therefore always be considered which probiotic will be used, depending on the patient's condition and the desired outcome. Another condition of the gastrointestinal tract in which probiotics have been shown to be beneficial is the colonization of *Helicobacter pylori*, which is a problem for about 50% of the world's population (Brown, 2000).

29.6.1.2 Hepatoprotective effect of probiotic bacteria

Toxic liver damage is of increasing interest due to its increasing frequency. The most widespread worldwide are drug-induced and alcoholic hepatotoxicity. Drug-induced hepatotoxicity is a leading cause of acute liver failure in Western Europe and the United States, associated with involuntary or targeted acetaminophen overdose (Suk & Kim, 2012; Yoon et al., 2016).

Standard therapy for liver disease in many cases is insufficiently effective and safe for the patient. The addition of probiotics can significantly improve the treatment of patients suffering from toxic liver damage, as well as to be used in the prevention of liver disease. From a physiological point of view, the close functional and two-way communication between the intestine and the liver is one of the most important connections between the HM and the extraintestinal organs. Due to its unique anatomy and vascular system, the liver receives about 70% of its blood supply from the intestines through the portal vein. Thus it is constantly exposed not only to the products of digestion and absorption, but also to adverse substances from the intestinal lumen derived from the intestine, including bacteria and bacterial components such as lipopolysaccharide (endotoxin) 23 (Ponziani et al., 2018). The liver is an important immunological organ and after the entry of these substances through the portal circulation, it reacts by activating the innate and adaptive immune system with its subsequent damage. A better understanding of the pathophysiological links between intestinal dysbiosis, intestinal barrier integrity, and hepatic immune response to intestinal-derived factors is essential for the development of new therapies for the treatment of chronic liver disease (Tripathi et al., 2018).

Experimental and clinical studies have demonstrated the possible use of probiotics to prevent liver damage, and that the probiotic may be an effective hepatoprotector in the treatment and prevention of liver disorders (Georgieva, 2006; Iannitti & Palmieri, 2010).

The main attention is paid to the mechanisms of the hepatoprotective effect. According to the literature, understanding these mechanisms is of paramount importance in the future, as a number of liver disorders (inflammation, adipose tissue infiltration, hepatitis, etc.) are likely to become more common due to high-fat and increase in obesity. The link between the positive effects of probiotics and liver health is not direct, but seems to be based on prevention (Georgieva et al., 2015).

29.6.1.3 The radiation protection effect of probiotics

There are data on the protective effects of probiotics in chemotherapy and radiation. Radiation therapy is used in almost all types of tumors (cancer of the prostate, cervix, bladder, intestine, etc.). The side effects of it are very severe, which requires its cessation. The therapy kills both cancer and completely healthy cells. The mucosa is damaged throughout the digestive system, leading to severe nausea, vomiting, and diarrhea. Studies have shown that probiotics protect the lining of the digestive system from the harmful effects of radiation. An important condition is that probiotics be taken preventively and not after the onset of complications (Ciorba et al., 2011).

Probiotics, as living microbial supplements, help the body regain normal levels of "good" bacteria and boost immunity. There are about 500 different types of "good" bacteria. The two most common groups of probiotic bacteria are *Lactobacillus* and *Bifidobacterium*. Scientists have found that they protect against radiation damage. The mechanisms by which probiotics exert their radiation protection effect are discussed. Most likely it is due to their immune-stimulating and antioxidant effect. There are numerous studies on the effect of probiotic bacteria as antioxidants.

29.6.1.4 Antitumor and antimutagenic effect of probiotic bacteria—a problem with a wide social response

Cancer is one of the leading causes of death worldwide. They are considered to be diseases of economically developed and rich societies. The tendency is for these diseases to affect an increasing number of people. Colorectal cancer (CRC) is the second highest cancer mortality in the world and the most common localization of cancer in the digestive system. It is known that high levels of carcinogens are released in the GIT through diet. Obviously, diet, nutrition, and intestinal flora are key factors in the onset and development of colon cancer. Cancer therapy is a challenge that may not be impossible. The answer may lie in the effectiveness of some bacteria, known as probiotics or functional foods. One of the biggest challenges in modern science is to develop an effective methodology for inhibiting tumor growth. Chemotherapy and radiation therapy (Milenic et al., 2004; Van Cutsem et al., 2009) are by far the best ways to stop tumor growth, but they have many limitations (Dean et al., 2005; Knox & Meredith, 2000). In this context, finding an intrinsic way to inhibit tumor growth is one of the biggest challenges.

Probiotics can modulate the actions of the intestinal microflora through various mechanisms and thus show their anticancer activity. Probably, probiotics have different effects at different stages of carcinogenesis, which can be summarized as: antigenotoxicity, inhibition of enzyme activity in the colon, control of the growth of potentially harmful bacteria, interaction with colonocytes, stimulation of the immune system, and production of physiologically active metabolites. In general, the main mechanisms manifested by probiotic bacteria to cancer inhibition can be explained by a group of effects that depend on the type of probiotic strain. Ouwehand et al. (1999) described as early as 1999 the possible mechanisms of probiotics for cancer inhibition (Ouwehand et al., 1999).

In an experimental in vitro and in vivo study, Ma et al. (2008) showed that the probiotic *Bacillus polyfermenticus* inhibits the growth of colon cancer cells by reducing ErbB2 and ErbB3 receptors (which are known to play a significant role in tumor development) (Ma et al., 2008).

A modern study on the antitumor effects of *Lactobacillus Delbruckei* sp. *bulgaricus* strain DWT1 (LDB) and *Streptococcus thermophilus* strain DWT4 (ST), an established probiotic cocktail (LDB-ST), was performed on colon cancer cell lines by our team in 2015 (Georgiev et al., 2015). The probiotic cocktail showed promising primary screening results—on the one hand, low direct cytotoxicity and on the other, dose-dependent inhibition of proliferation on the colon cancer cell line—with HT-29 (in high concentration) (250–1000 µg/mL). (Fig. 29.2A and B).

In 2019, Palock and colleagues reported that the same probiotic formula containing *Lactobacillus bulgaricus DWT1* and ST could inhibit tumor growth by activating the proinflammatory response in macrophages (Guha et al., 2019). The

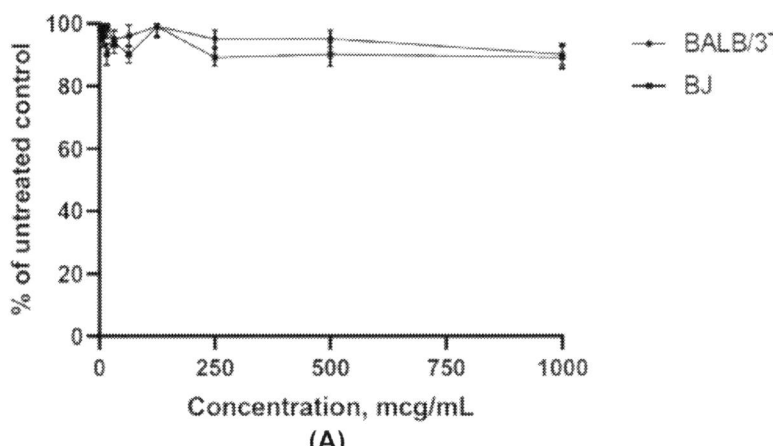
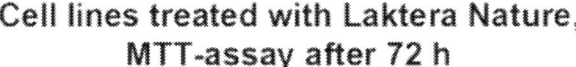
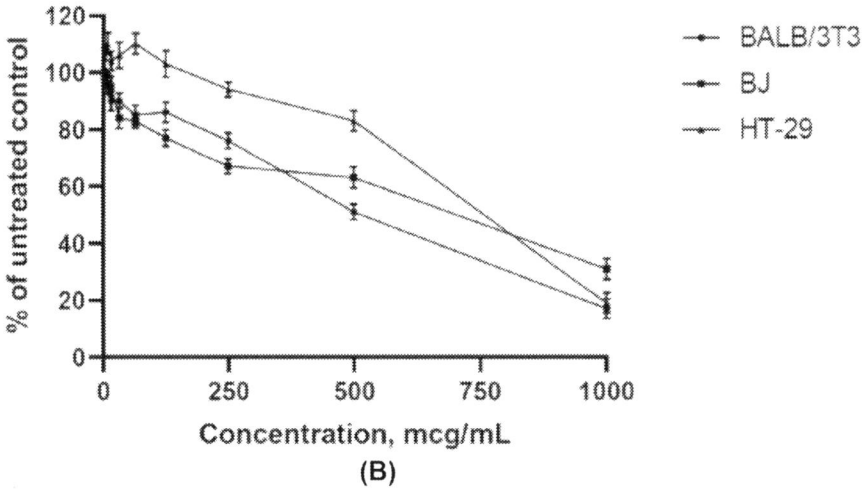

FIGURE 29.2 (A) BALB/3T3 and BJ cell lines treated with Laktera Nature in concentrations of 2–1000 μg/mL. MTT assay after 24 h. (B) Antiproliferative effects of probiotic food Laktera Nature used in concentrations of 2–1000 μg/mL on noncancerous (BALB/3T3 and BJ) and cancerous (HT-29, colon cancer) cell lines.

report revealed that after treatment with the established probiotic cocktail, the conversion of M2 to M1 state of macrophage cells of murine origin took place in vitro, ex vivo, and in vivo. The result of this study has the potential to develop newer strategies for inhibiting tumor growth.

29.7 Probiotics and metabolic syndrome

Metabolic syndrome is associated with an increased risk of cardiovascular disease and premature death. It is characterized by impaired glucose tolerance or type 2 diabetes, insulin resistance, as well as high blood pressure, dyslipidemia, decreased levels of high-density lipoprotein cholesterol (HDL-C), central obesity, and a body mass index > 30 kg/m^2. Many factors are involved in the pathogenesis of the metabolic syndrome and they determine the individual approach for both prevention and treatment.

In the process of co-evolution, the HM has transformed from an accompanying commensal into a "metabolic organ." Genetic diversity in the microbial community provides a variety of enzymes and biochemical pathways, making the HM able to take on metabolic functions that complement human physiology. As the metabolic capacity of HM is equal to that of the liver, HM can be considered as an additional (virtual) organ in the GIT (Gill et al., 2006). The full metabolic potential of the microbiome has only recently been established and the potential contribution of HM to metabolic status and human health, as well as the link with obesity and related disorders, has been assessed (Jandhyala et al., 2015).

Probiotics are products of living microorganisms, mainly derived from *Lactobacillus* and *Bifidobacterium*. They have been the subject of research in recent years, related to their influence on the metabolic syndrome. Convincing facts show that probiotic bacteria improve digestion, absorption of nutrients, modulate the immune system, and lower elevated cholesterol. Probiotics are a possible future for patients with insulin resistance and obesity.

29.8 Probiotics and urogenital infections

It is believed that in the near future probiotics can largely replace conventional antibiotic therapy without side effects. There is a lot of scientific evidence for the role and application of *Lactobacilli* in maintaining vaginal microbial balance, prevention, and treatment of various urogenital infections in response to exhaustion of conventional therapy (Ding et al., 2017; Macklaim et al., 2015; Reid & Bruce, 2006).

29.9 Probiotics and immunity

Hippocrates (460–370 BCE) stated: "All diseases begin in the intestines." Both the diversity and the abundance of microorganisms in the gut play an important role in maintaining human health.

The stimulation of the immune system by probiotics and their connection with the "second brain"—the immune system in the gastrointestinal tract—has been established.

More than 80% of the cells of the immune system are located in the intestinal lymphoid tissue. The billions of cells of the immune system in the abdominal cavity form the "second brain" of the body of each individual. This "second brain" has the task of protecting and defending the body from bacterial aggression of pathogenic microorganisms. Our knowledge of this "second brain" and how it works is another challenge and is at the very beginning of our study. As knowledge progresses, we will create more and more perfect means to protect and stimulate the body's naturally built defense systems.

Neural pathways and central nervous system (CNS) signaling systems, according to new research, can be activated by bacteria in the gastrointestinal tract, including commensal, probiotic, and pathogenic bacteria. In theory, any disease associated with damage to the intestinal microbiota can be affected by its therapeutic modulation. Of particular interest are probiotic genes and probiotic factors involved in the regulation of host immunity, as well as the role and mechanisms of probiotics in disease prevention and treatment.

As you can see in Fig. 29.3, probiotics play a role in defining and maintaining the delicate balance between necessary and excessive defense mechanisms, including innate and adaptive immune responses. The use of probiotics enhance the immune system by contributing with specific and nonspecific immune responses especially cytokines

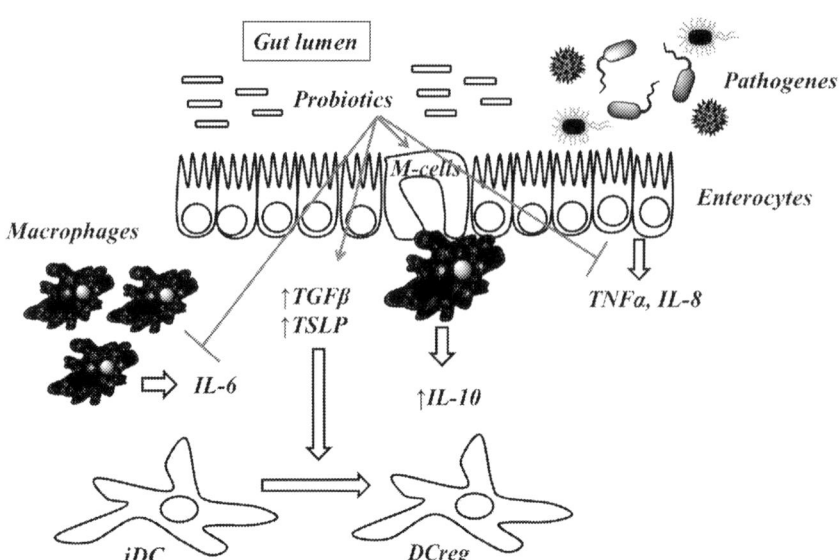

FIGURE 29.3 Probiotic modulation of the gastrointestinal mucosal immune system. While intestinal epithelial cells (IECs) exposed to pathogenic microbes or related stimuli produce proinflammatory mediators such as interleukin 8 (IL-8) and tumor necrosis factor α (TNF-α), probiotics suppress the production of these cytokines and instead induce antiinflammatory mediators such as transforming growth factor β (TGF-β) and thymic stromal lymphopoietin (TSLP), which can promote the differentiation of immature dendritic cells (iDCs) to regulatory dendritic cells (DCregs). Macrophages in the inflamed mucosa produce high amounts of IL-6, and probiotics can decrease their IL-6 production and increase IL-10 production.

release, natural killer, macrophage activation, and increased immunoglobulin levels. This immune reactions occur without a noticeable harmful inflammatory response (Ashraf & Shah, 2014; Ding et al., 2017).

The human body and the intestinal microflora are in a symbiotic relationship, and the hypothesis of a "superorganism" composed of body and microbes has recently been proposed. The intestinal microbiota performs important metabolic and immunological tasks and damage to its composition can alter homeostasis and lead to the development of various diseases.

There are new discoveries related to the effect of probiotics on immunity, thanks to the rapid development of metagenomic strategies. This knowledge will support treatment focused on the specific effects of different probiotics and prebiotics on the intestinal microbiota.

29.10 Probiotics and mental illness called Plus Ultra

The challenge and growing interest is to establish the link between microbiotic dysbiosis and the occurrence and/or course of major mental disorders, and to explore potential therapeutic options for microbiotic dysbiosis in psychiatric patients.

Microbiotic dysbiosis can negatively affect the functioning of the CNS through various intertwined pathways that collectively form the "brain–gut" axis. The brain–gut axis includes the CNS, the neuroendocrine and neuroimmune systems, the autonomic nervous system, the enteric nervous system, and intestinal microbiota. Experimental studies suggest that the brain–gut axis may play an important role throughout life in regulating stress, anxiety, and mood. The intestinal microbiota is increasingly seen as a symbiotic partner in maintaining good health. Metagenomic approaches could help to understand how the complex intestinal microbial ecosystem is involved in controlling the development and functioning of the brain.

Plus Ultra reflects the expectation that probiotics will most likely be used regularly in the complex treatment of anxiety, depression, Alzheimer's disease, and autism. There are some prospects for future developments of therapeutic substances, such as probiotics, prebiotics, and nutritional approaches in the treatment of mental disorders.

The study of the role of the human intestinal microbiota in the genesis and/or maintenance of psychiatric disorders is in its infancy, but is currently one of the most promising directions for research in psychiatry (Park et al., 2018; Slykerman et al., 2017). Today, autism is a psychiatric disorder in which the role of the microbiota is best studied. Some therapeutic options aimed at regulating microbiotic dysbiosis have already been studied as probiotic use or dietary modifications, but with conflicting results (Kushak et al., 2011).

29.11 The next 45 years

Predicting the future has never been easy and is usually based on what we know today. But it seems clear that probiotics will be used to treat depression and anxiety and potentially other forms of mental illness (Kushak et al., 2011; Puebla-Barragan & Reid, 2019). Of course, studies are underway using fecal microbiota transplantation for multiple sclerosis, Parkinson's disease, and dementia, so that in the coming years the strains that may have an effect will be identified, tested, and will be part of medical practice for microbial intervention. (Park et al., 2018; Slykerman et al., 2017).

A deeper step would be to implant probiotic strains directly into the brain, perhaps to counteract pathogens or to produce certain chemicals, such as γ-aminobutyric acid or serotonin, in certain places to try to improve function. This will require the ability to manipulate strains and control their spread outside the implanted site—all within the capabilities of molecular genetics and biomedical engineering. Disclosure of ethical issues may take longer, depending on what metabolites are produced and what functions they affect (Puebla-Barragan & Reid, 2019).

No more difficult ethical issues will be raised than if probiotics affect the development of the fetal organs and its life course. This is certainly possible, given that the risk of Alzheimer's disease can be reduced if the mother is treated. Whether probiotics will be implanted in the uterus, or their functions will be passed on through the mother's metabolism, remains to be seen, but both can happen. Apparently, there are compounds, including neurochemicals, vitamins, lipids, and peptides produced by microbes that already affect the development and functioning of the body (Gong et al., 2019; Lyte & Brown, 2018; Patel et al., 2013; Robertson et al., 2017; Wang et al., 2018).

There is already preliminary evidence of improved cognitive function in adults (Ceccarelli et al., 2017).

29.12 Summary

For the past 45 years, probiotic microbes have been identified, tested, and administered to patients and users worldwide. The market of more than US$40 trillion reflects not only interest in natural therapies and a desire to avoid drugs that are often ineffective or with serious side effects, but also due to rigorous research (Global Market Insights, Inc., 2017). There may never be enough large, randomized placebo-controlled trials to satisfy all critics, but the number of lives saved and improved by probiotics continues to grow. As future technology advances, it will be seen that different types of probiotics will be applied in new ways to further improve the well-being of humans, as well as other hosts from fish to honeybees, livestock, and wildlife.

29.13 Probiotics and Covid-19: data supporting the use of probiotics to prevent Covid-19

Of great interest is the link between Covid-19, gut microbiota, lung immunity, and probiotics. Would probiotics help?

Despite strategies based on social distancing, hygiene, and screening, Covid-19 is advancing rapidly around the world, with the risk of overloading health systems. For the time being, the establishment of effective drug therapies continues, vaccines are not yet available, so additional preventive strategies are urgently needed. Clinical data indicate that some probiotic strains help prevent bacterial and viral infections, including gastroenteritis, sepsis, and respiratory infections (RTIs). The reason for adding probiotic strains to the overall prevention and care strategy is based on science and clinical trials, although so far there have been no direct studies on the etiological agent of this pandemic (Baud et al., 2020; Su et al., 2020).

French Professor Jean Bousquet has examined the relationship between the consumption of fermented vegetables and mortality from Covid-19 in various European countries in 2020. Some of the countries with low mortality from Covid-19 are those with relatively high consumption of traditional fermented foods. He concluded that the consumption of fermented vegetables significantly reduced Covid-19 mortality for these countries. For each gram per day increase in the average national consumption of fermented vegetables, the risk of death from Covid-19 decreased by 35.4% (95% CI: 11.4%, 35.5%).

Jean Bousquet found that Bulgaria, Greece, and Romania had very low mortality rates. This can also be linked to diet, as cabbage (Romania) and fermented milk (Bulgaria and Greece) are common (frequently consumed there) foods. These foods are a known natural inhibitors of angiotensin-converting enzyme (Bousquet et al., 2020).

Two meta-analyses of randomized controlled trials (RCTs) in humans have shown that probiotics can reduce the frequency and duration of respiratory viral infections.

In two RCTs, one with 146 and the other with 235 patients on mechanical ventilation, probiotic administration improved pneumonia outcomes compared with placebo (Gu et al., 2020).

Other researchers are bolder "Probiotics are usually safe, even in the most vulnerable populations and intensive care units," said Professor David Baud and colleagues in a review paper in the *Frontiers of Public Health*. "Instead of considering intensive care patients too ill to receive probiotic and prebiotic therapy, RCTs (randomized clinical trials) with probiotics for the prevention of ventilator-associated pneumonia give reason to keep them in mind" (Baud et al., 2020).

In addition, these researchers listed the appropriate probiotics to consider, during the Covid-19 pandemic.

Covid-19 is being presented with a spectrum of disease severity, ranging from mild and nonspecific flu-like symptoms to pneumonia and life-threatening complications such as acute respiratory distress syndrome (ARDS) and multiorgan failure. While transmission of SARS-CoV-2 is thought to occur primarily through respiratory droplets, the gut may also contribute to the pathogenesis of Covid-19 (Ng & Tilg, 2020). SARS-CoV-2 RNA was detected in gastrointestinal and fecal samples from patients (Pan et al., 2020; Jin et al., 2020; Lin et al., 2020) and in sewage systems (Wu et al., 2020). Coronaviruses, including SARS-Cov-2, can invade enterocytes, thus acting as a reservoir for the virus (Lin et al., 2020). In fact, large clinical studies from China have shown that gastrointestinal symptoms are common in Covid-19 and are related to the severity of the disease (Jin et al., 2020; Lin et al., 2020).

As reports from China indicate that Covid-19 may be associated with intestinal dysbiosis (causing inflammation) and a weaker response to pathogens (Gao et al., 2020; Xu et al., 2020), these cases will require restoration of homeostasis (Di Pierro, 2020). Oral administration of probiotic strains may further affect this gut-lung axis, as some of them may migrate from the gut to distant sites, e.g. in the breast for the treatment of mastitis (Arroyo et al., 2010).

Mechanisms that could explain the clinical success of probiotics include improving the intestinal epithelial barrier, competing with nutrient pathogens and adhesion to the intestinal epithelium, antimicrobial production, and modulation of the host immune system (Bermudez-Brito et al., 2012). The intestinal microbiome has a critical effect on systemic immune responses and immune responses in distant sites, including the lungs (Abt et al., 2012; Zelaya et al., 2016). The administration of some *Bifidobacteria* or *Lactobacilli* has a beneficial effect on the clearance of influenza virus from the respiratory tract (Ichinohe et al., 2011; Zelaya et al., 2016). The application of probiotic strains improve the levels of type I interferons, increase the number and activity of antigen-presenting cells, NK (natural killer) cells, and T cells, as well as the levels of systemic and mucosal specific antibodies in the lungs (de Vrese et al., 2005; Ichinohe et al., 2011; Zelaya et al., 2016). There is also evidence that probiotic strains modify the dynamic balance between proinflammatory and immunoregulatory cytokines that allow viral clearance while minimizing immune-mediated lung damage. This may be particularly important in preventing ARDS, a major complication of Covid-19. Evidence for antiviral activity of probiotic strains against common respiratory viruses, including influenza, rhinovirus, and respiratory syncytial virus, is the result of clinical and experimental studies (Luoto et al., 2014; Namba et al., 2010; Turner et al., 2017). Although none of these effects or mechanisms have been tested on the new SARS-CoV-2 virus, this approach should be considered, especially when beneficial effects of probiotics against other coronavirus strains have been reported (Chai et al., 2013; Kumar et al., 2010; Liu et al., 2020; Wang et al., 2019).

Since the link between viral replication and gastrointestinal immunity is very close, the effect of probiotic bacteria can play an important role in stopping viral replication. New approaches to single-strain probiotic bacteria can be promising in terms of both vaccination and treatment models (Bozkurt, 2020).

29.14 Conclusion

From the first description to today's knowledge of probiotics, the thread of knowledge continues to unravel. In today's global society, where people are exposed to daily stress, the widespread use of antibiotics, poor nutrition, and a number of harmful external factors, the balance of the gastrointestinal flora suffers from constant disturbances. And the ingenious conjecture of Hippocrates that "all diseases begin in the intestinal tract" finds its modern confirmation. It is no coincidence that in Europe, probiotics and probiotic foods are among the most stable segments of the food market.

However, it should be noted that probiotics, although harmless, are not a magic panacea. Continuous and adequate supervision of their use is necessary to prevent even the slightest risk to human health. This supervision should be exercised strictly by the relevant health institutions, because the maxim of Hippocrates: "Primum non nocere!" (First, do no harm!) remains in force to this day. Despite the proven health benefits, a probiotic per se is not able to prevent or treat the whole huge range of human diseases. But the thread of our knowledge must continue to unravel.

The ability to control and predict the effects of probiotics, based on rigorous research, would allow both consumers and manufacturers to choose and offer products with proven healing properties and thus fully extend human life.

References

Abt, M. C., Osborne, L. C., Monticelli, L. A., Doering, T. A., Alenghat, T., Sonnenberg, G. F., et al. (2012). Commensal bacteria calibrate the activation threshold of innate antiviral immunity. *Immunity*, 37(1), 158–170.

Anukam, K., & Reid, G. (2007). Probiotics: 100 years (1907–2007) after Elie Metchnikoff's observations. *Communicating Current Research and Educational Topics and Trends in Applied Microbiology*, 1, 466–474.

Araya, M., Morelli, L., Reid, G., Sanders, M.E., Stanton, C., Pineiro, M., Ben Embarek, P. (2002). Guidelines for the evaluation of probiotics in food (pp. 1–11). Report of a Joint FAO/WHO Working Group on Drafting. Guidelines for the Evaluation of Probiotics in Food.

Arroyo, R., Martín, V., Maldonado, A., Jiménez, E., Fernández, L., & Rodríguez, J. M. (2010). Treatment of infectious mastitis during lactation: Antibiotics versus oral administration of Lactobacilli isolated from breast milk. *Clinical Infectious Diseases: An Official Publication of the Infectious Diseases Society of America*, 50(12), 1551–1558.

Ashraf, R., & Shah, N. P. (2014). Immune system stimulation by probiotic microorganisms. *Critical Reviews in Food Science and Nutrition*, 54(7), 938–956.

Baud, D., Dimopoulou Agri, V., Gibson, G. R., Reid, G., & Giannoni, E. (2020). Using probiotics to flatten the curve of coronavirus disease COVID-2019 pandemic. *Frontiers in Public Health*, 8, 186.

Bercik, P., Collins, S. M., & Verdu, E. F. (2012). Microbes and the gut-brain axis. *Neurogastroenterology and Motility: The Official Journal of the European Gastrointestinal Motility Society*, 24(5), 405–413.

Bermudez-Brito, M., Plaza-Díaz, J., Muñoz-Quezada, S., Gómez-Llorente, C., & Gil, A. (2012). Probiotic mechanisms of action. *Annals of Nutrition & Metabolism*, 61(2), 160–174.

Boukthir, S., Matoussi, N., Belhadj, A., Mammou, S., Dlala, S. B., Helayem, M., Rocchiccioli, F., Bouzaidi, S., & Abdennebi, M. (2010). Anomalies de la perméabilité intestinale chez l'enfant autiste [Abnormal intestinal permeability in children with autism]. *La Tunisie Medicale*, 88(9), 685–686.

Bousquet, J., Anto, J. M., Iaccarino, G., Czarlewski, W., Haahtela, T., Anto, A., et al. (2020). Is diet partly responsible for differences in COVID-19 death rates between and within countries? *Clinical and Translational Allergy*, 10, 16.

Bozkurt, H., (2020). Probiotic bacteria against the Covid-19.

Brown, A. C., & Valiere, A. (2004). Probiotics and medical nutrition therapy. *Nutrition in Clinical Care: An Official Publication of Tufts University*, 7(2), 56–68.

Brown, L. M. (2000). Helicobacter pylori: Epidemiology and routes of transmission. *Epidemiologic Reviews, 22*(2), 283–297.
Cai, J., Zhao, C., Du, Y., Zhang, Y., Zhao, M., & Zhao, Q. (2018). Comparative efficacy and tolerability of probiotics for antibiotic-associated diarrhea: Systematic review with network meta-analysis. *United European Gastroenterology Journal, 6*(2), 169–180.
Cani, P., & Delzenne, N. (2011). The gut microbiome as therapeutic target. *Pharmacology & Therapeutics, 130*(2), 202–212.
Carper, J. (1994). *Food-your miracle medicine*. New York: HarperCollins.
Ceccarelli, G., Fratino, M., Selvaggi, C., Giustini, N., Serafino, S., Schietroma, I., et al. (2017). A pilot study on the effects of probiotic supplementation on neuropsychological performance and microRNA-29a-c levels in antiretroviral-treated HIV-1-infected patients. *Brain and Behavior, 7*(8), e00756.
Chai, W., Burwinkel, M., Wang, Z., Palissa, C., Esch, B., Twardziok, S., et al. (2013). Antiviral effects of a probiotic Enterococcus faecium strain against transmissible gastroenteritis coronavirus. *Archives of Virology, 158*(4), 799–807.
Ciorba, M. A., Riehl, T. E., Rao, M. S., Moon, C., Ee, X., Nava, G. M., et al. (2011). Lactobacillus probiotic protects intestinal epithelium from radiation injury in a TLR-2/cyclo-oxygenase-2-dependent manner. *Gut, 61*(6), 829–838.
Dave, M., Higgins, P., Middha, S., & Rioux, K. P. (2012). The human gut microbiome: Current knowledge, challenges and future directions. *Translational Research, 160*(4), 246–257.
de Vrese, M., & Schrezenmeir, J. (2008). Probiotics, prebiotics, and synbiotics. *Advances in Biochemical Engineering/Biotechnology, 111*, 1–66.
de Vrese, M., Winkler, P., Rautenberg, P., Harder, T., Noah, C., Laue, C., et al. (2005). Effect of *Lactobacillus gasseri* PA 16/8, *Bifidobacterium longum* SP 07/3, B. bifidum MF 20/5 on common cold episodes: A double blind, randomized, controlled trial. *Clinical Nutrition (Edinburgh, Scotland), 24*(4), 481–491.
Dean, M., Fojo, T., & Bates, S. (2005). Tumour stem cells and drug resistance. *Nature Reviews Cancer, 5*(4), 275–284.
Derwa, Y., Gracie, D. J., Hamlin, P. J., & Ford, A. C. (2017). Systematic review with meta-analysis: The efficacy of probiotics in inflammatory bowel disease. *Alimentary Pharmacology & Therapeutics, 46*(4), 389–400.
Di Pierro, F. (2020). A possible probiotic (S. salivarius K12) approach to improve oral and lung microbiotas and raise defenses against SAR S-CoV-2. *Minerva Medica, 111*(3), 281–283.
Ding, Y. H., Qian, L. Y., Pang, J., Lin, J. Y., Xu, Q., Wang, L. H., Huang, D. S., & Zou, H. (2017). The regulation of immune cells by Lactobacilli: A potential therapeutic target for anti-atherosclerosis therapy. *Oncotarget, 8*(35), 59915–59928.
Driessen, F. M., Kingma, F., & Stadhouders, J. (1982). Evidence that *Lactobacillus bulgaricus* in yogurt is stimulated by carbon dioxide produced by *Streptococcus thermophilus*. *Netherland Milk and Dairy Journal, 36*, 135–144.
Gao, Q. Y., Chen, Y. X., & Fang, J. Y. (2020). 2019 Novel coronavirus infection and gastrointestinal tract. *Journal of Digestive Diseases, 21*(3), 125–126.
Georgieva, M. (2006). Toxicological and clinical pharmacological study of bulgarian low-lactose lactate probiotic biostim LBS [dissertation]. Sofia: Medical University.
Georgiev, K., Georgieva, M., Iliev, I., Peneva, M., & Alexandrov, G. (2015). Antiproliferative effect of Bulgarian spring water probiotics (Laktera Nature Probiotics), against human colon carcinoma cell line. *World Journal of Pharmaceutical Sciences, 4*(6), 130–136.
Georgieva, M., Georgiev, K., & Dobromirov, P. (2015). Probiotics and immunity. In K. Metodiev (Ed.), *Immunopathology and immunomodulation*. Intech Open.
Gibson, G. R., Scott, K. P., Rastall, R. A., Tuohy, K. M., Hotchkiss, A., Dubert-Ferrandon, A., et al. (2010). Dietary prebiotics: Current status and new definition. *Food Science and Technology Bulletin: Functional Foods, 7*(1), 1–19.
Gill, S. R., Pop, M., Deboy, R. T., Eckburg, P. B., Turnbaugh, P. J., Samuel, B. S., et al. (2006). Metagenomic analysis of the human distal gut microbiome. *Science (New York, N.Y.), 312*(5778), 1355–1359.
Global Market Insights, Inc., (2017). Probiotics market report 2024. Delaware. https://www.gminsights.com/industry-analysis/probiotics-market (Accessed 13.11.2018).
Gong, M., Hu, Y., Wei, W., Jin, Q., & Wang, X. (2019). Production of conjugated fatty acids: A review of recent advances. *Biotechnology Advances, 37*(8), 107454.
Gu, J., Han, B., & Wang, J. (2020). COVID-19: Gastrointestinal manifestations and potential fecal-oral transmission. *Gastroenterology, 158*(6), 1518–1519.
Guarner, F., & Malagelada, J. R. (2003). Gut flora in health and disease. *Lancet, 361*(9356), 512–519.
Guarner, F., Sanders, M. E., Eliakim, R., Fedorak, R., Gangl, A., Garisch, J., et al. (2017). *Global guidelines probiotics and prebiotics*. World Gastroenterology Organisation, http://medi-guide.meditool.cn/ymtpdf/24B36233-2CB9-27AE-C86B A55F6003C9AE.pdf (Accessed 16.10.2020).
Guha, D., Banerjee, A., Mukherjee, R., Pradhan, B., Peneva, M., Aleksandrov, G., et al. (2019). A probiotic formulation containing *Lactobacillus bulgaricus* DWT1 inhibits tumor growth by activating pro-inflammatory responses in macrophages. *Journal of Functional Foods, 56*, 232–245.
Hansen, E. B. (2002). Commercial bacterial starter cultures for fermented foods of the future. *International Journal of Food Microbiology, 78*(1–2), 119–131.
Herve-Jimenez, L., Guillouard, I., Guedon, E., Boudebbouze, S., Hols, P., Monnet, V., Maguin, E., & Rul, F. (2009). Postgenomic analysis of streptococcus thermophilus cocultivated in milk with *Lactobacillus delbrueckii* subsp. bulgaricus: Involvement of nitrogen, purine, and iron metabolism. *Applied and Environmental Microbiology, 75*(7), 2062–2073.
Hill, C., Guarner, F., Reid, G., Gibson, G. R., Merenstein, D. J., Pot, B., et al. (2014). Expert consensus document. The International Scientific Association for probiotics and prebiotics consensus statement on the scope and appropriate use of the term probiotic. *Nature Reviews Gastroenterology & Hepatology, 11*(8), 506–514.

Hooper, L. V., & Gordon, J. I. (2001). Commensal host-bacterial relationships in the gut. *Science (New York, N.Y.), 292*(5519), 1115–1118.

Human Microbiome Project Consortium. (2012). Structure, function and diversity of the healthy human microbiome. *Nature, 486*, 207–214.

Iannitti, T., & Palmieri, B. (2010). Therapeutical use of probiotic formulations in clinical practice. *Clinical Nutrition (Edinburgh, Scotland), 29*(6), 701–725.

Ichinohe, T., Pang, I. K., Kumamoto, Y., Peaper, D. R., Ho, J. H., Murray, T. S., & Iwasaki, A. (2011). Microbiota regulates immune defense against respiratory tract influenza A virus infection. *Proceedings of the National Academy of Sciences of the United States of America, 108*(13), 5354–5359.

Jandhyala, S. M., Talukdar, R., Subramanyam, C., Vuyyuru, H., Sasikala, M., & Nageshwar Reddy, D. (2015). Role of the normal gut microbiota. *World Journal of Gastroenterology, 21*(29), 8787–8803.

Jin, X., Lian, J. S., Hu, J. H., Gao, J., Zheng, L., Zhang, Y. M., et al. (2020). Epidemiological, clinical and virological characteristics of 74 cases of coronavirus-infected disease 2019 (COVID-19) with gastrointestinal symptoms. *Gut, 69*(6), 1002–1009.

Kalliomäki, M., Salminen, S., Arvilommi, H., Kero, P., Koskinen, P., & Isolauri, E. (2001). Probiotics in primary prevention of atopic disease: A randomised placebo-controlled trial. *Lancet, 357*(9262), 1076–1079.

Kennedy, P. J., Clarke, G., Quigley, E. M., Groeger, J. A., Dinan, T. G., & Cryan, J. F. (2012). Gut memories: Towards a cognitive neurobiology of irritable bowel syndrome. *Neuroscience and Biobehavioral Reviews, 36*(1), 310–340.

Knox, S. J., & Meredith, R. F. (2000). Clinical radioimmunotherapy. *Seminars in Radiation Oncology, 10*(2), 73–93.

Kumar, R., Seo, B. J., Mun, M. R., Kim, C. J., Lee, I., Kim, H., & Park, Y. H. (2010). Putative probiotic Lactobacillus spp. from porcine gastrointestinal tract inhibit transmissible gastroenteritis coronavirus and enteric bacterial pathogens. *Tropical Animal Health and Production, 42*(8), 1855–1860.

Kushak, R. I., Lauwers, G. Y., Winter, H. S., & Buie, T. M. (2011). Intestinal disaccharidase activity in patients with autism: Effect of age, gender, and intestinal inflammation. *Autism: The International Journal of Research and Practice, 15*(3), 285–294.

Lee, Y. K., & Salminen, S. (2009). *Handbook of probiotics and prebiotics* (2nd ed.). Hoboken, New Jersey, USA: John Wiley and Sons.

Lin, L., Jiang, X., Zhang, Z., Huang, S., Zhang, Z., Fang, Z., et al. (2020). Gastrointestinal symptoms of 95 cases with SARS-CoV-2 infection. *Gut, 69*(6), 997–1001.

Liu, Y. S., Liu, Q., Jiang, Y. L., Yang, W. T., Huang, H. B., Shi, C. W., et al. (2020). Surface-displayed porcine IFN-λ3 in *Lactobacillus plantarum* inhibits porcine enteric coronavirus infection of porcine intestinal epithelial cells. *Journal of Microbiology and Biotechnology, 30*(4), 515–525.

Lloyd-Price, J., Abu-Ali, G., & Huttenhower, C. (2016). The healthy human microbiome. *Genome Medicine, 8*(1), 51.

Luoto, R., Ruuskanen, O., Waris, M., Kalliomäki, M., Salminen, S., & Isolauri, E. (2014). Prebiotic and probiotic supplementation prevents rhinovirus infections in preterm infants: A randomized, placebo-controlled trial. *The Journal of Allergy and Clinical Immunology, 133*(2), 405–413.

Lyte, M., & Brown, D. R. (2018). Evidence for PMAT- and OCT-like biogenic amine transporters in a probiotic strain of Lactobacillus: Implications for interkingdom communication within the microbiota-gut-brain axis. *PLoS One, 13*(1), e0191037.

Ma, X., Hua, J., & Li, Z. (2008). Probiotics improve high fat diet-induced hepatic steatosis and insulin resistance by increasing hepatic NKT cells. *Journal of Hepatology, 49*(5), 821–830.

Macklaim, J. M., Clemente, J. C., Knight, R., Gloor, G. B., & Reid, G. (2015). Changes in vaginal microbiota following antimicrobial and probiotic therapy. *Microbial Ecology in Health and Disease, 26*, 27799.

Mattila-Sandholm, T., Blaut, M., Daly, C., Vuyst, L., Doré, J., Gibson, G., et al. (2002). Food, GI-tract functionality and human health cluster: PROEUHEALTH. *Microbial Ecology in Health and Disease, 14*(2), 65–74.

McFarland, L. V. (2015). From yaks to yogurt: The history, development, and current use of probiotics. *Clinical Infectious Diseases: An Official Publication of the Infectious Diseases Society of America, 60*(Suppl. 2), S85–S90.

Metchnikoff, E. (1907). Lactic acid as inhibiting intestinal putrefaction. In P. Chalmers Mitchell (Ed.), *The prolongation of life: Optimistic studies* (pp. 161–183). London: Heinemann.

Michaylova, M., Minkova, S., Kimura, K., Sasaki, T., & Isawa, K. (2007). Isolation and characterization of *Lactobacillus delbrueckii* ssp. bulgaricus and *Streptococcus thermophilus* from plants in Bulgaria. *FEMS Microbiology Letters, 269*(1), 160–169.

Milenic, D. E., Brady, E. D., & Brechbiel, M. W. (2004). Antibody-targeted radiation cancer therapy. *Nature Reviews Drug Discovery, 3*(6), 488–499.

Morelli, L., Vescovo, M., Cocconcelli, P. S., & Bottazzi, V. (1986). Fast and slow milk-coagulating variants of Lactobacillus helveticus HLM 1. *Canadian Journal of Microbiology, 32*(9), 758–760.

Namba, K., Hatano, M., Yaeshima, T., Takase, M., & Suzuki, K. (2010). Effects of *Bifidobacterium longum* BB536 administration on influenza infection, influenza vaccine antibody titer, and cell-mediated immunity in the elderly. *Bioscience, Biotechnology, and Biochemistry, 74*(5), 939–945.

Ng, S. C., & Tilg, H. (2020). COVID-19 and the gastrointestinal tract: More than meets the eye. *Gut, 69*(6), 973–974.

Ouwehand, A., Kirjavainen, P., Shortt, C., & Salminen, S. (1999). Probiotics: Mechanisms and established effects. *International Dairy Journal, 9*(1), 43–52.

Pan, Y., Zhang, D., Yang, P., Poon, L., & Wang, Q. (2020). Viral load of SARS-CoV-2 in clinical samples. *The Lancet Infectious Diseases, 20*(4), 411–412.

Park, C., Brietzke, E., Rosenblat, J. D., Musial, N., Zuckerman, H., Ragguett, R. M., et al. (2018). Probiotics for the treatment of depressive symptoms: An anti-inflammatory mechanism? *Brain, Behavior, and Immunity, 73*, 115–124.

Patel, A., Shah, N., & Prajapati, J. B. (2013). Biosynthesis of vitamins and enzymes in fermented foods by lactic acid bacteria and related genera—a promising approach. *Croatian Journal of Food Science and Technology, 5*(2), 85–91.

Peneva, D., & Alexandrov, A., (2015). Inventors; Daflorn LTD, assignee. Probiotics for dietary dairy product. US Patent 9,131,708B2. September 15.

Ponziani, F. R., Zocco, M. A., Cerrito, L., Gasbarrini, A., & Pompili, M. (2018). Bacterial translocation in patients with liver cirrhosis: Physiology, clinical consequences, and practical implications. *Expert Review of Gastroenterology & Hepatology, 12*(7), 641–656.

Puebla-Barragan, S., & Reid, G. (2019). Forty-five-year evolution of probiotic therapy. *Microbial Cell, 6*(4), 184–196.

Reid, G., & Bruce, A. W. (2006). Probiotics to prevent urinary tract infections: The rationale and evidence. *World Journal of Urology, 24*(1), 28–32.

Reid, G., Gadir, A. A., & Dhir, R. (2019). Probiotics: Reiterating what they are and what they are not. *Frontiers in Microbiology, 10*, 424.

Robertson, R. C., Seira Oriach, C., Murphy, K., Moloney, G. M., Cryan, J. F., Dinan, T. G., et al. (2017). Omega-3 polyunsaturated fatty acids critically regulate behaviour and gut microbiota development in adolescence and adulthood. *Brain, Behavior, and Immunity, 59*, 21–37.

Rusch, V. (2002). Probiotics and definitions: A short overview. In P. J. Heidt, T. Midtvedt, V. Rusch, & D. van der Waaij (Eds.), *Monograph 15: Probiotics bacteria and bacterial fragments as immunomodulatory agents* (pp. 1–4). Germany: Herborn Litterae, Herborn-Dill.

Salminen, S. (1996). Uniqueness of probiotic strains. *IDF Nutrition News Letter, 5*, 16–18.

Salminen, S., & Marteau, P. (1997). Safety of probiotic lactic acid bacteria and other probiotics. Lactic 97 (Proceedings). *Adria Normandie Caen*, 71–72.

Sanders, M. E. (2008). Probiotics: Definition, sources, selection, and uses. *Clinical Infectious Diseases: An Official Publication of the Infectious Diseases Society of America, 46*(2), S58–S151.

Simmering, R., & Blaut, M. (2001). Pro- and prebiotics—The tasty guardian angels? *Applied Microbiology and Biotechnology, 55*(1), 19–28.

Singh, V. P., Sharma, J., Babu, S., Rizwanulla., & Singla, A. (2013). Role of probiotics in health and disease: A review. *JPMA. The Journal of the Pakistan Medical Association, 63*(2), 253–257.

Slykerman, R. F., Hood, F., Wickens, K., Thompson, J., Barthow, C., Murphy, R., et al. (2017). Effect of *Lactobacillus rhamnosus* HN001 in pregnancy on postpartum symptoms of depression and anxiety: A randomised double-blind placebo-controlled trial. *EBioMedicine, 24*, 159–165.

Su, S., Shen, J., Zhu, L., Qiu, Y., He, J. S., Tan, J. Y., et al. (2020). Involvement of digestive system in COVID-19: Manifestations, pathology, management and challenges. *Therapeutic Advances in Gastroenterology, 13*, 1756284820934626.

Suk, K. T., & Kim, D. J. (2012). Drug-induced liver injury: Present and future. *Clinical and Molecular Hepatology, 18*(3), 249–257.

Tripathi, A., Debelius, J., Brenner, D. A., Karin, M., Loomba, R., Schnabl, B., & Knight, R. (2018). The gut-liver axis and the intersection with the microbiome. *Nature Reviews Gastroenterology & Hepatology, 15*, 397–411.

Turner, R. B., Woodfolk, J. A., Borish, L., Steinke, J. W., Patrie, J. T., Muehling, L. M., et al. (2017). Effect of probiotic on innate inflammatory response and viral shedding in experimental rhinovirus infection—a randomised controlled trial. *Beneficial Microbes, 8*(2), 207–215.

Ursell, L., Haiser, H., Van Treuren, W., Garg, N., Reddivari, L., Vanamala, J., Dorrestein, P., Turnbaugh, P., & Knight, R. (2014). The intestinal metabolome: An intersection between microbiota and host. *Gastroenterology, 146*(6), 1470–1476.

Vajro, P., Poeta, M., Pierri, L., Pizza, C., D'Aniello, R., Sangermano, M., et al. (2014). Chapter 33—Probiotics to treat visceral obesity and related liver disease. In R. R. Watson (Ed.), *Nutrition in the prevention and treatment of abdominal obesity* (pp. 363–380). London: Academic Press.

Van Cutsem, E., Köhne, C. H., Hitre, E., Zaluski, J., Chang Chien, C. R., Makhson, A., et al. (2009). Cetuximab and chemotherapy as initial treatment for metastatic colorectal cancer. *The New England Journal of Medicine, 360*(14), 1408–1417.

Veringa, H. A., Galesloot, T. E., & Davelaar, H. (1968). Symbiosis in yoghourt (II). Isolation and identification of a growth factor for *Lactobacillus bulgaricus* produced by *Streptococcus thermophilus*. *Netherland Milk and Dairy Journal, 22*, 114–120.

Wang, K., Ran, L., Yan, T., Niu, Z., Kan, Z., Zhang, Y., et al. (2019). Anti-TGEV miller strain infection effect of *Lactobacillus plantarum* supernatant based on the JAK-STAT1 signaling pathway. *Frontiers in Microbiology, 10*, 2540.

Wang, L., Guo, M. J., Gao, Q., Yang, J. F., Yang, L., Pang, X. L., & Jiang, X. J. (2018). The effects of probiotics on total cholesterol: A meta-analysis of randomized controlled trials. *Medicine, 97*(5), e9679.

Ward, R., & German, J. (2004). Understanding milk's bioactive components: A goal for the genomics toolbox. *The Journal of Nutrition, 134*(4), 962S–967S.

Wu, F., Zhang, J., Xiao, A., Gu, X., Lee, W. L., Armas, F., et al. (2020). SARS-CoV-2 titers in wastewater are higher than expected from clinically confirmed cases. *mSystems, 5*(4), e00614–e00620.

Xu, K., Cai, H., Shen, Y., Ni, Q., Chen, Y., Hu, S., et al. (2020). Management of corona virus disease-19 (COVID-19): The Zhejiang experience Zhejiang da xue xue bao. Yi xue ban = *Journal of Zhejiang University. Medical Sciences, 49*(1), 147–157.

Yoon, E., Babar, A., Choudhary, M., Kutner, M., & Pyrsopoulos, N. (2016). Acetaminophen-induced hepatotoxicity: A comprehensive update. *Journal of Clinical and Translational Hepatology, 4*(2), 131–142.

Zelaya, H., Alvarez, S., Kitazawa, H., & Villena, J. (2016). Respiratory antiviral immunity and immunobiotics: Beneficial effects on inflammation-coagulation interaction during influenza virus infection. *Frontiers in Immunology, 7*, 633.

Chapter 30

Probiotics: health safety considerations

Hemant Borase[1], Mitesh Kumar Dwivedi[1], Ramar Krishnamurthy[1] and Satish Patil[2]

[1]*C.G. Bhakta Institute of Biotechnology, Uka Tarsadia University, Maliba Campus, Bardoli, India*, [2]*School of Life Sciences, Kavayitri Bahinabai Chaudhari North Maharashtra University, Jalgaon, India*

30.1 Introduction

For a long time, human beings have admired the key role of microorganisms in the ecosystem, ranging from photosynthesis deep inside the ocean to nutrient recycling on the earth surface. Humans were using fermented food product as part of their diet many centuries ago, maybe without the awareness of the health benefits. Many of these fermented preparations are still in use today such as curd, yogurt, tempeh, kombucha, kefir, and sauerkraut in different parts of the world (Chilton et al., 2015). Ilya Ilyich Metchnikoff [Nobel Prize in Physiology or Medicine (1908)] working in Pasteur Institute, France, was a pioneer to propose that fermented milk has beneficial actions for human health. He also made important suggestions such as lower gut microflora of humans might be the cause of illness, and such adverse effects can be relieved by consumption of beneficial microorganisms. Metchnikoff correlated the longer life span of the human population residing in the Bulgar Mountains with consumption of yogurt harboring *Lactobacillus bulgaricus* (Gupta et al., 2021).

Over the past decades, microbes in the human intestine (human gut microbiome) have been reported in many vital functions such as homeostasis, normal intestinal functioning, and in psychology (Daliri & Lee, 2015; Lerner et al., 2017). This led to a rapid surge in interest towards consumption and medical prescriptions of traditional fermented products, commercial pharmaceuticals and nutraceuticals harboring useful microorganisms for disease prevention and treatment (Singh et al., 2019). The origin of the term "probiotic" (meaning "for life," originated from the Latin word *pro* and Greek word *bios*) was dated back to 1953, where Werner Kollath (a German physician) used it for dynamic substances that were important for human growth and development (Pace et al., 2020). The World Health Organization (WHO), Food and Agriculture Organization (FAO) and International Scientific Association for Probiotics and Prebiotics (ISAPP) defined probiotic as "live microorganisms that, when administered in adequate amounts, confer a health benefit on the host" (Pace et al., 2020).

Probiotic industry is a big business. In 2013, the worldwide probiotic business was US$32 billion (Byakika et al., 2019). The estimated global market value of probiotics was around US$49 billion in 2019 and expected to reach nearly twofold by 2027 with an annual growth rate of 5%–30%, depending upon product and country (Caselli et al., 2013). Apart from traditional fermented products, probiotics are now incorporated in food products such as ice cream, chocolate, cookies, fruits, meat, and cereals.

Probiotic microorganisms majorly consist of bacterial species of lactic acid synthesizing bacilli [lactic acid bacilli (LAB)] including species of genus *Lactobacillus*, *Bifidobacteria*, *Lactococcus*, *Enterococcus*. Representative probiotics strains are *Lactobacillus reuteri*, *Enterococcus faecium* SF68, *Escherichia coli* strain Nissle 1917, *Lactobacillus rhamnosus*, *Lactobacillus acidophilus*, *Lactobacillus plantarum* and *Bifidobacterium infantis* (2019). *Saccharomyces cerevisiae* and *Saccharomyces boulardii* are also a probiotic yeast strains.

Probiotics are mainly consumed for treatment of gastrointestinal imbalance, diarrhea, antibiotic-associated diarrhea, diabetes, control of serum cholesterol, allergies, bacterial vaginosis, atopia, irritable bowel syndrome, depression, and liver disorders to name a few (Cuello-Garcia et al., 2015; Pace et al., 2020; Zucko et al., 2020). Probiotics are reported to exhibit therapeutic benefits by multiple actions and includes modifying gut microbiota, empowering gut epithelial barrier, and improving immunity (Bermudez-Brito et al., 2012).

Despite the multiple health and therapeutic effects, as in the case of most of drugs, the probiotics are not entirely safe and have some inherent risks. Most of the existing literature highlights the beneficial role of probiotics, but its safety and adverse effects still need to be addressed properly (Fig. 30.1).

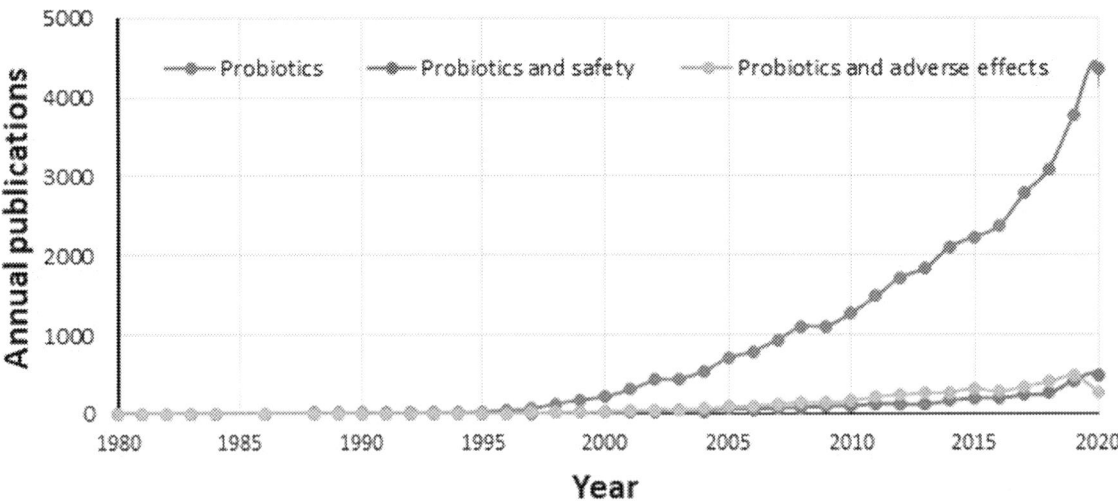

FIGURE 30.1 PubMed data on probiotics over the years. PubMed data clearly reflecting the fact that majority of research related to probiotic was focused on basic research and health benefits, but there is scarcity of data on safety and adverse effects of probiotics.

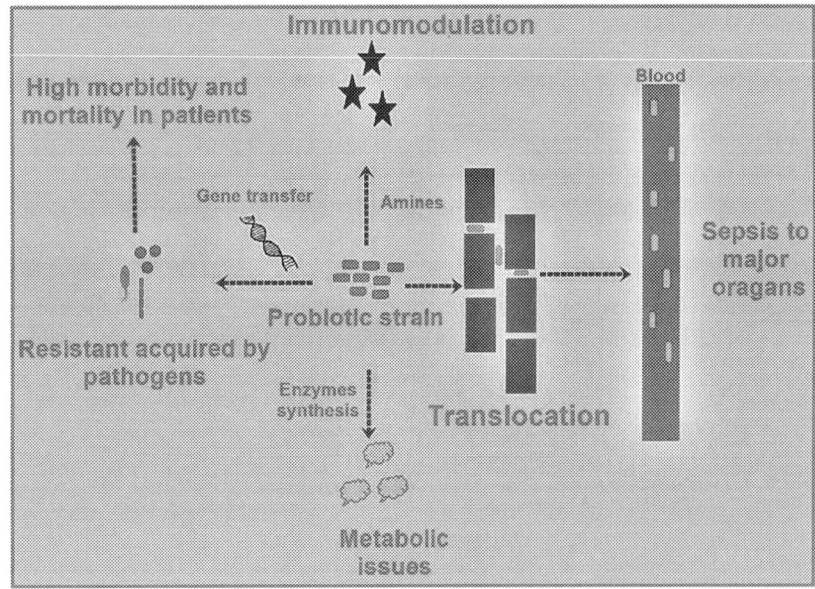

FIGURE 30.2 Schematic representation of reported adverse effects of probiotics.

One of the probable reasons behind this is might be that researchers as well as the probiotic industry are not willing to report negative finding on probiotics, owing to universally accepted perception of probiotics as panacea to cure multiple health issues. Another major reason is that today probiotics is very big business; there may be "pressure" on regulatory agencies to keep minimal regulation of scientific research for smooth transfer (without adequate safety assessment) into the consumer market (Fig. 30.2).

Multiple reports have suggested to address diverse health caveats regarding probiotics safety (Shanahan, 2012). The negative impacts of probiotics consumption are largely discussed in high-risk individuals such as patients recovering from surgery, below standard gastrointestinal mucosal barrier, and in immunocompromised patients (Didari et al., 2014).

The most commonly reported adverse effects of probiotics are fungemia and bacteremia, but in recent time the list is starting to increase and includes infectious/gastrointestinal diseases (meningitis, pneumonia, peritonitis, nausea, vomiting, taste alteration), allergic (D-lactic acidosis, rash, rhinitis, etc.), genetic (antibiotic resistance, virulence factor transfer) and pathotoxicogenetic (food poisoning, immune evasion/overstimulation, increased protein adhesion and aggregation, microbial conjugation) (Kothari et al., 2019; Lerner et al., 2019; Sotoudegan et al., 2019).

Unsatisfactory performance of most of the probiotic strains was revealed when challenged against intestinal dysbiosis (McFarland, 2014). Neurotransmitters and immune-modulating biogenic amines (histamine, tyramine, putrescine, cadaverine) are produce by LAB, and a population sensitive to these compounds complained about headaches and multiple side effects (Martin & Vij, 2016). Owing to recent literature questioning the safety of probiotics, detail and unbiased scientific evaluation of probiotics for "risk—benefit" ratio must be done before giving regulatory clearance and entry into the market in the best interest of consumer health and also protecting consumer rights (Sanders et al., 2010; Toscano et al., 2017).

However, several important issues must be addressed regarding enhancement of probiotic safety and effectiveness. One of the important requirements for probiotics to be beneficial is its ability (chemically or physically) to inhibit pathogenic microbes and promote growth of beneficial host microbiota (Hu et al., 2017). There is a rapid increase in new microbial strains claimed with probiotic properties, but each strain must separately and in combination be assessed for safety and efficacy, and it should not take for consideration with commonly established probiotic strains (Shanahan, 2012). How does a host recognize and distinguish pathogenic microorganisms and probiotics? Many are of the opinion that probiotics are familiar to human system, as fermented food have been consumed for a long time, but what about new probiotic strains? Another important issue arises with variable response of probiotics on different age groups such as pregnant woman and infants, and hence labeling probiotics as function of age groups should be made so that the consumer will be aware of this.

In this chapter, a relevant discussion is made regarding adverse effects of probiotic strains already found in probiotic-containing products and its impacts on different users (infant, pregnant, immunocompromised). Some burgeoning issues related to probiotics such as antibiotic resistance and gene transfer, synthesis of harmful metabolites, and genetically modified probiotics are highlighted. Finally, regulatory systems to ensure probiotics quality is described.

30.1.1 Risk of probiotic-originated infections

Safety studies of probiotics primarily based on information obtained from limited strains of *Lactobacilli* and *Bifidobacteria*, and reports of safety studies with other probiotic microbial strains (*Lactobacillus casei*, *S. cerevisiae*, *S. boulardii*) were less reported. Moreover, these are already available for consumers (Singh et al., 2019; Zielińska et al., 2018). Commonly reported adverse effects of probiotic strains are discussed below.

30.1.1.1 Adverse effects due to lactic acid bacteria

Lactobacillus belongs to Gram-positive, microaerophilic, nonspore-forming bacteria and are important components of human and animal digestive microflora. *Lactobacillus* is the most studied group of probiotic microbes with many useful properties ranging from assistance in food digestion, absorption to treatment of diarrhea, and cancer (Turpin et al., 2010). There is an increase in reports showing *Lactobacillus* infection in patient with dysfunctional gut barrier, organ failure, and weak immunity (Cuello-Garcia et al., 2015; Pace et al., 2020; Zucko et al., 2020). *Lactobacillus* is responsible for dental caries, bacterial endocarditis, neonatal sepsis, genital infections, and endometritis along with bacteremia (Salminen et al., 2004).

Commercial formulation of *L. rhamnosus* prescribed to prevent antibiotic-associated diarrhea and gastroenteritis (Salminen et al., 2004). A female patient is given antimicrobial therapy along with probiotic preparation containing *L. rhamnosus* before treatment of inflammatory perforation of valvular cusp. After valve implantation, the patient reported a high fever with other systemic inflammatory response syndrome (SIRS) symptoms.

L. rhamnosus-associated bacteremia is linked with immunosuppression, surgery, and antibiotic therapy (1996). A male infant with short gut syndrome was supplemented with *Lactobacillus* GG. After 4 weeks, the patient experience diarrhea along with fever. Subsequent blood culturing showed the presence of *Lactobacillus* that was given externally as probiotics (2004). Similar results were reported for infants with gastroschisis. Although antibiotic therapy (ceftriaxone and ampicillin) gets rid of *Lactobacillus bacteremia*, continuous monitoring and antiinflammatory drugs are needed when probiotics are used during treatment of short gut syndrome and gastroschisis to prevent probiotic-originated sepsis. Intestinal inflammation promoted migration/translocation of probiotics across intestinal mucosa; it also increases membrane permeability and lowers the attachment to intestine, leading to sepsis (Land et al., 2005). Liver abscess along with pleural empyema were observed in a female patient (74 years old) with type II diabetes mellitus. The patient had taken around 1.5 L/d dairy product containing *L. rhamnosus* GG for 4 months before onset. The liver pus sample was analyzed by pulsed-field gel electrophoresis (PFGE) and was positive for *L. rhamnosus* (Land et al., 2005). The above reports clearly reveal a another side of probiotics and should not discourage using probiotics, but serve as an early warning to identify risks for susceptible patients. In some reports, *Lactobacillus* isolated from a patient was not distinguishable from the probiotic strain, making molecular characterization an indispensable tool for strain identification (Abe et al., 2010).

30.1.2 Adverse effects due to *Bifidobacter*

Bifidobacterium is a genus of Gram-positive, anaerobic, and nonmotile bacteria. Similar to *Lactobacillus*, *Bifidobacterium* species are abundant occupants of the gastrointestinal tract. *Bifidobacterium breve*, *Bifidobacterium lactis*, *B. infantis* are some of the probiotic strains of *Bifidobacterium* with multiple health benefits ranging from colorectal cancer and enterocolitis inflammatory bowel disease to competitive elimination of pathogens (Abdollahi et al., 2016; O'Callaghan & van Sinderen, 2016). *Bifidobacterium* strains were isolated from breast milk directing its use towards infant formulas, but for most of commercial strains *Bifidobacterium* were not isolated from natural sources (Gueimonde et al., 2007).

A fetus was diagnosed with omphalocele and after birth (4 hours) an operation for omphalocele was performed followed by administration of antibiotics and *B. breve* BBG-01. After 12 days C-reactive protein and white blood cell count were found to increase and on day 14 (blood culture made on day 10) blood culture showed presence of *Bifidobacterium*. Immediately, therapy was stopped and antibiotics were changed accordingly. The patient recovered without any complications due to *Bifidobacterium* septicemia; however, strain-specific studies using specific primers and monoclonal antibodies identifies the same *Bifidobacterium* given as probiotics (Ohishi et al., 2010). Present study cites the need for risk assessment of *Bifidobacterium* under different physiological conditions.

Incidence of anaerobic meningitis are very low and most of the time the pathogens are *Bacteroides fragilis* and *Fusobacterium necrophorum*, but a few reports proved *B. breve* as causative agent of meningitis in neonates and infants. The strain showed resistant to penicillin and cephalosporins. The probable mechanism of invasion is from mucosa of the intestine to meninges via blood (Nakazawa et al., 1996). *Bifidobacterium animalis* subsp. *lactis* (one of the industrially used *Bifidobacterium* strain) reported presence of tetracycline resistance genes and some other commensal bifidobacteria strains found to be responsible for dental and pulmonary infections (Meile et al., 2008). Charteris et al. (1998) investigated antimicrobial susceptibility of *Bifidobacterium* isolates having probiotic potential from the gastrointestinal tract of human. Out of total isolate, many were resistant to different antibiotics (cefoxitin, aztreonam, vancomycin, streptomycin, fusidic acid, metronidazole, colistin sulfate) and they were susceptible to the six penicillins studied: cephalothin, cefuroxime, cefaclor, ceftizoxime, cefotaxime, bacitracin (Charteris et al., 1998).

30.1.3 Adverse effects due to *Saccharomyces boulardii*

Most of the probiotics are of bacterial origin but one strain of yeast, *S. boulardii* also emerged as promising probiotics. Henri Boulard during 1920 observed that some people were prevented from cholera infection due to drinking a special tea. The tea was prepared using the external skin of lychee and mangosteen fruits. He successfully isolated the active agent "yeast" responsible for cholera protection and named as *S. boulardii* (McFarland, 2014). The same strain was patented and used around the world as a probiotic. *S. boulardii* can be referred against antibiotic-associated diarrhea, as it is naturally resistant to antibiotics, and also against *Clostridium difficile* infection (Elmer et al., 1999). Multiple research reports highlighted efficacy of *S. boulardii* in different forms of diarrhea (Traveler's diarrhea, acute diarrhea in children, tube feeding-associated diarrhea) and inflammatory bowel diseases (Dinleyici et al., 2014).

Although use of *S. boulardii* as a probiotic is common in the entire world and it is generally regarded as safe, a few adverse reports are reported regarding the therapeutic administration of this yeast. Fungemia was commonly reported as adverse effects of *S. boulardii* to different age groups during postsurgery and chronic disorders apart from vaginitis and endocarditis (Hennequin et al., 2000). Sometime *S. boulardii* is transferred from patient receiving this probiotic to another patient admitted in close vicinity in intensive care units (ICUs). Migration of *S. boulardii* from defective gut into the blood and infected catheter are the most frequent reasons for yeast fungemia (Kralovicova et al., 1997). A diabetic patient (48 years old) with artery disease and necrosis in both feet was operated with femoropopliteal by-passes. During subsequent antibiotic therapy, patient developed diarrhea (*C. difficile*) and the same was treated with metronidazole and *S. boulardii*. Unfortunately, 8 days after bypass, patient develop sepsis due to *S. boulardii* and died later because of multiple organ failure (Lestin et al., 2003).

Muñoz et al. (2005) proved that *S. boulardii* was fatal to three immunosuppressed or critically ill patients (Muñoz et al., 2005). These patients had different medical status such as having undergone cardiac surgery, rheumatoid arthritis, and coronary artery bypass grafting that are all under broad spectral antibiotics to prevent different postoperative infections. *C. difficile*-associated diarrhea in these patients were treated with Ultralevura (commercial lyophilized *S. boulardii* culture). But after probiotics treatment, blood culture revealed fungemia due to *S. boulardii*, and all three patients died due to central nervous system stroke and bacteremia.

30.1.4 Use of probiotics in cancer patients

Cancer is group of diseases with genetic (oncogenes) and lifestyle (smoking, diet, and workplace) origins. During development of cancer, some body cells undergo uncontrolled proliferation without death leading to formation of a cell mass (tumor). Tumors may be restricted to one location (benign tumors) or can spread to nearby tissues via blood or lymph system (malignant tumors). There are multiple types of cancer depending on the organ or tissue where cancer arises, for example, brain cancer originates in the brain, blood cancer in blood, etc. Chemotherapy and radiotherapy are common treatments, having some side effects that lead to a weak immunity system, hair loss, etc. (National Cancer Institute, 2021). Chemotherapy-induced diarrhea is most common among cancer patients as these anticancer drugs disturb normal gut microflora. Such diarrhea reduces patient tolerance to chemo and radiotherapy and, hence, probiotics are used to prevent it (Redman et al., 2014). There are contradictory reports regarding use of probiotics during cancer treatment; some are suggesting beneficial effects while others find adverse effects of probiotic use in cancer. There is need for further research regarding interaction of probiotics with cancer patients and anticancer drugs. A diversity of studies performed on different age group cancer patients, having distinct types of cancer, suggest that general use of probiotics (*Lactobacillus*, *Bifidobacterium*, and *Saccharomyces*) have several adverse effects including alternation of chemotherapy agent, sepsis, allergy, and genotoxicity. Many times, due to low cost, easy administration, and the wide publicity of safety, probiotics were given to cancer patient without proper risk assessment (Ciernikova et al., 2017).

An 8-month-old infant was diagnosed with acute myeloid leukemia. Apart from chemotherapy, he was receiving probiotic *S. boulardii* capsules to prevent diarrhea. One day after completion of chemotherapy, a high fever was reported and blood culture analysis revealed the presence of *S. boulardii*. Although the infant recovered from infection after antifungal drugs, it raises safety issues of probiotic used (Cesaro et al., 2000). A patient with cell lymphoma develops endocarditis after administration of a probiotic *L. paracasei* by oral route. Another male with mantle cell lymphoma develops sepsis because of *L. acidophilus* (Di Cerbo et al., 2016). A case study report by Robin et al. (2010), was revealed a 10-year-old boy with acute lymphoblastic leukemia had not responded to treatment and, received cord blood transplant. Immunosuppressant antibiotics and steroids were given to prevent graft rejection. After few days, the patient developed a fever and sepsis. Subsequent blood cultures were positive for *L. acidophilus* and *L. rhamnosus*. Interestingly, no probiotics were used during the entire treatment. As a result, these organisms may enter from dairy products and are able to persist and emerge with a decrease in the patient's health status (Robin et al., 2010).

30.1.5 Use of probiotics in pregnant woman and infants

Diet plays a very important role during pregnancy. Recent reports suggested an increase in the occurrence of diabetes (gestational diabetes mellitus) and obesity among pregnant woman, leading to some deleterious effects such as hypertension, antenatal and intrapartum intervention, cesarean, infection, etc. (Linne, 2004; Rogozińska et al., 2015). Obesity was linked with alteration of the gut microbiota (Million et al., 2012). Contradiction is observed in literature as some claims link probiotics and obesity while others suggest probiotic use for lean body mass (Lahtinen et al., 2012; Shanahan, 2012). Host-specific (human and animal) variation was observed during meta-analysis of *Lactobacillus* and weight change (Million et al., 2012). Due to general assumptions of safety, probiotics are blindly given to infants and pregnant women. Sufficient reports suggested beneficial health effects of probiotics for pregnant woman and infant health, but an assessment of adverse effects on these populations are equally important, however, it is given less attention (Mantaring et al., 2018). A report pointed out a connection of consuming probiotic food with intrauterine growth restriction, leading to preterm delivery and high amounts of amniotic fluid in the amniotic sac (Quinlivan et al., 2011). In another study, 233 pregnant women were divided into three groups. The first group receive nutritional supplements, the second group receive nutritional supplements along with mixture of probiotics *L. rhamnosus*, and *B. lactis* and last group was devoid of both. The frequency of vomiting and nausea was reported to be higher in group two who received supplements and probiotics (Mantaring et al., 2018).

Initially in newborns, microflora is not well developed; however, the gut is immediately colonized by external microorganisms dominated by *E. coli* and *Enterococcus*. Diarrhea is a major health complication in infants. Species of *Lactobacillus* and *Bifidobacterium* are mostly recommended for infant diarrhea. However, ingestion of such live bacteria may be risky. Some reports found that use of probiotics in infants leads to sepsis, meningitis, nosocomial infections, and gastroschisis (Valenzuela-Grijalva et al., 2017). Sanders et al. (2010) suggested to analyze infant risk status before administering probiotic therapy to control diarrhea by considering weight, prematurity level, birth defect, hematological profile, inflammation, and an impaired mucosal barrier (Sanders et al., 2010). A detailed review by Sotoudegan et al. (2019) tabulated common to severe adverse effects in infants due to probiotics administration such as constipation, rash, chest pain, abdominal bloating, thirst, Kawasaki disease, epitasis, fungemia, and rhinitis (Sotoudegan et al., 2019).

30.1.6 Use of probiotics in immunocompromised patients and immunomodulation

Bacterial translocation and dysbiosis events are rare in healthy individuals; as such, bacteria are trapped by lymph nodes that produce different immune cells. This regular mechanism could be weakened in ill and immunocompromised individuals (Schlegel et al., 1998).

Individuals undergoing organ transplantation and receiving immunosuppressive drugs, HIV infected, ICU patients, heart defects, and cachectic are examples of critically ill and immunocompromised patients who have a higher risk of probiotic-originated infection as compared with healthy individuals (Zielińska et al., 2018). Bone marrow transplantation, liver cirrhosis, and other major surgeries increase gut permeability due to rapid inflammatory responses, resulting in dysbiosis with translocation. Administration of probiotics may increase translocation in such critically ill and immunocompromised patients and may give rise to septicemia (Leber et al., 2012). The situation may be further worsened if the probiotic strain has antibiotic resistance genes and virulent factors in its genome.

Inflammation in the pancreas is termed as pancreatitis. Besselink et al. (2008) revealed lethal effects of probiotics used during pancreatitis. Pancreatitis patients were divided into two groups, one group (144 patients) received freeze-dried, viable probiotic bacteria: *L. acidophilus*, *L. casei*, *L. salivarius*, *Lactococcus lactis*, *B. bifidum* and *B. lactis* and another group (144) received placebo. Infections occurred in 30% patient receiving probiotics and 16 % of them have died compared with only 6% deaths in placebo patients. Nine probiotic-receiving group patients also developed bowel ischemia while it did not occur in the placebo group. Based on these observations, the author not recommend prophylactic use of probiotics during treatment of pancreatitis (Besselink et al., 2008). A 53-year-old patient's bone marrow culture was found positive for *L. casei*. The patient has a history of rheumatic fever and also had a dental extraction. It was revealed that patient's daily diet consisted of yogurt, although there was no direct relation between yogurt and infection. But, maybe due to rheumatic fever there is an impaired resistance leading to the spread of *L. casei* (Zé-Zé et al., 2004).

The aging population (more than 65 years or older) treated with antibiotic therapy along with multistrain probiotic preparation (*Lactobacilli* and *Bifidobacteria*). It was observed that probiotics have no beneficial effect against antibiotic-associated diarrhea and *C. difficile* infection (Allen et al., 2013).

Effects of probiotics on the immune system is a result of multiple factors including the host's genetic makeup, abiotic factors, and probiotic signals leading to the generation of nonspecific immune responses. Various probiotics such as lactic acid bacteria and others are shown to modulate (upregulate or downregulate) immunological responses (Vaarala, 2003).

Production of type 1 cytokines (interferon γ, interleukin 6) increased by commonly used probiotics strains. There is indirect relationship between immunological alteration and clinical findings. The excessive activation of immune responses due to probiotics is possibly correlated with inflammation and autoimmune diseases (rheumatoid arthritis), hepatobiliary diseases, and cardioangilitis (Daliri & Lee, 2015; Singh et al., 2019). Dendritic cells play an important role in standardization of host immune responses; *L. rhamnosus*-stimulated dendritic cells produced low levels of chemokines and cytokines (Veckman et al., 2004). There is a need for a detailed investigation on contact between probiotics and host cells for immune response generation and it needs to connect with clinical findings for recommending further safety, efficacy, and approval.

30.1.7 Antibiotic resistance and horizontal gene transfer in probiotics

The lateral migration of mobile genetic elements between different organisms is a natural phenomenon called horizontal gene transfer (HGT). HGT is mediated by diverse mechanisms such as conjugation, transformation, and gene transfer agents. The gastrointestinal tract is a reservoir of microbial consortium with a huge number of microbes present in close proximity. As the gastrointestinal tract provides a favorable environment for HGT, and probiotics majorly reside in the gut, so the question arises about whether virulent, antibiotic-resistant genetic elements are transferred to and from probiotics and gut microbiome (Lerner et al., 2019). HGT is reported in several probiotics strains including *L. paracasei*,

L. rhamnosus, L. reuteri, L. gasseri, and *L. plantarum*, and therefore they may affect genetic stability and evolutionary conserved processes between microbiome and human leading to unbalancing human health (Ramakrishnan, 2018).

Beneficial and native bacteria harboring resistant genes are not pathogens, but may play part in supplying resistant to pathogenic and opportunistic pathogens. Microbial resistance to antibiotics is a serious issue leading to longer stays in the hospital, increase in morbidity, and mortality. Lactic acid bacteria contain plasmids encompassing genes convening resistance to a range of narrow- and broad-spectrum antibiotics such as chloramphenicol, erythromycin, tetracycline, macrolide, streptogramin, and streptomycin (Doron & Snydman, 2015).

Commercial strains of probiotics (*L. acidophilus*) acquired the vancomycin resistance gene (vanA) from *Enterococci* (Mater et al., 2008). Interestingly, this gene transfer is also observed in the gut of mice without antibiotic pressure at relatively high frequency. The author concluded that such incidence might happen in the human gut especially in immunocompromised patients or patients under antibiotic therapy. A plasmid (PAMβ1) encoding resistance to macrolides, lincosamides, and streptogramins occurred in *Enterococcus faecalis* and can transfer to bacteria belonging to *Lactobacillus, Bacillus, Staphylococcus*, and *Clostridium* (Sharma et al., 2014). A detailed study on vancomycin resistance in the *Lactobacillus* strain revealed that the antibiotic binds with D-alanine/D-alanine terminus present on the peptidoglycan of the cell wall and prevents polymerization of the peptidoglycan precursor. However, replacement of D-alanine with D-lactate prevents vancomycin binding and, hence, the bacteria generate a resistance to vancomycin (Gueimonde et al., 2013). In another study, the *Bifidobacterium* strain reflects a resistance to muciprocin (antibiotic) with the help of enzyme isoleucyl-tRNA synthetase which neutralizes the inhibitory effects of muciprocin (Serafini et al., 2011).

Like other organisms, probiotic microbes are also susceptible to genomic rearrangements due to the shift from their natural habitat (such as aquatic) to a new one (human gut). Effects of such genomic changes due to mutations, HGT, long-term preservation and storage need to be studied for its health promoting effects and safety. Lactic acid bacteria are small genome size (1.7–3.3 Mbp) with a variety of genes suggesting that they are highly adaptive in nature via both in gene loss and acquisition (Van Reenen & Dicks, 2011). The expert panel of WHO and FAO recommended a detailed study related to antibiotic resistance in *Lactobacilli* and *Bifidobacteria* used in powdered milk formulations containing probiotics (FAO/WHO, 2002). The panel also insisted that probiotic bacteria should not contain resistance encoding genes (Hill et al., 2014; Singh et al., 2019).

In summary, probiotics conserved resistant genes, plasmid, and transferable genetic material that can be transferred to other microbes, leading to an increase in resistance problems. Sequencing an entire genome of candidate probiotic strain may yield valuable information about antibiotic resistance, its control, and prevention for safe use of probiotics, particularly when using probiotics and antibiotics at same time.

30.1.8 Harmful metabolic activities of probiotics and production of host deleterious metabolites

As probiotics are live microbes, their metabolic activities in different therapeutic and food products during storage, as well as in the gut after probiotic consumption, is another vital safety aspect (Zielińska et al., 2018). Ideally, probiotics shouldn't synthesize harmful compounds from its metabolism; enzymes helping in colonization and invasion should also be absent, particularly for new strains (Gueimonde et al., 2004). As such, metabolic changes can cause obesity, diabetes, and other metabolic diseases (Kothari et al., 2019).

D-lactic acidosis is the most prevalent metabolic disease in patients with short bowel syndrome. In D-lactic acidosis, the balance between production and use of lactic acid is disturbed. A few cases reported the association of *Lactobacillus* spp. with D-lactic acid encephalopathy and it should be sidestepped in short bowel syndrome (Munakata et al., 2010). Colonization of high numbers of bacteria along with probiotic consumption in short bowel syndrome led to bacterial overgrowth. The probiotics then convert the host's primary bile salt to secondary bile acids, having carcinogenic potential or may behave as carcinogenesis promoters (Ridlon et al., 2014).

The process of bile salt deconjugation was reported for lowering cholesterol levels. However, excessive deconjugation resulted in reduced normal gut flora leading to diarrhea and mucosal inflammation (Althubiani et al., 2019; Singh et al., 2019).

Azoreductase and nitroreductase activity have been found among *Lactobacilli* and *Bifidobacteria*. Such enzymatic activity can cause toxic effects like the activation of carcinogens (O'Brien et al., 1999).

Biogenic amines such as histamine, tryptamine, tyramine, cadaverine, and putrescine are produced due to routine metabolic activity from their parent amino acids. They have several biological activities such as a hormonal precursor and food aroma. *Lactobacillus* and *Lactococcus* contain the enzyme amino acid decarboxylases which transforms amino acids to amines, leading to food toxicity (Stadnik & Dolatowski, 2012). Biogenic amines are also a neurotransmitter.

They can alter blood flow, initiate headaches, and cause allergic reactions (Martin & Vij, 2016). Biogenic amines are one of the factors responsible for food poisoning; lactic acid bacteria used in food products produces and releases biological amines into food (Kothari et al., 2019).

In an interesting study, Kuley et al. (2012) observed that *L. plantarum* (FI8595), *L. lactis* subsp. *cremoris* MG 1363) stimulate cadaverin (toxic biological amine) production in food borne pathogens (*E. faecalis, Staphylococcus aureus, and Listeria monocytogenes*) in fermented food products. Therefore there is need to use safe starter with negative amine activity (Kuley et al., 2012).

Mucin is a glycoprotein and a major component of the mucosal surface of gut; its primary function is protecting epithelial cells of the gut from acids and proteolytic enzymes. Hence, removal of mucin will facilitate entry of bacteria into different tissues, leading to translocation and septicemia (Ruseler-van Embden et al., 1989). Mucin degradation is recommended as a marker for safety of probiotic strains. No mucin degradation activity was found among three probiotic bifidobacteria strains; *Bifidobacterium longum* BB536, *B. breve* M-16V, and *B. infantis* M-63 (Abe et al., 2010). The author performed an *in vitro* study using mucin as the sole carbon source, SDS-PAGA, and degraded mucin residue analysis, but the *in vivo* study might have some different observations. In the same study, no translocation of *B. longum* BB536 was observed after oral administration in mice at high doses with no disturbance in the mucosal layer.

Probiotics species such as *L. rhamnosus* and *L. paracasei* subsp. *paracasei* associated with endocarditis secrete glycosidases and arylamidase which can breakdown human glycoproteins and can break gut barrier integrity (Oakey et al., 1995).

Neu et al. (2014) proposed marine bacterial isolates to be used as fish probiotics (Neu et al., 2014). They studied the toxicity of isolated microbes on two nontarget eukaryotic organisms, namely *Artemia* spp. and *Caenorhabditis elegans*. Among the different marine isolates (*Arthrobacter davidanieli* WX-11, *Pseudoalteromonas luteoviolacea* S4060, *Pseudoalteromonas piscicida* S2049, *Pseudoalteromonas rubra* S2471, *Photobacterium halotolerans* S2753, and *Vibrio coralliilyticus* S2052) under study, *P. luteoviolacea* produced pentabromopseudilin which was toxic to *Artemia* spp. and *C. elegans*. Although such findings have not yet been reported in mammals, the study shows the probability of probiotics to produce harmful secondary metabolites that may harm the host.

Hemolysis is the rupturing of erythrocytes, thereby liberating their content into the surrounding fluid. It is the unwanted physiological event in which β-hemolysis involve complete lysis by bacteria while α-hemolysis involve oxidation of hemoglobin to methemoglobin. *L. rhamnosus* strains isolated from clinical and food samples were shown positive α hemolysis in vitro while in recent studies, β-hemolysis has been reported in *L. paracasei* subsp. *paracasei* (Baumgartner et al., 1998; Pradhan et al., 2020). Therefore apart from analyzing production of harmful metabolites, new probiotic strains need to be evaluated for hemolytic potential to avoid harmful effects after consumption or administration of probiotics.

30.1.9 Ways of enhancing probiotics safety and some regulatory guidelines

Assessment of probiotics safety is a difficult task because there are considerable variations among different countries regarding safety assessment and regulatory guidelines for probiotic products (Gupta et al., 2021; Zucko et al., 2020). There are several in vitro and in vivo tests that should be followed for analyzing safety of the probiotic strain before introducing it into the consumer market. Primary importance should be given on complete identification of the strain using biochemical and genetic identification studies (16S rRNA sequencing, nucleic acid hybridization), followed by antibiotic resistance and gene transfer potential, resistance to gastric juice, and bile acid tolerance. Ample emphasis should also be given on any harmful metabolic activities and hemolytic potential (Lara-Villoslada et al., 2010). Followed by in vitro studies, animal models should be used to prove probiotic effectiveness in comparison with in vitro and before conducting human trials (FAO/WHO, 2002). Human trials need to be performed at different locations within the contexts of safety, physiology, and anatomy using enough volunteers of different age groups (healthy and diseased). The study is required to be robust, and the use of controlled placebo, double blind, and randomized control trial is a must.

Continual postmarket epidemiological vigilance for harmful incidences should continue to further improve the safety and quality of probiotics. Behavior of probiotics in critically ill and immunocompromised animal models needs to be analyzed in an unbiased fashion.

There are already many questions regarding the safety of the probiotic strain itself, but the safety issue of probiotic products is further magnified due to the presence of microbial contaminants, allergens, and excipients in over-the-counter probiotics formulations (Shanahan, 2012).

Microbiological analysis of several retail probiotic products were found to contain microorganisms that are not labeled on product. Analysis of ten commercially sold probiotic products in Europe were made to check the presence of genus and species provided on the label (Coeuret et al., 2004). Polymerase chain reactions and PFGE techniques were adopted for probiotic identification. Out of the ten total samples, five products did not match the number of probiotic bacteria, and three products had different species of *Lactobacilli* than was claimed on the label. Moreover, four products contained the same strain, but labeled differently. This present study demonstrated the requirement of stringent quality control and good manufacturing practices to ensure probiotic quality and consumer safety. Apart from detail (correct) labeling of probiotic strains and its number on the label, the label should also inform storage conditions, number of probiotic bacteria, and end of shelf life. The product should note if it is free from allergens or not, so that an allergic individual will be assured about offending allergens or even excipients having allergenic properties (Sanders et al., 2010). In many commercial probiotic products, the strain is encapsulated with calcium alginate beads. Do such chemicals lead to allergenic reactions in the host? (Kothari et al., 2019). Clear labeling of probiotic products on strain, safety, purity, and allergens is a basic consumer right.

Toscano et al. (2017) prepared a list of ten golden rules for correct use of probiotics; some of them are as follows. Probiotic strains must able to colonize in the gut and positively interact with gut microbiota. They need to be resistant to gastrointestinal environment. Further, probiotics that exhibiting health claims and disease prevention should be analyzed, regulated, and marketed as drugs rather dietary supplements (Toscano et al., 2017).

Except improvement in lactose maldigestion, the European Food Safety Authority (EFSA) denied all health benefits proposed for probiotics due to lack of justifiable evidence. On the other hand, the US Food and Drug Administration set minimum regulations for probiotic product may be due to market demands (Zucko et al., 2020). EFSA developed very strict protocols for microbe-based food products for human use. Qualified presumption of safety and Biosafety Evaluation of Probiotic Lactic Acid Bacteria for Human Consumption (PROSAFE) are examples of EFSA initiative for increasing efficacy and safety of probiotics. Some important guideline of PROSAFE are as follows: (1) need of genetic strain level characterization of lactic acid bacteria and its deposition in a culture collection center; (2) avoid *Enterococcus* and *Lactobacillus* probiotics having virulence genes; and (3) a gut colonization study and use of rat for endocarditis (Vankerckhoven et al., 2008).

The Canadian food and health safety authority is following FAO/WHO guidelines with requirements of strain-specific health benefits and harmful effects, according to claims made in safety dossier (Sanders et al., 2010). The food safety evaluation committee of Norway conducted studies on safety of *L. rhamnosus* GG in infants and children (4–36 months), and concluded that the evidence is not enough for the ability of this species to prevent disease and its long-term safety is also unknown. This study created concern on the probiotic species that is already present in multiple commercial products (http://www.vkm) (Risk Assessment on Use of *Lactobacillus Rhamnosus* (LGG) as an Ingredient in Infant Formula and Baby Foods (II), 2007). In India, the Indian Council of Medical Research in collaboration with the Department of Biotechnology formulated guidelines for the regulation of probiotic products in the country, which are very similar to multinational guidelines emphasizing strain identification, in vivo–in vitro studies, labeling, etc. (Ganguly et al., 2011). However, development of strict regulatory guidelines by the government on probiotics are negatively taken by industries that are expressing concern it will slowdown development of healthy functional foods (Table 30.1).

30.1.10 Adverse effects of probiotics on animals

Based on common agreements regarded as generally safe (without enough safety studies), probiotics are now globally consumed by the human population. Moving ahead, probiotics also enter into animal food, feed, and aquaculture industry with the purpose of overall growth and healthy improvements of economically important animals and aquatic organisms (Hai, 2015; Markowiak & Ślizewska, 2018). Ideally, the safety requirements for animal probiotics should be higher than probiotics used for human consumption, because from the animals, probiotics may enter into the food chain and eventually inside the human body. The Scientific Committee on Animal Nutrition of the EU made some recommendations on the safety of probiotics in animals (Gueimonde et al., 2004). The pigs were given *B. animalis* subsp. *lactis* Bb-12 starting from birth; this probiotic was found to remain in the gut without any detectable health effects. However, the next generation of the same pigs showed above normal levels of innate immunity markers (Solano-Aguilar et al., 2008). Basically, there is a significant difference in the microbiome of animals and human, but nevertheless it will yield valuable information due to multiple similarities with humans. Three strains of potentially probiotic bacteria (*L. rhamnosus* HN001, *L. acidophilus* HN017 and *B. lactis* HN019) were given to mice. The LD_{50} value of the *Lactobacilli* strain was found to be more than 50 g/kg/d (10^{11} cfu/mouse/d) which could be many times lower than the normal

TABLE 30.1 Recommendations for evaluating safety aspects of probiotics.

Factors related to safety for the intended use of probiotics in foods and drugs through safety assessment guidelines design by different regulatory agencies	*Identification of the exact probiotic strain*: Phenotypic tests, biochemical screening, genetic analysis (16S sequencing, nucleic acid hybridization)
	Translocation and gene transfer: Study of anatomy, physiology and hematological study of animal model genetic expression studies (proteomics, functional genomics)
	Antibiotic susceptibility/resistance: MIC values, probiotic performance in presence and absence of antibiotics, resistance profiling
	Metabolic activities: Production of amines, D-lactic acid; hemolytic activity, mucinolytic activity, deconjugation of bile acids, obesity
	Immunological activities: Immunomodulation and immunosuppression
	Sufficient types of in vivo and in vitro studies (efficacy and toxicological): Mice, rat, pigs, fishes, cattle, etc.; human trials on all types of consumers (infant, pregnant, immune compromised, etc.)
	Labeling: Name of strain(s), number, shelf life, excipients, specific instruction regarding allergenic reactions and under risk consumers
	Viability and sufficient number during production, storage and avoidance of contaminating bacteria: Good manufacturing practices
	New strain, genetically modified organism probiotics: All above and safety of recombinant products

MIC, Minimum inhibitory concentration.

amount of probiotics consumed by humans. Apart from this, no translocation was observed in blood and tissue samples (mesenteric lymph nodes, liver and spleen) of mice (Zhou et al., 2000). Different animals such as mice, ducks, and chickens gained abnormal weight after consumption of *L. fermentum* and *L. ingluviei*, although such studies have not been performed in humans. While another species, *L. plantarum*, causes weight loss in animals (Million et al., 2012). This report is an example of the need of strain and host dependent studied on multiple safety aspects of probiotics.

30.1.11 Safety of genetically engineered probiotics

Considerable debate is going on regarding genetically modified organisms (GMO) and products derived from them. Similar issues may arise by the use of genetic modifications tools to improve useful properties in probiotic bacteria. Interleukin-10 (IL-10) suppresses bowel inflammation, but is unstable in the gut and needed to be given in coated form. Lactococcus has been genetically modified to produce IL-10, but if such GMO is consumed by healthy subjects, it may altered their immune functions (Steidler et al., 2003), because the safety issue is not only related with GMO probiotic strain, but also recombinant products produced by them (Shanahan, 2012). In another study, *Bacteroides ovatus* (anaerobic commensal) was modified to synthesize the keratinocyte growth factor under the specific presence of dietary xylene, thereby ensuring biosafety and containment (Hamady et al., 2010).

30.1.12 Combination of probiotics and plant extracts for enhancing probiotics performance

Due to restrictions on the use of antibiotics as growth promoters, especially in animal feed, a combination of probiotics along with plant biologically active compounds is an emerging research area (Arowolo & He, 2018). Probiotics and plant extract synergistically stabilize rumen environment, enhance fermentation, and modulate immune response, it also prolongs the shelf life of a product as compared to either probiotics or plant extract (Valenzuela-Grijalva et al., 2017). An in vitro study on Caco-2 cells treated with combination of probiotic *L. reuteri* and *L. acidophilus* strains and herbal extracts of *Chamomilla recutita* was done. The above combination maintained intestinal integrity during inflammatory bowel diseases (Cocetta et al., 2019). In another study, symbiotic formulation of lactic acid bacteria and *Curcuma longa* rhizome extract strongly inhibit *Cutibacterium acnes* [causative agent of acne (an inflammatory skin disease)]. This observation leads authors to suggest use of this combination in cosmetics or as medicine (Kim et al., 2020). Probiotics restrict growth of pathogens while plant essential oils kill them and, hence, can be a new approach of treatment because of their complementary action against pathogens (Shipradeep et al., 2012). Dietary supplements containing grape seed extract, tea polyphenols, vitamin C, and *L. plantarum* CCFM8661 effectively relieve lead toxicity in blood by stimulating superoxide dismutase; catalase activities along with recovery of glutathione, zinc protoporphyrin, and malondialdehyde levels (Zhai et al., 2018). Researchers are working on the impact of phytochemicals on gene expression of probiotic strains such as *Lactobacilli* and *Bifidobacteria* to improve food safety and human health (Gyawali & Ibrahim, 2012). However, regulations of such combinations with respect to side effect and quality control is far away from being established (Zhai et al., 2018).

30.2 Conclusions

Due to the diversity of probiotic consumers (infant to elder, healthy to diseases, immunocompromised, pregnant woman) it is tedious to assess safety and adverse effects of probiotics. Since microbiota may differ in different individuals and their health status, application specific probiotics may be a more promising approach. Most of the time, commercial probiotic research intended for technological potential gives less importance to specific applications as well as a detailed study of probable adverse effects on intended users. Before introduction of novel probiotic strains or combination of more than one known probiotics strains in the consumer market, it should be tested for its metabolic activity, hemolytic activity, and toxin production as well as resistance to antibiotics. Equal importance should be given on the potential for sepsis and translocation, and gene transfer potential. Apart from these details, unbiased study is required for assessing safety of probiotics in infants, the immunocompromised, and recently operated individuals. International harmonium is also a need to regulate the highly unregulated probiotic market. Moreover, continuous long-term epidemiological surveillance needs to be undertaken for incidents of adverse effects of the postmarket introduced probiotics. The ultimate intention is not to declare probiotics as harmful microbes but to further increase its safety and efficacy.

Acknowledgments

Authors are thankful to the Uka Tarsadia University and Kavayitri Bahinabai Chaudhari North Maharashtra University for providing necessary facilities.

Declaration of competing interest

All authors of this chapter declare no conflicts of interest.

References

Abdollahi, M., Abdolghaffari, A. H., Gooshe, M., & Ghasemi-Niri, F. (2016). Safety of probiotic bacteria. In R. R. Watson, & V. R. Reedy (Eds.), *Probiotics, prebiotics and synbiotics. Bioactive foods in health promotion* (Vol. 1, pp. 227–243). Elsevier.

Abe, F., Muto, M., Yaeshima, T., Iwatsuki, K., Aihara, H., Ohashi, Y., & Fujisawa, T. (2010). Safety evaluation of probiotic bifidobacteria by analysis of mucin degradation activity and translocation ability. *Anaerobe*, *16*(2), 131–136. Available from https://doi.org/10.1016/j.anaerobe.2009.07.006.

Allen, S. J., Wareham, K., Wang, D., Bradley, C., Hutchings, H., Harris, W., Dhar, A., Brown, H., Foden, A., Gravenor, M. B., & Mack, D. (2013). Lactobacilli and bifidobacteria in the prevention of antibiotic-associated diarrhoea and *Clostridium difficile* diarrhoea in older inpatients (PLACIDE): A randomised, double-blind, placebo-controlled, multicentre trial. *Lancet*, *382*(9900), 1249–1257. Available from https://doi.org/10.1016/S0140-6736(13)61218-0.

Althubiani, A. S., Al-Ghamdi, S. B., Qais, F. A., & Khan, M. S. (2019). Plant-derived prebiotics and its health benefits. In M. J. A. Khan, I. Ahmad, & D. Chattppadhyay (Eds.), *New look to phytomedicine* (pp. 63–68). Academic Press.

Arowolo, M. A., & He, J. (2018). Use of probiotics and botanical extracts to improve ruminant production in the tropics: A review. *Animal Nutrition*, *4*(3), 241–249. Available from https://doi.org/10.1016/j.aninu.2018.04.010.

Baumgartner, A., Kueffer, M., Simmen, A., & Grand, M. (1998). Relatedness of *Lactobacillus rhamnosus* strains isolated from clinical specimens and such from food-stuffs, humans and technology. *LWT—Food Science and Technology*, *31*(5), 489–494. Available from https://doi.org/10.1006/fstl.1998.0395.

Bermudez-Brito, M., Plaza-Díaz, J., Muñoz-Quezada, S., Gómez-Llorente, C., & Gil, A. (2012). Probiotic mechanisms of action. *Annals of Nutrition and Metabolism*, *61*(2), 160–174. Available from https://doi.org/10.1159/000342079.

Besselink, M. G., van Santvoort, H. C., Buskens, E., Boermeester, M. A., van Goor, H., Timmerman, H. M., Nieuwenhuijs, V. B., Bollen, T. L., van Ramshorst, B., Witteman, B. J., Rosman, C., Ploeg, R. J., Brink, M. A., Schaapherder, A. F., Dejong, C. H., Wahab, P. J., van Laarhoven, C. J., van der Harst, E., van Eijck, C. H., ... Gooszen, H. G. (2008). Probiotic prophylaxis in predicted severe acute pancreatitis: A randomised, double-blind, placebo-controlled trial. *The Lancet*, *371*(9613), 651–659. Available from https://doi.org/10.1016/S0140-6736(08)60207-X.

Byakika, S., Mukisa, I. M., Byaruhanga, Y. B., & Muyanja, C. (2019). A review of criteria and methods for evaluating the probiotic potential of microorganisms. *Food Reviews International*, *35*(5), 427–466. Available from https://doi.org/10.1080/87559129.2019.1584815.

Caselli, M., Cassol, F., Calò, G., Holton, J., Zuliani, G., & Gasbarrini, A. (2013). Actual concept of "probiotics": Is it more functional to science or business? *World Journal of Gastroenterology, 19*(10), 1527–1540. Available from https://doi.org/10.3748/wjg.v19.i10.1527.

Cesaro, S., Chinello, P., Rossi, L., & Zanesco, L. (2000). *Saccharomyces cerevisiae* fungemia in a neutropenic patient treated with *Saccharomyces boulardii*. *Supportive Care in Cancer, 8*(6), 504–505. Available from https://doi.org/10.1007/s005200000123.

Charteris, W. P., Kelly, P. M., Morelli, L., & Collins, J. K. (1998). Antibiotic susceptibility of potentially probiotic Lactobacillus species. *Journal of Food Protection, 61*(12), 1636–1643. Available from https://doi.org/10.4315/0362-028X-61.12.1636.

Chilton, S. N., Burton, J. P., Reid, G., & Reid, G. (2015). Inclusion of fermented foods in food guides around the world. *Nutrients, 7*(1), 390–404. Available from https://doi.org/10.3390/nu7010390.

Ciernikova, S., Mego, M., Semanova, M., Wachsmannova, L., Adamcikova, Z., Stevurkova, V., Drgona, L., & Zajac, V. (2017). Probiotic survey in cancer patients treated in the outpatient department in a comprehensive cancer center. *Integrative Cancer Therapies, 16*(2), 188–195. Available from https://doi.org/10.1177/1534735416643828.

Cocetta, V., Catanzaro, D., Borgonetti, V., Ragazzi, E., Giron, M. C., Governa, P., Carnevali, I., Biagi, M., & Montopoli, M. (2019). A fixed combination of probiotics and herbal extracts attenuates intestinal barrier dysfunction from inflammatory stress in an in vitro model using caco-2 cells. *Recent Patents on Food, Nutrition and Agriculture, 10*(1), 62–69. Available from https://doi.org/10.2174/2212798410666180808121328.

Coeuret, V., Gueguen, M., & Vernoux, J. P. (2004). Numbers and strains of lactobacilli in some probiotic products. *International Journal of Food Microbiology, 97*(2), 147–156. Available from https://doi.org/10.1016/j.ijfoodmicro.2004.04.015.

Cuello-Garcia, C. A., Brozek, J. L., Fiocchi, A., Pawankar, R., Yepes-Nuñez, J. J., Terracciano, L., Gandhi, S., Agarwal, A., Zhang, Y., & Schünemann, H. J. (2015). Probiotics for the prevention of allergy: A systematic review and meta-analysis of randomized controlled trials. *Journal of Allergy and Clinical Immunology, 136*(4), 952–961. Available from https://doi.org/10.1016/j.jaci.2015.04.031.

Daliri, E. B. M., & Lee, B. H. (2015). New perspectives on probiotics in health and disease. *Food Science and Human Wellness, 4*(2), 56–65. Available from https://doi.org/10.1016/j.fshw.2015.06.002.

Di Cerbo, A., Palmieri, B., Aponte, M., Morales-Medina, J. C., & Iannitti, T. (2016). Mechanisms and therapeutic effectiveness of lactobacilli. *Journal of Clinical Pathology, 69*(3), 187–203. Available from https://doi.org/10.1136/jclinpath-2015-202976.

Didari, T., Solki, S., Mozaffari, S., Nikfar, S., & Abdollahi, M. (2014). A systematic review of the safety of probiotics. *Expert Opinion on Drug Safety, 13*(2), 227–239. Available from https://doi.org/10.1517/14740338.2014.872627.

Dinleyici, E. C., Kara, A., Ozen, M., & Vandenplas, Y. (2014). *Saccharomyces boulardii* CNCM I-745 in different clinical conditions. *Expert Opinion on Biological Therapy, 14*(11), 1593–1609. Available from https://doi.org/10.1517/14712598.2014.937419.

Doron, S., & Snydman, D. R. (2015). Risk and safety of probiotics. *Clinical Infectious Diseases, 60*, S129–S134. Available from https://doi.org/10.1093/cid/civ085.

Elmer, G. W., McFarland, L. V., Surawicz, C. M., Danko, L., & Greenberg, R. N. (1999). Behaviour of *Saccharomyces boulardii* in recurrent *Clostridium difficile* disease patients. *Alimentary Pharmacology and Therapeutics, 13*(12), 1663–1668. Available from https://doi.org/10.1046/j.1365-2036.1999.00666.x.

FAO/WHO, (2002). Report of a Joint FAO/WHO Working Group on Drafting Guidelines for the Evaluation of Probiotics in Food. London, Ontario, Canada. Available from: http://www.fda.gov/ohrms/dockets/dockets/95s0316/95s-0316-rpt0282-tab-03-ref-19-joint-faowho-vol219.pdf.

Ganguly, N. K., Bhattacharya, S. K., Sesikeran, B., Nair, G. B., Ramakrishna, B. S., Sachdev, H. P. S., Batish, V. K., Kanagasabapathy, A. S., Muthuswamy, V., Kathuria, S. C., Katoch, V. M., Satyanarayana, K., Toteja, G. S., Rahi, M., Rao, S., Bhan, M. K., Kapur, R., & Hemalatha, R. (2011). ICMR-DBT guidelines for evaluation of probiotics in food. *Indian Journal of Medical Research, 134*(7), 22–25. Available from http://icmr.nic.in/ijmr/2011/july/Policy%20Document.pdf.

Gueimonde, M., Laitinen, K., Salminen, S., & Isolauri, E. (2007). Breast milk: A source of bifidobacteria for infant gut development and maturation? *Neonatology, 92*(1), 64–66. Available from https://doi.org/10.1159/000100088.

Gueimonde, M., Ouwehand, A. C., & Salminen, S. (2004). Safety of probiotics. *Scandinavian Journal of Nutrition/Naringsforskning, 48*(1), 42–48. Available from https://doi.org/10.1080/11026480410026447.

Gueimonde, M., Sánchez, B., de los Reyes-Gavilán, C. G., & Margolles, A. (2013). Antibiotic resistance in probiotic bacteria. *Frontiers in Microbiology, 4*. Available from https://doi.org/10.3389/fmicb.2013.00202.

Gupta, R., Lall, R., Srivastava, A. A., Martínez-Larrañaga, M. R., & Martínez, M. A., (2021). *Probiotics: Safety and toxicity considerations* (pp. 1081–1105).

Gyawali, R., & Ibrahim, S. A. (2012). Impact of plant derivatives on the growth of foodborne pathogens and the functionality of probiotics. *Applied Microbiology and Biotechnology, 95*(1), 29–45. Available from https://doi.org/10.1007/s00253-012-4117-x.

Hai, N. V. (2015). The use of probiotics in aquaculture. *Journal of Applied Microbiology, 119*(4), 917–935. Available from https://doi.org/10.1111/jam.12886.

Hamady, Z. Z. R., Scott, N., Farrar, M. D., Lodge, J. P. A., Holland, K. T., Whitehead, T., & Carding, S. R. (2010). Xylan-regulated delivery of human keratinocyte growth factor-2 to the inflamed colon by the human anaerobic commensal bacterium *Bacteroides ovatus*. *Gut, 59*(4), 461–469. Available from https://doi.org/10.1136/gut.2008.176131.

Hennequin, C., Kauffmann-Lacroix, C., Jobert, A., Viard, J. P., Ricour, C., Jacquemin, J. L., & Berche, P. (2000). Possible role of catheters in *Saccharomyces boulardii* fungemia. *European Journal of Clinical Microbiology and Infectious Diseases, 19*(1), 16–20. Available from https://doi.org/10.1007/s100960050003.

Hill, C., Guarner, F., Reid, G., Gibson, G. R., Merenstein, D. J., Pot, B., Morelli, L., Canani, R. B., Flint, H. J., Salminen, S., Calder, P. C., & Sanders, M. E. (2014). Expert consensus document: The international scientific association for probiotics and prebiotics consensus statement on the scope and appropriate use of the term probiotic. *Nature Reviews Gastroenterology and Hepatology, 11*(8), 506–514. Available from https://doi.org/10.1038/nrgastro.2014.66.

Hu, S., Wang, L., & Jiang, Z. (2017). Dietary additive probiotics modulation of the intestinal microbiota. *Protein and Peptide Letters, 24*(5), 382–387. Available from https://doi.org/10.2174/0929866524666170223143615.

Kim, J., Kim, H., Jeon, S., Jo, J., Kim, Y., & Kim, H. (2020). Synergistic antibacterial effects of probiotic lactic acid bacteria with curcuma longa rhizome extract as synbiotic against cutibacterium acnes. *Applied Sciences (Switzerland), 10*(24), 1–6. Available from https://doi.org/10.3390/app10248955.

Kothari, D., Patel, S., & Kim, S. K. (2019). Probiotic supplements might not be universally-effective and safe: A review. *Biomedicine and Pharmacotherapy, 111*, 537–547. Available from https://doi.org/10.1016/j.biopha.2018.12.104.

Kralovicova, K., Spanik, S., Oravcova, E., Mrazova, M., Morova, E., Gulikova, V., Kukuckova, E., Koren, P., Pichna, P., Nogova, J., Kunova, A., Trupl, J., & Krcmery, V. (1997). Fungemia in cancer patients undergoing chemotherapy versus surgery: Risk factors, etiology and outcome. *Scandinavian Journal of Infectious Diseases, 29*(3), 301–304. Available from https://doi.org/10.3109/00365549709019047.

Kuley, E., Balikci, E., Özoğul, I., Gökdogan, S., & Özoğul, F. (2012). Stimulation of cadaverine production by foodborne pathogens in the presence of *Lactobacillus, Lactococcus,* and *Streptococcus* spp. *Journal of Food Science, 77*(12), M650–M658. Available from https://doi.org/10.1111/j.1750-3841.2012.02825.x.

Lahtinen, S. J., Davis, E., & Ouwehand, A. C. (2012). Lactobacillus species causing obesity in humans: Where is the evidence? *Beneficial Microbes, 3*(3), 171–174. Available from https://doi.org/10.3920/BM2012.0041.

Land, M. H., Rouster-Stevens, K., Woods, C. R., Cannon, M. L., Cnota, J., & Shetty, A. K. (2005). *Lactobacillus sepsis* associated with probiotic therapy. *Pediatrics, 115*(1), 178–181. Available from https://doi.org/10.1542/peds.2004-2137.

Lara-Villoslada, F., Olivares, M., & Xaus, J. (2010). Safety of probiotic bacteria. *Bioactive foods in promoting health* (pp. 47–58). Elsevier Inc. Available from https://doi.org/10.1016/B978-0-12-374938-3.00004-9.

Leber, B., Spindelboeck, W., & Stadlbauer, V. (2012). Infectious complications of acute and chronic liver disease. *Seminars in Respiratory and Critical Care Medicine, 33*(1), 80–95. Available from https://doi.org/10.1055/s-0032-1301737.

Lerner, A., Neidhöfer, S., & Matthias, T. (2017). The gut microbiome feelings of the brain: A perspective for non-microbiologists. *Microorganisms, 5*(4), 1–24.

Lerner, A., Shoenfeld, Y., & Matthias, T. (2019). Probiotics: If it does not help it does not do any harm. really? *Microorganisms, 7*(4). Available from https://doi.org/10.3390/microorganisms7040104.

Lestin, F., Pertschy, A., & Rimek, D. (2003). Fungämie nach oraler Gabe von *Saccharomyces boulardii* bei einem multimorbiden Patienten. *Deutsche Medizinische Wochenschrift, 128*(48), 2531–2533. Available from https://doi.org/10.1055/s-2003-44948.

Linne, Y. (2004). Effects of obesity on women's reproduction and complications during pregnancy. *Obesity Reviews, 5*(3), 137–143.

Mantaring, J., Benyacoub, J., Destura, R., Pecquet, S., Vidal, K., Volger, S., & Guinto, V. (2018). Effect of maternal supplement beverage with and without probiotics during pregnancy and lactation on maternal and infant health: A randomized controlled trial in the Philippines. *BMC Pregnancy and Childbirth, 18*(1). Available from https://doi.org/10.1186/s12884-018-1828-8.

Markowiak, P., & Ślizewska, K. (2018). The role of probiotics, prebiotics and synbiotics in animal nutrition. *Gut Pathogens, 10*(1). Available from https://doi.org/10.1186/s13099-018-0250-0.

Martin, V. T., & Vij, B. (2016). Diet and headache: Part 1. *Headache, 56*(9), 1543–1552. Available from https://doi.org/10.1111/head.12953.

Mater, D. D., Langella, P., Corthier, G., & Flores, M. J. (2008). A probiotic Lactobacillus strain can acquire vancomycin resistance during digestive transit in mice. *Journal of Molecular Microbiology and Biotechnology, 14*(1–3), 123–127.

McFarland, L. V. (2014). Use of probiotics to correct dysbiosis of normal microbiota following disease or disruptive events: A systematic review. *BMJ Open, 4*(8). Available from https://doi.org/10.1136/bmjopen-2014-005047.

Meile, L., Le Blay, G., & Thierry, A. (2008). Safety assessment of dairy microorganisms: Propionibacterium and bifidobacterium. *International Journal of Food Microbiology, 126*(3), 316–320. Available from https://doi.org/10.1016/j.ijfoodmicro.2007.08.019.

Million, M., Angelakis, E., Paul, M., Armougom, F., Leibovici, L., & Raoult, D. (2012). Comparative meta-analysis of the effect of Lactobacillus species on weight gain in humans and animals. *Microbial Pathogenesis, 53*(2), 100–108. Available from https://doi.org/10.1016/j.micpath.2012.05.007.

Munakata, S., Arakawa, C., Kohira, R., Fujita, Y., Fuchigami, T., & Mugishima, H. (2010). A case of D-lactic acid encephalopathy associated with use of probiotics. *Brain and Development, 32*(8), 691–694. Available from https://doi.org/10.1016/j.braindev.2009.09.024.

Muñoz, P., Bouza, E., Cuenca-Estrella, M., Eiros, J. M., Pérez, M. J., Sánchez-Somolinos, M., Rincón, C., Hortal, J., & Peláez, T. (2005). *Saccharomyces cerevisiae* fungemia: An emerging infectious disease. *Clinical Infectious Diseases, 40*(11), 1625–1634. Available from https://doi.org/10.1086/429916.

Nakazawa, T., Kaneko, K. I., Takahashi, H., & Inoue, S. (1996). Neonatal meningitis caused by *Bifidobacterium breve*. *Brain and Development, 18*(2), 160–162. Available from https://doi.org/10.1016/0387-7604(95)00149-2.

National Cancer Institute, (2021). https://www.cancer.gov.

Neu, A. K., Månsson, M., Gram, L., & Prol-García, M. J. (2014). Toxicity of bioactive and probiotic marine bacteria and their secondary metabolites in *Artemia* sp. and *Caenorhabditis elegans* as eukaryotic model organisms. *Applied and Environmental Microbiology, 80*(1), 146–153. Available from https://doi.org/10.1128/AEM.02717-13.

O'Brien, J., Crittenden, R., Ouwehand, A. C., & Salminen, S. (1999). Safety evaluation of probiotics. *Trends in Food Science and Technology, 10*(12), 418–424. Available from https://doi.org/10.1016/S0924-2244(00)00037-6.

O'Callaghan, A., & van Sinderen, D. (2016). Bifidobacteria and their role as members of the human gut microbiota. *Frontiers in Microbiology, 7*, 1−23. Available from https://doi.org/10.3389/fmicb.2016.00925.

Oakey, H. J., Harty, D. W. S., & Knox, K. W. (1995). Enzyme production by lactobacilli and the potential link with infective endocarditis. *Journal of Applied Bacteriology, 78*(2), 142−148. Available from https://doi.org/10.1111/j.1365-2672.1995.tb02834.x.

Ohishi, A., Takahashi, S., Ito, Y., Ohishi, Y., Tsukamoto, K., Nanba, Y., Ito, N., Kakiuchi, S., Saitoh, A., Morotomi, M., & Nakamura, T. (2010). *Bifidobacterium septicemia* associated with postoperative probiotic therapy in a neonate with omphalocele. *Journal of Pediatrics, 156*(4), 679−681. Available from https://doi.org/10.1016/j.jpeds.2009.11.041.

Pace, F., Macchini, F., & Massimo Castagna, V. (2020). Safety of probiotics in humans: A dark side revealed? *Digestive and Liver Disease, 52*(9), 981−985. Available from https://doi.org/10.1016/j.dld.2020.04.029.

Pradhan, D., Mallappa, R. H., & Grover, S. (2020). Comprehensive approaches for assessing the safety of probiotic bacteria. *Food Control, 108*. Available from https://doi.org/10.1016/j.foodcont.2019.106872.

Quinlivan, J. A., Lam, L. T., & Fisher, J. (2011). A randomised trial of a four-step multidisciplinary approach to the antenatal care of obese pregnant women. *Australian and New Zealand Journal of Obstetrics and Gynaecology, 51*(2), 141−146. Available from https://doi.org/10.1111/j.1479-828X.2010.01268.x.

Ramakrishnan, S. (2018). Prokaryotic horizontal gene transfer within the human holobiont: Ecological-evolutionary inferences, implications and possibilities. *Microbiome*. Available from https://doi.org/10.1186/s40168-018-0551-z.

Redman, M. G., Ward, E. J., & Phillips, R. S. (2014). The efficacy and safety of probiotics in people with cancer: A systematic review. *Annals of Oncology, 25*(10), 1919−1929. Available from https://doi.org/10.1093/annonc/mdu106.

Ridlon, J. M., Kang, D. J., Hylemon, P. B., & Bajaj, J. S. (2014). Bile acids and the gut microbiome. *Current Opinion in Gastroenterology, 30*(3), 332−338. Available from https://doi.org/10.1097/MOG.0000000000000057.

Risk assessment on use of Lactobacillus rhamnosus (LGG) as an ingredient in infant formula and baby foods (II), (2007). http://www.vkm.no/dav/63bb45d3eb.pdf.

Robin, F., Paillard, C., Marchandin, H., Demeocq, F., Bonnet, R., & Hennequin, C. (2010). *Lactobacillus rhamnosus* meningitis following recurrent episodes of bacteremia in a child undergoing allogeneic hematopoietic stem cell transplantation. *Journal of Clinical Microbiology, 48*(11), 4317−4319. Available from https://doi.org/10.1128/JCM.00250-10.

Rogozińska, E., Chamillard, M., Hitman, G. A., Khan, K. S., & Thangaratinam, S. (2015). Nutritional manipulation for the primary prevention of gestational diabetes mellitus: A meta-analysis of randomised studies. *PLoS One, 10*(2). Available from https://doi.org/10.1371/journal.pone.0115526.

Ruseler-van Embden, J. G. H., van der Helm, R., & van Lieshout, L. M. C. (1989). Degradation of intestinal glycoproteins by *Bacteroides vulgatus*. *FEMS Microbiology Letters, 58*(1), 37−41. Available from https://doi.org/10.1111/j.1574-6968.1989.tb03014.x.

Salminen, M. K., Rautelin, H., Tynkkynen, S., Poussa, T., Saxelin, M., Valtonen, V., & Järvinen, A. (2004). Lactobacillus Bacteremia, clinical significance, and patient outcome, with special focus on probiotic *L. Rhamnosus* GG. *Clinical Infectious Diseases, 38*(1), 62−69. Available from https://doi.org/10.1086/380455.

Sanders, M. E., Akkermans, L. M. A., Haller, D., Hammerman, C., Heimbach, J., Hörmannsperger, G., Huys, G., Levy, D. D., Lutgendorff, F., Mack, D., Phothirath, P., Solano-Aguilar, G., & Vaughan, E. (2010). Safety assessment of probiotics for human use. *Gut Microbes, 1*(3), 1−22. Available from https://doi.org/10.4161/gmic.1.3.12127.

Schlegel, L., Lemerle, S., & Geslin, P. (1998). Lactobacillus species as opportunistic pathogens in immunocompromised patients. *European Journal of Clinical Microbiology and Infectious Diseases, 17*(12), 887−888. Available from https://doi.org/10.1007/s100960050216.

Serafini, F., Bottacini, F., Viappiani, A., Baruffini, E., Turroni, F., Foroni, E., Lodi, T., van Sinderen, D., & Ventura, M. (2011). Insights into physiological and genetic mupirocin susceptibility in bifidobacteria. *Applied and Environmental Microbiology, 77*(9), 3141−3146. Available from https://doi.org/10.1128/AEM.02540-10.

Shanahan, F. (2012). A commentary on the safety of probiotics. *Gastroenterology Clinics of North America, 41*(4), 869−876. Available from https://doi.org/10.1016/j.gtc.2012.08.006.

Sharma, P., Tomar, S. K., Goswami, P., Sangwan, V., & Singh, R. (2014). Antibiotic resistance among commercially available probiotics. *Food Research International, 57*, 176−195.

Shipradeep., Karmakar, S., Sahay Khare, R., Ojha, S., Kundu, K., & Kundu, S. (2012). Development of probiotic candidate in combination with essential oils from medicinal plant and their effect on enteric pathogens: A review. *Gastroenterology Research and Practice*. Available from https://doi.org/10.1155/2012/457150.

Singh, R. B., Watsom, R. R., & Takahashi, T. (2019). *The role of functional food security in global. Safety of probiotics in health and disease* (pp. 603−622).

Solano-Aguilar, G., Dawson, H., Restrepo, M., Andrews, K., Vinyard, B., & Urban, J. F. (2008). Detection of *Bifidobacterium animalis* subsp. lactis (Bb12) in the intestine after feeding of sows and their piglets. *Applied and Environmental Microbiology, 74*, 6338−6347. Available from https://doi.org/10.1128/AEM.00309-08.

Sotoudegan, F., Daniali, M., Hassani, S., Nikfar, S., & Abdollahi, M. (2019). Reappraisal of probiotics' safety in human. *Food and Chemical Toxicology, 129*, 22−29. Available from https://doi.org/10.1016/j.fct.2019.04.032.

Stadnik, J., & Dolatowski, Z. J. (2012). Biogenic amines content during extended ageing of dry-cured pork loins inoculated with probiotics. *Meat Science, 91*(3), 374−377. Available from https://doi.org/10.1016/j.meatsci.2012.02.022.

Steidler, L., Neirynck, S., Huyghebaert, N., Snoeck, V., Vermeire, A., Goddeeris, B., Cox, E., Remon, J. P., & Remaut, E. (2003). Biological containment of genetically modified *Lactococcus lactis* for intestinal delivery of human interleukin 10. *Nature Biotechnology, 21*(7), 785−789. Available from https://doi.org/10.1038/nbt840.

Toscano, M., De Grandi, R., Pastorelli, L., Vecchi, M., & Drago, L. (2017). A consumer's guide for probiotics: 10 golden rules for a correct use. *Digestive and Liver Disease*, 49(11), 1177–1184. Available from https://doi.org/10.1016/j.dld.2017.07.011.

Turpin, W., Humblot, C., Thomas, M., & Guyot, J. P. (2010). Lactobacilli as multifaceted probiotics with poorly disclosed molecular mechanisms. *International Journal of Food Microbiology*, 143(3), 87–102. Available from https://doi.org/10.1016/j.ijfoodmicro.2010.07.032.

Vaarala, O. (2003). Immunological effects of probiotics with special reference to lactobacilli. *Clinical & Experimental Allergy*, 33(12), 1634–1640. Available from https://doi.org/10.1111/j.1365-2222.2003.01835.x.

Valenzuela-Grijalva, N., Pinelli-Saavedra, A., Muhlia-Almazan, A., Domínguez-Díaz, D., & González-Ríos, H. (2017). Dietary inclusion effects of phytochemicals as growth promoters in animal production. *Journal of Animal Science and Technology*, 59, 1–7.

Van Reenen, C. A., & Dicks, L. M. T. (2011). Horizontal gene transfer amongst probiotic lactic acid bacteria and other intestinal microbiota: What are the possibilities? A review. *Archives of Microbiology*, 193(3), 157–168. Available from https://doi.org/10.1007/s00203-010-0668-3.

Vankerckhoven, V., Huys, G., & Vancanneyt, M. (2008). Biosafety assessment of probiotics used for human consumption: Recommendations from the EU-PROSAFE project. *Trends in Food Science & Technology*, 19, 102–114.

Veckman, V., Miettinen, M., Pirhonen, J., Sirén, J., Matikainen, S., & Julkunen, I. (2004). Streptococcus pyogenes and *Lactobacillus rhamnosus* differentially induce maturation and production of Th1-type cytokines and chemokines in human monocyte-derived dendritic cells. *Journal of Leukocyte Biology*, 75(5), 764–771. Available from https://doi.org/10.1189/jlb.1003461.

Zé-Zé, L., Tenreiro, R., Duarte, A., Salgado, M. J., Melo-Cristino, J., Lito, L., Carmo, M. M., Felisberto, S., & Carmo, G. (2004). Case of aortic endocarditis caused by *Lactobacillus casei*. *Journal of Medical Microbiology*, 53(5), 451–453. Available from https://doi.org/10.1099/jmm.0.05328-0.

Zhai, Q., Yang, L., Zhao, J., Zhang, H., Tian, F., & Chen, W. (2018). Protective effects of dietary supplements containing probiotics, micronutrients, and plant extracts against lead toxicity in mice. *Frontiers in Microbiology*, 9, 1–11.

Zhou, J. S., Shu, Q., Rutherfurd, K. J., Prasad, J., Gopal, P. K., & Gill, H. S. (2000). Acute oral toxicity and bacterial translocation studies on potentially probiotic strains of lactic acid bacteria. *Food and Chemical Toxicology*, 38(2–3), 153–161. Available from https://doi.org/10.1016/S0278-6915(99)00154-4.

Zielińska, D., Sionek, B., & Kołożyn-Krajewska, D. (2018). Safety of probiotics. *Diet, microbiome and health* (pp. 131–161). Elsevier. Available from https://doi.org/10.1016/B978-0-12-811440-7.00006-5.

Zucko, J., Starcevic, A., Diminic, J., Oros, D., Mortazavian, A. M., & Putnik, P. (2020). Probiotic—friend or foe? *Current Opinion in Food Science*, 32, 45–49. Available from https://doi.org/10.1016/j.cofs.2020.01.007.

Chapter 31

Probiotics: current regulatory aspects of probiotics for use in different disease conditions

Maja Šikić Pogačar[1], Dušanka Mičetić-Turk[1,2] and Sabina Fijan[2]
[1]*University of Maribor, Faculty of Medicine, Maribor, Slovenia,* [2]*University of Maribor, Faculty of Health Sciences, Institute for Health and Nutrition, Maribor, Slovenia*

31.1 Introduction

Probiotics are defined as "live microorganisms that, when administered in adequate amounts, confer a health benefit on the host" (FAO/WHO, 2001, 2002; Hill et al., 2014). The most common probiotics are members of the *Lactobacillus* group, which has recently been divided into 25 genera (Zheng et al., 2020) (e.g., including but not limited to strains of the following species: *Lactobacillus acidophilus, Lactobacillus delbrueckii* subsp. *bulgaricus, Lactobacillus gasseri, Lacticaseibacillus rhamnosus, Lacticaseibacillus casei, Lactiplantibacillus plantarum, Limosilactobacillus reuteri, Levilactobacillus brevis, Ligilactobacillus salivarius*) and *Bifidobacterium* genera (e.g., *Bifidobacterium infantis, Bifidobacterium animalis* subsp. *lactis, Bifidobacterium longum, Bifidobacterium longum, Bifidobacterium bifidum*). Also, strains from other bacterial species (e.g., *Pediococcus acidilactici, Lactococcus lactis, Leuconostoc mesenteroides, Enterococcus faecium, Streptococcus thermophilus, Bacillus subtilis, Clostridium butyricum, Escherichia coli*) and strains from certain yeasts (e.g., *Saccharomyces cerevisiae* var. *boulardii*) qualify as probiotics (Fijan, 2014).

The definition of probiotics is also supported by the *International Scientific Association for Probiotics and Prebiotics* (ISAPP) as noted in the consensus statement (Hill et al., 2014). ISAPP, webpage https://isappscience.org/, is an international nonprofit organization that champions probiotic and prebiotic science. ISAPP brings together global leading scientific experts and has shifted the paradigm for how probiotics and prebiotics are studied and understood.

Another important organization is the *International Probiotics Association* (IPA), webpage https://internationalprobiotics.org/, which is also a global nonprofit organization bringing together academia, scientists, healthcare professionals, consumers, industry, and regulators of the probiotic sector. The IPA's mission is to promote the safe and efficacious use of probiotics throughout the world.

According to the online Oxford advanced learners' dictionary, the term "-biotic" is derived from the Greek word "biōtikos," meaning "pertaining to life" or from the Greek word "bios" meaning life and refers to the biological ecosystem made up of living organisms together with their physical environment strategies that can be utilized to direct the gut microbiota toward a more favorable state for host health (Wegh et al., 2019). According to the same dictionary the prefix "pro-" is derived from Latin and means "in front of, on behalf of, instead of, on account of." Thus probiotics are for life. This term was derived by Lilly and Stillwell (1965) as growth-promoting factors produced by microorganisms and was intended to etymologically contrast the term "antibiotic," although it is not a complete antonym.

Besides the term "probiotics," there are also other terms associated with beneficial microbes or their metabolites that may promote a health benefit to the host, including: prebiotics, synbiotics, live therapeutic products, psychobiotics, immunobiotics, pharmabiotics, postbiotics, and parabiotics. For some of these terms, there are consensus statements, while for other terms there are not. According to the consensus statements of the ISAPP the definition of "prebiotics" was updated as "a substrate that is selectively utilized by host microorganisms conferring a health benefit" (Gibson et al., 2017) and "synbiotics" were updated as "a mixture comprising live microorganisms and substrate(s) selectively utilized by host microorganisms that confers a health benefit on the host" (Swanson et al., 2020).

The US *Food and Drug Administration* (FDA) created the category "live biotherapeutic products" in 2012 (Cordaillat-Simmons et al., 2020; FDA, 2016). This category has also been added to the ninth edition of the *European Pharmacopoeia* (EDQM, 2019). "Live biotherapeutic products" are medicinal products for human use containing live microorganisms are applicable to the prevention, treatment, or cure of a disease or condition inhuman beings. These live biotherapeutic agents (LBP) can be administered orally or vaginally in different pharmaceutical forms as was highlighted for the first time in 2019 in the European Pharmacopoeia. LBP may contain one or multiple microbial strains from the same or different species of microorganisms.

"Pharmabiotics" have appeared in literature addressing products containing live microorganisms with the intention to prevent or treat disease. The term is an attempt to avoid confusion between the nature of the product and its regulatory status. However, this terminology had no legal ground and was not internationally recognized, mainly because it could include more than just living microorganisms. This term was replaced with the previously mentioned "live biotherapeutic products" (Cordaillat-Simmons et al., 2020).

"Psychobiotics" are defined as live bacteria, which when ingested in adequate amounts, and confer mental health benefits (Bambury et al., 2018) and "immunobiotics" are proposed to define microbial strains that are able to beneficially regulate the immune system of the host (Villena & Kitazawa, 2017).

There are several different terms, such as "postbiotics" and "parabiotics," that include versions of functional bioactive compounds, which may be used to promote health, but do not contain live microorganisms and therefore cannot fall into the category of probiotics. A recently published consensus statement of the ISAPP defines "postbiotics" as a preparation of inanimate microorganisms and/or their components that confers a health benefit on the host (Salminen et al., 2021). Synonyms for "postbiotics" are also "biogenics," "metabolites," "cell-free supernatants," or "cell-free extracts" (Cuevas-González et al., 2020). According to the same authors, "parabiotics" are termed as nonviable probiotics, inactivated probiotics, or ghost probiotics (Table 31.1).

TABLE 31.1 Overview of main terms for live microorganisms and supporting soluble or nonsoluble substrate that aid in conferring a health benefit.

Term	Definition	Live microorganism	Soluble or nonsoluble substrate	Consensus statement
Probiotics	Live microorganisms that, when administered in adequate amounts, confer a health benefit on the host	Yes	No	ISAPP
Prebiotics	A substrate that is selectively utilized by host microorganisms conferring a health benefit.	No	Yes	ISAPP
Synbiotics	A mixture comprising live microorganisms and substrate(s) selectively utilized by host microorganisms that confers a health benefit on the host	Yes	Yes	ISAPP
live biotherapeutic products	Medicinal products for human use containing live microorganisms applicable to the prevention, treatment, or cure of a disease or condition inhuman beings	Yes	No	FDA
Pharmabiotics	Products, containing live microorganisms with the intention to prevent or treat disease	Yes	No	No
Psychobiotics	Live bacteria, which when ingested in adequate amounts, confer mental health benefits	Yes	No	No
Immunobiotics	Microbial strains that are able to beneficially regulate the immune system of the host	Yes	No	No
Postbiotics	Preparation of inanimate microorganisms and/or their components that confers a health benefit on the host	No	Yes	ISAPP
Parabiotics	Nonviable probiotics, inactivated probiotics, or ghost probiotics	No	Yes	No

FDA, Food and Drug Administration; *ISAPP*, International Scientific Association for Probiotics and Prebiotics.

In any case all used probiotics must have a GRAS (generally regarded as safe) status. The status qualified presumption of safety is valid for individual probiotic strains, while the GRAS status is intended for the food product or food supplement containing probiotic microorganisms and is approved by the US FDA (Laulund et al., 2017).

According to the ISAPP consensus panel (Hill et al., 2014), probiotic mechanisms can be strain-specific (i.e., rare and present in only a few strains of a given species), species-specific (i.e., frequently observed among most strains of a probiotic species, e.g., *Lacticaseibacillus casei* or *Bifidobacterium bifidum*), and some mechanisms might be widespread among commonly studied probiotic genera. The use of probiotics has increased exponentially during the last three decades, both in hospitalized patients and by the general population (Zorzela et al., 2017). This is reflected in the dramatic increase in publications on probiotics and the increasing diversity of products available on the market. Decades of evidence-based efficacy and safety trials of particular strains of probiotics have made probiotics a useful and frequently used therapeutic option. In many countries, probiotics are available as dietary supplements or over-the-counter products and as such national drug regulatory agencies cannot provide the same level of clinical guidance that they do for prescription medications. The responsibility falls on healthcare providers and the public, who are faced with a wide range of probiotic products available on the market and health claims (Sniffen et al., 2018).

The beneficial health effects, as supported by results from clinical trials, include the prevention and treatment of intestinal diseases, such as infectious, antibiotic-associated and *Clostridium difficile-associated* diarrhea, inflammatory bowel disease (IBD), irritable bowel syndrome (IBS), *Helicobacter pylori* infection, lactose intolerance, and allergies in children, as well as anxiety, depression, wound healing, etc. (Bagga et al., 2018; Cuevas-González et al., 2020; Fijan et al., 2019; Lau & Chamberlain, 2016; Liu et al., 2018; Maldonado Galdeano et al., 2019; Reid et al., 2011).

Selecting an appropriate probiotic is often a difficult task, as a variety of factors have to be taken into account when considering a particular probiotic product, that is, the disease-specific efficacy of probiotic strain, the mechanisms of action for particular probiotic strain, differences in manufacturing processes, and quality of the products. In addition, international guidelines for infectious disease or pediatric disease organizations do not always agree with which probiotics should be used for particular disease condition but also distinctive regulatory and quality control issues make it difficult to interpret clinical data (Sniffen et al., 2018).

The aim of this review is to present the current evidence on probiotics' efficacy and current regulatory aspects of probiotics for use in different number of pathologies, including acute gastroenteritis, allergic diseases, and other disorders.

31.2 Current regulation bodies that include probiotics

The US FDA gives special instructions on using probiotics on food labels and the document "*Label Claims for Conventional Foods and Dietary Supplements*" describes the procedures for using health claims on food and dietary supplements (FDA, 2018). The US FDA generally regards probiotics as safe; they are marketed directly to consumers and generally do not require a prescription (Draper et al., 2017).

In Canada, the "*Guidance Document for the Use of Probiotic Microorganisms in Foods*," issued by Health Canada in 2009 gives similar instructions. It also provides guidance on the safety, quality (stability) and labeling aspects of food products containing probiotic microorganisms as well as describing therapeutic claims that bring a food into the definition of a drug or a natural health product (Government of Canada, 2009).

On the other hand, the efficiency of probiotics is questionable to important groups that manage policies for foods, which include food supplements and therefore most probiotics on the market in the European Union (EU) member states, such as the *European Food Safety Agency* (EFSA). ESFA even gone as far to decide that, since the term "probiotics" in itself is viewed as a health claim, it should not be used for food supplements in the EU as a term (EUR-Lex, 2006). The ESFA also states that there is not enough solid scientific evidence to substantiate any of the 350-plus health claims of probiotics, mostly due to insufficient characterization of microorganisms, nondefined claims, nonbeneficial claims or insufficient characterization of the claimed health effect (EU Register, 2021). Such a rigid approach to probiotics is seen only in the EU. However, discussions are now in progress with ESFA and IPA to work on obtaining a formal recognition of probiotics as a food category comparable to dietary fiber (EFSA, 2020).

The *European Medicines Agency* regulate drugs in the EU and some probiotics and live biotherapeutic products can fall into this category and need to be registered as medicinal products. Another regulation body includes the *International Council for Harmonization of Technical Requirements for Pharmaceuticals for Human Use*, which provides guidelines on common expectations of regular authorities (FDA in the United States, European Medicines Agency in the EU, the Japanese Health Authority in Japan) and the pharmaceutical industry regarding drug registration (Cordaillat-Simmons et al., 2020).

There are several medical organizations that include probiotic therapy in their guidelines. The *World Gastroenterology Organization* (WGO) issued WGO Global Guidelines: Probiotics and Prebiotics in 2017 that include the concept of probiotics and prebiotics, the products, health claims and commerce, clinical applications, and the summaries of evidence for probiotics and prebiotics in adult and pediatric conditions, as well as references supporting all above data (Guarner et al., 2017). The American Gastroenterological Association (AGA) has also prepared guidelines. The *European Society for Pediatric Gastroenterology, Hepatology and Nutrition* has prepared guidelines for the use of probiotics for children with selected clinical conditions (Hojsak et al., 2018). The *European Society for Pediatric Infectious Diseases* (ESPID) has included probiotics in their guidelines for the management of acute diarrhea in children (Ahmadi et al., 2015). Even the *World Allergy Organization* (WAO) mentions the use of probiotics (Hojsak et al., 2018). On the other hand, guideline recommendations of *Centers for Disease Control and Prevention* and *National Institute for Health and Care Excellence* do not recommend probiotics because as a dietary supplement they are not regulated by the federal government and therefore potential exists for great variability among the products, providing a challenge to the prescribing physician to recommend their use (Gibson et al., 2017; Kolaček et al., 2017; NIH, 2020).

31.3 Regulations for use of probiotics in gastrointestinal diseases

31.3.1 Probiotics and acute gastroenteritis

Acute gastroenteritis (AGE) has been defined by the ESPGHAN as a decrease in the consistency of stools (loose or liquid) and/or an increase in the frequency of evacuations (typically 3 in 24 hours), with or without fever or vomiting (Szajewska et al., 2014). Diarrhea typically lasts for less than 7 days depending on the pathogen that caused it. AGE in children is a leading cause of morbidity and mortality in developing countries and can be due to viral or bacterial etiologies (Freedman et al., 2018). *Campylobacter* or *Salmonella* strains are the most common cause of bacterial diarrhea worldwide and rotavirus has been recognized as the most frequent cause of severe diarrhea in children (Dinleyici et al., 2012; Guarino et al., 2014).

Worldwide, children younger than 5 years of age experience on average three episodes of AGE per year and in Europe up to two episodes per year in children younger than 3 years of age (Szajewska et al., 2014; Urbańska et al., 2016). Especially in children, AGE is a frequent cause for visiting emergency departments; however, healthcare providers, besides rehydration, have little to offer (Freedman et al., 2018). The treatment has remained almost unchanged over the last 35 years with oral rehydration, breastfeeding and early refeeding as the important approaches to which adjuvant therapy with probiotics was added in the late 1990s (Ahmadi et al., 2015). Probiotics, such as *Lacticaseibacillus rhamnosus* GG, also known as LGG (formerly known as *Lactobacillus rhamnosus*) and *Saccharomyces boulardii*, have also been included in the guidelines for the management of acute diarrhea in children of the ESPID and ESPGHAN (Ahmadi et al., 2015; Guarino et al., 2015; Szajewska, Guarino, et al., 2020).

Latin-American guidelines recommend probiotics, that is, *Bifidobacterium lactis*, LGG, *Limosilactobacillus reuteri* (formally known as *Lactobacillus reuteri*), and *S. boulardii*, which should be given along with oral rehydration therapy for the treatment of acute pediatric diarrhea (Cruchet et al., 2015). Recommendations for children with AGE of the Asia-Pacific region include the following probiotics, LGG, *S. boulardii*. and *L. reuteri* DSM 17938, as active therapy to reduce the duration and severity of symptoms (Cameron et al., 2017). According to evident-based recommendation of the WGO *S. boulardii*, *L. reuteri* ATCC 55730, LGG, and *L. casei* DN-114 001 are useful in reducing the severity and duration (approx. 1 day) of acute infectious diarrhea in children (Guarner et al., 2012). In India, due to the lack of evidence for developing countries, experts do not consider probiotics effective for the treatment of acute diarrhea (Lo Vecchio et al., 2016). On contrary, AGA suggests against the use of probiotics in children with acute infectious gastroenteritis in the United States and Canada (Su et al., 2020). Furthermore, clinical recommendation varies according to the availability of the products on the local market.

In general, recommendation for *Bacillus clausii* is lacking due to limited data even though results of several studies showed that it might represent an effective therapeutic option in acute childhood diarrhea (Ianiro et al., 2018; Lahiri et al., 2015).

Many studies during the last decade demonstrated potential benefit from the use of probiotics in reducing the duration and severity of AGE and also shedding of the pathogen (Maragkoudaki et al., 2018; Parker et al., 2013; Szajewska et al., 2014; Urbańska et al., 2016). The mechanisms responsible for the beneficial role of probiotic bacteria include direct antimicrobial effects, improvement of mucosal barrier function, and immune-modulating activities due to the effects of probiotics on both innate and adaptive immunities (Coqueiro et al., 2019). The exact mechanisms by which *S. boulardii* might exert its actions are not clear yet. The possible mechanisms include interference with pathogen attachment, interaction with gut microbiota, inactivation of toxins, immunomodulatory effects, both within the lumen and systemically, intestinal receptor modification, etc. (Dinleyici et al., 2012; Szajewska, Kołodziej, et al., 2020).

Regardless of the strain, the effects of *S. boulardii* on the duration of diarrhea are similar (Szajewska, Kołodziej, et al., 2020). In addition to rehydration therapy, strains of various lactobacilli and bifidobacteria and *S. boulardii* are the most commonly used probiotic strains in the treatment of diarrhea (Ahmadi et al., 2015). The probiotic dose that proved effectiveness is 10^{10} to 10^{11} cfu/day (Li et al., 2019). Mixtures of probiotics have been shown to have possible additional benefits over single-strain products, however, whether the greater efficacy of multistrain products compared with single-strain products is due to synergistic interactions between strains or a consequence of the higher probiotic dose used is not clear (Kluijfhout et al., 2020).

The systematic review with meta-analysis of Urbańska et al. (2016) confirmed the beneficial effect of *L. reuteri* DSM 17938 for the treatment of acute diarrhea. The above strain is tailored from the strain *L. reuteri* ATCC 55730 by removing two potentially transferable resistance traits for tetracycline and lincomycin (Maragkoudaki et al., 2018). In line with current European guidelines, the use of *L. reuteri* DSM 17938 might be considered in the management of AGE, although the quality of evidence is low. Administration of *L. reuteri* DSM 17938 when compared with placebo or no intervention shortened the duration of diarrhea by approximately 1 day and the effect was comparable to the effect of LGG and *S. boulardii* (Urbańska et al., 2016).

Combined data from 11 randomized controlled trials (RCTs) (>2400 children, both inpatients and outpatients from Europe) showed that administration of LGG, compared with placebo or no treatment, reduced the duration of diarrhea in children by approximately 1 day especially with a high daily dose of LGG ($\geq 10^{10}$ cfu/day) (Szajewska et al., 2013). However, it was found to be ineffective for the prevention of acute pediatric diarrhea (McFarland, 2006). Even though LGG treatment has been recommended by many experts, recent RCTs showed no evidence of a beneficial effect of LGG treatment (Freedman et al., 2018; Guarino et al., 2015; Schnadower et al., 2018; Szajewska et al., 2014). In two randomized, double-blind, placebo-controlled trials, Freedman et al. (2018) and Schnadower et al. (2018) showed that when compared the effectiveness of the probiotic LGG with that of placebo in a total of 1857 infants and children with acute infectious gastroenteritis in Canada and the United States, the probiotics did not significantly alter the course of disease or duration of diarrhea.

Another meta-analysis (29 RCTs) showed that administration of *S. boulardii* (with the daily dose between 250 and 750 mg/day) when compared to placebo reduced the duration of diarrhea caused by bacterial and viral pathogens by 1 day (Dinleyici et al., 2012; Szajewska, Kołodziej, et al., 2020). Interestingly, when *S. boulardii* was given along with the mixture of other bacterial probiotic strains, it was less effective (Sniffen et al., 2018) (Table 31.2).

TABLE 31.2 Selected clinical studies on the efficacy of probiotics for acute gastroenteritis.

References	Type of study	Population	Probiotic	Daily dose and duration	Outcome
Dinleyici, Dalgic, et al. (2015)	RCT, single blind study	Hospitalized children 3–60 months. Experiment/control (*n*): 64/63	*L. reuteri* DSM 17938	10^8 cfu (5 days)	24 h reduction in the duration of hospitalization for patients treated with *L. reuteri*
Dinleyici, Kara, et al. (2015)	Multicenter RCT, single blind	Hospitalized children, 3–60 months. Experiment/control (*n*): 148/72	*S. boulardii* CNCM I-745	250 mg/twice a day (5 days)	24 h reduction in duration of hospitalization for patients treated with *S. boulardii*
Lahiri et al. (2015)	Open-label, prospective, randomized, controlled study	Hospitalized children, 6 months to 12 years Experiment/control (*n*): 69/62	*Bacillus clausii*	2×10^9 cfu (5 days)	*Bacillus clausii* reduced the duration, frequency and hospital stay of diarrhea
Das et al. (2016)	RCT, single blind	Hospitalized children, 3 months to 5 years Experiment/control (*n*): 30/30	*S. boulardii*	250 mg/twice a day (5 days)	Duration of diarrhea was significantly shortened by approx. 17 h compared to the control group
Schnadower et al. (2018)	RCT, double-blind study	3 months to 4 years Experiment/control (*n*): 483/488	LGG	10^{10} cfu (5 days)	There were no significant differences between the LGG group and the placebo group

RCT, Randomized controlled trial.

31.3.2 Probiotics and inflammatory bowel diseases

The incidences of IBDs have risen over the last decade. Crohn's disease (CD) and ulcerative colitis (UC) are frequently described IBDs and are characterized by a chronic and exacerbated inflammation of the intestinal mucosa with diarrhea, abdominal pain, nutritional deficiencies, weight loss, and others (Coqueiro et al., 2019; Ferreira et al., 2014). The phases of chronic inflammation alternate from exacerbated inflammation (clinical relapse) to clinical remission (Coqueiro et al., 2019).

The incidence of UC is more commonly reported than that of CD, and prevalence of UC is higher in developed countries (Coqueiro et al., 2019). Both diseases (CD and UC) differentiate by the location of the inflammation in the gastrointestinal tract (GIT). The precise etiology is unknown, but it is thought to be a complex interplay of genetics, epigenetics, lifestyle, host immune system and the intestinal microbiota. Gut microbiota plays an important role in the pathogenesis of IBD as many investigators favor the altered microbiota as primary cause that leads to inflammation, which was observed in subsets of CD and UC patients (Ganji-Arjenaki & Rafieian-Kopaei, 2018). In general, the microbiota of IBD patients consists of lower number of protective bacteria (*Bifidobacterium* spp. and *Lactobacillus* spp.) and an increased number of pathogenic bacteria (*Escherichia coli* and *Clostridium* spp.) compared with the microbiota of healthy individuals (Di Cagno et al., 2011; Macfarlane et al., 2004).

Furthermore, differences in the microbiota were observed in those with active disease or in remission and many studies highlighted the manipulation of microbiota as an attractive approach for therapeutic interventions in IBD (Derwa et al., 2017). Having the capacity of modulating the composition of intestinal microbiota and influence immune response through regulation of cytokine synthesis and their action on both immune and epithelial cells, probiotics may represent an alternative therapeutic method for the treatment of IBDs (Vanderpool et al., 2008). Active treatments including probiotics, prebiotics, and synbiotics were intensively been studied in CD, UC and pouchitis with promising results. Therefore attempting the treatment for IBDs with probiotics presents a reasonable approach and guidelines recommend such therapy.

31.3.2.1 Crohn's disease

CD is a chronic inflammatory disorder of the GIT that can result in progressive bowel damage and disability and is believed to be partly influenced by the gut microbiome (Limketkai et al., 2020). CD can affect individuals of any age, from children to the elderly, and may cause significant morbidity and impact on quality of life (Torres et al., 2020). It has a discontinuous pattern, where inflammation potentially affects the entire GIT. The patient presents with recurrent diarrhea with or without bleeding, abdominal pain, fever, fatigue, malnutrition, weight loss, oral ulcers, and anemia (Limketkai et al., 2020). Most frequently, CD affects the colon and ileum (Coqueiro et al., 2019).

Several medical agents are available for the treatment of CD including mesalazine, locally active steroids, systemic steroids, immunosuppressive and biological therapies [such as antitumor necrosis factor, antiintegrins, and antiinterleukin (IL)] (Torres et al., 2020). An important outcome in the management of CD is improved quality of life, especially in children (Ruemmele et al., 2014). Given the association between dysbiosis and CD, there is a hypothesized role for probiotics in restoring intestinal eubiosis and potentially improving inflammation (Limketkai et al., 2020).

Research into using probiotics in the CD treatment started in 1997 when Malchow (Malchow, 1997) administered *E. coli* Nissle 1917, for 1 year, to patients with active CD, previously treated with prednisolone. The recurrence rate was 33% in the probiotic group and 64% in the placebo group. Following 6 months of treatment, patients from the probiotic group discontinued their medical therapy, demonstrating that probiotics supplementation was effective in reducing the inflammation. In the study (Schultz et al., 2004) that included 11 adult participants with active mild-to moderate CD, the efficacy of probiotic LGG was investigated. Participants were treated with an 1-week course of corticosteroids and antibiotics (ciprofloxacin 500 mg twice daily and metronidazole 250 mg three times a day), prior to the study. Probiotic group received two billion cfu per day of LGG or and placebo group corn starch. There was no difference between treated and placebo group in induction of remission.

Approximately 75% of people with CD undergo operative procedure at least once in their lifetime to induce remission. However, as there is no known cure for CD, patients usually experience a relapse of CD even after surgery (Iheozor-Ejiofor et al., 2019). Four placebo-controlled trials assessed the efficacy of probiotics compared to placebo in terms of preventing either clinical or endoscopic relapse of CD in remission during the postoperative period (Fedorak et al., 2015; Marteau et al., 2006; Prantera et al., 2002; Van Gossum et al., 2007). The supplementation with *L. johnsonii* LA1, for 6 months, to CD patients submitted to a bowel resection surgery, did not show important therapeutic effects, and there was no difference between groups in intestinal lesions evaluated by endoscopy (Marteau et al., 2006). All four trials demonstrated the ineffectiveness of probiotics, regardless of the probiotic used (LGG; *L. johnsonii* LA1,

E. coli Nissle 1917 or VSL#3), for prophylaxis in the postoperative relapse of CD (Fedorak et al., 2015; Marteau et al., 2006; Prantera et al., 2002; Van Gossum et al., 2007). However, the study (Fedorak et al., 2015) showed that CD patients who were immediately treated with VSL#3 after the surgery had lower proinflammatory cytokines, such as IL-8 and IL-1b, in the intestinal mucosa, as well as a lower recurrence rate than the patients who received late supplementation with probiotics (90 days after the surgery).

The study (Steed et al., 2010) revealed the improvement of immune and inflammatory parameters with probiotic supplementation in CD patients who were administered twice a day with symbiotic product Synergy 1, containing *B. longum* (2×10^{11} cfu), inulin, and oligofructose for 6 months. A reduced disease activity index and proinflammatory biomarkers, such as tumor necrosis factor-α (TNF-α), in the intestinal mucosa, as well as improved histological parameters, were observed in these patients after the experimental period.

The administration of *S. boulardii*, associated with mesalazine, to patients with CD in remission, for 6 months in the study (Guslandi et al., 2000) showed to be effective in reducing the recurrence rate by 6.25%, compared to the group that received only medical treatment (37.5%). The study showed that medical treatment together with probiotic supplementation, when taken together, presented higher therapeutic potential. However, the study (Bourreille et al., 2013) revealed that there is no evidence for *S. boulardii* to present significant therapeutic effect in the CD patients in the remission phase not in the number of relapses nor in the mean time for the relapse to occur. The authors also demonstrated there was no effect of *S. boulardii* on the disease activity index, although probiotic proved to be safe for the patients and well tolerated. A study that included 75 children with CD in remission (5–21 years) showed no therapeutic effect of administration of LGG for 2 years, when administered with other medicines (such as salicylates, azathioprine, 6-mercaptopurine, or corticosteroids) (Bousvaros et al., 2005).

Overall, although evidence suggests a potential immunomodulatory role of probiotics in CD patients, most of the studies have shown inconsistent results and did not demonstrate therapeutic effects of probiotic supplementation in CD, which remains controversial. In the last European Society for Parenteral and Enteral Nutrition (ESPEN) guidelines on clinical nutrition in IBD, probiotic supplementation was considered ineffective in inducing and maintaining remission in CD patients. The guidelines also advise not to use probiotics as a treatment in active CD due to the lack of efficacy and the possible risks of and from bacteremia in acute severe colitis (Forbes et al., 2017). As stated in the recent ECCO/ESPGHAN guidelines on pediatric CD, probiotics are also not recommended for maintenance of remission (Ruemmele et al., 2014). Accordingly, The Latin American Expert group consensus does not recommend probiotics in the treatment of CD (Cruchet et al., 2015). Guidelines for Asia-Pacific region note that probiotics are less effective for CD and due to the lack of beneficial effect of probiotics in the treatment of CD they do not recommend probiotic supplementation (Cameron et al., 2017). Similarly, the AGA does not recommend use of probiotics in children and adults with CD (Su et al., 2020).

31.3.2.2 Ulcerative colitis

In UC, inflammation usually starts in the rectal area and spreads throughout the large intestine, resulting in mucosal ulceration, rectal bleeding, frequent stools, mucus discharge from the rectum, tenesmus, and lower abdominal pain (Coqueiro et al., 2019). It rarely involves the upper digestive tract and small intestine but may be associated with extra-intestinal inflammatory sites. Antiinflammatory (5-aminosalicylic acid, sulfasalazine, or corticosteroids) and immune-modulating drugs are the main medical treatments used in UC (Derwa et al., 2017; Kaur et al., 2020).

E. coli Nissle 1917 (ECN), a nonpathogenic Gram-negative strain isolated in 1917, has been proposed for the maintenance therapy of UC. Three major double-blind RCT compared the efficacy of ECN to that of mesalazine (antiinflammatory medicine) to prevent the relapse of UC (Kruis et al., 1997, 2004; Rembacken et al., 1999) (Table 31.3). In these trials, placebo was not used and therefore the evidence for efficacy of ECN relies on the demonstration of statistical equivalence with mesalazine. In the first double-blind RCT, Kruis et al. (1997) included 120 patients with UC in remission, who were allocated in two groups and treated with either 2.0×10^9 cfu/day of ECN or 1.5 g/day of mesalazine for 12 weeks. At the end of the study period, 16% of the subjects in the ECN group had relapse of UC versus 11.3% in the mesalazine group. In this study, authors suggested that probiotic treatment might offer another option for maintenance therapy of UC. Another RCT (Kruis et al., 2004) included 327 patients with UC in remission. This study also included a follow-up period allowing to properly search for equivalence between the two treatments (ECN vs. mesalazine). The treatment with ECN was proved safe, and clinically equivalent to mesalazine in maintaining remission after an acute relapse of UC (Ghouri et al., 2014; Kruis et al., 2004). Also, the results (Rembacken et al., 1999) of RCT support the role of ECN in the therapy of UC. Furthermore, ECN is probiotic recommended in European Crohn's and Colitis Organization (ECCO) guidelines as effective alternative to mesalazine in the maintenance of remission in UC patients (Scaldaferri et al., 2016).

TABLE 31.3 Selected clinical studies on the efficacy of probiotics for inflammatory bowel diseases.

References	Type of study	Population	Probiotic	Daily dose and duration	Outcome
Induction of remission of UC					
Guslandi et al. (2003)	A pilot trial	25 adult patients with a mild to moderate UC, 19–47 years of age	S. boulardii	250 mg three times a day for 4 weeks during maintenance treatment with mesalazine	S. boulardii can be effective in the treatment of UC (induction of remission). All patients also received usual medical therapy
Kato et al. (2004)	Multicenter, randomized placebo-controlled trial.	20 adult patients with a mild to moderate UC, older than 18 years	B. breve, B. bifidum, L. acidophilus[a]	100 mL of probiotic fermented milk (1.0×10^{10} cfu/100 mL) plus standard therapy, 12 weeks	The addition of bifidobacteria proved to be safe and more efficient when compared to standard therapy. All patients also received usual medical therapy
Tursi et al. (2010)	Double-blind, randomized, placebo-controlled study	90 adult patients with a mild to moderate UC, 19–69 years of age	VSL#3	VSL#3 mixture—two sachets per day (9×10^{11} cfu/sachet) for 8 weeks. All patients also received usual medical therapy	Probiotics improved symptoms, remission time, and others. All patients also received usual medical therapy
Tamaki et al. (2016)	Multicenter, double-blinded, placebo-controlled, randomized trial	56 adult patients with a mild to moderate UC, older than 18 years	B. longum subsp. longum BB536	$2–3 \times 10^{11}$ freeze-dried viable, sachets 3 × daily for 8 weeks	VSL#3 improves rectal bleeding and seems to reinduce remission in relapsing UC patients after 8 weeks of treatment. All patients also received usual medical therapy
Maintenance of remission of UC					
Rembacken et al. (1999)	Double-blind, randomized, placebo-controlled study	116 adult patients (18–80 years) with active UC	E. coli Nissle 1917	1×10^{11} cfu daily for 1 year	As effective as mesalazine at maintaining remission of UC
Ishikawa et al. (2003)	Placebo-controlled, randomized trial	21 adult patients with UC	Lactobacillus and Bifidobacterium[a]	Fermented milk (100 mL) for 1 year	Reduced exacerbation of symptoms and successful in maintaining remission
Kruis et al. (2004)	Double-blind, randomized, placebo-controlled study	327 adult patients with UC in remission, (18–70 years)	E. coli Nissle 1917	200 mg ($2.5–25 \times 10^{9}$ cfu/100 mg) 1 × daily for 12 months	As effective as mesalazine at maintaining remission
Zocco et al. (2006)	Open label	187 patients with UC in remission; 33–40 years	L. rhamnosus LGG	1.8×10^{10} cfu/day	No difference in relapse rates at 12 months LGG more effective than mesalazine at prolonging relapse-free time

(Continued)

TABLE 31.3 (Continued)

References	Type of study	Population	Probiotic	Daily dose and duration	Outcome
Wildt et al. (2011)	Double-blind, randomized, placebo-controlled study	44 patients with UC in remission; 23–68 years	L. acidophilus LA-5 and B. animalis subsp. lactis Bb-12	1.25×10^{10} cfu/capsule; 52 weeks	No significant clinical benefit of probiotics was observed in comparison with placebo for maintaining remission in patients with left-sided UC
Induction of remission of CD					
Gupta et al. (2000)	Open-label study	4 children with mild-to-moderate CD	L. rhamnosus LGG	2×10^{10} cfu for 6 months	LGG could improve disease activity index compared with baseline
Schultz et al. (2004)	Double-blind, randomized, placebo-controlled study	11 adult patients with active mild-to moderate CD	L. rhamnosus LGG	2×10^{9} cfu for 6 months	No difference in remission rates
Marteau et al. (2006)	Double-blind, randomized, placebo-controlled study	98 adult patients with CD; 27–42 years	L. johnsonii[a]	2×10^{9} cfu/day, 6 months	No difference in remission rates
Maintenance of remission of CD					
Guslandi et al. (2000)	Randomized, placebo-controlled study	32 patients (23–49 years)	S. boulardii	1 g/day, 6 months	Compared to mesalamine there was a significant prolongation of remission
Prantera et al. (2002)	Randomized, placebo-controlled study	45 patients operated for CD; 22–71 years	L. rhamnosus LGG	12×10^{9} cfu/day, 1 year	No significant difference in remission, LGG did not prevent relapse of CD
Bousvaros et al. (2005)	Double-blind, randomized, placebo-controlled study	75 children with remission of CD; 5–21 years	L. rhamnosus LGG	2×10^{10} cfu for 2 years	No difference in time to relapse of CD
Fedorak et al. (2015)	Multicenter, randomized, double-blind, placebo-controlled trial	119 patients in postoperative period, 37.6 ± 12.4 years of age	VSL#3	6 g/day (9×10^{11})	Lower concentration of proinflammatory cytokines in the intestinal mucosa and lower relapse rate. However, there was no statistical differences in endoscopic recurrence rates at day 90 between patients who received VSL#3 and patients who received placebo
Treatment of acute pouchitis					
Kuisma et al. (2003)	Double-blind, randomized, placebo-controlled study	20 patients, with a previous history of pouchitis and endoscopic inflammation	L. rhamnosus LGG	1×10^{10} cfu for 3 months	When compared to placebo there was no difference in PDAI

(Continued)

TABLE 31.3 (Continued)

References	Type of study	Population	Probiotic	Daily dose and duration	Outcome
Treatment of chronic pouchitis					
Gionchetti et al. (2000)	Double-blind, randomized, placebo-controlled study	40 patients in in clinical and endoscopic remission	VSL#3	VSL#3, 6 g/day, or an identical placebo for 9 months	Results suggest that oral administration of VSL#3 is effective in preventing flare-ups of chronic pouchitis
Mimura et al. (2004)	Double-blind, randomized, placebo-controlled study	36 patients	VSL#3	6 g/day (9×10^{11}), 1 year or until relapse	Probiotics were efficient in maintaining the remission achieved with antibiotics when compared to placebo
Prevention of pouchitis					
Gionchetti et al. (2003)	Double-blind, randomized, placebo-controlled study	40 patients who underwent IPAA for UC	VSL#3	6 g/day (9×10^{11}), 1 year	Compared to placebo probiotics were efficient in increasing the remission time
Laake et al. (2004)	Open label	41 patients with UC and 10 patients with familial adenomatous polyposis	*L. acidophilus* LA-5 and *B. lactis* Bb-12	Fermented drink (500 mL), 4 weeks	The results did not demonstrate an effect of probiotics on histology, although a significant effect on the PDAI was achieved

CD, Crohn's disease; *IPAA*, ileal pouch-anal anastomosis; *LGG*, *Lacticaseibacillus rhamnosus* GG; *PDAI*, Pouchitis Disease Activity Index; *UC*, ulcerative colitis.
^aNo strains specified.

Hegazy and El-Bedewy (2010) reported that in UC patients who are undergoing treatment with sulfasalazine (an antiinflammatory medicine) supplementation with probiotics, such as *L. delbruekii* and *L. fermentum*, for 8 weeks reduced several proinflammatory indicators in the colon (i.e., IL-6, TNF-α, and NF-κB p65 expression), and also leukocyte recruitment, in comparison with the placebo and medical treatment groups.

S. boulardii also has been suggested as a way to control inflammation and to promote epithelial restoration (Coqueiro et al., 2019). In the study (Guslandi et al., 2003), *S. boulardii* was administered to patients with active UC, who were taking also their regular therapy (mesalazine) and concluded that *S. boulardii* helped with the induction of the remission. Similar conclusions were observed in the studies with VSL#3 probiotic mixture containing the *Lactobacillus* spp. (*L. casei*, *L. plantarum*, *L. acidophilus*, and *L. delbrueckii* subsp. *bulgaricus*), *Bifidobacterium* spp. (*B. longum*, *B. breve*, and *B. infantis*), and *Streptococcus salivarius* subsp. *thermophilus*. The latter probiotic mixture induced the remission and helped in reduced UC disease activity index by 60% and showed no side effects when administered in patients with active UC (Miele et al., 2009; Sivamaruthi, 2018; Tursi et al., 2010). Moreover, VSL#3 supplementation increased the load of *Bifidobacterium* spp., *Lactobacillus* spp., and *Streptococcus salivarius* ssp. *thermophilus*.

Zocco et al. (2006) evaluated the effect of LGG in the remission of UC. Patients were randomly allocated into three groups: (1) treated with probiotics; (2) treated with mesalazine; and (3) treated with probiotics and mesalazine over the period of 1 year. In the latter study, the probiotic group, without medical treatment, presented a longer maintenance of the remission period, indicating that the therapeutic effect was due to probiotics supplementation.

Overall, the effects of probiotics on inflammation and immunomodulation are associated with improvements in UC signs and symptoms (induction, maintenance, and increasing the period between relapse) as observed in growing number of clinical studies. Especially, the efficacy of probiotics in pediatric and adult UC trials had been demonstrated for VSL#3 and *E. coli* Nissle 1917 (Miele et al., 2009; Turner et al., 2012; Tursi et al., 2010; Zocco et al., 2006).

WGO global guidelines suggest that *E. coli* Nissle 1917 may be as effective as mesalazine in maintaining the remission of UC; and that VSL#3 has efficacy in the induction and maintenance of remission of mild to moderate UC

(Guarner et al., 2012). Joint ECCO and ESPGHAN Guidelines consider probiotics in children with mild UC intolerant to mesalazine, or as an adjuvant therapy in those with mild residual activity despite standard therapy. However, probiotics should be used with caution in severely immunocompromised patients or those with intravenous catheters due to the sepsis (Turner et al., 2012). ESPGHAN and North American Society for Pediatric Gastroenterology, Hepatology and Nutrition (NASPGHAN) recommend VSL#3 and *E. coli* Nissle 1917 to be considered in mild UC as an adjuvant therapy as well as in those intolerant to mesalazine (Turner et al., 2018). The ESPEN, in its most recent guidelines on clinical nutrition in IBD, recommended probiotics therapy with *E. coli* Nissle 1917 or VSL#3, as an adjuvant treatment, for the induction and maintenance of the remission period in patients with mild to moderate UC (Forbes et al., 2017). Latin-American Experts recommend VSL#3 for patients with UC (Cruchet et al., 2015). On the other hand, proposed recommendations from the expert panel for the Asia-Pacific region do not include probiotics for the treatment of IBD due to the limited evidence (Cameron et al., 2017). Similarly, the AGA does not recommend use of probiotics in children and adults with UC (Su et al., 2020).

31.3.2.3 Pouchitis

Pouchitis is a chronic inflammation of the ileal pouch that occurs in approximately 50% of the patients following ileal pouch-anal anastomosis (IPAA) for chronic UC (Nguyen et al., 2019). Therapeutic approaches include also manipulations of pouch microbiota composition for maintaining antibiotic-induced remission in patients with chronic pouchitis (Ewaschuk & Dieleman, 2006). The most frequent symptoms of pouchitis are increased number of liquid stools, abdominal cramping, and pelvic discomfort while fever and bleeding are rare. Medical treatment of pouchitis includes metronidazole or ciprofloxacin, although it is uncertain which method of treatment is best (Magro et al., 2017; Nguyen et al., 2019). Therapeutic treatment with probiotics in the treatment of pouchitis has been intensively studied on both the prevention of pouchitis as well as maintenance of remission (Nguyen et al., 2019).

Preventive effect of VSL#3 on the onset of pouchitis after restorative proctocolectomy was indicated in the RCT that included 40 participants by Gionchetti et al. (2003). The study showed that VSL#3 was efficient in preventing the development of acute pouchitis during the first year after the pouch surgery for UC and experienced a significant improvement in their quality of life. A Cochrane systematic review reports that VSL#3 was more effective than placebo for the prevention of pouchitis (Nguyen et al., 2019). Another double-blinded, prospective RCT included 20 patients who were given LGG treatment versus placebo for the period of 3 months. In contrast to VSL#3 treatment, no significant differences were observed in chronic pouchitis disease activity in LGG patients despite an increase in total counts of fecal *Lactobacillus* spp. (Kuisma et al., 2003).

When remission of pouchitis is induced by antibiotics, VSL#3 mixture can help maintain remission. Two double-blind, placebo-controlled studies have shown the high efficacy of VSL#3 to maintain remission in patients with chronic pouchitis (Gionchetti et al., 2000; Mimura et al., 2004). In the Cochrane systematic review, VSL#3 was shown to be more effective than placebo in maintaining remission of chronic pouchitis in patients who achieved remission with antibiotics (Nguyen et al., 2019).

WGO global guidelines conclude that probiotics (especially VSL#3 mixture) are recommended in preventing the initial episode of pouchitis and further relapses of pouchitis after induction of remission with antibiotics (Guarner et al., 2012). The guidelines for Asia and Pacific region suggest that in pouchitis probiotic therapy may be considered based on clinical evidence. Particularly recommended probiotic preparation is VSL#3, even though the quality of evidence is weak (Cameron et al., 2017). Next, despite growing incidence of pouchitis among Latin American children, Latin American Expert group consensus does not recommendation probiotics on this pediatric indication due to the lack of sufficient evidence in the literature among the pediatric population (Cruchet et al., 2015). On the other hand, ESPEN guidelines recommend probiotic mixture VSL#3 for prevention of pouchitis in patients with UC who have undergone colectomy and pouch-anal anastomosis (Forbes et al., 2017). Joint ECCO and ESPGHAN guidelines suggest the use of VSL#3 both for the maintenance of antibiotic-induced remission and for the prevention of pouchitis in adults (Biancone et al., 2008) and in pediatric UC (Turner et al., 2012). In adults and children with pouchitis, the AGA suggests the use of the 8-strain combination of *L. paracasei* subsp. *paracasei*, *L. plantarum*, *L. acidophilus*, *L. delbrueckii* subsp. *bulgaricus*, *B. longum* subsp *longum*, *B. breve*, *B. longum* subsp *infantis*, and *S. salivarius* subsp. *thermophilus* over no or other probiotics (Su et al., 2020).

31.3.3 Probiotics and irritable bowel syndrome

IBS is one of the most common gastrointestinal functional disorders characterized by abdominal discomfort or pain associated with alterations in bowel habits. It affects about 11% of people worldwide (Li et al., 2020; Zhang et al., 2016).

The diagnosis of IBS is based on exclusion of other severe gastrointestinal disorders and fulfilling of the Rome IV criteria, which were updated and were released in 2016 (Dale et al., 2019; Schmulson & Drossman, 2017). Major symptoms in IBS include: abdominal pain, stool pattern alteration, distention, bloating, straining, and abdominal discomfort (Didari et al., 2015). The precise cause of IBS is currently unknown. However, the pathogenesis of IBS is thought to be multifactorial and to involve chronic low-grade mucosal inflammation, alterations in gut epithelial and immune function, and visceral hypersensitivity. IBS has also been associated with alterations in intestinal microbiota and specific profiles have been associated with particular symptoms and severity of disease (Dale et al., 2019; Zhang et al., 2016). Particularly bifidobacteria counts are reportedly decreased in fecal samples from IBS patients (Niu & Xiao, 2020).

The current therapeutic options for IBS treatment include pharmacological (i.e., low-dose antidepressants, spasmolytics, and 5-hydroxytryptamine type-3 antagonists), psychological, and complementary approaches (Li et al., 2020; Zhang et al., 2016). Long-term use of medication in IBS patients is associated with adverse events and for that reason many patients turn to alternative treatments (Didari et al., 2015). New therapeutic options with the potential to alter intestinal microbiota and improve the intestinal dysbiosis have recently been identified and include the low fermentable, oligo-, di-, monosaccharides, and polyols diet, antibiotics, and probiotics (Connell et al., 2018; Staudacher, 2017). Probiotics may influence the IBS symptoms, including abdominal pain, bloating, distension, flatulence, and altered bowel movements, and alter the composition of gut microbiota (Zhang et al., 2016). Many clinical studies have investigated the effects of probiotics in IBS patients, and majority of those suggest symptom improvement (Begtrup et al., 2013; Guglielmetti et al., 2011; Staudacher, 2017; Urgesi et al., 2014; Wong et al., 2014). These improvements were observed with *L. plantarum* (DSM 9843) (Ducrotté et al., 2012), *S. boulardii* (Abbas et al., 2014), a four-strain probiotic (*B. animalis* subsp. *lactis* BB-12, *L. acidophilus* LA-5, *L. delbrueckii* subsp. *bulgaricus* LBY-27, and *S. thermophiles* STY-31) (Jafari et al., 2014), a six-strain probiotic (*B. longum*, *B. bifidum*, *B. lactis*, *L. acidophilus*, *L. rhamnosus*, and *Streptococcus thermophilus*) (Yoon et al., 2014), and others. Overall, supplementation with a multistrain probiotic demonstrated greater potential to improve IBS symptoms than a single strain (Niu & Xiao, 2020). The specific symptoms of IBS improved by probiotic supplementation were not consistent between studies. Some studies found a general improvement in IBS symptoms, whereas others reported improvement in particular symptoms (i.e., abdominal pain and bloating) (Dale et al., 2019). As shown, using a high dose of probiotics may reduce abdominal pain and bloating (Kim et al., 2018; Spiller et al., 2016; Sun et al., 2018; Yoon et al., 2014). However, despite numerous clinical trials, it is difficult to conclude in detail on which particular probiotic or combination is the most efficient in IBS patients (Dale et al., 2019). In addition, regardless to the probiotic products used, the improvement in all symptoms is unlikely.

According to the WGO global guidelines, several studies have demonstrated significant therapeutic relief with probiotics in the symptomatic treatment of IBS, although most trials were performed in adults and there is only limited evidence on the efficacy of probiotics in the treatment of IBS in children (Cruchet et al., 2015; Guarner et al., 2012). As a result of probiotic treatment, a reduction in abdominal bloating and flatulence was a consistent finding in published studies, and some strains may also reduce abdominal pain and provide systemic relief. However, due to the insufficient evidence there are no recommendations on probiotics, prebiotics or synbiotics in patients with IBS (Guarner et al., 2012). The AGA makes no recommendations for the use of probiotics in children and adults with IBS due to the significant heterogeneity in study designs, outcomes, and probiotics used in the clinical trials (Su et al., 2020). Studies on the epidemiology of IBS in the Asia-Pacific region suggest that the condition is common in that part of the world. However, based on the available data, there is insufficient evidence for the expert group to recommend probiotics in the treatment of IBS in Asia-Pacific region (Cameron et al., 2017). Likewise, due to the limitations of the available evidence, there are no recommendations on the use of probiotics for treating symptomatic children and adults with IBS made by ESPGHAN Working Group nor by AGA (Su et al., 2020). On contrary, Latin-American Experts recommend LGG and VSL#3 for improving the symptoms of IBS (Cruchet et al., 2015) (Table 31.4).

31.3.4 Probiotics and antibiotic-associated diarrhea including *C. difficile*-associated diarrhea

The use of probiotics to prevent diarrhea, a common adverse effect of antibiotic treatment, is based on the assumption that diarrhea is caused by a disruption of the ecology of the gut microbiota altering the diversity and numbers of the bacteria in the intestine (Guo et al., 2019). Antibiotic-associated diarrhea (AAD) occurs in up to a 30% of children and in up to 70% of adults treated with antibiotics, from just few hours after antibiotic administration to 2 months after the end of treatment (Blaabjerg et al., 2017). Any type of antibiotics can cause AAD, however, the risk is higher with the use of aminopenicillins, cephalosporins, and clindamycin that act on anaerobes (Szajewska et al., 2016). The symptoms range from mild and self-limiting diarrhea to severe diarrhea. In such cases, usually no pathogen is identified. However, in severe forms of AAD *C. difficile* is frequently identified (Guo et al., 2019).

TABLE 31.4 Selected clinical studies on the efficacy of probiotics for irritable bowel syndrome.

References	Type of study	Population	Probiotic	Daily dose and duration	Outcome
Bausserman and Michail (2005)	Double-blind, randomized, placebo-controlled study	Pediatric patients, N = 50	L. rhamnosus GG	6 weeks	Reduced abdominal distension otherwise negative
Guglielmetti et al. (2011)	Multicenter, double-blind, randomized, placebo-controlled study	182 adult patients with IBS	B. bifidum MIMBb75	10^9 cfu/day, 4 weeks	More than half reported reduced pain and bloating with probiotics
Begtrup et al. (2013)	Single-center, double-blind, randomized, placebo-controlled study	198 primary care patients with IBS	L. paracasei subsp. paracasei F19, L. acidophilus La5 and B. lactis Bb12	5×10^{10}, 24 weeks	Reduced pain and bloating symptoms
Wong et al. (2014)	Double-blind, randomized, placebo-controlled study	42 adult patients with IBS	VSL#3	6 weeks, 4 capsule (1×10^{11} cfu) twice per day	Reduced pain, bloating and bowel movement difficulty
Abbas et al. (2014)	Single-center, double-blind, randomized, placebo-controlled study	109 adult patients with IBS	S. boulardii	3×10^9, 6 weeks	S. boulardii group showed a significant decrease in blood and tissue levels of proinflammatory cytokines interleukin-8 (IL-8) and tumor necrosis factor-α and an increase in antiinflammatory IL-10 levels. Health-related quality of life improved in the probiotic group
Staudacher (2017)	Multicenter, double-blind, randomized, placebo-controlled study	104 adults with IBS	VSL#3	45×10^{10} cfu twice daily; 4 weeks	Significant symptom relief and increased numbers of Bifidobacterium spp.

IBS, Irritable bowel syndrome.

Numerous probiotic species have been tested, most commonly lactobacilli, bifidobacteria, and *Saccharomyces* strains (Agamennone et al., 2018; Blaabjerg et al., 2017). Evidence suggests that probiotics may have a positive effect on AAD, that is, may moderately reduce the duration of diarrhea (by almost 1 day), and both LGG and *S. boulardii* showed a similar reduction of the risk of AAD (Blaabjerg et al., 2017).

The most frequently recommended probiotics for the prevention of AAD are LGG with a minimal daily dose of 2×10^9 cfu, and *S. boulardii* (Szajewska & Kołodziej, 2015; Szajewska et al., 2016). In addition, other probiotics (such as *L. acidophilus* LA-5, *L. casei*, *L. plantarum*, *Bifidobacterium lactis*, *E. faecalis* SF68, and *Bacillus clausii*) or combination of different probiotic strains (i.e., *L. acidophilus*, *L. casei*, *Bifidobacterium longum*, *Bifidobacterium lactis* BB-12, and *Streptococcus thermophilus*) had been used (Blaabjerg et al., 2017; Sniffen et al., 2018). Probiotics were typically early with the antibiotic and continued for 1–4 weeks after antibiotics were discontinued (Sniffen et al., 2018). In the systematic review and meta-analysis of 12 RCTs, Szajewska and Kołodziej (2015) showed that LGG, compared with placebo or no treatment, is effective in preventing AAD in the overall population of adults and children treated with antibiotics for any reason. According to evidence, it is recommended to start LGG administration early, before modification of the gut microbiota and overgrowth of pathogens occur (Cameron et al., 2017).

A meta-analysis (Goldenberg et al., 2015) that included 23 RCTs testing various probiotics (either *Bacillus* spp., *Bifidobacterium* spp., *Clostridium butyricum*, *Lactobacillus* spp., *Lactococcus* spp., *Leuconostoc cremoris*, *Saccharomyces* spp., or *Streptococcus* spp., alone or in combination) for the prevention of AAD in children (0–18 years) found appropriate probiotic doses $>4 \times 10^9$ cfu/day. Strong evidence for efficacy of probiotics in preventing AAD was found for: *S. boulardii* I-745 or *L. casei* DN114001 or the multistrain formulation of *L. acidophilus* CL1285, *L. casei* LBC80R, and *L. rhamnosus* CLR2 (McFarland et al., 2018). The largest study conducted on AAD (Allen et al., 2013), included almost 3000 subjects (1493 probiotic and 1488 placebo group), and showed no significant effect of probiotic versus placebo. The subjects of the study were elderly people (>65 years of age) who were taking daily 6×10^{10} of two strains of *L. acidophilus* (CUL60 and CUL21) and two strains of bifidobacteria (*B. bifidum* CUL20 and *B. lactis* CUL34) for 21 days. The study of Allen et al. (2013) included elderly participants who may be more susceptible to adverse effects of antibiotics and for that reason the efficacy of probiotics was not observed (Allen et al., 2013).

The ESPGHAN working group provides strong recommendations for the use of LGG or *S. boulardii* CNCM I-745 for AAD prevention and a weak recommendation for the use of *S. boulardii* CNCM I-745 for the prevention of *C. difficile*-associated AAD (Szajewska et al., 2016). In Asia Pacific region as well as in the Latin America, based on clinical evidence, expert groups support probiotic administration (either LGG or *S. boulardii* CNCM I-745) for the prevention of AAD (Cameron et al., 2017; Cruchet et al., 2015). WGO recommendations for the prevention of AAD in adults include *L. acidophilus* CL1285 and *L. casei* ($\geq 10^{10}$ cfu daily); LGG (10^{10} cfu twice daily); *S. boulardii* CNCM I-745 (250 mg twice daily); *L. reuteri* DSM 17938 (10^8 cfu twice daily); and the mixture of probiotics *L. acidophilus* NCFM, *L. paracasei* Lpc-37, *Bifidobacterium lactis* Bi-07, and *B. lactis* Bl-04 (1.70^{10} cfu daily) (Guarner et al., 2017). The AGA makes no recommendations for the use of probiotics in the treatment of *C. difficile* infection (Su et al., 2020) (Table 31.5).

TABLE 31.5 Selected clinical studies on the efficacy of probiotics for AAD.

References	Type of study	Population	Probiotics	Daily dose and duration	Outcome
Wenus et al. (2008)	Randomized, placebo controlled, double blinded	Hospitalized adult patients	LGG, *L. acidophilus* LA-5, *Bifidobacterium* Bb-12	Patients were administered fermented milk drink containing LGG 10^8 cfu/mL, La-5 (10^7 cfu/mL) and Bb-12 (10^8 cfu/mL) or placebo with heat-killed bacteria, during a period of 14 days	A fermented multistrain probiotic milk drink may prevent four of five cases of AAD in adult hospitalized patients
Fox et al. (2015)	Randomized, placebo controlled, double blinded	Outpatients, Children, N = 72 (1–12 years)	LGG, *L. acidophilus* LA-5, *Bifidobacterium* Bb-12	LGG 5.2×10^9 cfu/day, Bb-12 5.9×10^9 cfu/day, La-5 8.3×10^9 cfu/day	Probiotics significantly reduced the risk of diarrhea due to the antibiotic administration
Wan et al. (2017)	Multicenter, randomized, placebo controlled, double blinded	Hospitalized children; N = 408;	*S. boulardii*	250 mg/day during antibiotic therapy	In patients treated with antibiotics for more than 5 days, the risk of diarrhea in *S. boulardii* group was reduced by 63%
Trallero et al. (2019)	Pilot, unicentric, randomized, double-blind, parallel group, placebo-controlled study	36 adult patient treated with amoxicillin-clavulanic acid (n): 18, 18	*L. acidophilus* NCFM, *L. rhamnosus* Lr-32, *B. breve* M-16V, *B. longum* BB536, *B. lactis* Bl-04, *B. bifidum* Bb-02	10^9 cfu/day 30 days	A beneficial effect of probiotics on AAD by delaying the onset of diarrhea and showed a tendency to decrease the number of daily stools versus placebo

AAD, Antibiotic-associated diarrhea; *LGG*, *Lacticaseibacillus rhamnosus* GG.

Antibiotics can disturb gastrointestinal microbiota, which might result with reduced resistance to pathogens, such as *C. difficile*, and lead to *C. difficile*-associated diarrhea (Goldenberg et al., 2017). ESPGHAN working group recommends physicians to first evaluate the patient's risk of developing AAD or *C. difficile*-associated diarrhea before deciding upon the use of probiotics. Whether the patient will develop AAD of *C. difficile*-associated diarrhea depends on various factors including class of antibiotic(s) used and duration of antibiotic treatment, age of the individual patient, need for hospitalization, comorbidities, and previous episodes of AAD or *C. difficile*-associated diarrhea (Szajewska et al., 2016).

A systematic review (Goldenberg et al., 2017) analyzed the efficacy and safety of probiotics for preventing *C. difficile*-associated diarrhea in adults and children. A complete case analysis (31 trials, 8672 participants who completed the study) showed that compared with placebo or no treatment, administration of probiotics reduced the risk of *C. difficile*-associated diarrhea by 60% in adults and children. The authors concluded that short-term use of probiotics showed to be effective and safe when used along with antibiotics in patients who are not immunocompromised or severely debilitated (Goldenberg et al., 2017). In preventing *C. difficile* infection administration of *S. boulardii* reduced the risk of developing diarrhea in children and in adults (Kotowska et al., 2005). The optimal dose of *S. boulardii* has not been established (Szajewska et al., 2016). A 2017 systematic review showed that various doses of *S. boulardii* were used with no clear dose-dependent effect (Goldenberg et al., 2017). For that reason, a daily dose of not less than 250 mg and not more than 500 mg in children and up to 1000 mg in adults could be used to match the positive effect showed in RCTs (Szajewska et al., 2016).

The working group of ESPGHAN suggests that in case if the use of probiotics for preventing *C. difficile*-associated diarrhea in children is considered, then using *S. boulardii* is recommended (Szajewska et al., 2016). The same is the recommendation in Asia-Pacific region (Cameron et al., 2017).

31.3.5 Probiotics and *Helicobacter pylori*

H. pylori infection is one of the most common chronic bacterial infections in humans, affecting about 50% of the world's population (Fontes et al., 2019; Saleem & Howden, 2020). However, the prevalence varies considerably between the regions, with greater prevalence in developing countries than in developed countries. The prevalence of *H. pylori* among European populations is between 20% and 40%, as high as 83% in Latin American countries and as low as 17% in North America (Fontes et al., 2019; Zamani et al., 2018). On the other hand, in the Eastern Mediterranean region, the prevalence of *H. pylori* is up to 80% (Eshraghian, 2014). Huge variations in country-based prevalence can be observed within Asia, from the extreme prevalence rates in Kazakhstan (79.5%) to low prevalence in Indonesia (10.0%) (Zamani et al., 2018).

H. pylori infection is usually acquired during the first year of life in both developing and developed countries (Koletzko et al., 2011). The bacterium colonizes human stomach and can lead to chronic gastritis, peptic ulcer, gastric adenocarcinoma and mucosa-associated lymphoid tissue lymphoma (Zamani et al., 2018). Approximately 20% of infected people will manifest disease; people at high risk include those who live in low- and middle-income countries with poor sanitary conditions since the mechanism of transmission seems to be oral–oral or fecal–oral (Fontes et al., 2019). There are several antibiotic regimens available to treat the infection along with proton-pump inhibitors; however, antibiotic resistance of *H. pylori* is increasing around the world shifting the focus from antibiotics to alternative therapies, such as probiotics, curcumin, statins, and *N*-acetylcystein, for the treatment of infection and enhancement of eradication (Fontes et al., 2019). Probiotics help to competitively inhibit the colonization of *H. pylori* and produce bacteriostatic compounds (Shi et al., 2019). In addition, probiotics, such as *Lactobacillus* spp., *Bifidobacterium* spp., and *Saccharomyces boulardii*, have been evaluated as an adjuvant of eradication treatment reducing the adverse side effects of antibiotic treatment (i.e., AAD, vomiting or abdominal pain). Boonyaritichaikij et al. (2009), Cruchet et al. (2003), Gotteland et al. (2007), McFarland et al. (2015, 2016), Shi et al. (2019), and Zhu et al. (2014) concluded in their meta-analysis that supplementary probiotic preparations during standard triple *H. pylori* therapy may improve the eradication rate and the incidence of total adverse effects.

Several clinical trials have evaluated the role of probiotics in adults and children colonized with *H. pylori*. Emerging evidence suggests an inhibitory effect of *Lactobacillus* spp. and *Bifidobacterium* spp. on *H. pylori* (Wang et al., 2013; Zhang et al., 2015). In a study (Lionetti et al., 2006) evaluating adjunctive probiotic supplementation, eradication of 82.5% was obtained from a group of 40 children receiving eradication therapy for *H. pylori* therapy. A study by Hurduc et al. (2009) showed that the incidence of side effects was significantly reduced when *S. boulardii* was used. Two probiotics have strong strength of efficacy evidence for preventing adverse events associated with treatments for *H. pylori* (*S. boulardii* I-745 and the mixture of *L. helveticus* R52 + *L. rhamnosus* R11), while LGG only showed moderate strength. In addition, the same three probiotics may be valuable in preventing side effects of therapy but may not be effective in eradicating *H. pylori* (Sniffen et al., 2018).

Studies on *L. johnsonii*, *S. boulardii* ± inulin or *L. acidophilus* LB, and *L. gasseri* OLL2716 (LG21) indicate that they help maintaining lower levels of the pathogen in the gastric mucosa but that they do not eradicate *H. pylori* (Boonyaritichaikij et al., 2009; Cruchet et al., 2003; Gotteland et al., 2007; Pacifico et al., 2014). However, in studies in which probiotics (i.e., LGG, *L. casei*, *B. animalis*, *S. boulardii*, or combination of *L. casei* DN-114001, *L. bulgaricus*, and *S. thermophilus*) were used together with proton pump inhibitors and antibiotics, eradication rates moderately increased (Goldman et al., 2006; Hurduc et al., 2009; Sykora et al., 2004; Sýkora et al., 2005).

Nonetheless, due to the heterogeneity of studies and use of different probiotic strains and concentrations, optimal dose, and the time of dosing, the duration of therapy remains unclear and the role of adjuvant probiotic therapy to reduce adverse side effects, improve adherence, and thereby, increase the efficacy of *H. pylori* eradication remains controversial (Ji & Yang, 2020; Jones et al., 2017; Losurdo et al., 2018).

Joint ESPGHAN/NASPGHAN Guidelines for the Management of *H. pylori* in Children and Adolescents do not recommend the routine addition of either single or combination probiotics to eradication therapy to reduce side effects and/or improve eradication rates due to the fact that it is not supported by current evidence (Jones et al., 2017). Likewise, due to the lack of sufficient evidence Latin-American Expert group consensus does not recommend the use of probiotics for the treatment of *H. pylori* infection (Cruchet et al., 2015). WGO global guidelines report that several *Lactobacillus* spp. appear to reduce the side effects of eradication therapies for *H. pylori* and improve patient compliance. However, there is insufficient evidence to recommend the approach of using probiotic alone, without antibiotic therapy, as effective therapy against *H. pylori* infection (Guarner et al., 2012). On the other hand, based on available data, the Asia-Pacific expert panel suggests that probiotic, such as *S. boulardii* CNCM I-745, may be considered for the prevention of side effects of antibiotic therapy for *H. pylori* and for improving eradication rates in children (Cameron et al., 2017) (Table 31.6).

31.3.6 Recommendations for the use of probiotics in intestinal diseases by geographic location

Table 31.7 includes the recommendations on probiotic use for gastrointestinal diseases according to geographic region. As obvious from Table 31.7 by far the most commonly recommended probiotics are LGG, *Limosilactobacillus reuteri* DSM 17938 and *Saccharomyces boulardii* as well as the probiotic dietary supplement VSL#3 (Danisco-Dupont USA). This probiotic supplement is also known as Vivomixx in Europe or Visbiome in the United States and the De Simone formulation (DSF). Claudio Simone, MD, is the inventor of this 8 strain—450 billion probiotic formulation or the DSF, containing: *L. plantarum* DSM24730, *S. thermophilus* DSM24731, *B. breve* DSM24732, *L. paracasei* DSM24733, *L. delbrueckii* subsp. *bulgaricus* DSM24734, *L. acidophilus* DSM 24735, *B. longum* DSM24736, and *B. infantis* DSM24737. According to De Simone, DSF has been referred to as VSL#3 in the main *Gastroenterology Association Guidelines*; however, the current brand of VSL#3 does not contain the DSF any longer and many clinical studies are using this name and citing the DSF (De Simone, 2018a,b). This stresses the importance of careful strain-specific selection of probiotics.

31.4 Regulations for use of probiotics in diseases other than gastrointestinal diseases

This chapter contains the results of a selection of clinical trials on the efficacy of probiotics and the regulations on the use of probiotics where applicable for allergies, anxiety, depression and other mood disorders, wound healing and wound infections, and common acute infections.

31.4.1 Probiotics and allergies

Allergic diseases represent a spectrum of health conditions and a worldwide burden in different populations. In the field of allergy and immunology, the focus on prevention has become as important as effective disease management (Fiocchi et al., 2015). Allergic diseases have been linked to genetic and/or environmental factors, such as antibiotic use and westernized high fat and low fiber diet, which lead to altered microbial exposure and early intestinal dysbiosis, and account for the rise in allergy prevalence, especially in western countries. Exposure to these factors in early life is critical, and prenatal exposure may provide the greatest protection. Allergic diseases have shown reduced microbial diversity, including fewer lactobacilli and bifidobacteria, within the neonatal microbiota, before the onset of atopic diseases

TABLE 31.6 Selected clinical studies on the efficacy of probiotics for the eradication of *Helicobacter pylori*.

References	Type of study	Population	Probiotic	Daily dose and duration	Outcome
Sýkora et al. (2005)	Multicenter, prospective randomized double-blind study	86 symptomatic *H. pylori*-positive children	*L. casei* DN-114 001	Children received either eradication therapy or eradication therapy supplemented with fermented milk with 10^{10} cfu/mL for 14 days	Supplementation with fermented milk enhanced therapeutic benefit on *H. pylori* eradication in children with gastritis on triple therapy
Goldman et al. (2006)	Randomized, placebo-controlled study	65 symptomatic *H. Pylori*-positive children	*Bifidobacterium animalis* and *Lactobacillus casei*	Children received either eradication therapy or eradication therapy supplemented with yogurt containing 10^7 cfu/mL for 3 months	Supplementation with yogurt did not demonstrate an adjuvant effect of probiotic to eradication therapy in treatment of *H. pylori* infection
Szajewska et al. (2009)	Double-blind, randomized, placebo-controlled study	83 children with *H. pylori* infection	LGG	10^9 cfu/day, 7 days together with triple eradication regimen of placebo with triple eradication regimen	In children with *H. pylori* infection, supplementation of standard triple therapy with LGG did not significantly alter the eradication rate or side effects
Seddik et al. (2019)	Open-label prospective, randomized study	199 patients positive for *H. pylori* infection	*S. boulardii* CNCM I-745	50% of patients received standard sequential therapy and 50% sequential therapy plus bid *S. boulardii* 250 mg daily for 4 weeks	Addition of *S. boulardii* to sequential therapy improved *H. pylori* eradication rate and reduced the incidence of treatment-associated adverse side-effects
Cárdenas et al. (2020)	Single-blind randomized trial	63 patients positive for *H. pylori* infection	*S. boulardii* CNCM I-745	34 patients received eradication therapy and 29 eradication therapy supplemented with 750 mg of *S. boulardii* CNCM I-745 daily, for 2 weeks	Addition of *S. boulardii* CNCM I-745 induced a lower frequency of gastrointestinal symptoms that could be related to changes in gut microbiota

LGG, Lacticaseibacillus rhamnosus GG.

(Boyle et al., 2011; Kasatpibal et al., 2017). The immunomodulatory properties of probiotics have been proposed as a preventive intervention for the development of allergic diseases (Ricci et al., 2016).

Eczema, as defined by the WAO, encompasses both atopic and nonatopic conditions and is commonly referred to as atopic eczema (AE) or atopic dermatitis (AD). The clinical characteristics are itching, skin inflammation, a skin barrier abnormality, and susceptibility to skin infection. Although not always recognized by healthcare professionals as being a serious medical condition, AE can have a significant negative impact on the quality of life for children and their parents and care takers (Lu et al., 2018). Asthma, the most common chronic inflammatory respiratory disease, can affect people of any age, especially children. As probiotics affect immune cells, such as macrophages, dendrite cells, T cells, and natural and killer cells, and suppress allergen induced in inflammatory response, their preventive effect in allergies is being intensively researched (Lin et al., 2018).

Several systematic reviews and meta-analysis have found benefits of probiotic supplementation for AD (Jiang et al., 2020) and allergic rhinitis (Güvenç et al., 2016), but not enough evidence for asthma incidence (Wei et al., 2020) or AE (Lu et al., 2018) in infants. With the ever rising pool of clinical studies, the most promising probiotic strains are being identified in specific allergies so that adjuvant therapies with probiotics can be recommended (Güvenç et al., 2016).

TABLE 31.7 Recommendations on probiotic use for intestinal diseases according to geographic region.

Disease	Europe	United States	Latin America	Asia-Pacific region
Acute gastroenteritis	L. rhamnosus GG, S. boulardii, L. reuteri DSM 17938	L. rhamnosus GG, S. boulardii	L. rhamnosus GG, S. boulardii, L. reuteri DSM 17938	L. rhamnosus GG, S. boulardii
AAD	L. rhamnosus GG, S. boulardii	L. rhamnosus GG, S. boulardii	L. rhamnosus GG, S. boulardii	L. rhamnosus GG, S. boulardii
C. difficile-associated diarrhea	S. boulardii			S. boulardii
IBD (CD, UC, pouchitis)	E. coli Nissle 1917, VSL#3		VSL#3	VSL#3
IBS	Insufficient evidence		L. rhamnosus GG, VSL#3	Insufficient evidence
HP	Insufficient evidence	Insufficient evidence	Insufficient evidence	S. boulardii

AAD, Antibiotic-associated diarrhea; *CD*, Crohn's disease; *HP*, Helicobacter pylori; *IBD*, inflammatory bowel disease; *IBS*, irritable bowel syndrome; *UC*, ulcerative colitis.

Various combinations of lactobacilli, such as *L. rhamnosus*, *L. acidophilus*, or *L. paracasei* strains, and bifidobacteria, such as *B. bifidum*, *B. longum*, or *B. lactis* strains, have successful in achieving protective effects against allergic diseases in infants after maternal or infant supplementation, (Kim et al., 2010; Rautava et al., 2012; Wickens et al., 2012). The immune effects necessary for eczema prevention in probiotic studies are not clear. Reduced cord blood IFN-γ is associated with increased risk for eczema in early life, suggesting prenatal interventions, such as probiotics, which modulate the developing fetal immune system may be effective for eczema prevention (Boyle et al., 2011).

The World Allergy Organization and McMaster University Guidelines (Fiocchi et al., 2015) in their abstract have noted that intestinal microbiota may modulate immunological and inflammatory systemic responses and that probiotic supplementation has been proposed as a preventive intervention. Based on current available evidence they therefore recommend the use of probiotics (1) in pregnant women who are carrying a child with a high risk of allergy, (2) in breast-feeding women when the infant faces a high risk of developing allergy, and (3) in infants at high risk of developing allergy (Fiocchi et al., 2015; Hojsak et al., 2018). However, the WAO did not find differences in the effects among probiotics but that does not imply that such a difference does not exist. Therefore further research of possible differences among the strains of the same species might be warranted. They also state that there is a need for rigorously designed and well-executed randomized trials of probiotics in breast-feeding women that would properly measure and report patient-important outcomes, including quality of life and adverse effects. Long-term follow-up of such studies to evaluate long-term effects is also needed (Fiocchi et al., 2015) (Table 31.8).

31.4.2 Probiotics and anxiety, depression, and other mood disorders

Depression is a common mental disorder that may lead to marked disabilities in affected patients and has become a leading cause of global burden of disease. Current pharmacological treatment includes antidepressants, whose mechanisms are based on modulating monoamine neurotransmitters. Depression and anxiety disorders are the two most common mental health conditions. Accumulating data indicate that the gut microbiota can influence brain function and behavior via the gut–brain axis, including mood symptoms (Goh et al., 2019; Liu et al., 2019). It is known that bacteria in the intestine and probiotics can produce many chemicals, including neurotransmitters, such as serotonin, melatonin, dopamine, norepinephrine, acetylcholine, and endocannabinoids. These may directly impact brain function and mental health. The neurons present in the enteric nervous system interact directly with the neurochemicals produced by microbiota of the gut, thereby influencing the signaling to central nervous system (Cerdó et al., 2017; Sharma et al., 2021; Smith & Wissel, 2019). An altered gut microbiota in the form of dysbiosis at the extremes of life, both in the neonate and in the elderly, can have a profound impact on brain function. Therefore consumption of probiotics, such as psychobiotics, to alter composition of gut microbiota may be a novel way to treat patients with various mood disorders (Dinan & Cryan, 2017; Goh et al., 2019; Liu et al., 2019).

TABLE 31.8 Selected clinical studies on the efficacy of probiotics for allergies.

References	Type of study	Population	Probiotic	Daily dose and duration	Outcome
Isolauri et al. (2000)	Randomized, double-blind, placebo-controlled trial	27 infants with atopic eczema (mean age 4.6 months)	LGG and B. lactis Bb-12	3×10^8 cfu LGG, 10^9 cfu BB12 (for 6 months)	After 2 months, a significant improvement in skin condition occurred in patients given probiotic-supplemented formulas, as compared to the unsupplemented group
Kalliomäki et al. (2007)	Randomized, placebo-controlled trial follow-up	116 mother–infant pairs (n): 53, 62.	LGG	10^{10} cfu (for weeks before delivery and 6 months postnatally)	The risk of eczema was significantly reduced in the LGG group compared with the placebo group
Kim et al. (2010)	Randomized, double-blind, placebo-controlled trial	112 pregnant women with a family history of allergic diseases (n: 57,55)	B. bifidum BGN4, B. lactis AD011, L. acidophilus AD031	Total 4.8×10^9 cfu (4–8 weeks before delivery until 6 months breastfeeding infants)	The cumulative incidence of eczema during the first 12 months was reduced significantly in probiotic group. Prenatal and postnatal supplementation is an effective approach in preventing the development of eczema in infants at high risk of allergy during the first year of life
Boyle et al. (2011)	Randomized control trial	250 pregnant women with high risk for allergic disease	LGG	1.8×10^{10} cfu (from 36 weeks gestation to delivery)	Prenatal treatment with LGG was not sufficient for preventing eczema. If probiotics are effective for preventing eczema, then a postnatal component to treatment or possibly an alternative probiotic strain is necessary
Wickens et al. (2012)	Randomized, double-blind, placebo-controlled trial	425 infants in follow-up	L. rhamnosus HN001	6×10^9 cfu (from 35 weeks gestation until 6 months breastfeeding infants)	The protective effect of HN001 against eczema, when given for the first 2 years of life, extended to at least 4 years of age. This suggests that this probiotic might be an appropriate preventative intervention for high risk infants
Rautava et al. (2012)	Parallel, double-blind placebo-controlled trial	241 mother–infant pairs. Mothers with allergic disease and atopic sensitization	(1) L. rhamnosus LPR and B. longum BL999 and (2) L paracasei ST11 and B longum BL999	Total 2×10^9 cfu (2 months before delivery and during the first 2 months of breast-feeding)	Prevention regimen with specific probiotics administered to the pregnant and breast-feeding mother, that is, prenatally and postnatally, is safe and effective in reducing the risk of eczema in infants with allergic mothers

LGG, Lacticaseibacillus rhamnosus GG.

Several reviews with meta-analyses were found on the efficacy of probiotics for depressive symptoms and anxiety (Chao et al., 2020; Goh et al., 2019; Huang et al., 2016; Liu et al., 2019). The main probiotics with a significant effect in reducing depression or anxiety, measured by Beck Depression Inventory scale, Beck Anxiety Inventory scale, Profile of Mood States, Hamilton Depression Rating Scale, and other rating scales in these studies included various strains of lactobacilli alone or in combination with bifidobacteria strains, although studies using *B. coagulans*, *S. thermophilus* strains were also found (Liu et al., 2019); however, some studies found that various species of lactobacilli alone did not have an effect on depression and that lactobacilli alone or in combination with other probiotics did not have an effect on anxiety (Liu et al., 2019); therefore strain selection is very important and future studies with clinically significant presentations are indicated and necessary adequately to evaluate the potential efficacy of probiotics for depression and anxiety. This is especially important given the increasing need for the development of novel psychopharmacological agents for these conditions (Liu et al., 2019).

The Royal Australian and New Zealand College of Physiatrists clinical practice guidelines published in 2020 (Malhi et al., 2021) have mentioned the gut–brain axis and clinical studies supporting the benefits of supplementing probiotics in the management of depressive disorders and suggest that probiotics might be helpful as one of the strategies for instituting a healthy diet but emphasize that further research is necessary. Differences in quantity of dose, type of strain, type of prebiotic, assessment of gut microbiota, duration of intervention, standardization of neurological measurements, variety and complexity of neurological symptoms, study design, and cohort size make it difficult to confirm evidence of efficacy (Chao et al., 2020). Accumulating evidence of high-quality clinical studies will therefore contribute to future clinical guidelines for probiotic supplementation for mood disorders (Table 31.9).

TABLE 31.9 Selected clinical studies on the efficacy of probiotics for anxiety, depression, and other mood disorders.

References	Type of study	Population	Probiotic	Daily dose and duration	Outcome
Steenbergen et al. (2015)	Triple-blind, randomized, controlled trial	40 young adults (n): 20/20	B. bifidum W23, B. lactis W52, L. acidophilus W37, L. brevis W63, L. casei W56, L. salivarius W24, L. lactis W19 and W58	2.5×10^9 cfu (4 weeks)	Participants with probiotics intervention showed a significantly reduced overall cognitive reactivity to but BDI total score revealed no main effect of time
Östlund-Lagerström et al. (2016)	Randomized, double-blind, placebo-controlled trial	290 senior citizens aged >65 years (n): 125/165	L. reuteri DSM 17983	10^8 cfu (12 weeks)	Probiotic treatment did not significantly affect depression score
Slykerman et al. (2017)	Randomized, double-blind, placebo-controlled trial	423 pregnant women at 14–16 weeks' gestation (n): 193/230	L. rhamnosus HN001	6×10^9 cfu (6 months)	Mothers in the probiotic treatment group reported significantly lower depression scores than those in the placebo group
Ghorbani et al. (2018)	Randomized multicenter trial	40 adults aged between 18 and 55 with major depressive disorder (n): 20/20	L. casei, L. acidophilus, L. bulgaricus, L. rhamnosus, B. breve, B. longum, S. thermophilus[a]	Total 4.3×10^9 cfu (6 weeks)	Probiotic group had a significantly decreased HDRS score
Kazemi et al. (2019)	Randomized control trial	74 patients with major depressive disorder (n): 38/36	L. helveticus R0052, B. longum R0175	2×10^9 cfu (8 weeks)	Probiotic supplementation resulted in a significant decrease in BDI score

BDI, Beck Depression Inventory; *HDRS*, Hamilton Depression Rating Scale.
[a] No strains specified.

Probiotics can affect mental state, sleep quality, or healthy adults under stressful conditions via changes in gut microbiota (Nishida et al., 2019). They also seem to effect cognitive functions as well as learning power and memory in people with Alzheimer's disease (Akbari et al., 2016). Children with autism spectrum disorder seem to have a dysbiosis disorder with a significantly higher abundance of the genera *Bacteroides*, *Parabacteroides*, *Clostridium*, *Faecalibacterium*, and *Phascolarctobacterium* and a lower percentage of *Coprococcus* and *Bifidobacterium* (Iglesias-vázquez et al., 2020). Thus the wide range of applications for probiotics seems limitless.

31.4.3 Probiotics and wound healing and wound infection

Skin damage can be caused by a variety of different reasons, such as trauma (including cuts, abrasions, chemical burns, fire burns, cold, heat, radiation, surgery), or as a consequence of underlying illnesses, such as diabetes. The most effective wound management strategy is to prevent infections, promote healing, and prevent excess scarring (Fijan et al., 2019; Mihai et al., 2018). However, possible use of live microorganisms on wounds, such as probiotics, represents a major shift in the paradigm of the current doctrine of wound treatment as well as the traditional teaching of "germ theory" where the idea of using bacteria to fight bacteria is not intuitive (Reid et al., 2003; Siddharthan et al., 2018). To achieve some the healing properties of probiotic metabolites some researchers recommend the use of cell-free supernatants or extracts (Bermudez-Brito et al., 2012; Guéniche et al., 2009; Lukic et al., 2017), but as mentioned in the introduction, this no longer refers to probiotics, which need to be live microorganisms.

Lactobacilli and bifidobacteria, such as strains of *L. reuteri*, *L. plantarum*, *L. rhamnosus*, and *B. longum*, have the proven ability to interact with various cells and to induce host mucosal defense systems as well as various tissue repair mechanisms and dermatological disorders, including nonhealing wounds; therefore they also make ideal probiotic candidates to directly inhibit pathogens' growth and promote healing of the skin. Other nonconventional probiotics, such as strains of *Streptococcus thermophilus* and *Staphylococcus epidermidis*, commonly associated with healthy skin microbiome, have also shown beneficial effects on cutaneous repair. The effects have been proven through the gut–skin axis as well as in topical form (Fijan et al., 2019; Lukic et al., 2017). The adjuvant role of probiotics together with antibiotics in the treatment of chronic wounds is also an emerging area (Kadam et al., 2019). The problem with chronic wounds is the formation of biofilms composed of a community of microorganisms in which the overall effect in the community unit is greater than the sum of its singular or specific parts, thus an important approach to promote wound healing could be to enable an "ecological shift" that increases growth of nonproblematic bacteria, possibly involving the use of probiotics (Fonseca, 2011).

The Organization for Economic Cooperation and Development emphasizes that it is necessary to strengthen the scientific evidence of alternative therapies and also states that probiotics are a promising alternative therapy to the topical use of antibiotics due to the increasing occurrence and transmission of antibiotic-resistant microorganisms (Cecchini et al., 2015). The European Wound Medical Association does not mention probiotics as adjuvant therapy in its regulations for chronic wounds as there are not enough yet rigorous clinical and scientific data to propose concrete recommendations. However, they are mentioned in their journal as one possible route in promoting wound healing (Fonseca, 2011).

There are no systematic reviews or meta-analyses on the effect of probiotics and wound healing, but there are 13 meta-analyses on the effect of probiotics and wound infections after hepatic resections, colorectal cancer surgery, gastrointestinal surgery, liver transplantation or resections, abdominal surgery, reducing postoperative complications, and elective surgery. Of these, it was found that probiotics were effective in reducing postoperative infections for colorectal cancer surgery patients (Chen et al., 2020; Ouyang et al., 2019; Wu, Xu, et al., 2018) and abdominal surgery patients (Pitsouni et al., 2009) as well as reducing general surgical site infections (Kasatpibal et al., 2017; Kinross et al., 2013; Lytvyn et al., 2016; Wu, Liu, et al., 2018) and shortening duration of hospitalization after liver resection (Gan et al., 2019). All these data indicate that probiotics taken together with prebiotics show great potential as adjunctive therapy in preventing wound infections and that current evidence suggests the probiotics in combination with antibiotics could be recommended, but that more rigorous, high-quality multicentered clinical studies are needed.

Only two clinical studies used topical application of *L. plantarum* ATCC 1024 on infected wounds: in one case, a burn wound (Peral et al., 2009) and, in the other case, chronic foot ulcers (Peral et al., 2010). In the clinical study on burns, it was found that the topical application of the *L. plantarum* ATCC 1024 on burns was as effective against pathogens as topical application of silver ions (Peral et al., 2009). In the second clinical study on diabetic patients with chronic ulcers, topical application of *L. plantarum* ATCC 1024, besides achieving a statistically significant decrease in pathogen load after 10 compared to day 1 with topical probiotic treatment, also improved healing; higher production of IL-8 and a reduction in the number of infected ulcers was furthermore achieved (Peral et al., 2010). There were two additional studies (El-Ghazely et al., 2016; Mayes et al., 2015) with oral use of probiotics. All these studies resulted in a decreased pathogenic load with probiotic administration.

The next five clinical trials noted in Table 31.10 (Aisu et al., 2015; Kanazawa et al., 2005; Kotzampassi et al., 2015; Rayes et al., 2005; Usami et al., 2011) involved investigation of the reduction of surgical site infections after various surgery using different combination of probiotics, including: *B. breve* Yakult, *B. lactis* BB-12, *B. mesentericus* TO-A, *C. butyricum* TO-A, *E. faecalis* T110, *L. acidophilus* LA-5, *L. casei* Shirota, *L. delbrueckii*, *L. fermentum*, *L. mesenteroides* LMG P-20607, *L. paracasei* subsp. *paracasei* LMG P-17806, *L. plantarum* LMG P-20606, LGG, *P. pentosaceus* LMG P-20608, and *S. boulardii*. All studies resulted in a reduction of the surgical site infection thus indirectly influencing wound healing.

31.4.4 Probiotics and common acute infections

Most common acute infections include upper respiratory tract infections (URTI) and AGE. They also cause more outpatient doctor and emergency care visits and higher antibiotic use (Haskins, 1989; Hojsak et al., 2018). Several common acute infections are viral illnesses, such as colds and influenza, where inappropriate antibiotic use is common (King et al., 2019). Evidence suggests that probiotic supplementation reduces episodes of common infectious diseases including respiratory tract infections through improvement of immune function (Hao et al., 2015). In addition, probiotic supplementation reduces the duration of symptoms in otherwise healthy children and adults with common acute respiratory conditions (King et al., 2014, 2019).

Infections occur in elderly as the immune system weakens with age (Hao et al., 2015). At least three randomized clinical studies have also been found on the effectiveness of probiotics for URTI in elderly (Fujita et al., 2013; Guillemard et al., 2010; Turchet et al., 2003). One study was a monocentric, randomized, stratified, open, pilot study, where 360 community residents over 60 years of age were randomized to receive (1) one 100-mL bottle of Actimel (a milk fermented with yogurt cultures and *L. casei* DN-114 001, containing 10^8 cfu/mL twice daily for 3 weeks) or (2) they were in the control group (Turchet et al., 2003). The study found no difference in the incidence of winter infections between groups. However, they found that the duration of all pathologies and maximal temperature was significantly lower in the treatment group than in the control group. The other study was also a multicentric, double-blind controlled trial, involving 1072 volunteers (median age 76 years) randomized to consumption of either probiotic strain *L. casei* DN-114 001 or control for 3 months (Guillemard et al., 2010). The probiotic group was associated with a decreased duration of common infectious diseases in comparison to the control group, especially URTI. The study considering the effect of probiotics among elderly people (mean age 83 years) (Fujita et al., 2013) was conducted with 76 participants in the probiotics group and 78 participants in the placebo group. The results showed that probiotics did not reduce the episode rates of acute URTI but did reduce their duration.

Common acute infections in children are a significant burden for health care, especially for children attending day care centers, who have a two to three times higher chance of acquiring common infections than children who stay at home (Hojsak et al., 2018; Silverstein et al., 2003). Probiotic treatment during infancy has been associated with other beneficial health effects, including reduced rates of infection and gastrointestinal symptoms (Boyle et al., 2011). If probiotics are considered for the prevention of URTI in children attending day care centers during winter months, only LGG could be a proposed probiotic as evidence is limited and meta-analyses confirming its efficacy are lacking (Hojsak et al., 2018).

Probiotics, provided to reduce the risk for common acute infections, may be associated with reduced antibiotic use in infants and children. Additional well-designed studies are needed to substantiate these findings in children and explore similar findings in other population groups (King et al., 2019). Their potential biological role against COVID-19 infection also warrants further clinical and laboratory investigation (Khaled, 2020).

In the systematic review and meta-analysis on the effect of probiotics on the duration of acute respiratory infections in healthy children and adults (King et al., 2014), it was found that in seven RCTs, a significantly fewer numbers of days of illness per person, shorter illness episodes by almost a day, and fewer numbers of days absent from day care/school/work were noted in participants who received a probiotic intervention than in those who had taken a placebo. The main probiotics used were LGG, *L. reuteri* ATCC 55730, *L. plantarum* DSM 15312, *L. delbrueckii* subsp. *bulgaricus*, *L. paracasei* DSM 13434, *L. paracasei* subsp. *casei* DN-114001, *L. acidophilus* NCFM, *B. lactis* BB-12, and *B. animalis* subsp. *lactis* Bi-07. This review included a large number of high-quality studies that demonstrate a consistent trend in favor of probiotics, the results are probably reliable. Further research and meta-analyses are recommended in different population groups to identify potential sources of variability in the results (Table 31.11).

TABLE 31.10 Selected clinical studies on the efficacy of probiotics for wound healing and wound infections.

References	Type of study	Population	Probiotic	Daily dose and duration	Outcome
Rayes et al. (2005)	Randomized, double blind	Liver transplant surgery (n): 33/33	P. pentosaceus LMG P-20608, L. mesenteroides LMG P-20607, L. paracasei subsp. paracasei LMG P-17806; L. plantarum LMG P-20606 (10^{10} cfu)	Oral (starting on the day of surgery for 2 weeks)	Lower incidence of wound infection, significantly lower overall postoperative bacterial infections. Significantly lower duration of antibiotic therapy
Kanazawa et al. (2005)	Randomized, controlled	Biliary cancer surgery (n): 21/23	L. casei Shirota, B. breve Yakult (2×10^8 cfu)	Oral (for 14 days after surgery)	Significantly lower incidence of overall infections. Lower, but not statistically significant, incidence of wound infections. Slightly lower duration of postoperative antibiotic therapy
Peral et al. (2009)	Prospective	Patients with second- and third-degree burns (n): 38/42	L. plantarum ATCC 10241 (10^5 cfu)	Daily topical application for 10 days	Topical probiotic treatment of second-degree burn patients was as effective as silver sulfadiazine in control group in decreasing pathogen load
Peral et al. (2010)	Prospective	Chronic infected leg ulcers (n): 34	L. plantarum ATCC 10241 (10^5 cfu)	Daily topical application for 10 days	Statistically significant decrease of pathogen load after 10 days ($P<.001$) compared to day 1 with topical probiotic treatment
Usami et al. (2011)	Two arm, randomized, controlled	Hepatic surgery (n): 32/29	L. casei Shirota, B. breve Yakult (2×10^8 cfu)	Oral (14 days before operation and 11 days allowed food intake)	No infectious complications after surgery in probiotic group resulting in a statistically significant difference ($P<.05$)
Mayes et al. (2015)	Randomized, blinded	Burn injury (n): 10/10	LGG (1.5×10^{10} cfu)	Oral (start within 10 days after burn and until 95% wound closure)	Trend of less requirement for antifungal agents ($P=.03$) in probiotic group. No significant difference in number of days of antibiotic therapy
Aisu et al. (2015)	Clinical trial	Colorectal cancer surgery (n): 75/81	E. faecalis T110, C. butyricum TO-A, B. mesentericus TO-A (no information on concentration)	Oral (15 days prior surgery, restarted the same day the patient started drinking water after surgery	Significant lower surgical superficial incisional site infection ($P=.016$)
Kotzampassi et al. (2015)	Randomized, double blinded, placebo controlled	Colorectal cancer surgery (n): 84/80	L. acidophilus LA-5, L. plantarum, B. lactis BB-12, S. boulardii (5.5×10^9 cfu)[a]	Oral (1 day prior to operation and 14 days after surgery)	Statistically significant decrease in surgical site infections ($P=.02$)
El-Ghazely et al. (2016)	Randomized, double blinded, controlled	Pediatric thermal burn (n): 20/20	L. fermentum and L. delbrueckii (2.0×10^9 cfu)[a]	Oral—during hospital stay	Trend toward decrease in infection incidence ($P=.113$)

[a] No strains specified.

TABLE 31.11 Selected clinical studies on the efficacy of probiotics for common infections, including respiratory tract infections.

References	Type of study	Population	Probiotic	Daily dose and duration	Outcome
Leyer et al. (2009)	Double-blind, placebo-controlled study	Children 3–5 years (n): 112, 110, 104	L. acidophilus NCFM, B. lactis Bi-07	(a) 10^{10} cfu L. acidophilus NCFM, (b) 10^{10} cfu L. acidophilus NCFM and B. lactis Bi-07 (6 months)	Daily dietary probiotic supplementation for 6 months was a safe effective way to reduce fever, rhinorrhea, and cough incidence and duration and antibiotic prescription incidence, as well as the number of missed school days attributable to illness
Hojsak et al. (2010)	Randomized, double-blind, placebo-controlled study	742 hospitalized children	LGG	10^9 cfu daily from day of admission until discharge from hospital	LGG administration can be recommended as a valid measure for decreasing the risk for nosocomial gastrointestinal and respiratory tract infections in pediatric facilities
Guillemard et al. (2010)	Randomized double-blind, placebo-controlled trial	1072 free living elderly	L. paracasei subsp. casei DN-114001, S. thermophilus, L. delbrueckii subsp. bulgaricus	3 months	Consumption of a fermented dairy product containing the probiotic strain L. casei DN-114 001 in elderly was associated with a decreased duration of common infectious diseases, especially upper respiratory tract infections, such as rhinopharyngitis
Berggren et al. (2011)	Randomized, double-blind, placebo-controlled study	272 subjects (n): 135, 137	L. plantarum DSM 15312, L. paracasei DSM 13434	10^9 cfu probiotics daily for 12 weeks	Intake of the probiotic strains reduced the risk of acquiring common cold infections
Smith et al. (2013)	Double-blind, placebo-controlled study	231 healthy college students (n): 101, 97	LGG, B. lactis BB-12	10^{10} cfu for 12 weeks	Probiotics group missed significantly fewer school days. LGG and BB-12 may be beneficial among college students with upper respiratory infections for mitigating decrements in health-related quality of life
Lazou Ahrén et al. (2020)	Randomized, double-blind, placebo-controlled study	106 children during common cold season	L. plantarum HEAL9 and L. paracasei 8700:2	10^9 cfu probiotics daily for 3 months	Intake of L. plantarum HEAL9 and L. paracasei 8700:2 once daily for a period of 3 months was beneficial to children and reduced the severity of common colds

LGG, Lacticaseibacillus rhamnosus GG.

31.5 Conclusions

This chapter focused on the prevention of a selection of diseases or pathologies for which various scientific evidence has proven that certain probiotic strains are effective. However, not all possible diseases or pathologies for which probiotics can be effective were included. Some examples include infantile colic, necrotizing enterocolitis, etc. For some of the investigated diseases, recommendations were not warranted despite several published clinical studies as not all clinical studies are without bias and high quality to be generalized for healthcare recommendations via meta-analyses.

With increasing knowledge about the essential role of gut microbiome in the human health, the gut microbiome is now considered an important ally, interacting with most human cells (Cani, 2018). The discovery of links, or axes, for instance, the "gut–brain" and "gut–brain-skin," has opened up new research dimensions. Besides mechanistic studies on fundamental topics (such as antimicrobial activity, competitive exclusion, immunomodulation, and strengthening of the intestinal epithelial barrier function), much research is focused on mechanisms of microbiome effects on the immune, the central nervous, and the endocrine systems (Clarke et al., 2014; Salem et al., 2018; Zhou & Foster, 2015). These revolutionary discoveries about the importance of the human microbiome for human health have also accelerated further development of the probiotic sector. Scientific evidence of probiotic benefits on human health is continuously expanding (Fijan et al., 2019).

In light of all this, more high-quality and well-designed double-blind, randomized, placebo-controlled clinical studies are warranted and will surely expand the already very diverse effectiveness of probiotics as important support to the human microbiome for the prevention of disease.

References

Abbas, Z., Yakoob, J., Jafri, W., Ahmad, Z., Azam, Z., Usman, M. W., Shamim, S., & Islam, M. (2014). Cytokine and clinical response to Saccharomyces boulardii therapy in diarrhea-dominant irritable bowel syndrome: A randomized trial. *European Journal of Gastroenterology and Hepatology*, 26(6), 630–639.

Agamennone, V., Krul, C. A. M., Rijkers, G., & Kort, R. (2018). A practical guide for probiotics applied to the case of antibiotic-associated diarrhea in The Netherlands. *BMC Gastroenterology*, 18(1), 103.

Ahmadi, E., Alizadeh-Navaei, R., & Rezai, M. S. (2015). Efficacy of probiotic use in acute rotavirus diarrhea in children: A systematic review and meta-analysis. *Caspian Journal of Internal Medicine*, 6(4), 187–195.

Aisu, N., Tanimura, S., Yamashita, Y., Yamashita, K., Maki, K., Yoshida, Y., Sasaki, T., Takeno, S., & Hoshino, S. (2015). Impact of perioperative probiotic treatment for surgical site infections in patients with colorectal cancer. *Experimental and Therapeutic Medicine*, 10(3), 966–972.

Akbari, E., Asemi, Z., Kakhaki, R. D., Bahmani, F., Kouchaki, E., Tamtaji, O. R., Hamidi, G. A., & Salami, M. (2016). Effect of probiotic supplementation on cognitive function and metabolic status in Alzheimer's disease: A randomized, double-blind and controlled trial. *Frontiers in Aging Neuroscience*, 8, 256.

Allen, S. J., Wareham, K., Wang, D., Bradley, C., Hutchings, H., Harris, W., Dhar, A., Brown, H., Foden, A., Gravenor, M. B., & Mack, D. (2013). Lactobacilli and Bifidobacteria in the Prevention of Antibiotic-Associated Diarrhoea and Clostridium Difficile Diarrhoea in Older Inpatients (PLACIDE): A randomised, double-blind, placebo-controlled, multicentre trial. *The Lancet*, 382(9900), 1249–1257.

Bagga, D., Reichert, J. L., Koschutnig, K., Aigner, C. S., Holzer, P., Koskinen, K., Moissl-Eichinger, C., & Schöpf, V. (2018). Probiotics drive gut microbiome triggering emotional brain signatures. *Gut Microbes*, 9(6), 1–11.

Bambury, A., Sandhu, K., Cryan, J. F., & Dinan, T. G. (2018). Finding the needle in the haystack: Systematic identification of psychobiotics. *British Journal of Pharmacology*, 175(24), 4430–4438.

Bausserman, M., & Michail, S. (2005). The use of Lactobacillus GG in irritable bowel syndrome in children: A double-blind randomized control trial. *Journal of Pediatrics*, 147(2), 197–201.

Begtrup, L. M., De Muckadell, O. B. S., Kjeldsen, J., Christensen, R. D., & Jarbol, D. E. (2013). Long-Term treatment with probiotics in primary care patients with irritable bowel syndrome—A randomised, double-blind, placebo controlled trial. *Scandinavian Journal of Gastroenterology*, 48(10), 1127–1135.

Berggren, A., Ahrén, I. L., Larsson, N., & Önning, G. (2011). Randomised, double-blind and placebo-controlled study using new probiotic Lactobacilli for strengthening the body immune defence against viral infections. *European Journal of Nutrition*, 50(3), 203–210.

Bermudez-Brito, M., Plaza-Díaz, J., Muñoz-Quezada, S., Gómez-Llorente, C., & Gil, A. (2012). Probiotic mechanisms of action. *Annals of Nutrition & Metabolism*, 61(2), 160–174.

Biancone, L., Michetti, P., Travis, S., Escher, J. C., Moser, G., Forbes, A., Hoffmann, J. C., Dignass, A., Gionchetti, P., Jantschek, G., Kiesslich, R., Kolacek, S., Mitchell, R., Panes, J., Soderholm, J., Vucelic, B., & Stange, E. (2008). European evidence-based consensus on the management of ulcerative colitis: Special situations. *Journal of Crohn's and Colitis*, 2(1), 63–92.

Blaabjerg, S., Artzi, D. M., & Aabenhus, R. (2017). Probiotics for the prevention of antibiotic-associated diarrhea in outpatients—A systematic review and meta-analysis. *Antibiotics*, 6(4).

Boonyaritichaikij, S., Kuwabara, K., Nagano, J., Kobayashi, K., & Koga, Y. (2009). Long-term administration of probiotics to asymptomatic preschool children for either the eradication or the prevention of Helicobacter pylori infection. *Helicobacter*, 14(3), 202–207.

Bourreille, A., Cadiot, G., Dreau, G. L., Laharie, D., Beaugerie, L., Dupas, J. L., Marteau, P., Rampal, P., Moyse, D., Saleh, A., Guern, M. E. L., & Galmiche, J. P. (2013). Saccharomyces boulardii does not prevent relapse of Crohn's disease. *Clinical Gastroenterology and Hepatology*, 11(8), 982–987.

Bousvaros, A., Guandalini, S., Baldassano, R. N., Botelho, C., Evans, J., Ferry, G. D., Goldin, B., Hartigan, L., Kugathasan, S., Levy, J., Murray, K. F., Oliva-Hemker, M., Rosh, J. R., Tolia, V., Zholudev, A., Vanderhoof, J. A., & Hibberd, P. L. (2005). A randomized, double-blind trial of Lactobacillus GG vs placebo in addition to standard maintenance therapy for children with Crohn's disease. *Inflammatory Bowel Diseases*, 11(9), 833–839.

Boyle, R. J., Ismail, I. H., Kivivuori, S., Licciardi, P. V., Robins-Browne, R. M., Mah, L. J., Axelrad, C., Moore, S., Donath, S., Carlin, J. B., Lahtinen, S. J., & Tang, M. L. K. (2011). Lactobacillus GG treatment during pregnancy for the prevention of eczema: A randomized controlled trial. *Allergy: European Journal of Allergy and Clinical Immunology, 66*(4), 509–516.

Cameron, D., Hock, Q. S., Kadim, M., Mohan, N., Ryoo, E., Sandhu, B., Yamashiro, Y., Jie, C., Hoekstra, H., & Guarino, A. (2017). Probiotics for gastrointestinal disorders: Proposed recommendations for children of the Asia-Pacific region. *World Journal of Gastroenterology, 23*(45), 7952–7964.

Cani, P. D. (2018). Human gut microbiome: Hopes, threats and promises. *Gut, 67*(9), 1716–1725.

Cecchini, M., Langer, J., & Slawomirski, L. (2015). Antimicrobial resistance in G7 countries and beyond: Economic issues, policies and options for action: OECD report.

Cerdó, T., Ruíz, A., Suárez, A., & Campoy, C. (2017). Probiotic, prebiotic, and brain development. *Nutrients, 9*(11).

Chao, L., Liu, C., Sutthawongwadee, S., Li, Y., Lv, W., Chen, W., Yu, L., Zhou, J., Guo, A., Li, Z., & Guo, S. (2020). Effects of probiotics on depressive or anxiety variables in healthy participants under stress conditions or with a depressive or anxiety diagnosis: A meta-analysis of randomized controlled trials. *Frontiers in Neurology, 11*, 421.

Chen, C., Wen, T., & Zhao, Q. (2020). Probiotics used for postoperative infections in patients undergoing colorectal cancer surgery. *BioMed Research International, 2020*.

Clarke, G., Stilling, R. M., Kennedy, P. J., Stanton, C., Cryan, J. F., & Dinan, T. G. (2014). Minireview: Gut microbiota: The neglected endocrine organ. *Molecular Endocrinology, 28*(8), 1221–1238.

Connell, M., Shin, A., James-Stevenson, T., Xu, H., Imperiale, T. F., & Herron, J. (2018). Systematic review and meta-analysis: Efficacy of patented probiotic, VSL#3, in irritable bowel syndrome. *Neurogastroenterology and Motility, 30*(12).

Coqueiro, A. Y., Raizel, R., Bonvini, A., Tirapegui, J., & Rogero, M. M. (2019). Probiotics for inflammatory bowel diseases: A promising adjuvant treatment. *International Journal of Food Sciences and Nutrition, 70*(1), 20–29.

Cordaillat-Simmons, M., Rouanet, A., & Pot, B. (2020). Live biotherapeutic products: The importance of a defined regulatory framework. *Experimental and Molecular Medicine, 52*(9), 1397–1406.

Cruchet, S., Obregon, M. C., Salazar, G., Diaz, E., & Gotteland, M. (2003). Effect of the ingestion of a dietary product containing *Lactobacillus johnsonii* La1 on *Helicobacter pylori* colonization in children. *Nutrition (Burbank, Los Angeles County, Calif.), 19*(9), 716–721.

Cruchet, S., Furnes, R., Maruy, A., Hebel, E., Palacios, J., Medina, F., Ramirez, N., Orsi, M., Rondon, L., Sdepanian, V., Xóchihua, L., Ybarra, M., & Zablah, R. A. (2015). The use of probiotics in pediatric gastroenterology: A review of the literature and recommendations by Latin-American experts. *Pediatric Drugs, 17*(3), 199–216.

Cuevas-González, P. F., Liceaga, A. M., & Aguilar-Toalá, J. E. (2020). Postbiotics and paraprobiotics: From concepts to applications. *Food Research International, 136*, 109502.

Cárdenas, P. A., Garcés, D., Prado-Vivar, B., Flores, N., Fornasini, M., Cohen, H., Salvador, I., Cargua, O., & Baldeón, M. E. (2020). Effect of Saccharomyces boulardii CNCM I-745 as complementary treatment of *Helicobacter pylori* infection on gut microbiome. *European Journal of Clinical Microbiology and Infectious Diseases, 39*(7), 1365–1372.

Dale, H. F., Rasmussen, S. H., Asiller, Ö. Ö., & Lied, G. A. (2019). Probiotics in irritable bowel syndrome: An up-to-date systematic review. *Nutrients, 11*(9).

Das, S., Gupta, P. K., & Das, R. R. (2016). Efficacy and safety of Saccharomyces boulardii in acute rotavirus diarrhea: Double blind randomized controlled trial from a developing country. *Journal of Tropical Pediatrics, 62*(6), 464–470.

De Simone, C. (2018a). Important warning and court decision regarding VSL#3 ®.

De Simone, C. (2018b). P884 no shared mechanisms among 'old' and 'new' VSL#3: Implications for claims and guidelines. *Journal of Crohn's and Colitis, 12*(Suppl. 1), S564–S565.

Derwa, Y., Gracie, D. J., Hamlin, P. J., & Ford, A. C. (2017). Systematic review with meta-analysis: The efficacy of probiotics in inflammatory bowel disease. *Alimentary Pharmacology and Therapeutics, 46*(4), 389–400.

Di Cagno, R., De Angelis, M., De Pasquale, I., Ndagijimana, M., Vernocchi, P., Ricciuti, P., Gagliardi, F., Laghi, L., Crecchio, C., Guerzoni, M., Gobbetti, M., & Francavilla, R. (2011). Duodenal and faecal microbiota of celiac children: Molecular, phenotype and metabolome characterization. *BMC Microbiology, 11*.

Didari, T., Mozaffari, S., Nikfar, S., & Abdollahi, M. (2015). Effectiveness of probiotics in irritable bowel syndrome: Updated systematic review with meta-analysis. *World Journal of Gastroenterology, 21*(10), 3072–3084.

Dinan, T. G., & Cryan, J. F. (2017). Brain-gut-microbiota axis and mental health. *Psychosomatic Medicine, 79*(8), 920–926.

Dinleyici, E. C., Eren, M., Ozen, M., Yargic, Z. A., & Vandenplas, Y. (2012). Effectiveness and safety of *Saccharomyces boulardii* for acute infectious diarrhea. *Expert Opinion on Biological Therapy, 12*(4), 395–410.

Dinleyici, E. C., Kara, A., Dalgic, N., Kurugol, Z., Arica, V., Metin, O., Temur, E., Turel, O., Guven, S., Yasa, O., Bulut, S., Tanir, G., Yazar, A. S., Karbuz, A., Sancar, M., Erguven, M., Akca, G., Eren, M., Ozen, M., & Vandenplas, Y. (2015). Saccharomyces boulardii CNCM I-745 reduces the duration of diarrhoea, length of emergency care and hospital stay in children with acute diarrhoea. *Beneficial Microbes, 6*(4), 415–421.

Dinleyici, E. C., Dalgic, N., Guven, S., Metin, O., Yasa, O., Kurugol, Z., Turel, O., Tanir, G., Yazar, A. S., Arica, V., Sancar, M., Karbuz, A., Eren, M., Ozen, M., Kara, A., & Vandenplas, Y. (2015). Lactobacillus reuteri DSM 17938 shortens acute infectious diarrhea in a pediatric outpatient setting. *Jornal de Pediatria, 91*(4), 392–396.

Draper, K., Ley, C., & Parsonnet, J. (2017). A survey of probiotic use practices among patients at a tertiary medical centre. *Beneficial Microbes, 8*(3), 345–351.

Ducrotté, P., Sawant, P., & Jayanthi, V. (2012). Clinical trial: Lactobacillus plantarum 299 v (DSM 9843) improves symptoms of irritable bowel syndrome. *World Journal of Gastroenterology, 18*(30), 4012–4018.

EDQM. (2019). *European pharmacopoeia* (9th ed.). Council of Europe.

EFSA. (2020). *Ad hoc meeting with industry representatives.* European Food Safety. Retrieved from http://www.efsa.europa.eu/en/events/event/190118.

El-Ghazely, M. H., Mahmoud, W. H., Atia, M. A., & Eldip, E. M. (2016). Effect of probiotic administration in the therapy of pediatric thermal burn. *Annals of Burns and Fire Disasters, 29*(4), 268–272.

Eshraghian, A. (2014). Epidemiology of *Helicobacter pylori* infection among the healthy population in Iran and countries of the Eastern Mediterranean Region: A systematic review of prevalence and risk factors. *World Journal of Gastroenterology, 20*(46), 17618–17625.

EU Register. (2021). *Nutrition and health claims—European Commission.* Retrieved from https://ec.europa.eu/food/safety/labelling_nutrition/claims/register/public/?event = search.

EUR-Lex. (2006). Regulation (EC) No 1924/2006 of the European Parliament and of the Council of 20 December 2006 on Nutrition and Health Claims Made on Foods. *OJ L 404*, December 30, 2006, pp. 9–25. Retrieved from https://eur-lex.europa.eu/eli/reg/2006/1924/oj.

Ewaschuk, J. B., & Dieleman, L. A. (2006). Probiotics and prebiotics in chronic inflammatory bowel diseases. *World Journal of Gastroenterology, 12*(37), 5941–5950.

FAO/WHO. (2001). *Health and nutritional properties of probiotics in food including powder milk with live lactic acid bacteria.* Cordoba, Argentina, 1-4 October, 2001. Retrieved from http://www.fao.org/3/a0512e/a0512e.pdf.

FAO/WHO. (2002). *Guidelines for the evaluation of probiotics in food.* London, Ontario, Canada, April 30 and May 1, 2002. Retrieved from https://www.who.int/foodsafety/fs_management/en/probiotic_guidelines.pdf.

FDA. (2016). *Early clinical trials with live biotherapeutic products: Chemistry, manufacturing, and control information; guidance for industry.* US Depratment of Health and Human Servies Food and Drug Administration. Retrieved from https://www.fda.gov/files/vaccines,%20blood%20&%20biologics/published/Early-Clinical-Trials-With-Live-Biotherapeutic-Products--Chemistry--Manufacturing--and-Control-Information--Guidance-for-Industry.pdf.

Fedorak, R. N., Feagan, B. G., Hotte, N., Leddin, D., Dieleman, L. A., Petrunia, D. M., Enns, R., Bitton, A., Chiba, N., Paré, P., Rostom, A., Marshall, J., Depew, W., Bernstein, C. N., Panaccione, R., Aumais, G., Steinhart, A. H., Cockeram, A., Bailey, R. J., ... Madsen, K. (2015). The probiotic Vsl#3 has anti-inflammatory effects and could reduce endoscopic recurrence after surgery for Crohn's disease. *Clinical Gastroenterology and Hepatology, 13*(5), 928–935.e2.

Ferreira, C. M., Vieira, A. T., Vinolo, M. A. R., Oliveira, F. A., Curi, R., & Martins, F. D. S. (2014). The central role of the gut microbiota in chronic inflammatory diseases. *Journal of Immunology Research, 2014*.

Fijan, S. (2014). Microorganisms with claimed probiotic properties: An overview of recent literature. *International Journal of Environmental Research and Public Health, 11*(5), 4745–4767.

Fijan, S., Frauwallner, A., Langerholc, T., Krebs, B., Haar, J. A. T., Heschl, A., Turk, D. M., Rogelj, I., ter Haar (née Younes), J. A., Heschl, A., Turk, D. M., & Rogelj, I. (2019). Efficacy of using probiotics with antagonistic activity against pathogens of wound infections: An integrative review of literature. *BioMed Research International, 2019*(7585486), 1–21.

Fiocchi, A., Pawankar, R., Cuello-Garcia, C., Ahn, K., Al-Hammadi, S., Agarwal, A., Beyer, K., Burks, W., Canonica, G. W., Ebisawa, M., Gandhi, S., Kamenwa, R., Lee, B. W., Li, H., Prescott, S., Riva, J. J., Rosenwasser, L., Sampson, H., Spigler, M., ... Schünemann, H. J. (2015). World Allergy Organization-McMaster University Guidelines for Allergic Disease Prevention (GLAD-P): Probiotics. *World Allergy Organization Journal, 8*(1), 4.

Fonseca, A. P. (2011). Biofilms in wounds: An unsolved problem? *European Wound Management Association Journal, 11*(2), 10–23.

Fontes, L. E. S., Martimbianco, A. L. C., Zanin, C., & Riera, R. (2019). N-acetylcysteine as an adjuvant therapy for *Helicobacter pylori* eradication. *Cochrane Database of Systematic Reviews, 2019*(2).

Forbes, A., Escher, J., Hébuterne, X., Kłęk, S., Krznaric, Z., Schneider, S., Shamir, R., Stardelova, K., Wierdsma, N., Wiskin, A. E., & Bischoff, S. C. (2017). ESPEN guideline: Clinical nutrition in inflammatory bowel disease. *Clinical Nutrition, 36*(2), 321–347.

Fox, M. J., Ahuja, K. D. K., Robertson, I. K., Ball, M. J., & Eri, R. D. (2015). Can probiotic yogurt prevent diarrhoea in children on antibiotics? A double-blind, randomised, placebo-controlled study. *BMJ Open, 5*(1).

Freedman, S. B., Williamson-Urquhart, S., Farion, K. J., Gouin, S., Willan, A. R., Poonai, N., Hurley, K., Sherman, P. M., Finkelstein, Y., Lee, B. E., Pang, X.-L., Chui, L., Schnadower, D., Xie, J., Gorelick, M., & Schuh, S. (2018). Multicenter trial of a combination probiotic for children with gastroenteritis. *New England Journal of Medicine, 379*(21), 2015–2026.

Fujita, R., Iimuro, S., Shinozaki, T., Sakamaki, K., Uemura, Y., Takeuchi, A., Matsuyama, Y., & Ohashi, Y. (2013). Decreased duration of acute upper respiratory tract infections with daily intake of fermented milk: A multicenter, double-blinded, randomized comparative study in users of day care facilities for the elderly population. *American Journal of Infection Control, 41*(12), 1231–1235.

Gan, Y., Su, S., Li, B., & Fang, C. (2019). Efficacy of probiotics and prebiotics in prevention of infectious complications following hepatic resections: Systematic review and meta-analysis. *Journal of Gastrointestinal and Liver Diseases, 28*(2), 205–211.

Ganji-Arjenaki, M., & Rafieian-Kopaei, M. (2018). Probiotics are a good choice in remission of inflammatory bowel diseases: A meta analysis and systematic review. *Journal of Cellular Physiology, 233*(3), 2091–2103.

Ghorbani, Z., Nazari, S., Etesam, F., Nourimajd, S., Ahmadpanah, M., & Jahromi, S. R. (2018). The effect of synbiotic as an adjuvant therapy to fluoxetine in moderate depression: A randomized multicenter trial. *Archives of Neuroscience, 5*(2).

Ghouri, Y. A., Richards, D. M., Rahimi, E. F., Krill, J. T., Jelinek, K. A., & DuPont, A. W. (2014). Systematic review of randomized controlled trials of probiotics, prebiotics, and synbiotics in infammatory bowel disease. *Clinical and Experimental Gastroenterology, 7*, 473–487.

Gibson, G. R., Hutkins, R., Sanders, M. E., Prescott, S. L., Reimer, R. A., Salminen, S. J., Scott, K., Stanton, C., Swanson, K. S., Cani, P. D., Verbeke, K., & Reid, G. (2017). Expert consensus document: The International Scientific Association for Probiotics and Prebiotics (ISAPP) consensus statement on the definition and scope of prebiotics. *Nature Reviews Gastroenterology & Hepatology, 14*(8), 491–502.

Gionchetti, P., Rizzello, F., Venturi, A., Brigidi, P., Matteuzzi, D., Bazzocchi, G., Poggioli, G., Miglioli, M., & Campieri, M. (2000). Oral bacteriotherapy as maintenance treatment in patients with chronic pouchitis: A double-blind, placebo-controlled trial. *Gastroenterology, 119*(2), 305–309.

Gionchetti, P., Rizzello, F., Helwig, U., Venturi, A., Lammers, K. M., Brigidi, P., Vitali, B., Poggioli, G., Miglioli, M., & Campieri, M. (2003). Prophylaxis of pouchitis onset with probiotic therapy: A double-blind, placebo-controlled trial. *Gastroenterology, 124*(5), 1202–1209.

Goh, K. K., Liu, Y. W., Kuo, P. H., Chung, Y. C. E., Lu, M. L., & Chen, C. H. (2019). Effect of probiotics on depressive symptoms: A meta-analysis of human studies. *Psychiatry Research, 282*.

Goldenberg, J. Z., Lytvyn, L., Steurich, J., Parkin, P., Mahant, S., & Johnston, B. C. (2015). Probiotics for the prevention of pediatric antibiotic-associated diarrhea. *Cochrane Database of Systematic Reviews, 2015*(12).

Goldenberg, J. Z., Yap, C., Lytvyn, L., Lo, C. K. F., Beardsley, J., Mertz, D., & Johnston, B. C. (2017). Probiotics for the prevention of Clostridium difficile-associated diarrhea in adults and children. *Cochrane Database of Systematic Reviews, CD006095*(12).

Goldman, C. G., Barrado, D. A., Balcarce, N., Cueto Rua, E., Oshiro, M., Calcagno, M. L., Janjetic, M., Fuda, J., Weill, R., Salgueiro, M. J., Valencia, M. E., Zubillaga, M. B., & Boccio, J. R. (2006). Effect of a probiotic food as an adjuvant to triple therapy for eradication of *Helicobacter pylori* infection in children. *Nutrition (Burbank, Los Angeles County, Calif.), 22*(10), 984–988.

Gotteland, M., Poliak, L., Cruchet, S., & Brunser, O. (2007). Effect of regular ingestion of Saccharomyces boulardii plus inulin or Lactobacillus acidophilus LB in children colonized by *Helicobacter pylori*. *Acta Paediatrica, 94*(12), 1747–1751.

Government of Canada. (2009). *Guidance document—The use of probiotic microorganisms in food—Canada.Ca*. Retrieved from https://www.canada.ca/en/health-canada/services/food-nutrition/legislation-guidelines/guidance-documents/guidance-document-use-probiotic-microorganisms-food-2009.html.

Guarino, A., Ashkenazi, S., Gendrel, D., Vecchio, A. L., Shamir, R., & Szajewska, H. (2014). European Society for Pediatric Gastroenterology, Hepatology, and Nutrition/European Society for Pediatric Infectious Diseases Evidence-Based Guidelines for the Management of Acute Gastroenteritis in Children in Europe: Update 2014. *Journal of Pediatric Gastroenterology and Nutrition, 59*(1), 132–152.

Guarino, A., Guandalini, S., & Vecchio, A. L. (2015). Probiotics for prevention and treatment of diarrhea. *Journal of Clinical Gastroenterology, 49*, S37–S45.

Guarner, F., Khan, A. G., Garisch, J., Eliakim, R., Gangl, A., Thomson, A., Krabshuis, J., Lemair, T., Kaufmann, P., Andres De Paula, J., Fedorak, R., Shanahan, F., Sanders, M. E., Szajewska, H., Ramakrishna, B. S., Karakan, T., & Kim, N. (2012). World gastroenterology organisation global guidelines: Probiotics and prebiotics October 2011. *Journal of Clinical Gastroenterology, 46*(6), 468–481.

Guarner, F., Khan, A. G., Garisch, J., Eliakim, R., Gangl, A., Thomson, A., & Lemair, J. (2017). *World Gastroenterology Organisation global guidelines: Probiotics and prebiotics*. World Gastroenterology Organisation. Retrieved from https://www.worldgastroenterology.org/guidelines/global-guidelines/probiotics-and-prebiotics/probiotics-and-prebiotics-english.

Guglielmetti, S., Mora, D., Gschwender, M., & Popp, K. (2011). Randomised clinical trial: Bifidobacterium bifidum MIMBb75 significantly alleviates irritable bowel syndrome and improves quality of life—A double-blind, placebo-controlled study. *Alimentary Pharmacology and Therapeutics, 33*(10), 1123–1132.

Guillemard, E., Tondu, F., Lacoin, F., & Schrezenmeir, J. (2010). Consumption of a fermented dairy product containing the probiotic Lactobacillus casei DN-114001 reduces the duration of respiratory infections in the elderly in a randomised controlled trial. *British Journal of Nutrition, 103*(1), 58–68.

Guo, Q., Goldenberg, J. Z., Humphrey, C., El Dib, R., & Johnston, B. C. (2019). Probiotics for the prevention of pediatric antibiotic-associated diarrhea. *Cochrane Database of Systematic Reviews, 4*(4).

Gupta, P., Andrew, H., Kirschner, B. S., & Guandalini, S. (2000). Is Lactobacillus GG helpful in children with Crohn's disease? Results of a preliminary, open-label study. *Journal of Pediatric Gastroenterology and Nutrition, 31*(4), 453–457.

Guslandi, M., Mezzi, G., Sorghi, M., & Testoni, P. A. (2000). Saccharomyces boulardii in maintenance treatment of Crohn's disease. *Digestive Diseases and Sciences, 45*(7), 1462–1464.

Guslandi, M., Giollo, P., & Testoni, P. A. (2003). A pilot trial of Saccharomyces boulardii in ulcerative colitis. *European Journal of Gastroenterology and Hepatology, 15*(6), 697–698.

Guéniche, A., Bastien, P., Ovigne, J. M., Kermici, M., Courchay, G., Chevalier, V., Breton, L., & Castiel-Higounenc, I. (2009). Bifidobacterium longum lysate, a new ingredient for reactive skin. *Experimental Dermatology, 19*(8), e1–e8.

Güvenç, I. A., Muluk, N. B., Mutlu, F. Ş., Eşki, E., Altintoprak, N., Oktemer, T., & Cingi, C. (2016). Do probiotics have a role in the treatment of allergic rhinitis? A comprehensive systematic review and meta-analysis. *American Journal of Rhinology and Allergy, 30*(5), e157–e175.

Hao, Q., Dong, B. R., & Wu, T. (2015). Probiotics for preventing acute upper respiratory tract infections. *Cochrane Database of Systematic Reviews, 2015*(2).

Haskins, R. (1989). Acute illness in day care: How much does it cost? *Bulletin of the New York Academy of Medicine: Journal of Urban Health, 65*(3), 319–343.

Hegazy, S. K., & El-Bedewy, M. M. (2010). Effect of probiotics on pro-inflammatory cytokines and NF-Kb activation in ulcerative colitis. *World Journal of Gastroenterology, 16*(33), 4145–4151.

Hill, C., Guarner, F., Reid, G., Gibson, G. R., Merenstein, D. J., Pot, B., Morelli, L., Canani, R. B., Flint, H. J., Salminen, S., Calder, P. C., & Sanders, M. E. (2014). The International Scientific Association for probiotics and prebiotics consensus statement on the scope and appropriate use of the term probiotic. *Nature Reviews Gastroenterology & Hepatology, 11*(8), 506−514.

Hojsak, I., Abdović, S., Szajewska, H., Milošević, M., Krznarić, Ž., & Kolaček, S. (2010). Lactobacillus GG in the prevention of nosocomial gastrointestinal and respiratory tract infections. *Pediatrics, 125*(5).

Hojsak, I., Fabiano, V., Pop, T. L., Goulet, O., Zuccotti, G. V., Çokuğraş, F. C., Pettoello-Mantovani, M., & Kolaček, S. (2018). Guidance on the use of probiotics in clinical practice in children with selected clinical conditions and in specific vulnerable groups. *Acta Paediatrica, 107*(6), 927−937.

Huang, R., Wang, K., & Hu, J. (2016). Effect of probiotics on depression: A systematic review and meta-analysis of randomized controlled trials. *Nutrients, 8*(8).

Hurduc, V., Plesca, D., Dragomir, D., Sajin, M., & Vandenplas, Y. (2009). A randomized, open trial evaluating the effect of Saccharomyces boulardii on the eradication rate of *Helicobacter pylori* infection in children. *Acta Paediatrica, International Journal of Paediatrics, 98*(1), 127−131.

Ianiro, G., Rizzatti, G., Plomer, M., Lopetuso, L., Scaldaferri, F., Franceschi, F., Cammarota, G., & Gasbarrini, A. (2018). Bacillus clausii for the treatment of acute diarrhea in children: A systematic review and meta-analysis of randomized controlled trials. *Nutrients, 10*(8).

Iglesias-vázquez, L., Van Ginkel Riba, G., Arija, V., & Canals, J. (2020). Composition of gut microbiota in children with autism spectrum disorder: A systematic review and meta-analysis. *Nutrients, 12*(3).

Iheozor-Ejiofor, Z., Gordon, M., Clegg, A., Freeman, S. C., Gjuladin-Hellon, T., Macdonald, J. K., & Akobeng, A. K. (2019). Interventions for maintenance of surgically induced remission in Crohn's disease: A network meta-analysis. *Cochrane Database of Systematic Reviews, 2019*(9).

Ishikawa, H., Akedo, I., Otani, T., Umesaki, Y., Tanaka, R., & Imaoka, A. (2003). Randomized controlled trial of the effect of bifidobacteria-fermented milk on ulcerative colitis. *Journal of the American College of Nutrition, 22*(1), 56−63.

Isolauri, E., Arvola, T., Sutas, Y., Moilanen, E., & Salminen, S. (2000). Probiotics in the management of atopic eczema. *Clinical and Experimental Allergy, 30*(11), 1605−1610.

Jafari, E., Vahedi, H., Merat, S., Momtahen, S., & Riahi, A. (2014). Therapeutic effects, tolerability and safety of a multi-strain probiotic in Iranian adults with irritable bowel syndrome and bloating. *Archives of Iranian Medicine, 17*(7), 466−470.

Ji, J., & Yang, H. (2020). Using probiotics as supplementation for *Helicobacter pylori* antibiotic therapy. *International Journal of Molecular Sciences, 21*(3).

Jiang, W., Ni, B., Liu, Z., Liu, X., Xie, W., Wu, I. X. Y., & Li, X. (2020). The role of probiotics in the prevention and treatment of atopic dermatitis in children: An updated systematic review and meta-analysis of randomized controlled trials. *Pediatric Drugs, 22*(5), 535−549.

Jones, N. L., Koletzko, S., Goodman, K., Bontems, P., Cadranel, S., Casswall, T., Czinn, S., Gold, B. D., Guarner, J., Elitsur, Y., Homan, M., Kalach, N., Kori, M., Madrazo, A., Megraud, F., Papadopoulou, A., & Rowland, M. (2017). Joint ESPGHAN/NASPGHAN guidelines for the management of *Helicobacter pylori* in children and adolescents (update 2016). *Journal of Pediatric Gastroenterology and Nutrition, 64*(6), 991−1003.

Kadam, S., Shai, S., Shahane, A., & Kaushik, K. S. (2019). Recent advances in non-conventional antimicrobial approaches for chronic wound biofilms: Have we found the 'chink in the armor'? *Biomedicines, 7*(2), 35.

Kalliomäki, M., Salminen, S., Poussa, T., & Isolauri, E. (2007). Probiotics during the first 7 years of life: A cumulative risk reduction of eczema in a randomized, placebo-controlled trial. *Journal of Allergy and Clinical Immunology, 119*(4), 1019−1021.

Kanazawa, H., Nagino, M., Kamiya, S., Komatsu, S., Mayumi, T., Takagi, K., Asahara, T., Nomoto, K., Tanaka, R., & Nimura, Y. (2005). Synbiotics reduce postoperative infectious complications: A randomized controlled trial in biliary cancer patients undergoing hepatectomy. *Langenbeck's Archives of Surgery, 390*(2), 104−113.

Kasatpibal, N., Whitney, J. D., Saokaew, S., Kengkla, K., Heitkemper, M. M., & Apisarnthanarak, A. (2017). Effectiveness of probiotic, prebiotic, and synbiotic therapies in reducing postoperative complications: A systematic review and network meta-analysis. *Clinical Infectious Diseases: An Official Publication of the Infectious Diseases Society of America, 64*(Suppl. 2), S153−S160.

Kato, K., Mizuno, S., Umesaki, Y., Ishii, Y., Sugitani, M., Imaoka, A., Otsuka, M., Hasunuma, O., Kurihara, R., Iwasaki, A., & Arakawa, Y. (2004). Randomized placebo-controlled trial assessing the effect of bifidobacteria-fermented milk on active ulcerative colitis. *Alimentary Pharmacology and Therapeutics, 20*(10), 1133−1141.

Kaur, L., Gordon, M., Baines, P. A., Iheozor-Ejiofor, Z., Sinopoulou, V., & Akobeng, A. K. (2020). Probiotics for induction of remission in ulcerative colitis. *Cochrane Database of Systematic Reviews, 2020*(3).

Kazemi, A., Noorbala, A. A., Azam, K., Eskandari, M. H., & Djafarian, K. (2019). Effect of probiotic and prebiotic vs placebo on psychological outcomes in patients with major depressive disorder: A randomized clinical trial. *Clinical Nutrition, 38*(2), 522−528.

Khaled, J. M. A. (2020). Probiotics, prebiotics, and COVID-19 infection: A review article. *Saudi Journal of Biological Sciences, 28*(1).

Kim, J. Y., Kwon, J. H., Ahn, S. H., Lee, S. I., Han, Y. S., Choi, Y. O., Lee, S. Y., Ahn, K. M., & Ji, G. E. (2010). Effect of probiotic mix (Bifidobacterium bifidum, Bifidobacterium lactis, Lactobacillus acidophilus) in the primary prevention of eczema: A double-blind, randomized, placebo-controlled trial. *Pediatric Allergy and Immunology, 21*(2 Part 2), e386−e393.

Kim, J. Y., Park, Y. J., Lee, H. J., Park, M. Y., & Kwon, O. (2018). Effect of Lactobacillus gasseri BNR17 on irritable bowel syndrome: A randomized, double-blind, placebo-controlled, dose-finding trial. *Food Science and Biotechnology, 27*(3), 853−857.

King, S., Glanville, J., Sanders, M. E., Fitzgerald, A., & Varley, D. (2014). Effectiveness of probiotics on the duration of illness in healthy children and adults who develop common acute respiratory infectious conditions: A systematic review and meta-analysis. *British Journal of Nutrition, 112*(1), 41−54.

King, S., Tancredi, D., Lenoir-Wijnkoop, I., Gould, K., Vann, H., Connors, G., Sanders, M. E., Linder, J. A., Shane, A. L., & Merenstein, D. (2019). Does probiotic consumption reduce antibiotic utilization for common acute infections? A systematic review and meta-analysis. *European Journal of Public Health*, *29*(3), 494−499.

Kinross, J. M., Markar, S., Karthikesalingam, A., Chow, A., Penney, N., Silk, D., & Darzi, A. (2013). A meta-analysis of probiotic and synbiotic use in elective surgery. *Journal of Parenteral and Enteral Nutrition*, *37*(2), 243−253.

Kluijfhout, S., Van Trieu, T., & Vandenplas, Y. (2020). Efficacy of the probiotic probiotical confirmed in acute gastroenteritis. *Pediatric Gastroenterology, Hepatology and Nutrition*, *23*(5), 464−471.

Kolaček, S., Hojsak, I., Canani, R. B., Guarino, A., Indrio, F., Orel, R., Pot, B., Shamir, R., Szajewska, H., Vandenplas, Y., Van Goudoever, J., & Weizman, Z. (2017). Commercial probiotic products: A call for improved quality control. A position paper by the ESPGHAN Working Group for Probiotics and Prebiotics. *Journal of Pediatric Gastroenterology and Nutrition*, *65*(1), 117−124.

Koletzko, S., Jones, N. L., Goodman, K. J., Gold, B., Rowland, M., Cadranel, S., Chong, S., Colletti, R. B., Casswall, T., Guarner, J., Kalach, N., Madrazo, A., Megraud, F., & Oderda, G. (2011). Evidence-based guidelines from ESPGHAN and NASPGHAN for *Helicobacter pylori* infection in children. *Journal of Pediatric Gastroenterology and Nutrition*, *53*(2), 230−243.

Kotowska, M., Albrecht, P., & Szajewska, H. (2005). Saccharomyces boulardii in the prevention of antibiotic-associated diarrhoea in children: A randomized double-blind placebo-controlled trial. *Alimentary Pharmacology and Therapeutics*, *21*(5), 583−590.

Kotzampassi, K., Stavrou, G., Damoraki, G., Georgitsi, M., Basdanis, G., Tsaousi, G., & Giamarellos-Bourboulis, E. J. (2015). A four-probiotics regimen reduces postoperative complications after colorectal surgery: A randomized, double-blind, placebo-controlled study. *World Journal of Surgery*, *39*(11), 2776−2783.

Kruis, W., Schütz, E., Fric, P., Fixa, B., Judmaier, G., & Stolte, M. (1997). Double-blind comparison of an oral Escherichia coli preparation and mesalazine in maintaining remission of ulcerative colitis. *Alimentary Pharmacology and Therapeutics*, *11*(5), 853−858.

Kruis, W., Frič, P., Pokrotnieks, J., Lukáš, M., Fixa, B., Kaščák, M., Kamm, M. A., Weismueller, J., Beglinger, C., Stolte, M., Wolff, C., & Schulze, J. (2004). Maintaining remission of ulcerative colitis with the probiotic Escherichia coli Nissle 1917 is as effective as with standard mesalazine. *Gut*, *53*(11), 1617−1623.

Kuisma, J., Mentula, S., Jarvinen, H., Kahri, A., Saxelin, M., & Farkkila, M. (2003). Effect of *Lactobacillus rhamnosus* GG on ileal pouch inflammation and microbial flora. *Alimentary Pharmacology and Therapeutics*, *17*(4), 509−515.

Laake, K. O., Line, P. D., Grzyb, K., Aamodt, G., Aabakken, L., Røset, A., Hvinden, A. B., Bakka, A., Eide, J., Bjørneklett, A., & Vatn, M. H. (2004). Assessment of mucosal inflammation and blood flow in response to four weeks' intervention with probiotics in patients operated with a J-configurated ileal-pouch-anal-anastomosis (IPAA). *Scandinavian Journal of Gastroenterology*, *39*(12), 1228−1235.

Lahiri, K., Jadhav, K., Gahlowt, P., Najmuddin, F., & Padmashree, D. Y. (2015). Bacillus clausii as an adjuvant therapy in acute childhood diarrhoea. *IOSR Journal of Dental and Medical Sciences (IOSR-JDMS) e-ISSN*, *14*(5), 74−76.

Lau, C. S., & Chamberlain, R. S. (2016). Probiotics are effective at preventing Clostridium difficile-associated diarrhea: A systematic review and meta-analysis. *International Journal of General Medicine*, *9*, 27.

Laulund, S., Wind, A., Derkx, P., & Zuliani, V. (2017). Regulatory and safety requirements for food cultures. *Microorganisms*, *5*(2), 28.

Lazou Ahrén, I., Berggren, A., Teixeira, C., Niskanen, T. M., & Larsson, N. (2020). Evaluation of the efficacy of Lactobacillus plantarum HEAL9 and Lactobacillus paracasei 8700:2 on aspects of common cold infections in children attending day care: A randomised, double-blind, placebo-controlled clinical study. *European Journal of Nutrition*, *59*(1), 409−417.

Leyer, G. J., Li, S., Mubasher, M. E., Reifer, C., & Ouwehand, A. C. (2009). Probiotic effects on cold and influenza-like symptom incidence and duration in children. *Pediatrics*, *124*(2), e172−e179.

Li, B., Liang, L., Deng, H., Guo, J., Shu, H., & Zhang, L. (2020). Efficacy and safety of probiotics in irritable bowel syndrome: A systematic review and meta-analysis. *Frontiers in Pharmacology*, *11*.

Li, Y. T., Xu, H., Ye, J. Z., Wu, W. R., Shi, D., Fang, D. Q., Liu, Y., & Li, L. J. (2019). Efficacy of Lactobacillus rhamnosus GG in treatment of acute pediatric diarrhea: A systematic review with meta-analysis. *World Journal of Gastroenterology*, *25*(33), 4999−5016.

Lilly, D. M., & Stillwell, R. H. (1965). Probiotics: Growth-promoting factors produced by microorganisms. *Science (New York, N.Y.)*, *147*(3659), 747−748.

Limketkai, B. N., Akobeng, A. K., Gordon, M., & Adepoju, A. A. (2020). Probiotics for induction of remission in Crohn's disease. *Cochrane Database of Systematic Reviews*, *2020*(7).

Lin, J., Zhang, Y., He, C., & Dai, J. (2018). Probiotics supplementation in children with asthma: A systematic review and meta-analysis. *Journal of Paediatrics and Child Health*, *54*(9), 953−961.

Lionetti, E., Miniello, V. L., Castellaneta, S. P., Magistá, A. M., De Canio, A., Maurogiovanni, G., Ierardi, E., Cavallo, L., & Francavilla, R. (2006). Lactobacillus reuteri therapy to reduce side-effects during anti-*Helicobacter pylori* treatment in children: A randomized placebo controlled trial. *Alimentary Pharmacology and Therapeutics*, *24*(10), 1461−1468.

Liu, R. T., Walsh, R. F. L., & Sheehan, A. E. (2019). Prebiotics and probiotics for depression and anxiety: A systematic review and meta-analysis of controlled clinical trials. *Neuroscience and Biobehavioral Reviews*, *102*, 13−23.

Liu, Y., Alookaran, J., & Rhoads, J. (2018). Probiotics in autoimmune and inflammatory disorders. *Nutrients*, *10*(10), 1537.

Lo Vecchio, A., Dias, J. A., Berkley, J. A., Boey, C., Cohen, M. B., Cruchet, S., Liguoro, I., Lindo, E. S., Sandhu, B., Sherman, P., Shimizu, T., & Guarino, A. (2016). "Comparison of recommendations in clinical practice guidelines for acute gastroenteritis in children. *Journal of Pediatric Gastroenterology and Nutrition*, *63*(2), 226−235.

Losurdo, G., Cubisino, R., Barone, M., Principi, M., Leandro, G., Ierardi, E., & Leo, A. D. (2018). Probiotic monotherapy and *Helicobacter pylori* eradication: A systematic review with pooled-data analysis. *World Journal of Gastroenterology*, *24*(1), 139−149.

Lu, C. L., Liu, X. H., Stub, T., Kristoffersen, A. E., Liang, S. B., Wang, X., Bai, X., Norheim, A. J., Musial, F., Araek, T., Fonnebo, V., & Liu, J. P. (2018). Complementary and alternative medicine for treatment of atopic eczema in children under 14 years old: A systematic review and meta-analysis of randomized controlled trials. *BMC Complementary and Alternative Medicine*, *18*(1).

Lukic, J., Chen, V., Strahinic, I., Begovic, J., Lev-Tov, H., Davis, S. C., Tomic-Canic, M., & Pastar, I. (2017). Probiotics or pro-healers: The role of beneficial bacteria in tissue repair. *Wound Repair and Regeneration*, *25*(6), 912–922.

Lytvyn, L., Quach, K., Banfield, L., Johnston, B. C., & Mertz, D. (2016). Probiotics and synbiotics for the prevention of postoperative infections following abdominal surgery: A systematic review and meta-analysis of randomized controlled trials. *Journal of Hospital Infection*, *92*(2), 130–139.

Macfarlane, S., Furrie, E., Cummings, J. H., & Macfarlane, G. T. (2004). Chemotaxonomic analysis of bacterial populations colonizing the rectal mucosa in patients with ulcerative colitis. *Clinical Infectious Diseases*, *38*(12), 1690–1699.

Magro, F., Gionchetti, P., Eliakim, R., Ardizzone, S., Armuzzi, A., Barreiro-de Acosta, M., Burisch, J., Gecse, K. B., Hart, A. L., Hindryckx, P., Langner, C., Limdi, J. K., Pellino, G., Zagórowicz, E., Raine, T., Harbord, M., & Rieder, F. (2017). Third european evidence-based consensus on diagnosis and management of ulcerative colitis. Part 1: Definitions, diagnosis, extra-intestinal manifestations, pregnancy, cancer surveillance, surgery, and ileo-anal pouch disorders. *Journal of Crohn's and Colitis*, *11*(6), 649–670.

Malchow, H. A. (1997). Crohn's disease and Escherichia coli: A new approach in therapy to maintain remission of colonic Crohn's disease?". *Journal of Clinical Gastroenterology*, *25*(4), 653–658.

Maldonado Galdeano, C., Cazorla, S. I., Dumit, J. M. L., Vélez, E., & Perdigón, G. (2019). Beneficial effects of probiotic consumption on the immune system. *Annals of Nutrition and Metabolism*, *74*(2), 115–124.

Malhi, G. S., Bell, E., Bassett, D., Boyce, P., Bryant, R., Hazell, P., Hopwood, M., Lyndon, B., Mulder, R., Porter, R., Singh, A. B., & Murray, G. (2021). The 2020 Royal Australian and New Zealand College of Psychiatrists Clinical Practice Guidelines for mood disorders. *Australian & New Zealand Journal of Psychiatry*, *55*(1), 7–117.

Maragkoudaki, M., Chouliaras, G., Moutafi, A., Thomas, A., Orfanakou, A., & Papadopoulou, A. (2018). Efficacy of an oral rehydration solution enriched with Lactobacillus reuteri DSM 17938 and zinc in the management of acute diarrhoea in infants: A randomized, double-blind, placebo-controlled trial. *Nutrients*, *10*(9), 1189.

Marteau, P., Lémann, M., Seksik, P., Laharie, D., Colombel, J. F., Bouhnik, Y., Cadiot, G., Soulé, J. C., Bourreille, A., Metman, E., Lerebours, E., Carbonnel, F., Dupas, J. L., Veyrac, M., Coffin, B., Moreau, J., Abitbol, V., Blum-Sperisen, S., & Mary, J. Y. (2006). Ineffectiveness of Lactobacillus johnsonii LA1 for prophylaxis of postoperative recurrence in Crohn's disease: A randomised, double blind, placebo controlled GETAID trial. *Gut*, *55*(6), 842–847.

Mayes, T., Gottschlich, M. M., James, L. E., Allgeier, C., Weitz, J., & Kagan, R. J. (2015). Clinical safety and efficacy of probiotic administration following burn injury. *Journal of Burn Care & Research: Official Publication of the American Burn Association*, *36*(1), 92–99.

McFarland, L. V. (2006). Meta-analysis of probiotics for the prevention of antibiotic associated diarrhea and the treatment of Clostridium difficile disease. *American Journal of Gastroenterology*, *101*(4), 812–822.

McFarland, L. V. (2015). Meta-analysis of single strain probiotics for the eradication of *Helicobacter pylori* and prevention of adverse events. *World Journal of Meta-Analysis*, *3*(2), 97.

McFarland, L. V., Huang, Y., Wang, L., & Malfertheiner, P. (2016). Systematic review and meta-analysis: Multi-strain probiotics as adjunct therapy for *Helicobacter pylori* eradication and prevention of adverse events. *United European Gastroenterology Journal*, *4*(4), 546–561.

McFarland, L. V., Evans, C. T., & Goldstein, E. J. C. (2018). Strain-specificity and disease-specificity of probiotic efficacy: A systematic review and meta-analysis. *Frontiers in Medicine*, *5*, 124.

Miele, E., Pascarella, F., Giannetti, E., Quaglietta, L., Baldassano, R. N., & Staiano, A. (2009). Effect of a probiotic preparation (VSL#3) on induction and maintenance of remission in children with ulcerative colitis. *American Journal of Gastroenterology*, *104*(2), 437–443.

Mihai, M. M., Preda, M., Lungu, I., Gestal, M. C., Popa, M. I., & Holban, A. M. (2018). Nanocoatings for chronic wound repair—Modulation of microbial colonization and biofilm formation. *International Journal of Molecular Sciences*, *19*(4), 1179.

Mimura, T., Rizzello, F., Helwig, U., Poggioli, G., Schreiber, S., Talbot, I. C., Nicholls, R. J., Gionchetti, P., Campieri, M., & Kamm, M. A. (2004). Once daily high dose probiotic therapy (VSL#3) for maintaining remission in recurrent or refractory pouchitis. *Gut*, *53*(1), 108–114.

NIH. (2020). *Probiotics—Health professional fact sheet*. Retrieved from https://ods.od.nih.gov/factsheets/Probiotics-HealthProfessional/.

Nguyen, N., Zhang, B., Holubar, S. D., Pardi, D. S., & Singh, S. (2019). Treatment and prevention of pouchitis after ileal pouch-anal anastomosis for chronic ulcerative colitis. *Cochrane Database of Systematic Reviews*, *2019*(5).

Nishida, K., Sawada, D., Kuwano, Y., Tanaka, H., & Rokutan, K. (2019). Health benefits of Lactobacillus gasseri CP2305 tablets in young adults exposed to chronic stress: A randomized, double-blind, placebo-controlled study. *Nutrients*, *11*(8), 1859.

Niu, H. L., & Xiao, J. Y. (2020). The efficacy and safety of probiotics in patients with irritable bowel syndrome: Evidence based on 35 randomized controlled trials. *International Journal of Surgery*, *75*, 116–127.

Östlund-Lagerström, L., Kihlgren, A., Repsilber, D., Björkstén, B., Brummer, R. J., & Schoultz, I. (2016). Probiotic administration among free-living older adults: A double blinded, randomized, placebo-controlled clinical trial. *Nutrition Journal*, *15*(1), 1–10.

Ouyang, X., Li, Q., Shi, M., Niu, D., Song, W., Nian, Q., Li, X., Ding, Z., Ai, X., & Wang, J. (2019). Probiotics for preventing postoperative infection in colorectal cancer patients: A systematic review and meta-analysis. *International Journal of Colorectal Disease*, *34*(3), 459–469.

Pacifico, L., Osborn, J. F., Bonci, E., Romaggioli, S., Baldini, R., & Chiesa, C. (2014). Probiotics for the treatment of *Helicobacter pylori* infection in children. *World Journal of Gastroenterology*, *20*(3), 673–683.

Parker, M. W., Schaffzin, J. K., Vecchio, A. L., Yau, C., Vonderhaar, K., Guiot, A., Brinkman, W. B., White, C. M., Simmons, J. M., Gerhardt, W. E., Kotagal, U. R., & Conway, P. H. (2013). Rapid adoption of Lactobacillus rhamnosus GG for acute gastroenteritis. *Pediatrics*, *131*(Suppl. 1).

Peral, M. C., Martinez, M. A., & Valdez, J. C. (2009). Bacteriotherapy with Lactobacillus plantarum in burns. *International Wound Journal*, 6(1), 73–81.

Peral, M. C., Rachid, M. M., Gobbato, N. M., Martinez, M. A. H., & Valdez, J. C. C. (2010). Interleukin-8 production by polymorphonuclear leukocytes from patients with chronic infected leg ulcers treated with Lactobacillus plantarum. *Clinical Microbiology and Infection: The Official Publication of the European Society of Clinical Microbiology and Infectious Diseases*, 16(3), 281–286.

Pitsouni, E., Alexiou, V., Saridakis, V., Peppas, G., & Falagas, M. E. (2009). Does the use of probiotics/synbiotics prevent postoperative infections in patients undergoing abdominal surgery? A meta-analysis of randomized controlled trials. *European Journal of Clinical Pharmacology*, 65(6), 561–570.

Prantera, C., Scribano, M. L., Falasco, G., Andreoli, A., & Luzi, C. (2002). Ineffectiveness of probiotics in preventing recurrence after curative resection for Crohn's disease: A randomised controlled trial with Lactobacillus GG. *Gut*, 51(3), 405–409.

Rautava, S., Kainonen, E., Salminen, S., & Isolauri, E. (2012). Maternal probiotic supplementation during pregnancy and breast-feeding reduces the risk of eczema in the infant. *Journal of Allergy and Clinical Immunology*, 130(6), 1355–1360.

Rayes, N., Seehofer, D., Theruvath, T., Schiller, R. A., Langrehr, J. M., Jonas, S., Bengmark, S., & Neuhaus, P. (2005). Supply of pre- and probiotics reduces bacterial infection rates after liver transplantation—A randomized, double-blind trial. *American Journal of Transplantation*, 5(1), 125–130.

Reid, G., Jass, J., Sebulsky, M. T., John, K., & Mccormick, J. K. (2003). Potential uses of probiotics in clinical practice potential uses of probiotics in clinical practice. *Clinical Microbiology Reviews*, 16(4), 658–671.

Reid, G., Younes, J. A., Van der Mei, H. C., Gloor, G. B., Knight, R., & Busscher, H. J. (2011). Microbiota restoration: Natural and supplemented recovery of human microbial communities. *Nature Reviews. Microbiology*, 9(1), 27–38.

Rembacken, B. J., Snelling, A. M., Hawkey, P. M., Chalmers, D. M., & Axon, A. T. R. (1999). Non-pathogenic Escherichia coli vs mesalazine for the treatment of ulcerative colitis: A randomised trial. *The Lancet*, 354(9179), 635–639.

Ricci, G., Cipriani, F., Cuello-Garcia, C. A., Brozek, J. L., Fiocchi, A., Pawankar, R., Yepes-Nuñes, J. J., Terraciano, L., Gandhi, S., Agarwal, A., Zhang, Y., & Schünemann, H. J. (2016). A clinical reading on 'World Allergy Organization-McMaster University Guidelines for Allergic Disease Prevention (GLAD-P): Probiotics. *World Allergy Organization Journal*, 9(1), 9.

Ruemmele, F. M., Veres, G., Kolho, K. L., Griffiths, A., Levine, A., Escher, J. C., Amil Dias, J., Barabino, A., Braegger, C. P., Bronsky, J., Buderus, S., Martín-de-Carpi, J., De Ridder, L., Fagerberg, U. L., Hugot, J. P., Kierkus, J., Kolacek, S., Koletzko, S., Lionetti, P., ... Phillips, A. (2014). Consensus guidelines of ECCO/ESPGHAN on the medical management of pediatric Crohn's disease. *Journal of Crohn's and Colitis*, 8(10), 1179–1207.

Saleem, N., & Howden, C. W. (2020). Update on the management of *Helicobacter pylori* infection. *Current Treatment Options in Gastroenterology*, 18(3), 476–487.

Salem, I., Ramser, A., Isham, N., & Ghannoum, M. A. (2018). The gut microbiome as a major regulator of the gut-skin axis. *Frontiers in Microbiology*, 9, 1459.

Salminen, S., Collado, M. C., Endo, A., Hill, C., Lebeer, S., Quigley, E. M. M., Sanders, M. E., Shamir, R., Swann, J. R., Szajewska, H., & Vinderola, G. (2021). The International Scientific Association of Probiotics and Prebiotics (ISAPP) consensus statement on the definition and scope of postbiotics. *Nature Reviews Gastroenterol Hepatol*. Available from https://doi.org/10.1038/s41575-021-00440-6.

Scaldaferri, F., Gerardi, V., Mangiola, F., Lopetuso, L. R., Pizzoferrato, M., Petito, V., Papa, A., Stojanovic, J., Poscia, A., Cammarota, G., & Gasbarrini, A. (2016). Role and mechanisms of action of Escherichia coli Nissle 1917 in the maintenance of remission in ulcerative colitis patients: An update. *World Journal of Gastroenterology*, 22(24), 5505–5511.

Schmulson, M. J., & Drossman, D. A. (2017). What is new in Rome IV. *Journal of Neurogastroenterology and Motility*, 23(2), 151–163.

Schnadower, D., Tarr, P. I., Casper, T. C., Gorelick, M. H., Dean, J. M., O'Connell, K. J., Mahajan, P., Levine, A. C., Bhatt, S. R., Roskind, C. G., Powell, E. C., Rogers, A. J., Vance, C., Sapien, R. E., Olsen, C. S., Metheney, M., Dickey, V. P., Hall-Moore, C., & Freedman, S. B. (2018). Lactobacillus rhamnosus GG vs placebo for acute gastroenteritis in children. *New England Journal of Medicine*, 379(21), 2002–2014.

Schultz, M., Timmer, A., Herfarth, H. H., Sartor, R. B., Vanderhoof, J. A., & Rath, H. C. (2004). Lactobacillus GG in inducing and maintaining remission of Crohn's disease. *BMC Gastroenterology*, 4.

Seddik, H., Boutallaka, H., Elkoti, I., Nejjari, F., Berraida, R., Berrag, S., Loubaris, K., Sentissi, S., & Benkirane, A. (2019). Saccharomyces boulardii CNCM I-745 plus sequential therapy for *Helicobacter pylori* infections: A randomized, open-label trial. *European Journal of Clinical Pharmacology*, 75(5), 639–645.

Sharma, R., Gupta, D., Mehrotra, R., & Mago, P. (2021). Psychobiotics: The next-generation probiotics for the brain. *Current Microbiology*.

Shi, X., Zhang, J., Mo, L., Shi, J., Qin, M., & Huang, X. (2019). Efficacy and safety of probiotics in eradicating *Helicobacter pylori*: A network meta-analysis. *Medicine*, 98(15), e15180.

Siddharthan, R., Chapek, M., Warren, M., & Martindale, R. (2018). Probiotics in prevention of surgical site infections. *Surgical Infections*, 19(8), 781–784.

Silverstein, M., Sales, A. E., & Koepsell, T. D. (2003). Health care utilization and expenditures associated with child care attendance: A nationally representative sample. *Pediatrics*, 111(4 Pt 1).

Sivamaruthi, B. S. (2018). A comprehensive review on clinical outcome of probiotic and synbiotic therapy for inflammatory bowel diseases. *Asian Pacific Journal of Tropical Biomedicine*, 8(3), 179.

Slykerman, R. F., Hood, F., Wickens, K., Thompson, J. M. D., Barthow, C., Murphy, R., Kang, J., Rowden, J., Stone, P., Crane, J., Stanley, T., Abels, P., Purdie, G., Maude, R., & Mitchell, E. A. (2017). Effect of Lactobacillus rhamnosus HN001 in pregnancy on postpartum symptoms of depression and anxiety: A randomised double-blind placebo-controlled trial. *EBioMedicine*, 24, 159–165.

Smith, L. K., & Wissel, E. F. (2019). Microbes and the mind: How bacteria shape affect, neurological processes, cognition, social relationships, development, and pathology. *Perspectives on Psychological Science, 14*(3), 397–418.

Smith, T. J., Rigassio-Radler, D., Denmark, R., Haley, T., & Touger-Decker, R. (2013). Effect of Lactobacillus rhamnosus LGG R and Bifidobacterium animalis ssp. lactis BB-12 R on health-related quality of life in college students affected by upper respiratory infections. *British Journal of Nutrition, 109*(11), 1999–2007.

Sniffen, J. C., McFarland, L. V., Evans, C. T., & Goldstein, E. J. C. (2018). Choosing an appropriate probiotic product for your patient: An evidence-based practical guide. *PLoS One, 13*(12).

Spiller, R., Pélerin, F., Decherf, A. C., Maudet, C., Housez, B., Cazaubiel, M., & Jüsten, P. (2016). Randomized double blind placebo-controlled trial of Saccharomyces cerevisiae CNCM I-3856 in irritable bowel syndrome: Improvement in abdominal pain and bloating in those with predominant constipation. *United European Gastroenterology Journal, 4*(3), 353–362.

Staudacher, H. M. (2017). Nutritional, microbiological and psychosocial implications of the low FODMAP diet. *Journal of Gastroenterology and Hepatology (Australia), 32*, 16–19.

Steed, H., MacFarlane, G. T., Blackett, K. L., Bahrami, B., Reynolds, N., Walsh, S. V., Cummings, J. H., & MacFarlane, S. (2010). Clinical trial: The microbiological and immunological effects of synbiotic consumption—A randomized double-blind placebo-controlled study in active Crohn's disease. *Alimentary Pharmacology and Therapeutics, 32*(7), 872–883.

Steenbergen, L., Sellaro, R., van Hemert, S., Bosch, J. A., & Colzato, L. S. (2015). A randomized controlled trial to test the effect of multispecies probiotics on cognitive reactivity to sad mood. *Brain, Behavior, and Immunity, 48*, 258–264.

Su, G. L., Ko, C. W., Bercik, P., Falck-Ytter, Y., Sultan, S., Weizman, A. V., & Morgan, R. L. (2020). AGA clinical practice guidelines on the role of probiotics in the management of gastrointestinal disorders. *Gastroenterology, 159*(2), 697–705.

Sun, Y. Y., Li, M., Li, Y. Y., Li, L. X., Zhai, W. Z., Wang, P., Yang, X. X., Gu, X., Song, L. J., Li, Z., Zuo, X. L., & Li, Y. Q. (2018). The effect of Clostridium butyricum on symptoms and fecal microbiota in diarrhea-dominant irritable bowel syndrome: A randomized, double-blind, placebo-controlled trial. *Scientific Reports, 8*(1).

Swanson, K. S., Gibson, G. R., Hutkins, R., Reimer, R. A., Reid, G., Verbeke, K., Scott, K. P., Holscher, H. D., Azad, M. B., Delzenne, N. M., & Sanders, M. E. (2020). The International Scientific Association for Probiotics and Prebiotics (ISAPP) consensus statement on the definition and scope of synbiotics. *Nature Reviews Gastroenterology and Hepatology*, 1–15.

Sykora, J., Valecková, K., Amlerová, J., Siala, K., Dedek, P., Watkins, S., Varvarovská, J., Stozický, F., Pazdiora, P., & Schwarz, J. (2004). P0900 supplements of one week triple drug therapy with special probiotic Lactobacillus casei Imunitass (strain DN-114 000) and Streptococcus thermophilus and Lactobacillus bulgaricus in the eradication of H. pylori-colonized children: A prospective randomised TR. *Journal of Pediatric Gastroenterology and Nutrition, 39*, s400.

Szajewska, H., & Kołodziej, M. (2015). Systematic review with meta-analysis: Lactobacillus rhamnosus GG in the prevention of antibiotic-associated diarrhoea in children and adults. *Alimentary Pharmacology and Therapeutics, 42*(10), 1149–1157.

Szajewska, H., Albrecht, P., & Topczewska-Cabanek, A. (2009). Randomized, double-blind, placebo-controlled trial: Effect of Lactobacillus GG SUPPLEMENTATION On *Helicobacter pylori* eradication rates and side effects during treatment in children. *Journal of Pediatric Gastroenterology and Nutrition, 48*(4), 431–436.

Szajewska, H., Skórka, A., Ruszczyński, M., & Gieruszczak-Białek, D. (2013). Meta-analysis: Lactobacillus GG for treating acute gastroenteritis in children—updated analysis of randomised controlled trials. *Alimentary Pharmacology and Therapeutics, 38*(5), 467–476.

Szajewska, H., Guarino, A., Hojsak, I., Indrio, F., Kolacek, S., Shamir, R., Vandenplas, Y., & Weizman, Z. (2014). Use of probiotics for management of acute gastroenteritis: A position paper by the ESPGHAN working group for probiotics and prebiotics. *Journal of Pediatric Gastroenterology and Nutrition, 58*(4), 531–539.

Szajewska, H., Canani, R. B., Guarino, A., Hojsak, I., Indrio, F., Kolacek, S., Orel, R., Shamir, R., Vandenplas, Y., Van Goudoever, J. B., & Weizman, Z. (2016). Probiotics for the prevention of antibiotic-associated diarrhea in children. *Journal of Pediatric Gastroenterology and Nutrition, 62*(3), 495–506.

Szajewska, H., Guarino, A., Hojsak, I., Indrio, F., Kolacek, S., Orel, R., Salvatore, S., Shamir, R., van Goudoever, J. B., Vandenplas, Y., Weizman, Z., & Zalewski, B. M. (2020). Use of probiotics for the management of acute gastroenteritis in children: An update. *Journal of Pediatric Gastroenterology and Nutrition, 71*(2), 261–269.

Szajewska, H., Kołodziej, M., & Zalewski, B. M. (2020). Systematic review with meta-analysis: Saccharomyces boulardii for treating acute gastroenteritis in children—A 2020 update. *Alimentary Pharmacology and Therapeutics, 51*(7), 678–688.

Sýkora, J., Valečková, K., Amlerová, J., Siala, K., Dědek, P., Watkins, S., Varvařovská, J., Stožický, F., Pazdiora, P., & Schwarz, J. (2005). Effects of a specially designed fermented milk product containing probiotic Lactobacillus casei DN-114 001 and the eradication of H. pylori in children: A prospective randomized double-blind study. *Journal of Clinical Gastroenterology, 39*(8), 692–698.

Tamaki, H., Nakase, H., Inoue, S., Kawanami, C., Itani, T., Ohana, M., Kusaka, T., Uose, S., Hisatsune, H., Tojo, M., Noda, T., Arasawa, S., Izuta, M., Kubo, A., Ogawa, C., Matsunaka, T., & Shibatouge, M. (2016). Efficacy of probiotic treatment with Bifidobacterium longum 536 for induction of remission in active ulcerative colitis: A randomized, double-blinded, placebo-controlled multicenter trial. *Digestive Endoscopy, 28*(1), 67–74.

Torres, J., Bonovas, S., Doherty, G., Kucharzik, T., Gisbert, J. P., Raine, T., Adamina, M., Armuzzi, A., Bachmann, O., Bager, P., Biancone, L., Bokemeyer, B., Bossuyt, P., Burisch, J., Collins, P., El-Hussuna, A., Ellul, P., Frei-Lanter, C., Furfaro, F., … Fiorino, G. (2020). ECCO guidelines on therapeutics in Crohn's disease: Medical treatment. *Journal of Crohn's and Colitis, 14*(1), 4–22.

Trallero, O. G., Serrano, L. H., Inglés, M. B., Vallés, D. R., & Rodríguez, A. M. (2019). Effect of the administration of a probiotic with a combination of Lactobacillus and Bifidobacterium strains on antibiotic-associated diarrhea. *Revista Espanola de Quimioterapia, 32*(3), 268–272.

Turchet, P., Laurenzano, M., Auboiron, S., & Antoine, J. M. (2003). Effect of fermented milk containing the probiotic Lactobacillus casei DN-114001 on winter infections in free-living elderly subjects: A randomised, controlled pilot study | Cochrane Library. *Jounral of Nutrition and Health*, 7 (2), 75−77.

Turner, D., Levine, A., Escher, J. C., Griffiths, A. M., Russell, R. K., Dignass, A., Dias, J. A., Bronsky, J., Braegger, C. P., Cucchiara, S., De Ridder, L., Fagerberg, U. L., Hussey, S., Hugot, J. P., Kolacek, S., Kolho, K. L., Lionetti, P., Pærregaard, A., Potapov, A., ... Ruemmele, F. M. (2012). Management of pediatric ulcerative colitis: Joint ECCO and ESPGHAN evidence-based consensus guidelines. *Journal of Pediatric Gastroenterology and Nutrition*, 55(3), 340−361.

Turner, D., Ruemmele, F. M., Orlanski-Meyer, E., Griffiths, A. M., De Carpi, J. M., Bronsky, J., Veres, G., Aloi, M., Strisciuglio, C., Braegger, C. P., Assa, A., Romano, C., Hussey, S., Stanton, M., Pakarinen, M., De Ridder, L., Katsanos, K., Croft, N., Navas-López, V., ... Russell, R. K. (2018). Management of paediatric ulcerative colitis, Part 1: Ambulatory care-an evidence-based guideline from European Crohn's and Colitis Organization and European Society of Paediatric Gastroenterology, Hepatology and Nutrition. *Journal of Pediatric Gastroenterology and Nutrition*, 67(2), 257−291.

Tursi, A., Brandimarte, G., Papa, A., Giglio, A., Elisei, W., Giorgetti, G. M., Forti, G., Morini, S., Hassan, C., Pistoia, M. A., Modeo, M. E., Rodino', S., D'Amico, T., Sebkova, L., Sacca', N., Di Giulio, E., Luzza, F., Imeneo, M., Larussa, T., ... Gasbarrini, A. (2010). Treatment of relapsing mild-to-moderate ulcerative colitis with the probiotic VSL3 as adjunctive to a standard pharmaceutical treatment: A double-blind, randomized, placebo-controlled study. *American Journal of Gastroenterology*, 105(10), 2218−2227.

United States FDA. (2018). *Label claims for conventional foods and dietary supplements*. FDA. Retrieved from https://www.fda.gov/food/food-labeling-nutrition/label-claims-conventional-foods-and-dietary-supplements.

Urbańska, M., Gieruszczak-Białek, D., & Szajewska, H. (2016). Systematic review with meta-analysis: Lactobacillus reuteri DSM 17938 for diarrhoeal diseases in children. *Alimentary Pharmacology and Therapeutics*, 43(10), 1025−1034.

Urgesi, R., Casale, C., Pistelli, R., Rapaccini, G. L., & De Vitis, I. (2014). A randomized double-blind placebo-controlled clinical trial on efficacy and safety of association of simethicone and Bacillus coagulans (Colinox®) in patients with irritable bowel syndrome. *European Review for Medical and Pharmacological Sciences*, 18(9), 1344−1353.

Usami, M., Miyoshi, M., Kanbara, Y., Aoyama, M., Sakaki, H., Shuno, K., Hirata, K., Takahashi, M., Ueno, K., Tabata, S., Asahara, T., & Nomoto, K. (2011). Effects of perioperative synbiotic treatment on infectious complications, intestinal integrity, and fecal flora and organic acids in hepatic surgery with or without cirrhosis. *Journal of Parenteral and Enteral Nutrition*, 35(3), 317−328.

Van Gossum, A., Dewit, O., Louis, E., De Hertogh, G., Baert, F., Fontaine, F., Devos, M., Enslen, M., Paintin, M., & Franchimont, D. (2007). Multicenter randomized-controlled clinical trial of probiotics (*Lactobacillus johnsonii*. LA1) on early endoscopic recurrence of Crohn's disease after ileo-caecal resection. *Inflammatory Bowel Diseases*, 13(2), 135−142.

Vanderpool, C., Yan, F., & Polk, D. B. (2008). Mechanisms of probiotic action: Implications for therapeutic applications in inflammatory bowel diseases. *Inflammatory Bowel Diseases*, 14(11), 1585−1596.

Villena, J., & Kitazawa, H. (2017). Editorial: Immunobiotics-interactions of beneficial microbes with the immune system. *Frontiers in Immunology*, 8.

Wan, C. M., Yu, H., Liu, G., Xu, H. M., Mao, Z. Q., Xu, Y., Jin, Y., Luo, R. P., Wang, W. J., & Fang, F. (2017). A multicenter randomized controlled study of Saccharomyces boulardii in the prevention of antibiotic-associated diarrhea in infants and young children. *Zhonghua Er Ke Za Zhi = Chinese Journal of Pediatrics*, 55(5), 349−354.

Wang, Z. H., Gao, Q. Y., & Fang, J. Y. (2013). Meta-analysis of the efficacy and safety of Lactobacillus-containing and Bifidobacterium-containing probiotic compound preparation in *Helicobacter pylori* eradication therapy. *Journal of Clinical Gastroenterology*, 47(1), 25−32.

Wegh, C. A. M., Geerlings, S. Y., Knol, J., Roeselers, G., & Belzer, C. (2019). Postbiotics and their potential applications in early life nutrition and beyond. *International Journal of Molecular Sciences*, 20(19).

Wei, X., Jiang, P., Liu, J., Sun, R., & Zhu, L. (2020). Association between probiotic supplementation and asthma incidence in infants: A meta-analysis of randomized controlled trials. *Journal of Asthma*, 57(2), 167−178.

Wenus, C., Goll, R., Loken, E. B., Biong, A. S., Halvorsen, D. S., & Florholmen, J. (2008). Prevention of antibiotic-associated diarrhoea by a fermented probiotic milk drink. *European Journal of Clinical Nutrition*, 62(2), 299−301.

Wickens, K., Black, P., Stanley, T. V., Mitchell, E., Barthow, C., Fitzharris, P., Purdie, G., & Crane, J. (2012). A protective effect of Lactobacillus rhamnosus HN001 against eczema in the first 2 years of life persists to age 4 years. *Clinical and Experimental Allergy*, 42(7), 1071−1079.

Wildt, S., Nordgaard, I., Hansen, U., Brockmann, E., & Rumessen, J. J. (2011). A randomised double-blind placebo-controlled trial with *Lactobacillus acidophilus* La-5 and Bifidobacterium animalis subsp. Lactis BB-12 for maintenance of remission in ulcerative colitis. *Journal of Crohn's and Colitis*, 5(2), 115−121.

Wong, R. K., Yang, C., Song, G. H., Wong, J., & Ho, K. Y. (2014). Melatonin regulation as a possible mechanism for probiotic (VSL#3) in irritable bowel syndrome: A randomized double-blinded placebo study. *Digestive Diseases and Sciences*, 60(1), 186−194.

Wu, X.-D., Liu, M.-M., Liang, X., Hu, N., & Huang, W. (2018). Effects of perioperative supplementation with pro-/synbiotics on clinical outcomes in surgical patients: A meta-analysis with trial sequential analysis of randomized controlled trials. *Clinical Nutrition*, 37(2), 505−515.

Wu, X.-D., Xu, W., Liu, M.-M., Hu, K.-J., Sun, Y.-Y., Yang, X.-F., Zhu, G.-Q., Wang, Z.-W., & Huang, W. (2018). Efficacy of prophylactic probiotics in combination with antibiotics vs antibiotics alone for colorectal surgery: A meta-analysis of randomized controlled trials. *Journal of Surgical Oncology*, 117(7), 1394−1404.

Yoon, J. S., Sohn, W., Lee, O. Y., Lee, S. P., Lee, K. N., Jun, D. W., Lee, H. L., Yoon, B. C., Choi, H. S., Chung, W. S., & Seo, J. G. (2014). Effect of multispecies probiotics on irritable bowel syndrome: A randomized, double-blind, placebo-controlled trial. *Journal of Gastroenterology and Hepatology (Australia)*, 29(1), 52−59.

Zamani, M., Ebrahimtabar, F., Zamani, V., Miller, W. H., Alizadeh-Navaei, R., Shokri-Shirvani, J., & Derakhshan, M. H. (2018). Systematic review with meta-analysis: The worldwide prevalence of *Helicobacter pylori* infection. *Alimentary Pharmacology and Therapeutics*, *47*(7), 868–876.

Zhang, M. M., Qian, W., Qin, Y. Y., He, J., & Zhou, Y. H. (2015). Probiotics in *Helicobacter pylori* eradication therapy: A systematic review and meta-analysis. *World Journal of Gastroenterology*, *21*(14), 4345–4357.

Zhang, Y., Li, L., Guo, C., Mu, D., Feng, B., Zuo, X., & Li, Y. (2016). Effects of probiotic type, dose and treatment duration on irritable bowel syndrome diagnosed by Rome III criteria: A meta-analysis. *BMC Gastroenterology*, *16*(1).

Zheng, J., Wittouck, S., Salvetti, E., Franz, C. M. A. P., Harris, H. M. B., Mattarelli, P., O'Toole, P. W., Pot, B., Vandamme, P., Walter, J., Watanabe, K., Wuyts, S., Felis, G. E., Gänzle, M. G., & Lebeer, S. (2020). A taxonomic note on the genus Lactobacillus: Description of 23 novel genera, emended description of the genus Lactobacillus beijerinck 1901, and union of Lactobacillaceae and Leuconostocaceae. *International Journal of Systematic and Evolutionary Microbiology*, *70*(4), 2782–2858.

Zhou, L., & Foster, J. A. (2015). Psychobiotics and the gut-brain axis: In the pursuit of happiness. *Neuropsychiatric Disease and Treatment*, *11*, 715–723.

Zhu, R., Chen, K., Zheng, Y. Y., Zhang, H. W., Wang, J. S., Xia, Y. J., Dai, W. Q., Wang, F., Shen, M., Cheng, P., Zhang, Y., Wang, C. F., Yang, J., Li, J. J., Lu, J., Zhou, Y. Q., & Guo, C. Y. (2014). Meta-analysis of the efficacy of probiotics in *Helicobacter pylori* eradication therapy. *World Journal of Gastroenterology*, *20*(47), 18013–18021.

Zocco, M. A., Zileri Dal Verme, L., Cremonini, F., Piscaglia, A. C., Nista, E. C., Candelli, M., Novi, M., Rigante, D., Cazzato, I. A., Ojetti, V., Armuzzi, A., Gasbarrini, G., & Gasbarrini, A. (2006). Efficacy of Lactobacillus GG in maintaining remission of ulcerative colitis. *Alimentary Pharmacology and Therapeutics*, *23*(11), 1567–1574.

Zorzela, L., Ardestani, S. K., McFarland, L. V., & Vohra, S. (2017). Is there a role for modified probiotics as beneficial microbes: A systematic review of the literature. *Beneficial Microbes*, *8*(5), 739–754.

Index

Note: Page numbers followed by "*f*" and "*t*" refer figures and tables, respectively.

A

Aberrant crypt foci (ACF), 194
ACF-producing sialomucin (SIM-ACF), 194–195
Acidophilus, 216
Acinetobacter, 131, 224
Acne vulgaris, 129–130
Actinobacteria, 41, 94, 150–151, 162, 191
Active probiotics, 188–189
Acute colitis, 63
Acute gastroenteritis (AGE), 468–469, 469*t*
Acylated homoserine lactone (AHL), 269
Adherence capacity, 369
Adipokine hypothesis, 321
Adjuvant potential
  of biosurfactants, 423–424
  of LAB ghost cells, 424
Aeromonas, 61–62
Aflatoxins (*AflR*), 371
Agouti-related protein (AgRP), 326
Akkermansia, 78–79, 134, 192
  A. muciniphila, 79
Albeit microbiota, 51
Alcanivorax, 202
Allergic diseases
  probiotics in prevention and management of, 139–143
Allergic disorders, 150–151
Allergic rhinitis
  probiotics for prevention of, 141–142
  probiotics for treatment of, 142–143
Allergies, 480–482
Alpha 7 nicotinic acetylcholine receptor (α7nAChR), 45–46
American Gastroenterological Association (AGA), 468
American Human Microbiome Project, 432
Amoxicillin, 73
Anaerostipes, 195
Anemia, 402
Angiotensin-converting enzyme (ACE), 200
Animal model studies, 119
Animal studies for prevention of asthma through probiotics, 140
Antibacterial chemotherapeutics, 70–74, 72*f*
Antibiotic-associated diarrhea (AAD), 110–112, 214, 266, 439, 476–479
  comparative table on role of probiotic strains, 111*t*
Antibiotics, 110, 254
  resistance in probiotics, 454–455
Antifungal drugs, 305–306, 313–314
Antigen-presenting cells (APCs), 419
Antimicrobial compounds, 243
Antimicrobial peptides (AMPs), 163–164
Antimicrobial potential of probiotics
  against foodborne pathogens, 367–368
    antifungal and antimycotoxin activities of probiotics, 368
    antiviral activity of probiotics, 368
    Campylobacter, 367
    Listeria monocytogenes, 367–368
    Salmonella, 367
    STEC, 367
Antimicrobial resistance (AMR), 265–266
Antiquorum sensing, 269
Anxiety, 482–485
Apolipoprotein (apo) B-containing lipoproteins, 337
5-ASA, 70
Asia-Pacific Economic Cooperation (APEC), 30
Asperger syndrome (AS), 360
Asthma, 139
  prevention of, 140–141
    animal studies for prevention of asthma through probiotics, 140
    human studies for prevention of asthma through probiotics, 141
  probiotics for treatment of, 141
Atherosclerotic plaques, 337–338
Atopic dermatitis (AD), 481
  etiology and pathophysiology of, 117–118
  future perspectives of probiotics in prevention and treatment of, 123
  intervention of probiotics in, 119–123
    animal model studies, 119
    human studies/clinical trials, 119–123
    mechanism of probiotics in amelioration of AD, 123
    overview of mechanisms of action of probiotics in atopic dermatitis, 124*f*
Atopic diseases, rationale for using probiotics in, 139–140
Atopic eczema (AE), 152, 481
Atopic skin diseases
  etiology and pathophysiology of atopic dermatitis, 117–118
  future perspectives of probiotics in prevention and treatment of AD, 123
  intervention of probiotics in atopic dermatitis, 119–123
  probiotics in prevention and treatment of, 117
  relationship between gut microbiota and atopic dermatitis, 118–119
  clinical trials for treatment, 122*t*
  studies of probiotics using animal model, 120*t*
Atopobium, 59
Attention-deficit/hyperactivity disorder (ADHD), 356–357, 360
Autism and probiotics, 354
Autism spectrum disorder (ASD), 353–355
  gut microbiota of children with, 357–358
  literature evidence in, 358
Autoaggregation, 270
Autoimmune diseases
  cystic fibrosis, 163
  future perspectives, 178
  gut microbiota associated with, 165–166
  multiple sclerosis, 163
  probiotics
    and prebiotics in suppression of, 161–163
    in suppression of autoimmune diseases, 167–178
  relationship between gut microbiota and immune system, 163–165
  link between gut microbiota and adaptive immunity, 165
  link between gut microbiota and innate immunity, 164–165, 164*f*
  rheumatoid arthritis, 162
  systemic lupus erythematosus, 162
  type-1 diabetes mellitus, 162–163
Autoinducers (AIs), 269
  AI-2, 269
  AI-3, 269

B

Bacilli, 94
Bacillus spp, 1, 78, 95–96, 107, 314
  B. amyloliquefaciens, 142–143
  B. cereus, 192
  B. clausii, 42–43, 107
  B. coagulans, 75, 102–103, 107, 167–172, 213

Bacillus spp (*Continued*)
  B. mesentericus, 107
  B. pumilus, 142–143
  B. subtilis, 107, 142–143, 225–226
    RZ001, 79
  B. subtilisnatto, 76
Bactereroides, 47–48
Bacteria, 65, 148–149
  bacteria–bacteria interaction, 370
Bacterial cells, 6–8
Bacterial communities, 224–225
Bacterial conversion of cholesterol, 342
Bacterial genera in human large intestine, 64–66
Bacterial ghosts (BGs), 424
Bacterial species, 130
Bacterial vaginosis (BV), 237–238, 243–244, 272–273
Bacterial viability, 6
Bacterioides, 73
Bacterium-like particles (BLPs), 417
  from LAB, 421–423
Bacteroides, 59, 62, 64, 66, 94, 134, 192
  B. caccae, 62
  B. faecis, 77
  B. fragilis, 47–48, 62, 67, 110, 150–151, 164–166
  B. ovatus, 62
  B. thetaiotaomicron, 64
  B. vulgates, 62
Bacteroidetes, 41, 43, 79, 150–151, 162, 176, 191, 195
Bacteroidia, 195
Bacterroides, 74
Basic Consumer Act (CBA), 27
Bcl-2-associated X-protein (BAX), 197
Bifidobacter, adverse effects due to, 452
Bifidobacteria, 73, 134, 148–149, 215, 224
Bifidobacteriaceae, 79, 175–176
Bifidobacterium, 1, 5, 42–43, 59, 64, 66–67, 74–75, 78, 94–96, 107, 121, 150–152, 161–163, 166–167, 174–176, 178, 188–189, 194, 200, 223–227, 229–231, 435, 452
  B. adolescentis, 42–43, 151–152
  B. animalis, 42–43, 119–121, 176, 194–195
    subsp. *lactis* HN019, 152
  B. bifidum, 42–43, 75, 107, 112, 123, 130, 167–172, 177–178, 192, 213
    YIT 10347, 192
  B. breve, 42–43, 64, 75, 95, 107, 112
    C50, 152–156
    M-16V, 102–103, 141
  B. infantis, 42–43, 75, 94, 107, 112, 131, 141, 192, 227
    M-63, 102–103
  B. lactis, 48–49, 75, 95, 102–103, 131, 140
    HN019, 121, 141
  B. longum, 42–43, 48, 75, 107, 131, 226
    BB536, 78, 102–103
    CECT 7347, 121–123
  B. thermophilus, 75
  BR03 DSM 16604, 121
  strains, 78

Bifidus, 216
Bile acids, 194
  synthesis, 343–344
Bile salt hydrolase (BSH), 341, 403–404
Bile salts, deconjugation of, 341–342
Bio-25, 405
Bioactive components, 1
Bioactive probiotic products, 399
Biogenic amines, 455–456
Biogenics, 6
Biologic Drugs, 25–27
Biological materials, 31
Biological medicinal products, 17–18
Biological Products, 30–31
Biological treatment, 70
Biosurfactants, 423–424
"Biotherapeutic" foods. *See* Functional foods
Biotics, 189
Blautia, 162
Blood-brain barrier, (BBB), 43
Body weight (BW), 325–326
Bowel diseases. *See also* Diarrheal diseases
  antibacterial chemotherapeutics, 70–74
  drugs used in pharmacological alleviation, 71f
  general characteristics of drugs used in, 70–74
  intestinal microbiota in development of, 61–70
Brain endothelial cellular (BEC), 43
Brain-derived neurotrophic factor (BDNF), 326, 353
Breast cancer (BC), 187
  probiotics and prebiotics in, 198–200
Bruguiera gymnorrhiza, 80
Burn patients, 132–133
Butyric acid, 405

C

C-reactive protein (CRP), 167–172
Campylobacter, 61–62, 73, 367
  C. jejuni, 110
Canada
  pharmaceutical regulatory framework in, 25–26
Canadian regulatory framework, 24–27
Cancer therapy, 440
Cancer therapy-induced diarrhea, 112
Candida spp., 118, 313
Candida vaginitis (CV), 243–244
Candidiasis, 306–312
Carbohydrate antigen 19-9 (CA19-9), 194–195
Carcinoembryonic antigen (CEA), 194–195
Carcinoembryonic cell adhesion molecule 6 (CEAM6), 197
Cardiovascular diseases (CVDs), 337, 403–404
Cathelicidins and related antimicrobial peptide (CRAMP), 324
Cell-free supernatants (CFS), 6, 196, 267–268, 399
Cell-wall protein, 196

Center for Diseases Control (CDC), 20, 243–244, 289–290
Central nervous system (CNS), 43, 163, 353, 442
Cervical cancer (CC), 190–191
  probiotics and prebiotics in, 200–202
Chemotherapy, 453
Children nutritional deficiencies, 400–402
Chlorhexidine, 226
Cholesterol
  bacterial conversion of, 342
  coprecipitation of, 342–343
  incorporation and assimilation of, 342
  inhibition of
    cholesterol transmembrane transporter expression, 343
    hepatic cholesterol synthesis, 343–344
Chronic diabetic foot ulcers, 132
Ciprofloxacin, 73
Clindamycin, 73
Clinical trials, 119–123
  authorisation, 15
Clostridia, 94, 150–151
Clostridiaceae, 150–151
Clostridium, 59, 61–62, 67, 150–151
  C. butyricum, 142, 197–198
  C. difficile, 94
    C. difficile-associated diarrhea, 476–479
  C. perfringens, 62, 73, 93–94
  C. ramosum, 62, 64
Clostridium difficile diarrhea (CDD), 112, 214
Clostridium difficile infection (CDI), 223, 228–231
  epidemiology, pathophysiology, and clinical presentation, 228–229
  probiotics in prevention and treatment, 229–231, 230t
Clotridiales, 195
Cocaine-and amphetamine-related transcript (CART), 326
Code of Federal Regulations (CFR), 20
Colon cancer, probiotics and prebiotics in, 193–198
Colonization of intestinal ecosystem, 353–354
Colony-forming units (CFU), 102, 119–121, 436–437
Colorectal cancer (CRC), 187, 193, 440
Combination therapies, 240
Commensal bacteria emergence, 161
Commensal microbial flora, 237
Commensal phylotypes, 129
Common Technical Document (CTD), 15
Compound Annual Growth Rate (CAGR), 408
Conjugated-linolenic acid (CLNA), 196
Consumer Affairs Agency (CAA), 27
Coprococcus, 195
  composition, 43
Coronary heart disease (CHD), 403–404
Corynebacterium, 130–131
Council of the European Union (CEU), 16
Covid-19, 43–44
Cow milk allergy (CMA), 214
Crohn's disease (CD), 41–42, 59–60, 62, 404, 470–471

Cryptophyta, 162
Cryptosporidium, 110
Cutaneous T-cell lymphoma (CTCL), 133
Cutibacterium, 130–131
  C. acnes, 129–130
Cyclin-dependent kinase 1 (CDK1), 194–195
Cyclooxygenase-2 (COX-2), 78, 194
Cyclospora, 110
Cystathionine-β-synthase (CBS), 69
Cystathionine-γ-lyase (CSE), 69
Cysteine, 69
Cystic fibrosis (CF), 161, 163
  probiotics in suppression of, 178
Cytochrome c (Cyto-c), 196
Cytokines, 41, 165
  storm syndrome, 43–44
Cytosine-phosphate-guanine (CpG), 289–290
Cytotoxic T lymphocyte (CTL), 173

D

D-lactic acidosis, 455
De Simone formulation (DSF), 480
Deconjugation of bile salts, 341–342
Delivery system of probiotics, 372
Dendritic cells (DCs), 163–164, 271–272, 387
Dental caries, probiotics in, 252–253
Deoxyribonucleases (DNases), 252
Depression, 482–485
Dermal infections, 312–313
Dermatophytosis, 312
Desulfobacter, 59, 66
Desulfobulbus, 59, 66
Desulfomonas, 59, 66
Desulfotomaculum, 59, 66
Desulfovibrio, 59–60, 63, 65–66, 193–194
  D. desulfuricans, 60
  D. vulgaris, 66–67
Dextran sulfate sodium (DSS), 63
Diabetes, 321
  probiotics for management of, 327–331
Diabetes mellitus (DM), 321–322
  pathophysiology and risk factors of, 322–327
Diabetic ulcers, 132
Dialister, 162
Diarrhea, 453–454
Diarrheal diseases, 109
  colony morphology, 108f, 109f
  list of Indian probiotic drugs marketed, 108t
  mode of action of probiotics, 113
  photographic images, 109f
  probiotics in prevention and treatment of, 109–113
Dietary management strategies, 216
Dietary prebiotics, 3
Dietary Supplement Health and Education Act (DSHEA), 21
2,3-dioxygenase, 45–46
Directives, 16
DNA-based methods, 129
Doren, 195
Dose of probiotics, 437

Drug
  classification in Japan, 30–31
  definition in Japan, 30
  drug-induced hepatotoxicity, 439
  status, 14f, 15
Dysbiosis, 93–94, 140, 166, 199, 325, 353, 355–356, 386, 397
  in critically ill patients, 225
Dyslipidemia, 337

E

Eggerthella, 162
Elderly nutritional deficiencies, 402–403
Encapsulation, 366–367, 372
  technology for development of functional ingredients, 405–408
Endoplasmic-reticulum (ER), 325
Endothelial dysfunction, 289
Energy deficiency, 65
Entamoeba histolytica, 110
Enteral tube feeding diarrhea (EFT), 113
Enterobacter, 94
  E. faecalis, 62
Enterobacteriaceae, 74, 77, 151–152
Enterococci, 134
Enterococcus spp., 59, 66, 95–96, 107, 195
  E. faecalis, 62, 73, 107, 192, 225–226, 314
  SL-5, 130
  E. faecium, 42–43, 76, 107, 188–189
  strains, 78–79
Enterohemorrhagic *Escherichia coli* (EHEC), 281–282, 288–291
  infection, 283–285
  origin, definition, and characteristics, 288–289
  probiotics on EHEC infection, 290–291
  treatment of EHEC infection, 289–290
Epidemiological studies, 139
Epithelial cells, 65
Epithelial growth factor (EGF), 94
Ergyphilus, 226
Escherichia, 59, 66, 78–79, 151–152
  E. coli, 1, 42–43, 61–62, 73, 96, 110, 150–151, 192–193, 216, 224, 364
Escherichia coli Nissle 1917 (ECN), 177, 471
Eubacteria, 150–151
Eubacterium, 59, 66, 162
Europe
  health claims made on foods, 18–19
  probiotic claims for foods in, 18–20
European Commission (EC), 16
European Crohn's and Colitis Organization (ECCO), 471
European Directorate for Quality of Medicines (EDQM), 16–17
European Food Safety Authority (EFSA), 16–17, 148–149, 457, 467
European Medicines Agency (EMA), 16
European Parliament (EP), 16
European Society for Parenteral and Enteral Nutrition (ESPEN), 471
European Society for Pediatric Infectious Diseases (ESPID), 468

European Union (EU), 16–17, 467
  food and pharmaceutical regulatory framework in, 17–20
Exopolysaccharides (EPSs), 193–194
Experimental autoimmune encephalomyelitis (EAE), 166
Extrusion method, 372

F

Faecal Microbial Transplantation (FMT), 266
Faecalibacterium, 59, 192
  composition, 43
  F. prausnitzii, 77, 167
Faecalobacterium, 162
FDA. *See* US Food and Drug Administration (FDA)
Fecal microflora transplantation (FMT), 76, 358
Federal lawmaking processes, 20
Fermentation, 431
Fermented milk product with probiotic (FMPP), 357–358
Firmicutes, 41, 94, 150–151, 191
Firmicutes/Bacteroidetes ratio (F/B ratio), 77, 323
Flavonifractor, 162
Follicular helper T cells (Tfh), 165
Food, 15, 31–36
  allergens, 214
  biologic drugs, 25–26
  Canadian regulatory framework, 24–27
  complementary recommendations, 16–17
  drug definition in Japan, 30
  drug regulatory statuses, 36
    identification of different legal international definitions, 32t, 33t
  drug status, 15
  drugs classification in Japan, 30–31
  food or dietary supplements regulatory statuses, 33
  general US regulatory framework, 20–24
  health claims in United States, 21–22
  intolerances, 405
  Japanese regulatory framework, 27–31
  manufacturing of biological products, 31
  Natural Health Products, 25
  pharmaceutical law in Japan, 30
  pharmaceutical regulatory framework
    in Canada, 25–26
    in EU, 17–20
    in Japan, 29–31
    in United States, 20–21
  pharmaceutical regulatory status for probiotics in United States, 23–24
  probiotics, 13–15, 433
    as medical foods, 22–23
    claims for foods in Europe, 18–20
    regulations at product level, 14
    regulatory framework, 24–25, 27–29
    regulatory statuses, 32–35
    for special dietary uses, 28
    for special medical purposes, 19–20
    for specific dietary use, 34–35

Food (*Continued*)
　　for specific health uses, 28–29
　　standards and constraints associated with pharmaceutical regulatory frameworks, 26–27
　　standards for biological materials, 31
　　status of probiotics in United States, 21–23
　　supplements, 16
　　various regulatory statuses applicable to products containing probiotics, 16–31
　　　general EU regulatory framework, 16–20
Food allergy, 152–156. *See also* Pediatric allergy
　　dietary management strategies, 216
　　future prospective of probiotic in food allergies, 217
　　intake of probiotics, 216
　　lactose intolerance, 214
　　probiotics
　　　and gut microbiome, 213
　　　in mitigation, 213–214
　　　role of, 214–216
　　　　mechanism of action of probiotics, 215
　　　　role of probiotics mitigation in lactose intolerance, 215–216
　　　therapeutic applications, 216
Food and Agriculture Organization (FAO), 107, 449
Food and drug association, 148–149
Food and pharmaceutical regulatory framework in United States, 20–21
　　food status of probiotics in, 21–23
　　health claims in, 21–22
　　pharmaceutical regulatory status for probiotics in, 23–24
Food for Special Dietary Uses (FOSDU), 28
Food for Special Medical Purposes (FSMP), 23
Food Sanitation Act (FSA), 27
Foodborne diseases, 281–282, 363–364
　　delivery system of probiotics, 372
　　foodborne pathogens, 365*t*
　　　antimicrobial potential of probiotics against, 367–368
　　　and diseases, 364
　　　pathogenicity mechanisms of, 364
　　health significance of probiotics, 373–374
　　probiotics, 364–367
　　　and bacterial pathogens interaction, 371
　　　and foodborne viruses interaction, 372
　　　and immune system interaction, 370
　　　bacteria–bacteria interaction, 370
　　　interference in signaling system, 371
　　　mechanisms of action, 368–372
　　　physical interaction with epithelium, 369
　　　preventing production of the toxin, 371
　　　secretion of antimicrobial substances, 370
　　safety of probiotic therapy, 372–373
　　supplementation of probiotics, 372
Foodborne pathogens, 365*t*
　　and diseases, 364
　　pathogenicity mechanisms of, 364
Foods with Function Claims (FFC), 27
Foods with Health Claims (FHC), 27
Foods with Nutrient Function claims (FNFC), 27
Foods with Specified Health Use (FOSHU), 27
Frailty syndrome (FS), 402–403
Free Fatty Acid Receptor-3 (FFAR3), 328–329
Fructo-oligosaccharides (FOS), 3, 148–149, 161
Fructosyltransferase (*ftf*), 268–269
Function health claims, 18
Functional foods, 432
Functional gastrointestinal disorders (FGIDs), 101, 215
Functional ingredients, 405–408
Fungal pathogens, 305
　　probiotics in fungal diseases, 305–314
　　　antifungal effects of, 310*t*
　　　for dermal infections, 312–313
　　　in oral fungal infections, 306–312
　　　in systemic fungal infections, 313–314
　　　in vaginal fungal infections, 313
Fusobacteria, 191
Fusobacterium, 62, 64
　　F. nucleatum, 151–152, 193–194

G

G-protein-coupled receptors (GPCRs), 388
Galacto-oligosaccharide (GOS), 3
Gamma-aminobutyric acid (GABA), 354, 399
Gammaproteobacteria, 202
Gastric cancer (GC), 191, 281
Gastrointestinal (GI), 101, 190, 252, 281
　　disorders, 354–355, 404–405
　　probiotics in, 468–480
Gastrointestinal tract (GIT), 161, 243, 282, 353, 470
　　probiotics and diseases of, 439
　　viability of probiotic bacteria in, 435–437
General EU regulatory framework, 16–20
　　legal requirements, 16
General Foods (GF), 27
　　law, 17
Generally regarded as safe (GRAS), 148–149, 467
Genetically engineered probiotics, 458
Genetically modified organisms (GMO), 458
Genome-wide association studies (GWASs), 322
Genotyping test (GT), 214
Germ-free mice (GF mice), 76, 150–151
Giardia lamblia, 110
Gingivitis, 251
Glucosyltransferases (*gtfs*), 268–269
Glutathione acts, 69–70
Golden age of microbiology, 431
Good manufacturing practices (GMP), 21, 31
Green banana-resistant starch (GBRS), 80–81
Gut dysbiosis, 41–42, 46–47
Gut microbiome, 213–215
Gut microbiota (GM), 43–44, 131, 161, 163–166, 353–354
　　and atopic dermatitis, 118–119
　　of children with ASD, 357–358
　　in T1D, 322–324
　　in T2D, 325
Gut-associated lymphoid tissues (GALT), 149–150
Gut-lung axis, 385–386
Gut-mediated resistant infections, 273–274
Gut–brain axis, 353, 355–356
　　attention-deficit/hyperactivity disorder, 360
　　autism spectrum disorder, 354–355
　　colonization of intestinal ecosystem, 353–354
　　gastrointestinal disorders, 354–355
　　gut microbiota, 354
　　gut microbiota of children with ASD, 357–358
　　neurodevelopmental disorders, 360
　　techniques in microbiota, 358–359

H

Haemophilus influenza, 62
Halitosis, 251–252, 255–259
Hardening of arteries, 337–338
Harmful bacteria, 190
Health disorders, malnutrition and, 404–405
Health Foods (HF), 27
Health safety of probiotics
　　adverse effects, 450
　　　due to *Bifidobacter*, 452
　　　of probiotics, 457–458
　　　due to *Saccharomyces boulardii*, 452–453
　　antibiotic resistance in probiotics, 454–455
　　combination of probiotics, 458–459
　　fermented food, 449
　　genetically engineered probiotics, 458
　　harmful metabolic activities of probiotics, 455–456
　　horizontal gene transfer in probiotics, 454–455
　　immunomodulation, 454
　　probiotics
　　　in cancer patients, 453
　　　in immunocompromised patients, 454
　　　in pregnant woman and infants, 453–454
　　　safety and regulatory guidelines, 456–457
　　risk of probiotic-originated infections, 451–452
Health-beneficial effects, 6–7
Health-promoting microbes, 7
Healthy microflora, 5
Healthy vaginal microflora, 244
Helicobacter pylori, 107, 191–193, 285–288, 479–480
　　infection, 283–285
　　vaccine delivery system for, 287–288
Helicobacteraceae, 195
Hemolysis, 456
Hemolytic uremic syndrome (HUS), 281–282, 289
High-density lipoprotein (HDL), 330–331
High-density lipoprotein cholesterol (HDL-C), 337, 441
Histone deacetylase (HDAC), 197–198
HMGCoA reductase (HMGR), 343

Homeostasis, 41
Horizontal gene transfer (HGT), 454–455
   in probiotics, 454–455
Hormone therapy (HRT), 198
Hospital-acquired pneumonia (HAP), 223.
   See also Ventilator-associated pneumonia (VAP)
Hospital-acquired pneumonia, 224–227
Human cancers
   fructooligosaccharides and galactooligosaccharides, 189f
   microorganisms used as probiotics, 188t
   probiotics and prebiotics
      in breast cancer, 198–200
      in cervical cancer, 200–202
      in colon cancer, 193–198
      in prevention and management of, 187–191
      in stomach cancer, 191–193
Human chorionic gonadotropin (hCG), 201
Human epidermal growth factor receptor (HER-2), 194
Human leukocyte antigen (HLA), 322
Human Microbiome Project Consortium, 432
Human microbiota, 432
Human milk, 140
Human papillomavirus (HPV), 194
Human studies, 119–123
   for prevention of asthma through probiotics, 141
Humoral immunity, 113
Hydrogel, 372
Hydrogen, 66
Hydrogen breath tests (HBT), 214
Hydrogen peroxide (H_2O_2), 305
Hydrogen sulfide effect on intestinal cells, 67–70
3-hydroxy-3-methylglutaryl-CoA (HMGCoA), 343
5 hydroxytryptamine (5HT). *See* Serotonin
Hygiene, 213–214
   hypothesis, 118, 139
Hypolipidemic mechanisms of action
   of probiotic bacteria, 340–344
      bacterial conversion of cholesterol, 342
      coprecipitation of cholesterol, 342–343
      deconjugation of bile salts, 341–342
      incorporation and assimilation of cholesterol, 342
      inhibition of cholesterol transmembrane transporter expression, 343
      inhibition of hepatic cholesterol synthesis, 343–344
      stimulation of bile acid synthesis, 343–344
Hypothalamic–pituitary–adrenal axis (HPA axis), 353

I

Immune homeostasis, 42, 47–48
Immune system, 163–165
Immunity, 149–150
Immunobiotic LAB, 417

probiotic LAB, 418–424
vaccine adjuvants, 417–418
Immunobiotics, 419, 466
   probiotic LAB as, 419–420
Immunocompromised patients, 450–451, 454
   probiotics in, 454
Immunoglobulin E (IgE), 117–118, 140
Immunomodulation, probiotics in, 454
Immunoregulatory functions, 148–149
Incretin effect, 328
Inducible NO synthase (i-NOS), 194–195
Infectious diarrhea, 110
Inflammation hypothesis, 321
Inflammatory bowel diseases (IBDs), 59, 149–150, 166, 467, 470–475
   clinical studies on, 472t
Inside-Out hypothesis, 118
Intake of probiotics, 216
Intensive care units (ICUs), 452
Interferon (IFN), 117–118
   IFN-γ, 132, 193
Interleukin (IL), 117–118, 287, 386
   IL-1, 164–165
   IL-13, 41
   IL-4, 140
   IL-5, 140
   IL-10, 458
International Clinical Trials Registry Platform (ICTRP), 27–28
International Council for Harmonisation (ICH), 15
International Probiotics Association (IPA), 465
International Research Group on New Antimicrobial Strategies (ISGNAS), 433
International Scientific Association for Probiotics and Prebiotics (ISAPP), 1, 449, 465
Intestinal cells, hydrogen sulfide effect on, 67–70
Intestinal ecosystem, colonization of, 353–354
Intestinal epithelial cells (IECs), 292
Intestinal microbiome, 74–81
Intestinal microbiota, 432
   in development of bowel diseases, 61–70
Intravaginal administration of probiotics, 239–240
Irritable bowel disease (IBD), 404
Irritable bowel syndrome (IBS), 101, 215, 467, 475–476
   probiotics in prevention and management, 102–103
Ischemic heart disease (IHD), 337

J

Japan
   drug definition in Japan, 30
   drugs classification in Japan, 30–31
   pharmaceutical law in Japan, 30
   pharmaceutical regulatory framework in, 29–31
   responsible authorities and structures, 29
Japanese regulatory framework, 27–31

K

Klebsiella, 94, 162, 224
   K. aerogenes, 62
   K. oxytoca, 110
   K. pneumoniae, 73
Kluyveromyces marxianus, 198
Kwashiorkor, 400

L

Lachnospira, 195
Lactic acid bacteria (LAB), 147–149, 192–193, 243, 266, 338–339, 363, 398, 433
   adverse effects due to, 451–452
   probiotic, 339
Lactic acidosis, 96
Lactobacillaceae, 175–176
Lactobacilli, 1, 73–74, 148–151, 161–162, 215, 224, 314
Lactobacillus acidophilus (LA), 42–43, 49, 75, 77, 94, 107, 111–112, 130, 167–172, 177–178, 192–193, 213, 223, 229–230, 291
   CICC 6074, 194–195
   LA-5, 119–121
   NCFM, 121
Lactobacillus rhamnosus GG (LGG), 102–103, 119–121, 140, 148–150, 178, 213, 225–226, 231, 439
Lactobacillus rhamnosus yoba 2012 (LRY), 192–193
Lactobacillus spp., 1, 5, 42–43, 59, 64, 66, 74–75, 77–78, 95–96, 102, 123, 132, 140, 162–163, 166–167, 174–175, 178, 188–189, 192–194, 224–227, 229–231, 237, 243, 435
   L. alimentarius NKUSS6, 78
   L. amylovorus, 42–43
   L. brev, 75
   L. brevis, 77
   L. buchneri, 47–48
   L. bulgaricus, 78, 107, 111, 147, 223, 226, 435
   L. casei, 42–43, 75, 77, 110, 112, 167–172, 177–178, 225–226, 229–230
      CECT 9104, 121–123
      DN-114 001, 231
   L. crispatus, 201
   L. cromoris, 201
   L. delbrueckii, 75, 107, 133, 173
      L. delbrueckii bulgaricus, 130
      L. delbrueckii subsp *ulgaricus*, 47–48
   L. fermentum, 75, 133, 140, 177–178
      K81, 201
      K85, 201
      TISTR, 196
      YL-11, 196
   L. gassei, 42–43
   L. gasseri, 48–49, 201
   L. helveticus, 42–43, 167
      HY7801, 119
   L. johnsonii, 42–43, 123
      N6.2, 176

Lactobacillus spp. (*Continued*)
  L. kefiranofaciens, 202
    L. kefiranofaciens M, 174–175
  L. kefiri
    L. kefiri K, 174–175
    MSR101, 197
  L. lactis, 47–48, 75
  L. mucosae K76, 201
  L. paracasei, 47–48, 75, 107, 112
    06TCa19, 193
    GMNL-32, 162, 173
    LP-33, 142
    Lpc-37, 121
    NCC2461, 140
    ST11, 132
  L. pentosus, 42–43
    KCA, 130
  L. plantaris, 227
  L. plantarum, 42–43, 47–49, 77, 107, 112, 130, 140, 167, 192–193
    5BL, 202
    229V, 74
    299, 226
    A7, 176
    C70, 199–200
    CJLP133, 121–123
    MBTU-HK1, 196
    WCFS1, 130, 132–133
    ZDY 2013, 193
  L. reuteri, 9, 42–43, 49, 75, 96, 110, 177, 197
    ATCC 55730, 231
    DSM 122460, 152–156
    DSM 17938, 102–103
    GMNL-89, 162, 167–173
    GMNL-263, 173
    I5007, 77
    K97, 201
    K99, 201
  L. rhamnosus, 42–43, 48, 75, 77–78, 95–96, 107, 110–113, 192–193, 229–230
    19070-2, 152–156
    GG, 130–131
    GR-1, 140
    HN001, 121, 141
  L. salivarius, 75, 140
    LS01 DSM 2275, 121
  strains, 77–78
Lactococci, 148–149
Lactococcus sp.
  HY 449, 130
  L. lactis, 42–43
    NZ9000, 140
Lactose intolerance (LI), 214–216
  induced diarrhea, 113
Laribacter hongkongensis, 110
Leaky gut syndrome, 354–355
Levilactobacillus brevis, 47–48
Limnobacter, 195
Lipid overflow hypothesis, 321
Lipopolysaccharides (LPS), 46–47, 77, 196, 273–274
Lipoteichoic acid (LTA), 134
Listeria monocytogenes, 367–368

Live Biotherapeutic Products (LBPs), 18, 23, 466
Live microorganisms, 147–149, 216
Liver X receptors (LXR), 343
Llactose tolerance test (LTT), 214
Lonicera japonica, 80
Low-density lipoprotein (LDL), 330–331
Low-density lipoprotein cholesterol (LDL-C), 337
Lower respiratory tract infections (LRTIs), 383
Lupus, 162
Lysine motifs (LysM), 421–423

M
Major depressive disorder (MDD), 49
Malassezia spp, 131
  M. globosa, 131
  M. restricta, 131
Malnutrition and health disorders, 404–405
Manage human disease, 13
Matrix metalloproteinase-2F (MMP2F), 197
MCF-7 cells, 200
Medical food, 22–23
Medical probiotic, 433
Melanocortin-4 receptor (MC4R), 326
Mercaptopyruvate sulfur transferase (MST), 69
Mesenchymal stem cells (MSC), 255
Meta-analysis, 293
Metabiotics, 6
Metabolic disorders, 404
Metabolic syndrome (Ms), 404, 441–442
Metabolic waste of activity of probiotic, 6
Metabolomics, 432
Methanobrevibacter smithii, 66–67
Methanogenic microorganisms, 66
Methionine, 69
Metronidazole, 72–73
  gel, 239
Microbial deoxyribonucleic acid, 140
Microbial surface components recognizing adhesive matrix molecules (MSCRAMMs), 270
Microbiome, 93–94, 140, 150–151, 223, 266
Microbiota, 41–42, 59, 150–151, 282
  and gut-lung axis, 385–386
    pulmonary microbiota in diseases, 386
    during respiratory disorders, 386
Microbiota transfer therapy (MTT), 358
Microbiotic dysbiosis, 443
Microencapsulation, 406
Microflora, 282
Microorganisms, 1, 42–43, 66
Ministry of Health, Labour, and Welfare (MHLW), 29
Mitogen-activated protein kinase (MAPK), 194–195
Molecular hydrogen as universal electron donor in intestinal SRB metabolism, 66–67
Mollicutes, 162
Mood disorders, 482–485
Mother's microbiome and child health, 151–152
Mucin, 64, 456
Mucispirillum, 193–194

Mucosa-associated lymphoid tissue (MALT), 283
Mucus, production of, 369
Multidrug-resistant (MDR) bacteria, probiotics against, 267–272
  antibacterial action, 267–268
  antibiofilm action, 268–269
  antidrug resistance property, 272
  antiinvasion actions, 270
  antiquorum sensing, 269
  antitoxic property, 269–270
  antivirulence property, 269
  bacterial colonization interference, 270–271
  immunomodulation, 271–272
  interbacterial aggregation, 270
  intrabacterial aggregation, 270
Multiple sclerosis (MS), 161, 163
  probiotics in suppression of, 176–178
Muribaculaceae, 195
MyD88, 150–151, 164–165
Mysterious disease. *See* Hemolytic uremic syndrome

N
N-acetylcysteine, 70
6-*N*-hydroxyaminopurine, 133
N-nitrosodimethylamine (NDMA), 192
Nanoparticles (NPs), 192
National Cholesterol Education Program (NCEP), 337
National Institute of Health (NIH), 20
National Institute of Health Sciences (NIHS), 29
Natural Health Products (NHP), 25–26
Natural killer cells (NK cells), 370
Necrotizing enterocolitis (NEC), 405
  mechanisms of probiotic action in preterm, 94
  microbiome, dysbiosis, and NEC, 93–94
  probiotics and prevention of, 94–96
  probiotics in prevention and management of, 93
  safety aspects of probiotics, 96
Neonatal intensive care units (NICUs), 93
Neurodevelopmental disorders, 356–357, 360
Neuropeptide Y (NPY), 326
Next generation of probiotics, 5
Next-generation sequencing technology, 161
Niemann–Pick type-C1 Like-1 (NPC1L1), 340–341
Nitric oxide (NO), 78
Nitric oxide synthase (iNOS), 78
NLEA authorized health claims, 21
Nod-like receptors (NLRs), 149–150
Nonviable microbial cells, 8–9
Norovirus (NoV), 364
North American Society for Pediatric Gastroenterology, Hepatology and Nutrition (NASPGHAN), 474–475
Nosocomial diarrhea (ND), 110–112, 214
  antibiotic-associated diarrhea, 110–112
  Clostridium difficile diarrhea, 112
Nosocomial infections
  Clostridium difficile infection, 228–231
  description of probiotics, 223–224
  hospital-acquired pneumonia and ventilator-associated pneumonia, 224–227

dysbiosis in critically ill patients, 225
  epidemiology, pathophysiology, and
      clinical presentation, 224−225
  probiotics in, 225−226
  probiotics in prevention and treatment of
      VAP in pediatrics, 226−227
  probiotics in prevention and treatment of,
      223−224
NSP4 protein, 294
Nuclear factor kappa B (NF-kB), 370
Number needed-to-treat (NNT), 102
Nutribiotics, 7, 397−399
Nutrition, 44−45
Nutritional health benefits
  of postbiotics and probiotics, 400−405
      overnutrition situations, 403−405
      undernutrition situations, 400−403
Nutritional status, 397−399

O

Obesity, 321, 453
  gut microbiota and, 326−327
  pathophysiology and risk factors of,
      322−327
  probiotics for management of, 327−331
Odds ratio (OR), 141−142
Odoribacter, 193−194
Oligosaccharides, 3, 161, 189
"One Health" approach, 266
Oral administration of probiotics, 239
Oral cavity, 251
Oral diseases, 251
  dental caries, 252−253
  halitosis, 255−259
  oral cavity, 251
  periodontal diseases, 253−255
Oral fungal infections, 306−312
Oral malodor, 251−252
Oral probiotics, 133
Organ-specific resistant infections
  in gut-mediated resistant infections,
      273−274
  probiotics in, 272−274
  in resistant pulmonary infections, 274
  in resistant skin and wound
      infections, 273
  in urogenital infections, 272−273
Organisation for Economic Co-operation and
    Development (OECD), 15
Oscillospira, 195
Outer membrane protein A (OmpA), 289
Outside-in hypothesis, 118
Over-The-Counter (OTC), 30
Overnutrition situations, 403−405
  cardiovascular diseases, 403−404
  malnutrition and health disorders,
      404−405
  metabolic disorders, 404

P

Pancreatitis, 454
Parabacteroides, 79
  composition, 43
Parabiotics, 466

Parkinson's disease, 42
Pathogens, 107
Pathogens infection, 405
Patient-Oriented Eczema Measure (POEM),
    117
Pattern recognition receptors (PRRs), 149−150
PCR-denaturing gradient gel electrophoresis
    (PCR-DGGE), 246
Pediatric allergy
  clinical studies, 152−156
    atopic eczema, 152
    food allergy, 152−156
  microbiota and allergic disorders, 150−151
    outcome of some clinical studies, 153t
  mother's microbiome and child health,
      151−152
  prenatal and neonatal probiotic intake in,
      147−148
  probiotics, prebiotics, and immunity,
      149−150
  safety of probiotics and prebiotics, 148−149
Pediococcus, 192−193
  P. acidilactici TISTR 2612, 196
  P. pentosaceus LI05, 79−80
Peptostreptococcus, 64, 191
Periodontal diseases, 253−255
Periodontitis, 251
Pharma status of probiotics, 17−18
Pharmabiotics, 7−9, 466
Pharmaceutical and Medical Devices Agency
    (PMDA), 29
Pharmaceutical Inspection Cooperation Scheme
    (PIC/S), 31
Pharmaceutical probiotic, 433
Pharmaceutical regulatory framework
  in Canada, 25−26
  pharmaceutical regulatory framework,
      29−31
  standards and constraints associated with,
      26−27
    biologic drugs, 26−27
    NHP, 26
  in United States, 20−21
Pharmaceutical regulatory framework in EU,
    17−20
  pharma status of probiotics, 17−18
Pharmaceutical regulatory status for probiotics
    in United States, 23−24
Pharmaceutical Safety and Environmental
    Health Bureau (PSEHB), 29
Pharmaceutical standards, 18
Pharmaceuticals and Medical Devices
    Evaluation Centre (PMDE), 29
Pichia kudriavzevii, 198
Pistacia atlantica, 192
Plaque, 337−338
Plasma glucose test (PGT), 214
Plectranthus amboinicus, 110
Plus Ultra, 443
Pneumococcal surface protein A (PspA),
    421−423
Polyphenols, 3
Polysaccharide A (PSA), 164−165
Polysaccharides, 165
Polyunsaturated fatty acids (PUFAs), 3, 191

Porphyromonas, 150−151
Postbiotics, 6−7, 397, 399, 466
  main groups, 6t
  nutritional health benefits of, 400−405
  pharmabiotics and specific health claim, 8t
  probiotics categorized as nutribiotics, 8t
  and sources, 7t
Postnatal period, 148
Pouchitis, 475
Prebiotics, 3−5, 75−80, 148−150, 161, 239,
    354, 465
  probiotic species, 77−80
  effect of probiotics on UC, 76
  and sources, 4t
Pregnant women nutritional deficiencies, 402
Prevotella, 150−151, 191
Probioceuticals, 9
Probiotic(s), 1−3, 2f, 7, 13−15, 74−75, 93,
    107, 119, 147−150, 188−189, 213,
    223−224, 237, 266−267, 281, 305,
    338, 354, 363−367, 397−399,
    431−432, 465
  action in preterm, 94
  in amelioration of AD, 123
  and antibiotic-associated diarrhea, 476−479
  autism and, 354
  bacteria, 338−344
    antitumor and antimutagenic effect of,
        440−441
    hepatoprotective effect of, 439−440
    hypolipidemic mechanisms of action of,
        340−344
    probiotic LAB, 339
    probiotic non-LAB, 340
    safety of, 437
  clinical translation of probiotic investigation,
      49−53
    clinical trials focusing, 50t
    role of probiotic in Covid-19, 52t
  concept, 1
  confusion, 13
  current market of, 408−409
  current microorganisms used as probiotics, 3t
  definition and classification of, 432−435
  different terminologies related to, 2f
  dose of, 437
  food status of probiotics in United States,
      21−23
  in fungal diseases, 305−314
  in gastrointestinal diseases, 468−480
  gut microbiota and Covid-19, 43−44
    innate and adaptive immunity against
        Covid-19 infection, 44f
  gut microbiota regulates potent
      immunoregulators, 42f
  health effects of, 437−441
  and health implications, 282−283
  and *Helicobacter pylori*, 479−480
  history of, 386−387
  and immunity, 442−443
  importance of, 44−47
    influence of gut microbiota, 45f
    probiotic nutritional interconnections, 46f
  and inflammatory bowel diseases, 470−475
  in intestinal diseases, 480

Probiotic(s) (*Continued*)
  and irritable bowel syndrome, 475–476
  LAB, 418–424
    adjuvant potential of biosurfactants, 423–424
    adjuvant potential of LAB ghost cells, 424
    adjuvant properties of, 421
    bacterium-like particles from, 421–423
    immunobiotics, 419
    as immunobiotics, 419–420
    as novel vaccine adjuvants, 420–421
  lactobacilli, 244
  in maintaining immune homeostasis, 42, 47–48
  mechanism of action of, 215
  as medical foods, 22–23
  and mental illness, 443
  and metabolic syndrome, 441–442
  mitigation in lactose intolerance, 215–216
    mechanism by which probiotics protect our health, 215f
  mode of action of, 113
    BV, 238
    commensal microbial flora, 237
    evidence, 240
    modes of administration of, 239–240
    preventing UTI, 237
    UTI, 238
    vaginal microbiota, 237
    yeast vaginitis, 238–239
  non-LAB, 340
  nutritional health benefits of, 400–405, 401t
  in organ-specific resistant infections, 272–274
  pharma status of, 17–18
  in prevention and management of IBS, 102–103
  in prevention and treatment of CDI, 229–231, 230t
  in prevention and treatment of diarrheal diseases, 109–113
    cancer therapy-induced diarrhea, 112
    enteral tube feeding diarrhea, 113
    infectious diarrhea, 110
    lactose intolerance induced diarrhea, 113
    nosocomial diarrhea, 110–112
    travelers' diarrhea, 110
  in prevention and treatment of oral diseases
    dental caries, 252–253
    halitosis, 255–259
    periodontal diseases, 253–255
  for prevention of allergic rhinitis, 141–142
  probiotic claims for foods in Europe, 18–20
  probiotic interlink with immunization efficacy, 49
  probiotic mechanism of action, 47–49
  probiotic-derived factors, 9
  regulation bodies that include probiotics, 467–468
  regulations for, 480–487
    allergies, 480–482
    anxiety, 482–485
    common acute infections, 486–487
    depression, 482–485
    mood disorders, 482–485
    wound healing, 485–486
    wound infection, 485–486
  role on EHEC infection, 290–291
  roles in vaginal infection, 245–246
  on RV infection, 294
  safety of probiotic bacteria, 437
  species, 77–80
    bacillus strains, 78–79
    bifidobacterium strains, 78
    lactobacillus strains, 77–78
    other species, 79–80
  strains, 434–435
  supplementation in food materials, 372
  in suppression of autoimmune diseases, 167–178
    probiotics in suppression of cystic fibrosis, 178
    probiotics in suppression of multiple sclerosis, 176–178, 177f
    probiotics in suppression of rheumatoid arthritis, 167–172, 172f
    probiotics in suppression of systemic lupus erythematosus, 172–174, 173f
    probiotics in suppression of type 1 diabetes mellitus, 174–176, 175f
    studies depicting role of, 168t
  therapy, 252
  treatment, 103
  for treatment of allergic rhinitis, 142–143
  for treatment of asthma, 141
  for treatment of skin conditions
    acne vulgaris, 129–130
    psoriasis, 130–131
    seborrheic dermatitis, 131–132
    skin cancer, 133–134
    wound healing, 132–133
  and urogenital infections, 442
  usage and safety, 387–388
  various regulatory statuses applicable to products containing, 16–31
  viability of probiotic bacteria in gastrointestinal tract, 435–437
  yeasts, 344–345
    hypocholesterolemic mechanisms of action for, 345
Product level, 14
Proopiomelanocortin (POMC), 326
Propionate, 343–344
Propionibacterium, 151–152, 162
  P. acnes, 129
  P. freudenreichii, 79–80, 141, 197–198
PROSAFE, 457
Prostaglandin E2 (PGE2), 78
Prostaglandin-endoperoxide synthase 2 (PTGS-2), 194
Proteobacteria, 41, 79, 94, 150–151, 202
Proteus mirabilis, 73
Proton-pump inhibitors (PPIs), 283
Pseudomonas, 224
  P. aeruginosa, 132, 195–196, 226
Psuedobutyvibrio, 162
Psychobiotics, 354, 466
Pulmonary microbiota in diseases, 386
  microbiota during respiratory disorders, 386
Pulsed-field gel electrophoresis (PFGE), 451–452
Pyridoxal-5′-phosphate-dependent enzymes, 69

Q

Qualified health claim, 22
Qualified Presumption of Safety (QPS), 148–149
Quorum sensing, 269

R

Radiation protection effect of probiotics, 440
Radiotherapy, 453
Randomized controlled trials (RCTs), 95, 141, 469
Reactive oxygen species (ROS), 194
Recurrent respiratory tract infection (RRTI), 390
Reinforcement of intestinal barrier, 369
Remnant lipoprotein particle (RLP-P), 344
Resistant pulmonary infections, 274
Resistant skin and wound infections, 273
Respiratory diseases, 383–384
  history of probiotics, 386–387
  microbiota and gut-lung axis, 385–386
  probiotic usage and safety, 387–388
  pulmonary microbiota in diseases, 386
Respiratory disorders, microbiota during, 386
Respiratory infections
  probiotic administration in, 388–392
    methodological and clinical aspects, 388–389
    probiotic and respiratory infections, 389–390
    probiotic and respiratory viral infections, 390–392
Respiratory tract infections (RTIs), 383–385
  treatment, 384–385
Rheumatoid arthritis (RA), 161–162
  probiotics in suppression of, 167–172
Rhodococcus, 162
Ribosomal RNA (rRNA), 323
Rifaximin, 73
Rikenellaceae, 195
Risk reduction claims, 18
ROR-γt, 150–151
Roseburia, 134, 162, 195
  composition, 43
  R. intestinalis, 77
Roseomonas mucosa, 123
Rotavirus (RV), 282, 291–294
  infection, 283–285
    efficacy of probiotics, 293–294
    treatment of, 293
  probiotics on RV infection, 294
Ruminococcaceae, 195
Ruminococci, 134
Ruminococcus, 150–151

S

16S rRNA gene, 150–151
Saccharomyces, 1, 95, 224, 229–230
  S. boulardii, 96, 213, 231
    adverse effects due to, 452–453
  S. cerevisiae, 42–43, 198, 239–240
    S. cerevisiae var. *boulardii*, 75
Salmonella, 61–62, 73, 110, 364, 367
  S. boulardii, 111–113

S. thermophilus, 111, 175–176
S. typhimurium, 110
Scaling and root planning (SRP), 254–255
Scientific Committee on Animal Nutrition (SCAN), 148–149
Scoring for Atopic Dermatitis (SCORAD), 119
Seborrheic dermatitis, 131–132
Selective digestive decontamination (SDD), 273–274
Serotonin, 354
Severe acute malnutrition (SAM), 400
Severe acute respiratory syndrome coronavirus 2 (SARS-CoV-2), 41–42, 385
Shiga toxin-producing *E. coli* (STEC), 284, 367
Shiga toxins (Stx), 281–282, 364, 371
Shigella, 61–62, 73, 78–79, 110, 151–152
Short interfering RNA (siRNA), 343
Short-chain fatty acids (SCFAs), 44–45, 65, 121, 149–150, 161, 192, 286, 324, 338, 388, 399
Simulator of the Human Intestinal Microbial Ecosystem (SHIME), 192
Skin cancer, 133–134
Skin microbiome, 129
Skin microbiota, 312
"Split-mouth" design, 254–255
Sporolac, 237
Staphylococcus, 52, 94, 118, 131, 151–152
   S. aureus, 117, 130–131, 133, 192–193, 216, 224
   S. epidermidis, 62, 118, 130, 133
Stomach cancer
   beneficial effects of probiotics on human health, 190f
   probiotics and prebiotics in, 191–193
Streptococci, 130, 150–151, 162, 215
Streptococcus, 74, 107, 131, 151–152, 191–192, 225–226, 229–230
   S. mobilis, 62
   S. pneumonia, 148–149
   S. pyogenes, 130
   S. salivarius, 95–96, 174–175
   S. thermophiles, 42–43, 226
   S. thermophilus, 75, 95–96, 107, 112, 123, 130, 147, 174–175, 177, 188–189, 223
   S. thermophilus 06, 152–156
Streptococcus faecalis, 107
Streptomycetes, 197
Substance, 14
Sucrose gel, 239
Sulfate-reducing bacteria (SRB), 59
Superoxide dismutase (SOD), 194–195
Synbiotics, 5, 5t, 75, 80–81, 189–190, 354, 465
   treatment, 103
Synthetic prebiotic oligosaccharides, 189
Systemic fungal infections, 313–314
Systemic inflammation, 327
Systemic inflammatory response syndrome (SIRS), 451
Systemic lupus erythrematosus (SLE), 161–162
   probiotics in suppression of, 172–174

T

T cells, 43
T helper 1 cells (Th1 cells), 117–118
T helper 2 cells (Th2 cells), 117–118
T helper 17 cells (Th17 cells), 47, 164–165
T regulatory cells (Tregs), 324
Therapeutic pharmabiotics, 7–8
Thiosulfate sulfur transferase (TST), 69
Thrombotic thrombocytopenic purpura (TTP), 283
TNF-related apoptosis inducing ligand (TRAIL), 195–196
Toll-like receptors (TLRs), 94, 149–150, 164–165, 324, 421
   TLR2, 47
Topical probiotic, 129–130
Transforming growth factor (TGF), 327
   TGF-3, 119–121
      TGF-beta 1, 273
Travelers' diarrhea (TD), 110, 214
Triacylglycerol (TAG), 337
Trichophyton, 118
Trinitrobenzenesulfonic acid (TNBS), 70–71
Tumor necrosis factor (TNF), 76
   TNF-α, 41, 192–193
Turicibacterales, 195
Type 1 diabetes (T1D), 321
   gut microbiota in, 322–324
   pathophysiology and risk factors of, 322
   probiotics for management of, 327–328
Type-1 diabetes mellitus (T1DM), 132, 161–163
   probiotics in suppression of, 174–176
Type-1 T-helper cells, 43
Type 2 diabetes (T2D), 321
   gut microbiota in, 325
   pathophysiology and risk factors of, 324–325
   probiotics for management of, 328–330

U

Ulcerative colitis (UC), 59–60, 404, 470–475
   general characteristics of drugs used in bowel diseases, 70–74
   intestinal microbiome, antibiotics, and probiotics in prevention and management of, 59–61
   main factors affecting, 61f
   modification of intestinal microbiome, 74–81
      probiotics, 75–80
      synbiotics, 80–81
   role of intestinal microbiota in development of bowel diseases, 61–70
      bacterial genera in human large intestine, 64–66
      hydrogen sulfide effect on intestinal cells, 67–70
      molecular hydrogen as a universal electron donor in intestinal SRB metabolism, 66–67
Unconjugated bile salt, 341–342

Undernutrition situations, 400–403
   children nutritional deficiencies, 400–402
   elderly nutritional deficiencies, 402–403
   pregnant women nutritional deficiencies, 402
Universal electron donor in intestinal SRB metabolism, 66–67
University Hospital Medical Information Network—Clinical Trials Registry (UMIN-CTR), 27–28
Upper respiratory tract infections (URTIs), 383, 486
Urinary tract infection (UTI), 49, 237–238
   preventing, 237
Urogenital infections, 272–273, 442
US Food and Drug Administration (FDA), 20, 224, 466
US regulatory framework, 20–24

V

Vaccination, 417–418
Vaccine adjuvants, 417–418
Vaginal fungal infections, probiotics in, 313
Vaginal infection, 244–245
   probiotic roles in prevention and treatment of, 245–246
Vaginal microbiota, 237
Vaginitis, 244–245
Vagococcus, 195
Vancomycin, 73
Ventilator-associated pneumonia (VAP), 223–227
   in adults, 225–226
   in pediatrics, 226–227
Very low birth weight (VLBW), 93
Virgi bacillus, 202
Vitamin-D deficiency (VDD), 213–214, 388
Vitreoscilla filiformis, 123, 132
Vivomixx, 358, 480
Volatile sulfur compounds (VSCs), 251–252
Vulvovaginal candidiasis (VVC), 239, 305, 313

W

World Allergy Organization (WAO), 468
World Gastroenterology Organization (WGO), 468
World Health Organization (WHO), 42–43, 107, 251, 265–266, 337, 449
Wound healing, 132–133, 485–486
   burn patients, 132–133
   diabetic ulcers, 132
Wound infection, 485–486

X

Xyloglucans, 161

Y

Yeast vaginitis, 238–239
Yersinia, 61–62

Printed in the United States
by Baker & Taylor Publisher Services

Probiotics in the Prevention and Management of Human Diseases
A Scientific Perspective